Nursing
Practice

This title is also available as an e-book.
For more details, please see
www.wiley.com/buy/9781118481363
or scan this QR code:

Nursing Practice

Knowledge and Care

Edited by

Ian Peate
Visiting Professor of Nursing
Head of School
School of Health Studies
Gibraltar

Muralitharan Nair
Visiting Lecturer
Department of Adult Nursing and
Primary Care
School of Health and Social Work
University of Hertfordshire
UK

Karen Wild
Senior Lecturer; Lead in Student
Opportunity
School of Nursing, Midwifery, Social
Work and Social Sciences
University of Salford
UK

WILEY Blackwell

This edition first published 2014 © 2014 by John Wiley & Sons, Ltd.

Registered office: John Wiley & Sons, Ltd, The Atrium, Southern Gate, Chichester, West Sussex, PO19 8SQ, UK

Editorial offices: 9600 Garsington Road, Oxford, OX4 2DQ, UK
The Atrium, Southern Gate, Chichester, West Sussex, PO19 8SQ, UK
350 Main Street, Malden, MA 02148-5020, USA

For details of our global editorial offices, for customer services and for information about how to apply for permission to reuse the copyright material in this book please see our website at www.wiley.com/wiley-blackwell

Library of Congress Cataloging-in-Publication Data

Nursing practice (Peate)
   Nursing practice : knowledge and care / edited by Ian Peate, Karen Wild, Muralitharan Nair.
      p. ; cm.
   Includes bibliographical references and index.
   ISBN 978-1-118-48136-3 (pbk.)
   I. Peate, Ian, editor.   II. Wild, Karen, 1959– editor.   III. Nair, Muralitharan, editor.   IV. Title.
   [DNLM: 1. Nursing Care–methods.   2. Nursing Process.   WY 100.1]
   RT41
   610.73–dc23
                                          2014020576

A catalogue record for this book is available from the British Library.

Wiley also publishes its books in a variety of electronic formats. Some content that appears in print may not be available in electronic books.

Cover image: Science Photo Library/LTH NHS Trust
Cover design by Design Deluxe

Set in 9.5/11 MinionPro by Toppan Best-set Premedia Limited
Printed and bound in Singapore by Markono Print Media Pte Ltd

1   2014

Brief Contents

Contents

Preface

The way in which health and social care is delivered continues to change and this is appropriate as these changes occur in order to respond to the needs of people. The changes bring with them a range of challenges for nurses and other health and social care professionals. The needs of people in relation to their health and well-being demand that nurses are knowledgeable and up to date with contemporary practice and this is absolutely right, the public need to know that the people providing care are fit for purpose and fit for practice. This is a tall order given the transformations that are occurring within the ever widening sphere of health and social care (wherever this may be) and the amount of knowledge the nurse needs to possess in order to be able to say confidently and competently that they are up to date are changing on a daily basis.

The content of this book is derived from a variety of sources, for example, the Nursing and Midwifery Council's (NMC) (2010) Standards for Pre registration and the Royal College of Nursing's (RCN) (2012) Principles of Nursing Practice. There are a number of themes and trends that are driving strategic direction and change within and without of the nursing profession and these too have had an impact on the chapters within the book.

- The UK population is set to rise to 65.6 million over ten years to 2018
- Infant and mortality is at its lowest rate ever.
- Premature mortality is still poor compared to some other European countries
- There are different health outcomes between socioeconomic groups
- Black and ethnic minority groups experience worse health outcomes than white communities
- The population is ageing
- There will be more people living with long term conditions and dementia
- Lifestyle choice continues to hinder good health i.e. obesity, heavy drinking and sexually transmitted infections are not improving
- Expectations of health and social services amongst the public are rising
- Users and Carers are a more focused part of health and social care delivery systems
- Patient centred healthcare and self-management has led to a growth in service user involvement
- Movement of care into the community is a growing policy theme
- There is an increased emphasis on patient safety and adverse incidents
- Experiences of poor health care dominates public discourse
- The majority of nurses work in the NHS

- There are a growing number of nurses working in voluntary and independent health care settings
- Nurses continue to take on and develop more advanced roles
- There is and will continue to be an increase in the use of assistant practitioners and health care assistants across the health and social care sectors.

Nursing Practice: Knowledge and Care provides you with much information to enable you to develop a deeper understanding of issues that impact on the health and well-being of the people that nurses serve. The book has been written by a number of expert practitioners and academics who are passionate about the art and the science of nursing, dedicated to the health and well-being of the public and committed to nurse education and the notion of lifelong learning.

The book is presented to you in five units:

Unit 1 Contextualising the Art and Science of Nursing
Unit 2 The Elements of Care
Unit 3 The Principles of Care
Unit 4 Scientific Nature of Disease
Unit 5 The Art and Science of Nursing Care.

It is intended that the book be used as a reference book at home or in the classroom. The art and science of nursing has been intertwined in the chapters and each unit is interrelated. The focus will be on the adult field of nursing; however, where appropriate, each chapter provides examples of how content can be applied to the other fields of nursing.

The first four chapters are "scene setting" chapters and we would suggest you read these first. The remaining chapters have been arranged in such a way that they can be read at random, for example, if you are caring for people with cardiovascular conditions it would be useful to delve into the chapter that address issues concerning cardiovascular disorders and then go on to other chapters such as the discussion of diabetes mellitus in the endocrinology chapter as related to cardiovascular disease. We are aware however that we all have our own learning styles and you will use whatever approach appeals to you.

In general we have used a systems approach, we understand that people are not systems and we have chosen this approach in order to make learning and application easier. There are 37 chapters. Each chapter is preceded by learning outcomes related where appropriate to the NMC's (2010) Standards for Pre registration Nurse Education.

There are a range of learning features and activities within the chapters and these are discussed in the "How to Use Your Textbook" in the next pages.

Our overriding intention is to offer you information and in so doing help you understand the impact you can have on the health and well-being of people. Nursing requires many skills, a large number of them are common to the care of people in hospitals and the community (primary care) setting. In the book we indicate this aspect of commonality and in other places it should be apparent on reflection. At all times it is understood that the provision of nursing care requires special adaptation of a general principle to meet individual, family or communities needs.

We have very much enjoyed writing this text and we sincerely hope that you find it of value in helping you become the best possible nurse, who provides care in a confident, competent and compassionate manner.

Ian Peate
Karen Wild
Muralitharan Nair

References

Nursing and Midwifery Council (2010) "Standards for Pre registration Nurse Education"
http://standards.nmc-uk.org/PublishedDocuments/Standards%20for%20 pre-registration%20nursing%20education%2016082010.pdf   last accessed October 2013
Royal College of Nursing "Principles of Nursing Practice" RCN. London

Acknowledgements

Ian would like to thank his partner Jussi Lahtinen for his unrelenting support. To Mrs Frances Cohen for her continued encouragement and kindness and the staff at the RCN Library London for their assistance and expertise.

Karen wishes to thank her husband Gary for his constant loving patience and presence, and also Norma, her friend and mentor and the woman who constantly exemplifies what good nursing should be.

Muralitharan would like to thank his wife, Evangeline, and his daughters, Samantha and Jennifer, for their continued support and patience.

About the Editors

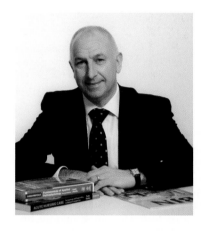

Ian Peate

EN(G) RGN DipN (Lond) RNT BEd (Hons) MA (Lond) LLM
Visiting Professor of Nursing, Editor in Chief British Journal of Nursing, Head of School, School of Health Studies, Gibraltar
Ian began his nursing a career in 1981 at Central Middlesex Hospital, becoming an Enrolled Nurse working in an intensive care unit. He later undertook three years student nurse training at Central Middlesex and Northwick Park Hospitals, becoming a Staff Nurse then a Charge Nurse. He has worked in nurse education since 1989. His key areas of interest are nursing practice and theory, men's health, sexual health and HIV. Ian has published widely; he is Visiting Professor of Nursing, Editor in Chief British Journal of Nursing and Head of School of the School of Health Studies Gibraltar.

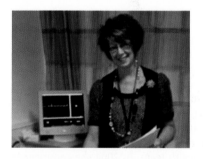

Karen Wild

SRN, HV, RNT, MA (Manchester), Cert Ed.
Senior Lecturer; and Lead in Student Opportunity, School of Nursing, Midwifery and Social Work, College of Health and Social Care, University of Salford
Karen commenced her career in nursing in 1978 in her local general hospital. Initially working within a surgical unit as a staff nurse, she embarked upon a career in health visiting, with a specific interest in family support and women's health. From 1989 she has worked in nurse education, where she has focused on the field of Adult nursing. She is particularly interested in health promotion, adult health and illness and the development of self-awareness. As an admissions tutor and Lead for widening participation within the school, she is a keen advocate for recruiting the best candidates into the nursing profession.

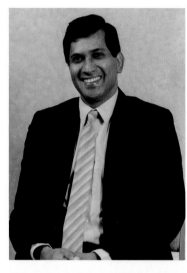

Muralitharan Nair

SRN, RMN, DipN (Lond) RNT, Cert Ed., BSc (Hons) MSc (Surrey), Cert in Counselling, FHEA
Visiting Lecturer, Department of Adult Nursing and Primary Care, School of Health and Social Work, University of Hertfordshire
Muralitharan commenced his nursing a career in 1971 at Edgware General Hospital becoming a Staff Nurse. In 1975 he commenced his mental health nurse training at Springfield Hospital and worked as a Staff Nurse for approximately 1 year. He has worked at St Mary's Hospital Paddington and Northwick Park Hospital returning to Edgware General Hospital to take up the post of Senior Staff Nurse and then Charge Nurse. He has worked in nurse education since 1989. His key interests include physiology, diabetes, surgical nursing and nurse education. Muralitharan has published widely in journals, and co-edited in a number of textbooks. He has now retired as full a time lecturer but still works as a visiting lecturer at University of Hertfordshire.

Contributors

Wasiim Allymamod

Staff Nurse, Central and North West London NHS Foundation Trust. He began his career in nursing in 1999 and in 2008 studied for his Bachelor of Science Honours with the University of West London and was awarded a first class honours in Mental Health. He worked for the West London Mental Health NHS trust for 10years. Wasiim has contributed in articles relating to Mental Health. The key area of interest is working towards a more holistic approach to Mental Health and Health Promotion.

Mary E. Braine

RGN, DipN (Lond), BSc (Hons), MSc, PGCE, D Prof.
Senior Lecturer, School of Nursing, Midwifery, Social Work and Social Sciences, University of Salford
Mary began her nursing career at University College Hospital, London working on an orthopaedic ward then moving into gastro-enterology. After completing her specialist training in neuroscience practice she specialised in neuroscience nursing working for many years at Salford Royal Hospital. She has over 20 years of experience in neuroscience, has published in various journals and books and has presented nationally and internationally on topics related to neuroscience nursing practice. Mary is on the editorial board of the British Journal of Neuroscience Nursing, board member of the British Association of Neuroscience Nurses and the national lead for Neuroscience Nursing Benchmarking group. Her key interests include acquired brain injury, personal development planning and reflective practice.

Carl Clare

RN DipN BSc (Hons) MSc (Lond) PGDE (Lond)
Senior Lecturer, Department of Adult and Primary Nursing, University of Hertfordshire
Carl began his nursing a career in 1990 as a Nursing Auxiliary. He later undertook three years student nurse training at Selly Oak Hospital (Birmingham), moving to The Royal Devon and Exeter Hospitals, then Northwick Park Hospital, and finally The Royal Brompton and Harefield NHS Trust as a Resuscitation Officer and Honorary Teaching Fellow of Imperial College (London). He has worked in nurse education since 2001. His key areas of interest are physiology, sociology, cardiac care and resuscitation. Carl has previously published work in cardiac care, resuscitation and pathophysiology.

Nigel Davies

MSc, BSc (Hons), RN, Cert Ed
Visiting Professor, University of West London
Healthcare Education and Management Consultant
Nigel graduated with a first class honours degree from South Bank Polytechnic in 1990. His clinical practice, across several London hospitals was in general medicine, cardiothoracic surgery and critical care. He became a Lecturer Practitioner and then Senior Lecturer in the late 1990s and was appointed as a visiting professor at the University of West London in 2010. He moved into nursing management roles with responsibility for practice development and quality improvement and for over ten years has been a director of nursing combined with a lead as Director of Infection Prevention and Control. He has over 20 publications in peer reviewed journals. Nigel currently works as a healthcare education and management consultant combining this with study for a doctorate in education.

Ann Foley

RGN/RSCN RNT Bsc [Hons] MA FHEA
Ann commenced her dual training of adult and children's nursing in 1985 at Booth Hall Children's Hospital Manchester working between Booth Hall and North Manchester General Hospital qualifying in 1989 . Her early career was spent in Paediatric Burns and plastic surgery undertaking staff nurse and sister positions . In 1994 she commenced a Lecturer Practitioner Position working for Pennine Acute NHS Trust and The Northern College of nursing. She entered full time education from 1998 working for Salford University within the child health team. In 2004 she commenced a Principal Lecturer position leading child health at the University of Central Lancashire and in 2008 took over the Pre registration provision of Adult, Children's and Mental Health Nursing. Her key interests relate to safeguarding, parenting child development and children's surgery.

David Garbutt

RGN, Bsc (Hons), RNT, MA (University of Wales) PGCE
School of Nursing, Midwifery, Social Work and Social Sciences, University of Salford
David is a Nursing Lecturer in Long Term Conditions and End of Life Care. He has a 20 year clinical background in cancer, hospice and palliative care nursing as a Lead Cancer Nurse, Macmillan Palliative Care Clinical Nurse Specialist and End of Life Care

Education Facilitator. His academic interests focus on the facilitation of learning of healthcare professionals when caring for dying patients and those close to them particularly through the use of the use of the arts and humanities. His research interests include the impact and effectiveness of healthcare interventions on the experience of dying for individuals and their families

Frances Gascoigne

RGN, PG Diploma Intensive nursing care, BSc (Hons), MSc, RNT, Med in Human Relations, PhD (University of Nottingham)

Frances qualified as an adult and children's nurse at the Johannesburg General Hospital (South Africa) and Harare Maternity Hospital (Zimbabwe). After working in intensive care and cardio thoracic units in Southern Africa and New Zealand she moved to the UK and worked at Papworth and Killingbeck Hospitals. Frances entered nurse education in 1993 where her key interests are the teaching of physiology and applied physiology. Her research has focused on the use of mental imagery for the teaching of the biological sciences.

Laureen Hemming

RGN, DipN London, RCNT, BA(open), PGCEA, BPhil Complementary Health Studies

Visiting Lecturer, School of Adult Nursing and Primary Health Care, University of Hertfordshire

Laureen commenced her nursing career at Addenbrooke's Hospital, Cambridge in 1966. After a few posts in gynaecology, medicine, radiotherapy and emergency nursing, Laureen became a ward sister of an acute elderly care ward at Guy's Hospital. In 1982 Laureen moved into nurse education, initially as a clinical teacher, but later as a nurse tutor and then Senior Lecturer at the University of Hertfordshire delivering degree courses in Cancer Nursing and Palliative Care. She has contributed to nursing journals and written chapters for a variety of professional textbooks and presented work at international palliative care conferences. Although retired from full time teaching, Laureen continues to contribute to in-service education at local healthcare trusts on pain management for people with dementia.

Ann Jewell

RGN, BSc (Hons)

Practice Education Facilitator, Lecturer Practitioner, Pennine Care NHS Foundation Trust

Ann began her nursing career in 2000, undertaking an Adult Nurse Degree Programme at Salford University. Ann worked on a busy Elective Surgery Ward, before taking a District Nursing post at Oldham Community Health Services in 2004. Ann moved into her current role of Practice Educator in 2009, following her great interest in facilitating the learning of pre registration student nurses and other healthcare professional students.

Michael Lappin

RN, EN(G), BSc (Hons), MSc, PGCE

Lecturer in Adult Nursing, School of Nursing, Midwifery, Social Work and Social Sciences, University of Salford

Mike began his career in 1976 at North Ormesby Hospital, Middlesbrough, becoming an Enrolled Nurse working in General Medicine, Respiratory Medicine and Coronary Care. He moved to Manchester in 1988 to complete the conversion course at Trafford General Hospital. Deciding to stay in Manchester he continued to work in Coronary Care as a Staff Nurse and then as a Charge Nurse at Salford Royal Hospital. He then joined the Professional Development team in Salford before moving to the University of Salford as a full time lecturer. His key areas of interest include leadership, change management, action learning and the professional development of staff. He is also an international link lecturer with the University of Technology, Cyprus

Paul Maloret

RNLD, Dip (HE), BA (hons), MA, PG Cert, PG Dip.

Professional Lead for Learning Disability Studies; Principal Lecturer, School of Nursing and Social Work, University of Hertfordshire

Paul commenced his nursing a career in 1996 at Harperbury Hospital becoming a Staff Nurse within an assessment and treatment unit. In 1999 he commenced in a role as a Community Learning Disability Nurse and lead a team to provide service to many people with learning disabilities and mental health problems. He has worked in nurse education since 2004, his key interests include Autism, learning disabilities and mental health. Paul has published widely in journals and textbooks. He is currently the Professional Lead for Learning Disabilities at the University of Hertfordshire.

Jean Mason Mitchell

RGN RM PGCHER MSc

Lecturer in Midwifery, School of Nursing, Midwifery, Social Work and Social Sciences, University of Salford

Jean began a nursing career in 1980 at Leigh Infirmary in Lancashire and worked on the medical and orthopaedic wards. She commenced midwifery education in 1984 at the Royal Bolton Hospital and worked there as a staff midwife and subsequently team leader until 2003. She then became a lecturer practitioner with the University of Salford and Salford Royal NHS Trust and became a full time lecturer in midwifery at the University of Salford in 2011. Her key areas of interest are clinical skills and simulation, safeguarding, mentorship and preceptorship for newly qualified midwives. She has been published in the British Journal of Midwifery and in Evidence based Midwifery.

Rosemary McCarthy

RM, RN, PGCE, MSc

Lecturer in Midwifery, School of Nursing, Midwifery, Social Work and Social Sciences, University of Salford

Rose commenced her nursing career in 1985 working across South Manchester University Hospitals becoming a Staff Nurse and working on a female renal/medical ward at Withington hospital. In 1991 she qualified as a midwife and worked as a rotational midwife in several units until 2003 when she became a Delivery Suite Coordinator at Wythenshawe Hospital. Rose became a Clinical Teaching Fellow at the University of Manchester in 2005 and held a dual role as an educator and clinician until 2010 when she became a full time Midwifery Lecturer at the University of Salford. She continues to work as a midwife at the University Hospitals of South Manchester NHS FT, where she is also a Supervisor of Midwives. Her key interests are in Maternal Critical Care and Acute Illness Management. She also has an interest in Maternal Global health and teaches an Acute Illness Management course in Uganda. Rose has published in a number of journals and has co-authored a Maternal Acute Illness management training course manual.

Louise McErlean

RGN, BSc (Hons) MA (Herts),
Senior Lecturer, Department of Adult Nursing and Primary Care, University of Hertfordshire

Louise commenced her nursing career in Glasgow in 1986 and specialised in intensive care nursing. She worked a Staff Nurse in Intensive care and then as a Sister in London. A move to Nurse Education followed in 2005. Louise has focused on adult nursing and her interests include physiology, clinical skills, simulation and nurse education.

Iain McGregor

RN(A), BN, CertHE
Deputy Manager, Millington Springs Care Home
Elder Homes Group

Iain began his nursing career in a care home for Older People in Scotland, before progressing through the ranks and becoming involved in the training and education of staff members within the care homes across Scotland and North East England. Iain then moved onto becoming the Quality Assurance Manager of a large independent health and social care training company, before the call of clinical practice beckoned and returning him to be a Deputy Manager of a medium sized care home in Nottinghamshire. Iain's passions in nursing are all around improving the quality of care delivered within care home environments and has been regularly involved in the National Older People's Forum.

Helen Paterson

EN, RN, Dip (N), BSc (Gerontological Nursing)
Matron for Specialist Medicine, Royal Berkshire NHS Foundation Trust, Reading

Helen commenced her career in nursing in 1980 at Forres Community hospital Morayshire, Scotland as an Enrolled Nurse. Having been being married to someone in the Forces, she has moved every 2-3yrs which as enabled her to gain a wealth of experience through working in various areas such as Nursing homes, Maternity, Pharmacy technician, Private hospitals and a community hospital. In 2000 she completed her conversion course to RN, and went to work as a staff nurse in Frimley Park Hospital for a year on a Care of the Elderly ward. In 2004 she completed a BSc in Gerontological Nursing whilst working at Royal Surrey County Hospital as a Discharge Co- ordinator. She then went on to work for Surrey community Health as a Falls Co ordinator for SW Surrey, Matron for Care of the Elderly at Hampshire Hospital , Basingstoke and is currently Matron of Specialist Medicine managing the 5 Elderly care wards, Neuro rehabilitation ward, and four specialist teams, Neurology Specialist Nurses, COCOC team (supporting older people with a diagnosis in Cancer), Pain team and Palliative Care Team. Helen is very passionate about nursing Older People, and hopes the chapter she has written enhances your knowledge and skills and will hopefully encourage more nurses to develop a career in elderly care.

Alicia Powell

RMN, BBehSc (Psychology), BSc Mental Health Nursing (Hons)
Community Mental Health Practitioner – Hounslow Mental Health Assessment Team, West London Mental Health NHS Trust

Alicia began her nursing career at West London Mental Health Trust in 2003 after emigrating from Australia. Prior to this she graduated with a Bachelor of Behavioural Science in Psychology from Griffith University, Brisbane in 2001. In the UK, Alicia began as a Health Care Assistant working in secure forensic units at St Bernard's, Ealing Hospital. This was followed by a 3 year secondment to undertake student nurse training at Thames Valley University where she graduated in 2008 with First Class Honours. As a Registered Mental Health Nurse she initially worked as a staff nurse in an Acute ward, followed by several years as a Community Mental Health Nurse. She currently works as a Mental Health Practitioner in a Mental Health Assessment Team. Alicia has particular interests in recovery and social inclusion, health promotion, student development and education. Alicia has been involved in the publication of another textbook focussing on mental health nursing.

Linda Sanderson

MSc, RSCN, RGN, RNT
Senior Lecturer, Pre-registration Children's nursing, School of Health, University of Central Lancashire

I qualified as a RGN with BSc (Hons) nursing in 1985. I worked with adults in a variety of settings until RSCN training was commenced in 1989. When qualified as a children's nurse I began working on the Yorkshire Regional Centre for Paediatric and Adolescent Oncology and Haematology Unit in Leeds. I worked on the oncology unit for 14 years in total, as a staff nurse, senior sister and lecturer practitioner. As the lecturer practitioner I was seconded to the University of Leeds to run the Paediatric and Adult Oncology courses.

In 2004 I left the clinical area of oncology and worked as a sister on a busy general Paediatric ward at Airedale General Hospital.

In 2006 I commenced as Senior Lecturer Child Health at the University of Central Lancashire (UCLan). During my time at UCLan I have been a module leader for a variety of modules across the pre-registration nursing and post registration nursing courses, a course leader for the Diploma (HE) Children's nursing and most recently the Admissions tutor for Childrens nursing. I thoroughly enjoy facilitating the learning of student nurses in all fields of nursing but particularly Children's nursing.

Melanie Stephens

RGN, DipnN, BSc (Hons), MA.
Senior Lecturer in Adult Nursing, School of Nursing, Midwifery, Social Work and Social Sciences, University of Salford

Melanie began her nursing career at Manchester Royal Infirmary, before moving on to various positions from nursing in medicine, gynaecology, burns and plastic surgery, intensive care and as a tissue viability nurse specialist. Melanie now works in higher education leading the schools tissue viability modules and her key interests are simulation, blended learning and internationalisation.

Steve Trenoweth

PhD, MSc, PGDipEA, BSc (Hons), RMN, MBPsS, FHEA
Associate Professor and Research Academic, University of West London

Steve is a qualified mental health nurse and has particular experience of working in acute and forensic mental health areas. His previous research involved the use of personal construct psychology to explore personal change and his current teaching and research interests include positive and holistic health. He is currently engaged on a project exploring the neurpsychology of stress and cognitive failure.

Jo Welch

RNMH, MA, BA (Hons), PGCE, PGDE, PG Dip (Applied Psychology)
Senior Lecturer, Centre for Learning Disability Studies, University of Hertfordshire

Jo commenced her nursing a career in 1985 in Surrey and has moved around the South East in various roles working with people who have a learning disability before becoming a Community Learning Disability Nurse. Having worked in clinical and managerial roles both in the NHS and Private Sector Jo returned to Hertfordshire as a Community Nurse and entered the world of Nurse Education in 2006. Jo is a facilitator of the Positive Choices Network and has interests in Offenders with a Learning Disability and the Physical Health of individuals and the role of Nurses as leaders and managers. Jo is currently working with the Learning Disability team at the Centre for Learning Disability Studies at the University of Hertfordshire.

Anthony Wheeldon

MSc (Lond), PGDE, BSc(Hons), DipHE, RN
Department of Adult Health and Primary Care, University of Hertfordshire

After qualification in 1995 Anthony worked as a staff nurse and senior staff nurse in the Respiratory Directorate at the Royal Brompton and Harefield NHS Trust. He began teaching on post-registration courses in 2000 before moving into full time nurse education at Thames Valley University in 2002. Anthony has a wide range of nursing interests including Cardiorespiratory nursing, anatomy and physiology, respiratory assessment and nurse education. He is currently an Associate Subject Lead for Adult Nursing at the University of Hertfordshire.

How to Use Your Textbook

Features Contained within your Textbook

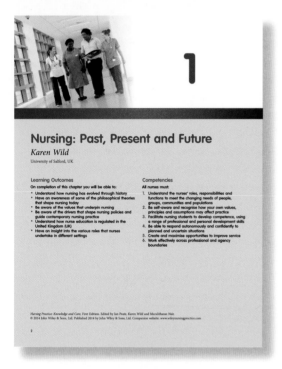

Nursing: Past, Present and Future

Karen Wild
University of Salford, UK

Learning Outcomes
On completion of this chapter you will be able to:
- Understand how nursing has evolved through history
- Have an awareness of some of the philosophical theories that shape nursing today
- Be aware of the values that underpin nursing
- Be aware of the drivers that shape nursing policies and guide contemporary nursing practice
- Understand how nurse education is regulated in the United Kingdom (UK)
- Have an insight into the various roles that nurses undertake in different settings

Competencies
All nurses must:
1. Understand the nurses' roles, responsibilities and functions to meet the changing needs of people, groups, communities and populations
2. Be self-aware and recognise how your own values, principles and assumptions may affect practice
3. Facilitate nursing students to develop competence, using a range of professional and personal development skills
4. Be able to respond autonomously and confidently to planned and uncertain situations
5. Create and maximise opportunities to improve service
6. Work effectively across professional and agency boundaries

Nursing Practice: Knowledge and Care, First Edition. Edited by Ian Peate, Karen Wild and Muralitharan Nair.
© 2014 John Wiley & Sons, Ltd. Published 2014 by John Wiley & Sons, Ltd. Companion website: www.wileynursingpractice.com

2

The overview page gives a summary of the topics covered in each part.
Every chapter begins with a list of **learning outcomes** and **competencies** contained within the chapter.

Jot this down boxes are short exercises and reflective questions to get you thinking.

> **Jot This Down** Exercise 1
> 1. Convert 550 mg to g
> 2. Convert 0.1 g to mg
> 3. Convert 50 mcg (or μg) to mg
> 4. Convert 100 mL to litres
> 5. Convert 0.125 g to mg
>   Answers to Exercise 1: **1.** 0.55 g; **2.** 100 mg; **3.** 0.5 mg; **4.** 0.1 litres; **5.** 125 mg

Medicines management boxes provide information about drugs and medicines.

> **Medicines Management**
>
> The medications given to patients for MRSA de-colonisation typically include:
> - Either: **Mupirocin** (often referred to by its trade name of Bactroban), which is a cream applied to the anterior nares of both nostrils two–three times daily for 5 days, or: **Neomycin** (often referred to by its trade name of Naseptin), which is a cream or ointment applied to both nostrils four times a day for 10 days.
> - **Chlorhexidine 4%** skin wash/bath, daily for 5 days. Patient should be told to pay particular attention to washing the axillae, groin and skin folds and skin should be moistened with water before applying the chlorhexidine to reduce the likelihood of reactions. Hair should also be washed with the Chlorhexidine, at least three times during the 5 days, if possible. A normal shampoo can be used after the Chlorhexidine each time.
>
> Treatment should be prescribed or follow a patient group direction, and practitioners should note guidance in the British National Formulary (BNF 2013).

Fields boxes give further insight into the other key areas of nursing: Learning Disabilities, Children's and Mental Health.

> **Nursing Fields** Children's Nursing
>
> *Every Child Matters* (Department for Education and Skills 2003)
>
> Common assessments and information sharing will be a major step forward...professionals will increasingly work alongside each other in the same team...clear lines of professional accountability should ensure that multi-disciplinary teams are able to benefit from a wide range of professionals working together, without losing the advantages of those professionals' individual specialisms.

What to do if boxes give extra information on a specific topic.

> **What To Do If...**
>
> Student nurse, Gemma, was attending a baby clinic with her mentor, an HV. Gemma noticed a mum and baby at the clinic who were sat quietly on their own, so she went to talk to them. The conversation moved to the baby, who was 6 months old. The mum told Gemma that she was very worried about her baby as he was not taking notice of his environment like other babies were and also not smiling much.

Link to/Go to boxes provide website addresses for further resources.

> **Link To/Go To** Nursing field: Adult
>
> You can access the results of the Care Quality Commission inpatient surveys by NHS Trust to see how your area compares with others in the UK:
> http://www.cqc.org.uk/surveys/inpatient

What the Experts Say

One of the guiding principles for me is that I need to gain permission from my patients prior to any care related activity, whether it is sitting and listening to patient's feelings or something more invasive, for example, the administration of intra-venous fluids. I always gain verbal consent from those in my care. The 'code' helps guide this principle, and I will often use this as an aide memoire when mentoring student nurses.

(Staff Nurse, Orthopaedic Surgical ward)

What the experts say are real-life quotes from family members, nurses and others to give insight into real situations.

Care, Dignity and Compassion

Maintaining patient dignity while they are wearing a surgical gown is difficult – as they are worn backwards (with the opening to the patient's rear) and patients often complain that the gowns do not keep them covered. Wherever possible, the patient may keep on their underwear until the moment they are to be transferred. Patients who have a dressing gown should be encouraged to wear it and those who do not have a dressing gown with them should be given a second surgical gown to wear in the place of a dressing gown.

Care, dignity and compassion boxes remind you to think about the patient.

The Evidence

The speech-mangling, cucumber-guzzling, gin-tippling, patient-brutalising Mrs Gamp could well be Dickens's finest grotesque, although he thought of her as highly realistic. In his preface to Chuzzlewit, Dickens wrote that Mrs Gamp was, "four-and-twenty years ago, a fair representation of the hired attendant on the poor in sickness," and she was so popular with Victorian readers that it took Florence Nightingale's efforts in the Crimea to steer the public perception of nurses away from the Gamp stereotype. Even her weirdest quirks came from real life: her habit of standing by the fireplace and rubbing her nose on the fender, for example, came from a description of a nurse given to him by his friend Angela Burdett-Coutts.

(Collin 2012)
http://www.telegraph.co.uk/culture/charles-dickens/9044813/Sarah-Gamp-My-favourite-Charles-Dickens-character.html

Evidence boxes provide background information and evidence.

Primary Care

Chemotherapy is usually administered while the person is an outpatient and most of the side-effects can occur once they have returned home, so they may feel vulnerable and alone.

Primary care boxes give information about how to manage issues in the primary care setting.

Red flags highlight important points that must not be overlooked.

Red Flag

Although student nurses may not be called to account by the NMC for any acts or omissions in practice, this does not mean that they are immune from blame and can be called to account both in law and by Universities via the 'fitness for practice' route.

Key points at the end of each chapter remind you of important points to remember.

Key Points

- Nursing practice is structured by codes of ethics and standards, with which an individual can be held accountable in a court of law.
- The standards set help define the roles of nursing and are critical to moral decision-making.

Glossary is where to go for an explanation of any terms in the chapter.

Glossary

Advocacy: individuals have the right to choose treatment options without coercion, based on information about the outcome of accepting or rejecting the treatment
Applied ethics: describes an approach to ethical decision-making, which uses moral theories and principles to examine and address practical issues in everyday professional life

Your textbook is full of **photographs, illustrations and tables.**

Self-assessment review questions help you test yourself after each chapter.

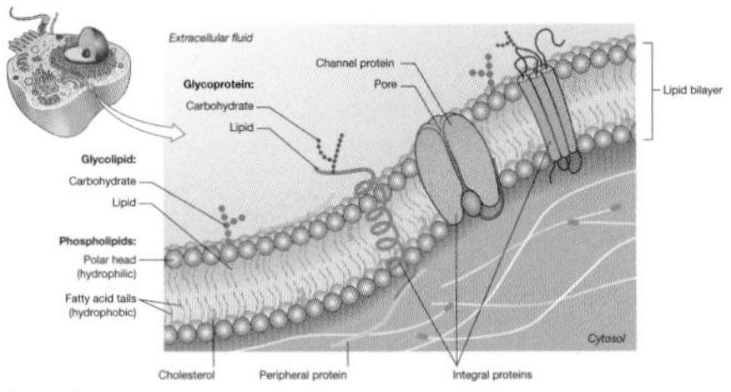

Figure 19.6 Cell membrane.

The Anytime, Anywhere Textbook

Wiley E-Text

For the first time, your textbook comes with free access to a **Wiley E-Text: Powered by VitalSource** version – a digital, interactive version of this textbook which you own as soon as you download it.

Your **Wiley E-Text** allows you to:

Search: Save time by finding terms and topics instantly in your book, your notes, even your whole library (once you've downloaded more textbooks)

Note and Highlight: Colour code, highlight and make digital notes right in the text so you can find them quickly and easily

Organize: Keep books, notes and class materials organized in folders inside the application

Share: Exchange notes and highlights with friends, classmates and study groups

Upgrade: Your textbook can be transferred when you need to change or upgrade computers

Link: Link directly from the page of your interactive textbook to all of the material contained on the companion website

The **Wiley E-Text** version will also allow you to copy and paste any photograph or illustration into assignments, presentations and your own notes.

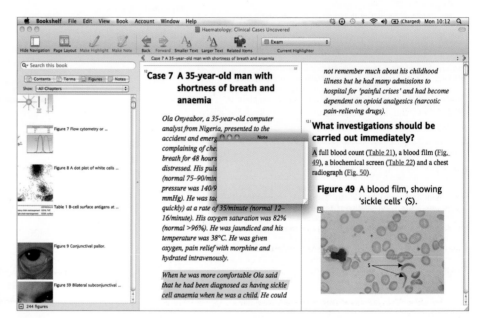

Wiley E-Text
Powered by VitalSource®

To access your Wiley E-Text:

- Find the redemption code on the inside front cover of this book and carefully scratch away the top coating of the label. Visit **www.vitalsource.com/software/bookshelf/downloads** to download the Bookshelf application to your computer, laptop, tablet or mobile device.
- If you have purchased this title as an e-book, access to your **Wiley E-Text** is available with proof of purchase within 90 days. Visit **http://support.wiley.com** to request a redemption code via the 'Live Chat' or 'Ask A Question' tabs.
- Open the Bookshelf application on your computer and register for an account.
- Follow the registration process and enter your redemption code to download your digital book.
- For full access instructions, visit **wileynursingpractice.com**.

The VitalSource Bookshelf can now be used to view your Wiley E-Text on iOS, Android and Kindle Fire!

· **For iOS:** Visit the app store to download the VitalSource Bookshelf: **http://bit.ly/17ib3XS**
· **For Android and Kindle Fire:** Visit the Google Play Market to download the VitalSource Bookshelf: **http://bit.ly/BSAAGP**
  You can now sign in with the email address and password you used when you created your VitalSource Bookshelf Account.

Full E-Text support for mobile devices is available at: **http://support.vitalsource.com**

CourseSmart

CourseSmart gives you instant access (via computer or mobile device) to this Wiley-Blackwell e-book and its extra electronic functionality, at 40% off the recommended retail print price. See all the benefits at **www.coursesmart.com/students**.

Instructors…receive your own digital desk copies!

CourseSmart also offers instructors an immediate, efficient, and environmentally-friendly way to review this textbook for your course.

For more information visit **www.coursesmart.com/instructors**.

With **CourseSmart**, you can create lecture notes quickly with copy and paste, and share pages and notes with your students. Access your **CourseSmart** digital textbook from your computer or mobile device instantly for evaluation, class preparation, and as a teaching tool in the classroom.

Simply sign in at **http://instructors.coursesmart.com/bookshelf** to download your Bookshelf and get started. To request your desk copy, hit 'Request Online Copy' on your search results or book product page.

We hope you enjoy using your new textbook. Good luck with your studies!

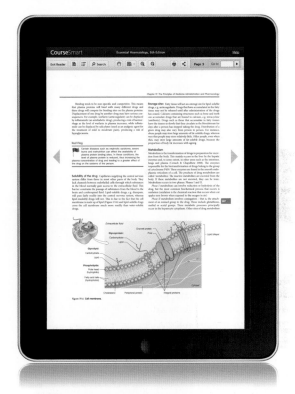

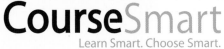

About the Companion Website

Don't forget to visit the companion website for this book:

 www.wileynursingpractice.com

There you will find valuable material designed for both students and instructors:

- Interactive flashcards for self-test
- Interactive multiple-choice questions
- Glossary of useful terms from the book
- Chapter key points from the book
- Chapter references from the book
- Useful website links from the book

There is an instructor-only section of the website containing:

- Figures from the book in PowerPoint format
- Worksheets to enhance learning and revision

Unit 1

Contextualising the Art and Science of Nursing

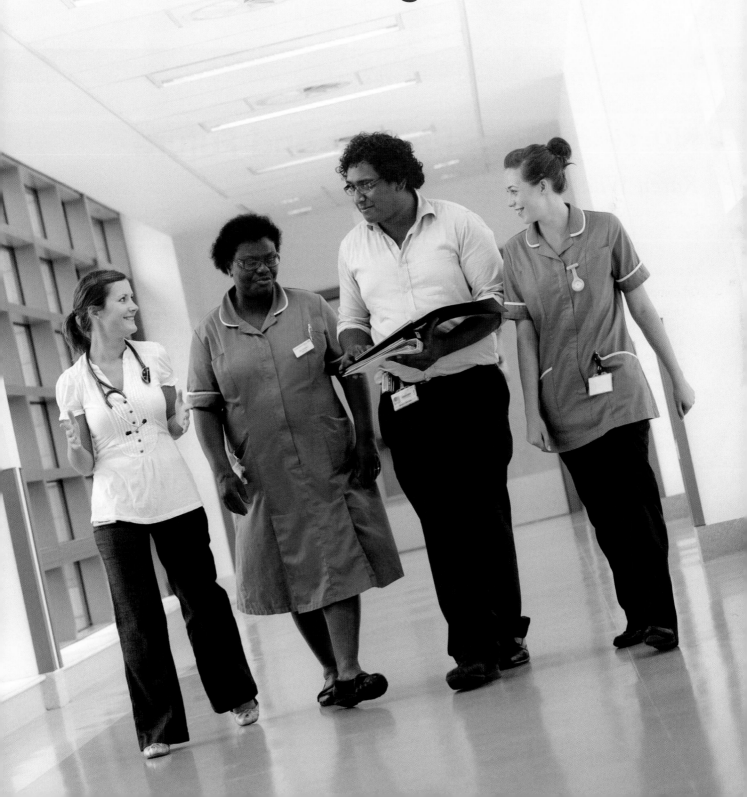

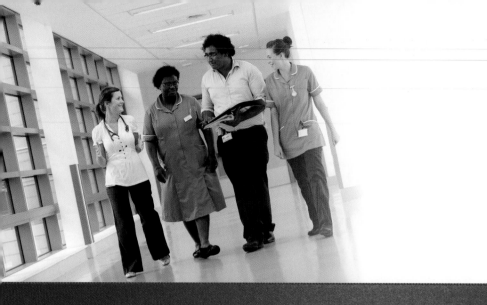

1

Nursing: Past, Present and Future

Karen Wild

University of Salford, UK

Learning Outcomes

On completion of this chapter you will be able to:

* Understand how nursing has evolved through history
* Have an awareness of some of the philosophical theories that shape nursing today
* Be aware of the values that underpin nursing
* Be aware of the drivers that shape nursing policies and guide contemporary nursing practice
* Understand how nurse education is regulated in the United Kingdom (UK)
* Have an insight into the various roles that nurses undertake in different settings

Competencies

All nurses must:

1. Understand the nurses' roles, responsibilities and functions to meet the changing needs of people, groups, communities and populations
2. Be self-aware and recognise how your own values, principles and assumptions may affect practice
3. Facilitate nursing students to develop competence, using a range of professional and personal development skills
4. Be able to respond autonomously and confidently to planned and uncertain situations
5. Create and maximise opportunities to improve service
6. Work effectively across professional and agency boundaries

 Visit the companion website at **www.wileynursingpractice.com** where you can test yourself using flashcards, multiple-choice questions and more.

Unit 1 image source: LTH NHS Trust / Science Photo Library
Nursing Practice: Knowledge and Care, First Edition. Edited by Ian Peate, Karen Wild and Muralitharan Nair.
© 2014 John Wiley & Sons, Ltd. Published 2014 by John Wiley & Sons, Ltd. Companion website: www.wileynursingpractice.com

Introduction

In their report to the Prime Minister (DH 2010), the Commission on the Future of Nursing and Midwifery stated that:

> England's nurses and midwives are the lifeblood of the NHS and other health services and have always been at the heart of good health care. In 2009 there were well over half a million nurses and midwives on the Nursing and Midwifery Council (NMC) register residing in England. As the largest group of registered professionals in the NHS, they are a huge workforce with great power and potential to influence health and health care. They are ideally placed to improve the experiences of service users and families, and they influence health in a wide range of health, social care and community settings.
>
> In the last decade nurses have acquired greater responsibility as autonomous interdependent practitioners: they lead programmes of care, act as partners and employers in general practice, and also lead their own services and run their own clinics.
>
> (Department of Health 2010, p. 16)

This chapter will explore the evolution of nursing as described earlier and highlight the unique roles that nurses play in contemporary society. It will look at past and current structures of the NHS and health provision in the UK and describe the legislation that supports the professional status of Nursing.

> ### Jot This Down
> When you reflect on your role as a nurse, what would you say was your motivation to care?

In the 'Jot This Down' exercise, you may have identified certain traits in your behaviour or personality that motivate you to care. The need to help others and to respect an individual's dignity and independence can influence the desire to care. You may see yourself as a naturally caring person, so-called altruistic traits. Work that is challenging and varied might appeal to you; job satisfaction and the ability to work in a team may also help to motivate you as a nurse. You may have considered the characteristics of the role that you have, such as autonomy, feedback (people saying thank you), the variety of skills that you have developed and satisfaction in seeing the completion of an aspect of care. You may also relate your motivation to care in terms of the value that you hold in society and the opportunities you have for personal development and growth within the profession. Some may relate the motivation to the relative job security that nursing brings; its salary and peer support may be significant too. The intellectual basis of nursing and the continued development of knowledge, skills and proficiency may also feature on your list.

The fundamental basis of nursing is associated with caring and helping, and nursing can be described as both an art and a science. Caring defines nurses and their work, and as such, there are many facets associated with the role and function of the nurse. The role is constantly evolving and is difficult to classify.

Recent developments have influenced the guidance developed by the chief nursing officer's (CNO) 6Cs (DH 2012) and the RCN's (2010) *Principles of Nursing Practice* (**rcn.org.uk/nursing** principles). In Table 1.1 you can see the links that can be mapped between the 6Cs and the RCN's *Principles of Nursing Practice*.

In Table 1.1, there is clear evidence from both the RCN and the CNO that nursing encompasses many roles, and it serves to high-

Table 1.1 Mapping the 6Cs against the basics of the RCN's *Principles of Nursing Practice*. (Source: Watterson 2013)

THE 6CS OF NURSING	RCN'S PRINCIPLES OF NURSING PRACTICE
Compassion • relationships based on empathy, respect and dignity	**Principle A** • dignity, equality, diversity and humanity
Courage • doing the right thing, speaking up if concerned, strength and vision to innovate	**Principle B** • ethical and legal integrity, accountability, responsibility **Principle C** • safety, the environment, organisational health and safety, risk management
Care • the core business of nursing, which helps the individual and improves the health of the whole community • caring defines nursing	**Principle D** • advocacy, empowerment and patient-centred care • patient involvement in care
Communication • central to successful caring relationships; listening is as important as what is said and done. *'No decision about me without me'*; communication key with patients and staff	**Principle E** • communication, handling feedback, recording, reporting and monitoring **Principle G** • interdisciplinary and multi-agency working; teamworking, continuity of care
Competence • the ability to understand an individual's health and social needs • expertise, clinical and technical skill to deliver effective care based on research and evidence	**Principle F** • evidence-based practice, education, technical skill, clinical reasoning
Commitment • to patients and populations • to build on and improve care and patient experiences	**Principle H** • leadership which contributes to an open and honest culture • nurses leading by example

light the core professional values and behaviours that underpin nursing. The CNO is the government's most senior nursing adviser and has the responsibility to ensure that the government's strategy for nursing is delivered. The CNO leads over 597 625 nurses, midwives, health visitors, other allied health professionals.

This chapter is concerned with the professional values that underpin nursing practice. An overview is provided of the development of nursing, from what was an unstructured, *ad hoc* approach to caring, to a regulated profession.

Care has been claimed to be an essential human need for the full development, health maintenance and survival of human beings in all world cultures (Leininger 2002), yet care throughout history has not been awarded the same importance as cure. Leininger poses the question: does cure gain more attention because of the public recognition of dramatic new technologies, and because it is associated with males? In contrast, the tradition of caring has tended to be a female activity, focussing on the individual, the family and groups of people. She asserts that there can be no curing without caring, and that the culture of care can be embedded in our history, through examples such as religious (or spiritual), social, political, educational and economic contexts. The next section will provide a snapshot of that history and tradition.

A Glance at the History of Nursing

Almost unanimously, the history of nursing will tend to focus on the works and publications of Florence Nightingale; however, nursing has been shaped and formed throughout history and has been influenced by a global perspective. To appreciate the development of contemporary nursing in the UK, it helps to take a look at where nursing has come from, and how it continues to develop and grow.

Health and disease is a constant factor of the human state, and the need for some form of support and care of individuals and populations throughout history varies greatly. What follows is a review of the evidence that supports the idea of people helping other people in times of need, through history, and the development of systems of care and the fundamental beginnings of nursing as we know it today.

Pre-history

Paleopathology is the study of diseases in past populations, and archaeologists have retrieved ancient human remains which demonstrate that fractured limbs have been healed; this signifies that some form of care provision occurred. In addition, evidence of infectious diseases such as tuberculosis and syphilis has also been identified in bone remains. Indicators that some form of treatment was given exists in the skull evidence of ancient man, where the practice of trepanation (or drilling holes in the cranium) has been seen. In some skulls, there is evidence of more than one hole with partial healing, indicating that the treatment was often survived.

Cave paintings illustrate life events such as birth and death, and there are images that suggest female interaction. Those who lived in the prehistoric period suffered similar conditions to those experienced by society today, and according to Hallett (2010), tribes in those early years took part in caring for their sick and wounded. The role of spirituality and health linked to strange occurrences, such as sudden flooding or times of drought, have helped shape beliefs around supernatural interventions, for example the visitation of evil spirits. Healers or *Shamans* would employ various brews and magical potions to heal the sick. Those responsible for feeding and cleaning the sick were predominantly females.

Evidence to support the evolution of nursing has been gathered and interpreted from hieroglyphic inscriptions, cuneiform writings, papyri and documented histories in the forms of drawings, ancient objects and oral traditions.

Ancient History

In Ancient Greece, temples were erected to honour the goddess of health, Hygeia. Care at the temples was related to bathing and this activity was overseen by priestesses. No mention is made of nurses as a separate entity, but temple attendants probably assisted the physicians by 'caring' for their patients. Babylonian civilisations from around 3000 BC acknowledged the role of public health measures, such as large stone drains, to cope with human waste.

The foundation of modern medicine was laid down by Hippocrates in Ancient Greece, who is credited with the belief that diseases were caused naturally and not because of superstition or the intervention of gods.

The first hospitals were established in the Byzantine Empire, which was the first part of the Roman Empire. As the Roman Empire expanded, hospitals were erected. It was Fabiola, a wealthy Roman, who was responsible for the introduction of hospitals in the West. She dedicated her immense wealth to the sick and served as a role model, nursing the sick herself, despite the repulsive wounds and sores of the inmates. The primary carers in these hospitals were young men on the verge of adulthood, who were called *contubernales*. After the Roman invasion in approximately ad2, slave girls were known to assist Roman physicians. *Valetudinariums* – civilian hospitals – were kept clean and aired by bailiffs' wives, who would also watch over the sick.

In the Middle Ages, medical knowledge and development slowed and many of the influences of the Ancient Greeks and in particular the Romans in this country were destroyed. Rome and the Catholic Church dominated the direction of medicine, and throughout the Middle Ages, military, religious and lay orders of men provided most of the health care. Some of these orders of men included the Knights Hospitallers, the Order of the Holy Spirit and Teutonic Knights. While these men provided care, charlatans and 'quacks' provided treatment for money; examples are diagnoses made by the use of astrology and the widely practised treatment of bloodletting, often doing more harm than good. The Black Death was to kill two-thirds of England's population between 1348 and 1350, and the commonly held doctrine from the church that disease was a punishment from God for sinful behaviour did little to help the poor and uneducated. Figure 1.1 depicts the experience of birth and the support given to a woman in labour during this time.

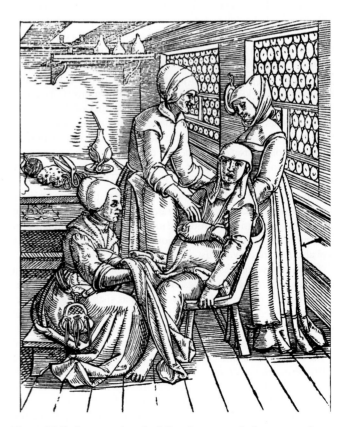

Figure 1.1 Early engraving depicting the support of a woman in labour. Reproduced with permission of Everett Collection Historical/Alamy.

Several hospitals were opened during this period, for example St Thomas's, St Bartholomew's and Bethlem. Care that had been provided by nuns was now provided by local women, whose efforts were overseen by matrons. Their duties centred on domestic chores.

The second half of the 18th century saw the evolution of scientific method, the so-called 'Age of Enlightenment'. Its purpose was to reform society using reason, challenging tradition and advancing knowledge. Scientific endeavour flourished during the Enlightenment and philanthropists provided the means to open charity hospitals around the UK. These hospitals employed nurses, who may have been paid or unpaid, who carried out domestic duties. It was not unusual for so-called nurses to drink alcohol and take money from patients in order to pay for their alcohol. Charles Dickens, in his 1843 novel *Martin Chuzzlewit*, developed the main theme related to 'selfishness'. One of the characters, the nurse, Mrs Gamp, was an odious individual who was a midwife and 'layer-out of the dead' (perhaps one of the first health visitors: 'from cradle to the grave').

The Evidence

The speech-mangling, cucumber-guzzling, gin-tippling, patient-brutalising Mrs Gamp could well be Dickens's finest grotesque, although he thought of her as highly realistic. In his preface to Chuzzlewit, Dickens wrote that Mrs Gamp was, "four-and-twenty years ago, a fair representation of the hired attendant on the poor in sickness," and she was so popular with Victorian readers that it took Florence Nightingale's efforts in the Crimea to steer the public perception of nurses away from the Gamp stereotype. Even her weirdest quirks came from real life: her habit of standing by the fireplace and rubbing her nose on the fender, for example, came from a description of a nurse given to him by his friend Angela Burdett-Coutts.

(Collin 2012)
http://www.telegraph.co.uk/culture/charles-dickens/9044813/Sarah-Gamp-My-favourite-Charles-Dickens-character.html

Sarah Gamp was immoral, self-indulgent, sloppy and generally drunk. A notorious stereotype of untrained and incompetent nurses of the early Victorian era, before the reforms of campaigners such as Florence Nightingale. Mrs Gamp is everything we least expect of a good nurse: she was selfish, untrustworthy, a bully, nasty to patients and slothful.

Parish nurses and their supposed inadequacies were justification of the need to change the way that nurses were employed and governed, and in 1727, two pamphlets were published to support the creation of a workhouse. Workhouses were established to employ and maintain the poor, and nursing duties were generally performed by elderly female inmates who were illiterate, fond of a drink and inept in the demands of caring for the sick. The development of the workhouse infirmaries saw a move to the more familiar set-up of providing a separate annex to the workhouse building; this allowed segregation of the sick according to the nature of their illness. It is difficult to differentiate what history tells us about the nature of nursing: that is the difference between 'nursing work' and the 'work done by nurses'. Nurses began to be employed by workhouse guardians and in 1865, William Rathbone, with the help of Florence Nightingale, financed the introduction of trained nurses to the Brownlow Hill Infirmary in Liverpool. Interestingly, the employment of pauper nurses continued under the supervision of a trained nurse (White 1978).

Alongside the Poor Law acts of the 19th century, medical schools began to emerge, as medical knowledge grew. The Royal College of Surgeons was formed in 1800 and at this time, doctors were required to carry out some aspects of their training in hospitals.

The year 1800 brought about the era of social and political revolution, and many of the great philosophers, such as Emanuel Kant brought radical intellectualism into the minds of many. In 1784, Kant challenged society to: 'Dare to know! Have the courage to use your own understanding', which became the motto of the Enlightenment. Science and technical development reached new heights and the Victorian era from 1831 saw the biggest developments in social and scientific engagement. During 1853 to 1856, Britain and France became involved in the Crimean war against Russia, and the American Civil war started in 1861.

Jot This Down

The American Civil War of 1861 was regarded as the first 'modern war' because of the large scale use of what was then considered modern technology.

- Make a list of the developments in health care that you think have been influenced by wars and conflict throughout history

In the 'Jot This Down' exercise above, you may have thought about more recent developments that you are aware of, such as the hospital at Camp Bastion in Afghanistan, with its innovations in trauma surgery and nursing care; or the development of triage, to assess those most in need of emergency care. Interestingly, triage was developed in the First World War in France to treat mass casualties. You may have included the use of the tourniquet to limit blood loss; this was known in Roman times and has been adapted by the military today to be applied, if needed, with one hand. Ultrasound is a product of war, first used to detect cracks in armour in the Second World War, by tank engineers. Your list may also include infection control and the use of antibiotics to treat infections. Modern infection control has been influenced by the work of Florence Nightingale during the Crimean War, as she pioneered the cleaning and ventilation of the Scutari hospital, thus reducing mortality rates among the sick and wounded.

Florence Nightingale (1820–1910)

Known for her pioneering work in the Crimean War, Florence Nightingale (Figure 1.2) opened the way to bring respectability to nursing. Born in Italy in 1820, she is now celebrated as a social reformer and statistician. From a professional viewpoint, Nightingale is seen as the founder of modern nursing; she spoke with firm conviction about the nature of nursing as a distinct profession, allowing young middle-class women an opportunity to make a meaningful contribution to society. At the time, nursing in the middle and upper classes was defined as caring for sick and elderly relatives, for example, a daughter might nurse her ageing and sick father. Nightingale was concerned with what she saw as the all-encompassing plight of the Victorian woman – on the one hand redundant wives of the wealthy, and on the other women who were poverty stricken and forced to toil for long hours at tedious and unskilled work.

Born to a wealthy upper-class family herself, the expectation was that she would marry well and produce a family. However, she defied the wishes of her family and in the first decade of her adult life, fought to use her talents in a productive and helpful way in order to benefit society.

In March 1853, Russia invaded Turkey, and Britain, concerned about the growing power of Russia, went to Turkey's aid. This conflict occurred in and around Scutari and became known as the Crimean War. Soon after British soldiers arrived in Turkey, they began to fall ill with malaria and cholera. Florence Nightingale volunteered her services to the war effort and was given permission to take a group of nurses to a hospital in Scutari based several miles from the front. Here, she was faced with mass infections, lack of medical supplies and poor hygiene.

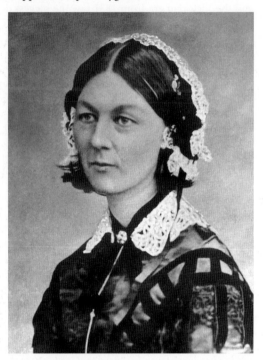

Figure 1.2 **Florence Nightingale.** Reproduced with permission of Superstock/David Cole.

After the war, she wrote *Notes on Nursing*, where she set out the basic foundation on which nursing was to be based, and expressed the proper functions of nursing. These functions in Nightingale's view included improving the environment of the sick room with clean air and ventilation, making and recording astute observations of the sick and their environment and developing knowledge around the process of recovery.

The Evidence How to Ventilate without a Chill

…with a proper supply of windows, and a proper supply of fuel in open fire places, fresh air is comparatively easy to secure when your patient or patients are in bed. Never be afraid of open windows then. People don't catch colds in bed. This is a popular fallacy. With proper bed-clothes and hot water bottles, if necessary, you can always keep a patient warm in bed, and well ventilate him at the same time.

(Nightingale 1859)

Florence Nightingale was seen by many historians as 'The Lady with the Lamp' after a report in *The Times* newspaper from the Crimea, which depicted her as a lone figure in the night, a small lamp in her hand, checking on the welfare of the wounded soldiers. Interestingly, the lighting of lamps is documented in the *Nursing Mirror* pocket diary of 1913, shown in Figure 1.3, which gives specific times for lamps to be lit throughout the year.

After returning to England as a national heroine, she began reforming conditions in British hospitals (in the first instance, this was confined to military hospitals). Nightingale was able to raise £45 000 in funds to improve the quality of nursing. In 1860, she used these funds to found the Nightingale School and Home for Nurses at St Thomas's Hospital.

Her philosophy of nursing was based on the belief that there should be a theoretical basis for nursing practice and that nurses should be formally educated. Resolute in her desire to professionalise nursing, she insisted that nursing schools should be controlled and staffed by women who were trained nurses. She also wanted to

TIMES FOR LIGHTING LAMPS.

JANUARY.		FEBRUARY.	
Sat. 4	5. 3	Sat. 1	5.45
,, 11	5.11	,, 8	5.57
,, 18	5.20	,, 15	6.11
,, 25	5.33	,, 22	6.22

MARCH.		APRIL.	
Sat. 1	6.38	Sat. 5	7.37
,, 8	6.50	,, 12	7.49
,, 15	7. 2	,, 19	8. 0
,, 22	7.14	,, 26	8.12
,, 29	7.26		

MAY.		JUNE.	
Sat. 3	8.24	Sat. 7	9.11
,, 10	8.34	,, 14	9.16
,, 17	8.45	,, 21	9.19
,, 24	8.56	,, 28	9.19
,, 31	9. 4		

1913.

JULY.		AUGUST.	
Sat. 5	9.17	Sat. 2	8.45
,, 12	9.12	,, 9	8.33
,, 19	9. 5	,, 16	8.20
,, 26	8.56	,, 23	8. 6
		,, 30	7.51

SEPTEMBER.		OCTOBER.	
Sat. 6	7.35	Sat. 4	6.31
,, 13	7.19	,, 11	6.15
,, 20	7. 3	,, 18	6. 0
,, 27	6.47	,, 25	5.46

NOVEMBER.		DECEMBER.	
Sat. 1	5.33	Sat. 6	4.50
,, 8	5.20	,, 13	4.49
,, 15	5.10	,, 20	4.51
,, 22	5. 1	,, 27	4.55
,, 29	4.53		

Figure 1.3 **Lighting the lamps in 1913.**

develop a systematic approach to the assessment of patients where an individual approach to care provision based on individual patient needs was required. She strongly believed in the maintenance of patient confidentiality.

The philanthropist, William Rathbone, worked with Nightingale to develop the first district nursing service. This was acknowledged by Queen Victoria with the title 'Queen's Nurses' being awarded to nurses caring for people at home. In the late 1800s, courses were provided to teach women to develop an insight into sanitation in homes. These women had a duty to care for the health of adults, children and pregnant women (pre- and antenatal), and the first health visitor was employed in Salford in 1862 (Adams 2012).

In the 1870s, America's first trained nurse, Linda Richards was mentored by Nightingale. Richards went on to pioneer the development of nursing in both America and Japan (Doona 1996). In 1883, Nightingale was awarded the Royal Red Cross by Queen Victoria, and became the first woman to receive the Order of Merit. In 1873, Nightingale wrote, 'Nursing is most truly said to be a high calling, an honourable calling'. She died in London in 1910.

Mary Seacole (1805–1881)

Daughter of a Scottish soldier with a Jamaican mother, Seacole (Figure 1.4) learned her nursing skills in the family boarding house for invalid soldiers. She was well travelled, visiting the Bahamas, Central America and Britain. Despite the War Office in England refusing her application to be an army nurse in the Crimean War Seacole funded her own visit and arrived in Scutari to offer her services to Nightingale, but these were refused. Undeterred, Seacole set up her own services and established the British Hotel near Balaclava. Here, she provided comfort and convalescence to the British and Russian soldiers, often at the battle front (Anionwu 2005).

Seacole also became involved in the training of nurses for employment in the workhouses. Her contribution to nursing has not always been recognised, and unlike Nightingale, she does not feature significantly in the established nursing literature until the 1970s. It is most certainly the case that Seacole's work in the Crimean War was overshadowed at the time by that of Florence Nightingale; however, there has been a revival of interest in her contribution, with an introduction to her life and works added to the school national curriculum in the UK.

The development of education and regulation for nurses

Throughout the 1890s, pressure grew for the registration of nurses, and leaders within the profession were debating the need to pass a public examination just as medical practitioners had been required to do since 1858. However, Florence Nightingale was opposed to this notion, worried that central examination might undermine her philosophy of nursing. In 1887, Ethel Bedford-Fenwick (a former Matron at St Bartholomew's Hospital, London) formed the British Nurses' Association, which sought to provide for the registration of British nurses, based on the same terms as physicians and surgeons, as evidence of their having received systematic training. Bedford-Fenwick was a staunch supporter of professional regulation. Up until this time, nurses remained relatively free from external regulation. In 1902, the Midwives Registration Act established the state regulation of midwives, and midwives undertook training in order to register with the Central Midwives Board. A House of Commons Select Committee was established in 1904 to consider the registration of nurses, and in 1909, the Central Committee for the State Registration of Nurses was formed.

The First World War (1914–1918) provided the final stimulus to the creation of nursing regulation, partly because of the contributions made by nurses to the war effort. The College of Nursing (this later became the Royal College of Nursing in 1928) was established in 1916. Its principal functions were to:

- *Advance the profession of nursing through improved education and training*
- *Promote consistency of nursing curricula*
- *Recognise approved nursing schools*
- *Create and maintain a register of nurses who were certified proficient through training*
- *Promote Parliamentary Bills in any way connected with the interests of nursing, education of nurses and the professional recognition of nursing.*

(Baly 1995)

Eventually in 1919, the Nurses Registration Acts were passed for England, Wales, Scotland and Ireland. The General Nursing Council (GNC) for England, Wales, Scotland and Ireland and other bodies were established as a result of these Acts. The Councils were established in 1921, with clearly agreed duties and responsibilities for the training, examination and registration of nurses and the approval of training schools for the purpose of maintaining a Register of Nurses for England and Wales, Scotland and Ireland.

The GNC Register of qualified nurses included a number of 'parts': one part contained the names of all nurses who satisfied the rules of admission, and there were also supplementary parts for:

- Male nurses
- Nurses trained in caring for people with mental diseases
- Nurses trained to care for sick children.

Later additions to the parts of the register included nurses trained to care for 'mental defectives' (people with learning difficulties) and nurses of infectious diseases.

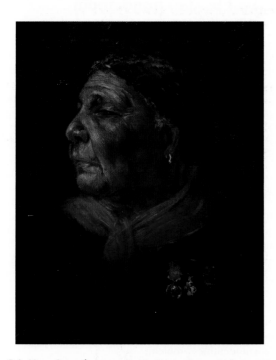

Figure 1.4 Mary Seacole. Reproduced with permission of Nils Jorgensen/Rex.

The GNC had powers to undertake disciplinary procedures and remove the names of State Registered Nurses (SRNs) from the register if they were deemed 'not fit and proper persons' having committed an act of misconduct or 'otherwise' – conduct unbecoming of a nurse.

Progressively, nursing began to emerge as acceptable work for the middle-class woman, no longer labelled as menial duties but now seen as work that was professional, respectable and valued. In the inter-war years, the image of nursing was associated with courage and heroism; the First World War had enabled women to enter new areas of freedom and independence.

The Register of Nurses was first published in 1922. The GNC and the other bodies survived intact until changes were made in 1979. These resulted in the creation of the United Kingdom Central Council (UKCC) and the four National Boards for the UK.

The development of modern nursing

Despite the TV and media image of the nurse as an attractive female, who falls in love with the doctor, the 1960s heralded a seed change in the way that nurses viewed their role in terms of accountability and the consequences of their actions. Theories to support the art and science of nursing began to emerge, and models of nursing were introduced to help describe nursing in a variety of care settings and roles. Chapter 7 within this book explores these developments in detail.

Many of the theories that relate to nursing have a philosophical foundation and will include ideas about the nature of nursing, the nature of the person, the nature of society and the environment and the nature of health. Some examples of the key influencers in relation to this are highlighted in the next section.

Virginia Henderson (1897–1996)

Known as the 'modern day mother of nursing', upon graduation, Virginia Henderson began her nursing career in Washington DC in 1921, working as a nurse in the community. She soon entered the education arena and wrote about her early experience as a nurse teacher. In the 1940s, she began to develop her personal definition of nursing, her so-called 'concept', which focussed on the importance of independence for the patient, helping with rehabilitation and progress from hospital to home. She identified 14 nursing components based on human need and geared towards the nurses' role:

- Substitutive – doing for the person
- Supplementary – helping the person
- Complementary – working with the person.

The Evidence   Henderson's Definition of Nursing

The unique function of the nurse is to assist the individual, sick or well, in the performance of those activities contributing to health or its recovery (or to peaceful death) that he would perform unaided if he had the necessary strength, will or knowledge and to do this in such a way as to help him gain independence as rapidly as possible.

(Henderson 1966)

The 14 components are, in the main, physiological and focus on physical aspects such as breathing, eliminating, maintaining hygiene and nutrition. However, Henderson also acknowledged the importance of spiritual, moral and sociological needs of the individual. Henderson (1966) implies that nursing is more than a matter of carrying out doctors' orders. Instead, nursing involves a special relationship with the person (and often the family). According to Henderson, the nurse intervenes with knowledge and skills to meet those needs that individuals and family would not normally be able to provide.

Her concept highlights **what** the nurse ought to focus on; however, it has been criticised for its lack of in-depth guidance as to **how** the nurse assists in meeting the individual components (Wills & McEwen 2002). She saw nurses as functioning independently from the physician, promoting the treatment plans prescribed. Her concept encompassed the notion of the life continuum, with nurses helping both sick and healthy people from the newborn to those who are dying. Nurses, according to Henderson, should be knowledgeable in biological and social sciences and must have the ability to assess basic human need.

With human need as the central component of Henderson's concept, it has paved the way for further theories as to individual needs and how nurses can help in meeting these needs.

Dorothea Orem (1914–2007)

Orem developed the 'Self-Care Theory' based on the premise that people should be self-reliant and responsible for their own care and the care of others in their family. Her philosophy focussed on the distinct individuality of the person, and the interaction of the person with the nurse, based on the need to meet self-care. In this way, she developed the idea of a health continuum, where the patient moves from dependency to independency. The nurses' role in the continuum is to help the achievement of independence, act as an advocate, redirector, supporter and teacher, and to provide an environment that contributes to the therapeutic environment. Orem's philosophy is that nursing is the ability to care for another, especially when they are unable to care for themselves (Orem 1991).

Hildegard Peplau (1909–1999)

Peplau was the first published nurse theorist since Florence Nightingale. Her work focussed on the therapeutic nature of nursing, asserting that the nurse–patient relationship is the foundation of nursing practice. She wanted to revolutionise the established approach to care, where the nurse passively acted out the doctor's orders and the patient passively received the treatment. She saw a human dynamic in the shared experience of caring and being cared for, where each party experiences personal growth through learning and coping.

This dynamic is achieved through developmental stages in the nurse–patient relationship, and relies on the distinct character roles typical of the nurse. Typical character roles include: the nurse as a resource, answering questions and interpreting data; nurse as a technical expert, providing physical care through clinical skills; nurse as a teacher, providing instruction and facilitating understanding (Peplau 1952).

The developmental stages are mapped out as follows:

Orientation Phase
- Establish rapport
- Set parameters
- Understand roles and begin to establish trust

Identification Phase
- Patient identifies problems
- Nurse helps patient to recognise their own role in self-care

Exploitation Phase
- Patient trust is established, makes full use of nursing service
- Problem-solving
- Setting future goals

Resolution Phase
- Patient needs met
- Relationship ends on mutual basis
- Patient less reliant on nurse, more self-reliant.

Patricia Benner

Benner was contemporary theorist who introduced the concept that expert nurses develop skills and understanding of their craft through the experience and education of caring. She described five levels of nursing experience and coined the phrase: 'from novice to expert' in her publication in 1982. Her work is significant, as it changed the perception of the term 'expert nurse' from the most highly paid and prestigious, to encompass the notion of the expert as one who provides the 'most exquisite care', and that practise itself could inform the theory of care (Benner 1982).

Margaret Newman

In 1979, Newman presented her 'theory of expanding consciousness'. She presents the notion that disease (ill health) and the absence of disease (health) in the individual are equally important in the human lifespan. She asserts that consciousness is a healthy state; the more individuals interact with their environment and the world around them, the more conscious they are. Crisis such as health breakdown increases consciousness – she relates to this as the total response that the individual makes to that crisis: physiological, psychological and social. In this way, no matter how disordered or hopeless a situation may seem, the process of becoming more of oneself and finding meaning in the situation is a demonstration of expanding consciousness (Newman 1979).

The theoretical and conceptual philosophies of nursing promoted by the theorists are highlighted in Table 1.2.

The Beginnings of the NHS and Nursing

The National Health Service was established on 5 July 1948 with the aim of health care being free at the point of delivery. The 1949 Nurses Act allowed that the constitution of the GNC be amended; the general and male nurse parts of the register were amalgamated. Nurses welcomed the development of the NHS, as they recognised through first-hand experience of caring, the suffering that resulted from having to pay for medical care.

Figure 1.5 shows a copy of the state examination that was taken in 1963 to demonstrate the principles and practice of nursing. Interestingly, there is no reference to any evidence base to underpin the answers that are given, nor are the candidates asked to critically analyse the care that they give.

Workforce planning was crude and with the development of new hospitals and services came the need for a greater number of nurses. Sadly at the time of the development of the NHS, no real provision for the education of nurses had been established *en-masse*, and there was no recognition for nurses to help shape the development of services. Services were isolated, in particular the provision of mental health care. Children were isolated from their families with visiting restricted to weekends only in many wards.

Table 1.2 Theoretical and conceptual philosophies of nursing.

THEORIST	CONCEPTUAL PHILOSOPHY
Florence Nightingale	**Concepts of society and environment:** major emphasis on the environment of care, light, noise, smell and warmth
Virginia Henderson	**Concepts of the person:** the mind and body are inseparable; individuals are unique; individual needs are mirrored in 14 components of basic nursing care **Concepts of health:** values independent function
Dorothea Orem	**Concepts of the person:** the individual as a whole made up of physical, psychological and social structures with an element of self-care ability
Hildegard Peplau	**Concepts of the person:** the human dynamic and therapeutic relationship; the stages of that relationship
Patricia Benner	**Concepts of the person:** person is self-interpreting and engaged, learning, concern, cultural appreciation, direct involvement in caring
Margaret Newman	**Concepts of health:** expanding consciousness through the experience of illness

Child and Family Nursing The Platt Report 1959

Acknowledged that:
- *The emotional care of children was important and that separation could be damaging*
- *Children should not be admitted to adult wards*
- *Physical environment should be cheerful*
- *Nurse in charge should be a trained children's nurse*
- *Paediatricians should have concern for all admitted*
- *Nursery nurses for children under 5*
- *Children should be prepared for admission*
- *Education provision should where possible continue*
- *Parents should be able to visit freely and to stay with children under 5 years*
- *All staff should be trained in the emotional needs of children*

(Davies 2010)

Some significant dates in the history of the NHS are shown in Figure 1.6.

Early Nursing Research

The Briggs Committee, a working group, was set up in 1976 to review the training of nurses and midwives, and set the expectation that nurse education would incorporate the latest findings of evidence to underpin practice. The work of this committee led to the Nurses, Midwives and Health Visitors Act of 1979, which dissolved the GNC. The GNC was replaced by the UKCC for Nursing, Midwifery and Health Visiting, with four National Boards for England, Wales, Scotland and Northern Ireland. The UKCC had a specific responsibility for the quality of education of nurses, the

THE GENERAL NURSING COUNCIL FOR ENGLAND AND WALES

The Board of Examiners by whom this paper was set is constituted as follows:—

MISS D. ODLUM, M.A., M.R.C.S., L.R.C.P., D.P.M.   MISS E. W. M. CLARE, S.R.N.

F. G. ELLIS, ESQ., M.S., F.R.C.S.   J. FAIRBANK, ESQ., S.R.N., R.M.N.

MISS A. G. NOTMAN, S.R.N., R.S.C.N.

PRELIMINARY STATE EXAMINATION—PART II.

Tuesday, 1st October, 1963.

PRINCIPLES & PRACTICE OF NURSING
(including BACTERIOLOGY & PRINCIPLES OF ASEPSIS AND FIRST AID).

Physiology   *PHYSIOLVG*   *Physiolic*   *Physiol*   *PHYSIOL*

Time allowed 2 hours.

IMPORTANT.—*Read the questions carefully, and answer only what is asked, as no marks will be given for irrelevant matter.*

NOTE.—Candidates MUST attempt FOUR questions and not more than four.

1. How would you care for the hands, feet and hair of a very ill patient? Indicate why the measures you mention are important.

2. What observations does the nurse make of the patient's pulse and respiration? Choose any one patient you have nursed and show why you thought these observations were important.

3. You find an elderly neighbour unconscious at the foot of the stairs. What would you do? Give reasons for your actions.

4. What factors do you consider important in the maintenance of harmonious relationships in the ward?

5. For what reasons is oxygen given to patients? Describe any one method which may be used for its administration.

6. The practice today is to keep the patient in bed as little as possible. What are the advantages of this?

7. What precautions may be taken to prevent the spread of infection in a hospital ward?

Figure 1.5 Copy of the state examination taken in 1963.

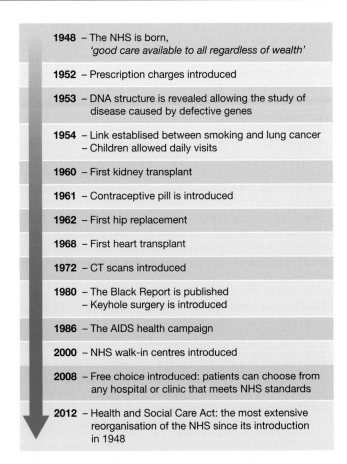

Figure 1.6 Some significant dates in the history of the NHS.

The timeline shows:

- **1948** – The NHS is born, *'good care available to all regardless of wealth'*
- **1952** – Prescription charges introduced
- **1953** – DNA structure is revealed allowing the study of disease caused by defective genes
- **1954** – Link established between smoking and lung cancer – Children allowed daily visits
- **1960** – First kidney transplant
- **1961** – Contraceptive pill is introduced
- **1962** – First hip replacement
- **1968** – First heart transplant
- **1972** – CT scans introduced
- **1980** – The Black Report is published – Keyhole surgery is introduced
- **1986** – The AIDS health campaign
- **2000** – NHS walk-in centres introduced
- **2008** – Free choice introduced: patients can choose from any hospital or clinic that meets NHS standards
- **2012** – Health and Social Care Act: the most extensive reorganisation of the NHS since its introduction in 1948

Table 1.3 Comparison of Project 2000 curriculum to traditional nurse training.

PROJECT 2000	TRADITIONAL NURSE TRAINING
Education in Higher Educational Institutions (HEIs)	Took place in schools of nursing, most likely hospital-based
Supernumerary status, not counted as 'numbers' on wards	Part of the workforce, included on the team 'off duty' rota
Increase of theory content to represent 50% of the three-year course	Practice component significantly outweighs time spent in classroom
Includes a minimum HEI award (Diploma) along with nurse registration	No final award but eligible for nurse registration
Focus on health rather than ill health with emphasis on the life sciences	Illness model focus
Common Foundation Programme (CFP) of 18 months for all student nurses	No foundation programme
Four specialist pre-registration branches of 18 months to follow CFP: Adult Child health Mental health Learning disabilities	No branches, nurses start on specific programme at beginning of three-year training

maintenance of student training records, the provision of professional guidance and a remit to handle professional misconduct.

The first code of conduct for nurses, midwives and health visitors was developed in 1984 by the UKCC, setting out standards of professional behaviour and accountability. This was an effort at transparency to provide the public with standards that they could expect and to guide the profession with regard to their duty of care to their patients and clients.

Much of the work of Briggs in the 1970s paved the way for reform in relation to nurse education. In 1984, the UKCC set up a project to consider reforming nurse education, which became known as Project 2000. The UKCC's report, published in 1986, provided the Council's strategy (UKCC 1986). The strategy was implemented by the mid-1990s and up to this point, nurse education worked on the apprenticeship model, where students were salaried, part of the workforce and in the majority of cases, had their education based in one local hospital. Examinations were both hospital and nationally set. Until Project 2000, the whole model of education for nurses was geared towards the needs of the local health services and provided hands on, practical approaches to clinical practice (RCN 2007).

Project 2000

Project 2000 introduced a framework for pre-registration nurse programmes which was to radically change the experience of student nurses in practice and in education. Table 1.3 shows a comparison between the traditional style of nurse education and the revolution in education that was introduced with Project 2000.

While presenting a radical change to the way that nurses were educated, Project 2000 had many critics, not least from the established workforce in nursing in the wards and departments. Many found the transition from students as part of the workforce to supernumerary status difficult to adapt to.

Jot This Down

The introduction of Project 2000, while embraced by some, was a cause of concern to many nurses.

- Why would this radical change in the way that nurses were educated cause so much anxiety?

In the 'Jot This Down' exercise above, you may have made the same conclusions that the professional bodies and nurse educators were investigating as Project 2000 began to develop.

Researchers began to look at the experience from Project 2000 (Hamill 1995), and just as importantly the outcome, in relation to newly qualified nurses (UKCC 1999). What they found was concern over the fitness to practise of some qualified nurses following the first round of Project 2000.

The Peach Report was published in response to the UKCC's desire to conduct a detailed examination of the effectiveness of pre-registration nurse education and determine if students were 'fit for practice' and 'fit for purpose' (UKCC 1999). The report outlined several recommendations, for example:

- A reduction in the common foundation programme from 18 months to one year
- An increase in the branch programme from 18 months to two years

- To ensure that students experienced at least three months' supervised clinical practice towards the end of the programme
- Longer student placements
- The introduction of practice skills and clinical placements early on in the common foundation programme
- Greater flexibility in entry to nursing programmes.

Subsequent revisions included more focus on clinical skills acquisition, a closer link between theory and practice, and the development of roles that support mentors in practice such as practice education facilitators (PEFs).

Drivers for Change

Nurse education can be seen as an organic element, responding to changes within society, the healthcare setting and the educational system. As such, there are a number of so-called 'drivers' that have been identified to help identify the kind of health care that will be needed in the future and subsequently, the type of nurse needed to support that health care (RCN 2004).

Examples of the drivers include:

- Demographic changes, we live in an ever-ageing population
- People living longer with chronic disease and long-term illness
- Lifestyle dictating health, e.g. obesity
- The public expectation of quality care
- Focus on prevention and health promotion
- Primary care and a move away from hospital care delivery towards a community focus
- Supporting patients and carers to self-manage their conditions.

Such drivers influence the type of care that can be expected in the future and determine the preparation of the future nursing workforce.

Technological advances continue to shape the way that nurses work, and the need to be computer literate to cope with managing patients' records and data is a constant feature of the nurses' role. Advances in telehealth and remote patient monitoring are being developed, particularly in the community setting, and telehealth has been seen as an effective tool for telephone triage, an example being 'NHS 111' in England.

Telecare is the use of electronic equipment, sensors and aids in a person's home to support independent living. Geared towards home care, the technology can help people with a range of long-term conditions to avoid unnecessary hospital admissions. Technological developments will continue, with an increased understanding and use of new applications associated with bio-technology, bioengineering and robotics.

The Evidence Telehealth, the Use of Florence (Flo)

Practice nurses can use the 'Flo telehealth system' to convey interactive and positive health messages to selected patients to enhance clinical management. An example is an interactive mobile phone texting service with blood pressure (BP) management. Patients measure their BP, text their readings to Florence, receive an immediate automatic response and have their results reviewed by the GP or practice nurse at least weekly.

(Cottrell et al. 2012)

The demographic pattern of the UK population also has an influence on nursing today. According to UK National Statistics, life expectancy at birth in the UK in 2008–2010 was 78.1 years for males and 82.1 years for females. The population is calculated to increase from 62.3 million in 2010 to 73.2 million in 2035; this is in part due to the projected natural increase based on more births than deaths: people are living longer and surviving the chronic illnesses that at one time would prove fatal. The provision of care will see a continued growth and an increasingly diverse role for the Third Sector, as well as reliance on the commercial sector to make available considerable aspects of secondary care provision (Longley et al. 2007).

International migration has necessitated health care to adapt ways of working to support cultural differences. Isolation of the elderly is a common feature; stress and the breakdown of the extended family are examples of factors affecting the population's health.

Patterns of health and disease are influenced by lifestyle, less physical activity and sedentary lifestyles, and coupled with the 'fast food' culture have contributed to a rise in the incidence of obesity. Cigarette smoking accounts for around 18% of all deaths of adults over the age of 35 years (The Health and Social Care Information Centre 2012). The same study highlighted that in England in 2010/2011, there were approximately 1.5 million hospital admissions with a primary diagnosis of a disease that can be caused by smoking. This is a steady rise from 1996/1997, when the number was 1.1 million admissions.

The rise of consumerism has led to a more informed user of healthcare services. Expectations of the care received are high, for example in Islington in 2009, 40% of respondents to the Citizens Panel that investigated Health and Social Care, said that better provision of opportunities to take up health screening, e.g. breast cancer, would improve the health of residents.

The ethical component of care is another example of the drivers for development in nursing. Acknowledgement of individual rights and nursing responses to this and the consideration of mental capacity are discussed in Chapter 3 of this book. Diversity and equity and the maintenance of a fair and non-discriminatory health service in which everybody can participate to reach their potential are important drivers for nursing.

Jot This Down

From examples of the 'drivers' in health care above, what would you say were the important components of nursing programmes of study to equip the nurse of the future to support excellent health care?

From the 'Jot This Down' exercise above, you may have considered the need to include a significant placement within the community setting, the ability to assess complex needs and to respond appropriately, work effectively within teams, work in partnership with people and their families to promote health and support self-care, and to recognise opportunities for health promotion.

Modernising Nursing Careers

In 2006, the four UK chief nursing officers created a vision for the nursing profession in the 21st century, setting the direction for modernising nursing careers (DH 2006). Similar to the RCN in 2004, it too considered the drivers for change in relation to:

The context of nursing: diversity in society, demographics, health patterns, inequalities, expectations of health care, advances in technology, economics of care.

Changing health care: putting the patient first, integrated care, patient choice, care of people with long-term conditions, health promotion, community focus of care, new ways of working.

The report highlighted that wherever nurses work, there are four elements that are key to the role.

The Evidence Elements for All Nurses
- Practice
- Education, training and development
- Quality and service development
- Leadership, management and supervision

(DH 2006)

The vision for the future is for nurses to be able to respond to the complexity of a modern society with all of its demands for quality, cost-effective, technological care. The report identified a need for nurses to be able to meet the elements identified in the evidence box: in practice, the ability to work in diverse care settings; in development, be able to pursue education and training when needed; in service development, be both generalist and specialist skilled as required; in leadership, be able to take on changed roles and responsibilities.

The Nursing and Midwifery Council (NMC) and Nurse Education

In 1998, the government initiated a major review of how the nursing profession was regulated. The outcome of this review resulted in consultation with nurses and midwives regarding professional regulation and areas that needed to be addressed. Recommendations were suggested and acted upon regarding self-professional regulation, regulatory mechanisms and procedural rules. The United Kingdom Central Council (UKCC) and the four national boards were abolished; quality assurance elements were incorporated into the work of the Nursing and Midwifery Council (NMC).

The NMC was set up by Parliament to safeguard the public and to ensure that nurses and midwives provide high standards of care to their patients. The Nursing and Midwifery Order 2001 (SI 2002/253) established the Council and it came into being on 1 April 2002.

Professional and Legal Issues

 The NMC maintains a register of nurses and midwives, setting standards for education and practice and offering guidance and advice to the professions. An overarching aim is to inspire confidence by ensuring that those on the professional register are fit to practise and by dealing speedily and fairly with those who are not.

The Council for Healthcare Regulatory Excellence (CHRE) promotes the health, safety and well-being of patients and other members of the public in the regulation of health professionals and has the job of scrutinising the work of the nine health profession regulators:

- General Chiropractic Council
- General Dental Council
- General Medical Council
- General Optical Council
- General Osteopathic Council

- General Pharmaceutical Council
- Health Professions Council
- Nursing and Midwifery Council
- Pharmaceutical Society of Northern Ireland

Under the NHS Reforms and Health Care Professions Act 2002 and the Health and Social Care Act 2008, the CHRE has a number of powers, for example it carries out checks on how healthcare regulators carry out their work as well as providing advice to the regulators concerning policy.

The fundamental concern of the NMC is the protection of the public. Its duties to society are to serve and protect by:

- Maintaining a register listing all nurses and midwives
- Setting standards and guidelines for nursing and midwifery education, practice and conduct
- Providing advice for registrants on professional standards
- Ensuring quality assurance related to nursing and midwifery education
- Setting standards and providing guidance for local supervising authorities for midwives
- Considering allegations of misconduct or unfitness to practise due to ill health.

In maintaining the professional register, the NMC provides the profession and public with a database of all registered nurse and midwives. The information shared includes the name and registration status of the nurse on one or more of the three parts of the register; nursing, midwifery and/or community public health nurse. There are currently over 650 000 qualified nurse registrants in the UK.

Professional and Legal Issues

 To stay on the professional register, the nurse must renew their registration every three years. This is known as periodic renewal. An annual retention fee is also required at the end of the first and second year of the registration period.
- Nurses must be able to demonstrate that their skills and knowledge are suitable for their work. Currently, a nurse is required to undertake a minimum of 35 hours of learning relevant to practice over a three-year period.

When in 2002 the UKCC ceased to exist, its function was taken over by the NMC which looked to the future of nurse education in the UK. The NMC mapped the standards of proficiency for pre-registration nursing education, producing its latest version in 2010.

As established earlier, as health care changes, so too does the role of the nurse and as such, so must the education required to prepare the student for the new roles and responsibilities (Carvalho *et al.* 2011). After extensive consultation, the NMC have introduced new standards for nurse education (NMC 2010) and students must meet these standards to be eligible to enter the professional register. The standards help to ensure parity throughout the UK for any field of nursing (fields replace branches).

The standards identify what students must demonstrate at the point of registration with the NMC, and guide the Approved Education Institutions (AEIs) and partners in the delivery of nurse education programmes. Registration conveys a message to the public that the nurse who is admitted to the register has reached and possesses a satisfactory level of competence along with a certain standard of behaviour – good character and good health.

The latest NMC 2010 guidelines are specifically geared to new programmes of study, which began in September 2011, and set out standards for competence and standards for education.

Standards for competence identify the specific knowledge, skills and attitudes the student must acquire by the end of the programme within the context of their particular field of nursing, and are arranged in four domains:

- Professional values
- Communication and interpersonal skills
- Nursing practice and decision-making
- Leadership management and teamworking.

The first domain, *Professional values*, emphasises the need for holistic, non-judgemental caring and sensitive practice. Here, the nurse is reminded of the obligation to respect the rights of individuals, with particular attention to equality and diversity and the needs of an ageing population.

> **Nursing Field** Mental Health: Professional Values
>
> Mental health nurses must work with people of all ages, utilising values-based mental health frameworks. They must use different methods of engaging people, and work in a way that promotes positive working relationships focussed on social inclusion, human rights and recovery, that is, a person's ability to live a self-directed life, with or without symptoms, that they believe is meaningful and satisfying.
>
> (NMC 2010)

The *Communication and interpersonal skills* domain, highlights the need for excellence, making safe and effective, compassionate and respectful communication with people. The use of communication technologies to inform patient choice, and the skilled use of therapeutic principles to engage in caring relationships is emphasised. In addition, maintaining accurate records and supporting confidentiality features in the competencies.

> **Nursing Field** Learning Disabilities: Communication and Interpersonal Skills
>
> Learning disabilities' nurses must use complex communication and interpersonal skills strategies to work with people of all ages who have learning disabilities and help them to express themselves. They must also be able to communicate and negotiate effectively with other professionals, services and agencies, and ensure that people with learning disabilities, their families and carers, are fully involved in decision-making.
>
> (NMC 2010)

The third domain, *Nursing practice and decision-making*, reminds the nurse that practice should be autonomous, compassionate, skilful and safe and must be dignified and promote health and well-being. The competency stresses the need for evidence-based care delivered through systematic nursing assessments, recognising risk and evaluating care.

> **Nursing Field** Child and Family: Nursing Practice and Decision-Making
>
> Children's nurses must be able to care safely and effectively for children and young people in all settings, and recognise their responsibility for safeguarding them. They must be able to deliver care to meet the essential and complex physical and mental health needs informed by deep understanding of biological, psychological and social factors throughout infancy, childhood and adolescence.
>
> (NMC 2010)

The last domain is comprised of *Leadership, management and teamworking* competency, which highlights the importance of accountability in practice and endeavour for improving nursing practice and standards of health care. Self-management and the management of others is also a feature alongside ongoing leadership skills development.

> **Nursing Field** Adult: Leadership, Management and Teamworking
>
> Adult nurses must be able to provide leadership in managing adult nursing care, understand and coordinate interprofessional care when needed and liaise with specialist teams. They must be adaptable and flexible, and able to take the lead in responding to the needs of people of all ages in a variety of circumstances, including situations where immediate or urgent care is needed. They must recognise their leadership role in disaster management, major incidents and public health emergencies, and respond appropriately according to their levels of competence.
>
> (NMC 2010)

Standards for education provide the framework from which programmes of study are approved and delivered. There are 10 standards that institutions and service providers must meet.

Professional and Legal Issues The 10 Standards for Pre-registration Nursing

1. **Safeguarding the public:** nursing and midwifery education must be consistent with *The code: Standards of conduct, performance and ethics for nurses and midwives* (NMC 2008)
2. **Equality and diversity:** education must address key aspects of equality and diversity and comply with current legislation
3. **Selection, admission, progression and completion:** must be open and fair
4. **Support of students and educators:** programme providers must support students to achieve the programme outcomes, and support educators to meet their own professional developmental needs
5. **Structure design and delivery of programmes:** to meet NMC standards and requirements, e.g. 4600 hours in no less than three years
6. **Practice learning opportunities:** must be safe, effective, integral to the programme and appropriate to programme outcomes
7. **Outcomes:** must ensure that NMC standards for competence are met and that students are fit for practice and for award on completion

8. **Assessment:** programme outcomes must be tested using valid and reliable assessment methods
9. **Resources:** the educational facilities in academic and practice settings must support delivery of the approved programme
10. **Quality assurance:** programme providers must use effective assurance processes in which findings lead to quality enhancement.

(NMC 2010)

Essential Skills Clusters

In addition to the standards set, students must engage in essential skills clusters that are incorporated into the programme of study throughout the three years; these are common to all fields and include:

- Care, compassion and communication
- Organisational aspects of care
- Infection prevention and control
- Nutrition and fluid management
- Medicines management.

Professional and Legal Issues Essential Skills Clusters

Care, compassion and communication
People can trust a newly registered graduate nurse to:
- Provide collaborative care based on the highest standards, knowledge and competence
- Engage in person-centred care empowering people to make choices about how their needs are met when they are unable to meet them for themselves
- Respect them as individuals and strive to help them to preserve their dignity at all times
- Engage with them or their family or carers within their cultural environments in an acceptant and anti-discriminatory manner free from harassment and exploitation
- Engage with them in a warm, sensitive and compassionate way
- Engage therapeutically and actively listen to their needs and concerns, responding using skills that are helpful, providing information that is clear, accurate, meaningful and free from jargon
- Protect and keep as confidential all information relating to them
- Gain their consent based on sound understanding and informed choice prior to any intervention and that their rights in decision making and consent will be respected and upheld.

Organisational aspects of care
People can trust a newly registered graduate nurse to:
- Treat them as partners and work with them to make a holistic and systematic assessment of their needs; to develop a personalised plan that is based on mutual understanding and respect for their individual situation, promoting health and well-being, minimising risk of harm and promoting their safety at all times
- Deliver nursing interventions and evaluate their effectiveness against the agreed assessment and care plan
- Safeguard children and adults from vunerable situations and support and protect them from harm
- Respond to their feedback and a wide range of other sources to learn, develop and improve services
- Promote continuity when their care is to be transferred to another service or person
- Be an autonomous and confident member of the multidisciplinary or multiagency team and to inspire confidence in others

- Safely delegate to others and to respond appropriately when a task is delegated to them
- Safely lead, coordinate and manage care
- Work safely under pressure and maintain safety of service users at all times
- Enhance the safety of service users and identify and actively manage risk and uncertainty in relation to people, the environment, self and others
- Prevent and resolve conflict and maintain a safe environment
- Select and manage medical devices safely.

Infection prevention and control
People can trust a newly registered graduate nurse to:
- Identify and take effective measures to prevent and control infection in accordance with local and national policy
- Maintain effective standard infection control precautions and apply these to needs and limitations in all environments
- Provide effective nursing interventions when someone has an infectious disease, including the use of standard isolation techniques
- Comply with hygiene, uniform and dress codes in order to limit, prevent and control infection
- Safely apply the principles of asepsis when performing invasive procedures and be competent in aseptic technique in a variety of settings
- Act in a variety of environments including the home care setting, to reduce risk when handling waste, including sharps, contaminated linen and when dealing with spillages of blood and other body fluids.

Nutrition and fluid management
People can trust a newly registered graduate nurse to:
- Assist them to choose a diet that provides an adequate nutritional and fluid intake
- Assess and monitor their nutritional status and in partnership, formulate and effective plan of care
- Assess and monitor their fluid status and in partnership with them, formulate an effective plan of care
- Assist them in creating an environment that is conducive to eating and drinking
- Ensure that those unable to take food by mouth receive adequate fluid and nutrition to meet their needs
- Safely administer fluids when fluid cannot be taken independently.

Medicines management
People can trust a newly registered graduate nurse to:
- Correctly and safely undertake medicines calculations
- Work within legal and ethical frameworks that underpin safe and effective medicines management
- Work as part of a team to offer holistic care and a range of treatment options of which medicines may form a part
- Ensure safe and effective practice in medicines management through comprehensive knowledge of medicines, their actions, risks and benefits.

Link To/Go To

The full document of the 2010 NMC Standards for Nurse Education can be accessed at:

nmc-uk.org/PreRegNursing/statutory/background/Pages/introduction.aspx

Current Nurse Education

From September 2013, all programmes of study in nursing became degree level only, and diploma entry study in the UK has been phased out nationally as a move towards this development. The NMC sees the future nurse as a leader, delegator, supervisor and person who can challenge other nurses and healthcare professionals. In order to develop and sustain change in practice, graduate (degree level) nurses need to:

- *Think analytically*
- *Use problem-solving approaches*
- *Utilise best evidence in decision-making*
- *Keep up with technological advances.*

(NMC 2010)

In the UK, student nurses qualify in a specific **field** of nursing, and enter the NMC register as a nurse in one or more of the four fields. The education programme is full time and consists of 4600 hours of combined theoretical and clinical instruction distributed equally.

Nursing Fields

Child and family nursing
The fundamentals of child and family nursing are addressed in Chapter 11. Nurses working in this field understand the developmental needs of children, in particular those who are acutely ill or suffering long-term debilitating conditions. Children's nurses are skilled in working alongside parents and families.

Learning disabilities nursing
The fundamentals of learning disabilities nursing are addressed in Chapter 10.

In essence, these nurses care for people with a wide range of physical and mental health conditions. The work is demanding and the skills needed include: assertiveness to advocate against discrimination; an awareness of legislation and support mechanisms to promote independence; the ability to work in a specialist support team in a variety of settings that might include schools, workplaces, residential care homes and community centres.

Mental health nursing
The fundamentals of mental health nursing are addressed in Chapter 12.

Nurses in this field are skilled in supporting patients and families, forming therapeutic relationships and enabling recovery from mental health breakdown where possible.

The range of mental health problems is vast, and mental health nurses understand the many dimensions that can impact upon a person's mental well-being.

The work is predominantly focussed in the community, with some aspects of acute care hospital-based.

Adult nursing
Specifically focussed on work with adults, but by its nature will cover all areas of care, from the community to the hospital setting. This is working with adults who have long-term chronic illness or acute illness and also with well adults as promoters of health.

Nurses working with adults need to be skilled in communication, understanding of the sciences on which nursing is based, knowledge of ethics and principles of health. They also need technical and clinical competence.

Adults will present with mental health problems and learning difficulties, and as such, awareness of these fields is essential.

The appropriateness of the four nursing fields has been examined with a concern that future health services may require a more generic worker, who would be helpful when meeting general health needs. The provision of degree-level programmes has the potential to enhance the status of nursing even further, providing nurses with skills that go beyond diploma level, with the aim of ensuring that the care of the patient is improved and enhanced. The new standards have been aligned with European Union Directive 2005/36/EC *Recognition of Professional Qualifications*. This sets out the requirements for training nurses responsible for general care and provides the baseline for general nursing in the EU. The Directive includes detailed requirements on programme length, content and ratio of theory to practice, as well as the nature of practice learning and range of experience.

The Francis Report

Between 2005 and 2008, there was growing concern over the unusually high mortality rate at the Mid Staffordshire NHS Foundation Trust; this prompted an initial investigation in 2010. Chaired by Robert Francis QC, this first inquiry considered individual cases of patient care, in an effort to learn lessons and prevent mistakes in the future, not just at the Mid Staffordshire Trust but across the NHS. His final report, a public inquiry, was published in February 2013. This report builds on the work and conclusions of the first inquiry. It tells of a culture of secrecy and defensiveness, which led to appalling suffering by many patients and their families (Mid Staffordshire NHS Foundation Trust 2013).

In his findings, Francis highlights a culture of care that failed in its primary concern of protecting patients and upholding the public's confidence in the system of care provided. In both reports, he sends a clear message that 'it should be patients, not numbers, which count'. Although focussed on one organisation, the report highlights a whole system failure, which has major implications for all healthcare systems across the UK. The 1782 page report has 290 recommendations, calling for a re-emphasis on what is important in care and not, as some might have expected, a total re-organisation of the system. What Francis wanted to do was to use the evidence to focus on the positive values of care and to learn from this so that the failings identified are not repeated. His recommendations focus on a series of themes based around:

- Openness, transparency and candour throughout the healthcare system
- Fundamental standards for healthcare providers
- Improved support for compassionate caring, committed nursing and stronger healthcare leadership.

There is recognition that the focus of compassion and caring in nursing should be emphasised right from recruitment into nursing, through education and continuous professional development (CPD). Francis makes the point that training and CPD in nursing should apply at all levels from student nurse to director of nursing. The challenge will be in resourcing this development.

The message from the inquiry strongly promotes the culture of putting patients first and protecting them from avoidable harm. It also strongly advocates an open and honest approach to patient care, where patients share in the decision-making of their care based on the best information available. In addition, the report identifies the need for a greater role for families and carers of older people.

In response to the Francis report, the NMC has highlighted the core theme of 'the Code' (NMC 2008), which states 'make the care of people your first concern, treating them as individuals and respecting their dignity'. The chief executive of the NMC recommends that 'this needs to be the core principle of the whole healthcare system'.

The RCN has also responded to the report, supporting the notion of transparency and the importance of speaking out in defence of patients in poor care. It supports the notion that poor leadership creates a culture of poor care and is critical of the lack of guidance into safe levels of staffing. Support for the recruitment of the right students who possess the values identified in the review has been made; however, like the NMC, the RCN does not support the recommendation that student nurses should have an extended period of direct patient care as a pre-requisite to training. The RCN believes that the current system of 2300 hours in practice for student nurses is sufficient, but emphasises the need to support mentors in practice to ensure positive learning experiences.

The Cavendish Review released in July 2013 looked at the complexity of caring roles within health care carried out by non-regulated and trained individuals. It found over 1.3 million frontline staff that are not registered nurses, but are responsible for the delivery of the majority of hands-on care both in hospitals and in the community. It highlights the confusion that patients feel when approached by different carers, the assumptions made by patients that all carers are nurses, the bureaucracy of employment, and the lack of consistency of approach to training and development. It proposes a 'certificate of fundamental care' linked to nurse training among its many recommendations (DH 2013).

Link To/Go To

The Cavendish Review is an independent review into Healthcare assistants and Support Workers in the NHS and care settings and can be accessed at:

www.gov.uk/government/uploads/attachment_data/file/12732/Cavendish_Review_ACCESSIBLE_-_FINAL_VERSION_16–7-13.pdf

---

The Care Quality Commission (CQC) is an independent regulator of health and adult social care services in England. It ensures that the care provided by hospitals, dentists, ambulances, care homes and home-care agencies meets government standards of quality and safety. In addition, it protects the interests of vulnerable people, including those whose rights are restricted under the Mental Health Act.

By putting the views, experiences, health and well-being of people who use services at the centre of its work, it has a range of powers to take action if people are getting poor care. Table 1.4 gives an overview of the standards and desired outcomes, which the CQC applies to measure care within health and social care settings, and relates to the quality and safety of care. Providers must have evidence that they meet the outcomes (CQC 2010).

In addition, public interest in the quality of nursing education and practice has prompted the NMC to review its Quality Assurance and publish its latest framework (NMC 2013).

The New Framework for Nursing and Midwifery

Launched by the NMC in July 2013, the new framework sets out a three-year strategy for assuring the quality of nursing and midwifery education, and the supervision of midwives. The Quality Assurance (QA) framework's principal aim is to ensure patient safety.

Professional and Legal Issues

The Quality Assurance (QA) framework (2013) aims to:
- Increase lay involvement through the increased use of reviewers who are neither nurses nor midwives
- Increase the proactive management of emerging risk by ensuring that education institutions (HEIs) and local supervising authorities (LSAs) have approved safeguards in place
- Over the three-year cycle, reduce the burden of regulation on well performing education institutions and LSAs
- Ensure that quality assurance focusses on outcomes of education and midwifery supervision as opposed to dictating how standards should be met.

(NMC 2013)

The target audience for the framework is primarily the public, and the NMC sees this as a means to transparency, clarity, utility, accountability and improvement. The term 'public' encompasses the population of nurses, service users and carers, and the specific community of educators and service providers. Changes to the framework have been informed by a number of factors, not isolated to the response to the Francis inquiry report into the Mid Staffordshire Foundation Trust, but the use of data from nurses, service users and carers, educational institutions and service providers.

The QA sets out its approach as follows:

PUBLIC PROTECTION:
- Ensure new entrants to the register are capable of safe, effective practice
- Ensure the profession knows how and when to raise a concern
- Ensure swift and effective response to fitness for practice concerns.

'RIGHT TOUCH' REGULATION:
- Encourage stakeholder feedback, and comment on, for example, the transparency and accountability of the framework.

FOCUSSING ON OUTCOMES:
- Shift of emphasis from how standards are achieved towards focus on outcomes of education to better protect the public
- More discretion for the interpretation and meeting of standards in diverse settings.

RISK-BASED:
- More scrutiny and support for the practice-based element of the course
- Proposed publication of guidance for educational audit of practice placements.

INVOLVING STAKEHOLDERS:
- Build on the theme of engagement with service users and carers to develop programmes of education
- Seek direct student feedback as a mechanism for quality

Table 1.4 Outcomes applied by the CQC in relation to the quality and safety of care.

TITLE AND SUMMARY OF OUTCOME
Care and welfare of people who use healthcare services People experience effective, safe and appropriate care, treatment and support that meets their needs and protects their rights.
Assessing and monitoring the quality of service provision People benefit from safe, quality care because effective decisions are made and because of the management of risks to people's health, welfare and safety.
Safeguarding people who use services from abuse People are safeguarded from abuse, or the risk of abuse, and their human rights are respected and upheld.
Cleanliness and infection control People experience care in a clean environment, and are protected from acquiring infections.
Management of medicines People have their medicines when they need them, and in a safe way. People are given information about their medicines.
Meeting nutritional needs People are encouraged and supported to have sufficient food and drink that is nutritional and balanced, and a choice of food and drink to meet their different needs.
Safety and suitability of premises People receive care in, work in or visit safe surroundings that promote their well-being.
Safety, availability and suitability of equipment Where equipment is used, it is safe, available, comfortable and suitable for people's needs.
Respecting and involving people who use services People understand the care and treatment choices available to them. They can express their views and are involved in making decisions about their care. They have their privacy, dignity and independence respected, and have their views and experiences taken into account in the way in which the service is delivered.
Consent to care and treatment People give consent to their care and treatment, and understand and know how to change decisions about things that have been agreed previously.
Complaints People and those acting on their behalf have their comments and complaints listened to and acted on effectively, and know that they will not be discriminated against for making a complaint.
Records People's personal records are accurate, fit for purpose, held securely and remain confidential. The same applies to other records that are needed to protect their safety and well-being.
Requirements relating to workers People are kept safe, and their health and welfare needs are met, by staff who are fit for the job and have the right qualifications, skills and experience.
Staffing People are kept safe, and their health and welfare needs are met, because there are sufficient numbers of the right staff.
Supporting workers People are kept safe, and their health and welfare needs are met, because staff are competent to carry out their work and are properly trained, supervised and appraised.
Cooperating with other providers People receive safe and coordinated care when they move between providers or receive care from more than one provider.

- Educators feedback on the application of standards in practice.

All of the criteria set out as shown are focussed on responding to the strength of public interest in the quality of nursing and midwifery education and practice, and an acknowledgment from our professional body that high profile failures in care undermine the public's trust in nursing. The process of raising concerns is addressed in Chapter 3 of this book.

Role of the Nurse

The role and function of the nurse has evolved and developed over the years and were explored in the first part of this chapter. In order to meet the healthcare needs of the nation, political and professional pressures have transformed the role of the nurse and other healthcare professionals, with the aim of developing their full potential. Roles are described as both generic and specialist.

Registered nurses working in clinical settings can carry out roles such as:

- Managing caseloads
- Administering and prescribing medications (if qualified as a non-medical prescriber)
- Delivering care which is evidence-based and which follows an agreed pathway or model of care
- Managing teams
- Discharge planning
- Documentation and communication of care.

As society changes, coupled with rapid and important advances in science and technology, so too does the role and function of the nurse and other health and social care practitioners. A reduction in doctors' hours saw the rise of the nurse practitioner and the specialist nurse (McGee & Castledine 2004). Nurses are advancing their skills and their practice, underpinned by an evidence base and further education. It is not unusual for nurses to undertake roles traditionally seen as medical, for example the nurse endoscopist, specialist ophthalmic nurses performing cataract surgery and surgical practitioners skilled in vascular surgery and hernia repair.

Many of the new nursing roles identified here exist today because, over time, the nursing profession has sought to advance its professional practice and status. The key issues of clinical competence, clinical decision-making and the awareness of boundaries and limitations are central to the safety of the patient and the success of such roles.

Other key roles that are part of the scope of practice and can influence the career pathway of the nurse include:

- Mentoring and teaching in practice
- Taking on leadership roles: ward sister/charge nurse
- Specialist public health nurse
- Nurse consultant
- Nurse prescriber
- Nurse educator
- Nursing researcher.

The Evidence The Intellectual Properties of the Nurse

- A body of knowledge on which professional practice is based
- A specialised education to transmit this body of knowledge to others
- The ability to use the knowledge in critical and creative thinking.

(Hood 2010)

In order to develop and sustain the caring perspective of nursing, there has to be a theoretical basis from which they practice. Nurses draw upon the scientific and theoretical perspectives of other disciplines to enhance the nature and safety of the care that they provide.

Jot This Down

In order to provide evidence-based safe and effective care, nursing draws information from a number of disciplines.

- Make a list of the disciplines that you think support the theoretical and practice base of nursing.

In the 'Jot This Down' exercise above, you may have considered disciplines such as the life sciences: sociology, psychology and biology. Other disciplines include pharmacology, physiology and microbiology. Themes such as economics and budget management, leadership skills and teaching are influential theoretical principles for the registered nurse. The combination of knowledge related to science and experience has the potential to enable the nurse to make reliable clinical decisions. Professional nursing practice is also based on a body of knowledge that is derived from experience – expertise. The use of expertise should never be undervalued however; having experience may not always be enough to help provide safe care. Nurses derive knowledge through intuition, tradition and experience.

Benner (1982) discusses the subject of intuition as a form of expertise. Intuition can be described as 'just knowing' and the 'just knowing' comes from the individual. It is internal and can occur independently of experience or reason. It can become validated by experience and interaction with other nurses.

What the Experts Say

Within this Trust we have initiated hourly patient communication from senior nursing staff. An adult male had been admitted early one morning with a severe asthma attack, he was wheezing and exhausted and we commenced medications and regular monitoring of his saturation levels. Later that day whilst on my hourly rounds, the staff nurse communicated that the patient had suddenly improved; she knew this because he had stopped wheezing and was dropping off to sleep. As soon as I caught sight of him my intuition told me that something was wrong: the patient had stopped wheezing from sheer exhaustion and his saturation levels were low, he was unresponsive and I immediately called the emergency team.

(Clinical Matron, Medical Unit)

Nurses use their body of knowledge in order to provide care that has undergone critical scrutiny, or a systematic approach has been used to provide that care. Care becomes creative and innovative and provides nurses with new ways of thinking and addressing the problems that people may have. Advancing nursing practice ensures that nurses have the knowledge base and practical skills to provide specialist nursing care. Critical thinking allows nurses to see different approaches to clinical situations, and can occur when nurses are faced, for example, with people who have complex needs. Specialist nursing roles and professional development are considered in Chapter 2.

The NHS and Healthcare Reform

On 1 April 2013, the NHS saw its biggest reform in its 65-year history. Hundreds of NHS organisations were abolished and hundreds of others were created, transforming the provision, commissioning and regulation of health care.

The Health and Social Care Act 2012 has abolished 153 primary care trusts responsible, up until the new Act, for commissioning health care, and the nine strategic health authorities responsible for performance managing the NHS. In their place are 211 Clinical Commissioning Groups (CCGs) led by GPs. Under the plans, GPs and other clinicians have much more responsibility for spending the budget in England, while greater competition with the private sector will be encouraged. The CCGs are held to account by NHS England, who will commission specialist services and Primary Care operating regionally through 27 local area teams. Originally, the commissioning groups were to be led by GPs, but other professionals, including hospital doctors and nurses, will also now be involved.

The reforms are designed to help ensure the long-term sustainability of the NHS, by achieving value for money and shifting care out of hospital and into the community. The CCGs are expected to use their expertise and clinical knowledge to purchase the most efficient services and the hope is that tendering for these services will drive up competition and so improve quality and standards.

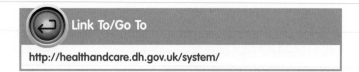

Link To/Go To

http://healthandcare.dh.gov.uk/system/

Figure 1.7 gives an overview of the health and care system from April 2013. It illustrates the statutory bodies that make up the system, oriented around people and communities and where they will receive their local health and care services. Clicking on any of the organisations will provide you with more information about their specific role.

In addition to the changes at NHS Trust level, local authorities have a much larger role in the responsibility for budgeting public health activities. Health, social care, public health and children's services are integrated. Local authorities are charged with the role of working closely with health and care providers and to use their local knowledge to take on challenges such as alcohol and drug misuse, obesity and smoking.

None of the changes in this latest reform changes the way that patients access services, nor do they alter the long-established position that in the main, health care will remain free at the point of delivery, funded from taxation and based on need and not an ability to pay.

Conclusion

Being a competent registered nurse with the core values at the centre of care brings with it many privileges, not least is the privilege of working with the public and providing them with a service that is safe and of a high quality. From a historical perspective, nurses have come a long way and are now seen as being professionals working comfortably and confidently alongside other healthcare professionals, with levels of education that match many of the allied professions in health care.

With regards to the demand for health care, there are many drivers, including the kind of and main causes of disease. Many of these will change over time, for example obesity levels and health inequalities are important factors that must be taken into account at present. There will be a continued need to support the self-care of the growing numbers of people who experience long-term health conditions. The continuing demand from the public to meet

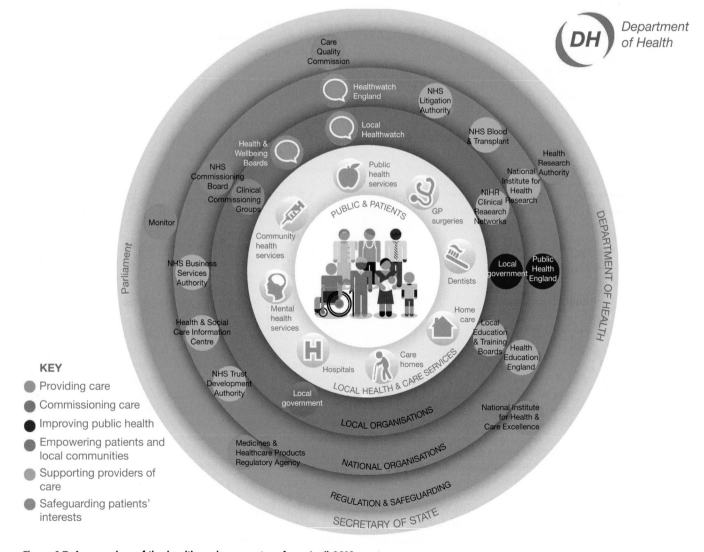

Figure 1.7 An overview of the health and care system from April 2013. Source: Department of Health, used under the Open Government Licence v2.0.

health needs will remain high, as well as patient demand for choice, including care packages and treatment options, and access to care provision. All of these factors play a part in the modernisation of nursing and the key areas to address within nurse education.

Government reform of health care will continue to concentrate on measuring effectiveness, ensuring value for money, reducing disparity in performance (locally and nationally, individually and corporately), improving safety and quality, enhancing productivity and engaging clinicians and recipients of care in all of this. NHS managerial structures are changing and this will continue, along with the provision closer to home for the more generalist services and consideration being given to specialist services. Regulation of the professions is continuing to come under scrutiny and this is focussing on quality and safety.

There is an increase in specialist and advanced roles and with this comes a blurring of professional and sector boundaries (i.e. health and social care sectors). Care provision will increasingly follow the patient pathway, with an emphasis on community care closer to home and multidisciplinary teamworking.

GNC: General Nursing Council (no longer in existence)
NHS: National Health Service
Paleopathology: the study of diseases in past populations
Project 2000: a framework for pre-registration nurse programmes, which was to radically change the experience of student nurses in practice and in education
RCN: Royal College of Nursing
Standards for competence: identify the specific knowledge, skills and attitudes the student must acquire by the end of the programme within the context of their particular field of nursing
Standards of proficiency: identify what students must demonstrate at the point of registration with the NMC and guide the Approved Education Institutions (AEIs) and partners in the delivery of nurse education programmes
Telecare: the use of electronic equipment, sensors and aids used in a person's home to support independent living
UKCC: United Kingdom Central Council for nursing, midwifery and health visiting (no longer in existence).

Key Points

- The fundamental basis of nursing is associated with caring and helping, and nursing can be described as both an art and a science.
- Caring defines nurses and their work, and as such, there are many facets associated with the role and function of the nurse. The role is constantly evolving and is difficult to classify.
- Care has been claimed to be an essential human need for the full development, health maintenance and survival of human beings in all world cultures.
- Many of the theories developed through the 20th century that relate to nursing have a philosophical foundation, and include ideas about the nature of nursing, the nature of the person, the nature of society and the environment and the nature of health.
- With regards to the demand for health care, there are many drivers, including the kind and main causes of disease.
- Project 2000 introduced a framework for pre-registration nurse programmes, which was to radically change the experience of student nurses in practice and in education. New developments have seen the revision of nursing curriculums from 2013 onwards.
- On 1 April 2013, the NHS saw its biggest reform in its 65-year history. Hundreds of NHS organisations were abolished and hundreds of others created, transforming the provision, commissioning and regulation of health care.

Glossary

Essential skills clusters: are incorporated into the programme of study throughout the three years. These are common to all fields and include: care, compassion and communication; organisational aspects of care; infection prevention and control; nutrition and fluid management and medicines management
Fields of nursing: identifies which area of expertise the nurse possesses at the point of entry onto the professional register, i.e. Child, Mental health, Learning disabilities and Adult fields of nursing

References

Adams, C. (2012) The history of health visiting. *Nursing in Practice*, 68.

Anionwu, E.N. (2005) *A Short History of Mary Seacole: a resource for nurses and students*. Royal College of Nursing, London.

Baly M.E. (1995) *Nursing and Social Change*, 3rd edn. Routledge, London.

Benner, P. (1982) From novice to expert. *American Journal of Nursing*, 82(3), 402–407.

Carvalho, S., Reeves, M., Orford, J. (2011) *Fundamental Aspects of Legal, Ethical and Professional Issues in Nursing*, 2nd edn. Quay Books, London.

Collin, R. (2012) Sarah Gamp: My favourite Charles Dickens character. *Daily Telegraph*, 14 February 2012. http://www.telegraph.co.uk/culture/charles-dickens/9044813/Sarah-Gamp-My-favourite-Charles-Dickens-character.html

Cottrell, E., Chambers, R. & O'Connell, P. (2012) Using simple telehealth in primary care to reduce blood pressure: a service evaluation. *British Medical Journal*, 2, 6.

CQC (2010) *Essential Standards of Quality and Safety*. Care Quality Commission, London.

Davies, R. (2010) Marking the 50th anniversary of the Platt Report: from exclusion to toleration and parental participation in the care of the hospitalised child. *Journal of Child Health Care*, 14(1), 6–23.

DH (2006) *Modernising Nursing Careers: setting the direction*. TSO, London.

DH (2010) *Front Line Care. Report by the Prime Minster's Commission on the Future of Nursing and Midwifery in England 2010*. COI. TSO, London.

DH (2012) *Compassion in Practice. Nursing, Midwifery and Care Staff, Our Vision Our strategy*. TSO, London.

DH (2013) *The Cavendish Review: an Independent Review into Healthcare and Support Workers in the NHS and Social Care Settings*. TSO, London.

Doona M.E. (1996) Linda Richards and Nursing in Japan, 1885–1890. *Nursing History Review*, 4, 99–128.

Hallett C.E. (2010) *Celebrating Nurses. A Visual History*. Fil Rouge Press, London.

Hamill, C. (1995) The phenomenon of stress as perceived by Project 2000 student nurses: a case study. *Journal of Advanced Nursing*, 29(5), 1256–1264.

Henderson, V. (1966) *The Nature of Nursing: a definition and its implications for practice, research, and education*. McMillan Publishing, New York.

Hood (2010) *Conceptual Bases of Professional Nursing*, 7th edn. Lippincott, Philadelphia.

Leininger M (2002) *Transcultural Nursing: concepts, theories and practices*, 3rd edn. John Wiley and Sons, New York.

Longley, M., Shaw & C. Dolan, G. (2007) *Nursing: Towards 2015: alternative scenarios for healthcare, nursing and nurse education in the UK in 2015*. University of Glamorgan, Pontypridd.

McGee, P. & Castledine, G. (2004) *Advanced Nursing Practice*, 2nd edn. Blackwell Publishing, Oxford.

Newman, M.A. (1979) *Theory Development in Nursing*. Davis, Philadelphia.

Nightingale, F. (1859) *Notes on Nursing: what it is and what it is not*. Blackie & Son Ltd., Glasgow.

NMC (2008) *The Code: Standards of Conduct, Performance and Ethics for Nurses and Midwives*. Nursing and Midwifery Council, London.

NMC (2010) *Standards for Pre-Registration Nursing Education*. Nursing and Midwifery Council, London.

NMC (2013) *The Quality Assurance Framework for Nursing and Midwifery Education and Local Supervising Authorities for Midwifery*. Nursing and Midwifery Council, London.

Orem, D. (1991) *Self-care Deficit Theory*. Sage, California.

Peplau, H.E. (1952) *Interpersonal Relations in Nursing: a conceptual framework of reference for psychodynamic nursing*. Putnam, New York.

RCN (2004) *The Future Nurse: The RCN Vision Explained*. Royal College of Nursing, London.

RCN (2007) *Pre-registration Nurse Education. The NMC review and the issues*. Policy Briefing 14/2007. Royal College of Nursing Policy Unit, London.

RCN (2010) *The Principles of Nursing Practice*. Royal College of Nursing, London. www.rcn.org.uk/nursingprinciples (accessed July 2013).

The Mid Staffordshire NHS Foundation Trust (2010) *Independent Inquiry into care provided by Mid Staffordshire NHS Foundation Trust January 2005 – March 2009*. TSO, London.

The Mid Staffordshire NHS Foundation Trust (2013) *Report of the Mid Staffordshire NHS Foundation Trust Public Inquiry*. TSO, London.

The Health and Social Care Information Centre (2012) *Statistics on Smoking: England, 2012*. TSO, London.

UKCC (1986) *Project 2000 – A New Preparation for Practice*. United Kingdom Central Council, London.

UKCC (1999) *Fitness for Practice: The UKCC Commission for Nursing and Midwifery Education*. United Kingdom Central Council, London.

Watterson, L. (2013) 6Cs + principles = care. *Nursing Standard* 27(46), 24–25.

White R. (1978) *Social Change and the Development of the Nursing Profession. A Study of the Poor Law Nursing Service 1848–1948*. Henry Kimpton, London.

Wills, M.E. & McEwen M. (2002) *Theoretical Basis for Nursing*. Lippincott Williams & Wilkins, Philadelphia.

Test Yourself

1. Nursing forms the largest body of registered professionals employed within the NHS
   (a) True
   (b) False

2. Paleopathology is:
   (a) a way of carbon dating skeletal remains
   (b) the study of diseases in past populations
   (c) what historians rely on to interpret longevity
   (d) the study of food and diet in ancient civilisations

3. The first health visitor was:
   (a) Virginia Henderson
   (b) Linda Richards
   (c) Employed in Salford in 1862
   (d) Ethel Bedford-Fenwick

4. The Register of Nurses was first published in:
   (a) 1922
   (b) 1902
   (c) 1942
   (d) 1890

5. Hildegard Peplau was the first published nurse theorist since Florence Nightingale
   (a) True
   (b) False

6. The Nurses, Midwives and Health Visitors Act was established in:
   (a) 1948
   (b) 1952
   (c) 1990
   (d) 1979

7. What percentage of all deaths of adults over the age of 35 years are attributed to cigarette smoking?
   (a) 18%
   (b) 32%
   (c) 43%
   (d) 20%

8. The Cavendish Review is:
   (a) An independent review into the quality of care homes
   (b) An independent review into Healthcare Assistants and Support Workers in the NHS and care settings
   (c) A review into the way overseas visitors access UK health care
   (d) An inquiry into Government leadership within the NHS

9. In the new NHS Reforms, Clinical Commissioning Groups are made up of:
   (a) Primary care trusts
   (b) GPs only
   (c) GPs and other health professionals such as nurses
   (d) Charitable organisations allied to health

10. NHS England's main aim is to:
    (a) Purchase services such as dental and family planning for the people of England
    (b) Regulate the way that hospitals run
    (c) Ensure that all nurses are registered
    (d) Improve health outcomes for people in England

Answers

1. a
2. b
3. c
4. a

5. a
6. d
7. a
8. b
9. c
10. d

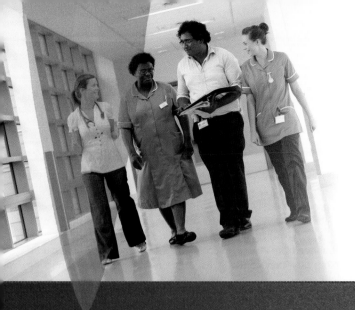

2

The Professional Nurse and Contemporary Health Care

Karen Wild

University of Salford, UK

Learning Outcomes

On completion of this chapter you will be able to:

- Review the RCN's Principles of Nursing Practice and apply these to aspects of the nurse as a professional
- Demonstrate a knowledge of the NMC's code of professional conduct; standards for conduct, performance and ethics
- Summarise the theories of learning
- Be aware of the concept of evidence-based practice
- Understand leadership styles and theories
- Have an understanding of the nurse's role in interprofessional working

Competencies

All nurses must:

1. Practise in confidence according to the NMC's code of professional conduct; standards for conduct, performance and ethics
2. Work in partnership with service users, carers, families, groups, communities and organisations
3. Appreciate the value of evidence in practice, be able to understand and appraise research, apply theory to work and identify areas for investigation
4. Act as change agents and provide leadership through quality enhancement
5. Work effectively across professional and agency boundaries, referring and communicating with others to support and respect choice in service users
6. Manage personal and professional development, learn from experience through supervision, reflection, evaluation and feedback

 Visit the companion website at **www.wileynursingpractice.com** where you can test yourself using flashcards, multiple-choice questions and more.

Nursing Practice: Knowledge and Care, First Edition. Edited by Ian Peate, Karen Wild and Muralitharan Nair.
© 2014 John Wiley & Sons, Ltd. Published 2014 by John Wiley & Sons, Ltd. Companion website: www.wileynursingpractice.com

Introduction

A profession can be defined by a number of key determinants; however, when asked to consider what is meant by the term 'professional' many individuals might find this a daunting task. Take, for example, the idea that a footballer may describe themselves as professional; equally, a member of the clergy will no doubt assert their professional standing within society. When considering the two examples given, it is clear to see how difficult defining the idea of what the term 'professional' might be. In general terms, professionals are considered to be individuals who have acquired a level of expertise or skill through formal education or training. This can be a useful starting point when describing nursing as a profession, however, it is only a small part of the criteria that can describe professional status, and the debate continues as to whether nurses fall into the true description of professional, or if they fall into the category of 'semi-professional'. Salvage (2002) describes the 'true' professions as male dominated, elitist and powerful and gives the examples of medicine and law. However, new professions and contemporary ways of working are changing how society views professional roles. An example of this is the medical profession, which is experiencing a shift in the gender balance with more equal female to male ratios emerging in practice. This supports the idea that ways of defining the term 'profession' are constantly shifting focus. In general, to claim professional status or membership to a profession, certain qualities should be met and these can include:

- Being subject to a code of rigorous ethics and moral obligations
- Being governed by a regulating body with a defined membership
- The ability to perform a specialist role that requires expert skill and/or knowledge
- Being responsible for advancing knowledge and research to support the profession
- Having a minimum standard entry qualification leading to a recognised practice and academic training
- Having continuous educational development with a recognised career structure
- Having an established body of theory and evidence to underpin practice
- Commanding a salary proportionate to the level of professional responsibility.

The purpose and function of nursing has developed over time, as have the characteristics of the nurse in contemporary society. When the above criteria are mapped against the status of nursing and some of the emerging specialist roles nurses hold, then the perception of nursing as being professional in nature is clear. Examples of specialist nurses that have developed alongside technological scientific advancement include nurse endoscopists, specialist nurse practitioners, community matrons, consultant nurses, nurse prescribers and advanced nurse practitioners. This chapter explores some of the professional functions of the nurse and highlights the main issues that are important themes to the nurse as a 'professional'.

The Nurse as a Professional

The Royal College of Nursing (2003) defines nursing as 'the use of clinical judgement in the provision of care to enable people to improve, maintain, or recover health, to cope with health problems, and to achieve the best possible quality of life, whatever their disease or disability, until death' (p. 5). This definition draws on what are perceived as the purposes of nursing as follows:

- To promote and maintain health
- To care for people when their health is compromised
- To assist recovery
- To facilitate independence
- To meet needs
- To improve/maintain well-being/quality of life.

In Chapter 1, you were introduced to *The Principles of Nursing Practice* as set out by the RCN in 2010, and these were mapped in that chapter against the values of nursing as described by the 6Cs. The RCN (2010) highlighted the full definitions of the Principles of Practice from **A** to **H**. Seen as the framework for excellence in nursing care, they address what everyone can expect from nursing practice.

Professional and Legal Issues RCN's Principles of Nursing Practice (2010)

Principle A	Nurses and nursing staff treat everyone in their care with dignity and humanity – they understand their individual needs, show compassion and sensitivity, and provide care in a way that respects all people equally
Principle B	Nurses and nursing staff take responsibility for the care they provide and answer for their own judgements and actions – they carry out these actions in a way that is agreed by their patients, and the families and carers of their patients, and in a way that meets the requirement of their professional bodies and the law
Principle C	Nurses and nursing staff manage risk, are vigilant about risk, and help to keep everyone safe in the places they receive health care
Principle D	Nurses and nursing staff provide and promote care that puts people at the centre, involves patients, service users, their families and their carers in decisions and helps them make informed choices about their treatment and care
Principle E	Nurses and nursing staff are at the heart of the communication process: they assess, record and report on treatment and care, handle information sensitively and confidentially, deal with complaints effectively, and are conscientious in reporting the things they are concerned about
Principle F	Nurses and nursing staff have up-to-date knowledge and skills, and use these with intelligence, insight and understanding in line with the needs of each individual in their care
Principle G	Nurses and nursing staff work closely with their own team and with other professionals, making sure patients' care and treatment is co-ordinated, is of high standard and has the best possible outcome
Principle H	Nurses and nursing staff lead by example, develop themselves and other staff, and influence the way care is given in a manner that is open and responds to individual needs

(Reproduced with permission of the Royal College of Nursing.)

In addition to the clarity given in the definition of nursing and *The Principles of Nursing Practice* as a guide, nurses also have a focussed code of practice from which to drive practice and form a professional framework from which nursing practice can be judged. The next section will focus on the code of professional conduct for nurses.

The NMC Code of Professional Conduct

The Professional Standards Authority (PSA) promotes the health, safety and well-being of patients and other members of the public in the regulation of health professionals and has the job of scrutinising the work of the nine health profession regulators:

- General Chiropractic Council
- General Dental Council
- General Medical Council
- General Optical Council
- General Osteopathic Council
- General Pharmaceutical Council
- Health Professions Council
- Nursing and Midwifery Council
- Pharmaceutical Society of Northern Ireland.

Under the NHS Reforms and Health Care Professions Act 2002 and the Health and Social Care Acts of 2008 and 2012, the Professional Standards Authority (PSA) for Health and Social Care (previously known as the Council for Healthcare and Regulatory Excellence, CHRE) has a number of powers:

- It oversees the statutory bodies that regulate healthcare professions
- It advises on issues of professional standards in health and social care
- It is accountable to UK parliament.

In addition, it shares good practice, promotes research, and introduces new ideas and guidance.

 Link To/Go To

Access the PSA website and search for guidance on maintaining clear sexual boundaries for healthcare workers and for patients and carers. You can utilise this information to support your essential skills clusters.

www.professionalstandards.org.uk

Professional nursing practice is not only judged by the recipient of care – the patient – but also by the profession itself. Professionals judge other professionals with regard to the quality and the appropriateness of the care that they provide. One of the key ways of making such judgements is through the Nursing and Midwifery Council (NMC). People receiving nursing care must be able to trust nurses with their well-being. To justify that trust, the nursing profession has a duty to maintain a good standard of practice and care, and to support this aim, the NMC has a 'Code' of standards of conduct, performance and ethics for nurses and midwives.

Professional and Legal Issues The Code: (NMC 2008a)

 The people in your care must be able to trust you with their health and well-being
To justify that trust, you must:

- make the care of people your first concern, treating them as individuals and respecting their dignity
- work with others to protect and promote the health and well-being of those in your care, their families and carers, and the wider community
- provide a high standard of practice and care at all times
- be open and honest, act with integrity and uphold the reputation of your profession.

As a professional, you are personally accountable for actions and omissions in your practice, and must always be able to justify your decisions.

You must always act lawfully, whether those laws relate to your professional practice or personal life.

Failure to comply with this code may bring your fitness to practise into question and endanger your registration.

This code should be considered together with the NMC's rules, standards, guidance and advice available from **http://www.nmc-uk.org**

Make the care of people your first concern, treating them as individuals and respecting their dignity

Treat people as individuals

1. You must treat people as individuals and respect their dignity.
2. You must not discriminate in any way against those in your care.
3. You must treat people kindly and considerately.
4. You must act as an advocate for those in your care, helping them to access relevant health and social care, information and support.

Respect people's confidentiality

5. You must respect people's right to confidentiality.
6. You must ensure people are informed about how and why information is shared by those who will be providing their care.
7. You must disclose information if you believe someone may be at risk of harm, in line with the law of the country in which you are practising.

Collaborate with those in your care

8. You must listen to the people in your care and respond to their concerns and preferences.
9. You must support people in caring for themselves to improve and maintain their health.
10. You must recognise and respect the contribution that people make to their own care and well-being.
11. You must make arrangements to meet people's language and communication needs.
12. You must share with people, in a way they can understand, the information they want or need to know about their health.

Ensure you gain consent

13. You must ensure that you gain consent before you begin any treatment or care.
14. You must respect and support people's rights to accept or decline treatment and care.
15. You must uphold people's rights to be fully involved in decisions about their care.
16. You must be aware of the legislation regarding mental capacity, ensuring that people who lack capacity remain at the centre of decision making and are fully safeguarded.
17. You must be able to demonstrate that you have acted in someone's best interests if you have provided care in an emergency.

(Continued)

Maintain clear professional boundaries

18. You must refuse any gifts, favours or hospitality that might be interpreted as an attempt to gain preferential treatment.
19. You must not ask for or accept loans from anyone in your care or anyone close to them.
20. You must establish and actively maintain clear sexual boundaries at all times with people in your care, their families and carers.

Work with others to protect and promote the health and well-being of those in your care, their families and carers, and the wider community

Share information with your colleagues

21. You must keep your colleagues informed when you are sharing the care of others.
22. You must work with colleagues to monitor the quality of your work and maintain the safety of those in your care.
23. You must facilitate students and others to develop their competence.

Work effectively as part of a team

24. You must work cooperatively within teams and respect the skills, expertise and contributions of your colleagues.
25. You must be willing to share your skills and experience for the benefit of your colleagues.
26. You must consult and take advice from colleagues when appropriate.
27. You must treat your colleagues fairly and without discrimination.
28. You must make a referral to another practitioner when it is in the best interests of someone in your care.

Delegate effectively

29. You must establish that anyone you delegate to is able to carry out your instructions.
30. You must confirm that the outcome of any delegated task meets required standards.
31. You must make sure that everyone you are responsible for is supervised and supported.

Manage risk

32. You must act without delay if you believe that you, a colleague or anyone else may be putting someone at risk.
33. You must inform someone in authority if you experience problems that prevent you working within this code or other nationally agreed standards.
34. You must report your concerns in writing if problems in the environment of care are putting people at risk.

Provide a high standard of practice and care at all times

Use the best available evidence

35. You must deliver care based on the best available evidence or best practice.
36. You must ensure any advice you give is evidence-based if you are suggesting healthcare products or services.
37. You must ensure that the use of complementary or alternative therapies is safe and in the best interests of those in your care.

Keep your skills and knowledge up to date

38. You must have the knowledge and skills for safe and effective practice when working without direct supervision.
39. You must recognise and work within the limits of your competence.
40. You must keep your knowledge and skills up to date throughout your working life.
41. You must take part in appropriate learning and practice activities that maintain and develop your competence and performance.

Keep clear and accurate records

42. You must keep clear and accurate records of the discussions you have, the assessments you make, the treatment and medicines you give, and how effective these have been.
43. You must complete records as soon as possible after an event has occurred.
44. You must not tamper with original records in any way.
45. You must ensure any entries you make in someone's paper records are clearly and legibly signed, dated and timed.
46. You must ensure any entries you make in someone's electronic records are clearly attributable to you.
47. You must ensure all records are kept securely.

Be open and honest, act with integrity and uphold the reputation of your profession

Act with integrity

48. You must demonstrate a personal and professional commitment to equality and diversity.
49. You must adhere to the laws of the country in which you are practising.
50. You must inform the NMC if you have been cautioned, charged or found guilty of a criminal offence.
51. You must inform any employers you work for if your fitness to practise is called into question.

Deal with problems

52. You must give a constructive and honest response to anyone who complains about the care they have received.
53. You must not allow someone's complaint to prejudice the care you provide for them.
54. You must act immediately to put matters right if someone in your care has suffered harm for any reason.
55. You must explain fully and promptly to the person affected what has happened and the likely effects.
56. You must cooperate with internal and external investigations.

Be impartial

57. You must not abuse your privileged position for your own ends.
58. You must ensure that your professional judgement is not influenced by any commercial considerations.

Uphold the reputation of your profession

59. You must not use your professional status to promote causes that are not related to health.
60. You must cooperate with the media only when you can confidently protect the confidential information and dignity of those in your care.
61. You must uphold the reputation of your profession at all times.

(NMC 2008a, pp. 1–9)

The code of conduct is not law; there is no legal imperative. It is, however, a guide which informs the general public and other professionals of the standard of conduct that they should expect from a registered nurse. You will have noticed the use of the word 'must' in the opening line of the code. Avery (2013) suggests that if the word 'must' was substituted for the word 'should', then this would have created a bias for negotiation and compromise, a situation on which the NMC was unwavering. Codes of conduct do not solve problems, they reflect professional morality. They operate in such a way as to remind the practitioner of the standards required by the profession. However, breaching the code of conduct is in effect a breach of registration and may lead to removal of the nurse's name from the register, and consequently of the right to practise.

The NMC was set up by Parliament to safeguard the public and to ensure that nurses and midwives provide high standards of care to their patients. The Nursing and Midwifery Order 2001 (SI 2002/253) established the Council and it came into being on 1 April 2002.

Safeguarding of the public is the key concern of the NMC. It protects the public by:

- Maintaining a register listing all nurses and midwives
- Setting and monitoring standards and guidelines for nursing and midwifery education, practice and conduct
- Ensuring that registrants keep their skills and knowledge up-to-date
- Ensuring quality assurance related to nursing and midwifery education
- Setting standards and providing guidance for local supervising authorities for midwives
- Considering allegations of misconduct or unfitness to practise.

In March 2013, there were 673 567 nurses and midwives on the register, and only those who have demonstrated that they meet the NMC standards can be registered and therefore legally allowed to practise in the UK. A review of the code and related standards is due in 2013–2014 (NMC 2013b).

Fitness to Practise

In addition to its regulatory powers, the NMC can also initiate investigations into a nurse's fitness to practise if they pose a risk to public safety.

The Evidence

Our fitness to practise cases involve only a very small number of nurses and midwives: 0.6 per cent of those on our register, with less than 0.1 per cent receiving a sanction.

(NMC 2013b)

When a nurse is called before the NMC as a result of concerns for fitness to practise, there is likely to be an initial assessment of the nature of the concern to determine whether urgent action is required. An investigation can help determine if there is a case to answer and this would necessitate a hearing to adjudicate a decision. In cases where there is a serious and immediate risk to patient or public safety, an interim order to suspend or restrict the nurse from practice can be made immediately.

Fitness to practise is the nurse's suitability to be on the register without restrictions; this may mean:

- Failing always to put the patient's interests first
- Not being properly trained, qualified and up-to-date
- Failing to treat patients with respect and dignity
- Not speaking up for patients who cannot speak for themselves.

Jot This Down

Make a list of the reasons why you think a nurse can be investigated for fitness to practise.

From the 'Jot This Down' exercise above, you may have thought about physical, sexual, emotional or verbal abuse; significant failure to provide adequate care; significant failure to keep proper records; failure to administer medicines safely; deliberately concealing unsafe practice; committing criminal offences; continued lack of

competence despite being given opportunities to improve; theft or a person's ill health. The NMC (2010a) considers these to be the most common examples of allegations of unfitness to practise.

A lack of competence relates to a lack of knowledge, skill or judgement of such a nature that the nurse is unfit to practise in a safe and effective manner (NMC 2010a). Some examples of lack of competence can include:

- A persistent lack of ability in correctly and/or appropriately calculating and recording the administration or disposal of medicines
- A persistent lack of ability in properly identifying care needs and accordingly, planning and delivering appropriate care
- Inability to work as part of a team
- Difficulty in communicating with colleagues or people in their care.

 Link To/Go To

For more information about fitness to practise, visit the NMC website at:

www.nmc-uk.org

Teaching and Learning in Practice

All registered nurses have a role to play in the development and facilitation of teaching and learning in the clinical learning environment. The NMC acknowledges that there is a strong public interest in the quality of nursing education and practice, where 'nurses who are about to enter the register have the knowledge, skills and behaviours to offer safe and effective care, and have regard for the health and well-being of service users' (NMC 2013a, p. 6). In addition, the Code (NMC 2008a) reminds us that nurses must be willing to share skills and experience for the benefit of colleagues, and must keep their knowledge and skills up-to-date throughout their working life. This can be attained by effective leadership, supervision, peer support and teaching.

The seminal work of Fretwell (1983) and Pembrey (1980) introduced us to the idea that the ward sister was a truly influential leader in the education and development of qualified nurses. The research focussed on the traits of the leader in relation to their:

- interest in the learner when starting on the ward
- ability to promote good learner/staff relationships
- ability to encourage staff to be approachable, available and pleasant
- ability to promote a good staff/patient relationship and quality of patient care
- skills in inviting questions and giving answers
- help and encouragement towards learners in their work
- ability to promote teamworking.

This work concluded that the ward sister is the key in establishing and maintaining a ward atmosphere conducive to learning. It also highlighted that the ward sister is key to the organisation and attitudes of the staff, not only for the learning environment but also patient care. While the work appears dated and uses out of fashion titles, the essence of the message remains: where you have effective clinical leadership, then it usually follows that you tend to have an effective clinical learning environment coupled with excellence in the delivery of care.

Jot This Down

Reflect on the situations that you have found yourself in as a learner.

- What was it in practice that made your learning experience a good one?

Teaching and learning in clinical practice takes place in a variety of settings, commonly in the acute setting, in the primary care environments, in someone's home, or more diverse settings, such as the prison service, hospices, etc. Wherever practice is placed, the learning environment that is fostered can influence the quality and the experience of all staff and patients involved. Teaching in the clinical area is one of the most important ways that nurses learn (Barton & Le May 2012).

In the 'Jot This Down' exercise above, you may have considered what makes an effective learning environment. The Irish Nursing Board (An Bord Altranais 2003) makes the following suggestions:

- Dynamic structures and processes
- Staff feel valued, are highly motivated and deliver quality patient care
- Good communication and interpersonal relationships between qualified nurse and student
- Acceptance of the student as a learner who can contribute to the delivery of quality patient care.

The Evidence

- The clinical education setting is the most influential in the development of nursing skills, knowledge and professional socialisation; stressing the learning climate within the clinical setting (Cheun-Heung & French 1997).
- The clinical environment also plays an important role in developing students' confidence, organisational skills and preparedness for practice (Edwards et al. 2004).

The creation of a positive learning environment is vital to enable meaningful and safe education and development for all staff in the clinical setting. The purpose of a planned clinical experience is to enable students to develop clinical skills, integrate theory with practice, apply problem-solving skills, develop interpersonal skills and become socialised into the formal and informal norms, protocols and expectations of the nursing profession and healthcare system (Conway & McMillan 2000; Hutchings & Sanders 2001; Jackson & Mannix 2001).

What the Experts Say

When I am aware that a new student is being allocated to the unit, I think about the systems that are in place to make their experience more welcoming. I remember too well how it feels to be in a new clinical setting, and how daunting this can be. So I run a kind of checklist through my head, which includes:

- Checking my off-duty to coordinate it with the student start time
- Making sure I have an orientation pack that is up-to-date with the names of all staff working on the unit
- Giving the student clear information about what they can expect from supervision
- Valuing the student's action plan and negotiating how best they learn
- Agreeing times for meetings and reviews
- Thinking about how best to give feedback on progress
- Opportunities to discuss any learning or health needs and reasonable adjustments.

(Staff Nurse and mentor, Thoracic medicine.)

The Nurse as a Mentor

Current NMC approved programmes of pre-registration nursing require students to engage in 50% theory and 50% practice. This puts a huge responsibility on nurses in practice to support and educate nurses of the future to enable them to be fit for practice. The role of the mentor and the associate mentor in teaching, supervising and assessing can never be understated; they are accountable to the NMC for their decision about a student's ability to apply knowledge, skills and competence that befit a newly qualified nurse. Mentors are required to be on the same part of the register that the students they assess are studying, and they must be registered for at least one year before taking on this role. Students should spend at least 40% of their allocated time in practice under the direct supervision of their allocated mentor (NMC 2008b). The nature of supervision can be direct or indirect dependent upon a number of variants, including:

- The type of activity that the student is engaged in
- Their current level of competence
- The need to assess the achievement of NMC competencies to progress on programmes of study
- Protected time for final placement students in addition to the 40% supervision time.

Mentors must have developed their own knowledge, skills and competency beyond that at the point of registration. They are skilled clinical decision-makers, act as role models and enable students to have a broad view of professional roles. Mentors help students make sense of their practice in a variety of ways, but it is useful to think of the skills that are needed in order to be an effective mentor.

Jot This Down

When you think about the role of the mentor, what are the people factors that affect their ability to facilitate teaching and learning in practice?

In the 'Jot This Down' exercise above, you will have no doubt reflected on the skills you have experienced when being mentored in practice. Those mentors show a genuine interest in the student, acknowledging that each student is an individual, with individual learning needs, preferred learning styles and skills dependent upon their past experience. In addition to this, they are excellent role models, they make you feel valued as a member of the team and give feedback in an open and honest way.

What the Experts Say

Comments from student nurses about mentors at the end of their second year of study ...

'She was what I would call a critical friend ... not afraid to tell me when I needed to stop and think situations through'

'A good mentor sets out their stall right from the start of placement, you know where you stand and feel comfortable to ask for help'

'My mentor on my last placement was really good at making sure that my portfolio was up-to-date, he brought his own in to show me and it really focussed my attention on how to get it right'

'I have mixed feelings, up to my last placement, mentors had always been supportive and willing to teach. This time was different, so I had to find other avenues of support within the nursing team'

'He (my mentor), showed me around and let me know where the tea and coffee was kept, I felt less anxious and able to relax right from the first day'.

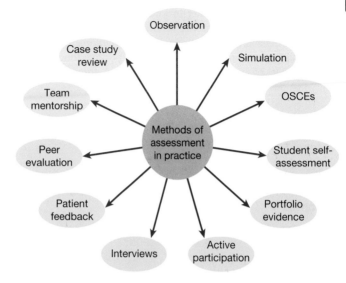

Figure 2.1 **Methods of assessment in clinical practice.**

Mentors are responsible for:

- Directing student learning experiences in practice
- Supervision of learning and the provision of feedback
- Supporting the achievement of objectives
- Assessing skills, attitudes and behaviours
- Gaining feedback from the wider care team on student progress
- Identifying concerns in student performance and setting action plans to address this
- Signing off outcomes and achievements.

There is a variety of ways that mentors can assess students or others within the practice setting and Figure 2.1 demonstrates some of these methods.

Red Flag Failing a Student

Duffy (2003) outlines the importance of good assessment and why this is essential in the role of the mentor. She states:

There has to be a recognition that some students need to fail. Potentially clinical assessment of student nurses can safeguard professional standards, patients and the general public. It is inevitable that some students will not be able to meet the required level of practice and it is essential that mentors do not avoid the difficult issue of having to fail these students.

(Duffy 2003, p. 83)

Clearly there will be occasions where mentors require support and guidance in order to ensure the best outcomes for the student and the care delivery that they are accountable for. Mentors can expect collaboration and guidance from the Higher Education Institutions (HEIs) who provide established communication systems to help deal with issues or questions regarding student progression. HEIs are responsible for evaluating and auditing the learning environment and for communicating changes to programmes of study. Link Lecturers can support both students and mentors in practice. In addition, placement providers in collaboration with HEIs have a role in developing mentors, supporting the learning environment and providing mentors with their own lines of supervision.

Theoretical Frameworks for Teaching and Learning

Teaching can be described as a system of activities with the intention of educating or instructing. It is a deliberate and methodological activity with a controlling element. This definition is often seen as a mechanistic definition of teaching. Schön (1987) uses a more reflective approach and emphasises the coaching analogy, whereby the learner is encouraged to seek explanations and the teacher provides advice and clarification.

Learning may be defined as a relatively permanent change of behaviour, what Kolb (1984, p. 38) expressed as a 'process whereby knowledge is created through the transformation of experience'. It is an outcome, an end-product. The processes by which learning occurs are complex and over time, psychologists have tried to describe them; however, none of the theories in isolation can provide a full understanding. There are a range of theories to support how we learn, and the next section will explore the most common theories of learning.

Behaviourism

This is a theory made popular by the works of Skinner, an American behavioural psychologist in the 1940s, and Pavlov, a Russian psychologist in the 1960s. They demonstrated that if a repeated incentive – for example, a negative stimulus such as an electric shock, or a positive stimulus such as the provision of food – is used often enough to reward or punish, then eventually the subject learns. They developed the theories around 'conditioned response' and 'operant conditioning', which can be seen in Table 2.1.

Behaviourist theory is associated with the reinforcement of punishment or reward and rehearsal of a task over time. If there is a positive outcome, this can result in perfection and is linked to:

- Activities that support learning
- Repetitive activity and continued practice
- Small bite-size steps
- Reinforcement.

The approach puts the learner in a passive situation, responding only when there is the presence of environmental stimuli. When relating the behaviourist theories to humans, reinforcement can be very subtle; a smile, frown, gentle phrases, positive touching can all be examples of social reinforcement. Social reinforcement works well when teaching and learning social skills.

> ### Jot This Down
> Reflect on types of social reinforcements that you see parents use with their children.

Table 2.1 Operant conditioning and conditioned response.

SKINNER'S 'OPERANT CONDITIONING'	PAVLOV'S 'CONDITIONED RESPONSE'
Skinner's experimental work involved rats and pigeons, and later, humans. He found that rats and pigeons when placed in a box containing a food tray and a lever to operate the release of the food, over time would learn the connection between pressing the lever and releasing the food.	In his experiment, Pavlov found that if he rang a bell at the same time as giving food to dogs, the dogs began to associate the bell with food. In time, the dogs began to salivate at the sound of the bell in the absence of food, demonstrating a conditioned response.

Social reinforcement can be a useful teaching tool in clinical practice; for example, where a student nurse is being supervised carrying out a skill which is relatively new to them, as a teacher or facilitator of learning, you will make positive comments to reinforce effective skills.

Cognitive theories of learning

This type of learning relies on the mental processes involved in thinking, perception, organisation of thoughts, memory and insight. The learner comes with knowledge, skills and related experience to the learning situation, and their role in the leaning process is to construct their personal understanding of the information they are exposed to. According to Quinn and Hughes (2007), the term 'cognition' refers to the internal mental processes of humans and encompasses the domains of memory, which allow people to store experience from the past and use it in the present. Perception associated with mental organisation and the interpretation of sensory information and thinking is a cognitive process comprising internal mental representations of the world and that involves problem-solving, reflecting and making decisions.

The three main champions of cognitive theory (see Table 2.2) are:

- Piaget
- Bloom
- Ausubel.

Gestalt learning theory is a form of cognitive theory which emphasises the importance of totality in learning, i.e. the need to

Table 2.2 The focus of the three main theorists in cognitive learning.

THEORIST	COGNITIVE FOCUS
Jean Piaget 1896–1980	Constructed models of child development and the learning process identified four developmental stages: **1.** Sensory motor – the child understands his environment through the basic senses **2.** Intuitive pre-operational – memory and imagination play a part in learning, capable of more creativity **3.** Concrete operational – can go beyond the basic information given, but still relies on concrete examples to support reasoning **4.** Formal operational – here abstract reasoning becomes possible
Bloom's Taxonomy	Describes in hierarchical order, the cognitive processes involved in learning, the so-called cognitive domain. HIGHER ORDER THINKING SKILLS 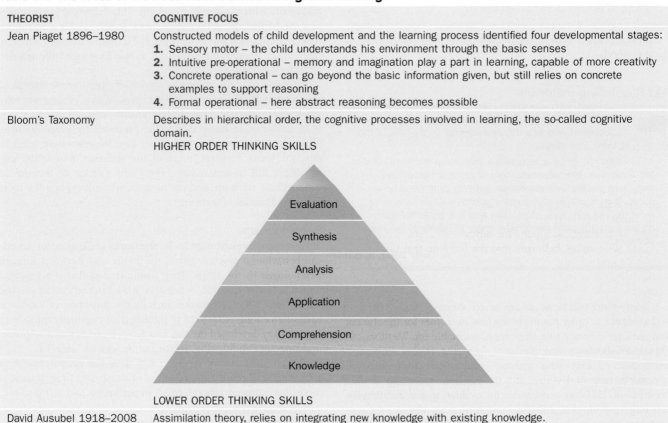 LOWER ORDER THINKING SKILLS
David Ausubel 1918–2008	Assimilation theory, relies on integrating new knowledge with existing knowledge. *If I had to reduce all of educational psychology to just one principle, I would say this: the most important single factor influencing learning is what the learner already knows. Ascertain this and teach him accordingly*

view things as a whole when learning rather than the reductionist approach of learning by stages. This is particularly helpful when teaching a skill in clinical practice, as it helps the learner focus on the expected outcome of the whole procedure done at normal pace before breaking it down into smaller tasks. Cognitive theory accepts that individuals have different needs and concerns at different times. Those who subscribe to cognitive theory believe that:

- Learning comes from understanding one's environment and one's experiences
- The structure of teaching will aid learning
- Feedback aids learning
- Individual differences and prior learning must be considered and taken into account.

Humanistic theories of learning

Humanistic theories focus on the individual and reject the behaviourist theories that people are unthinking and can be shaped by patterns of reward and punishment. Based on the work of Maslow (1954), Rogers (1983) and Knowles *et al.* (2011), the theories focus on the individuals' potential, their life experiences and prior knowledge, and their individual personalities in order to reach the highest level of personal achievement.

Maslow developed the hierarchy of needs, and this is important to consider from a teaching and learning perspective. Learning (or growth) takes place when feelings and experiences have been taken into consideration. Learning will only take place, however, if the learner feels comfortable and safe (elements at the base of the pyramid). An example often associated with this is the need for refreshment, or a comfort break during teaching session. As a learner moves up the hierarchy, other more complex needs arise, for example the need for esteem. Imagine a situation where you have been ridiculed for wrongly answering a question in class. Self-esteem in the learning situation can be met by providing acceptance, praise, and acknowledgement of another's views. Achievement of the full potential of the learner lies at the top of the pyramid (see Figure 11.3).

Carl Rogers (1983) is more commonly known for his work in the development of 'client centered therapy', where he aimed to offer his clients the knowledge and skills necessary to find their own solutions to their problems. This was in direct contrast to the paternalistic approach that told patients and clients how to deal with problems. Rogers argues that individuals learn best when they are active in the process and when they perceive that what is being learned is relevant. As such, he advocated a student-centred approach to learning, believing that the learning that takes place must be significant and meaningful, incorporating both thoughts and feelings. Rogers supports a shift in focus from what the teacher does to what is happening in the student's mind; the student becomes self-directed and is motivated to explore information at their own pace and in their own time.

Humanistic theories work well if the teacher understands that he/she can only facilitate learning, and that the learner will only respond positively if they perceive the activity will be self-enhancing. In order to learn, the learner needs to be ready for the activity, and be able to feel safe and supported. The humanist approach contrasts to the behaviourist idea of operant conditioning (arguing that all behaviour is the result of the application of consequences) and cognitivism, where the belief is that discovering knowledge or constructing meaning is central to learning. Humanists believe that it is important to study the person as a whole,

Table 2.3 The different approaches to learning, andragogy and pedagogy.

ANDRAGOGY	PEDAGOGY
• Learners are self-directed and responsible • Motivation is internally focussed • The teacher facilitates • Student-centred • Problem-solving as opposed to subject-centred • Life experience of learner is a rich source of information	• The teacher is the expert • Learners dependent on teacher for transfer of knowledge • Learners told what they have to learn • Motivation for learning is teacher led

particularly as the person grows and develops over the lifespan. The study of the self, motivation, goal setting and attainment are areas of specific interest. Humanism can be expressed as the development of self-actualised, autonomous people where learning is student centred and personalised; the role of the teacher is that of a facilitator. Affective and cognitive needs are central and the aim is to develop self-actualised people in a cooperative, supportive environment.

Andragogy describes an approach to teaching and learning that is adult focussed, and is the direct opposite to the notion of *pedagogy*, which relates to how children learn. Table 2.3 lists the different approaches to teaching and learning of andragogy and pedagogy.

Andragogy has been popularised by the American educator Malcolm Knowles who makes six assumptions about how adults are motivated to learn:

1. *Need to know the reason for learning*
2. *Experience and making mistakes is the foundation for learning*
3. *Responsibility and involvement in planning and evaluating learning supports self-concept*
4. *Learning is most interesting when immediately relevant to individuals and supports readiness*
5. *Learning is problem-centred to provide orientation*
6. *Response to learning is internal as a means of motivation.*

(Knowles *et al.* 2011)

In support of the principle of adult learning or pedagogy, Kolb (1984) presented a model of learning that asserts learning to be the process of transformating experience. His experiential learning cycle as shown in Figure 2.2 develops the notion that people learn more effectively when they are encouraged to be active in the process.

Concrete experience is where the learner experiences something new or re-interprets an existing experience. Learners are actively involved and in this phase, they tend to rely on their feelings and the senses to interpret what is happening. The learner is invited to feel and watch, what Kolb describes as *diverging*.

Reflective observation looks back at the event and evaluates any inconsistencies between what was felt and what is understood from the experience. The learner is invited to think and watch, what Kolb describes as *assimilating*.

Abstract conceptualisation involves making sense of what has happened, utilising past experiences and thinking about or visualising what to do next. The learner is invited to think and do, what Kolb describes as *converging*.

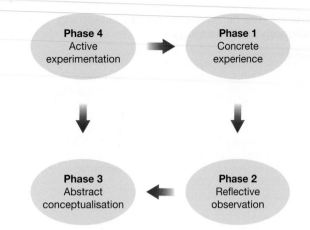

Figure 2.2 Kolb's experiential learning cycle. *Source:* Kolb 1984.

Active experimentation is when the learner considers what they have learned and how to apply this to practice. The learner is invited to feel and do, what Kolb describes as *accommodation*.

Jot This Down
Kolb's experiential learning cycle is a useful tool to apply to teaching and learning skills within the clinical setting.
• Think about how the cycle can be applied when teaching a clinical skill to a new student nurse.
• How important is it to understand the preferred learning style of the student when teaching a clinical skill?

Learning styles

Knowing a person's learning style helps to focus teaching and learning in a way that makes the learner feel more comfortable. A number of models exist but the most common are Honey and Mumford's (1992) learning styles and the VARK learning preference model.

Peter Honey and Alan Mumford worked together to develop Kolb's cycle of learning to identify four distinct learning styles or preferences:

1. Activist
2. Reflector
3. Theorist
4. Pragmatist.

   Activists are associated with getting involved in doing things. They typically enjoy practical activities, where there is an element of energy and fun. They will respond less comfortably to activities that require sitting and listening (long lectures), and working alone.

   Reflectors are associated with reviewing the experience. They typically enjoy time to think, to observe and take things in. Reflectors can be cautious and slow to make decisions but usually act on sound knowledge. They respond less comfortably to being dragged into activities, with no time to prepare and lack of privacy to think.

   Theorists are associated with analysing and drawing conclusions from experiences. They feel comfortable when they have an understanding of their observations, when they know how concepts fit in. They like logical processes and will easily work with frameworks and models. They are least comfortable when faced with time-wasting, unstructured timetables and not being able to ask a question.

   Pragmatists are associated with planning and setting targets to create a link between what they are involved in and what the outcome should be. They enjoy practical problem-solving, like to work quickly, respond well to problems and will work with things that interest them. They are least comfortable with anything theoretical and with too much focus on past events not related to the here and now.

The VARK learning style inventory designed by Neil Fleming in 1987 aims to help individuals understand their learning preferences:

- **V**isual
- **A**ural
- **R**ead/write
- **K**inaesthetic.

It is estimated that 50–70% of individuals are multimodal (i.e. have more than one preference when it comes to learning). In Table 2.4, the VARK learning style inventory identifies the key preferences for learning in each domain.

According to Fleming and Baume (2006), VARK is designed to be a starting point for a conversation between the teacher and the learner. It can also act as a catalyst for staff development and stimulate variety in teaching and learning.

 Link To/Go To

http://www.VARK-learn.com/english/page.asp?p=questionnaire

to access the VARK learning styles questionnaire.

Nurses often tend to be practical or experiential learners. They may learn best from doing, as opposed to reading about something. Remember when supporting teaching and learning to relate theory to everyday life, use practice or real-life scenarios, bringing facts and theory to life. Where possible allow people to work in groups, sharing ideas and learning from each other.

The Adult Learner

If you are engaged in teaching fellow healthcare professionals, the approach you use will need to acknowledge the specific needs of the adult learner. The methods used will be very different from those employed when teaching children. The following features are associated with adult learners (Rogers & Horricks 2010; Quinn & Hughes 2007):

- They are adults by definition
- Their process of growth is continuing as opposed to just starting
- They bring to the learning situation a set of experiences and values
- They come with intentions and expectations
- They have competing interests
- They already hold established patterns of learning.

Effective teaching in higher education demands that the individual teacher, the organisational culture and the policies and procedures in place meet the needs of the learner.

Table 2.4 The VARK domains.

DOMAIN	KEY PREFERENCES FOR LEARNING
Visual	In order to facilitate learning, the student prefers to: · Use picture, videos, posters, slides · Listen to lecturers who use gestures and picturesque language · Follow flowcharts · Underline key points, use colour and highlighting · Use texts with lots of diagrams and pictures · Analyse graphs To perform well in any test or examination: · Highlight and underline when revising · Use of mind maps · Order notes in a flowchart and write essays around this.
Aural	In order to facilitate learning, the student prefers to: · Attend classes · Attend discussions and tutorials · Discuss topics with others (including teachers) · Explain new ideas to other people · Use a recording device · Remember the interesting examples, stories, jokes, etc. · Describe the overheads and other visuals to somebody who was not there · Leave spaces in notes for later recall To perform well in any test or examination: · Imagine talking with the examiner · Spend time in quiet places recalling the ideas · Practise writing answers to old exam questions.
Read/Write	In order to facilitate learning, the student prefers to: · Make lists and headings · Use dictionaries, glossaries, definitions, handouts, textbooks, notes. · Listen to teachers who use words well and provide lots of information verbally and in notes To perform well in any test or examination: · Write exam answers · Practise with multiple choice questions · Write paragraphs, beginnings and endings · Write lists (a,b,c,d; 1,2,3,4) · Arrange words into hierarchies and points.
Kinaesthetic	In order to facilitate learning, the student prefers to: · Use all of their senses, i.e. clinical laboratories, clinical practice · Listen to teachers who give examples of real-life applications, and who use hands-on approaches To perform well in any test or examination: · Write practice answers · Role play the exam situation or experience a mock exam so that they can understand it · Any study ideas are only valuable if they sound practical, real, and relevant to you.

Teacher factors:

- Being there – availability of people to teach and help others learn
- Characteristics of the effective teacher – recognition of need
- Use an adult-centred approach
- Knowledge of the student – their learning needs
- Knowledge of the subject – learning theory, nursing theory and practice, curriculum outcomes, learning needs, objectives, etc.
- The most appropriate person to teach
- Adequately prepared to teach and help others learn, planning in advance or on 'the hoof' using theory to inform teaching
- Acknowledgement of learning style – appropriate method of teaching used
- Being able to share knowledge
- Valuing the teaching role.

By acting as a teacher you also become a role model to other staff (this may include other members of the healthcare team, not only nurses), as well as patients. Teaching as a skill, along with all the other skills cited in this text, can be learned and developed. Good teachers are created, not born. The skills listed above reflect the skills required by the nurse who engages in teaching. Teaching strategies to facilitate learning – those of direct observation, role modelling, professional socialisation and peer learning – are all skills that support the nurse who teaches in practice.

The factors above should be taken into account when preparing to teach. The following five steps can be used as a framework to help you with your teaching in the clinical area:

1. Create a positive learning environment
2. Know who your learners are
3. Know what it is that you want them to know
4. Prepare
5. Ask for feedback.

Students learn in a variety of settings, and nurse education leading to a professional qualification combined with an academic achievement takes place in diverse environments. Healthcare environments can be fast-paced and demanding of nurses' time and focus; mentors need to respond effectively to meet the needs of patients. Learning is shared with other students, ideally with students from other disciplines to encourage teamworking and interprofessional integration. The NMC (2010b, p. 9) states that students should become increasingly self-directed and independent, and able to make use of a variety of resources.

> **Jot This Down**
> Reflect on a recent learning experience that you have had. What resources did you use to support your learning in practice?

In the 'Jot This Down' exercise above, you may have thought about some of the following resources:

- Utilise practice placement assessment documents
- Additional action plans, significant event reporting, key skills (self-assessment)
- Individual placement objectives
- Role clarification
- Responsibility clarification
- Clear about what learner wants from student/mentor relationship
- Integrate evidence-based practice (EBP) into everyday practice
- Knowledge of local/national policies, procedures.

This is by no means an exhaustive list. Learning opportunities undoubtedly occur in direct contact with patients and clients, as well as in simulated practice, which allows students to learn in a safe situation that mimics reality. Chapter 1 provides information with regard to the competency framework in nurse education.

In addition to the learning environment and the variety of learning experiences, learners are also influenced by:

- Motivational factors
- Readiness to learn
- Individual learning difficulties.

The Evidence

Ewan and White (1996) suggest the following conditions for learning (Student factors):

- Motivation to learn, intrinsic and extrinsic factors
- Interest in the topic – meaningfulness
- General ability – e.g. consider where they are in the programme, intelligence, practice level – novice to advanced beginner
- Aptitude or skills development
- Learning style or preferred learning style.

Motivational factors are the key to successful learning and as demonstrated earlier in this chapter, are important features in many learning theories. Motivation occurs both *internally* and *externally,* and helps the learner focus attention on what is being taught.

Internal or intrinsic motivation is the personal desire to understand and make sense of learning. It is a strong motivational factor and tends to be associated with self-esteem, job satisfaction and quality of life (Knowles *et al.* 2011). By comparison, external or extrinsic motivation to learn is more associated with behaviourist theories that incorporate reward and stimulus from an external source. Here, individuals take reward from praise and acknowledgement of achievement.

Motivation can also be associated with the need to know or acquire new knowledge and skills, or the usefulness of this. As facilitators of learning, nurses need to be aware of factors that can stimulate or suppress motivation in others.

Jot This Down

A number of barriers are often associated with a person's motivation to learn, for example tiredness and lack of time.

- What factors do you think create barriers to your motivation to learn?

In the 'Jot This Down' exercise above, you may have considered barriers to motivation that link to your intrinsic or extrinsic triggers, such as the pace of teaching, the amount of feedback that you receive, your level of self-confidence, stress, etc. In a study conducted by the Department for Business, Innovation and Skills (DBIS 2013, p. 24), over three-fifths of young people who want to learn in the future identified course content and format; cost and finances; and family, partners and peers as barriers to learning. They also cited lack of motivation or direction as a barrier to future development.

Readiness to learn encompasses several dimensions or prerequisites to learning, including experiential, emotional and a person's physical and mental ability. Where the prerequisite is missing or has not evolved, then learning is diminished.

Experiential readiness to learn is based on the learner's experience as demonstrated in Figure 2.3. In this domain, cultural, developmental and prior education and learning all have an impact on a person's learning experience, either negatively or positively.

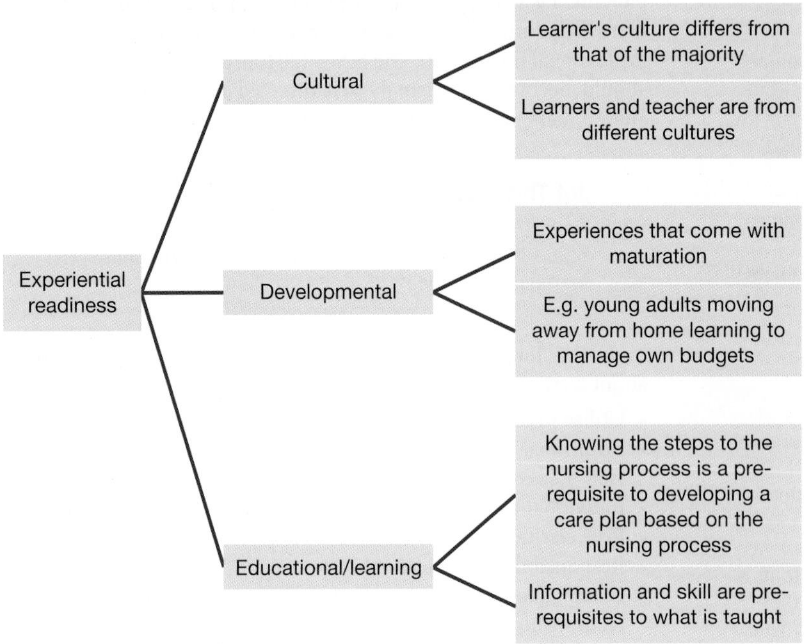

Emotional readiness to learn can be linked to motivation, for example anxiety can either switch people on or off learning. Emotional readiness can be seen in nursing students who may have high levels of anxiety in, for example, their ability to react effectively in an emergency situation.

Physical and/or mental readiness to learn relates to structure and functional abilities in the learner. A level of dexterity, fine motor skill and visual acuity is required to perform certain clinical skills, for example wound care. Moving and handling patients and clients with safety requires motor skills and physical strength.

Readiness to learn can be affected by visual, hearing and mobility problems that necessitate reasonable adjustments to be offered to support learning.

Lifelong Learning and PREP

Post-registration education and practice (PREP) is a set of standards and guidance produced by the NMC (2010c) designed to enhance practice and patient care. PREP helps the nurse to enhance practice and care by keeping up-to-date with

Figure 2.3 Experiential readiness to learn.

developments in practice, encouraging practitioners to be reflective and supporting the development of professional portfolios as a way of recording and evaluating ongoing education and learning. Continuing professional development (CPD), although not a guarantee of competence, is a key component of clinical governance (discussed later in this chapter) and affects all health and social care professionals. Continuing professional development is associated with lifelong learning that will enable nurses to meet the needs of the public.

Professional and Legal Issues Requirements for Periodic Renewal of Registration with the NMC

- Every three years you are legally required to renew your registration and pay a fee for this (an annual retention fee collected every 12 months)
- You are required to sign a notification of practice form, accompanied by the registration fee
- The notification of practice form requires that you make a declaration relating to the details on the form
- This declaration in effect states that the information you have provided is a true and accurate statement of your current practice and continuing professional development status
- You also declare that your health and character are sufficiently good to enable you to continue to practise safely and effectively
- There is a second section of the form concerned with the 'Police cautions and convictions declaration'. Registration (and therefore your ability to practise) will not be renewed until the completed and signed form and payment have been received.

The NMC's PREP requirements

You must demonstrate the ability to meet PREP requirements. These are legal requirements and you will not be able to register unless you meet them. There are two PREP standards that affect registration:

- The PREP practice standard that requires nurses and midwives to have worked for a minimum of 450 hours in practice over the last three years. This can be both paid and unpaid work. Practitioners who have had a gap in practice and who do not meet the standard will need to successfully complete a return to practice course in order to re-register
- The PREP continuing professional development standard that requires the registrant to have recorded CPD activities during the three-year period prior to renewal of registration. Completion of the Notification of Practice (NoP) form is mandatory. In order to meet this standard the nurse must:
  - Undertake at least 5 days or 35 hours of learning activity relevant to his/her practice during the three years prior to renewal of registration
  - Maintain a personal professional portfolio of learning activity
  - Comply with any request from the NMC to audit how those requirements have been met.

The way in which this standard is met is up to the individual nurse. The person who is required to demonstrate CPD activities is the best person to decide what learning activities are needed to comply with the standard. There is no such thing as an approved PREP (CPD) learning activity. It is essential that learning activities are documented in a way that conveys evidence that the learning activity you have undertaken has informed and influenced your practice. Having developed skills in professional portfolio management as students, many nurses continue to use this format as ongoing

evidence that can be provided if requested by the NMC. In this scenario, you must be able to provide documentation regarding the learning activities that you have completed within the three years prior to renewal of your registration. You will need to demonstrate where, what and how:

- *Where* you were practising when the learning activity took place
- *What* the learning activity was concerned with
- *How* the learning influenced or informed your practice, how it related to your practice.

An element of reflection is called for when considering what you have learned and how this has informed and developed your practice. The next section will highlight some of the processes that support the reflective practitioner.

Reflective Practice

Nursing is predominantly a practice-based discipline, where the aim of care is to be effective and competent; reflection can be a tool through which practice and knowledge about practice is communicated and validated. Reflecting on practice can provide nurses with an opportunity to learn from it, and has the potential to help the nurse become, among other things, a lifelong learner. In addition, the learning that occurs through the process of reflection supports knowledge, skills and behavioural development and ultimately augments care provision.

In support of the process of reflection, a number of models have been produced to support the framework of reflection. Such models provide the nurse with a structure to reflect in a systematic and logical way. The ultimate goal of reflection is to help the nurse bring meaning to situations both 'in' and 'on' practice. To be able to reflect on and in practice, the nurse must engage in an active and conscious process when encountering problematic aspects of care provision and attempting to make sense of them. Reflective practice is a process that can be used to engage in lifelong learning.

The Evidence The Two Constituents of Reflection

According to Schön (1983) there are two constituents to reflection:

- Reflection-in-action: this type of reflection is created from an experience and involves thinking about what is occurring while actually doing it
- Reflection-on-action: this type of reflection evolves when the nurse revisits the experience after the event.

In addition to the two constituents of reflection identified by Schön (1983), there is the notion of a third component: that of 'reflecting before action' to reduce the risk of errors prior to engaging in practice, as identified by Greenwood (1993). There have been many attempts at defining the concept of reflection. Reflective learning is learning from experience formally or informally, allowing the learner to consider his/her practice honestly and critically (Moon 2004). The outcome may be the development of a deeper understanding of personal skills, enhanced self-awareness and individual learning needs. Nurses can develop further and enhance their understanding of practice through reflection by questioning what they do and more importantly, why things are done, whether the outcome is as intended, and how things might be done more effectively next time.

There are a number of definitions of reflection within the nursing and wider literature and because of this, there may be confusion about what constitutes reflection.

- Boud *et al.* (1985) suggest that reflection occurs when individuals engage in activities that aim to explore their experiences in order to lead to new understanding and appreciation of the situation(s). The suggestion here is that you must learn through practice
- Johns (2000) states that reflection is a window allowing practitioners to view themselves within the context of their own lived experience. By doing this, practitioners can confront, understand and work towards resolving issues that arise in practice.

Models of reflection

A range of models exist to support the process of reflection, and just as there are a number of definitions of reflection, so too are there a number of reflective frameworks or models. While they are similar in the overall principle that they promote, they differ in the level of complexity and detail.

Driscoll (2007) considers three stages in his approach to reflection:

- *What?* – describes the event by returning to the situation
- *So what?* – analyses the event, by understanding the context
- *Now what?* – proposes actions after the event to modify future outcomes.

Driscoll's model represents a very simple framework from which to order reflection. In Figure 2.4, the more detailed Gibbs Reflective Cycle is shown.

Gibbs reflective cycle

Gibbs (1998) enables those who engage in reflective activity to consider events in a cyclical manner. Gibbs' model is one that promotes a simple approach to reflection in sequential steps. Gibbs (1998) points out that deep learning takes place when reflective practice is used. The starting point is a description of an event, and through the process of reflection, the nurse produces an action plan for future practice.

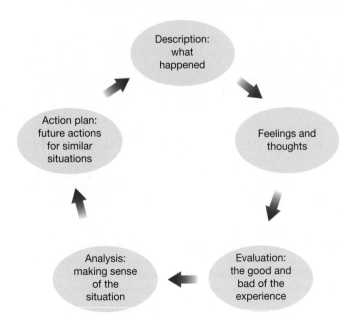

Figure 2.4 Gibbs Reflective Cycle.

Jot This Down

What would you say are triggers as a stimulus for your personal reflection?

In the 'Jot This Down' exercise above, you may have thought about some of the events in your nursing experience that have triggered some kind of thought process. These are often called 'significant events' or 'critical incidents'. Triggers for such events might include:

- A negative/positive experience
- A crisis or emergency situation
- Feedback from a mentor or patient
- Learning experience.

The analysis of an event or incident helps the nurse to make sense of their role within the healthcare setting and the many therapeutic and working relationships that take place there.

Johns' model of structured reflection (1994)

This model of reflection offers cues to the nurse to support the concept of accessing, making sense of, and learning from the experiences they have. To achieve this, the nurse is encouraged to 'look in' on thoughts and emotions about events and 'look out' at the situation experienced. In time, Johns has revised his model in an attempt to offer more in-depth reflection.

Leadership Styles and Theories

Nurses lead in a variety of ways, and in a variety of settings, and as a consequence, there are a number of differing styles and theories that underpin the way that individuals as leaders direct, plan and influence the behaviour of other people. In nursing, we often use the phrase 'ward manager' when referring to the so-called leader of a team in the clinical setting. But can we use the term 'manager' to truly reflect the meaning of leader? Consider the following quote from Grohar-Murray and DiCroce (2003): 'The authority of leadership is derived from the ability of the leader to influence others to accomplish goals, whereas the authority of management is derived from the manager's position in the organisation' (p. 17). The quote implies that managers can hold authority from a hierarchical perspective, whereas leaders possess innate qualities to support their abilities as a leader. Leadership can be thought of in terms of an individual's ability to maintain relationships with others in a way that constructively influences the way that they work.

Leadership is a complex subject, with a wealth of definitions that have been presented in the literature to illustrate what is meant by the term. Many view the leader as a charismatic, powerful individual with followers at a subordinate level. More modern concepts of leadership see it as something that is shared and distributed and can be identified at all levels within organisations. Not everyone is a leader, but everyone can contribute to the leadership process.

The Evidence

Very few people now adhere to the Platonic view about the great leader who is set apart from everybody else, but nevertheless there are important ways in which our leadership theories haven't changed. I think actually we're still very much bogged down in the idea of leaders as great individuals and people who are set apart from the group. And by, if you like, putting leaders on a pedestal and treating them as special and different we lose what really is special about leadership, which is that it is the best of us, and we – everybody – [are] a part of great leadership.

(Haslem *et al.* 2011)

Leadership styles can be said to be context dependent, and in Table 2.5 you can see the characteristics of many of the common styles and their potential impact on the teams or people in the work environment.

Nurses can apply leadership styles and adapt them to the ever-changing situations with which they are faced on a regular basis. An understanding of the theories that underpin leadership can guide nurses in adopting the most effective ways of working in practice.

Transactional leadership is also known as managerial leadership, which focusses on the leader as supervisor, organiser and someone interested in group performance. Classically, this type of leadership is synonymous with reward and punishment. Transactional leaders are happy to keep things on an even keel, and are thus not specifically looking for change or development. Typically, this type of leader will keep an eye on followers to praise or to find fault in ways of working. When leaders who adopt this way of leading perform poorly, then there is an associated link with poor standards of patient care (Basset & Westmore 2012).

Transformational leadership aims to enhance the development of others in the team through a number of mechanisms:

- Establishing direction
- Aligning people
- Motivating and inspiring
- Producing change
- Where you are going (vision)
- Effective communicators.

These types of leaders are inspirational, and act as role models to their followers. They are very much in tune with the skills of their followers and they take a genuine interest in them as people and can align tasks that enhance their performance. Followers are encouraged to identify with the organisation, taking ownership for the parts that they play.

What the Experts Say Working for a Transformational Leader

 For a long time I have had an interest in developing a media based learning tool for staff and students to develop skills in communicating with people who have dementia. My manager is really supportive, as a transformational leader, he has encouraged me to go ahead with this. He recognises my skills, not just in relation to teaching and learning, but also in time management and self direction. He shares the vision that I have, and is a real motivator. His democratic style has encouraged the involvement and enthusiasm of the ward team, who are behind me all the way.

(Band 6 Staff Nurse, Medical Unit)

Table 2.5 Leadership styles, characteristics and potential impact.

STYLE OF LEADERSHIP	CHARACTERISTICS	POTENTIAL IMPACT
Authoritarian	Decision-maker Task-orientated High standards Planning and expecting others to follow In control, maintains power over others	Positive: when instructions need to be clear and directed, e.g. in an emergency situation or when working with a novice Negative: may encourage staff dependency, and can demotivate others and stifle creativity
Democratic	Team player Sharing ideas Mutual respect of others' ideas Delegates as a means of developing others Interacts and seeks opinions of others	Positive: team approach can elicit more effective solutions Respect from team members who feel developed Negative: in emergency situations where delay in decision-making might be seen as lack of competence
Bureaucratic	Adheres to the rule book Governed by policy and regulations Follows close set of values and standards Strict disciplinarian	Positive: in situations where exact and precise ways of working are needed, e.g. high risk areas Negative: teams may feel apathetic, powerless and frustrated
Laissez-faire	Allows others to make decisions Enables others to manage and control their own work Expects others to work autonomously, and to ask for help if needed 'Hands-off' approach	Positive: in environments where the team is highly skilled, motivated and capable of working independently Negative: in environments where the team is inexperienced. The team can become demotivated, miss opportunities for development and fall behind with deadlines
Situational	Adapts style to manage particular situations Identifies the performance, competencies and commitment of others Flexible Acknowledges the relationship between the leader's supportive and directive behaviour and the follower's competence Provides emotional support and is a good communicator	Positive: allows for contingencies, and can be effective when supporting newly qualified nurses and students Negative: focusses too much on leaders and not enough on group interaction

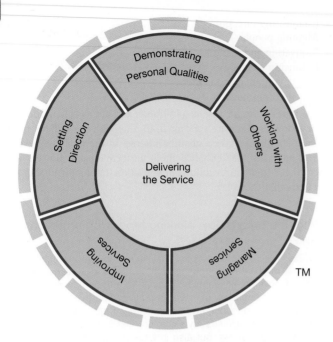

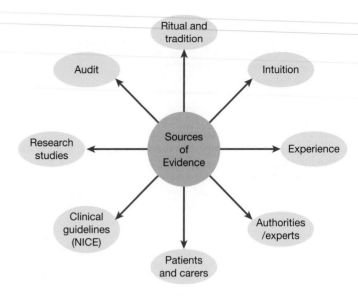

Figure 2.6 Sources of evidence.

Figure 2.5 The five domains of the Clinical Leadership Competency Framework (CLCF). (The CLCF and associated graphics are ©NHS Leadership Academy, 2011. All rights reserved.)

Other forms of guidance in the development of leadership skills are available through the Leadership Academy of the NHS. A Leadership Framework supports the development of all staff in health care irrespective of their role or discipline. They provide an online facility for self-assessment and modules of study.

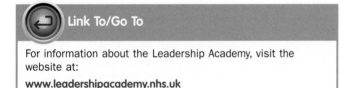

Link To/Go To

For information about the Leadership Academy, visit the website at:

www.leadershipacademy.nhs.uk

The Clinical Leadership Competency Framework (CLCF) (NHS 2011) (Figure 2.5) describes the competencies that clinicians need to become more actively involved in planning, delivery and transformation of health and social care services.

The CLCF model emphasises the need for all clinicians to be involved in the development of leadership skills and to empower leadership in others. Each of the five domains supports improving the quality and safety of healthcare services and staff, and seeks to enable clinicians to be competent in each domain. From student, up to experienced practitioner, it is expected that all competencies within the framework can be achieved to varying degrees, depending on the context in which they relate to practice.

Evidence-Based Practice

As a practitioner working within health care, you will probably hear the term 'evidence-based practice' (EBP) on a regular basis; in fact many will claim that their practice is 'evidence-based' and that they adhere to the NMC's code, which asserts that nurses should provide a high standard of practice and care at all times, using the best available evidence to deliver that care (NMC 2008a). The term 'evidence-based' is a concept that infers the use of the best information available to inform and question contemporary nursing practice.

Evidence-based medicine was first introduced in 1972 by Archie Cochrane, who believed that the influence of tradition and custom did little to enhance health care, at a time when research development was providing proof that practice was in many instances outdated and harmful. In 1997, the NHS Modernisation Agenda set out a 10-year plan to improve and standardise practice, with an emphasis on EBP and clinically effective care (DH 1997). The challenge for excellence in care does not end with the government, it also comes from the public, patients and their carers and the healthcare professions. Healthcare workers use evidence from a variety of sources (Figure 2.6); many are rooted in tradition and the perception of what evidence is will differ from person to person.

EBP has been described as 'doing the right things right' (Muir Gray 1997). Other descriptions include EBP as a method of problem-solving to elicit the best solution, and a combination of clinical expertise with application to provide the best available evidence from systematic research. EBP is key to promoting clinical effectiveness, and clinical effectiveness is synonymous with practitioners' understanding of the effectiveness of their interventions in practice.

There are clear stages to the process of EBP, which always begins with a question.

This is an important step of the process, as it helps to explore the subject and focus on the right information to provide answers to the question. However, it is not straightforward. An initial starting point might be questioning one's own practice, and a starting point might be to consider **why** and **how** a decision about the treatment or care that is provided is made. There is an art to developing questions in order to elicit a meaningful answer, and the evidence-based process flows from the question.

PICO is a framework for formulating questions and was developed by Sackett *et al.* in 1997, as a way of making questions more focussed:

P – Population or Patient – it may be useful to specify gender, age, disease type, morbidity. It may be useful here to stipulate the setting, for example in-patient or surgical care for information that relates to the clinical environment

I – Intervention, define what you are interested in – this may be a test or exposure to something (e.g. sunlight)

C – Comparison – define an alternative intervention by means of comparison

O – Outcomes – define the meaningful outcome, beneficial or harmful.

Jot This Down Structuring a Search Question Using PICO

Jill suffers from recurring bouts of cystitis (inflammation of the urethra) and when attending for her regular cervical smear (PAP) test, she asks you about the effectiveness of cranberry juice in reducing the symptoms of this nagging complaint.

· Using the PICO framework, think of search terms that you might use to find information for Jill that represents the best evidence.

In the 'Jot This Down' exercise above, you may have included search areas such as:

P – Population or Patient: *cystitis women*
I – Intervention: *cranberry juice*
C – Comparison: *water*
O – Outcomes: *reduced symptoms of cystitis.*

Where is the evidence base found?

Finding out about best practice requires finding out what has been written about it in the literature. There are many sources of literature including:

- Books
- The internet
- Journals
- Reports
- Bibliographic/electronic databases.

It would be an impossible task to think that a manual search of the thousands of journals available in health and social care alone would provide answers. Electronic databases store the converted journal indexes to help find relevant studies and research papers. Bibliographic databases theme articles into subject categories, where an abstract of the article can be viewed. In Box 2.1 a number of useful databases are provided.

When trying to find evidence, the best source is a systematic review, which will summarise the results from a large quantity of high quality research studies. The Cochrane Library is the first place to check for reviews in health care. The Cochrane Library is not a standard bibliographic database; it is a collection of a number of separate databases and is available as a CD-ROM and can be accessed via the internet. Most HEIs and NHS Trusts have access to the internet version.

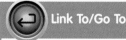 **Link To/Go To**

For information and step-by-step guidance on the use of the Cochrane Library, go to:

www.thecochranelibrary.com/view/0/HowtoUse.html

Box 2.1 Useful Databases for Literature Searching

Internurse
· Internurse is the online archive of peer-reviewed nursing articles from 13 high-quality journals, including the *British Journal of Nursing* and the *Journal of Wound Care*.

CINAHL
· Designed specifically for academic institutions, Academic Search Premier and CINAHL are multidisciplinary full-text databases containing the full text for more than 4600 journals, including nearly 3900 peer-reviewed titles.

Science Direct
· Science Direct contains over 25% of the world's science, technology and medicine, full text and bibliographical information.

Medline (Ovid)
· Medline is a bibliographical database of life sciences and biomedical information. It includes bibliographical information for articles from academic journals covering medicine, nursing, pharmacy, dentistry and health care.

The value of the evidence found

Nursing exists in a complex and constantly evolving healthcare system and not all published evidence is applicable to practice. Sorting through and reviewing the wealth of evidence is complex and requires the process of critical appraisal. Critical appraisal can be used to determine whether the quality of the study is robust enough to make the results useful; what the results of the study are and what they will mean to patients; whether the results are applicable to specific clinical settings.

Evidence can be appraised in a number of ways to take into account some of the following, as suggested by Burns and Grove (2011) and Polit and Beck (2011):

- The report structure – is it logical in its progression?
- The abstract – does it give you an insight into the theme of the study, how it was carried out and the key findings?
- The introduction – does it explain the **how** and **why** aspects of the study?
- The purpose of the research – is this established from the outset, with a rationale that is specific to address the study question?
- The literature review – how up-to-date is the literature that supports the study and is it broad enough to provide a wide review?
- Methodology – does this provide a step-by-step approach to the processes involved in the study?
- The analysis of the data – is a complete discussion of the data provided?
- The discussion – is this critically presented?
- The conclusions and limitations – are the implications for practice identified?
- References and bibliography – do these reflect the literature review and are they relevant to the study?

Change Management

Health care in the UK operates in a continuous cycle of change, most recently demonstrated in the Health and Social Care Act (2012). Nurses have a key role to play in the management of change; they are equipped to ensure that the principles of care in addition to the principles of access, equity and efficiency remain at the heart of any changes to service provision. One of the difficulties faced by

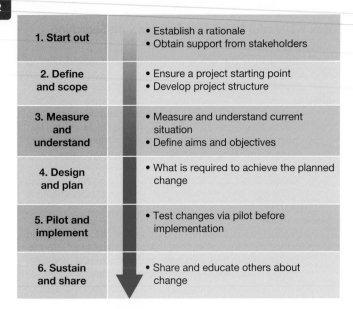

1. Start out	• Establish a rationale • Obtain support from stakeholders
2. Define and scope	• Ensure a project starting point • Develop project structure
3. Measure and understand	• Measure and understand current situation • Define aims and objectives
4. Design and plan	• What is required to achieve the planned change
5. Pilot and implement	• Test changes via pilot before implementation
6. Sustain and share	• Share and educate others about change

Figure 2.7 The six-stage framework for service improvement.
Source: NHS Institute for Innovation and Improvement 2010.

nurses when challenged with change in the workplace is that, like all people, they may be reluctant to modify the way they work. Hewitt-Taylor (2013) cites two aspects of altering practice: change and transition (Austin & Currie 2003; McLean 2011) and concludes that both need to be considered for change to be effectively managed:

Change – things that can be observed to be done differently
Transition – the experience and the way people feel about the importance of change.

It is natural for people to resist change, and this is multiplied in the workplace if the reason for change is not communicated effectively. Good nurse leadership is crucial to implementing change in the clinical setting, and as demonstrated earlier in this chapter, leadership is complex and multifaceted, and not limited to the nurses' grade or position within the team. The NHS Institute for Innovation and Improvement (2010), highlighted in Figure 2.7, provides a six-stage framework to guide staff in the management of change.

The Institute's framework encourages from the outset, the support and encouragement from strategic and operational stakeholders, ideally a senior member of the organisation, the so-called project sponsor, whose area of work or management will be positively affected by the change that you are proposing. Stakeholders may be patients or clients, as these are people who can be directly affected by changes in care, and it is increasingly important to recognise the involvement of such groups as users and carers in the planning and design of projects within the care setting. Often the language that is adopted in the initial planning stages can influence the way that the project is interpreted, and any proposal for change should be communicated in a simple and persuasive manner to engage interest and enable others to see the benefits of change immediately. Often a brief overview or case study can help to illustrate the points raised.

Scoping the project and creating a structure in stage two helps interested parties to understand where the starting point is in the proposed change, and how they will be involved in the delivery of

the change. Involvement of others at this stage can help with the delivery because you have listened to their ideas and hopefully incorporated them into the process, so you might think about the usefulness of focus groups and workshops. Much of this will depend on the size of the project and the numbers of people involved in the process of change; large projects might require a number of ways to engage staff over a longer period of time.

One of the challenges to change management is how to measure the effectiveness of what has been changed. In stage three, it is useful to establish a baseline from which you can demonstrate or quantify the effectiveness of changes made. Gage (2013) advises consideration of measurements which are: well defined; allow comparison; are easy to collect and integrate into daily work patterns; and are specific and sensitive, i.e. measure what you think you are measuring. Quantitative (numerical) data is easier to measure than qualitative (descriptive) data.

SMART is an acronym for Specific, Measurable, Achievable, Realistic and Time-oriented objectives, and stage four of the framework requires clarity in what is expected of the changes to be implemented. An action plan helps to identify who, what and when objectives are to be undertaken. Revisiting and refining action plans keep the momentum going and help those involved structure their progress.

Stage five of the framework involves testing and implementing the change to be made. A variety of tools to support the analysis of the changes made are available. If numerical data has been collected, a statistical tool can be used to demonstrate changes in trends.

Dissemination of the outcomes of the project supports stage six of the framework, which requires project leaders to sustain and share. Outcomes are the differences between 'what we did' and 'what we do now' as a result of the change that has taken place. Opportunities to share the experience and outcome of developments in practice are numerous and in organisations that embrace a culture of improvement, nurses can share developments though meetings, teaching sessions, conference presentations and publications. Initiatives that support the quality and enhancement of care are pivotal to the notion of clinical governance, which is discussed later.

Clinical Governance

Clinical governance is focussed on reducing the risk and improving the quality of care for patients. It is integral to health care, and patient safety is a top priority for all staff. There are other terms that are synonymous with clinical governance, such as:

- Quality assurance
- Clinical audit
- Quality enhancement
- Clinical effectiveness
- Evidence-based practice.

The 21st century NHS aspires to be a service that is responsive to individual and local needs and as such, must decentralise its provision and be devolved. One way of making this move towards devolution is to change the way health services are managed and run. Centralised services fail to provide care that is patient-centred, and do not recognise that patients are individuals with local and individual needs. Care needs to be delivered in a meaningful manner to the people who pay for it – the patients and the public. The current government is putting patients at the heart of the NHS, through an information revolution and greater choice and control;

shared decision-making will become the norm: *no decision about me without me* (DH 2012).

The introduction of clinical governance in the late 1990s was seen as one way of achieving this meaningful approach to health-care provision. In 1997, *The New NHS: Modern and Dependable* (DH 1997) was produced with a plan to modernise healthcare provision. Clinical governance was an integral part of the ten-year plan to improve the quality of care (DH 1999). One key component of this document (a White Paper) was to bring about major improvements in the quality of care delivered to patients from a clinical perspective. For the first time, statutory duties were enforced on NHS providers regarding the quality of care they offer (DH 2000). A formal responsibility for quality has now been placed on every health organisation in the UK through arrangements for clinical governance at local level.

Quality improvement within health and social care remains high on the political agenda, and there have been high profile cases which demonstrate failings in care, such as those at the Mid Staffordshire NHS Foundation Trust (2013), where an inquiry chaired by Sir Robert Francis heard evidence that an inadequately risk-assessed reconfiguration of services resulted in a complete breakdown in fundamental nursing care and the Trust's wider governance. The National Quality Board (2013) defines quality as safe, effective care that provides as positive an experience as possible for patients. Clinical governance is central to quality. There are many different interpretations of what clinical governance means, and it has been described as making each patient's experience the best it can be, enhancing and making quality in health care better, and doing the right thing at the right time to the right person in the right way.

The Evidence Clinical Governance Is:

A framework through which NHS organisations are accountable for continuously improving the quality of their services and safeguarding high standards of care by creating an environment in which excellence in clinical care will flourish.

(Scally & Donaldson 1998)

The overall aim of clinical governance is to continuously improve, strengthen and build on existing systems of quality assurance across a range of services. There are a range of activities that come under the umbrella of clinical governance, including:

- Clinical audit
- Risk management
- Significant event audit
- Evidence-based practice
- Reviewing complaints
- The involvement of users and carers
- Professional development.

In order for clinical governance to be effective, a number of points must be considered: first and foremost, it must focus on the improvement of the quality of patient care, and it applies to all areas where care is delivered. Consideration should be given to the nature of interprofessional working and the partnerships that exist not just between staff, but also between staff and patients. Public and patient involvement is an essential requirement for effective clinical governance; feedback from users of the services can support a culture that acknowledges mistakes, and shares positive feedback. Although it applies to all healthcare staff, nurses have a unique role to play because of their evidence-based professional practice and their prime role in influencing the patient's experience to be the best it can be. Nurses should be focussed on the needs of patients and be able to use the many facets of clinical governance to constantly evaluate and improve patient care.

It is not possible to achieve clinical governance in isolation. Structures need to be in place to support it, as well as ensuring that there are common standards and the common public ethos is ensured. National structures are in place to underpin local clinical governance initiatives, an example in England is the Care Quality Commission. The Care Quality Commission in England has put forward its strategy for 2013–2016, to ensure health and social care services provide people with safe, effective, compassionate, high quality care, and to encourage services to improve. The Care Quality Commission's role is predicted to be to inspect and regulate services in order to apply performance ratings to enhance patient choice (CQC 2013).

Interprofessional Working

The nurse as a professional is continuously working in partnership and collaboration with others to support the RCN (2010) Principle G 'Nurses and nursing staff work closely with their own team and with other professionals, making sure patients' care and treatment is co-ordinated, is of a high standard and has the best possible outcome'. This approach incorporates:

- Working in collaboration with patients and their informal carers
- Collaboration within the nursing team
- Partnership and collaboration with other professionals and inter-professional teams.

Effective interprofessional working can have the potential to improve and develop care, and where teams work well, they learn and support each other in this aim. Similar to clinical governance, the philosophy underpinning interprofessional working puts emphasis on the patient at the centre of care, and acknowledges that patients often move from one professional group to another, depending on need. This is not a new phenomenon, as far back as the 1970s the British Medical Association (BMA 1974) referred to the term 'primary health care team'. Contemporary health care, with the modernisation agenda, puts the enhancement of interprofessional working at the forefront. In the wider context of health care, demographic changes to the UK population mean an older generation of patients bring with them multiple health associated problems. In this scenario, the need for interprofessional collaboration and teamwork becomes more significant. The aim is to provide the patient with a service that is seamless and joined up; there is need for coordination of care between groups, and continuity for the individuals who receive care.

  Link To/Go To

http://www.kingsfund.org.uk/audio-video/joined-care-sams-story

This short video explores how joined-up care can transform the experience of care in a positive way.

'Interprofessional working' does not have a universally recognised definition; the term is often used synonymously with 'integrated care' or 'multidisciplinary teams'. The more recent term 'care coordination' has been defined by the National Coalition on Care Coordination in America.

The Evidence

'Care Coordination' is a person-centred, assessment-based, interdisciplinary approach to integrated health care and social support services in a cost-effective manner, in which an individual's needs and preferences are assessed, a comprehensive care plan is developed, and services are managed and monitored by an evidence-based process which typically involves a designated lead care coordinator.

(National Coalition on Care Coordination 2011)

Other language used to describe interprofessional working includes 'interdisciplinary teams', 'multiagency or interagency working' and 'multiprofessional teams'. The term interprofessional and interagency collaboration (IPIAC) was developed by Whittington *et al.* (2009) to express the importance of collaboration at professional and agency level. Whatever terminology is used, teams who work together to provide effective care are characterised by the following:

- Care is given to a common group of patients
- Teams share common goals or outcomes of care
- Roles are clearly defined and each member understands the role of others in the team
- Information is shared among the team
- Mechanisms exist to review care and to assess and adjust outcomes.

Jot This Down

Which agencies and health professionals are you likely to work with as an interprofessional team member? Make a list of the most common professional groups in health care.

In the 'Jot This Down' exercise above, you will probably have made a list of the most common healthcare groups: physiotherapists, paramedics, GPs, police, pharmacists, to name only a few. Each of the individual groups of health professionals has its own professional culture and unique educational programme to prepare it for practice. Just as nursing has a values system (the 6Cs), so too will the individual professions of medicine and those allied to medicine. To work effectively within teams, nurses have to be aware of the cultures and values of other professionals. This has been highlighted in recent child protection cases, where there has been sharp criticism levelled at the poor use of interagency working and communication.

Nursing Fields Children's Nursing

Every Child Matters (Department for Education and Skills 2003)

Common assessments and information sharing will be a major step forward...professionals will increasingly work alongside each other in the same team...clear lines of professional accountability should ensure that multi-disciplinary teams are able to benefit from a wide range of professionals working together, without losing the advantages of those professionals' individual specialisms.

Working in Collaboration with Patients

The development of the NHS Constitution, was one of several recommendations following Lord Darzi's report (DH 2008). It is the responsibility of all healthcare providers and commissioners of NHS care to take the Constitution into account in decisions affecting care. The constitution is made up of seven key principles that spell out the core values of the NHS. Principles 4 and 5 articulate the patient at the heart of care and joint working across agencies to deliver that care (DH 2013a). A 'seamless service' is the ideal; however, barriers continue to exist to fragment care, as health and social care are in a continuous state of change. In recognition of this, the government has released an initiative to support and encourage integrated care (DH 2013b).

What the Experts Say National Voices: An Individual's Viewpoint on Fragmented Care

"We are sick of falling through gaps. We are tired of organisational barriers and boundaries that delay or prevent our access to care. We do not accept being discharged from a service into a void. We want services to be seamless and care to be continuous.

Integrated Care and Support: Our Shared Vision (DH 2013b, p. 11)

Where seamless care works effectively: a case history

Alf is 86 years old and until recently had a clean bill of health. 'I had just turned 80 and my daughter persuaded me to go and see the doctor because of pain in my knee joints'. Alf's records showed that his last medical intervention was as a young lad; he had appendicitis and was admitted for surgery at the age of 11!

Alf was prescribed non-steroidal anti-inflammatory drugs for his joint pain and referred to the practice nurse for routine health screening. 'That was the turning point for me, until then, I assumed that I was well!', reports Alf. Routine screening revealed that Alf had Type 2 diabetes and an uncommon benign disorder of the liver: Gilbert's syndrome. Over the past 5 years Alf has really got to know the diabetic team that monitors his health, and despite feeling at times that he is on a merry-go-round of appointments, the service provides him with support and advice from the specialist dietician, annual retinal screening from the ophthalmic services, referrals to the podiatry service and meetings with specialist nurses to review his blood glucose levels and adjust his medications accordingly. Six months ago, Alf was admitted to hospital with acute retention of urine caused by enlargement of his prostate. While there, he developed a urinary tract infection and was really disoriented for a number of days. Communication from the primary care setting meant that nursing and medical staff in hospital were able to compare his normal state and to organise intermediate care as a step down from hospital. Here, the liaison District Nurse was able to review his case, discuss the prospect of a trial without catheter (TWOC) with the urologist, and as a result, speed Alf's return home. He was assessed by the occupational therapist who came home with him on discharge to gauge his need for adjustments to his home environment. He is now the proud owner of a perching stool in his kitchen, an adapted chair for his shower, a rail to help him in and out of bed and a walking stick, which he carries to the surgery! His care is now managed between the GP and specialist diabetic care team, and he has a range of drug therapies, which the local pharmacist arranges and delivers in blister packs that are easy to read and help ensure the right dosage of drug is administered at the right time. Most importantly, he feels involved in the decisions about his care and he is able to express his anxieties about his prostate problem. Communication and information about who and when to contact the service for help have supported Alf's transition from semi-dependency within the intermediate care setting, to independency within his own home.

 Link To/Go To

www.nationalvoices.org.uk
Review the narrative for coordinated care, commissioned by the NHS Commissioning Board.

Conclusion

The professional nature of nursing is constantly under scrutiny and, as health professionals, nurses make every effort to inspire confidence in the people for whom they care and other healthcare professionals. Patients expect nurses to provide the best care they can and this expectation is supported through the governing body for nurses, the NMC. In addition, the RCN has put forward its view of what professional nursing should be in its Principles of Practice guide (RCN 2010).

Professional nursing has a long tradition of supporting and developing learners in practice, and as such, students in nursing can expect professional and expert facilitation of learning in practice through the development of positive learning environments and the support of mentors who are specifically trained for the role.

Teaching and learning are important factors in the development of positive learning environments, and an understanding of the theories that underpin the facilitation of knowledge, skills and attitudes has become a feature of the profession. Intertwined with this is the need for the professional nurse to question and challenge practice; this requires skills in the use of evidence-based activities to interpret information and to engage in the process of change. Change to promote quality is supported within the NHS in the form of clinical governance. The Care Quality Commission in England has put forward its strategy for 2013–2016, to ensure health and social care services provide people with safe, effective, compassionate, high quality care, and to encourage services to improve.

Healthcare organisations must promote the development of professionalism with opportunities to develop individual professional identity and to value the professional contribution made by all within health and social care settings. Interprofessional working and learning aims to support the positive experience of patients and clients in health care through collaboration and placing patients at the core of that activity.

Key Points

- Professional nursing practice is not only judged by the recipient of care – the patient – but also by the profession itself. Professionals judge other professionals with regard to the quality and the appropriateness of the care that they provide.

- All registered nurses have a role to play in the development and facilitation of teaching and learning in the clinical learning environment.
- The processes by which learning occurs are complex and over time, psychologists have tried to describe them; however, none of the theories in isolation can provide a full understanding.
- Nurses can apply leadership styles and adapt them to the ever changing situations that they are faced with on a regular basis. An understanding of the theories that underpin leadership can guide nurses in adopting the most effective ways of working in practice.
- Nurses have a key role to play in the management of change; they are equipped to ensure that the principles of care, in addition to the principles of access, equity and efficiency, remain at the heart of any changes to service provision.
- Nurses should be focussed on the needs of patients and be able to use the many facets of clinical governance to constantly evaluate and improve patient care.
- Effective interprofessional working can have the potential to improve and develop care, and where teams work well, they learn and support each other in this aim. Similar to clinical governance, the philosophy underpinning interprofessional working puts emphasis on the patient at the centre of care, and acknowledges that patients often move from one professional group to another, depending on need.

Glossary

Andragogy: focus on adult learning through focus of experience
Behaviourism: a term used to describe a particular approach to teaching, which acknowledges that behaviour can be conditioned
Clinical governance: a systematic approach to maintaining and improving the quality of patient care within a system
Competence: the ability to practise with insight, skill and knowledge, while applying the values of nursing
Conditioned response: famous for his experiments on dogs, Pavlov created a learned response to set conditions
EBP: evidence-based practice
Fitness to Practice: ensures a nursing workforce that is competent
Humanistic learning theory: viewed as an act to fulfil one's potential, can be based on need and motivation to learn
Interprofessional working: working, learning and collaborating with other health and social care professionals with the aim of providing seamless care
Learning environment: in nursing, this usually describes the quality of the environment in which nurses learn, and can be related to any practice placement
Lifelong learning: the notion that, in nursing, there is a continued need to update and learn new and established bodies of knowledge, in order to meet the conditions of professional registration
Mentor: a qualified nurse who has undergone extra education and development in order to teach and assess students in practice
Operant conditioning: describes the work of Skinner who conditioned animals and humans to behave in a certain way for reward

(Continued)

Pedagogy: the art of learning through instruction, associated with the way children learn

PREP: post-registration education and practice

Professional: term used to describe a person belonging to/ qualified in a profession

Reflective practice: reviewing actions with a view to making sense and learning from situations

Sign-off mentor: makes the final end of programme assessment of students in practice having undergone sign-off supervision by an existing sign-off mentor or practice teacher

Standards of Practice: a code which sets the foundation of what is good practice to uphold the safety and well-being of patients

The Code: a set of shared values which guide good practice for nurses and midwives

Transactional leader: also known as managerial leadership, which focusses on the leader as supervisor, organiser and someone interested in group performance

Transformational leaders: are inspirational, and act as role models to their followers

VARK: an inventory which describes and categorises learning styles (**V**isual, **A**ural, **R**ead/Write, **K**inaesthetic)

References

An Bord Altranais (Irish Nursing Board) (2003) *Guidelines on the Key Points That May be Considered When Developing a Quality Clinical Learning Environment*. An Bord Altranais, Dublin.

Austin, J. & Currie, B. (2003) Changing organisations for a knowledge economy: the theory and practice of change management. *Journal of Facilities Management*, 2(3), 229–243.

Avery, G. (2013) *Law and Ethics in Nursing and Healthcare. An Introduction*. Sage, London.

Barton, D. & Le May, A. (2012) *Adult Nursing. Preparing for Practice*. Hodder and Arnold, London.

Bassett, S. & Westmore, K. (2012) How nurse leaders can foster a climate of good governance. *Nursing Management*, 19(5), 22–24.

BMA (1974) *Primary Health Care Teams*. British Medical Association, London.

Boud, D., Keogh, R. & Walker, D. (1985) Promoting reflection in learning: a model. In D. Boud, R. Keogh, & D. Walker (eds), *Reflections: turning experience into learning*. Kogan Page, London.

Burns, N. & Grove, S.K. (2011) *Understanding Nursing Research*, 4th edn. Philadelphia,: Elsevier.

Cheun-Heung, L. & French, P. (1997) Education in the practicum: a study of the ward learning climate in Hong Kong. *Journal of Advanced Nursing*, 26(3), 455–462.

Conway, J. & McMillan, M.A. (2000) Maximising learning opportunities and preparing for professional practice. In: J. Daly *et al.* (eds) *Contexts of Nursing: an introduction*, MacLennan and Petty, Sydney.

CQC (2013) *Raising Standards, Putting People First. Our Strategy 2013–2016*. Care Quality Commission, Newcastle upon Tyne.

DBIS (2013) *Motivation and Barriers to Learning for Young People not in Education, Employment or Training*. Department for Business, Innovation and Skills, London.

Department for Education and Skills (2003) *Every Child Matters*. HMSO, London.

DH (1999) *Clinical Governance: quality in the new NHS*. Department of Health, London.

DH (1997) *The New NHS: modern, dependable*. Department of Health, London.

DH (2000) *The NHS Plan: a plan for investment, a plan for reform*. Department of Health, London.

DH (2008) *High Quality Care for all: NHS next stage review final report*. Department of Health, London.

DH (2012) *Equality Analysis. Government Response to: liberating the NHS - no decision about me, without me*. Department of Health, London.

DH (2013a) *The NHS Constitution: the NHS belongs to us all*. Department of Health, London.

DH (2013b) *Integrated Care and Support: our shared commitment*. Department of Health, London.

Driscoll, J. (2007) Supported reflective learning: the essence of clinical supervision. In: Driscoll, J. (ed.) *Practising Clinical Supervision: a reflective approach for healthcare professionals*, 2nd edn. pp. 27–50. Elsevier, Edinburgh.

Duffy, K. (2003) *Failing Students: a qualitative study of factors that influence the decision regarding assessment of student's competence in practice*. www.hsc.uwe.ac.uk/practicesupport/data/sites/1/failingstudents2.pdf (accessed November 2013).

Edwards, E., Smith, S., Courtney, M., Finlayson, K. & Chapman, H. (2004) The impact of clinical placement location on students' competence and preparedness for practice. *Nurse Education Today*, 24, 248–255.

Ewan, C.E. & White, R. (1996) *Teaching Nursing: a self instructional handbook*, 2nd edn. Chapman & Hall, London.

Fleming, N. & Baume, D. (2006) Learning Styles Again: VARKing up the right tree. *Educational Developments*, 7(4), 4–7.

Fretwell, J. (1983) Creating a ward-learning environment: the sister's role. *Nursing Times Occasional Papers*, 79 (21, 22).

Gage, W. (2013) Using service improvement methodology to change practice. *Nursing Standard*, 27(23), 51–57.

Gibbs, G. (1998) *Learning by Doing: a guide to teaching and learning*. Further Education Unit, London.

Greenwood, J. (1993) The apparent desensitization of student nurses during their professional socialization: a cognitive perspective. *Journal of Advanced Nursing*, 18(9), 1471–1479.

Grohar-Murray, M.E. & DiCroce, H.R. (2003) *Leadership and Management in Nursing*, 3rd edn. Prentice Hall, New Jersey.

Haslem, A., Reicher, S. & Platow, M.J. (2011) *The New Psychology of Leadership. Identity, Influence and Power*. Psychology Press, Hove.

Hewitt-Taylor, J. (2013) Planning successful change incorporating process and people. *Nursing Standard*, 27(38), 35–40.

Honey, P. & Mumford, A. (1992) *The Manual of Learning Styles*, 3rd edn. Peter Honey, Maidenhead.

Hutchings, A. & Sanders, L. (2001) Developing a learning pathway for student nurses. *Nursing Standard*, 15(4), 38–41.

Jackson, D. & Mannix, J. (2001) Clinical nurses as teachers; insights from students of nursing in their first semester of study. *Journal of Clinical Nursing*, 10(2), 270–277.

Johns, C. (ed.) (1994) A philosophical basis for nursing practice. In: *The Burford NDU Model: caring in practice*. Blackwell Scientific Publications, Oxford.

Johns, C. (2000) *Becoming a Reflective Practitioner: a reflective and holistic approach to clinical nursing, practice development and clinical supervision*. Blackwell Scientific Publications, Oxford.

Knowles, M., Horton, E.F. & Swanson, R.A. (2011) *The Adult Learner: the definitive classic in adult education and human resource development*, 11th edn. Butterworth, Oxford.

Kolb, D.A. (1984) *Experiential Learning: experiences as the source of learning and development*. Prentice Hall, Upper Saddle River.

Maslow A. (1954) *Motivation and Personality*. Harper & Row, New York.

McLean, C. (2011) Change and transition: what is the difference? *British Journal of School Nursing*, 6(2), 78–81.

Mid Staffordshire NHS Foundation Trust (2013) Report of the Mid Staffordshire NHS Foundation Trust Public Inquiry. TSO, London.

Moon, J. (2004) *A Handbook of Reflective and Experiential Learning*. Routledge, London.

Muir Gray, J.A. (1997) Evidence-based practice is about 'doing the right things right'. In: *Evidence-based Healthcare: how to make health policy and management decisions*. Churchill Livingstone, Edinburgh.

National Coalition on Care Coordination (2011) *Implementing Care Coordination in the Patient Protection and Affordable Care Act* [online]. *Policy Brief.* www.nyam.org/social-work-leadrship-institute/docs/publications/N3C-Implementing-Care-Coordination.pdf (accessed November 2013).

National Health Service (2011) *Clinical Leadership Competency Framework.* NHS Leadership Academy, London.

National Quality Board (2013) *Quality in the New Health System – maintaining and improving quality from April 2013.* Department of Health, London. http://webarchive.nationalarchives.gov.uk/20130107105354/https://www.wp.dh.gov.uk/publications/files/2012/08/Quality-in-the-new-system-maintaining-and-improving-quality-from-April-2013-FINAL-2.pdf (accessed February 2014).

NHS (2010) *Quality and Service Improvement Tools: project management guide.* Institute for Innovation and Improvement. National Health Service, London.

NMC (2008a) *The Code: Standards of Conduct, Performance and Ethics for Nurses and Midwives.* Nursing and Midwifery Council, London.

NMC (2008b) *The Standards to Support Learning and Assessment in Practice.* Nursing and Midwifery Council, London.

NMC (2010a) *Guidance for Professional Conduct for Nursing and Midwifery Students.* Nursing and Midwifery Council, London.

NMC (2010b) *Standards for Pre-Registration Nursing Education.* Nursing and Midwifery Council, London.

NMC (2010c) *The PREP handbook.* Nursing and Midwifery Council, London.

NMC (2013a). *Quality Assurance Framework for Nursing and Midwifery Education and Local Supervising Authorities for Midwifery.* Nursing and Midwifery Council, London.

NMC (2013b) *Annual Report and Accounts 2012–2013 and Strategic Plan 2013–2016.* Nursing and Midwifery Council, London.

Pembrey, S. (1980) *The Ward Sister – Key to Care.* Royal College of Nursing, London.

Polit, D.F. & Beck, C.T. (2011) Nursing *Research: generating and accessing evidence in nursing practic*e, 9th edn. Philadelphia: Lippincott.

Quinn, F.M. & Hughes, S.J. (2007) *Quinn's Principles and Practice of Nurse Education*, 5th edn. Nelson Thornes, Cheltenham.

RCN (2003) *Defining Nursing.* Royal College of Nursing, London.

RCN (2010) *The Principles of Nursing Practice.* Royal College of Nursing, London. www.rcn.org.uk/nursingprinciples (accessed July 2013).

Rogers, C.R. (1983) *Freedom to Learn.* Merril, Columbus, OH.

Rogers, A. & Horricks, N. (2010) *Teaching Adults*, 4th edn. Open University, Maidenhead.

Sackett, D.L., Richardson, W.S., Rosenburg, W. & Haynes, R.B. (1997) *Evidence-Based Medicine: how to practise and teach EBM*, 2nd edn. Churchill Livingstone, London.

Salvage, J. (2002) *Retinking Professionalism: the first step for patient focussed care.* Institute for Public Policy Research, London.

Scally, G. & Donaldson, L.J. (1998) Clinical governance and the drive for quality improvement in the new NHS in England. *British Medical Journal* 317, 61–65.

Schön, D. (1983) *The Reflective Practitioner: how professionals think in action.* Basic Books, New York.

Schön, D. (1987) *Educating the Reflective Practitioner.* Jossey-Bass, San Francisco, CA.

Whittington, C., Thomas, J. & Quinney, A. (2009) *An Introduction to Interprofessional and Inter-Agency Collaboration.* http://www.scie.org.uk/assests/elearning/ipiac/ipiac01/resource/text/index.htm (accessed November 2013).

Test Yourself

1. The Professional Standards Authority (PSA) is:
   (a) Accountable to the government
   (b) A division of the NMC
   (c) An independent charity
   (d) Responsible to the RCN

2. The 'Code' is:
   (a) A legal document
   (b) A set of professional values
   (c) Applied to all healthcare workers
   (d) Used to protect the nurse

3. The NMC is:
   (a) A voluntary organisation
   (b) Controlled by the Department of Health
   (c) Available to all health workers for the purpose of registration
   (d) An organisation set up by Parliament to ensure that nurse and midwives provide high standards of care

4. Which one of the following is associated with humanistic theories of learning?
   (a) Pavlov
   (b) Skinner
   (c) Gestalt
   (d) PREP

5. A transformational leader is one who:
   (a) Is interested in the personal development of staff
   (b) Always has to be in control
   (c) Is not interested in the personal aspects of staff
   (d) Is disappointed when work is delayed

6. The framework through which NHS organisations are accountable for continuously improving the quality of their services and safeguarding high standards of care is known as:
   (a) Safeguarding
   (b) Clinical governance
   (c) The 'Code'
   (d) Clinical audit

7. EBP is an abbreviation of:
   (a) Everything best for patients
   (b) Evidence-based performance
   (c) Evidence backed by performance
   (d) Evidence-based practice

8. The Cochrane Library is:
   (a) A standard bibliographical database
   (b) A collection of a number of separate databases
   (c) Only available from a library
   (d) A small collection of archived material

9. SMART is an acronym for:
   (a) Specific, Measurable, Achievable, Realistic and Time-oriented objectives
   (b) Specific, Meaningful, Accessible, Realistic and Time-orientated objectives
   (c) Special, Mindful, Achievable, Robust and Teaching-focussed objectives
   (d) Specific, Measurable, Accessible, Reasonable and Time-oriented objectives

10. Interprofessional working is most closely associated with which of the RCN Principles of Nursing Practice (2010)?
    (a) F
    (b) G
    (c) A
    (d) D

Answers

1. a
2. b
3. d
4. c
5. a
6. b
7. d
8. b
9. a
10. b

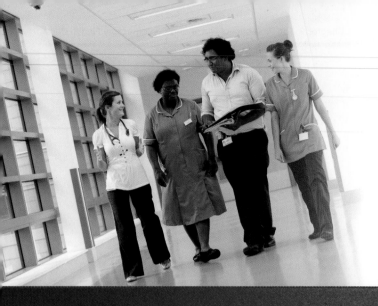

3

Health Promotion

Karen Wild

University of Salford, UK

Learning Outcomes

On completion of this chapter you will be able to:

- Gain an insight into the nurse's role as a health promoter
- Consider how health promotion is applied to nursing practice
- Be introduced to models of health promotion
- Gain an insight into the application of models to promote health in practice
- Be aware of contemporary approaches to health through the lifespan
- Have an insight into travel health promotion

Competencies

All nurses must:

1. Support and promote the health and well-being of people
2. Promote health to empower choices that promote self-care and safety
3. Encourage health-promoting behaviour through education, role modelling and effective communication
4. Secure equal access to health screening, health promotion and health care
5. Ensure people receive all the information they need in a language and manner that allows them to make informed choices and share decision-making
6. Recognise and respond to the major causes and social determinants of health, illness and health inequalities

 Visit the companion website at **www.wileynursingpractice.com** where you can test yourself using flashcards, multiple-choice questions and more.

Nursing Practice: Knowledge and Care, First Edition. Edited by Ian Peate, Karen Wild and Muralitharan Nair.
© 2014 John Wiley & Sons, Ltd. Published 2014 by John Wiley & Sons, Ltd. Companion website: www.wileynursingpractice.com

Introduction

The art of nursing demands that we support the health and well-being of those for whom we care, and the integration of health promotion activities into the everyday aspects of the care that nurses deliver is fundamental to this art. Whether it is a controlled measurement of health status, for example measuring blood pressure, or the more subtle art of listening and responding to a patient's thoughts and feelings, health promotion lies at the heart of nursing. This chapter will help you to develop that art and make links from the theories presented to the practice that you engage in. A key component of the nurse's role is to deliver high quality health care and support to all patients, regardless of the setting in which this takes place.

An important outcome from the Modernising Nursing Careers project (DH 2006b) was in relation to the challenges for nurses in response to the changing demands of society's health needs. It states that future nursing workforces will need to 'be able to use preventive and health promotion interventions' (DH 2006b, p. 10).

Health promotion is the process of enabling people to increase control over, and to improve, their health. It becomes an essential guide for health professionals in addressing the major health challenges faced by developing and developed nations. Health promotion is a process directed towards enabling people to take action, and as such, it is not something that is done on or to people; it is done by, with and for people, either as individuals or as groups. This chapter will explore health promotion from both the individual's perspective and the nurse's role in supporting the people for whom they care, through the processes of health promotion.

Health Promotion

Often confused with the label of 'health education', 'health promotion' involves empowerment of individuals and seeks to alter attitudes so that people might change their health behaviours.

In considering health promotion, nurses need to be able to understand the health education focus which:

- Is directed predominantly at healthy people
- Aims to prevent ill health arising in the first place
- Includes such aspects as:
  - Contraception
  - Nutrition
  - Hygiene
  - Sexual health education.

Health education has a focus mainly on giving information to change people's health behaviour, e.g. propaganda and instruction. It is only one aspect of health promotion, which acknowledges external factors that influence people's lifestyles, e.g. poverty, environment, social isolation.

In contrast to health education, health promotion aims:

- To prevent disease
- To ensure that people are well informed and able to make choices
- To change behaviour
- To help people acquire skills and confidence to take greater control over factors influencing their health
- To change policies and environments to facilitate health choices.

Health promotion began to take hold from a public health perspective in the 19th century, with work very much focussed on addressing poverty and overcrowding. Victorian philanthropists recognised the need to address the burden of industrialisation, where typically poverty was synonymous with overcrowding, open sewers, a lack of sanitation and fresh water, lack of resources for medical care and the occupational hazards of industrial work.

The Evidence

In the new industrial towns, cholera was even more dangerous because many of the houses had been built quickly with no attempts at planning. There was often no sanitation and no fresh water. In one street in Bolton, the people used a trench at the back of the houses as a toilet, which was cleared out and the mess stacked up against the end wall of the last house. The mess was taken away every 6 months.

(Account from the National Archives: **http://nationalarchives.gov.uk** (accessed 8 November 2012)

In 'The Evidence' account, there is proof of epidemic health problems and much of the focus was on public health as a way forward. This aspect of health will be addressed in detail in Chapter 4.

During the First and Second World Wars in 20th century Britain, the propaganda delivered to the public and to armed service members included techniques of 'shock horror' to address such health issues as sexually transmitted infections.

The Central Council for Health Education set up in 1927 shifted emphasis from disease to personal behaviour. The Central Council was principally concerned with propaganda and instruction, and this method of health promotion continued to exist until the Health Education Council was set up in 1968. It focussed mainly on the production of mass publicity campaigns. By the 1970s, health promotion moved responsibility for health from the government towards the individual's lifestyle.

The time line in Figure 3.1 shows the movement of emphasis from health education, through health promotion to the current emphasis on the public health agenda. Within the last few years, there has been a gradual change of healthcare policy within the UK to focus on prevention of illness and disease through the active promotion of health. In his review of the NHS in 2008, Lord Darzi highlighted a healthcare model that views health promotion as a key component of health care (DH 2008a). Historically, the emphasis in nursing was on care of the acutely ill in the hospital setting. With changes in society and radical developments in

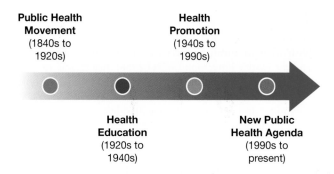

Figure 3.1 Historical journey of health promotion.

health care, this emphasis has shifted towards preventive interventions in health provision, and a greater focus on community-based care. The importance of teaching individuals and groups health-promoting behaviours is an essential component of health and ill-health nursing.

Promoting healthy lifestyles for people in England and Wales is an important governmental responsibility. The Department of Health runs initiatives to help people quit smoking, eat better and exercise more, as well as health screening projects and training and skills programmes. As such, the Department of Health is committed to tackling obesity, sexually transmitted infections, alcohol and substance misuse and smoking.

The government's success in these campaigns may be reflected in the actual picture of, for example, obesity in this country. England has the highest levels of obesity in the European Union (EU), and a direct consequence of this may be related to an increase in UK levels of diabetes. However, premature mortality rates from the two biggest killers (cancer and circulatory disease) are reducing faster in England than the average for the EU (DH 2007). A variety of government initiatives have influenced current health improvement strategies and health promotion activities within the UK over the last decade.

The government's health agenda (Healthy Lives; Healthy People: our strategy for public health in England (DH 2010a), Choosing Health (DH 2004) and Health Challenge England (DH 2006a)) has made the practice of health promotion everybody's business. The health agenda encourages nurses to develop skills that enable the prevention of ill health and to promote positive health. Initially, health promotion focussed upon changing an individual's behaviour; however, it now includes influencing and implementing health policies and promoting community action.

The terms 'health promotion' and 'health education' are inter-linked and are often used inappropriately when discussing prevention of ill health and promoting positive health. Health education represents one aspect of health promotion; it focusses upon the provision of information to enable individuals to change their behaviour and to adopt health-enhancing activities, while health promotion involves empowering individuals to alter their attitudes and change their behaviours in order to adopt health-enhancing activities. Health promotion also acknowledges the external forces that can influence an individual's attitude, behaviour and lifestyle choices, for example poverty and social isolation. *World Class Education and Training, for World Class Healthcare* (PHE 2012) introduces the Health Education England proposal, which aspires to excellence in shaping the public health workforce in the UK.

Defining Health

In any discussion around health promotion, there is a need to establish what we mean by the term 'health'. In the first *Ottawa Charter for Health Promotion* (WHO 1986), health was seen as a resource for everyday life, and not, as some might think, the objective of living. As such, health is seen as a positive concept, not merely limited to one's physical capacities, but intrinsically linked to, for example, where a person might live and to aspects of their social networks. In supporting health, nurses must understand the variety of dimensions and factors that will impact upon an individual's health status, and the ability of individuals to make choices with regard to their future health.

Jot This Down

- Take some time to think about what health means to you
- Now think about an older, more dependent person who you know, and consider what health might mean to them.

  Are there differences in the types of perception that you have for the two exercises?

Health is a subjective concept, and you will find from completing the 'Jot This Down' exercise above, that health can be seen in the light of one's experiences, self-esteem, social status and level of individual control. An older, more dependent individual may view health differently from a younger independent individual, based on, for example, their level of physical need.

Health is commonly defined in terms of measurable parameters. The World Health Organization (WHO) stated that 'health is a state of complete physical, mental and social well-being and not merely the absence of disease or infirmity' (WHO 1946). More recent definitions include the aspects of emotional, sexual, societal and spiritual health. Table 3.1 makes reference to the domains of health (Naidoo & Wills 2009).

What follows is an example of how the domains of health can be linked to an individual's health within the child and family field of nursing.

Nursing Fields Child and Family

Molly is 15 and is diagnosed with anorexia nervosa. When we look at the domains of her health, we can see:

Physically – she is underweight with a BMI of 12.4; her skin is dry and prone to cracking with sores that do not easily heal. Her hair is thinning and she is small for her age. She often purges herself following eating, making herself vomit and, as a result, her dental health is in decline.

Emotionally – Molly has an obsession with her calorie intake and efforts from her parents to try to introduce 'normal foods' result in Molly becoming upset, throwing things around and shutting herself away in her room for hours.

Mentally – Molly is intensely obsessed with her GCSE studies and any small criticism of her coursework makes her withdraw to her room after school. Her self-esteem is negatively reinforced and this becomes a reason not to eat. She secretly feels a sense of satisfaction and achievement if she does not eat, and believes that dieting is something that she does really well.

Socially – she withdraws from social activities, has few friends and resists any attempts to be involved with her peers.

Societally – Molly expresses a desire to belong, but cannot accept herself as being acceptable socially because of her self-perception, based on her weight. She expresses her feelings by saying that 'I feel out of step with the others at school'.

Spiritually – her beliefs are strongly influenced by pro-anorexia messages available online.

Sexually – she is not interested in developing a sexual relationship and shies away from any physical loving contact. Molly does not menstruate.

Table 3.1 Domains of Health (adapted from Naidoo & Wills 2009).

Physical	How your body functions; this can often be in terms of measuring physical parameters, e.g. blood pressure monitoring, body mass index (BMI) measurement, developmental assessment of motor development in children
Emotional	Recognition and appropriate expression of feelings, plus the ability to cope with stress
Mental	Clear and coherent thinking; here cognitive abilities can be measured, for example in children's developmental assessment, and in the elderly who may be suffering dementia
Social	The ability to make and maintain relationships with others
Societal	Being valued within society, regardless of religion, race, age, gender, etc.
Spiritual	Being at peace with oneself through a system of beliefs
Sexual	The acceptance and ability to achieve a satisfactory expression of one's sexuality

Factors Affecting Health

Many different factors affect a person's health or level of wellness. These factors often interact to promote health or to become risk factors for alterations in health. Factors that can contribute to health are numerous, here are just a few:

- Age
- Gender
- Education
- Religion
- Culture
- Social circumstances
- Lifestyles (partly determined by income)
- Social inequalities (can affect choices).

Other influences:

- Media
- Peers
- Own experience
- Knowledgeable others
- Significant happenings in our own or others' health careers.

Factors that can affect health can be demonstrated by considering the broader determinants of health, as seen in Figure 3.2.

Factors that affect health can be broadly divided into two areas:

1. Intrinsic or non-modifiable factors
2. Extrinsic or modifiable factors.

Jot This Down

Think of two individuals whom you have cared for recently in the clinical setting. Jot down a list of intrinsic (non-modifiable) and extrinsic (modifiable) factors that you think have influenced their health status.

You may have considered how each person's genetic make-up influences health status throughout life. Figure 3.2 has this kind of intrinsic factor at the centre. Genetic make-up affects personality, temperament, body structure, intellectual potential and susceptibility to the development of hereditary alterations in health, and in

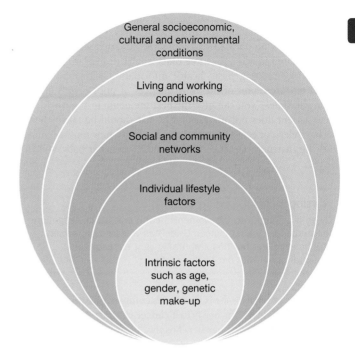

Figure 3.2 Determinants that influence health. *Source:* Adapted from Dahlgren & Whitehead 1991.

the main, these kinds of intrinsic influences are non-modifiable. Examples of chronic illnesses that are associated with genetic make-up include sickle cell disease, haemophilia, diabetes mellitus and cancer.

Other intrinsic factors might include age, gender and developmental factors. Cardiovascular disorders are relatively uncommon in young adults, but the incidence increases after the age of 40. Myocardial infarctions (MIs) are more common in men than women until women are past the menopause. Some diseases occur only in one gender or the other (e.g. prostate cancer in men and cervical cancer in women). The older adult often has an increased incidence of chronic illness and increased potential for serious illness or death from infectious illnesses, such as influenza and pneumonia.

Although cognitive abilities (our ability to understand, reason and perceive information) are determined prior to adulthood, the level of cognitive development affects whether people view themselves as healthy or ill; cognitive levels may also affect health practices. Injuries to and illnesses affecting the brain may alter cognitive abilities, an example of this might be the inability to sense hot or cold, leading to burn injuries. Educational levels affect the ability to understand and follow guidelines for health. For example, if an individual is functionally illiterate (cannot read or write), written information about healthy behaviours and health resources can be of little use.

The Evidence Health Literacy

The ability to read and understand health information has been characterised over the last 20–30 years as 'health literacy'. However, recent thinking has linked health literacy to other negative health behaviours, such as restricted access to health care and barriers to patient understanding and involvement.

(Raynor 2012)

54

In 'The Evidence' box above, poor literacy skills are seen to become a factor that can influence health. The evidence links poor literacy skills with poorer health outcomes and increased mortality. It is estimated that one in three older adults in England has difficulty understanding basic health information. Trueland (2012) quotes two examples of the consequences of poor health literacy when she states, 'you can give the best medicine in the world, but if the patient does not understand how it should be taken then it can be useless, or even dangerous. Similarly, if a new mother cannot read the instructions on mixing formula, then her baby will not thrive'.

Nursing Fields Learning Disabilities

Gwen is admitted to the women's health unit for investigations for suspected breast cancer. Gwen has a learning disability and has brought her hospital 'traffic light assessment' (hospital book) with her to the ward.

In Gwen's scenario, she is faced with complex investigations and a treatment regimen for her breast cancer. As part of the learning disability toolkit, Gwen has her 'hospital book' with her.

Jot This Down Nursing Practice and Decision-Making/Communication and Interpersonal Skills

What elements of Gwen's life do you think will be highlighted in the traffic light assessment booklet?

· **Red** signals issues that staff must know
· **Amber** signals things that are important to Gwen
· **Green** signals Gwen's likes and dislikes

Why might this be important in your role as a promoter of health?

In the above 'Jot This Down' exercise, you may have highlighted aspects in the amber signal that can help you to support Gwen's understanding of her treatment and care while she is being investigated and treated. There will be information about how to communicate with her and importantly, how to help her understand things.

What the Experts Say

Even the smallest thing can have an impact on the experience of my daughter while in hospital, for example she won't eat if she doesn't have her "special" adapted knife and fork. The traffic light assessment document is really helpful to give the nurses and staff a real insight into her daily activities, and to prevent any upset or further complications in her health and well-being.

(Ruth, a carer for her grown-up daughter with learning difficulties.)

Certain diseases occur at a higher rate of incidence in some races and ethnic groups than in others. For example, in the UK, cancer of the prostate is more prevalent in older men and those from the Afro-Caribbean communities. This is an example of an intrinsic factor that may not be modified.

The components of a person's lifestyle that affect health status include: patterns of eating, use of chemical substances (alcohol, nicotine, caffeine, legal and illegal drugs), exercise and rest patterns

and coping methods. Examples of altered responses are: the relationship of obesity to hypertension; cigarette smoking to chronic obstructive pulmonary disease; a sedentary lifestyle to heart disease; and a high-stress career to alcoholism. The environment has a major influence on health. Occupational exposure to toxic substances (such as asbestos and coal dust) increases the risk of pulmonary disorders. Air, water and food pollution increase the risk of respiratory disorders, infectious diseases and cancer. Environmental temperature variations can result in hypothermia or hyperthermia, especially in the older adult.

Socioeconomic background

Both lifestyle and environmental influences are affected by a person's level of income. Poverty, which crosses all racial and ethnic boundaries, negatively influences health status, and living at or below the poverty level often results in crowded, unsanitary living conditions or homelessness. Housing can be overcrowded and have poor heating or cooling. Crowded living conditions increase the risk of transferring communicable diseases. Other problems include lack of infant and child care, lack of medical care for injuries or illness, inadequate nutrition, use of addictive substances and violence.

 Link To/Go To

http://www.bristol.ac.uk/poverty/downloads/keyofficialdocuments/Tackling%20Health%20Inequalities.2007status.pdf

Tackling Health Inequalities: 2007 Status Report on the Programme for Action (DH 2007)

This report highlights the challenging nature of the health inequalities public service agreement target for 2010.

The social influences on health are well established:

· Ill health is not just a matter of chance or bad luck
· The existence of social inequalities in health is generally accepted
· Income is a key factor affecting health
· Employment is a key factor affecting health
· A social network can protect people against stress.

The Evidence

The geographic area in which one lives influences health status.

Among the population of working age within the UK in 2005:

· In Wokingham, Windsor and Maidenhead, one half of the population were in higher managerial and professional occupations, whereas in Blaenau Gwent, half of the population were in routine and manual occupations.

(Hall 2009; *Source*: Labour Force Survey, Office for National Statistics)

This is further illustrated by the gap between the best and the worst areas for life expectancy.

Life expectancy – Females
· Living in Kensington and Chelsea = 87.2 years
· Living in Liverpool = 78.3 years

Life expectancy – Males
· Living in Kensington and Chelsea = 83.1 years
· Living in Manchester = 73 years

(DH 2007)

Health beliefs and individual behaviour

Nurses and people working within health care should have an understanding of how a person's behaviour and attitude can directly influence the choices made about health, and it becomes important to understand why some individuals opt for more healthy behaviours than others. For example, if a person believes that exercise is good for them, then we may suppose it follows that a person will increase their physical activity. However, individual behaviour is complex and is driven by a mix of social and psychological factors. Our understanding of health changes continuously, with a huge flood of mixed information that is presented to us, which can affect our beliefs and behaviours through time. Once considered 'fattening', potatoes are now considered a healthy option; red wine can have health-related properties; in the 1940s, smoking was thought to be good for us and, as a result, was actively promoted.

Jot This Down

What behaviours in life do we consider to be unhealthy in contemporary society?

Health behaviour is mediated by the circumstances and environments in which individuals live: in their community, work, school or other settings. Lifestyle choices are not made in isolation; other factors may limit either the availability of healthy options in the first place or the skills of individuals to make and carry out healthy choices. In the 'Jot This Down' exercise above, you may have considered behaviours, such as smoking, alcohol consumption, poor diet and 'at risk' sexual behaviour, as highly significant unhealthy behaviours.

It is has been suggested that 50% of all deaths from the leading causes results from individual behaviour (Ogden 2001). The Health Survey for England (DH 2010b) states that between the 16-year period of 1993–2009, there has been a marked increase in the proportion of people who fall into the category of obesity. The proportion of obese men increased from 13% to 22% of the population. For women, the proportion increased from 16% to 24% (DH 2010b).

Jot This Down

You have seen the data showing a rise in obesity. Think about the health behaviour that might account for this trend in the figures over the 16-year period. How might people's beliefs about health and their subsequent behaviour have had an impact?

You may have thought about a variety of reasons why obesity levels are increasing in this country; many will be around our social habits, economics, inequality of choice of diet, and perhaps, the move towards a culture of eating convenience and fast foods.

Our beliefs about health can thus influence the way we react to health care and the way we adopt lifestyle behaviours. For example, a strong belief in the risk of certain behaviours might in turn alter our actions in relation to them. In a survey conducted by the Food Standards Agency in February 2007, 88% of people in the UK said that they believe that parents should be strict with children and make them eat healthily. In the same study, 89% of people claim that healthy eating is important to them (*Consumer Attitudes to Food Standards*, FSA 2007). If this is true, then it begs the question why obesity levels continue to rise. It is important to understand that beliefs about health-related behaviours do not always mean positive actions from individuals.

What the Experts Say

My mum always said not to sit on public toilets 'coz you can get infections like AIDS from them. It wasn't until the school nurse gave a talk about Sexually Transmitted Infections, that I realised my mum was old fashioned about things like that!

(Jenna, aged 14)

Individual beliefs about health and illness are a significant factor in the way our patients and clients behave in relation to their health status. Beliefs imply that there are certain assumptions that we trust to be true or accept as truth. A belief can be thought of as a 'convinced opinion'. Placebo effects (the positive response to medication simply because the recipient believes it will work) can arise not only from a conscious belief in a drug, but also from subconscious associations between recovery and the past experience of being treated. Such subconscious thoughts can control our bodily processes without us being aware, such as immune responses and the release of hormones to make us feel better.

Smoking-related behaviour and attitudes surveyed by the Office for National Statistics (ONS) were described in the *Opinions Survey Report No. 40: Smoking-related Behaviour and Attitudes 2008/09* (ONS 2009). The survey was carried out on behalf of the Department of Health and the NHS Information Centre for Health and Social Care. The survey monitors changes in the general attitude towards smoking and towards smoking in public places, as well as smoking behaviour and habits, and stopping smoking. Key findings from the report show that 67% of smokers said they would like to give up, which was significantly lower than in 2007 (74%). It also demonstrated that the proportion of those polled who supported the smoking ban in restaurants was 93%, compared with 75% who agreed with the ban in pubs. This suggests that the attitude of drinkers is proportionately different from the attitudes of those enjoying a restaurant environment, when it comes to smoking in public.

In western medicine, there has been a tendency to view health and illness in a very structured way. The body may be treated almost as a machine, with a clear distinction made between the physical aspects of health and illness, and psychological ill health. Illness and disease are treated by experts with elite scientific knowledge, and a person's health behaviour can be influenced by this quick, cure all approach. The expectation might be that an individual can get health problems sorted quickly and effectively by the NHS, with the belief that the doctor will have a prescription at the ready. The broad perception that illness and disease cause the body to malfunction or be invaded by pathogens, e.g. bacteria, can lead individuals to expect a cure, e.g. antibiotic therapy to clear infections.

However, cultural influences may affect the way people behave in relation to their health, as demonstrated in Figure 3.3. An example might be that illness is perceived as the 'will of God', or viewed as a punishment for past misdemeanours.

Individuals, therefore, might want the focus of health provision to be based on activities, e.g.:

- Prayer
- Waiting

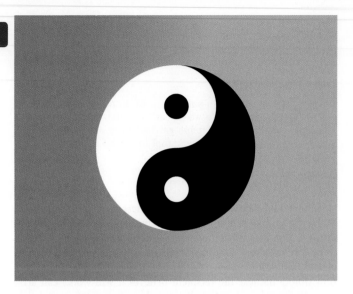

Figure 3.3 Health may be viewed in relation to balance of the 'humours' as in Yin and Yang.

- Fatalism
- Complementary therapies
- Making offerings in worship
- Eating special foods or taking special potions.

Jot This Down
Think of when you were a child and you were ill.
What sort of things did your family do to comfort you?
• Any special foods?
• Drinks?
• Activities?

Some behaviour may be determined by our traditions and values about health and illness, as in the 'What the Experts Say' account.

What the Experts Say

When I was a little girl and had to stay off school (say I had a throat infection), mum used to make a special bed for me on the couch in front of the telly; I would always be given hot blackcurrant drinks. Grandma used to bring me stewed apples which I hated but had to eat to make me better! Mum always said, 'we can go to the doctors for medicine (antibiotics) and it will be gone in a week; or we can leave well alone and it will disappear in 7 days'! She was right, and when my son was a child, I would do the same for him ..., but not the stewed apples!

(Linda, aged 53)

In the 'What the Experts Say' box above, Linda is describing illness behaviour and attitudes towards the treatment of illness, based on family traditions. Interestingly, Linda's mother's perception about the body's ability to fight minor infection is true, and when Linda was a child in the 1960s, the tradition was

to treat the most minor infections with antibiotics. Contemporary treatment has recognised the problems with this kind of approach, and now shies away from the over prescribing of antibiotic therapy (McNulty & Francis 2010).

Illness beliefs can have a framework which individuals use to understand their illness. In Linda's story five cognitive dimensions, as described by Leventhal *et al.* (1980), can be identified:

1. *Identity* – the label or medical diagnosis: 'I have a throat infection'
2. *The perceived cause of the illness* – may be biological or psychosocial: 'my throat infection was caused by a virus' or 'my throat infection was caused because I am run down, and haven't been eating well'
3. *Time line* – beliefs about how long the illness will last: 'my throat infection will be gone in a week'
4. *Consequences* – how the illness might impact upon the person's life, socially and emotionally: 'my throat infection means that I am off school'; 'I will miss the contact with my friends'
5. *Curability and controllability* – how an individual believes their illness can be controlled and cured: 'my throat infection will run its course naturally' or ' with medication, my throat infection will be cured'.

It is important for nurses to understand that:

- Many major causes of ill health are preventable and are the result of people's lifestyles
- The individual has some responsibility for their health
- Healthy behaviour is not evenly distributed across the population
- Lifestyles are partly determined by income
- People's behaviour can be a response to social circumstances
- There is a danger of 'victim blaming'.

The Evidence Type 1 and 2 Diabetes and Religious Fasting at Ramadan

'Ramadan' is a significant religious event, which requires all Muslims from puberty onwards to observe a complete fast (no food, drink, oral medications) between the hours of dawn and sunset. Food and drink is allowed between sunset and dawn and most will consume two meals a day: one at sunset and one before dawn.

Muslims with diabetes are exempt from fasting, but the underpinning belief of fasting is that it teaches self-control and discipline, and is a way to seek closeness to Allah. In a study of Ramadan practices in 13 countries, almost half (42.8%) of those suffering type 1 diabetes and more than three-quarters (78.7%) of those suffering type 2 diabetes fasted for at least 15 days during Ramadan. The evidence demonstrated that severe hypoglycaemic episodes were significantly more frequent during Ramadan compared with other months of the year.

(Sati *et al.* 2004)

As nurses, we need to be aware of the views and attitudes of those in our care, no matter how bizarre or odd they appear to others. Individual beliefs (as in the example given in 'The Evidence' box, above) need to be understood if nurses are to engage in supporting, caring and nurturing health and healthy choices in our patients and clients. The following section looks in more detail at how this can be developed.

Interpersonal Skills for Nursing and Health Promotion

Health promotion has been described as 'the process of enabling people to increase control over, and to improve their health' (WHO 1986), which implies a level of interpersonal involvement between the individual and someone in a position to enable change. Helping people to make healthy choices and lifestyle changes can be difficult. The motivation for change should ideally come from the individual, and telling people to do things rarely works. Nurses need to collaborate with patients to help and support their health strategies to enable changes to lifestyles.

Health teaching relies on the effective use of interpersonal skills in nursing care, and the quality of information that patients receive can influence the experience of care (DH 2003). To underpin good patient communication, five basic principles should be followed:

1. *Improve health*
2. *Provide the best care*
3. *Act professionally*
4. *Work efficiently*
5. *Treat everybody equally.*

(DH 2003)

Motivational Interviewing and Brief Interventions

Opportunities of raising awareness and addressing lifestyle issues with patients occur in nursing practice situations all of the time. The use of a brief, evidence-based intervention has been a theme in mental health nursing for some time and is widely accepted as a method of motivating individuals to think about their health behaviour. In the 'The Evidence' box below, you will see the FRAMES acronym as described by Miller and Spilker (2003), which serves as a useful reminder of the key components of a brief interview.

The Evidence FRAMES Acronym

· **F**eedback – should incorporate positive and negative consequences of behaviour
· **R**esponsibility – emphasis on the personal responsibility the individual has for any change in behaviour
· **A**dvice – helpful guidance to support the individual in the change process
· **M**enu – provide alternatives or options to support the change
· **E**mpathic interviewing – be supportive and respectful, listen without judging or confronting
· **S**elf-efficacy – help to build confidence and motivation, a positive approach to enhance the individual's belief in their ability to change

(Miller & Spilker 2003)

When discussing health-related behaviours, emphasis should be placed on the style of communication that is used, for example the attitude and approach that is taken when engaging with patients.

Jot This Down Communication and Interpersonal Skills

You are supporting a person in practice who has had a number of transient ischaemic attacks. What is evident to you is that the person visibly displays a number of the key modifiable risk factors that are linked to the possibility of a stroke (CVA), i.e. smoking, obesity and lack of exercise. Write down the approach that you might take in relation to the way you discuss the individual's lifestyle issues.

Communication about lifestyle change requires a different approach than, for example, communication around medications or explaining a test that is to be taken. In the above Jot This Down exercise, you may have thought about how you could best develop your relationship to address the individual's behaviour. Rollnick *et al.* (2008) described three communication styles used by health practitioners to support behaviour change in patients:

• Following
• Directing
• Guiding.

They suggest that guiding is the best form of communication to support behaviour change in patients. In order to guide effectively, the nurse must have an understanding of the behaviour from the patient's perspective. By active listening, reflecting and summarising, the nurse can clarify an individual's strengths and weaknesses and support their decisions and motivation for change.

It is important to raise issues in non-confrontational ways, and nurses need to take the right approach to discussing lifestyle issues with individuals. Focussing on the individual's 'problems' from the outset might create a negative response, and make the patient deny or be defensive about their health-related issues.

In the Jot This Down exercise above, you may have also considered your non-verbal skills that can facilitate good communication in this scenario, for example how attentive is your posture: Do you lean forward and nod approval? Do you smile and use appropriate eye contact? Can you remain silent and listen?

The Evidence

As professionals, we can often assume an approach which is authoritarian, paternalistic, confrontational, forceful or guilt inducing. There is evidence that such attitudes will not only limit progress, but actually are correlated with negative behavioural and clinical outcomes.

(Dennison & Hughes 2011)

Health promotion in the care setting will inevitably take account of lifestyle assessment, health teaching, effective communication, information giving and providing opportunistic health promotion strategies in everyday clinical practice.

As practitioners you may be engaged in:

• Advice and information giving
• Education and training
• Policy work and lobbying
• Community development
• Interagency collaboration
• Research profiling and monitoring
• Media development and campaigns.

Table 3.2 *Ottawa Charter for Health Promotion – terminology.*

Advocate	Acknowledges that the domains of health can be both supportive and harmful to individuals. Advocacy through health promotion aims to make conditions for health favourable. Here nurses can actively represent the interests of disadvantaged groups, or speak on the behalf of individuals (see 'What the Experts Say – Advocacy')
Enable	Focusses on equality of opportunity and resources. Examples of this might include supporting access to information, enhancing life skills to support people's choices, allowing equality in the control of factors that influence health. The role of the health promoter is to act as a catalyst and then to step back, enabling groups or individuals to take over
Mediate	Coordinated action to support health by the government, media, social and health services. Health strategies to meet the needs of the local community, adapting to special circumstances and cultural needs. Here, health promoters mediate by providing a sound evidence base or advice to local groups, by influencing policy, campaigning, participating in working groups

Understanding the approaches to health promotion is a key element of developing the skills needed to guide and support individuals to develop and maintain healthy lifestyles. Table 3.2 highlights the terminology that was introduced by the 1986 Ottawa Charter to describe health promotion activities (WHO 1986).

What the Experts Say Advocacy

> I couldn't get my point across to the doctor, I felt embarrassed to talk about something so personal and private. The nurse really helped me get my message across and also made me less embarrassed to talk about my problems. Having somebody with me to speak for me made a huge difference.

(Service user. Women's Health Care)

The Code (NMC 2008) highlights the nurse's role in advocacy to help individuals access relevant health care, information and support.

Models of Health Promotion

There are a variety of theories that guide health promotion interventions, and most theories are based in the social sciences, which include sociology, education, psychology and social policy studies. As such, different approaches to health promotion tap into different theoretical perspectives and academic disciplines. Nurses need to have an understanding of the theories that underpin health promotion activities. Theory becomes an important focus to help nurses select the most effective and acceptable strategies for promoting health. It helps nurses achieve transparency and accountability in approaches to health promotion and makes explicit the choices and strategies selected.

The Evidence Nurses' Perception, Understanding and Experiences of Health Promotion

This study highlighted that nurses were limited in their understanding of health promotion.

- Health promotion is considered the remit of every nurse
- Nurses should engage in health promoting practice
- Nurses need to understand the term 'health promotion' clearly
- Nurses should be less prescriptive (e.g. health education approach)
- More empowerment of patients.

The study demonstrated that health promotion activity was infrequent, being addressed only if the nurse had time.

(Casey 2007)

There are a variety of established approaches to promoting health, which have been described by Ewles and Simnett (2003) and Scriven (2010), including:

Medical approach – relies on patients and clients adhering to regimes of preventive behaviour, early detection of disease through screening and adherence to treatment. There is an emphasis on the medical review of a person's health through primary, secondary and tertiary prevention.

Behavioural change approach – is based on the notion of encouragement, with the health promoter providing healthy lifestyle choices. There are many different models of how to achieve behavioural change, including using media coverage, as described in the 'The Evidence' box (Change4life, DH 2008b). Use of role models, information and supportive environments can influence behaviour. This is a popular approach because it focusses on individuals and retains a role for the professional who gives the information and advice.

The Evidence

The 'Change4life' campaign focusses on promoting healthy behaviours in a 'Swap it – don't stop it' message aimed at overweight adults. The idea behind the message is not to give up the things you enjoy eating, but to consider a healthier option. There is a direct link between health promotion and preventive health care, where adults are supported because of their associated risk factors for ill health.

http://www.dh.gov.uk/health/2011/10/c4l-strategy (accessed November 2012).

Educational approach – this approach is respectful of the individual's right to an informed choice. The health promoter provides information and supports choices based on the individual's beliefs and attitudes.

Empowerment approach – this is a patient-centred approach, and the health promoter acts as a facilitator to help the individual gain knowledge and skills for healthy living. This approach is seen as ethically sound because it supports autonomy.

Social change approach – is focussed on society and the creation of a culture of care, through social and political action, and service provision that supports the rights of individuals to health.

Jot This Down

The UK has a diverse cultural and ethnic population. Try to identify the health picture and ethnic mix in the area in which you work, and then analyse the social and healthcare provision to meet the needs of individuals within these groups. Information can be gained from a variety of resources, including the annual statistical analysis from Directors of Public Health within your local area.

The Code (NMC 2008) requires nurses to consider all aspects of the above in the care they give. Aspects of the Code make this explicit:

- *You must act as an advocate for those in your care, helping them to access relevant health and social care, information and support*
- *You must support people in caring for themselves to improve and maintain their health*
- *You must share with people, in a way they can understand, the information they want or need to know about their health*
- *Work with others to protect and promote the health and well-being of those in your care, their families and carers, and the wider community.*

(NMC 2008, pp. 1–8)

Frameworks for Supporting Health

As seen earlier, a variety of approaches to health promotion exist, often drawing emphasis from each other. In the section that follows, you will be able to explore the ways in which education, behaviour change, social change and empowerment are used as a framework for supporting health.

In Figure 3.4, the model of health promotion as proposed by Tannahill visualises the overlapping spheres to illustrate the variety of approaches to promoting health. In this model:

Health education is a strategy used to provide positive information with regard to healthy lifestyles. Its focus is to empower individuals to make healthy choices by raising awareness of health issues and providing information to support those choices. Examples in practice might be health education in schools, the use of health promotion literature to support lifestyle choices or media

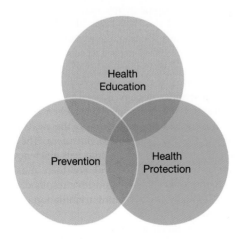

Figure 3.4 Tannahill's model of health promotion (cited in Downie *et al.* 1996).

campaigns to raise awareness about health issues. It is only one aspect of health promotion, and acknowledges that there are external forces that influence an individual's lifestyle, such as the environment, social status, poverty and social isolation.

Health protection aims to support the health of individuals or groups through policy and legislation. This can be interpreted through the number of health-related policies that are familiar to nurses in practice. Health and Safety regulations are a good example of this, as are COSHH guidelines aimed at the control of substances in the workplace that are harmful to health.

Health education and health protection overlap in Figure 3.4, and this demonstrates the relationship between the two approaches within the model. Education for health can be aimed at positive health protection and recent examples of this include lobbying for a ban on tobacco that is visibly on sale in shops and supermarkets in the UK.

Examples of policies and legal aspects of health may include, for example:

- The Clean Air Act
- Health and safety legislation
- Road safety
- Environmental issues
- Sale of alcohol restrictions.

Prevention centres on the services and provision of health care, based on the established understanding of the major illnesses that are present in the UK. The focus of prevention is broken down into three stages:

Primary prevention – when all the activities are geared towards preventing the onset of disease. Health education plays a significant role in informing the public about healthy lifestyles. For example, healthy eating can have a significant impact on the outcome of long-term health. Primary prevention aims to empower people to make healthy dietary choices and thus prevent the onset of illnesses, such as diabetes and heart disease. Immunisation is another example of primary prevention to reduce the incidence of morbidity from common infections, such as measles.

Nursing Fields Child and Family: Nursing Practice and Decision-Making, Communication and Interpersonal Skills

Primary prevention

Immunisation session in a secondary school for girls aged 14 against the Human Papilloma Virus (HPV)

The School Health Advisor (school nurse) sees each girl individually and there is an opportunity to give opportunistic health information; she connects with the girls at their level, explaining the terminology, and using a diagram to support the understanding of how HPV can affect the cervix in the long term.

The health promotion role of the nurse here includes:

- Primary prevention in the form of the provision of immunisation
- The opportunity to discuss health issues, such as healthy eating
- Acting as a source of information
- Listening and talking (generally finding out how well the girls are)
- Picking up on cues related to ill health or risky health behaviour

60

Secondary prevention – the strategies here are to identify individuals or groups at risk of disease with an aim of detecting and curing illnesses before they cause irreversible ill health. Examples commonly include screening those who are identified at risk through national screening programmes. Cervical screening is aimed at all sexually active women to detect the early stages of cell changes and cervical cancers.

Nursing Fields Adult Health: Nursing Practice and Decision-Making, Communication and Interpersonal Skills

Secondary prevention

Patient on a surgical ward

The nurse is engaged in assessing the patient who is 'at risk' and is involved in supporting the patient to prevent the risk of deep vein thrombosis (DVT) postoperatively. Risk factors for developing DVT include decreased mobility following surgery, a history of circulatory problems, especially to the peripheries, abdominal, pelvic or cardiovascular surgery.

The health promotion role of the nurse here includes:

- Teaching the person to perform leg exercises to shorten or reduce the impact of disease
- Adhering to local policy in applying anti-embolic stockings
- Building up coping skills in the patient, for example how to recognise early signs of DVT
- Acting as a source of information

Tertiary prevention – aims to minimise or reduce the progression of an already established disease. The focus here is to enable quality of life within the constraints of illness and disease. A good example of this is end of life care (see Chapter 20).

Nursing Fields Mental Health: Nursing Practice and Decision-Making, Communication and Interpersonal Skills

Tertiary prevention

People with established mental health problems may neglect their health; they may not notice symptoms of physical disease and may be reluctant to seek help. The unwanted side-effects of medication can also affect the person's health, for example weight gain.

Nurses can support tertiary prevention by understanding the links between psychological health and physical health.

The health promotion role of the nurse here includes:

- Monitoring the persons health, e.g. nutritional assessment, BMI measurement, and exploring the use of coping strategies to maintain health
- Encouraging the person not to ignore physical symptoms, and to seek support and diagnosis
- Carefully monitoring of the side-effects of medications
- Exploring lifestyle issues, such as alcohol use, smoking, exercise, etc.

Prevention and health protection are seen in Figure 3.4 to overlap. Both areas on the model can work together to support public health; an example of this is fluoridation of water in certain areas of the UK with higher than average dental decay.

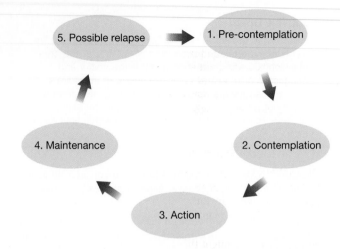

Figure 3.5 Prochaska and DiClemente's transtheoretical (stages of change) approach.

Behaviour Change

Models of behaviour change are a popular choice for nurses engaging in health promotion interventions. This approach is supported by literature that suggests inspiring confidence and motivation in individuals supports behaviour change (Dixon 2008).

The transtheoretical approach to promoting health was developed through observation of individual responses on healthy behaviour. People were seen to pass through a series of stages (Figure 3.5) when trying to make adjustments to their health behaviour (Prochaska & DiClemente (2005).

The transtheoretical (stages of change) model is an influential psychological model used in the design of approaches to health behaviour change. There are several stages.

At the *Pre-contemplation* stage, the individual is not aware of their dependency. This could be due to ambivalence, denial or selective exposure to information. When the individual becomes aware of a problem, they progress to the next stage, *Contemplation*. At this stage, the individual admits that something is wrong and starts to think seriously about change. This may last for a few weeks or several years. Some people may never progress past this stage. However, if they do, they begin the stage of *Preparation*; this combines intention to take action and behavioural criteria. Individuals who are prepared for action report some small behavioural change, such as smoking five cigarettes less in a day. The effect is a reduction in the problem behaviour. The next stage is *Action*, where a commitment is made to alter the problematic behaviour. This is a much shorter stage; when the decision has been made, the individual progresses to the next phase in the change process. The final stage is *Maintenance*. The new behaviour is strengthened and develops into self-efficiency. The individual's feelings of being in control are then maximised; the person feels better and can see the positive results of their behaviour change. Eventually, the exit point, termination of the problem cycle, is reached.

The model is cyclical, as shown in Figure 3.5, and can be bi-directional, i.e. people can move backwards and forwards from one stage to the next.

What the Experts Say

I was one of those yo-yo dieters, you know, lost a few kilos 1 month and then put it all back on the next month. I was good at losing weight for that special occasion, a holiday or family wedding, and then I would go back to my old ways.

(Jo, a 43-year-old Housing Officer)

In the 'What the Experts Say' box above, Jo is expressing the way she moves through the stages of *Contemplation, Preparation* and *Action* in the transtheoretical (stages of change) model.

- *Pre-contemplation* – in this stage Jo would be perfectly happy with her weight and plan to continue to eat and behave in her normal way
- *Contemplation* – Jo might think about losing weight based on a trigger, for example a family wedding
- *Preparation* – here, Jo makes a conscious decision to alter her behaviour towards food and possibly exercise
- *Action* – Jo eats healthily and builds in a routine of daily exercise
- *Maintenance* – Jo feels good about her new self, enjoys clothes and going out more
- *Possible relapse* – Jo may go back to her pre-contemplation stage, something she admits she has done often in the past.

The stages of change model can be applied to a variety of health-related behaviours, such as alcohol use, smoking and exercise. It is particularly suited to primary care settings because of its ease of use (Bennett *et al.* 2009). Assessing a person's readiness to change can be acted upon, as in the 'Primary Care' clinic session example.

Primary Care

Jo (from the previous scenario) has a routine cervical screening appointment with the practice nurse. During initial assessment, Jo is asked to step onto the scales for assessment of her BMI. The practice nurse calculates Jo's weight in kilograms ÷ by her height in metres². Jo has a BMI of 37.3, which indicates that she is clinically obese. The practice nurse talks to Jo about her BMI and the implications this can have on her long-term health. She asks Jo how she feels about her weight and whether she would agree to some support from the GP services. Jo expresses her history of yo-yo dieting in the past, and says that she would seriously like some professional support. The nurse offers Jo a prescription for a 12-week free subscription to a local slimming club, and 12 weeks' free access to a local authority gym. The nurse makes an appointment to see Jo in 6 weeks to review her progress.

In the above situation, the practice nurse is supporting Jo through the contemplation and preparation stages of the change model. With a BMI of 37.3, the practice nurse can demonstrate to Jo the classification of grade II obesity, identified in 'The Evidence' box. By making arrangements to review Jo's progress, the nurse is actively supporting and motivating Jo to alter her behaviour. She acts as an advocate by prescribing free slimming club and gym vouchers. She is also linking her interventions to other behavioural models of health promotion.

The Evidence Classification of Overweight and Obese Adults (NICE 2006)

Classification	Body Mass Index (BMI) kg/m²
Healthy weight	18.5–24.9
Overweight	25–29.9
Obesity grade I	30–34.9
Obesity grade II	35–39.9
Obesity grade III	40 or more

Obesity is defined as a chronic condition which is associated with an excess of body fat. This is diagnosed in adults by use of the BMI, identified above. However, BMI in isolation may not accurately identify the obesity. Imagine assessing an athlete who regularly works out and engages in body building: a BMI of 32 may not accurately indicate obesity grade I. Waist circumference measurement and body shape assessment are becoming more important predictors of long-term health problems. So-called 'apple' shapes in men with a waist circumference of more than 104 cm carry a four-fold risk of developing cardiovascular disease (Peate 2005).

Behaviour Models

The Health Belief Model (Becker 1974) predicts that behaviour is a result of core beliefs (or factors, see Figure 3.6) connected to:

- *Susceptibility to illness* ('if I continue to be obese, I will be more at risk of diabetes')
- *The seriousness of illness* (diabetes is a serious illness and can lead to heart disease)
- *The 'costs' involved in carrying out the behaviour* (dieting and attending a slimming club will be costly in terms of both finance and time)
- *The benefits of carrying out the behaviour* ('as I lose weight I will begin to feel more energised and happier with my self image')
- *Cues to action, which can be internal* (such as fatigue) *or external* (opportunistic screening and health promotion advice).

Health action or the theory of reasoned action (Fishbien & Ajzen 1975) and the later revised theory of planned action (Ajzen 1988) rely on individual attitudes about health and the values that others place on health. Past success or experience can play a role.

- *Attitude* towards behaviour – Jo may perceive dieting as boring but worth it in the long run
- *Subjective norm* – Jo may feel that she will be more attractive, 'my partner will be happy that I am losing weight'

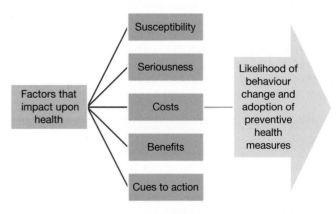

Figure 3.6 The Health Belief Model.

62

- *Perceived behavioural control* – Jo may relate to past experience, 'I am good at losing weight, I need to be motivated to continue to eat healthily, and not to put all of the weight back on again'.

In the above examples, the nurse's use of health promotion models has demonstrated how beliefs, motivation to change, empowerment to act and alter behaviour can have a positive impact on health. The next section explores examples of contemporary approaches to supporting health promotion throughout the lifespan.

The Contemporary Focus of Health Promotion

Government policies actively support and encourage nurses to use every available opportunity to promote an individual's health and well-being. The NMC acknowledges the role nurses play in supporting health and well-being, regardless of the setting, as a key standard of the Code (NMC 2008).

In its White paper, *Healthy Lives, Healthy People* (DH 2010), the government comments on opportunities for health across the lifespan:

- Improvements in maternal health give a better start to children, reduce infant mortality and reduce numbers of low birth-weight babies
- Better child health and development may improve educational outcomes, reduce risks of mental illness, unhealthy lifestyles and admissions to hospital from, for example, tooth decay
- Being in work is linked to improved physical and mental health
- Changing health behaviour could reduce premature death, dementia, heart disease and cancers
- Winter deaths could be significantly reduced through full take up of seasonal flu vaccines.

Five categories of healthy living:

- Starting well – includes advice on pregnancy, birth and the very young
- Developing well – children growing up, from 5 to 18 years
- Living well – supporting the health of adults from 18 years
- Working well – health in people of working years
- Ageing well – health in people from 45 years onwards.

Some examples of health promotion activities in these identified groups are discussed below.

Starting Well

There is a wealth of opportunities in nursing practice to support health promotion before, during and after pregnancy. (A more detailed account can be found in Chapters 11 and 13.)

Nurses, midwives and health visitors are ideally placed to support and promote family health and healthy lifestyles. Typically, the areas that are addressed in relation to health promotion during pregnancy are: healthy eating, smoking cessation, alcohol and drug abuse, physical activity and mental health.

 Link To/Go To

Information for healthy behaviour during and after pregnancy is provided at:

http://www.nhs.uk/conditions/pregnancy-and-baby/pages/pregnancy-and-baby-care.aspx

In the early years of childhood, a common theme of health promotion is healthy eating. Recently, there has been a reappearance of the 19th century nutritional problem of vitamin D deficiency and this has been attributed to lifestyle changes over the last two decades. Behaviour, related to lack of outdoor activity, obesity and poor diets are all thought to be contributory factors in vitamin D deficiency. Vitamin D is important for the growth and maintenance of healthy teeth and bones, and for the absorption of calcium. Low levels of vitamin D in the diet are associated with long-term problems, such as rickets and osteoporosis. Foods rich in vitamin D include butter, eggs, oily fish, fortified margarines and fortified breakfast cereals. An important source is sunshine.

In the 'What the Experts Say' box below, the health visitor is making the most of her opportunities to promote healthy eating at an early age; a good example of primary prevention. Nurses working in specialist units, for example children's orthopaedics, school nurses and nurses working in outpatients and Accident and Emergency environments are ideally suited to look out for risk factors associated with vitamin D deficiency. In the UK, risk factors for vitamin D deficiency include Afro-Caribbean or South Asian origin; darker skin colour causes poorer absorption of vitamin D from sunlight. People who cover themselves for cultural reasons may also be more at risk. This secondary prevention can initiate screening to assess for deficiency and promote the 'Healthy Start' scheme to provide free supplements for low income families.

What the Experts Say Primary Health Care: Leadership, Management and Team Working

" Through negotiation, I persuaded the GP to hold a lunchtime open surgery specifically for parents with new babies. For me, the rationale behind this is clear. Parents and infants are not exposed to sitting in a busy waiting room with susceptibility to respiratory infections: there is an opportunity for parents to meet with both the health visitor and the GP for advice and help (often this will focus on infant nutrition, breast feeding and weaning); developmental screening and vaccinations can be carried out on time; opportunities for postnatal checks can be facilitated. Parents can chat and share experiences. It also takes place on market day and the health centre is just across the road!

(Jen, Health Visitor)

In the example, Jen is responding to the health needs of new parents. She recognises the opportunity to provide this marginalised group with primary and secondary preventive measures, such as immunisation and screening activities. The fact that she is holding the sessions on market day taps into the social domain of health and recognises the possible difficulties of access to health promotion.

Developing Well – Children Aged 5–18

Nurses working with children and adolescents have a key role in providing health education and promoting healthy behaviour. Below is an example of the importance of primary prevention when addressing the issue of alcohol abuse among school children. Primary prevention in this situation aims to target current alcohol misuse behaviour in order to prevent future dependence.

Alcohol misuse in adolescence has far reaching consequences, and in 'The Evidence' box below, you can get an idea of the picture of alcohol behaviours in school children in England.

The Evidence

Alcohol-related behaviours in children and adolescents

- Less than half (45%) of school children aged between 11 and 15 have had at least one alcoholic drink in their lifetime
- A similar proportion of boys and girls drank alcohol in the past 7 days
- Younger pupils are less likely to have drunk alcohol than their older peers (from 1% of 11 year olds to 28% of 15 year olds)
- White pupils were more likely to have drunk alcohol recently than pupils of black or Asian ethnicity

http://www.hscic.gov.uk/catalogue/PUB11334
Smoking, Drinking and Drug Use Among Young People in England – 2011 (HSCIC 2012)

The number of adolescents consuming alcohol has shown a reduction from 65% between 1988 and 1998, to 54% in 2007, but the amount consumed by those drinking doubled over the same period, to 12.7 units per week. The recommendation for alcohol consumption in adults is clear (as shown in 'The Evidence' box below), yet, there is currently no guideline in the UK for alcohol consumption in adolescents. The UK has the third highest prevalence in Europe of 15 year olds who have reported being drunk on ten or more occasions over the previous year (Drinkaware 2012).

The Evidence Recommended Units of Alcohol Consumption Per Day

MEN – should not regularly drink more than 3–4 units per day
WOMEN – should not regularly drink more than 2–3 units per day

A unit is equal to half a pint of bitter (beer); a bottle of wine is equal to 10 units of alcohol.
NHS Choices
http://www.nhs.uk/Livewell/alcohol/Pages/Effectsofalcohol.aspx

The effects of alcohol on adolescent health may be physical, psychological or social.

Jot This Down

When promoting healthy lifestyles around alcohol consumption, what aspects of physical, psychological and social health would you be sharing with adolescents?

Regular alcohol consumption in adolescence is associated with increased accidents, risky behaviour (including violence, antisocial behaviour and unprotected sex), as well as a marked decrease in social educational and family functioning. There is growing evidence to support the link between early alcohol consumption and increased level of alcohol dependence in adulthood (Pitcänen *et al.* 2006). In the 'Jot This Down' exercise above, you may have considered the following effects of alcohol misuse:

Physical effects – the most obvious short-term effects relate to sleep disturbance; accidental trauma as a result of falling; vomiting and in some cases, aspiration of vomit as the gag reflex is inhibited; fainting or 'blacking out' as a result of 'binge drinking'. Gastrointestinal problems such as mouth ulcers, oesophagitis, gastritis and pancreatitis are all associated with alcohol misuse. Long-term effects of alcohol misuse are associated with the toxic effect of alcohol. Adolescent brains are still in the developmental phase and have an increased susceptibility to memory loss and a reduction in reasoning skills (IAS 2007).

Psychological effects – the Institute for Alcohol Studies (IAS 2007) clearly makes the link between alcohol misuse and co-morbid psychiatric disorders such as anxiety and neurosis, and more long-term mental health problems such as depression, psychosis, memory loss and self-harm. Teenagers may rationalise the reason for drinking is as a coping mechanism to reduce stress.

Social effects – you might be familiar with the acronym ASBO to describe the problem of antisocial behaviour, which can be synonymous with alcohol misuse. Others who do not abuse alcohol may be affected in a passive way; these so-called passive drinkers suffer socially from the effects of alcohol misuse. Drinkaware (2112) reports one in ten adolescents between the ages of 15 and 16 admitted to having been in trouble with the police as a result of alcohol. Drinking can be seen as a way of engaging socially and engaging in sexual relationships.

What the Experts Say Adolescent Alcohol Misuse

> Darren's mum had contacted the school because she was concerned about the gradual lack of social engagement Darren (aged 15) was having within the family. On a couple of occasions he had come home late from school, smelling of alcohol and behaving 'out of sorts', what his mum described as "angry behaviour, shouting accusations at me if I try to ask him what he is up to". Darren's mum is a lone parent and she has two younger children to care for. Darren spends a lot of time with his peers – a group of teenagers on the estate where they live. Darren has been a good achiever in his studies, but recently he has been failing to make the grades. His mum wants help. Last week Darren had broken down in tears begging his mum to help him stop drinking.

(School Health Advisor, School Nurse)

In the above 'What the Experts Say' Darren scenario, there are a number of factors identified that can alert the nurse to intervene, and prevention can be targeted at encouraging and supporting behaviour change. Risk factors for alcohol misuse in young people can include many of the factors in Darren's life, such as low parental supervision – his mother is a single parent; he may be associating with peers who take risks and be influenced by peer pressure to consume alcohol; his academic work is in decline. The strongest indication that he may respond to intervention from the School Nurse is his request to his mum for help.

You might want to reflect on the models of health that target behaviour change to address health promotion intervention for Darren. The theory of health action or the theory of reasoned action (Fishbien & Ajzen 1975) can be tools for addressing Darren's motivation to change.

64

- *Attitude* toward behaviour – Darren may perceive drinking as a way of fitting in with his peers, but is scared of the way it makes him angry towards his mum
- *Subjective norm* – Darren will have a strong sense that his mum will favour the behaviour he will show if he stops drinking
- *Perceived behavioural control* – Darren may feel that giving up drinking will help him to deal better with his GCSE studies.

For nurses to provide support in this scenario, they will work in conjunction with the individual, his family, the school staff and social support networks. Motivational interviewing and reviewing behaviour beliefs in relation to alcohol misuse can be an effective health promotion strategy when supporting adolescents.

Living Well

Health promotion in the adult aged 18 and above covers a wealth of subject areas; examples include information about lifestyles to prevent the common diseases such as heart disease, cancers and sexual health promotion (see Unit 5 on the range of disease processes and illness) and mental health promotion as identified in Chapter 12.

One of the most common themes to address is that of smoking and health. NICE (2006) recommends that the duty of every nurse should be to encourage patients to stop smoking. Smoking tobacco increases the risk of cardiovascular problems, cancer and respiratory diseases. Smoking is a popular habit, despite the well publicised health risks, which is partly due to the addictive nature of nicotine. However, smoking is a complex lifestyle behaviour that is difficult to understand. In 'The Evidence' box below, we can get an appreciation of the percentage of the adult population who engage in smoking tobacco. However, this is just a snapshot of the general picture and does not show the demographics of smoking. An example of the bigger picture is consideration of the gender pattern issues such as the ease in which men and women can give up smoking can be an important factor when establishing health promotion activities to support smoking cessation. The demographics of tobacco misuse are looked at in detail in Chapter 4.

The Evidence

The single biggest preventable cause of early death and illness is smoking and 21% of the adult population currently smoke.

(Robinson & Bulger 2010)

When we considered health promotion models earlier in the chapter, we established them as a useful means to conceptualise health promotion and create a way forward to plan and establish interventions. In smoking cessation, a taxonomy of need approach helps the nurse to assess what the patient needs to become healthier (Naidoo & Wills 2009).

What the Experts Say Communication and Interpersonal Skills, Nursing Practice and Decision-Making

I was caring for a woman who had surgery for a gynaecological condition, she was in her early 40s and a very heavy smoker (30–40 cigarettes a day). Her recovery was somewhat lengthy, partly due to her chronic cough and subsequent delay in wound healing. We talked about her smoking habit and she asked me for help in quitting. I was able to access the 'smokefree' website for her and, with help, download a 'quit app' onto her mobile phone. I then liaised with the medics to consider a prescription for nicotine replacement therapy. I was also able to make contact with the local smoking cessation group in the area and to pass the information on to her.

(Sophie, second year student nurse)

In the 'What the Experts Say' scenario above, the student nurse, Sophie, is responding to the expressed needs of the patient. In seeking interdisciplinary support, she is also tapping into the so-called normative needs, as defined by the experts, e.g. the need for nicotine replacement therapy. The approach taken by Sophie helps to empower the patient by providing information and choices to promote health. Empowerment in this context seeks to enable people to take charge of their health and the consequences of their lifestyles, and to feel in control of their circumstances.

Link To/Go To Communication and Interpersonal Skills

http://www.smokefree.nhs.uk

This is an interactive website that would be ideal to share with your patients and clients. You can quickly access your local NHS stop smoking services.

As well as substance misuse, such as smoking and alcohol consumption, the maturing adult is at risk from changes in health from cardiovascular disease, obesity, cancers and psychological stressors.

Cardiovascular disease in the adult is associated with the major risk factors of age, vascular changes, physical inactivity, male gender, smoking, hypertension and elevated blood cholesterol levels. Other factors, including obesity, and stress, can contribute to cardiovascular disease.

Obesity can affect all of the major organ systems of the body, increasing the risk of atherosclerosis, diabetes, hypertension and raised cholesterol levels. Obesity in the adult is associated with osteoarthritis and gallbladder disease, as well as heart disease.

Cancers of the breast, lung and colon are common in the middle years of adulthood and is thought to be associated with length of exposure to environmental carcinogens and to tobacco and alcohol use.

Physical and psychological stresses are numerous in the adult. Physical stressors might include work-related hazards, environmental pollutants or exposure to external risks, e.g. sunburn. Psychological stressors can develop as the adult ages. Examples might include adapting to life changes, work, unemployment, having children, divorce, being a carer for elderly relatives. Reaching retirement can have both a positive and a negative impact upon the psychological health of the adult.

Working Well

Flu vaccine for health workers, an example of primary prevention.

Around 4700 people die every year after getting flu. People in at-risk groups are 11 times more likely to die than someone who is not in an at-risk group (HPA 2012).

The Cold Weather Plan, jointly run with the Met Office and Health Protection Agency, advises people on how to stay healthy and supports local communities and professionals to better prepare for and respond to severe cold weather events.

According to the Department of Health, frontline healthcare workers are more likely to be exposed to the influenza virus, particularly during winter months, when some of the people in their care will be infected. It has been estimated that up to 1 in 4 healthcare workers may become infected with influenza during a mild influenza season; a much higher incidence than expected in the general population.

Flu (influenza) is a respiratory illness associated with the influenza virus, occurring more often in the winter months, between December and March. Three strains of influenza commonly exist: A, B and C. Influenza A is usually more severe and new strains of the illness are emerging, which is one of the reasons why vaccination is so important.

The campaign for 2012, which launched in November, a key time to get vaccinated, was carried out to:

- improve on the previous year's vaccination rates (rates for some at-risk groups are behind where they were at the same point in the previous year)
- guard against any possible false sense of security following a mild winter in the previous year
- build on local campaigns.

In the winter of 2011/2012, 44.6% of frontline health service workers involved in direct patient care in England were reported to have received the seasonal influenza vaccine (HPA 2012), the highest recorded uptake since the programme began in 2001. The highest uptake of the vaccine in this study was from practice nurses (58.1%) and the lowest uptake was among qualified nurses (39.3%).

Jot This Down Professional Values

You may have heard nurses talking about the flu vaccine and debating whether or not to go ahead and be vaccinated.

Think about the reasons for and against vaccination that the nurses might discuss.

In the above 'Jot This Down' exercise, you may have wondered why, in a workforce that is so well informed, the uptake of the influenza vaccine (a key example of primary prevention) is so poor. In Table 3.3 you can see some of the reasons why health workers might resist taking up the offer of vaccination.

In addition to the need for health workers to be vaccinated, there is a significant group of the population who need guidance to help prevent the serious complications of flu.

The at-risk groups for seasonal flu are:

- Patients aged 65 years and older
- Patients aged 6 months to under 65 years in an at-risk group (e.g. if they have chronic respiratory disease, chronic heart disease, chronic kidney disease, chronic liver disease, chronic neurological disease, diabetes or immunosuppression)
- Pregnant women
- Carers
- Those living in long-stay residential care homes.

The above at-risk groups are those most commonly in contact with nurses. The annual flu vaccine is determined by the pattern of flu globally and the previous year's pandemics, for example the 2012/2013 vaccine protected against: H1N1, the strain that caused swine flu in 2009; H3N2 flu that can infect birds and mammals, active in 2011; and B/Wisconsin/1, a strain active in 2010.

Table 3.3 The reasons why health workers might resist flu vaccination.

FALSE	TRUE
'I can't remember the last time I got flu, so I don't really need the vaccine'.	Vaccination is about protecting your colleagues or patients who may be more susceptible to the virus, as well as protecting you. Just because you've not had flu before doesn't mean you won't get it this year.
'I'm OK because I've already had flu this year, so I don't need the vaccine'.	You may think that you have had influenza, but unless laboratory testing confirmed you definitely had flu, you should still have the vaccination.
'People say that the vaccine will give me flu'.	The vaccines contain inactivated flu viruses so they cannot give you flu. You may experience a mild fever and a few aches and pains immediately after immunisation, but this can be a sign your immune system is responding.
'In my role in practice, I don't really treat anyone who has flu, so I don't need the vaccine'.	Health professionals are more likely to be exposed to the virus. Do not take the risk of passing it on to your patients, they may become seriously ill.
'I am worried that I will be infectious after having the jab, so I shouldn't have close contact with anyone for a period of time after I have been immunised'.	The vaccine does not contain a live virus and will not make you infectious to anyone, so it is safe to carry on as normal.

Link To/Go To

To find out more about the flu vaccine, who is at risk, the side-effects and contraindications, go to:

http://www.nhs.uk/conditions/flu/Pages/Introduction.aspx

Ageing Well

According to the data published by the Office of National Statistics (ONS) in 2009, there are almost 10 million people in the UK aged 65 and above, with the number of over 60s set to rise more than 50% in the next 25 years (ONS 2009). To get an idea of what this means in your geographical area, have a look at the link below.

Link To/Go To

http://www.ons.gov.uk/ons/interactive/theme-pages-1-2/age-interactive-map.html

The above link invites you to see patterns of ageing in the UK, from 1992 right up to 2033.

Have a look at your own location to see the development of the ageing population in your area.

Given the emerging pattern of a rise in the numbers of older people in society, nurses are ideally placed to promote evidence-based healthy ageing in practice. Chapter 9 develops the themes related to ageing and disease. As health promoters, nurses need to be aware of the preventative aspects of care that can support those with lifestyles associated with risk of the five major age-dependent illnesses of heart disease, malignancies, diabetes, osteoarthritis and Alzheimer's disease. According to Mazoro (2006), all of these have some association with lifestyle.

Promoting health in the older adult aims to deal with the largest lifestyle-related problems faced by the general population and to extend healthy life expectancy. The evidence to link healthy lifestyles to healthy ageing is mounting, and this supports nurses in providing effective health promotion advice and encouraging healthy lifestyle choices.

The Evidence Preventing Falls in Older People

A Cochrane review of interventions to prevent falls in older people found evidence in support of muscle strengthening and balance retraining programmes as effective preventive tools in reducing the number of age-related falls.

Gillespie (2004)

'The Evidence' box above substantiates the data underpinning the NICE (2004) guidance on falls prevention in older people.

What the Experts Say Communication and Interpersonal Skills, Nursing Practice and Decision-Making

" I regularly assess a number of older adults who have minor injuries following a fall, and my health promotion role is to actively address what might be the underlying cause. So I will ask the patient if they have ever fallen before, and I will look to see how well they walk and balance. It may be that the older patient has difficulty with their vision, or may be rushing to get to the toilet. Whilst chatting with the patient I can get an idea of their cognitive abilities too. Because of the complexity of ageing, there can be a number of underlying problems that I can address to prevent falls in the future.

(Deepan, Staff Nurse, NHS Walk-in Centre)

In the 'What the Experts Say' box above, Deepan, the staff nurse, is identifying the possible causes of falls in the older person. In this way, he is applying the NICE guidelines on falls prevention. Physical activity in the elderly can be impaired for a number of reasons; however, with support and motivation, older people can take steps to improve physical function, and, in turn, this can be associated with reducing the risks of such age-related problems as cardiovascular disease and cancer. Hydration plays a major role in falls prevention, and older people may fear drinking adequate amounts of fluid and not getting to the toilet on time. Dehydration can exacerbate the risk of postural hypotension as a person moves from a sitting to a standing position.

Modifiable lifestyle opportunities such as improved physical activity can encourage healthy ageing and improve quality of life for older people, and the above example is typical of an integrated approach to health promotion in nursing care.

Travel Health

According to the Health Protection Agency (HPA 2012), in 2007 nearly 70 million UK residents travelled abroad. Travel to different climates and environments can expose the individual to different diseases and health risks than those at home. Diseases such as yellow fever, malaria, dengue fever and rabies are common in some areas of the world. However, most travellers abroad will be exposed to more common health problems, such as intestinal infections causing diarrhoea and vomiting; overexposure to the sun; insect bites; accidents and injuries; and sexually transmitted infections.

People with chronic illness who embark on travel abroad may need extra advice and support, for example a person on oxygen therapy, who is flying to reach their destination, will need to contact the airline to establish their policy; some airlines will not allow oxygen on the plane. Some airlines will ask for a GP letter, or a 'fitness to fly' declaration.

Travellers to high-risk destinations need to:

- be aware of the disease risks associated with contaminated food and water, disease spread by animals and insects and infectious diseases spread by close personal contact
- be aware of the increase of sexually transmitted infections from unprotected sex both in the UK and abroad
- be educated regarding malaria tablets and bite prevention for travel to areas of the world where malaria is a problem.

Health promotion advice and support can broadly fall into two categories: primary prevention to provide protection in the form of immunisation; and secondary prevention to provide advice and support to those 'at risk' from the health hazards of travelling abroad.

Establishing information in the form of a travel risk assessment can help prepare the traveller for their trip and identify any special prophylaxis and immunisations they may need.

 Link To/Go To

https://www.rcn.org.uk/__data/assets/pdf_file/0006/78747/003146.pdf

Travel Health Nursing: career and competence development, RCN guidance 2012.

Travel assessment and advice should ideally be carried out by a practitioner who is competent in the specifics of travel health.

Jot This Down Travel Health Risk Assessment

What do you think a practice nurse should identify in the traveller during a travel risk assessment?

In the Jot This Down exercise above, you might have considered gathering information from two broad categories: the traveller and the travel details. Both of the categories are advocated by Stringer et al. (2002), as shown in the Table 3.4.

All of the categories in Table 3.4 can have an impact on the type and level of support and health promotion intervention that is needed for the traveller. Assessing a medical history can establish what, if any, protection is needed, for example in people with

Table 3.4 Information needed for a travel health risk assessment. Stringer *et al.* (2002)

TRAVELLER DETAILS	TRAVEL (DESTINATION) DETAILS
· Age	· Destination including
· Medication	stopovers
· Medical history	· Departure date
· Allergies	· Length of stay
· Vaccination history	· Mode of transport
· Pregnancy or breast-feeding	· Planned activities
· Special needs	· Type of accommodation
· Current health status	· Location

impaired immunity, some live vaccines might be contraindicated; in those with severe heart disease, extra attention to the effects of dehydration in hot climates may be considered. According to the HPA (2007), the most common cause of death abroad in UK travellers is due to coronary heart disease.

Pregnancy increases the risk from malaria and from deep vein thrombosis (DVT) and certain travel agencies will restrict travel for women in the final trimester of pregnancy. Women who are breast-feeding may be advised not to have live vaccines as prophylaxis prior to travel. The type of vaccine and immunisation required can be ascertained by accessing the 'Green Book'.

Jot This Down The 'Green Book'

This is a resource produced by the Department of Health to aid practitioners who are immunising against infectious diseases. Some areas of practice will have a copy to hand, for example specialist TB nurses, practice nurses, those working with children in the community and those with specialist responsibility for supporting homeless families.

· Have a look to see if this resource is available in your area of practice.

Travellers' diarrhoea is a common phenomenon caused by the ingestion of food or water contaminated with faeces either by humans or animals. Most episodes will last 3–5 days; however, more severe cases (5–10%) can last for 2 weeks or longer (NHS Choices, NHS 2011) and can be life-threatening if left untreated. Cruise travel is increasingly popular, but is also associated with outbreaks of food poisoning or norovirus. On the mainland, many illnesses such as cholera, hepatitis and typhoid are spread by food and water contaminated with human waste. Potentially unsafe foods include:

- Salads
- Raw fruit and vegetables (unless you wash and prepare them yourself)
- Buffet type foods that are shared with others
- Foods left exposed to flies
- Unpasteurised dairy products
- Undercooked meat and fish (especially shellfish)
- Re-heated or 'warmed up' prepared foods, e.g. street foods, takeaways.

Some areas of the world will have safe tap water, but travellers should be guided with regard to adding ice to drinks and using tap water for cleaning their teeth in areas where the water is considered

unsafe. People should always be advised to wash their hands before handling food.

Red Flag

 A woman on the oral contraceptive pill could lose contraceptive effectiveness if she suffers from travellers' diarrhoea. Advise women who are sexually active to take precautionary barrier methods of contraception if they have any bouts of diarrhoea and vomiting while travelling.

Another common complication of travel is sun damage and for some the ultimate goal of a golden sun tan is the reason for travel abroad. Nurses can provide useful tips on preventing the ageing and carcinogenic effects of sun, and the potential damage to unprotected eyes. Skin cancer is now one of the most common cancers seen in this country and begins when the cells' genetic material (DNA) changes because of ultraviolet (UV) damage. These cells reproduce independently and in severe cases, spread into nearby tissues and organs.

One annoying aspect of travel is exposure to insect bites and ticks. Serious illnesses, such as dengue fever, yellow fever and malaria, are spread by biting insects. For many insect-borne diseases, avoiding bites is the only way to prevent them. Advise travellers to:

- Avoid areas associated with insects, for example swamps, woods, jungles
- Dusk to dawn is the time when insects bite the most
- Good air conditioning and meshed windows can reduce the chance of being bitten
- Loose fitting clothes, long sleeves and trousers; avoid bare feet in heavily infested areas
- Clothes can be sprayed with insecticides
- DEET containing repellents are the most effective
- Plug-ins and lit coils can help
- Mosquito nets that are intact and treated with repellents are best.

Blood-borne infections such as HIV (Human Immunodeficiency Virus) and hepatitis B and C (associated with liver cirrhosis and primary liver cancer) are more common in some countries than the UK, and travellers can find themselves more at risk from dental therapy, tattooing and body piercing when abroad. Information for travellers can include:

- The use of condoms for sex, which should have been purchased in the UK with the British Standard Kitemark or the European Standard CE mark to ensure the greatest safety and protection
- Advise to have a dental check and any treatment before travel to reduce the need while away. If medical or dental treatment is required, ensure that equipment is sterilised
- The possibility of vaccination to protect against Hepatitis B
- The provision of anti-malarial prophylaxis prior to travel to reduce the risk of blood-borne infection.

Conclusion

Health promotion is an important aspect of nursing care, and as such, it is highlighted as an integral part of the NMC's Code of practice. Nurses have a role in supporting people to make healthy choices and in developing strategies to help people attain their choices. By learning how to approach people to support health,

68

nurses can develop their competence in health promotion activities. This chapter has introduced the reader to the concept of health promotion and the ways in which practitioners may approach health promotion activities. It has highlighted models of health promotion with examples of how these can be applied in a number of scenarios. Contemporary health issues have been given using a lifespan approach, with examples from the fields of nursing to illustrate this. In addition, travel health has been included to recognise the diversity of health promotion in today's society.

 Useful Links

Smoking:
http://www.canstopsmoking.com
http://www.nice.org.uk/PH1

Diet:
http://www.eatwell.gov.uk
http://www.nationalobesityforum.org.uk

Alcohol:
http://www.drinkaware.co.uk
http://www.drinking.nhs.uk

Exercise:
http://www.nhs.uk/LiveWell/Fitness

General health:
http://www.nhs.uk/Livewell

Child and family
http://www.chimat.org.uk

Travel health
http://www.fitfortravel.nhs.uk
http://www.hpa.org.uk

Key Points

- Health promotion is the process of enabling people to increase control over, and to improve, their health. It becomes an essential guide for health professionals in addressing the major health challenges faced by developing and developed nations. Health promotion is a process directed towards enabling people to take action and, as such, it is not something that is done on or to people; it is done by, with and for people either as individuals or as groups.
- Health is seen as a positive concept, not merely limited to one's physical capacities, but intrinsically linked to, for example, where a person might live and to aspects of their social networks. In supporting health, nurses must understand the variety of dimensions and factors that will impact upon an individual's health status, and the ability of individuals to make choices with regard to their future health.
- Individual beliefs about health and illness are a significant factor in the way our patients and clients behave in relation to their health status.
- Individual beliefs need to be understood if nurses are to engage in supporting, caring and nurturing health and healthy choices in our patients and clients.
- Health promotion in the care setting will inevitably take account of lifestyle assessment, health teaching, effective communication, information giving and providing opportunistic health promotion strategies in everyday clinical practice
- There is a variety of theories that guide health promotion interventions, and most theories are based in the social sciences, which include sociology, education, psychology and social policy studies.
- When discussing health-related behaviours, emphasis should be placed on the style of communication that is used, for example the attitude and approach that is taken when engaging with patients.
- Models of behaviour change are a popular choice for nurses engaging in health promotion interventions.

Glossary

BMI: calculation of an individual's body mass index
Domains of health: include physical, mental, emotional, social, sexual and societal health
Emotional health: recognition and appropriate expression of feelings, plus the ability to cope with stress
Green Book: a resource produced by the Department of Health to aid practitioners who are immunising against infectious diseases
Health education: has a focus mainly on giving information to change people's health behaviour, e.g. propaganda and instruction
Health promotion: involves empowerment of individuals and seeks to alter attitudes in order that people might change their health behaviours
Mental health: clear and coherent thinking; here cognitive abilities can be measured, for example in children's developmental assessment and in the elderly who may be suffering from dementia
Motivational interviewing: a method of motivating individuals to think about their health behaviour
Physical health: how your body functions, which can often be in terms of measuring physical parameters, for example blood pressure monitoring, body mass index measurement, assessment of motor development in children
Primary prevention: geared towards preventing the onset of disease
Secondary prevention: identifies individuals or groups at risk of disease with the aim of detecting and curing illnesses before they cause irreversible ill health
Sexual health: the acceptance and ability to achieve a satisfactory expression of one's sexuality
Social health: the ability to make and maintain relationships with others
Societal health: being valued within society, regardless of religion, race, age, gender, etc.
Spiritual health: being at peace with oneself through a system of beliefs
Tertiary prevention: aims to minimise or reduce the progression of an already established disease

References

Ajzen, I. (1988) *Attitudes, Personality and Behaviour*. Dorsey Press, Chicago.
Becker, M.H. (1974) *The Health Belief Model and Personal Health Behaviour*. Slack Thorofare, New Jersey.

Bennett, C., Perry, J. & Laurence, Z. (2009) Promoting health in primary care. *Nursing Standard*, 23(47), 48–56.

Casey, D. (2007) Nurses' perceptions, understanding and experiences of health promotion. *Journal of Clinical Nursing*, 16:1039–1049.

Dahlgren, G. & Whitehead, M. (1991) *Policies and Strategies to Promote Social Equity in Health*. Institute of Futures Studies, Stockholm.

Dennison, C.R. & Hughes, S. (2011) Motivating our patients to adopt and maintain healthy lifestyles. *Journal of Cardiovascular Nursing*, 26(1), 5–6.

DH (2003) *Toolkit for Producing Patient Information*. Department of Health, London.

DH (2004) *Choosing Health: making healthier choices easier*. Department of Health, London.

DH (2006a) *Health Challenge England*. Department of Health, London.

DH (2006b) *Modernising Nursing Careers – Setting the Direction*. Department of Health, London.

DH (2007) *Tackling Health Inequalities: 2007 Status Report on the Programme for Action*. Department of Health, London.

DH (2008a) *High Quality Care for All, NHS next Stage Review Final Report*. Department of Health, London.

DH (2008b) Change4life. Department of Health, London.

DH (2010a) *Healthy Lives: Healthy People*. Department of Health, London.

DH (2010b) *The Health survey for England 2009: trend tables*. Department of Health, London.

Dixon, A. (2008) *Motivation and Confidence: what does it take to change behaviour?* King's Fund, London.

Downie, R.S., Tannahil, C. & Tannahill, A. (1996) *Health Promotion: Models and Values*. 2nd ed. Oxford University Press.

Drinkaware (2012) *Alcohol and Young People*. http://tinyurl.com/ybf3kq8 (accessed November 2012).

Ewles, L. & Simnett, I. (2003) *Promoting Health: a practical guide*, 5th edn. Baillière Tindall, London.

Fishbien, M. & Ajzen, I. (1975) *Belief, Attitude, Internal Behaviour: an introduction to theory and research*. Addison-Wesley, Reading, MA.

FSA (2007) *Consumer Attitudes to Food Standards*, London Food Standards Agency, London.

Gillespie, L. (2004) Preventing falls in elderly people. Editorial. *British Medical Journal*. 328, 653.

Hall, C. (2009) *A Picture of the United Kingdom using the National Statistics Socio-economic Classification*. Office for national Statistics, London.

HPA (2007) *Foreign Travel-associated Illnesses: England, Wales and Northern Ireland – 2007 Report*. Health Protection Agency, London. http://www.hpa.org.uk/webc/HPAwebFile/HPAweb_C/1204186182561 (accessed November 2012).

HPA (2012) *Travel Health*. Health Protection Agency, London. http://www.hpa.org.uk/Tropics/InfectiousDiseases/InfectionsAZ/TravelHealth (accessed November 2012).

HSCIC (2012) *Smoking, Drinking and Drug Use Among Young People in England – 2011*. Health and Social Care Information Centre, Leeds.

IAS (2007) *Binge Drinking: medical and social consequences*. Institute of Alcohol Studies, Cambridgeshire.

Leventhal, H., Meyer, D. & Nerenz, D. (1980) The common sense representation of illness danger. In: S. Rachman (ed.) *Medical Psychology*, Vol. 2, pp. 7–30. Pergamon, New York.

Mazoro, E.J. (2006) *Handbook of the Biology of Ageing*, 6th edn. Academic Press, London.

McNulty, C. & Francis, N. (2010) Optimising antibiotic prescribing in primary care settings in the UK: findings of a BSAC multidisciplinary workshop 2009. *Journal of Antimicrobial Chemotherapy*, 65(11), 2278–2284.

Miller, E.T. & Spilker, J. (2003) Readiness to change and brief educational interventions: successful strategies to reduce stroke risk. *Journal of Neuroscience Nursing*, 35(4), 215–222.

Naidoo, J. & Wills, J. (2009) *Foundations of Health Promotion*. Saunders, Oxford.

NHS Choices (2011) *Traveller's Diarrhoea: Introduction*. http://www.nhs.uk/conditions/travelersdiarrhoea/Pages/Introduction.aspx (accessed November 2012).

NICE (2004) *Clinical Practice Guideline for the Assessment and Prevention of Falls in Older People*. National Institute for Clinical Excellence, London.

NICE (2006) *Brief Interventions and Referral for Smoking Cessation in Primary Care and Other Settings*. National Institute for Health and Clinical Excellence, London.

NMC (2008) *The Code: Standards of Conduct, Performance and Ethics for Nurses and Midwives*. Nursing and Midwifery Council, London.

Ogden, J. (2001) Health psychology. In: J. Naidoo & J. Wills (2009) *Health Studies. An Introduction*. Palgrave, Basingstoke.

ONS (2009) *Opinions Survey Report No. 40: Smoking-related Behaviour and Attitudes, 2008/09*. Office for National Statistics, Newport.

Peate, I. (2005) Male obesity: a gender specific approach to nurse management. *British Journal of Nursing*, 14(3), 134–138.

Pitcänen, T., Lyyra, A. & Pulkkinen, L. (2006) Age of onset of drinking and use of alcohol in adulthood: a follow up study from age 8–42 for females and males. *Addiction* 100(5), 652–661.

PHE (2012) *World Class Education and Training for World-Class Health Care*. Public Health England, London.

Prochaska, J.O. & DiClemente, C.C. (2005) The transtheoretical approach. In: J.C. Norcross & M.R. Goldfried (eds.) *Handbook of Psychotherapy Integration*, 2nd edn. Oxford University Press, New York.

Raynor, D.K. (2012) Is it time to shift our focus from patient to provider? Editorial. *British Medical Journal*, 344, e2188.

Robinson, S. & Bulger, C. (2010) *General Lifestyle Survey 2008. Smoking and Drinking Among Adults, 2008*. Office for National Statistics, Newport.

Rollnick, S., Miller, W.R. & Butler, C.C. (2008) *Motivational Interviewing in Health Care; helping patients change behaviour*. Guilford Press, New York.

Sati, I., Bernard, E., Detournay, B. et al. (2004) A population based study of diabetes and its characteristics during the fasting months of Ramadan in 13 countries: results of the Epidemiology of Diabetes and Ramadan 1422/2001 (EPIDIAR) study. *Diabetes Care*, 27(10), 2306–2311.

Scriven, A. (2010) *Promoting Health: A practical guide*, 6th edn. Bailliere Tindall, Edinburgh.

Stringer, C., Chiodni, J. & Zuckerman, J. (2002) International travel and health assessment. *Nursing Standard*, 16(39), 49–54.

Trueland, J. (2012) Read this carefully. *Nursing Standard*, 27(8), 20–21.

WHO (1946) *Constitution of the World Health Organization*. World Health Organization, Geneva.

WHO (1986) *Ottawa Charter for Health Promotion*. World Health Organization, Geneva.

Test Yourself

1. Health promotion in the early 19th century came about because of:
   (a) Lack of resources to medical care
   (b) The development of industrialisation
   (c) Open sewers and overcrowded living conditions
   (d) All of the above

2. The historical journey of health promotion followed this pattern:
   (a) Health promotion; new public health agenda; public health movement; health education
   (b) New public health agenda; health promotion; public health movement; health education
   (c) Public health movement; health education; health promotion; new public health agenda
   (d) Health promotion; public health movement; health education; new public health agenda

3. The domains of health include:
   (a) Not smoking, drinking alcohol or engaging in risky behaviour
   (b) Seeking advice on how to maintain the optimum height for weight ratio
   (c) Physical, emotional, mental, social, societal, spiritual, sexual health
   (d) The physical absence of disease

4. An intrinsic factor that can influence health can include:
   (a) Genetic make-up
   (b) Gender
   (c) Age
   (d) All of the above

5. Extrinsic factors of health are sometimes referred to as:
   (a) Weather dependent
   (b) Treatable
   (c) Modifiable
   (d) Unchangeable

6. The term 'health literacy' has been characterised as:
   (a) The ability to read and understand health information
   (b) People not being able to read or write
   (c) Dyslexia in 10% of the population
   (d) Difficulty understanding health information

7. The following is considered to be unhealthy behaviour in contemporary society:
   (a) Healthy eating
   (b) Uptake of immunisation
   (c) At-risk activities, such as binge drinking
   (d) Dental screening

8. Body mass index is calculated in the following way:
   (a) Kilogrammes divided by height in metres squared
   (b) Metres squared × height in centimetres
   (c) Kilogrammes divided by height
   (d) Height × kilogrammes squared

9. Primary prevention is described as:
   (a) Screening to prevent the onset of disease
   (b) The recognition of symptoms that complicate illness
   (c) The investigation period of health promotion
   (d) Geared towards the prevention of disease

10. Travel health risk assessment can be focussed on these two areas of concern:
    (a) Diet abroad and sun exposure
    (b) Traveller details and travel (destination) details
    (c) Traveller destination and facilities for health care
    (d) Traveller details and current passport/visa application

Answers

1. d
2. c
3. c
4. d
5. c
6. a
7. c
8. a
9. d
10. b

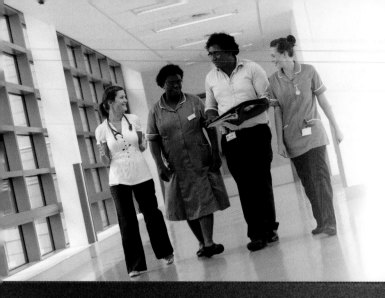

4

Public Health

Karen Wild[1] and Ann Jewell[2]

[1]University of Salford, UK
[2]Pennine Care NHS Foundation Trust

Learning Outcomes

On completion of this chapter you will be able to:

- Summarise the standards of proficiency for community public health nurses
- Have an insight into the development of the public health movement in the UK
- Demonstrate a knowledge of the role of Public Health England (PHE)
- Be aware of the significance of deprivation and inequalities in health on nursing
- Have an understanding of the causes of health inequalities
- Understand the public health role of the nurse in the community primary care setting

Competencies

All nurses must:

1. Support health and well-being
2. Understand how illness, ageing, disability, death and dying affect lives and public health
3. Encourage health promoting behaviour through education and role modelling
4. Understand public health principles and recognise and respond to the major causes and social determinants of health, illness and health inequalities
5. Secure equal access to health screening, health promotion and health care
6. Promote social inclusion to improve health, well-being and the experience of health care

 Visit the companion website at **www.wileynursingpractice.com** where you can test yourself using flashcards, multiple-choice questions and more.

Nursing Practice: Knowledge and Care, First Edition. Edited by Ian Peate, Karen Wild and Muralitharan Nair.
© 2014 John Wiley & Sons, Ltd. Published 2014 by John Wiley & Sons, Ltd. Companion website: www.wileynursingpractice.com

Introduction

A useful starting point to the understanding of this chapter is to explore the meaning of public health and primary care nursing. For many nurses working within the care setting, care delivery is primarily focussed on the individual and their immediate family or network of support. This focus on individualised care will more commonly encompass the medical traditions of curing disease and providing rehabilitation, with some acknowledgement of health promotion. Public health, on the other hand, is focussed towards the needs of larger groups and populations, with a strong emphasis on positive health outcomes, health improvement and protection, and disease prevention. Some elements of this chapter will mirror the themes that have been explored in Chapter 3.

Nurses working within the primary care setting will be involved with a combination of individualised care and the more specialised focus on public health. The creation of a third part to the Nursing and Midwifery Council (NMC) register, that of specialist community public health nursing, recognises the contribution of nurses working, for example, as health visitors, school health advisors, practice nurses, sexual health nurses and public health nurses. These specialist nurses are required to respond to the changing health needs of the communities and public with which they work. The NMC identifies standards of proficiency to underpin the principles of public health practice. These can be grouped into four domains:

- *Search for health needs*
- *Stimulation of awareness of health needs*
- *Influence on policies affecting health*
- *Facilitation of health-enhancing activities.*

(NMC 2004)

In some areas of the UK, the title 'Health Visitor' is still used; in other areas, there has been a change of focus and the term 'specialist community public health nurse' is used. In Scotland, the term 'family health nursing' is associated with public health. These specialist nurses are described by the Department of Health (DH 2011) as being public health nurses educated to work at community, family and individual level. In addition, the NMC (2004) defines the community public health nursing service as one that:

> ... *aims to reduce health inequalities by working with individuals, families, and communities promoting health, preventing ill health and in the protection of health. The emphasis is on partnership working that cuts across disciplinary, professional and organisational boundaries that impact on organised social and political policy to influence the determinants of health and promote the health of whole populations.*

As such, the NMC has set standards for proficiency of public health nursing, as demonstrated in Table 4.1.

Public health is an overarching term which covers aspects of health promotion and disease prevention. In general, many of the activities that nurses engage in may not be interpreted as public health at all: examples such as immunisation and screening for health form only part of the nurse's public health role. Knowledge of the causes and patterns of disease helps nurses to understand why people or groups of populations become affected by poor health.

Red Flag

The government intends to strengthen the public health function of nurses (DH 2010a). As a nurse you need to be aware that, even if you are not registered on the specialist NMC register, you still need to develop your skills and understanding around public health.

Setting the Scene for Public Health in the UK

A glance back to the previous chapter will remind you of the historical focus of public health and sanitary reforms of the industrial Victorian era. As industrial Britain flourished in the 19th and 20th centuries, populations grew and the health and welfare of its workforce deteriorated. Between 1801 and 1841, the population of London doubled. The industrial North, with its trade in textiles, saw the population of the city of Leeds in Yorkshire triple. With the increase in population numbers, combined with poor living conditions, disease and poor health became widespread. Figure 4.1 highlights some of the important landmarks that heralded the development of public health in the 19th century.

The Evidence The Broad Street Pump: Dr John Snow

During the 19th century, severe cholera epidemics posed a threat to the people of London. It was generally believed that the spread of this infection was due to London fogs and 'bad air'. Dr John Snow suggested that cholera was spread by poisons in the vomit and stools of cholera patients. In 1854, around 500 people died in the Soho area of London.

By plotting a map, Snow identified that a water pump on Broad Street was a common denominator and that the majority of the deaths occurred in people living close by, who frequently used the water pump. In addition, a workhouse nearby with some 535 inmates was spared, and Snow found that the workhouse had its own water pump.

Snow ordered that the handle be removed from the Broad Street water pump, and this resulted in a reduced incidence of the disease.

Snow was the first to demonstrate the importance of mapping mortality and morbidity to support the study of epidemiology.

Florence Nightingale championed the principle of public health to inform the practice of nursing when she published *Notes on Nursing*, which detailed her views on healthcare reform gained from her experience during the Crimean War (Nightingale 1859).

The early 20th century saw an increased interest in public health and sanitary reform. There was an increasing body of evidence to support the idea that epidemic disease, spread through inadequate water and sanitary provision, coupled with poor housing, affected all layers of the social spectrum. As a result, state reform and intervention saw the development of public health policies.

In Britain, community health care in the early part of the 20th century focussed its attention on the welfare of mothers and

Table 4.1 Standards of proficiency for entry to the NMC register for specialist community public health nurses.
Reproduced with permission of the NMC.

PRINCIPLE	DOMAIN
Search for health needs	
Surveillance and assessment of the population's health and well-being	Collect and structure data and information on the health and well-being and related needs of a defined population. Analyse, interpret and communicate data and information on the health and well-being and related needs of a defined population. Develop and sustain relationships with groups and individuals with the aim of improving health and social well-being. Identify individuals, families and groups who are at risk and in need of further support. Undertake screening of individuals and populations and respond appropriately to findings.
Stimulation of awareness of health needs	
Collaborative working for health and well-being	Raise awareness about health and social well-being and related factors, services and resources. Develop, sustain and evaluate collaborative work.
Working with and for communities to improve health and well-being	Communicate with individuals, groups and communities about promoting their health and well-being. Raise awareness about the actions that groups and individuals can take to improve their health and social well-being. Develop capacity and confidence of individuals and groups, including families and communities, to influence and use available services, information and skills, acting as advocate where appropriate. Work with others to protect the public's health and well-being from specific risks.
Influence on policies affecting health	
Developing health programmes and services and reducing inequalities	Work with others to plan, implement and evaluate programmes and projects to improve health and well-being. Identify and evaluate service provision and support networks for individuals, families and groups in the local area or setting.
Policy and strategy development and implementation to improve health and well-being	Appraise policies and recommend changes to improve health and well-being. Interpret and apply health and safety legislation and approved codes of practice with regard for the environment, well-being and protection of those who work with the wider community. Contribute to policy development. Influence policies affecting health.
Research and development to improve health and well-being	Develop, implement, evaluate and improve practice on the basis of research, evidence and evaluation.
Facilitation of health-enhancing activities	
Promoting and protecting the population's health and well-being	Work in partnership with others to prevent the occurrence of needs and risks related to health and well-being. Work in partnership with others to protect the public's health and well-being from specific risks.
Developing quality and risk management within an evaluative culture	Prevent, identify and minimise risk of interpersonal abuse or violence, safeguarding children and other vulnerable people, initiating the management of cases involving actual or potential abuse or violence where needed.
Strategic leadership for health and well-being	Apply leadership skills and manage projects to improve health and well-being. Plan, deliver and evaluate programmes to improve the health and well-being of individuals and groups.
Ethically managing self, people and resources to improve health and well-being	Manage teams, individuals and resources ethically and effectively.

children, and the health of school children. With this focus, public health nursing began to emerge. In 1909, a government examination of the Poor Law brought about the introduction of a unified State Medical Service. This important change in the way that medicine and health care were provided led to the development of the National Health Service Act of 1946.

Jot This Down

Imagine working as a nurse during the development of the NHS in 1946. What kind of public health problems do you think that you might have been involved in supporting?

In the 'Jot This Down' exercise above, you may have thought about some of the serious communicable diseases at the time and these would include common infections, such as diphtheria, polio and measles. Now, thanks to the development of vaccination, these infections, once life-threatening to the post-war population, are rare and treatable. However, we can still see pockets of populations not heeding campaigns to prevent outbreaks of infections. A prime example of this is a measles outbreak in Wales in 2013, highlighted in 'The Evidence' box.

> ### The Evidence
>
> The rise in the cases of measles may be attributed to the lower uptake of the MMR vaccine in recent years in the wake of negative publicity surrounding unfound claims of a link between MMR and Autism...currently one in eight children enter primary school not fully protected against measles (or mumps or rubella) at a time when the UK is experiencing an increased number of measles cases.
>
> (Public Health Wales 2013)
> (**http://www.wales.nhs.uk/sitesplus/888/page/43749**)

In 'The Evidence' box above you can see a link between the public concern about the possible (yet unfounded) risks associated with vaccination and a subsequent poor uptake of primary prevention activities. This helps to demonstrate that the NHS of the 21st century faces a different set of challenges in public health, and these include:

- *An increase in public expectation*
- *Demographic changes*
- *The development of an information-based society*
- *Changing patterns of health and disease*
- *Developments in treatment*
- *Changes in the health workplace.*

(Owen & Reilly 2011, p. 5)

> ### The Evidence
>
> People in the 21st century expect services to be fast, high quality, responsive and fitted around their lives. All public health services should put the person who uses them at their heart. This applies especially to health and social care because all care is personal.
>
> (DH 2006)

The first contemporary public health strategy in the UK was published in 1992 by the then Conservative government. *The Health of the Nation* (DH 1992) highlighted the major health concerns of the time, including cancers, accidents, smoking, heart disease and sexual health. Subsequent strategies of the Labour government included: *Saving Lives, Our Healthier Nation* (DH 1999); and *Choosing Health: Making Healthier Choices Easier* (DH 2004a). These strategies proposed targets for reducing the incidence of morbidity and mortality, and specifically used health promotion to facilitate health improvement and enable individuals to make healthy choices. These targets also addressed the wider issues of inequalities in health and environmental issues.

The current Coalition government has acknowledged the need for individuals to make healthy choices and take more responsibility for their own health. *Healthy Lives, Healthy People: Our Strategy for Public Health in England* (DH 2010b) heralds the move away from the notion of the so-called 'nanny state' where people expect the state to take care of their health.

Alongside the many policies that govern our approach to public health, nurses have seen the development of a variety of agencies and support networks, as set out in Figure 4.2.

In December 2011, the first Director of Nursing for Public Health was appointed. The role was created to provide high quality

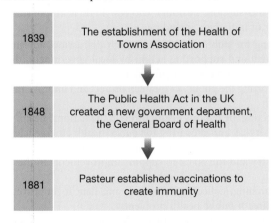

Figure 4.1 Some important public health interventions of the 19th century.

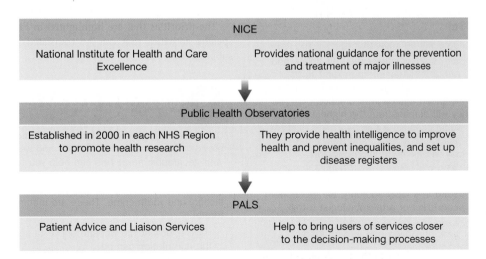

Figure 4.2 Examples of agencies and services to support contemporary public health activities.

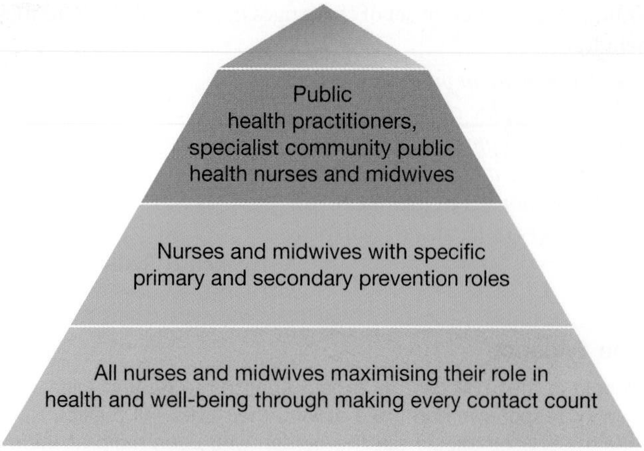

76

Figure 4.3 Three levels of nursing and midwifery practice: improving and protecting the public's health. (PHE 2013.)

independent nursing advice to the government, and to coordinate nursing policy development in relation to public health, and the development of social care. On her Department of Health blog, the Director states that:

> *...every nurse and midwife can become a health promoting practitioner by using their knowledge and skills to make a personal and professional impact. In addition to the nurses, midwives and health visitors working in specialist public health roles, we all have the potential to make a difference to the public's health throughout our interactions with patients, families and communities – "making every contact count" for improved health and well-being.*

> **(http://vivbennett.dh.gov.uk/health-promoting -practitioners/** (accessed July 2013)).

Public Health England recognises three levels of nursing and midwifery practices, as shown in Figure 4.3.

In 2013, the government set out a public health workforce strategy (*Healthy Lives, Healthy People* DH 2013a), which acknowledges the significant changes made to the public health system and the introduction of specialised public health workers to support them.

The Evidence **The Vision for the Public Health Workforce (DH 2013a)**

The public health workforce will be known for its:

- **Expertise** – public health staff, whatever their discipline and wherever they work, will be well-trained and expert in their field, committed to developing and maintaining that expertise and using an evidence-based approach to practice
- **Professionalism** – they will demonstrate the highest standards of professional conduct in their work
- **Commitment** to the population's health and well-being – in everything they do, they will focus on improving and protecting the health and well-being of their populations, taking account of equality and rights, whether their role is as a director of public health in a local authority, an infection control nurse in an acute trust or a microbiologist within Public Health England
- **Flexibility** – they will work effectively and in partnership across organisational boundaries.

The Health and Social Care Act of 2012 provides a new focus for public health. 'The Government's commitment to put the public's health centre stage has been applauded by those we have heard from...at a local level, the move of public health services into local authorities is widely supported' (NHS Future Forum Report, NHS 2011).

One of the biggest changes that the 2012 Act has made is the shift of public health services from the NHS to local government. It is acknowledged that the reason people suffer health inequalities is not wholly down to the provision of health care, but in its widest context, is a combination of factors that impinge on individuals' or communities' lifestyles. Control at local government level is seen as an important way of developing a streamlined public health service based on targeting local health needs.

The 2012 Act also makes it the duty of the Secretary of State to take steps to protect the health of the people of England. As a result, the Health Protection Agency was abolished to make way for the development of Public Health England.

Public Health England

Public Health England (PHE) is an executive agency of the Department of Health. It was set up in 2013 to bring together public health specialists from over 70 organisations into a single public health service. The aim of the service is to protect and improve the nation's health and support healthier choices. PHE is responsible for a number of initiatives, including:

- Making the public healthier through discussion, advising government and supporting action by local government, the NHS and other people and organisations
- Supporting the public, so they can protect and improve their own health
- Protecting the nation's health through the national health protection service, and preparing for public health emergencies
- Sharing information and expertise with local authorities, industry and the NHS, to support improvements in the public's health
- Researching, collecting and analysing data to improve understanding of public health problems
- Reporting on improvements in the public's health, so everyone can understand the challenge and the next steps
- Helping local authorities and the NHS to develop the public health system and its specialist workforce.

The priorities that are highlighted in Figure 4.4 identify field-specific activities that can be translated into nursing care and support.

Link To/Go To Child and Family Nursing Field

Child Health Profiles at: **http://www.chimat.org.uk/profiles** provides a snapshot of the health and well-being of children in your geographic area. This can help you to establish data on wide ranging topics, including, for example, immunisation levels, rates of teenage pregnancy, hospital admissions and alcohol and youth crime. These are instantly available in app format.

- Have a look at the website above to see how accessible the information can be.

Helping people to live longer and more healthy lives by reducing preventable deaths and the burden of ill health associated with smoking, high blood pressure, obesity, poor diet, poor mental health, insufficient exercise and alcohol
(Adult Field Specific)

Reducing the burden of disease and disability in life by focussing on preventing and recovering from the conditions with the greatest impact, including dementia, anxiety, depression and drug dependency
(Mental Health Field Specific)

Protecting the country from infectious diseases and environmental hazards, including the growing problem of infections that resist treatment with antibiotics

Supporting families to give children and young people the best start in life, through working with health visiting and school nursing, family nurse partnerships and the troubled families programme
(Child and Family Field Specific)

Improving health in the workplace by encouraging employers to support their staff, and those moving into and out of the workforce, to lead healthier lives

Figure 4.4 Public Health England priorities for 2013/2014.

Jot This Down

- How might a specialist community public health nurse benefit from this kind of information?

In the 'Jot This Down' exercise above, you may have thought about how comparsion with health indicators nationally can support specialist community public health nurses in their role by enabling them to utilise evidence-based resources to improve public health services locally. The profiles allow comparison so that expertise and insights into better care management can be shared.

The most recent Department of Health strategy has a vision which aims to improve and protect the nation's well-being, and improve the health of the poorest fastest (DH 2012a,b). This latest policy focusses on two outcomes:

1. Increased healthy life expectancy
2. Reduced differences in life expectancy and healthy life expectancy between communities.

This latest strategic approach to public health is focussed around achieving positive health outcomes for the population and reducing inequalities in health. What emerges is a shift away from the target-driven performance-managed policies of the past, to a more process-oriented approach that acknowledges inequalities in health. The next section explores the impact that inequalities have on public health.

Health Inequalities

Health inequalities are real and are an established fact of the general picture of disease and the causes of mortality in this country. What the measurement of health aims to establish is:

- The extent of the inequalities and whether they are on the rise or falling
- The causes of inequalities
- How to measure and monitor them
- What can be done about them.

The picture of health on a global scale can be said to be improving, and in the UK, it is generally accepted that in contemporary society on average, a person can expect to live longer, be healthier and be in a financially better position than a person 50 years ago. However, these patterns of improvement are not equally distributed, and the gap between rich and poor communities and groups has widened, as demonstrated in 'The Evidence' box.

The Evidence

...in the UK despite the creation of the Welfare State and the virtual abolition of absolute poverty, although the health of the poorest has improved over time this has not occurred at such a quick rate as the health of the richest, thus the gap between rich and poor has widened
(Evans 2007)

Poor health is linked to social and economic disadvantage. An example is the link between smoking and income. NICE (2012) states that in the UK, three out of four families that receive income support spend one-seventh of their disposable income on cigarettes. It also highlights concerns with the rise in the state pension age, to 66 by 2026 and 68 by 2046, which means that many people who are disadvantaged will have to continue working while experiencing ill health or disability.

Health inequalities can be described as:

- *Health differences between individuals*
- *Health differences between population groups*
- *Health differences between groups occupying unequal positions in society.*

(Graham 2007)

As such, health inequalities are concerned with the gap or gradient in health, usually measured by differences in illness (morbidity) and death (mortality) between population groups that can be identified by a number of social characteristics. These include social class, ethnic group, wealth and income, gender, educational achievement, housing and geography (Noble & Wright 2000).

Jot This Down

You will recall from Chapter 3 the information around factors that influence health.

- Jot down as many factors that you can think of that affect our health and well-being.
- Which of the factors from your list might be influenced by **social** determinants, such as poor housing, unemployment or having an affluent well-educated lifestyle?

From the 'Jot This Down' exercise above, you may have identified a whole list of factors, such as age, education, where you live, etc. As nurses, we should be aware that a person's social and economic position is directly linked to health. Because of this, an individual's ability to withstand stressors may be adversely affected.

- Stressors can be biological, social, psychological and economic
- Social and economic conditions can prevent people from changing their behaviour to improve their health
- An individual's social position can reinforce behaviours that damage their health
- Health inequalities result from a complex set of interactions that can include:
  - Long-term effects of a disadvantaged social position
  - Differences in access to information, resources and services
  - Differences in exposure to risk
  - Lack of control over life circumstances
  - Care systems that may reinforce inequalities.

What the Experts Say A Head Teacher Says:

We are constantly reminded of the impact of poor nutrition on the health and educational ability of our pupils, and are surprised at the number of children at both ends of the scale: those underweight for their age and height, and those who are clearly obese. Most of the children who attend this school are from disadvantaged social backgrounds, a high proportion of the parents are unemployed and live in council flats or rented property. Indeed, many of the parents were pupils themselves not that long ago; they too had similar backgrounds and associated poor nutrition. There are currently no children's play areas in the immediate area, and we are conscious of the fact that many children are sent to school without having breakfast.

(Head Teacher, inner city Primary School)

In the Head Teacher's statement, the link between socioeconomic, geographical and biological health is clear, and this is a classic example of health inequalities that exist within contemporary Britain. In 1998, the government commissioned a report into health inequalities, which was carried out by Sir Donald Acheson. The report emphasised the importance of the social and economic environment as a factor in health inequalities (Acheson 1998).

There are a number of organisations that support research and development to investigate the causes of health inequalities. While many are government-led and supported, some are independent charitable organisations.

Link To/Go To

http://www.jrf.org.uk/

The Joseph Rowntree Foundation and Housing Trust is a dual charity that aims to:

Search out the underlying causes of poverty and inequality, and identify solutions – through research and learning from experience

Demonstrate solutions – by developing and running services, stewardship of our land and buildings, innovating and supporting others to innovate

Influence positive and lasting change – publishing and promoting evidence, and bringing people together to share ideas

In order to deliver appropriate health services to local communities, it is important that the make-up and need of the population are understood. It is widely recognised that health status is dependent upon the 'wider determinants of health', which are measured using indicators of deprivation.

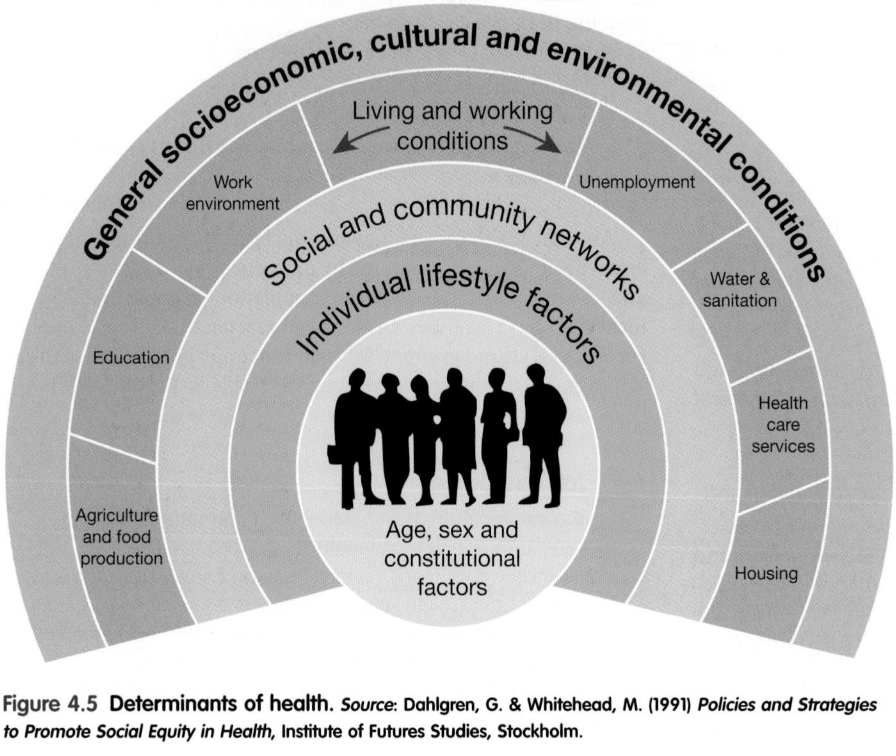

Measuring Deprivation

As established above, health inequalities may be influenced by several different factors, such as poverty, inadequate housing, transport, education and employment. These factors are described as the *wider determinants of health* and can be seen in Figure 4.5.

Figure 4.5 demonstrates one way of representing the interaction between lifestyle, cultural and socioeconomic conditions, crime, education, housing, transport, employment issues and health.

Some of the wider determinants of health are:

- *Poverty*
- *Employment*
- *Education*
- *Housing*
- *Accidents*
- *Social capital.*

(DH 2003)

Determinants of health provide a useful way of understanding why a population is likely to have good or poorer health, and also to determine the pre-

Figure 4.5 Determinants of health. *Source:* Dahlgren, G. & Whitehead, M. (1991) *Policies and Strategies to Promote Social Equity in Health,* Institute of Futures Studies, Stockholm.

dicted incidence of ill health in a given population. Risk factors are a useful tool to determine who is likely to suffer ill health, and to help support the individual to address such factors.

The Marmot Review

In November 2008, Professor Sir Michael Marmot was asked by the Secretary of State for Health to chair an independent review to set objectives for the most effective evidence-based strategies for reducing health inequalities in England from 2010.

Published on 11 February 2010, it proposes an evidence-based strategy to address the social determinants of health, the conditions in which people are born, grow up, live, work and age, and which can lead to health inequalities. It draws further attention to the evidence that most people in England are not living as long as the best off in society and spend longer in ill health. The detailed report contains many important findings, some of which are summarised below.

- People living in the poorest neighbourhoods in England will on average die seven years earlier than people living in the richest neighbourhoods
- People living in poorer areas not only die sooner, but spend more of their lives with disability – an average total difference of 17 years.

The Review highlights the social gradient of health inequalities – put simply, the lower one's social and economic status, the poorer one's health is likely to be. Health inequalities arise from a complex interaction of many factors – housing, income, education, social isolation, disability – all of which can be strongly affected by one's economic and social status.

Health inequalities are largely preventable. Not only is there a strong social justice case for addressing health inequalities, there is also a pressing economic case. It is estimated that the annual cost of health inequalities is between £36 billion and £40 billion through lost taxes, welfare payments and costs to the NHS. Action on health inequalities requires action across all the social determinants of health, including education, occupation, income, home and community.

The objectives propose six interventions that address the social determinants of health inequalities:

1. *Give every child the best start in life*
2. *Enable all children, young people and adults to maximise their capabilities and have control over their lives*
3. *Create fair employment and good work for all*
4. *Ensure a healthy standard of living for all*
5. *Create and develop healthy and sustainable places and communities*
6. *Strengthen the role and impact of ill health prevention.*

(The Marmot Review, Marmot 2010)

Link To/Go To

http://www.lho.org.uk/LHO_Topics/national_lead_areas/marmot/marmotindicators.aspx

Click on the links for the area in which you live and look at the male and female life expectancy. Compare this with the UK average. What does this tell you about the determinants of health in your area?

Future challenges for the NHS concern the demand for healthcare and provision and the supply of health and social services. The demand for healthcare is increasing because of an ageing society, a rise in the incidence of long-term conditions, and an increase in the expectations of the public. The supply of healthcare is challenged because of increasing costs of providing care combined with constraints on public resources.

The Causes of Health Inequalities

Current debates about the underlying causes of health inequalities are divided, but their common aim is to explain the reasons why groups in society might be affected. In Table 4.2, you can see the arguments that are put forward to demonstrate two ideas around the causes of inequality: the psychosocial and neo-material perspectives.

A third explanation is offered by the *lifecourse* account of inequality; it provides an alternative viewpoint as to why there are such differences in health. If you go back to the Head Teacher's 'What the Experts Say' box, you will recall the Head Teacher saying that many of the parents of his current pupils were once in a similar position of poor nutrition. This supports the notion that health effects of adverse socioeconomic circumstances accumulate throughout the lifecourse. The idea that the effects of poverty can be seen to be strongest in those who are born, grow up in, and remain in material hardship, and this is manifest in the next generation, is the so-called 'cycle of poverty'.

People in the UK have traditionally been classified socially as being upper-, middle- or lower-class, and defined by occupation, wealth and education. The Registrar General's social classification was based on occupation and ranged from professional occupations, such as doctors, to unskilled occupations, such as labourers.

These stereotypes of the 20th century are seen as outdated, and sociologists are inclined to view class in relation to cultural and social activities, as well as wealth. New research from the BBC Lab UK (2013) suggests that class has three dimensions:

- Economic capital – which considers such aspects as a person's income, savings and house value

Table 4.2 Psychosocial and neo-material causes of health inequalities.

THE PSYCHOSOCIAL PERSPECTIVE	THE NEO-MATERIAL PERSPECTIVE
• Emphasises the negative emotional experiences of living in an unequal society • Analyses the impact that stress, shame and powerlessness have on health • Considers how unequal access affects the impact of the above through physical changes to cardiovascular, endocrine and immune systems, e.g. the effects of chronic stress on a person due to lack of control and low social status	• Health is influenced by material factors, most importantly income and employment • Emphasises unequal distribution of resources, e.g. housing and education • The above leads to unequal consumption of a healthy lifestyle, e.g. unequal access to food, transport, housing, health care and education

Box 4.1 The Proposed Seven Social Classes

Elite	Most privileged group in the UK and has the highest levels of all three capitals
Established middle-class	The second wealthiest and the largest group: make-up 25% of the population. They score high on cultural capital
Technical middle-class	A small group who are prosperous but score low on the cultural and social capitals
New affluent workers	A young-in-age class group, socially and culturally active with mid-levels of economic capital
Traditional working-class	Scores low on all levels of capital, but is not deprived. This group has the oldest average age at 66 years, and makes up 14% of the population
Emergent service workers	Young, urban group who are relatively poor but have high social and cultural capital
Precariat, or precarious proletariat	The poorest, most deprived class, scoring low for social and cultural capital

- Social capital – which looks at the number and status of people that a person knows socially
- Cultural capital – defined as the extent and nature of cultural interests and activities that a person engages in.

What emerges is the suggestion of a revision of the established way of classifying people socially, as shown in Box 4.1.

Compare Box 4.1 with the Office for National Statistics Classification, which has its categories aggregated to produce approximate social classes I–V, as follows:

I. Professional occupations
II. Managerial and technical occupations
III. Skilled occupations
IV. Partly skilled occupations
V. Unskilled occupations.

Whatever method of classification is used to determine social class, one constant remains: those who are socioeconomically less well off tend to have poorer health, and this can be because of their living or working conditions, resources and their social effect, lifestyle issues or any combination of these factors.

 Link To/Go To

http://longerlives.phe.org.uk/

This interactive map demonstrates the best and worst geographical locations for risk of premature death in the UK. Click on the map to see the ranking out of 150 for your area. The highest scores relate to the worst areas for risk of premature death.

Poverty is a central concern of public health, not only in this country, but worldwide. People living in poverty (this can equate to poor housing, overcrowding, poor sanitary conditions) have a reduced life expectancy and experience poorer health than the rest of the population.

The Evidence

The housing conditions that are proven to be important for health include:

- overcrowding (linked to infectious/respiratory disease)
- damp and mould (linked to respiratory disease, eczema, asthma, and rhinitis), indoor pollutants and infestation (linked to asthma)
- low temperature (linked to respiratory infection, hypothermia, bronchospasm and heart disease)
- homelessness (linked to a range of conditions)
- unpopular, stigmatised or poor housing and neighbourhood conditions (linked to poor mental health).

(Marsh et al. 2000)

While poverty is synonymous with health breakdown, it does not always follow that pattern.

Jot This Down

Can you think about the types of health problems that might not follow the assumption that poverty equates to ill health?

In the 'Jot This Down' exercise above, you will be excused from assuming that most health-related problems can be directly associated with poor housing, poor educational achievement and limited access to services.

The evidence on drug use and alcohol consumption suggests that both are widespread in society; for the most part, consumption bears little relationship to social class or income. Marmot (1997) presents evidence for 'heavy' drinking (those regularly drinking above the recommended daily allowance), which shows lower levels of heavy consumption among unemployed people than among those in work, with the greatest incidence among those in professional and managerial occupations. He concludes that survey evidence does not 'lend support to the popular conception that it is the poor and unemployed who are disproportionately represented among heavy drinkers'.

Similarly, data on drug use shows that, while experimentation with drugs is widespread among young people (one half of all 16–24-year-olds report having used drugs at some time), there is little variation by socioeconomic circumstances or correlation with poverty and social exclusion.

The Health and Social Care Act (2012) acknowledges the causes of inequalities in health are wide and diverse. As such, actions to reduce inequalities are being taken across the system.

Nursing Fields Learning Disabilities

Case study: collaboration and innovation to help the most vulnerable.

Walsall Integrated Learning Disabilities service, in partnership with the DH Pacesetters programme, has successfully addressed the historically low take-up of breast screening by women with learning disabilities. Through a combination of user engagement and raising self-awareness of the needs of this group, the project has improved screening rates from 62% to 100% for those women who are able to be screened.

(Tackling Inequalities Fact sheet, DH 2012b)

Epidemiology and Public Health

Epidemiology is concerned with the study of how diseases are dispersed between groups of populations and the factors that influence this distribution. As such, the rate of disease, its timing and place, and the people that are affected can suggest a pattern to epidemiologists who will be involved in predicting the development of disease amongst the wider population.

Jot This Down

Think about the factors that an epidemiologist might consider when an outbreak of influenza spreads within a community.

In the 'Jot This Down' exercise above, you will have probably thought about the key risk factors (or conditions) that might lead to an outbreak of influenza, and in particular those for whom the infection will be most risky. Epidemiologists will want to establish such things as:

- Does the outbreak coincide with climate conditions/seasonal changes?
- Are there certain geographical patterns?
- Which age groups are most commonly affected?
- Does lifestyle and habit affect the vulnerability to contracting the illness?
- What preventive strategies might there be available?

The Evidence

In its letter to address the 2013/2014 influenza immunisation programme, the Department of Health made the following announcement:

Last year, the NHS was asked to plan to reach uptake of 70% for people aged under 65 years in clinical risk groups, as the second of a three year trajectory to reaching uptake of 75% by 2013/14. This is important because people in these groups are at increased risks from severe complications of flu. It is disappointing that overall vaccine uptake for the under 65 years in clinical risk groups has apparently stalled and has only been around 50% for several years now.

In 2013/14 we are asking local areas to ensure that they offer flu vaccine to everyone at risk so we

- *reach or exceed 75% uptake for people aged 65 years and over; and*
- *reach or exceed 75% uptake for people under 65 years in risk groups, including pregnant women.*

'The majority of flu vaccinations are given in primary care and general practice is key to the success of the flu vaccination programme. It remains the responsibility of GPs to order sufficient flu vaccine for eligible patients in 2013/14'.

(DH & PHE 2013)

In 'The Evidence' box above, there is a link to the epidemiological data that informs the best practice for the prevention of influenza in vulnerable groups; here the target is those people over the age of 65 and those in high-risk groups, such as pregnant women. Both the Department of Health and Public Health England see the

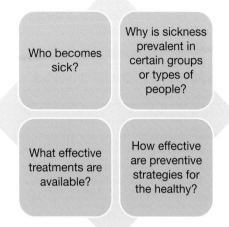

Figure 4.6 The questions that drive epidemiology. *Source:* Mullhall 2001.

GP (and in all likelihood the practice nurse), as being key to supporting this public health initiative.

Epidemiologists are interested in the health experiences of groups, as opposed to the health of individuals. The nature and cause of disease (the aetiology) is the focus of attention, alongside the study and distribution of disease. Data derived from population studies, the incidence of birth and death, lifestyles and the health behaviours of populations, alongside the sociological determinants of health, all contribute to the study of epidemiology. In Figure 4.6, according to Mullhall (2001), four main questions drive epidemiology.

The Evidence

Smoking in pregnancy rates vary ten-fold between local authorities in England:

- 3% of women in Westminster smoked in pregnancy compared with 30% in Blackpool during 2011/2012.
- The overall figure for England (13%) remains largely unchanged.

However, the variation between local authorities shows inequalities persist.

(*Source:* Calculated by the East of England Public Health Observatory (ERPHO) from the Health and Social Care Information Centre's return on Smoking Status at Time of Delivery (SSATOD) for inclusion in the Local Tobacco Control Profiles for England).

Epidemiologists categorise information in relation to patterns of health and disease in two ways:

- **Descriptive** epidemiology, which describes the patterns of distribution of health and disease, as well as the determinants of disease
- **Analytical** epidemiology, which explores the 'cause and effect' relationship between determinants and health/disease (often multiple causes and multiple effects).

An example of descriptive epidemiology can be seen in Box 4.2.

For both the determinants (causes) and distribution (who acquires diseases and where), there are a number of ways in which the evidence is collated. The public health system in the UK is

Box 4.2 Mortality Rates

Crude mortality rate	Number of deaths per 1000 of the population
Age-specific mortality rate	Number of deaths per 1000 people in a specific age range
Infant mortality rate	Number of deaths in the first year of life per 1000 live births

geared towards this type of disease surveillance. Doctors in both the community and hospital setting are responsible for notifying the occurrence of the most communicable diseases. Directors of public health collate the evidence to support the planning of health services in response to trends.

Jot This Down

Which disease do you think are notifiable in this country?

Write down a list and compare this with the information at:

(**http://www.hpa.org.uk/Topics/InfectiousDiseases/InfectionsAZ/NotificationsOfInfectiousDiseases/ListOfNotifiableDiseases/**)

Health Protection

Public Health England's health protection teams work alongside the NHS, local authorities and emergency services, providing specialist support in communicable disease, infection control and emergency planning.

The agency provides local services through a network of health protection teams, supported by regional offices and laboratories. Northern Ireland, Scotland and Wales provide their own public health support. The agency is responsible for advice in the following areas:

- Health Protection Services, based in health protection units, provide specialist advice and operational support for the local NHS, local authorities and other agencies during health protection incidents
- Specialist microbiology service, a network of laboratories operating across England, providing clinical and public health microbiology tests for both the NHS and clinical health sector, or testing food, water and environmental samples (FW&E) for local authorities and other stakeholders
- Emergency response designs and delivers exercises and training across England for the NHS to improve preparedness for incidents, such as infectious disease outbreaks, natural hazards, CBRN events and new or re-emerging health threats.

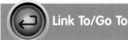 **Link To/Go To**

http://www.hpa.org.uk/Topics/TopicsAZ/

Have a look at the A–Z listings on the PHE website, click on to 'M' and find MRSA. Now have a look at the resources that are available for health workers, patients, and other interested groups (e.g. Nursing homes).

Primary Care Nursing

'Primary care nursing' refers to all the health services that are provided in the community setting and community nursing care is focussed on all aspects of health. Community nursing services provide the public with essential evidence-based nursing, which enables the public to remain in their own home and environment whenever possible, and receive health care and health education according to their individual needs. Primary care nursing focusses on all aspects, ages, conditions and healthcare requirements that are able to be delivered safely and effectively in the patient's own environment. Here, we will look at the different nursing professions that work in primary care, empower and enable patients and their families to sustain health and promote well-being within their own community.

Jot This Down

The range of services that Primary Care Nursing covers is vast. List the services you think are delivered within primary care.

The services you may have thought of in the 'Jot this Down' exercise above may include: District Nursing, Health Visiting and School Nursing. The exact parameters for community nursing are dependent on individual NHS Trusts and commissioned services (**http://www.england.nhs.uk**). Communities have differing requirements and nursing needs, and the services commissioned and delivered can vary greatly from one geographical area to another. In order to maintain patient care delivery within the primary care setting, there are several other services and these include: community matrons, tissue viability nursing, learning disability nursing, dieticians, weight management clinics and intermediate care.

Primary care and community nursing have a strong focus on health promotion, health improvement and patient empowerment. Due to this, the services provided within primary care will ensure that a patient's healthcare delivery is holistic. When we consider the Public Health White Paper of 2010, *Healthy Lives, Healthy People* (DH 2010b), we can see the emphasis on public health. The 2012 Health and Social Care Bill puts the onus on clinical commissioning groups (CCGs) to draw up plans of care provision for local services across England.

The Evolution of Primary Care Nursing

In 1858, William Rathbone, employed a nurse to care for his terminally ill wife. After her death, Rathbone continued to employ the nurse, and tasked her to visit the poor areas of the city of Liverpool to promote health care to the poor, who could not access health care due to the costs. The rest of Rathbone's life was dedicated to building up a community healthcare system, and with the help of Florence Nightingale, the Liverpool Model of Community Nursing was introduced, and soon spread to other cities throughout the country.

With the creation of the National Health Service in 1946, district nursing within the community setting, working to this Liverpool model with contributions from the Queens Nursing Institute, continued to develop as local authorities funded more District Nurses. By 1959, a nurse training programme became nationalised,

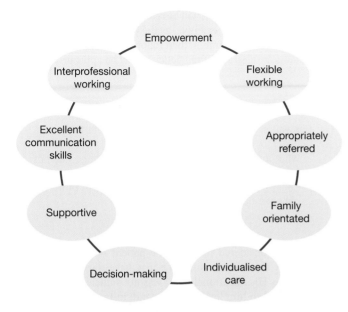

Figure 4.7 **Basic principles of Community Nursing.**

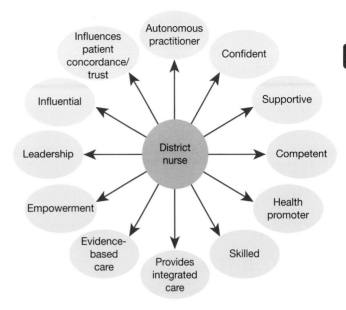

Figure 4.8 **The many roles of the District Nurse.**

rather than training on the job, and consequently, modern community nursing evolved as an important sector of the NHS.

Jot This Down

In contemporary nursing, the Community Nurse is experienced in working autonomously, utilising skills, competencies and knowledge for nursing patients in their home environment.

· What would you consider to be the basic principles of community nursing and management of the patient in their own home?

In the 'Jot This Down' exercise above, you may have considered the assessment process, the implementation of realistic care plans, and the need for excellent communication skills to support the delivery of care. Other principles might include aspects shown in Figure 4.7, the ability to work independently, having flexibility and the skill of problem-solving (an example might be maintaining asepsis in difficult surroundings).

District Nursing

District nursing within the community setting has become diverse, and the District Nurse has become more autonomous and flexible to meet patients' needs, and more adaptable to nurse a variety of patients within their own environment. They are increasingly independent as their roles grow and develop.

More and more technical nursing skills and procedures are undertaken within a patient's own home environment, and due to this, the role of the District Nurse has become highly skilled, diverse and important in ensuring that patients are adequately supported at home and therefore not admitted into the acute hospital setting. Up-to-date, relevant education is important to meet the ever-growing clinical requirements of patients and to support the growing body of carers at home.

Recent government agendas have shown the growing need to nurse patients within their own home, as this reduces the ever-increasing strain on hospital admissions. To add to this, evidence has suggested that a patient's health will improve more quickly when nursed in their own home environment (**http://www.nice.org.uk**).

As we are living in a diverse society that has a growing number of older people, an increasing number of patients who have diagnosed long-term conditions, and more patients who wish to die in their own home, the role of the District Nurse, as demonstrated in Figure 4.8, has become more and more important. Other community nursing disciplines are paramount to ensure that best patient care is delivered. Consideration should also be given to the prevention of hospital admissions, and provider organisations have to ensure that District Nurses are confident caseload holders and provide an effective service (RCN 2013).

Jot This Down

Have a look at the RCN website 'Harnessing the Potential'. How do demographic changes affect healthcare requirements?

There are over 10 000 specialised qualified District Nurses in England (Information Centre for Health and Social Care 2007), who see patients in their own home setting. They provide full holistic assessments and can therefore refer patients to the correct health discipline. Excellent communication and interpersonal skills are important in order to develop a successful therapeutic relationship with patients, and to maintain professional relationships within the interdisciplinary team. Some of the skills undertaken by the District Nurse are shown in Figure 4.9.

As District Nurses work autonomously, and problem-solve continually, 'looking outside the box' is important, to provide effective rationales and different care pathways to guide and ensure excellent patient care delivery.

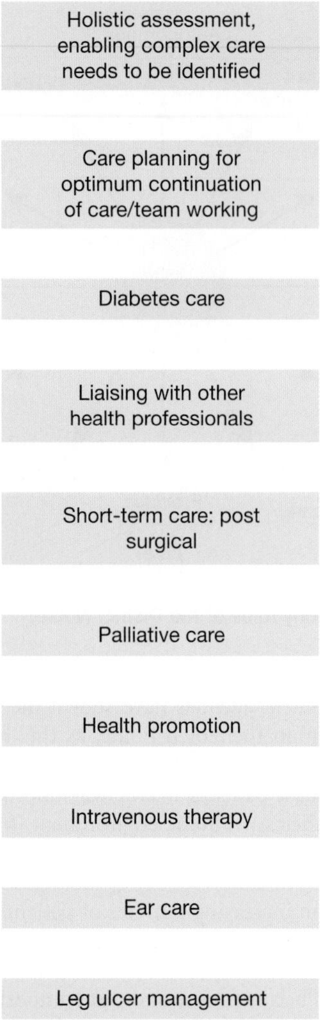

Holistic assessment, enabling complex care needs to be identified

Care planning for optimum continuation of care/team working

Diabetes care

Liaising with other health professionals

Short-term care: post surgical

Palliative care

Health promotion

Intravenous therapy

Ear care

Leg ulcer management

Figure 4.9 Clinical skills undertaken by District Nurses.

What the Experts Say

> I am 83 years old, and I try to be as independent as I possibly can. I had a nasty fall putting my bin out, and banged my shin. I managed to put plasters on for a few days, but it wasn't healing so I went to see the doctor, as it was getting me down and I was feeling poorly. The doctor advised me to go home, and he would ask the District Nurses to call and see me, as I didn't feel able to make another appointment for the clinic. My age is getting to me I think! A District Nurse called and said she thought I had an infection in my wound. The nurse asked me lots of questions, and sorted out some antibiotics with my doctor. She then said she was going to weigh me, and asked if I was eating OK. I was honest, and told her my appetite was poor, and some days it was an effort to cook. I can't thank the District Nurses enough, as its 6 weeks down the line now, and my leg feels better, I have been prescribed supplementary diet drinks, and a pressure relieving cushion on my favourite chair!

The District Nurse will carry out a full assessment of nursing needs, as well as wound assessment and treatment; this will include activities of daily living (Roper *et al.* 1980). As a result of this assessment, the District Nurse will determine if other nursing needs are evident, and if so, the patient will be referred on to other disciplines within primary care. For example, as the patient showed signs and symptoms of malnourishment, then following an assessment of his dietary status, a referral to the Dietician may be appropriate.

Jot This Down

Can you see how the assessment can benefit the patient?
- What may have happened if the District Nurse had not assessed the patient's nutritional status?
- Could this have affected the healing process of the patient's tibial wound?

It may be considered that had the patient not been assessed holistically by the District Nurse, he may have started to lose his independence. His nutritional input was not sufficient, and consequently, this led to him losing weight, and, in turn, this can cause problems such as pressure ulcers. The patient was independent prior to his fall, and through evidence-based nursing care and health education by the District Nurse and other primary care health professionals, he should regain some, if not all, of his independence. The services available within the primary care setting enabled the patient to get help and support without the need of acute hospital input.

Community Matrons

Community Matrons and their contribution to primary care nursing are important in reducing the number of chronically ill patients being admitted into hospital. There are approximately 15 million people in England with at least one long-term condition (DH 2013b). The role of the Community Matron is to manage these patients in their own home environment, and empower patients to be able to be in control of their illness, and to recognise when the condition worsens.

Jot This Down

Think about long-term conditions.
- What is a chronic illness?
- Why is it important to nurse and support these patients in the primary care setting?

  Have a look at media reports regarding the amount of NHS money that can be saved managing long-term conditions in the primary care setting.

Long-term conditions and chronic illness, such as heart disease, diabetes, respiratory disease, and strokes, would typically in the past involve the patient being admitted to hospital at the onset of the illness. However, it is beneficial to the patient to be nursed in the primary care setting, by Community Matrons. This is supported by the evidence, which has shown that patients' health improves and the level of autonomy is greater when nursed in the home setting (DH 2013b).

Health Visitor and School Health Advisor

Health Visitors and School Health Advisors (school nurses) are two distinct nursing roles, and as such, have a different focus and approach towards their respective client groups in practice. Despite this, their roles can be thought of as complementary, bringing together family and child health issues to improve health outcomes and to address inequalities.

In community settings, where the population ranges across all ages and social strata, the Health Visitor is a qualified nurse who has undertaken further training around child health, public health and health promotion. The Health Visitor plays an important role with regard to encouraging health and well-being in families. The Public Health Paper, *Healthy Lives, Healthy People* (DH 2010b) sets out actions that enable the Health Visitor to engage with parents of young children and empower them.

From a historical perspective, health visiting has been around in various formats for the last 150 years. Victorian philanthropists recognised the benefits of supporting families with young children, particularly those in poor living and social conditions. Health visiting gradually moved into local government by the end of the 19th century, and became a state sponsored provision with the establishment of the Notification of Births Acts of 1907 and 1915. Once thought of as the 'woman from the welfare', the health visitor in contemporary Britain can be seen as a professional who holds a qualification in nursing and has undergone further education and training to enable them to lead on the Healthy Child Programme (HCP) implemented by the Department of Health and Department for Children, Schools and Families (DH & DCSF 2009). In particular, their work with children under 5 years is the main focus of their activities. As such, health visitors work closely with NHS services such as maternity services, and with children's social care provision.

Jot This Down

Think about areas of health and well-being that the Health Visitor will address in the community setting, and how these link with public health?

In the 'Jot This Down' exercise above, you may have thought about Health Visitors addressing health and well-being in the following areas:

- Preventing childhood illness
- Encouraging healthy lifestyles
- Health education
- Immunisation programmes from birth
- Supporting children of vulnerable mothers.

Much of the focus of health visiting has an impact on public health. One example is the child immunisation programme to reduce the number of incidents of the common preventable childhood diseases. Encouraging healthy lifestyles is an important part of the Health Visitor role, as this links closely to well-being and can be of great benefit to community health (DH 2010a).

Jot This Down

Consider which group of people Health Visitors predominantly support in the primary care setting.

In the 'Jot This Down' exercise above, you will have identified that Health Visitors provide advice, support and health education in a nurturing, empathetic way to new parents and their children, up to school age. Through training, the Health Visitor, like all nurses, is skilled at enabling parents to be empowered through evidence-based practice and rationales, and work in accordance with the NMC guidelines.

It is the Health Visitor who often is the first healthcare professional to recognise parents in need of further input regarding the health and well-being of their child. At this stage, it is important to liaise with other healthcare professionals and the safeguarding team as necessary.

The Evidence

Lord Laming's report on The Protection of Children in England: A Progress Report (Lord Laming 2009) discusses practitioners' responsibilities for safeguarding and promoting the welfare of children, while still supporting the parents and children.

When thinking about the social classes identified earlier in this chapter, it is evident that the role of the Health Visitor is diverse, and can be complex. Promoting health and well-being is important, and can be introduced in several ways. This can be achieved by developing initiatives that include a whole community, such as the Sure Start programme. This government-led initiative that commenced in the late 1990s is aimed at ensuring every child in the UK has the opportunity for the best start in life (Sure Start 2013). The immunisation programme for babies and young children is undertaken by the Health Visitor. This provides essential health protection, ensuring the protection of the whole community from infectious diseases.

It is important that the Health Visitor forges a professional relationship with parents, in order to understand and empathise with difficult situations. The Department of Health's Health Visiting programme offers an insight into the different initiatives throughout the country, providing health and well-being structures for parents and young children that are well planned, ethical, constructive and helpful to parents and their young children. It is important to consider that the Health Visitor must ensure that any concerns regarding the health and well-being of a young child can be addressed in a professional way, and that ultimately the cases of child neglect are reduced. The RCN's 2011 report on the UK position on health visiting in the early years acknowledges that the majority of Health Visitors are working almost exclusively in the area of child health: child protection and safeguarding and working with vulnerable and at-risk families (RCN 2011). The various roles of the Health Visitor can be seen in Figure 4.10.

 ### Link To/Go To

The Department of Health's 'Health Visiting programme', and some case studies are available at: **www.nhsconfed.org**

Sir Ian Kennedy's review of NHS services for children (Public Health Outcomes Framework 2012) highlights the many problems that can arise.

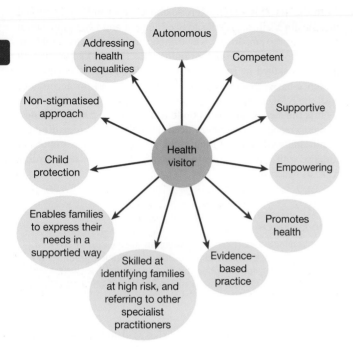

Figure 4.10 The various roles of the Health Visitor.

The Health Visitor Implementation Plan (DH 2011) was drawn up by the Department of Health in an effort to strengthen and expand Health Visitor services. It recognises that good health visiting services combined with effective working partnerships with GPs and maternity care can help ensure that families have a positive start. Under the plan, all families can expect access to support from the health visiting service in the following ways:

- **A range of services** targeted at young families, including Sure Start provision. Health Visitors work to support the development of these and other voluntary sector arrangements
- **Universal services** provided by the Health Visitor under the guidance of the Healthy Child Programme to ensure a healthy start, for example, immunisations, health and development checks, support and access for parents to a range of community services and resources
- **Universal Plus** to provide a rapid response from the health visitor team when specific expert help or advice is needed, e.g. postnatal depression, advice on weaning or concerns about parenting
- **Universal Partnership Plus** to give ongoing support from the health visiting team in partnership with other services to support more complex issues over longer periods of time. Examples might include: Sure Start Children's Centres and the Family Nurse Partnership.

The Evidence Health Visitors in Sure Start Children's Centres

Sure Start Children's Centres are accessible to all families with young children, and have an important role in identifying and supporting families in greatest need. Local authorities have statutory duties under the Childcare Act 2006 to secure sufficient provision of children's centres to meet local need, as far as is reasonably practicable. Every children's centre should

have access to a named Health Visitor. Health Visitors have unique professional expertise to:

- Deliver universal child and family health services through children's centres (the Healthy Living Programme)
- Lead health improvement through children's centres on subjects such as healthy eating, accident prevention and emotional well-being
- Help families stay in touch with wider sources of support through children's centres, including from the community and other parents
- Be leaders of child health locally, including fostering partnerships between GPs, midwives and children's centres.

Many Health Visitors work closely with local children's centres, often using them as a base: work with their local children's centre leader and are members of the management team; share information appropriately; review local cases; and share skills and experience.

(The Health Visitor Implementation Plan, DH 2011)

School Health Advisor (School Nurse)

When a child reaches school age, the School Health Advisor (sometimes known as the school nurse) will provide several different services within the school setting, to ensure health education and healthy children. This is achieved by working in collaboration with teachers, parents and other healthcare professionals in the community setting. The School Health Advisor is a qualified nurse, who has undertaken specialist training around public health and health education; this along with essential nursing skills will ensure that all children have access to a professional practitioner focussing on health and well-being and also contributing to the different cultural needs of communities.

What the Experts Say Some 11-Year-Old Children's Perceptions of Their School Nurse:

'To have someone to talk to about health problems'
'So that you can get information about not smoking'
'In case you get hurt or are frightened'
'Someone to talk to but not my teacher'

The School Health Advisor is the only NHS professional who works exclusively to meet the health needs of children at school and their families, and ideally all secondary schools in England should have a named nurse to support:

- *Children with complex health needs*
- *Health promotion around sexually transmitted infections*
- *Prevention of teenage pregnancies*
- *Health information around smoking, obesity, alcohol*
- *Promoting positive mental health*
- *Immunisation*
- *Dental health*
- *Improved health literacy.*

(Thomas 2012; cited in Barton and Le May 2012)

Jot This Down

When you look at the list above, can you think of additional ways a School Health Advisor can support school-aged children, from 5 to 19?

In the Jot This Down exercise above, you may have thought about more diverse support, such as for bullying problems and emotional issues. In addition, the role can extend to advocating for the school child, ensuring that their rights to health and social care are met. School nurses provide several different services, depending on the community requirements. Through government and local health authority agendas, the School Health Advisor will provide the necessary training to teachers and parents, which will benefit school communities.

In the primary care setting, it is important that Health Visitors and School Health Advisors understand their position when dealing with vulnerable children. Throughout their specialised education, they undertake training to make professional judgements regarding care delivery, and ensuring that children and young people's well-being is maintained in a secure environment, and that they are safe. Every nurse is accountable to the NMC regarding the care they deliver and Health Visitors and School Health Advisors see safeguarding as a key aspect in their role.

Lord Laming's report in 2003 discussed that there should be certain criteria in place to protect children from any form of abuse and neglect (Lord Laming 2003). The National Service Framework for England, Every Child Matters (DH 2004b) sets out specific outcomes that are very important to all children and young people within the UK:

- Be healthy…enjoy good physical and mental health
- Stay safe…be protected from harm
- Enjoy and achieve…get the most out of childhood years
- Make a positive contribution…being involved in the community
- Achieve economic well-being…no disadvantages to prevent meeting full potential.

When reviewing the role of the Primary Care Nurse, specialist education and development within the specific field of work is the key to providing excellent evidence-based practice and care delivery. Communication skills are important in all assessments, irrespective of age, gender, culture or social status of the person being assessed. Health promotion is an area of work in the community where nurses have an influential and supportive role. When we look back to the 1860s and William Rathbone's dedication to building a community healthcare system for all, and the creation of the NHS in 1946, we can see that primary care nursing has evolved and is now strongly linked with public health, the eradication of life-threatening disease, healthy environments within the community setting and excellent nurse relationships within the community, to support the health of both young and old, and of all cultures and ethnicities.

Conclusion

Public health and primary care nursing is concerned with the health, well-being and care of all people across the lifespan. Levels of public health are measured using the determinants of health as a guiding principle. Determinants of health help to guide government policy related to health and health improvement and to focus strategies geared to improve the health of individuals, communities and populations.

Health inequalities focus attention on the health differences between individuals, population groups and groups occupying different positions in society. They are concerned with the gap or gradient in health, usually measured by incidences of mortality or morbidity between population groups. Such gaps or gradients can be measured by analysing social class, ethnic group, wealth and income, gender, education, etc.

Epidemiologists study the distribution and determinants of disease in human populations, and apply this data to the control of health problems. In doing so, epidemiologists identify the patterns and distribution of disease, and explore the cause and effect of disease.

Specialist community public health nurses are recognised by the introduction of a third part to the NMC register. Community nursing services provide the public with essential evidence-based nursing, that enables people to remain in their own home and environment whenever possible, and receive health care and health education according to their individual needs.

Key Points

- Public health is focussed on the needs of large groups and populations, with a strong emphasis on positive health outcomes, health improvement and protection, and disease prevention.
- In 2013, the government set out a public health workforce strategy (*Healthy Lives, Healthy People*, DH 2013a), which acknowledges the significant changes made to the public health system to support these changes with specialised public health workers.
- Public Health England (PHE) is an executive agency of the Department of Health set up in 2013 to bring together public health specialists from over 70 organisations into a single public health service. The aim of the service is to protect and improve the nation's health and support healthier choices.
- The picture of health on a global scale can be said to be improving, and in the UK it is generally accepted that in contemporary society on average, a person can expect to live longer, be healthier and be in a financially better position than a person 50 years ago. However, these patterns of improvement are not equally distributed, and the gap between rich and poor communities and groups has widened.
- Poverty is a central concern of public health, not only in this country, but worldwide. People living in poverty (this can equate to poor housing, overcrowding, poor sanitary conditions) have a reduced life expectancy and experience poorer health than the rest of the population.
- Epidemiology is concerned with the study of how diseases are dispersed between groups of populations and the factors that influence this distribution. As such, the rate of disease, its timing and place, and the people affected can suggest a pattern to epidemiologists who will be involved in predicting the development of disease among the wider population.
- Primary care nursing refers to all the health services that are provided in the community setting and community nursing care is focussed on all aspects of health. Community nursing services provide the public with essential evidence-based nursing, which enables people to remain in their own home and environment wherever possible, and receive health care and health education according to their individual needs.

88

Glossary

Director of Nursing for Public Health: appointed in 2011 to advise the government on nursing policy and development in relation to public health

District Nurse: a registered nurse with an extra specialist practitioner qualification

Epidemiology: analyses the way diseases are spread between populations and the factors that influence that distribution

Health inequalities: an analysis of the gap or gradient in health between population groups that can usually be measured by a number of social characteristics

Health protection: teams work alongside the NHS to provide information, advice and expertise, as well as emergency response during disease outbreaks

Health Visitor: a qualified nurse who has undergone extra education on the recognised Health Visitor programme of study

NICE – the National institute for Health and Care Excellence: provides national guidance for the prevention and treatment of major illnesses

Primary care nursing: focussed in the community setting to support all people who need nursing support in their home environment

Public health: an overarching term that covers aspects of health promotion and disease prevention

Public Health England: an executive agency of the Department of Health

Specialist community public health nurse: a registered nurse who has undergone specialist post-qualification education in community public health nursing

School Nurse: registered nurse who specialises in supporting the health and well-being of school-aged children. May have an extra qualification as a Specialist Community Public Health Nurse

References

Acheson, D. (1998) *Independent Inquiry Into Inequalities in Health.* HMSO, Department of Health, London.

DH (1992) *The Health of the Nation.* Department of Health, London.

DH (1999) *Saving Lives, Our Healthier Nation.* Department of Health, London.

DH (2003) *Tackling Health Inequalities: a programme for action.* Department of Health, London.

DH (2004a) *Choosing Health: making healthier choices easier.* Department of Health, London.

DH (2004b) *Every Child Matters.* Department of Health, London.

DH (2006) *Our Health, Our Care, Our Say: a new direction for community services.* Department of Health, London.

DH (2010a) *Our Health and Well-being Today.* Department of Health, London.

DH (2010b) *Healthy Lives, Healthy People: our strategy for public health in England.* Department of Health, London.

DH (2011) *Health Visitor Implementation Plan 2011–2015. A Call to Action.* Department of Health, London.

DH (2012a) *A Public Health Outcomes Framework for England, 2013–2016.* Department of Health, London.

DH (2012b) *Tackling Inequalities in Healthcare Fact Sheet.* Department of Health, London. www.gov.uk/government/uploads/system/uploads/attachment_data/file/138267/C2.-Factsheet-Tackling-inequalities-in-healthcare-270412.pdf (accessed 27 June 2013).

DH (2013a) *Healthy Lives, Healthy People: a public health workforce strategy.* Department of Health, London.

DH (2013b) *Improving Quality of Life for People with Long Term Conditions.* Department of Health, London. www.gov.uk/government/policies/improving-quality-of-life-for-people-with-long-term-conditions (accessed on 1 July 2013).

DH & DCSF (2009) *Healthy Child Programme: the two year review.* Department of Health & Department for Children Schools and Families, London.

DH & PHE (2013) *The Flu Immunisation Programme 2013/14.* Letter. Gateway reference number: 00157. Department of Health & Public Health England, London.

Evans, D. (2007) New directions in tackling inequalities in health. In: J. Orme, J. Powell, P. Taylor & M. Grey (eds.) *Public Health for the 21st Century: new perspectives on policy, participation and practice,* 2nd edn. Ch. 9. Open University Press, Berkshire.

Graham, H. (2007) *Unequal Lives. Health and Socioeconomic Inequalities.* Open University Press, Maidenhead.

Information Centre for Health and Social Care (2007) See: http://www.hscic.gov.uk/pubs/hse07healthylifestyles.

Lord Laming (2009) *The Protection of Children in England*: a progress report. The Stationery Office, London.

Lord Laming (2003) *The Victoria Climbié Inquiry.* The Stationery Office, London. http://www.official-documents.gov.uk/document/cm57/5730/5730.pdf (accessed 1 July 2013).

Marmot, M. (1997) Inequality, deprivation and alcohol use. *Addiction,* 92(3 suppl 1), 13–20.

Marmot, M. (2010) *Fair Society Healthy Lives.* The Marmot Review. Institute of Health Equity, London.

Marsh, A.D., Gordon, D., Heslop, P. & Pantazis, C. (2000) Housing deprivation and health: a longitudinal analysis. *Housing Studies,* 15(3), 411–428.

Mullhall, A. (2001) Epidemiology. In: J. Naidoo & J. Wills (eds) *Health Studies. An Introduction.* Ch. 2. Palgrave, Basingstoke.

NHS (2011) *Future Forum Report: summary report on proposed changes to the NHS.* https://www.gov.uk/government/uploads/system/uploads/attachment_data/file/135149/dh_127540.pdf (accessed 1 July 2013).

NICE (2012) Health inequalities and population health. *Local Government Public Health Briefing PHB4.* National Institute for Health and Care Excellence, London.

Nightingale, F. (1859) *Notes on Nursing: what it is and what it is not.* Wilder Publications, Virginia.

NMC (2004) *Standards of Proficiency for Speciality Community Health Nurses. Standards.04.04.* Nursing and Midwifery Council, London.

Noble, M. & Wright, G. (2000) Identifying poverty in rural England. *Policy and Politics,* 28(3), 293–308.

Owen, S. & Reilly, R. (2011) The context and direction of health care. In: P. Linsky, R. Kane & S. Owen (eds) *Nursing for Public Health: promotion, principles and practice.* Ch.1. Oxford University Press, Oxford.

PHE (2013) *Nursing and Midwifery Contribution to Public Health. Improving health and well-being.* Public Health England. London.

Public Health Outcomes Framework (2012) See: https://www.gov.uk/government/publications/healthy-lives-healthy-people-improving-outcomes-and-supporting-transparency (accessed 1 July 2013).

RCN (2011) *The RCN's Position on Health Visiting in the Early Years.* Royal College of Nursing, London.

RCN (2013) *District Nursing, Harnessing the Potential.* Royal College of Nursing, London.

Roper, N., Logan, W.W. & Tierney, A.J. (1980) *The Elements of Nursing.* Churchill Livingstone, London.

Sure Start (2013) http://www.education.gov.uk/childrenandyoungpeople/earlylearningandchildcare/delivery/surestart/a0076712/sure-start-children's-centres (accessed 1 July 2013).

Thomas, J. (2012) Public health and primary care. In: D. Barton & A. Le May (2012) *Adult Nursing Preparing for Practice.* Ch. 10. Hodder Arnold, London.

Test Yourself

1. On which part of the NMC register will you find the specialist community public health nurse?
   (a) Part 4
   (b) Part 1
   (c) Part 3
   (d) Not on any of the above

2. In what year was the first Director of Nursing for Public Health appointed?
   (a) 1998
   (b) 2000
   (c) 1948
   (d) 2011

3. Public Health England (PHE) is:
   (a) An executive agency of the Department of Health
   (b) Based in the north of England
   (c) Concerned with the distribution of health promotion leaflets
   (d) Looks after the welfare of children in school

4. In which two ways do epidemiologists classify the information they gather in relation to patterns of health and disease?
   (a) Analytical and cultural
   (b) Analytical and data-based
   (c) Descriptive and analytical
   (d) Descriptive and data-based

5. Social and economic conditions can prevent people from changing their behaviour to improve their health.
   (a) True
   (b) False

6. The infant mortality rate is a measurement of:
   (a) The number of still births in the year
   (b) Number of deaths in the first year of life per 1000 live births
   (c) An estimate of predicted deaths of infants in a geographical location
   (d) An account of illness in the first year of life per 1000 infants

7. Community nursing support can positively influence the number of people with long-standing health problems who are nursed at home.
   (a) True
   (b) False
   (c) No difference

8. Health Visitors are:
   (a) Social workers with an interest in child health
   (b) Qualified nurses with no extra expertise
   (c) Always dual qualified as children's nurses and adult nurses
   (d) Qualified nurses who have undergone extra education and training in specialist health visiting or public health nursing courses

9. The Health Visitor Implementation Plan (2011) was drawn up by the Department of Health in an effort to:
   (a) Strengthen and expand health visitor services
   (b) Develop better GP services
   (c) Impact upon the Public Health England
   (d) Swap the role of Health Visitor for that of community specialist

10. The role of the Community Matron is to:
    (a) Manage patients in their own home environment
    (b) Empower patients to be able to be in control of their illness
    (c) Encourage patients to be aware of there condition becoming worse
    (d) All of the above

Answers

1. c
2. d
3. a
4. c
5. a
6. b
7. a
8. d
9. a
10. d

Unit 2

The Elements of Care

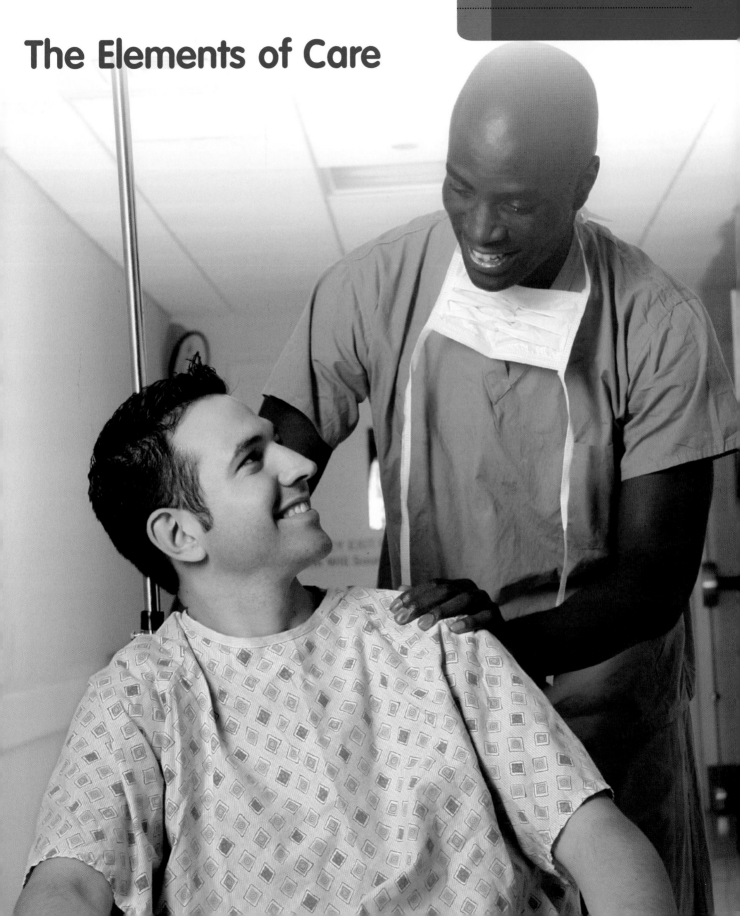

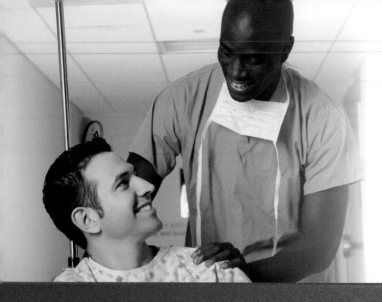

5

Ethics, the Law and the Nurse

Karen Wild

University of Salford, UK

Learning Outcomes

On completion of this chapter you will be able to:

- **Understand 'The Code' (NMC 2008a) and how it translates to ethical situations in practice**
- **Be aware of ethical values and morals that underpin care**
- **Consider the approaches and theories that contribute to ethical care**
- **Be mindful of the ethical principles and how they relate to the care that nurses provide**
- **Discuss how the law is established and operates both in the UK and in Europe**
- **Provide an overview of human rights and European Directives in nursing**

Competencies

All nurses must:

1. **Practice with confidence according to *The code: Standards of conduct, performance and ethics for nurses and midwives***
2. **Act to care for and safeguard the public**
3. **Be accountable for safe, compassionate and person-centred, evidence-based nursing that respects dignity and human rights**
4. **Promote the rights, choices and wishes of patients**
5. **Work within recognised professional, ethical and legal frameworks**
6. **Respect individual rights to confidentiality and keep information secure and confidential in accordance with the law and relevant ethical and regulatory framework**

 Visit the companion website at **www.wileynursingpractice.com** where you can test yourself using flashcards, multiple-choice questions and more.

Unit 2 image source: JSmith/iStock
Nursing Practice: Knowledge and Care, First Edition. Edited by Ian Peate, Karen Wild and Muralitharan Nair.
© 2014 John Wiley & Sons, Ltd. Published 2014 by John Wiley & Sons, Ltd. Companion website: www.wileynursingpractice.com

Introduction

The legal and ethical issues in nursing are complex and varied. What this chapter aims to do is provide the reader with an introduction to the legal and ethical context in which nursing takes place. As such, it will endeavour to explore the theories that can be used in decision-making when nurses face complex dilemmas in caring, and provide opportunities to think about and develop skills in ethical practice. A number of the chapters in this book will relate specifically to ethical aspects of care that focus on the themes within that chapter. For example, Principles of Caring for People with Mental Health Problems (Chapter 12) will pick up on the Mental Health Acts, and the chapter dealing with end of life care (Chapter 20) will pick up on Advance Directives.

Imagine that you are an older person who suddenly becomes ill and needs critical care. You are admitted to an environment in which you are surrounded by high tech gadgets, with people in uniform who appear very young to you. The language used is often unfamiliar and because an assumption is made that you are deaf, most people shout at you. A number of different healthcare practitioners approach you, many ask you the same questions, and they expose your body and handle your naked flesh; sometimes this is painful, but you do not feel your requests are being taken seriously.

Although the above commentary sounds a little dramatic, this can be the experience of individuals who are in our care. As such, nurses need to demonstrate that they understand and can apply codes of professional behaviour that support all patients and clients, including the most vulnerable people in society. These can include those with complex needs as a result of ageing, cognitive impairment and long-term conditions and those people who are approaching the end of life (NMC 2010a). This is further supported by the Chief Nursing Officer for England when she states: 'the context of health care is changing. Most significantly, with people living longer…many with multiple and complex needs and with higher expectations of what health, care and support can and should deliver' (DH & NHS Commissioning Board 2012, p. 7).

Jot This Down

Individuals who are in need of care, and their carers, expect, and are entitled to, safe and competent care.

- Which attitudes and behaviours do you think are most valued by the people for whom you care?

In the 'Jot This Down' exercise above, you will no doubt have thought about the importance of caring and compassion. Other attributes that patients expect of nurses are:

- Putting patients first
- Having common sense
- Being willing to help
- Being self-motivated and knowledgeable
- Honesty
- Being emotionally intelligent
- Being competent.

Being competent includes technical competence, professional competence and ethical competence (Quallington 2012). The

Box 5.1 Standards of Conduct, Performance and Ethics for Nurses and Midwives

'The Code' states that:

The people in your care must be able to trust you with their health and well-being

To justify that trust, you must:

- Make the care of people your first concern, treating them as individuals and respecting their dignity
  - Treat people as individuals
  - Respect people's confidentiality
  - Collaborate with those in your care
  - Ensure you gain consent
  - Maintain clear professional boundaries
- Work with others to protect and promote the health and well-being of those in your care, their families and carers, and the wider community
  - Share information with your colleagues
  - Work effectively as part of a team
  - Delegate effectively
  - Manage risk
- Provide a high standard of practice and care at all times
  - Use the best available evidence
  - Keep your skills and knowledge up to date
  - Keep clear and accurate records
- Be open and honest, act with integrity and uphold the reputation of your profession
  - Act with integrity
  - Deal with problems
  - Be impartial
  - Uphold the reputation of your profession

(*Source*: NMC 2008a)

As a professional, you are personally accountable for actions and omissions in your practice and must always be able to justify your decisions.

You must always act lawfully, whether those laws relate to your professional practice or personal life.

attribute of nurses in relation to ethical competence is the focus of this chapter.

Nursing practice is structured by codes of ethics and standards (shown in Box 5.1) that guide nursing practice and protect the public. Individual nursing practice can be held to these standards in a court of law. The guidelines are especially important because nurses encounter legal and ethical problems almost daily. The large number of ethical issues facing nurses in clinical practice makes the standards for nurses and midwives critical to moral and ethical decision-making. These standards also help to define the roles of nurses.

What the Experts Say

One of the guiding principles for me is that I need to gain permission from my patients prior to any care related activity, whether it is sitting and listening to patient's feelings or something more invasive, for example, the administration of intravenous fluids. I always gain verbal consent from those in my care. The 'code' helps guide this principle, and I will often use this as an aide memoire when mentoring student nurses.

(Staff Nurse, Orthopaedic Surgical ward)

A 'standard' is a statement or criterion that can be used by a profession and by the general public to measure quality of practice. Established standards of nursing practice make each individual nurse accountable for practice. This means that each nurse providing care has the responsibility or obligation to account for his or her own behaviours within that role. Professional nursing organisations develop and implement standards of practice to help clarify the nurse's responsibilities to society. In the UK, the Nursing and Midwifery Council (NMC 2008a) identifies standards of conduct (as set out in Box 5.1). It also identifies standards of performance and ethics for nurses and midwives.

One of the key components for competency in pre-registration education in nursing is the importance of ethical practice. It recognises that an established code of ethics is one criterion that defines a profession, and acknowledges that an ethical code is an essential feature of nursing care. The 'Code' provides an excellent frame of reference to support nurses in ethical behaviour. Ethics are principles of conduct, and ethical behaviour is concerned with values, moral duty, obligations and the distinction between right and wrong.

Values

Often described as principles and standards, values are a collection of our personal beliefs and attitudes about all aspects of our life and experiences. Values can influence a person to make decisions or behave in a certain way, and are useful in nursing to inform ethical decisions.

Jot This Down

Think about the values that you hold to be important. Where have these come from, and what influences your values?

Values are a part of who you are and what makes you worthwhile (Hendrick 2004). In the 'Jot This Down' exercise above, you may have considered the many influences that have shaped your value system. Examples such as your education, family values, your religion and the views of important people in your life may have emerged for you. Other influences may have come from the law, media or as a result of your personal life experiences. Values have the potential to motivate and guide a person's choices and decision-making abilities – understanding your own value system may help when making an ethical decision regarding nursing practice.

The Evidence

Professional values in nursing have been established by the Chief Nursing Officer for England, who in December 2012 launched a three-year vision and strategy for nursing and midwifery and care staff.

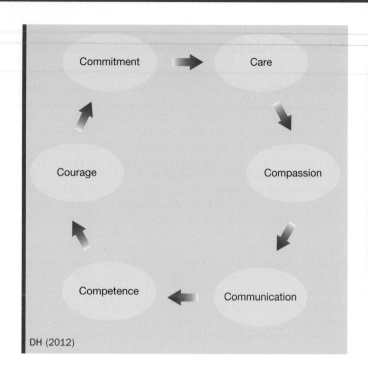

DH (2012)

Putting the values (the 6Cs) together, as in 'The Evidence' box above, helps to define a vision for nursing. As the Chief Nursing Officer points out, the values and behaviours covered by the 6Cs are not a new concept; however, presenting them together in this way helps to define a vision and is an opportunity to reinforce the values that underpin care.

Our individual value systems are shaped over time and just as you as a nurse will have a system of values, so too will your patients and clients. They may be similar in their values or can differ significantly, opening up potential for conflict. When this conflict does arise, the nurse must respect the values of others, ensuring that a balance has been achieved between the patient's rights and the nurse's professional duties (Fry & Johnstone 2008).

What the Experts Say

A starting point when meeting a new patient is to establish what their values are about their mental health problem, this will allow people to make informed choices about treatment options, and the types of care available. I have been in situations where the patients' values are very different from my values as a nurse. A recent example of this is a patient who refused medication and as a result attempted to take his own life.

(Community Mental Health Nurse)

Approaches to Ethics

The actions taken by nurses on a daily basis have a direct influence on the well-being of those in their care and it is often a challenge to identify all actions as being morally significant or morally neutral. An example might be of the nurse carrying out a simple urinalysis: that act of measuring urine output and testing urine for, e.g. the presence of albumin, may be considered a psychomotor skill and morally neutral. However, the interpretation of the information can have a radical effect on the care and treatment of an individual and so be considered morally significant.

Applied Ethics

Applied ethics is the term used to describe an approach to ethical decision-making which uses moral theories and principles to examine and address practical issues in everyday professional life. This approach acknowledges that ethics is not just about the big issues, such as life and death. In nursing, everyday approaches to care should reflect an ethical stance. Just as nurses are encouraged to reflect on the care that they deliver, they are also encouraged to reflect ethically on actions that they engage in on an ongoing basis.

Jot This Down

An outpatients department is extremely busy, time is limited for each patient contact and nurses find themselves doing 'routine' tasks with little time for rapport with patients who often have to wait for long periods of time.

- List what you perceive to be caring behaviours in an environment like this
- How satisfied would you feel if you were a nurse in this situation?
- How satisfied would the patients feel in this kind of environment?

In the 'Jot This Down' exercise above, you may recognise examples of caring behaviours: good communication, staff accessibility and kindness, staff keeping promises and following up on patient anxieties by returning to the patient and providing information and help. By reflecting on this, you can apply your value system in relation to caring. Have a look at the 'What the Experts Say' box:

What the Experts Say Patient at the Haematology Outpatient Department

It was my first visit and I really struggle to walk, and I am slightly deaf. I thought that the nurse called my name, so I stood and walked toward her. She just disappeared around a corner and I couldn't keep up with her. I was faced with a number of corridors and doors and had no idea where she had gone or what I should do, so I just stood for what seemed an age. Eventually she appeared and seemed really annoyed with me, saying that I was keeping the consultant waiting! I stood my ground and pointed out that she had disappeared from view. She tried to diffuse the situation by saying in a jokey way, 'Oh I am always doing that!'

(Patient with leukaemia, aged 86 years.)

In the scenario at the Haematology outpatient department, you can see examples of an uncaring approach. In this scenario, the nurse is hurried; she belittles the patient, provides negative communication, is disrespectful, lacks compassion, is inattentive and made the person feel uncared for…the list can go on. However, this kind of approach is thankfully not that common, based on the evidence presented by the Care Quality Commission.

The Evidence

The Care Quality Commission provides some positive thoughts on the caring behaviour of nurses in its 2012 survey.

Of the patients who responded (51% response rate):

- 70% said nurses always answered their questions in a way that they could understand
- 81% of respondents said that nurses did not talk in front of them as if they were not there
- 76% said that they 'always' had trust and confidence in the nurses that were treating them.

(CQC 2012 Inpatients survey)

Applied ethics helps us to find the moral ground from which we can view the issues in public life. It helps us to identify morally correct approaches (and therefore recognise when actions are not ethical) in the care environment.

 Link To/Go To Nursing field: Adult

You can access the results of the Care Quality Commission inpatient surveys by NHS Trust to see how your area compares with others in the UK:

http://www.cqc.org.uk/surveys/inpatient

There are three common approaches to the process of ethical thinking:

1. Rules based (Deontology)
2. Outcomes based (Utilitarian)
3. Virtue based.

Deontology

Rules-based ethics is often described as 'duty-based' and is concerned with the idea that some acts are right and some are wrong. As a result of this, people have a duty to act accordingly, regardless of the consequences of the act; whether an action is ethical depends on the intentions behind the decisions, rather than the outcomes. Deontological ethics (deontology) considers what actions are right, and has fundamental moral rules, such as: it is wrong to kill, to steal, to tell lies, and it is right to keep promises.

Generally, deontologists are bound by constraints, for example the prerequisite not to kill, but they are also given options, for example the right not to donate money to a charity if they do not wish to. There are however, complexities to the notion of deontology, because ideas of duty and what is right can vary among individuals from a variety of cultural backgrounds.

What the Experts Say Student Nurses Discuss Conscientious Objection

We were debating in class the other day about a woman's right to terminate her pregnancy, and her right to care in this situation. But then a colleague said that they had a strong belief in the preservation of human life, and as such was against termination of pregnancy and would object to involvement in care that brought about loss of life in this situation. So we concluded that our obligations or duty to care can sometimes be in conflict with our beliefs.

Strict utilitarians, in contrast, recognise neither constraints nor options, and the aim of the utilitarian is to maximise the good by any and all means necessary.

Outcomes-Based Ethics – Utilitarianism

A useful way of describing the utilitarian perspective is 'the greatest good for the greatest number' – this can be interpreted as always acting in such a way that will produce the greatest overall amount of good in the world. The value of the act is determined by its usefulness, with the main emphasis on the outcome or consequence. The focus or the moral position arising from utilitarianism is to put aside our own self-interests for the sake of all. It is often referred to as consequentialism, and is based on the notion that in ethical decision-making, the person should choose the action that maximises good consequences.

Utilitarianism can be considered as 'cost and benefit' and deciding which of alternative courses of action can produce the best overall outcomes. If a nurse uses a utilitarian approach with regard to truth telling for example, he/she would have to take into account, when making a decision, the consequence or the outcome of truth telling, and whether the act (telling the truth) would produce more happiness than unhappiness. In this circumstance, even if a decision is made to tell the truth in order to arrive at the greatest good for the greatest number, this may not necessarily be the morally correct theory to justify the action. A deontological approach may prove to be more appropriate (Peate 2012).

The attraction of a utilitarian approach within large organisations such as the NHS lies in its ability to apply the greatest benefits to the greatest numbers, i.e. to address the health needs of the majority of the population. This can be problematic as it does not necessarily allow for individual differences. An example of this may be the need for treatment of a rare condition, which may not be included in the resource allocation that is geared to the more common health problems.

Jot This Down

A person in your care requires drug therapy. The prescription says to administer this by injection, but you know that the drug can be just as effectively administered orally.

- What would be the difference of approach from a deontological and a utilitarian stance on this?

In the 'Jot This Down' exercise above, the deontological approach would be to follow the rule of the prescription and to administer the injection, regardless of the consequences (e.g. fear of injections, pain and risk of infection). The utilitarian stance would be to consider the ethically right choice based on the most happiness and the least unhappiness for the people concerned, and the nurse would be justified in requesting a change to the prescription on this basis.

Virtue Ethics

The ideology behind virtue ethics lies in the idea that it is person rather than action based; it is not so much about what you should do but more focussed on how you should be. Thus, it is not the consequences of actions or the duties and rules that govern actions, but rather the moral character of the person carrying out the actions that is important. The great philosophers such as Plato and Aristotle would ponder over how a virtuous person would act in certain circumstances to draw conclusions about the nature of moral behaviour.

The traditional list of cardinal virtues includes: prudence, justice, bravery and self-control. However, simply adopting these virtues to behave in an ethical way is criticised because, although it sends out positive messages about how to be a good person, it does not provide clear guidance on what to do in certain situations where dilemmas occur.

A combination of intellectual and moral ethics is required for what Aristotle termed 'practical wisdom' (Thompson *et al.* 2006). Practical wisdom comes with experience, and is concerned with how to act in certain circumstances. An example is honesty; knowing how to be honest without causing pain or offence requires experience, the ability to reflect and the social skills to practise in ways that are suitable in each situation.

Morals and Ethics

Nursing ethics is about asking ourselves whether something that can be done, should be done or should not be done. Some answers can be considered more socially or morally acceptable than others, depending on the context in which they exist. When applied to the care setting, this subconscious decision-making can be influenced by our opinions and personal values, a sense of what is right or wrong, our understanding of our obligations and duties as a nurse, and the subsequent consequences of our actions. Normative ethics is the branch of philosophy which studies morality in this sense.

Just as an individual has values, it is sensible to assume that he or she will have some kind of moral code underpinning behaviour. The complexity of moral development, the means of learning what is right and wrong and what should or should not happen, begins in childhood and continues through life. An example of a moral code is the 'golden rule' that is a common message in religious texts throughout the ages: that of treating others as you would want to be treated yourself.

Morals can be thought of as standards of conduct that reflect ideal human behaviour, for example an expectation that in society, truth and honesty will apply to all situations, regardless of negative consequences. In nursing this can be challenging; however, an insight into the ethical principles and how these relate to nursing ethical frameworks can guide nurses in difficult moral situations.

Ethical Principles

Ethics is relevant to all areas of nursing practice and the wider aspects of research, management and education fall under this umbrella. Active involvement in ethical decision-making is an integral part of being a nurse, because the primary aims of caring are to do good and to minimise harm. These two fundamental considerations when engaging in caring are significant overarching ethical principles, and are linked together with justice and the belief in a person's individual rights, as demonstrated in Figure 5.1.

Autonomy

The term 'autonomy' is derived from the Greek and is broadly defined as self-determination or self-rule (Dickeson *et al.* 2010). It is the ability to make one's own decisions and have the right to choose. It recognises the uniqueness of individuals and that the person has the right to self-determination.

In Chapter 2, autonomy was discussed in relation to the autonomous practice of the nurse. Patient autonomy and the principle of

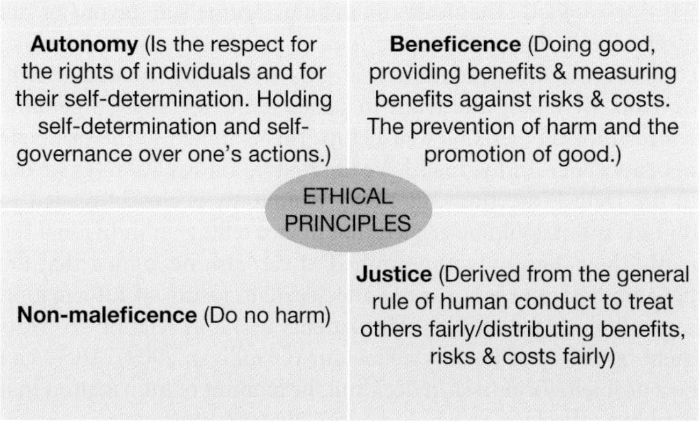

Figure 5.1 **Ethical principles.** *Source*: Beauchamp and Childress 2008.

respect for a patient's autonomy is central to the nurse–patient relationship. As such, respecting a person's autonomy means that the nurse values a patient's right to make choices, even if the nurse feels that a choice may not be in the patient's best interest. It also recognises the need to seek consent from an individual for treatment and care. A patient should always be allowed to choose, based on the best information given: the notion of informed consent. (We will visit this aspect of law later in the chapter.)

Autonomy is a counterpoint of paternalism. Paternalism can be said to be acting for another person without their agreement or consent. The person acting paternalistically is assuming that he/she knows best and that his/her actions are in the patient's best interests. Autonomy can be overridden or not respected when a person acts paternalistically.

What the Experts Say Respecting a Person's Autonomy

Ian was worried a lumbar puncture to take a spinal fluid sample would hurt.

I watch 'House' and they're always doing lumbar puncture on 'House' so no, I know what it's all about and if there was a better way of getting into the spinal fluids then I would consider it. The minute I showed any concern about it, they dropped it. They made it absolutely clear that we were all there to help one another and if there's any aspect of testing that I was uncomfortable with then they wouldn't even go there. http://www.healthtalkonline.org/medical_research/Biobanking/Topic/4191/

Beneficence

The principle of 'doing good' in a healthcare context can be linked to a duty to avoid doing harm. Nurses have an obligation to do good for patients and individuals in their care and to support and act in a way that benefits patients. It can be argued then that beneficence is a duty of care.

Jot This Down

Review 'The Code' (NMC 2008a) to identify which statements relate specifically to the principle of beneficence.

The principle of beneficence means acting in the best interest of patients and clients, based on a professional skilled assessment of them. It can be said to encompass the need to:

- work within a competency framework, providing care which is skilled and evidence-based
- ensure the best interest of individuals in our care acknowledges the need to systematically monitor practice and outcomes
- use regular and ongoing supervision and a commitment to continuous professional development.

An obligation to act in the best interest of a person may become paramount when the nurse is working with individuals whose capacity for autonomy is compromised, for example by immaturity, extreme distress and mental or physical incapacity.

Non-maleficence

Non-maleficence means to 'do no harm' and works with the principle of beneficence. At face value, this seems a simple mantra to follow, but in reality, it can be complicated. However, nurses should never intentionally cause harm. Beauchamp and Childress (2008) point out the difficulty in defining the nature of harm. There are many types, ranging from physical and emotional injury to deprivation of property or violation of rights. In health care, harm can have a narrower definition, including pain, disability, emotional harm or death. Harm is a subjective entity and can mean different things to different people. Harm may have to be accepted in order to bring about good, for example administering painful injections to deliver life-saving medications.

Justice

Justice is often referred to as fairness, and being fair and right is something most people would aim for. Patients may be forgiven for asking the question, 'is it fair that I have to wait for this or that treatment?' When justice is discussed in a healthcare arena, there are many factors that will influence whether we are being fair and right, and the above example of inequalities in access to health care is just one.

Other terms that are associated with justice are:

- Justice as a means of punishment or retribution (an eye for an eye). Punishment or retribution has more to do with the law than health. Crime is punishable by society through the judicial system.
- Justice as fairness (fair distribution)
- Justice as entitlement.

In defining the term justice, Beauchamp and Childress (2008) suggest that justice is the fair, equitable and appropriate treatment of all people. The underpinning principle associated with justice, therefore, is that everyone is valued equally and treated alike. Being fair and equitable will also depend on what society feels is owed to others – it is therefore subjective and can be loaded with values and judgements. Justice to individuals also implies care that does not discriminate on the basis of sexual orientation, gender, race or religion, age or illness (physical and psychological).

There are three perspectives associated with justice:

- ***Egalitarian***, *concerned with the distribution of healthcare resources in accordance with individual need. In this perspective individual need should be met by equal access to services*
- ***Libertarian*** *perspective relates to liberty and choice and is associated with how hard an individual has worked in order to earn health care; they are judged on merit.*

- *Rights imply that the state has an obligation to provide care and that the patient should suffer no harm as a result of that provision. People's rights have to be upheld in order to meet the criteria associated with a rights perspective.*

(Seedhouse 2002)

Fidelity

The principle of fidelity is a simple one: it means to be faithful to agreements and promises.

What the Experts Say

When I was a student nurse (all those years ago!) I distinctly remember my tutor saying to me, 'never break a promise, if you say you will get back to someone, you must always do this'. He (my tutor) expressed the scenario of a patient waiting for the nurse to return with some information that the patient feels important. By not going back, the trust and belief that the patient has in you and other nurses can be negatively affected. It's something that I now discuss with my students.

(A senior lecturer in nursing)

In the 'What the Experts Say' scenario, you can see how fidelity can be viewed as the basis for the nurse–patient relationship. Gastmans (2002) acknowledges this by suggesting that fidelity is to do with faithfulness. Two ethical issues arise from this: confidentiality and advocacy, and these will be explored in more detail later in the chapter.

Jot This Down

Tim is admitted to the surgical unit for abdominal surgery, he also suffers from the early stages of MS (multiple sclerosis). He admits that he needs a bit of support to get in and out of bed, and you negotiate with him to use the call button to alert the nursing team to assist in this. That evening Tim falls as he tries to get out of bed unassisted.

- Tim has agreed with the nurse how to protect himself from accidental injury
- He does not follow the agreement to get help before getting out of bed.

  How has the principle of fidelity been compromised here?

In the 'Jot This Down' scenario, the nurse–patient relationship has been affected by the action of the patient, who has not followed up on his promise. The difficulty for the nurse here is to understand the behaviour behind this, and to make allowances for individual constraints and contradictions that can manifest in the patients we care for. A person might agree to alert the nurse to his needs, but continue to behave in a way that does not allow this. Fidelity always involves an agreement and vice versa.

Veracity

The principle of veracity is the need to tell the truth and to avoid misinterpretation and deception. In nursing and health care, this is not as straightforward as it may seem.

Some healthcare workers feel uncomfortable about revealing the truth of a person's condition, saying that the truth may do more harm than good. The most compelling argument in favour of full disclosure is that patients are then in the best position to make choices (exercise autonomy) about how their treatment will develop. By telling the truth to patients, nurses imply a genuine concern for the person's well-being. This is linked to the principle of beneficence. Individuals have the right to information (as set out in the Data Protection Act 1998). Autonomy is closely related to dignity and it could be argued that by not telling an individual the truth, their dignity is undermined. It can also be argued that the person's best interests can be affected. Disclosure of information can influence the choices that patients make in relation to treatment options and healthy behaviour (O'Sullivan 2009). There can be a problem for nurses in deciding the amount of information that is right to disclose, to whom and in what circumstances.

Legal and Ethical Dilemmas in Nursing

A dilemma is a choice between two unpleasant, ethically troubling alternatives. Nurses face dilemmas almost daily, many commonly experienced dilemmas involve confidentiality; a person's rights and issues of dying and death. The nurse must use ethical and legal guidelines to make decisions about moral actions when providing care in these and in many other situations. However, it should be acknowledged that no one profession is responsible for ethical decisions, and it is important in a complex care situation for all caregivers to be involved in decisions.

Confidentiality

'The Code' (NMC 2008a) states that:

- *You must respect people's right to confidentiality*
- *You must ensure people are informed about how and why information is shared by those who will be providing their care*
- *You must disclose information if you believe someone may be at risk of harm, in line with the law of the country in which you are practising.*

Nurses are responsible for protecting the confidentiality and security of the individual's health information. A duty of confidence (derived from common law and statute law) arises when one person (a patient) discloses information to another party (a nurse) where it is reasonable to expect that the information shared will be held in confidence. In this way, the nurse is protecting the rights of the individual. This is identified in Article 8 of the 1998 Human Rights Act, which asserts that we all have a right to privacy, and that right can only be overruled in the interest of national security, public safety, prevention of crime, the protection of health and morals or the protection of the rights and freedom of others.

Red Flag Some Examples of How Confidentiality Can Be Breached

It is not acceptable for nurses and midwives to:

- Discuss matters related to the people in their care outside the clinical setting
- Discuss a case with colleagues in public where they may be overheard
- Leave records unattended where they may be read by unauthorised persons

In 2013, Dame Fiona Caldicott carried out a government review (known as the Caldicott review) into the sharing of information (what she described as information governance), stating that every citizen should feel confident that information about their health is securely safeguarded and shared appropriately. She highlighted that everyone working in the healthcare system should see information governance as part of their responsibility.

The Evidence The Caldicott Review 2013: Revised List of the Caldicott principles

1. **Justify the purpose(s):** every proposed use or transfer of personal confidential data should be defined, scrutinised and documented
2. **Don't use personal confidential data unless it is absolutely necessary:** the need for patients to be identified should be considered
3. **Use the minimum necessary personal confidential data:** when this is deemed essential, consider and justify so the minimum amount of personal data is transferred
4. **Access to personal confidential data should be on a strict need-to-know basis**
5. **Everyone with access to confidential data should be aware of their responsibilities**
6. **Comply with the law:** organisations must comply with legal requirements
7. **The duty to share information can be as important as the duty to protect patient confidentiality:** this supports the notion of the best interests of the patient in line with professional, employer and regulatory bodies.

(DH 2013)

Patient/client records hold a great deal of personal information that can easily identify them. Data such as name, date of birth and so on are necessary components to apply care within a safe framework. Records also contain additional information about a person's health, lifestyle, past and current health issues. Figure 5.2 demonstrates the legislation that has been developed to support confidentiality in the UK.

Jot This Down

Disclosure means the giving of information

- Under what circumstances can the nurse be required to disclose patient/client information?

In the 'Jot This Down' exercise above, you may have considered the following as reasons to disclose information about those in your care:

- *Disclosure with consent* – explicit consent is either verbal or written; implied consent is when there is an assumption that information can be shared within the care team. As a nurse you should make people in your care aware of the need to share information within the team.
- *Disclosure without consent* – this is when exceptional circumstances overrule the right to a person's confidentiality. Under common law, if a person is deemed a threat to the public, disclosure can be an option.

The Data Protection Act 1998	• Governs the processing of information that identifies individuals • Applies to all forms of data, paper and electronic
The Human Fertilisation and Embryology Act 1990	• Places a statutory ban on disclosure relating to gamete donors and people receiving treatment • Healthcare workers have been prosecuted under this act
The National Health Service Venereal Disease Regulations (SI 1974 No.29)	• The non-disclosure of persons treated for STIs
The Mental Capacity Act (2005)	• Empowers and protects people to make decisions for themselves
The Freedom Of Information Act 2000 (Scotland 2002)	• Grant people rights of access to information not covered by the Data Protection Act 1998
The Computer Misuse Act 1990	• Secures data against unauthorised access

Figure 5.2 **UK legislation related to confidentiality.**

- *Disclosure to third parties* – information is shared to others not directly involved in the person's care. Individuals should be made aware of this and give their consent.
- *Nurse acting as a witness in a court case* – if summoned, nurses are compelled to give evidence. Refusal to disclose information can render them in contempt of court.

Red Flag

 One of the fundamental areas of good practice associated with disclosure is for the nurse to keep a clear documented account of the decision-making process and the advice sought in any situation.

Consent

All adults must be presumed to have the mental capacity to agree to or refuse treatment. As such, any competent patient can decline any examination, any investigation or any proposed treatment, even if this treatment is considered 'life-saving'. It is imperative that the person consents before any treatment, care or examination. If a person refuses intervention, but it still goes ahead, then this is a civil or criminal wrong, so-called 'trespass against the person', and practitioners could see themselves falling foul of assault and battery, and be called to account by the NMC. Harm in this situation can result in an accusation of negligence on the part of the nurse.

Patients and clients may give what is known as *implied consent*, as in the primary care scenario.

What the Experts Say Implied Consent

Patients attending the clinic, by the very nature of them turning up for their appointment, implies that they are willing to discuss and consider the treatments that can take place. Nonetheless, it is my responsibility to respect their right to autonomy. A patient might roll up their sleeve for a blood test, but it is always important to provide information and to make sure that the patient is happy to go ahead with investigations or treatment.

(District Nursing Sister)

For consent to be valid, there are three key principles that have to be satisfied:

1. Consent is *informed*
2. The individual is *competent*
3. Consent is *voluntary*.

Informed Consent

The process of obtaining consent is important and is underpinned in 'The Code' (NMC 2008a). Individuals need to be given clear information about the nature and purpose of even basic treatments, and failure to provide sufficient information would invalidate consent. Where consent has been given, then no charge of trespass of the person can take place. Appreciations of legal cases that illustrate past examples are useful to understand the consequences of consent.

The Evidence

The courts (Sidaway v. Bethlam Royal Hospital Governors and Others 1985) have clearly demonstrated that when a competent individual has given consent (uncoerced) for a procedure to be performed, an action for trespass to the person cannot proceed.

The patient should receive information about the nature of care that they will receive. This is supported by 'The Code' (NMC 2008a), which states that 'you must uphold people's rights to be fully informed in decisions about their care'; for example how treatment might be administered; for what time frame; if treatment will involve inpatient care; the expected outcome of treatment; and any side-effects that may be experienced, etc. The difficulty that many nurses face is in deciding the level and amount of information that should be given or offered.

One of the key reasons for providing the patient with information is to enable him/her to make a balanced judgement on whether to provide or withhold consent. The nurse is advised to provide the patient with any information that is 'material' or 'significant' (DH 2009) in relation to the risks for the patient.

Mental Capacity and the Right to Refuse Treatment

All adults are said to have the capacity to consent. However, there may be situations where doubt exists and an assessment of capacity should be made.

Jot This Down

What factors do you think might affect the person's capacity to consent to treatment?

In the 'Jot This Down' exercise above, you may have considered a number of factors that can affect an individual's capacity to make choices. Imagine the patient that you were introduced to right at the start of the chapter, the one who is admitted to a critical care environment. It is reasonable to assume that the patient in this scenario may be suffering:

- Fear and /or anxiety
- Pain
- The influence of medication
- Confusion
- Shock/panic.

Competent Patients

The starting point here is the assumption that all competent adults have the absolute right to refuse or to withdraw from treatment, even if this decision means that the individual will suffer or die as a result of this. The 'Code' reinforces this for nurses and midwives when it states, 'You must respect and support people's rights to accept or decline treatment and care'. In 'The Evidence' box below, you can see a famous case from 2002, which highlighted the right to refuse treatment.

The Evidence Ms B v. an NHS Hospital Trust [2002]

Ms B sustained a spinal injury, which over the course of 2 years left her paralysed from the neck down. Although fully conscious and alert, she was only able to breathe with the support of a ventilator. It was her wish to have the ventilator switched off, as she had no desire to keep on living in that way. Her doctors refused and she subsequently brought a court action against the NHS Trust. The court was satisfied that Ms B was competent and her decision was not influenced by mental health breakdown. Continued ventilation in this case was ruled as battery and so the ventilator was removed and Ms B was allowed to die.

In 'The Evidence' box, Ms B was asking for medical support to be withdrawn and Dame Elizabeth Butler-Sloss made the ruling that Ms B had the mental capacity to refuse treatment; that is, she was deemed competent. If a person is to be considered competent, then he or she must be able to understand and retain information that is shared in order to make decisions. Alongside this, individuals need to be aware of and understand the consequences of refusing treatment. Three elements emerge associated with capacity:

- Understanding and the ability to retain information
- Knowledge of the consequences of refusing treatment
- Evaluation of the facts in making a decision.

A person's control over their life when their competency or mental capacity has been altered is through the use of advanced directives (referred to as an advanced decision to refuse treatment in the Mental Capacity Act 2005).

The NMC (2008a) demands that nurses are aware of the legislation regarding mental capacity, ensuring that people who lack capacity remain at the centre of decision-making and are fully safeguarded. The Mental Capacity Act of 2005, which came into force in 2007, defines mental capacity. It sets out the legal requirements for assessing whether or not a person lacks the capacity to make a decision. Where a person lacks the capacity to make a decision for themselves, any decision must be made in that person's best interests. The Mental Capacity Act (2005) is enforced in England and Wales and is applicable to all those working in health and social care, who are involved in the care, treatment and support of those aged 16 or over who may lack the capacity to make decisions for themselves.

The Evidence The Mental Capacity Act (2005)

The Act sets out five principles to apply where decisions relating to mental capacity have to be made:

1. A person must be assumed to have capacity unless it is established that he lacks capacity.
2. A person is not to be treated as unable to make a decision unless all practicable steps to help him to do so have been taken without success.
3. A person is not to be treated as unable to make a decision merely because he makes an unwise decision.
4. An act done, or decision made, under this Act for or on behalf of a person who lacks capacity must be done, or made, in his best interests.
5. Before the act is done, or the decision is made, regard must be had to whether the purpose for which it is needed can be as effectively achieved in a way that is less restrictive of the person's rights and freedom of action.

(Dimond 2009)

Under The Mental Capacity Act (2005), a person lacks capacity if:

- they have an impairment or disturbance (e.g. a disability, condition or trauma or the effect of drugs or alcohol) that affects the way their mind or brain works, and
- that impairment or disturbance means that they are unable to make a specific decision at the time it needs to be made.

Nursing Field Learning Disabilities: The Mental Capacity Act (2005)

The patient must be able to communicate his/her decision to the healthcare team. The nurse should never underestimate the patient's ability to communicate regardless of physical or psychological condition. For example, in the case of a patient with learning disabilities, the nurse must make use of all resources available to facilitate communication, and this may include taking time to explain to the individual the issues in simple language, employing visual aids and if appropriate, signing. It may be advisable for the nurse to engage the support of those who know the patient, for example the family, carers and staff from statutory and non-statutory agencies.

Voluntary Consent

Consent must be given freely and voluntarily, without any pressure or undue influence being exerted on the patient. If the nurse feels the patient is being pressurised into agreeing to (or refusing) treatment, he/she should arrange to see the patient alone to ascertain if the decision is truly that of the patient.

Coercion invalidates consent. If a patient is being treated in an environment where he/she is being involuntarily detained, for example a psychiatric hospital, a psychiatric unit or a prison, care must be taken to ensure that the patient is not being coerced (DH 2009).

Consent in Children

Nurses working with children and young people must work within the legal framework for consent and capacity. When obtaining consent, the nurse should consider whether the child is legally competent, and children as a rule should be involved in decisions about their care as much as possible. Gaining consent from this age group will be the same as it is for adults. However, in this age group the refusal of treatment despite the person being aged over 16 years and competent, can be overridden by a person with parental responsibility or the order of a court.

Nursing Field Children's Nursing

In England and Wales, children under the age of 16 are generally considered to lack the capacity to consent or to refuse treatment. The onus in this situation is on the parents or those with parental responsibility.

Young people aged 16 and 17 are presumed able or competent to give consent, although it is deemed good practice to involve parents in the discussions.

In Scotland, The Age of Legal Capacity Act (1991) has one important difference – that parents cannot override the refusal of consent by a competent child. It states that the decision of competence lies with the qualified medical practitioner based on the child's capability to understand the nature and consequences of treatment and procedures.

Red Flag

 Childminders, teachers and others who are caring for children cannot give consent on behalf of those in their care.

Those under 16 years of age who have sufficient understanding and intelligence to enable them to fully understand what is involved in the proposed intervention may have the capacity to consent to that intervention (DH 2009) Children who possess these abilities are said to be 'Gillick competent'.

The Evidence Gillick Competence, Fraser Guidelines

The term 'Gillick competent' comes from a court case, Gillick v. West Norfolk and Wisbech Area Health Authority [1985] 3 All ER HL. This concerned a teenage girl's right to consent to medical treatment without her parents' knowledge.

The questions that need to be considered are:

- Does the child understand the proposed treatment, his/her medical condition, the consequences that may emerge if he/she refuses or agrees to treatment?
- Does he/she understand the moral, social and family issues involved in the decision he/she is to make?
- Does the mental state of the child fluctuate?
- What treatment is to be performed – does the child understand the complexities of the proposed treatment and potential risks associated with it?

The Nurse as Advocate

Individuals who are receiving care may be unable or unprepared to make independent decisions. However, patients as consumers are better educated about options for care, and may have very definite opinions. The nurse as an advocate actively promotes the person's rights to autonomy and freedom of choice. By speaking for the person, she/he mediates between the person and others, and/or protects the person's right to self-determination or autonomy. Advocacy, empowerment, patient-centred care and patient involvement in their care are principal themes of the Royal College of Nursing (**http://www.rcn.org.uk/principles**).

What the Experts Say

> Often after the consultant surgeon has spoken to our patients, there can be a need to revisit the information that has been shared. Patients will often say, 'I didn't like to bother the doctor about silly concerns, but I would like you to help me with something'. I feel that by listening and guiding patients in this way helps to explore any concerns the individual might have. This allows them to make independent choices.

(Charge Nurse, GI Surgical unit)

As a nurse, you must practise advocacy founded on the belief that individuals have the right to choose treatment options without coercion, based on information about the outcome of accepting or rejecting the treatment. The nurse must also accept and respect the decision of the individual, even although it may differ from the decision the nurse would make. According to MIND, the National Association for Mental Health – 'An advocate is someone who can both listen to you and speak for you in times of need' (Mind 2010).

The goals of the nurse as advocate are to:

- *Assess the need for advocacy*
- *Communicate with other healthcare team members*
- *Provide individual and family teaching*
- *Assist and support individual decision-making*
- *Serve as a change agent in the healthcare system*
- *Participate in health policy formulation.*

(Peate 2012)

Legal Perspectives

It is important that as a nurse you are aware of how the law impinges on your everyday practice. A range of legal issues need to be considered by the nurse when working with patients in any setting. Few areas of health care are untouched by the law, and it is often only when something adverse occurs that nurses consider the legal implications. Involvement with the legal process may occur at any time during the course of a nurse's career.

Legal Frameworks

Orderly behaviour in a collective society is governed by rules, and these rules are referred to in this context as laws. UK law has evolved over hundreds of years based on tradition, social morals and politics.

As children, we learn the rules of what is generally considered acceptable and unacceptable behaviour, and just as our ethical stance is governed by our values, so too is our respect for the authority of the law. In the care setting, patients are legally pro-

European Court of Human Rights (The Strasbourg Court)	• Enforces the Convention on Human Rights • Hears appeals against the House of Lords judgements that are against the Convention
House of Lords	• Highest court, makes judgements on points of law • Is the supreme court of appeal
Court of Appeal	• Criminal and civil divisions • Hears appeals from the Crown, County and High Court
High Court	• 3 divisions: Family, Queen's Bench and Chancery • Judges preside over decisions from Crown and County court and consider high value civil cases
Crown Court	• Will consider appeals from Magistrates Court. Deals with serious cases committed for trial or sentence
County Court	• Deals with family matters and disputes between individuals
Magistrates Court	• Deals with mostly criminal cases (96%) and some civil cases

Figure 5.3 The Court system, England and Wales.

tected because of their rights, and as nurses, we have a responsibility to be aware of how the law protects patients' rights and how to safeguard them from others who may encroach on them. (Safeguarding is discussed in detail in Chapter 8.)

Law can be viewed as a system of rules that aim to regulate the behaviour of groups or individuals, as well as defining the rights and obligations that arise as a consequence of those rules.

For the law to be effective, there has to be a system to punish those who fail to adhere to the set rules. In England and Wales, there is a well established court system whose hierarchy is shown in Figure 5.3.

Sources of Law

The principal source of law is Parliament. There are two primary forms of law: statute and common law. Acts of Parliament (or directives) and regulations of the European community are known as statute law. Common law is judge-made or case-made law in response to rulings laid down by UK law courts, the European Court of Justice or by the Court of Human Rights in Strasbourg.

- *Statute law* is established through Acts of Parliament, also known as primary legislation. Most English law is developed in this way. The law-making abilities are given to Parliament by society. There are various stages proposed and legislative law must pass through these prior to becoming enforceable. It usually starts with a Green Paper issued for consultation; following feedback, a White paper is produced that sets out government policy. An Act of Parliament does not become statute until it has passed through both Houses of Parliament (the House of Commons and the House of Lords) and received Royal assent. Secondary legislation is the making of regulation by statutory instruments.

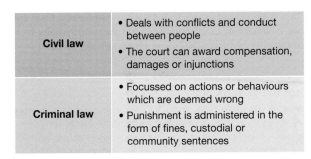

Civil law	• Deals with conflicts and conduct between people • The court can award compensation, damages or injunctions
Criminal law	• Focussed on actions or behaviours which are deemed wrong • Punishment is administered in the form of fines, custodial or community sentences

Figure 5.4 The legal system is divided into civil and criminal law.

> **The Evidence Articles of the Human Rights Act 1998**
>
> Article 2: Right to life
> Article 3: Prohibition of torture
> Article 4: Prohibition of slavery and enforced labour
> Article 5: Right to liberty
> Article 6: Right to a fair trial
> Article 7: No punishment without law
> Article 8: Respect for private and family life
> Article 9: Freedom of thought, conscience and religion
> Article 10: Freedom of expression
> Article 11: Freedom of assembly and association
> Article 12: Right to marry
> Article 14: Prohibition of discrimination.

- *Common law*, also known as case law or judge-made law, is law that is decided through the court system. This type of law comes into play when the courts cannot turn to a relevant statute. This may be because a particular Act of Parliament concerning the specific area of law under deliberation has not been made. In case law, the courts look to precedent, considering previous cases to determine how a decision has been made and how statute has been interpreted.

The legal system is divided into two parts: civil and criminal law, as identified in Figure 5.4.

The Law and NHS Provision

The National Health Service Act in 1946 was the initial starting point for the establishment of the NHS on 5 July 1948. The legislation was revisited in 1977 and again in 2006 and placed a range of duties on the Secretary of State and set out the structure of the NHS in England. The latest Act of Parliament to influence the organisation and provision of care in this country is the Health and Social Care Act 2012.

> **The Evidence The Health and Social Care Act 2012**
>
> • To safeguard its future, the NHS needs to change to meet the challenges it faces – only by modernising can the NHS tackle the problems of today and avoid the crisis of tomorrow
> • The Health and Social Care Act 2012 puts clinicians at the centre of commissioning, frees up providers to innovate, empowers patients and gives a new focus to public health.

European Law

European law can also influence English law. European laws are equally binding and applicable to all countries of the UK. The UK parliament may change laws, but it is subject to EU Court of Justice interpretation. The European Court of Human Rights in Strasbourg was developed to consider cases of human rights.

The Human Rights Act 1998

The primary aim of this Act is to give the courts greater powers to protect some fundamental rights. It introduces the European Convention on Human Rights (1950) into British domestic law. The most important principle of the legislation is that everyone's life shall be protected by law.

Articles of the Human Rights Act can influence the way that care is delivered by nurses and the principles underpinning human rights apply to all nurses in that they should:

- Maintain dignity
- Promote and protect autonomy
- Practice in a non-discriminatory manner.

A number of the specific articles of the 1998 Act impinge on nursing, for example, **Article 8** – *the right to respect for private and family life*. The article states that 'there shall be no interference by a public authority with the exercise of his rights except which in accordance with the law'. An example of how this can be interpreted can be in relation to a person's autonomy or choice around treatments that might interfere with this right.

> **Jot This Down**
>
> A District Nurse is refused entry to an elderly person's home by the son who lives there on a semi-permanent basis. He says that he is fed up of the intrusions of the so-called 'authorities' and that he can adequately care for his elderly parents if they need it.
>
> • Which article of the Human Rights Act (1998) is at play here?
> • Who has the right to refuse care in this situation?

In the 'Jot This Down' exercise above, you will have pinpointed Article 8, *The right to respect for private and family life*. This is a complicated scenario, however the Human Rights Act makes it clear that one person in a family home cannot use their right to privacy to the detriment of the rights of another person living in the home.

European Directives and Nurse Education

The European Union adopts legislation in the form of Directives and Regulations. European Directives require member states to implement their provisions for the benefit of Europe as a whole. Progammes of study at educational institutions across the country for registration as an adult nurse must comply with the requirements of two European Directives, in particular 77/453/EEC and 89/595/EEC. These requirements are mandatory and require that awards (certificates, diplomas and degrees) be granted before registration. Article 1 of 77/453/EEC requires that the qualifications of adult nurses guarantee that the person has acquired:

- Adequate knowledge of the sciences on which general nursing is based, including sufficient understanding of the structure,

104

physiological functions and behaviour of healthy and sick persons, and of the relationship between the state of health and physical and social environment of the human being

- Sufficient knowledge of the nature and ethics of the profession and of general principles of health and nursing
- Adequate clinical experience; such experience should be selected for its training value and should be gained under the supervision of qualified nursing staff in places where the number of qualified staff and the equipment are appropriate for the nursing care of patients
- The ability to participate in the training of health personnel and experience of working with such personnel
- Experience of working with members of other professions in the health sector.

This Directive also specifies that nursing programmes comprise a programme of three years with 4600 hours of training, with a balance between theory and practice. Practical instruction must include nursing in relation to:

- General and specialist medicine
- General and specialist surgery
- Child care and paediatrics
- Maternity care
- Mental health and psychiatry
- Care of the older person
- Home nursing.

Directive 89/595/EEC makes clear the balance of theory and practice and dictates that this must be not less than one-third theory and one-half practice. The Directive also defines theoretical and clinical instruction. The NMC (2010a), however, has dictated that a programme should contain 2300 hours of practice.

Duty of Care

Nurses have a duty of care. This is explicitly spelled out within The Code when it states:

> You have a duty of care at all times and people must be able to trust you with their lives and health. You are personally accountable for acts or omissions in your professional practice and must always be able to justify your decisions. You must always act lawfully, whether those laws relate to your practice or personal life.

(NMC 2008a)

This is a legal obligation to take reasonable care to avoid a breach of duty. In determining the standard of care that should be adopted, the courts have used the Bolam test. The Bolam test sets the standard that dictates how a nurse should practice in relation to other nurses; a nurse will be deemed negligent if he/she falls short of the standards expected of the 'reasonable' nurse. In summary, the nurse is judged against other reasonable nurses, how those reasonable nurses practice, and how they would act in the same or a similar situation. Below is an extract from the Bolam case that sets the expected standard:

The Evidence The Bolam test

The test is the standard of the ordinary skilled man exercising and professing to have that special skill. A man need not possess the highest expert skill at the risk of being found negligent...it is sufficient if he exercises the skill of an ordinary competent man exercising that particular art.

Once a nurse volunteers to help in an emergency, then a duty of care is assumed. Employers bind nurses contractually to safeguard patients and to maintain standards of care.

What the Experts Say

I will often hear of the anxieties that newly appointed staff and students have about their role in an emergency situation. They are worried about 'not being experienced to cope' or 'feeling out of their depth'.

The question here is – what would be reasonably expected of them in an emergency given their training and experience within the clinical setting?

(Resuscitation Specialist Nurse)

There is no precise answer to address the above concern, however a general principle would be to expect the nurse to follow the reasonable standard of approved practice referred to as the Bolam test (Bolam *v*. Friern Barnet 1957). Although this test concerns a doctor, the Bolam test is often used to judge the 'reasonableness' of any healthcare professional's actions. The final arbiter of what reasonable means will be the courts (DH 2009).

Negligence

Negligence relates to any act or omission on the part of the nurse which results in injury, harm or loss. Such acts or omissions can result in a civil claim for compensation or a criminal prosecution.

The NMC recommends that all registrants caring for patients or clients have professional indemnity insurance. This is in the interest of clients, patients and registrants in the event of a claim for professional negligence. Most employers will have various liability clauses to protect their employees in the event of negligent acts or omissions, but this cover does not usually extend to activities undertaken outside the registrant's employment. This means that independent practice would not be covered. In general, within the NHS, it is the NHS Trust that will be sued by the courts; however, a claim may also be brought against the nurse. For a successful claim of negligence, the following must be proven in a court of law:

- A duty of care is owed
- The duty of care is breached
- The breach of that duty has caused harm
- Damage or other losses have resulted from that harm.

Jot This Down

It does not matter what kind of treatment is undertaken by the individual; if all the elements of negligence above are present, there is a potential claim for damages.

- Think of examples of clinical negligence that can occur in practice.

In the 'Jot This Down' exercise above, you may have considered negligence as a result of errors in surgery, medication or diagnosis. What about less obvious negligence, such as a delay in treatment, not giving an individual the treatment they need or failing to disclose the side-effects of treatment.

The Evidence

The number of clinical claims recorded under the Clinical Negligence Scheme for Trusts (CNST) rose by more than 30% between 2009/10 and 2010/11.

NHSLA (2012)

In 'The Evidence' box above, what is demonstrated may be a reflection of the culture that is emerging with regard to compensation, combined with an increase of media coverage on cases of unacceptable levels of care and errors being made within the NHS setting. A negligence claim can be a lengthy process, and the nurse may be accountable or answerable to employers, the NMC, the civil courts and to the criminal court.

Accountability

The Code (NMC 2008a) states that:

As a professional, you are personally accountable for actions and omissions in your practice and must always be able to justify your decisions.

Nurse and midwives are involved in decision-making on a constant basis, in a wide variety of settings and often under pressure to do so. Nurses are responsible for making the best decisions based on the evidence for best practice and can be called to account to justify the decisions that they make. As such, accountability is seen as integral to professional practice. If a nurse is asked to deliver care which he or she considers is unsafe or harmful to the individual, they should carefully consider options and raise concerns with the appropriate person.

 Link To/Go To

Access the NMC website at: **http://www.nmc-uk.org**

Look at the current guidelines relating to:

- Regulation in Practice Topics – this information helps nurses and midwives apply professional judgement across a range of topics including:
  - Delegation of duties
  - Social networking sites
  - Gifts and gratuities from patients.

Accountability in Practice

The need for nursing staff to demonstrate accountability is paramount. To support accountability in practice, nurses and other healthcare staff can show:

- Evidence of competence
- Working to the range of duties as described in job descriptions
- Ongoing professional development
- Sharing of good practice
- Adherence to protocols and procedure manuals.

(RCN 2011a)

The Royal College of Nursing has developed the Principles of Nursing Practice, which guide the profession in relation to what people can expect from nursing practice, whether they are colleagues, patients or the families or carers of patients.

The Evidence The RCN Principles, Principle B

Nurses and nursing staff take responsibility for the care they provide and answer for their own judgments and actions – they carry out these actions in a way that is agreed with their patients, and the families and carers of their patients, and in a way that meets the requirements of their professional bodies and the law.

(The Principles, RCN 2011b)

Professional accountability involves assessment of the best interests of the patient, and the use of professional judgement and nursing skills to make the best decision and to enable you to account for that decision based on the best evidence available to you. Occasionally, and on behalf of the public interest, the NMC will investigate complaints made about the professional conduct or the fitness to practise of nurses and midwives on the professional register.

Accountability for Mentors

Mentors are qualified nurses who support the education and development of student nurses in practice. This mandatory requirement of the NMC ensures that all students on approved programmes of study have a mentor in practice. The mentor makes judgements about the performance of the student, their fitness for practice and ultimately for registration. As such, they are involved in determining a student's competence and ability to practise safely. Any delegation of duties to a student by the mentor must take place under supervision. As a mentor, the registered nurse's accountability is to ensure that the individual who undertakes the work is able to do so (RCN 2009). The professional guidelines to support this principle are highlighted in 'The Evidence' box below.

The Evidence Responsibilities of an NMC Mentor

Mentors are responsible and accountable for:

- Organising and coordinating student learning activities in practice
- Supervising students in learning situations and providing them with constructive feedback on their achievements
- Setting and monitoring achievements of realistic learning objectives
- Assessing total performance – including skills, attitudes and behaviours
- Providing evidence as required by programme providers of student achievement or lack of achievement
- Liaising with others (e.g. mentors, sign-off mentors, practice facilitators, practice teachers, personal tutors, programme leaders) to provide feedback, identify any concerns about the student's performance and agree action as appropriate
- Provide evidence for, or acting as, sign-off mentors with regard to making decisions about achievement of proficiency at the end of a programme.

(NMC 2008b, p. 21)

Accountability as a Student Nurse

Student nurses are exposed to a variety of practice settings and are involved in observation and participation in care activities. Over time, the expectation is that the student will become more involved in providing care. Students have a responsibility to work only within their level of understanding and competence (NMC 2002). This should always be under the supervision of a registered nurse of midwife.

What the Experts Say

I was asked to pass a urinary catheter on a woman who was having gynaecological surgery, but I had only seen this done in the simulation lab at university. I expressed my concern to my mentor, and she was great, talking me through the principles and allowing me to observe her when she passed the catheter. She had assumed that as a second year student, I would have the skills needed, but I had not yet come across this in practice.

(Student nurse, year 2, semester 3)

Although the student is supernumerary (they are additional to the workforce requirement and staffing figures), they must make an active contribution to the work of the practice area to enable them to learn how to care for patients (RCN 2007). This in itself implies accountability, but it is the registered nurse who supervises or mentors the student who is professionally responsible for the consequences of any acts or omissions on the student's part.

Red Flag

Although student nurses may not be called to account by the NMC for any acts or omissions in practice, this does not mean that they are immune from blame and can be called to account both in law and by Universities via the 'fitness for practice' route.

Delegation

The ability to delegate, assign tasks and supervise are essential competencies for all registered nurses and midwives. Decisions relating to delegation by registered nurses or midwives must be based on the fundamental principles of safety and public protection, which are the underlying principles of regulation, and according to the NMC, the following should be considered:

- The needs of the people in their care
- The stability of the people being cared for
- The complexity of the task being delegated
- The expected outcome of the delegated task
- The availability of resources to meet those needs
- The judgement of the nurse.

Registered nurses are accountable for the decision to delegate care and care should be delegated only to a person who has had appropriate training and is deemed competent to perform the task. An example might be the delegation of care to a support worker.

Red Flag

If an aspect of care is delegated, the nurse or midwife remains accountable for the overall management of the person in their care.

Where another, such as an employer, has the authority to delegate an aspect of care, the employer becomes accountable for that delegation. However, in accordance with the Code, the nurse or midwife must act without delay if they believe a colleague or anyone else may be putting someone at risk.

Raising Concerns in Practice

Because of the duty of care that nurses and midwives have for their patients, they are obligated to put the interests of the people in their care first and to act to protect them if they are considered to be at risk (NMC 2008a). No matter in what care environment nurses work, they must make themselves aware of the local policy for raising concerns and for whistle-blowing in practice. Local safeguarding policies should also be considered in order to protect patients and clients from abuse.

Raising and escalating concerns early can prevent minor issues becoming major ones (Figure 5.5) (NMC 2010b).

Red Flag

Speaking up on behalf of people in your care and clients is an everyday part of your role; failure to do so will lead you to be called to account for your actions or omissions.

The key points to consider when faced with concerns about care are clear; you must:

- Take immediate action
- Protect client confidentiality
- Refer to policy
- Record concerns and actions taken.

Concerns might include aspects related to the delivery of care to individuals or groups of people. There may be risks to health and safety with, for example, the incorrect use of harmful substances. Nurses might find themselves in an environment of care that they feel is harmful to patients, such as one that presents a risk of infection or the use of outdated, deficient clinical equipment to support care.

The Public Interest Disclosures Act of 1998 provides protection for those who honestly raise genuine concerns about wrong-doing or malpractice in the workplace. The protection extends to employees who, as a result of escalating genuine concerns, are victimised or dismissed for doing so.

All senior staff and clinical leaders in nursing should make available appropriate systems for raising concerns in practice, and should ensure that concerns are investigated promptly with a full objective assessment of the situation. Senior staff who investigate concerns should protect staff who raise concerns from unwarranted criticisms, and keep them informed of the progress and outcomes (NMC 2010b).

Conclusion

Nursing practice is structured by codes of ethics and standards, and an individual can be held accountable in a court of law for failure to comply. The standards set help define the roles of nursing and are critical to moral decision-making. A helpful resource for the nursing profession is 'The Code' (NMC 2008), which highlights standards of conduct, performance and ethics for nurses and midwives.

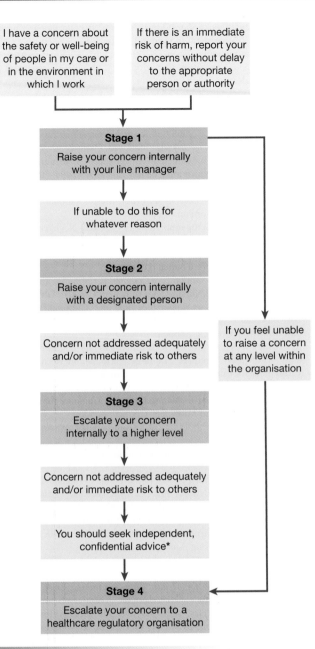

Seeking advice

If you are unsure about whether or how to raise a concern at any stage, you should seek advice.

* Independent, confidential advice is available from your professional body, trade union or PCaW. Students can also speak to their university tutor or mentor.

This flowchart should be used in conjunction with the full guidance available at www.nmc-uk.org/guidance.

Figure 5.5 Stages in raising and escalating concerns. (Reproduced with permission of the Royal College of Nursing and NMC: http://www.nmc-uk.org)

Values underpin our decisions as nurses. Values and behaviour are demonstrated in the 6Cs (caring, compassion, competence, communication, courage, commitment).

A variety of approaches in nursing underpin ethical decision-making. These include the rules that we believe to be right, the consequences of our actions and the moral codes that we live by.

Ethical principles of not harming, doing good, allowing choice and being fair also underpin nursing approaches. Legal dilemmas exist in nursing and nurses are responsible by law for their actions. In addition, people have the right to refuse treatment and to complain if treatment is poor or puts them at risk. To support this, the UK and European Law influences people's rights in healthcare situations. To meet the rights of individuals in their care, nursing staff are accountable for their actions when delivering care to patients, their families and carers, in a way that meets the requirements of their professional body and the law.

The duty of care that nurses have extends to alerting others in positions of management to situations where they have concerns. To that end, the professional body in nursing (NMC) sets clear guidelines for the escalation of concerns.

Key Points

- Nursing practice is structured by codes of ethics and standards, with which an individual can be held accountable in a court of law.
- The standards set help define the roles of nursing and are critical to moral decision-making.
- The Code (NMC 2008) highlights standards of conduct, performance and ethics for nurses and midwives.
- Values underpin our decisions and behaviours and are demonstrated in the 6Cs (caring, compassion, competence, communication, courage, commitment).
- A variety of approaches underpin ethical decision-making; these include the rules that we believe to be right, the consequences of our actions and the moral codes that we live by.
- Ethical principles of not harming, doing good, allowing choice and being fair also underpin nursing approaches.
- Legal dilemmas exist in nursing and nurses are responsible by law for their actions.
- People have the right to refuse treatment and to complain if treatment is poor or puts them at risk.
- The UK and European Law influences people's rights in healthcare situations.
- Staff are accountable for their actions when delivering care to patients, their families and carers and their actions must meet the requirements of their professional body and the law.

Glossary

Advocacy: individuals have the right to choose treatment options without coercion, based on information about the outcome of accepting or rejecting the treatment

Applied ethics: describes an approach to ethical decision-making, which uses moral theories and principles to examine and address practical issues in everyday professional life

Autonomy: respect for the rights of individuals and for their self-determination; holding self-determination and self-governance over one's actions; the ability to make one's own decisions; have the right to choose

Beneficence: doing good, providing benefits and measuring benefits against risks and cost; the prevention of harm and the promotion of good

(Continued)

Bolam test: the standard of the ordinary skilled man exercising and professing to have that special skill. A man need not possess the highest expert skill at the risk of being found negligent…it is sufficient if he exercises the skill of an ordinary competent man exercising that particular art

Common law: also known as case law or judge-made law, is law that is decided through the court system

Confidentiality: keeping personal information about others safe from disclosure to non-interested parties

Consent: the mental capacity to agree to or refuse treatment

Consequentialism: the consequences of an action is the ultimate judgement about the rightness of that action (see utilitarianism)

Deontological ethics (deontology): considers what actions are right, and has fundamental moral rules such as: it is wrong to kill, to steal, to tell lies, and it is right to keep promises

Ethics: principles of conduct; ethical behaviour is concerned with values, moral duty, obligations and the distinction between right and wrong

Fidelity: to be faithful to agreements and promises

Informed consent: where a person is fully involved in decisions about their care

Justice: derived from the general rule of human conduct to treat others fairly/distributing benefits, risks and costs fairly distributed

Mental capacity: the patient is able to communicate his/her decision to the healthcare team

Non-maleficence: do no harm

Statute law: established through Acts of Parliament, also known as primary legislation

Utilitarianism: acting in a way that brings about the greatest good for the greatest number

Values: a collection of our personal beliefs and attitudes about all aspects of our life and experiences

Veracity: to tell the truth and to avoid misinterpretation and deception

Virtue ethics: is person- rather than action-based, that is not so much about what you should do but more focussed on how you should be

References

B v. an NHS Trust (2000). EWHC 429 (Fam).

Beauchamp, T.L. & Childress, J.F. (2008) *Principles of Biomedical Ethics*, 6th edn. Oxford University Press, Oxford.

Bolam *v.* Friern Barnet *HMC* (1957) 1 All ER 118.

CQC (2012) *In-patients Survey*. http://www.cqc.org.uk/public/news/results-latest-inpatient-survey (accessed June 2013).

DH (2009) *Reference Guide to Consent for Examination or Treatment*, 2nd edn. Department of Health, London.

DH (2013) *Information: To Share Or Not To Share? The Information Governance Review*. Department of Health, London.

DH & NHS Commissioning Board (2012) *Compassion in Practice. Nursing, Midwifery and Care Staff. Our vision and strategy*. Department of Health, London.

Dickeson, D., Huxtable, R. & Parker, M. (2010) *The Cambridge Medical Ethics Workbook*, 2nd edn. Cambridge University Press, Cambridge.

Dimond, B. (2009) *Legal Aspects of Consent*, 2nd edn. Quay Books, London.

Fry, S. & Johnstone, M.J. (2008) *Ethics in Nursing Practice: A Guide to Ethical Decision Making*, 3rd edn. Blackwell, Oxford.

Gastmans, C. (2002) A fundamental ethical approach to nursing. Some proposals for ethics education. *Nursing Ethics*, 9(5), 494–507.

Hendrick, J. (2004) *Law and Ethics*. Nelson Thorne, Cheltenham.

Mind (2010) *The MIND Guide to Advocacy*. Mind (National Association for Mental Health), London.

NHSLA (2012/13) NHS Litigation Authority Clinical Negligence Scheme for Trusts. NHS Litigation Authority, London.

NMC (2002) *An NMC Guide for Students of Nursing and Midwifery*. Nursing and Midwifery Council, London.

NMC (2008a) *The Code: Standards of Conduct, Performance and Ethics for Nurses and Midwives*. Nursing and Midwifery Council, London.

NMC (2008b) *Standards to Support Learning and Assessment in Practice. NMC Standards for Mentors, Practice Teachers and Teachers*. Nursing and Midwifery Council, London.

NMC (2010a) *Standards for Pre registration Nursing Education*. Nursing and Midwifery Council, London. http://standards.nmc-uk.org/PublishedDocuments/Standards%20for%20pre-registration%20nursing%20education%2016082010.pdf (accessed June 2013).

NMC (2010b) *Raising and Escalating Concerns. Guidance for Nurses and Midwives*. Nursing and Midwifery Council, London.

O'Sullivan, E. (2009) Withholding truth from patients. *Nursing Standard*, 23(48), 35–40.

Peate, I. (2012) *The Student's Guide to Becoming a Nurse*. Wiley-Blackwell, Chichester.

Q“allington, J. (2012) *Ethics, Values and the Role of the Nursing Student. Nursing 2012 and Beyond*. http://www.rcn.org.uk/__data/assets/pdf_file/0005/445217/Ethics,_Values_and_the_Role_of_the_Nursing_Student_Jan_Quallington.pdf (accessed June 2013).

RCN (2007) *Helping Students Get the Best from Their Practice Placements*. Royal College of Nursing, London.

RCN (2009) *Guidance for Mentors of Nursing Students and Midwives*. 2nd edn. RCN Toolkit. Royal College of Nursing, London.

RCN (2011a) *First Steps for Health Care Assistants*. Royal College of Nursing, London. http://www.rcn.org.uk/__data/assets/pdf_file/0004/387265/RCN_23930_First_steps_A5_flyer.pdf (accessed June 2013).

RCN (2011b) *The Principles of Nursing Practice*. Royal College of Nursing, London.

Seedhouse, D. (2002) An ethical perspective – how to do the right thing. In: J. Tingle, A. Cribb (eds.) *Nursing Law and Ethics*, 2nd edn, pp 150–158. Blackwell, Oxford.

Sidaway v. Bethlam Royal Hospital Governors and Others (1985) 1 All ER 643.

Thompson, I.E., Melia, K.M., Boyd, K.M. & Horsburgh, D. (2006) *Nursing Ethics*, 5th edn. Churchill Livingstone, Edinburgh.

Test Yourself

1. What is the publication that guides the ethical framework for nurses and midwives and protects the public?
    (a) Standards for medicines management (2007)
    (b) Standards for specialist education in practice (2001)
    (c) The code: Standards of conduct, performance and ethics for nurses and midwives (2008)
    (d) Standards to support learning and assessment in practice (2008)

2. The Chief Nursing officer for England set the vision for nursing in the 6Cs. These are:
    (a) Capability, caring, consideration, compassion, compliance, competence
    (b) Caring, compassion, competence, communication, courage, commitment
    (c) Communication, courage, caring, capability, commitment, conversation
    (d) Caring, compassion, courage, communication, capability, commitment

3. Applied ethics means an approach to ethical decision-making that:
    (a) Is based on rules-based thinking
    (b) Is concerned with the best outcome for the biggest group
    (c) Is nothing to do with the decisions that nurses face in care
    (d) Is based on practical issues in everyday professional life

4. The Quality Care Commission provides inpatient surveys and in 2012, it demonstrated that the percentage of nurses that did not talk in front of them as if they were not there was:
    (a) 20%
    (b) 70%
    (c) 81%
    (d) 76%

5. There are three approaches to the process of ethical thinking. These are:
    (a) Seeing, thinking, doing
    (b) Rules based, outcomes based, virtue based
    (c) Thinking based, rules based, application based
    (d) Rules, application and virtue ethics

6. The term deontology means
    (a) Duty-based ethics
    (b) Outcome-based ethics
    (c) Consequential ethics
    (d) Applied ethics

7. The notion in ethics of the 'greatest good for the greatest number' relates directly to:
    (a) Virtue ethics
    (b) Deontology
    (c) Values
    (d) Utilitarian ethics

8. Justice as an ethical principle is concerned with:
    (a) Avoiding harm
    (b) Fairness
    (c) Doing good
    (d) Virtue ethics

9. For consent to be valid in this country, there are three principles that have to be satisfied. These are that the patient is:
    (a) Informed, competent and awake
    (b) Competent, volunteers and informed
    (c) Informed, aware and competent
    (d) Competent, alert and volunteers

10. Childminders, teachers and others who are caring for children can normally give consent for those in their care. True or False?
    (a) True
    (b) False

Answers

1. c
2. b
3. d
4. c
5. b
6. a
7. d
8. b
9. b
10. b

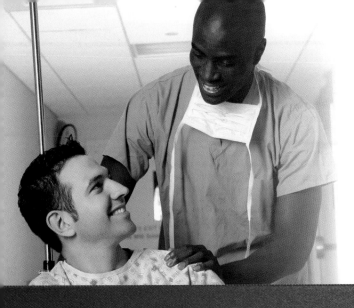

6

The Nursing Process

Mike Lappin

University of Salford, UK

Learning Outcomes

On completion of this chapter you will be able to:

- Summarise the many definitions of nursing
- Demonstrate a knowledge of the history of the Nursing Process and gain an insight into the concept (philosophy/principles) of the Nursing Process
- Consider the philosophy and relate it to the practice of nursing, and consider the organisational models of care
- Have an understanding of the stages of the Nursing Process: assessment, diagnosis, planning, implementation and evaluation (ADPIE)
- Gain an insight into the importance of the nursing diagnosis
- Have an understanding of how 'intentional rounding' and compassion link to the concept of individualised care

Competencies

All nurses must:

1. Appreciate the value of evidence in practice, be able to understand and appraise research, apply relevant theory and research findings to their work and identify areas for further investigation
2. Build partnerships and therapeutic relationships through safe, effective and non-discriminatory communication. They must take account of individual differences, capabilities and needs
3. Use the full range of communication methods, including verbal, non-verbal and written, to acquire, interpret and record their knowledge and understanding of people's needs. They must be aware of their own values and beliefs and the impact this may have on their communication with others. They must take account of the many different ways in which people communicate and how these may be influenced by ill health, disability and other factors, and be able to recognise and respond effectively when a person finds it hard to communicate
4. Maintain accurate, clear and complete records, including the use of electronic formats, using appropriate and plain language

(Continued)

Nursing Practice: Knowledge and Care, First Edition. Edited by Ian Peate, Karen Wild and Muralitharan Nair.
© 2014 John Wiley & Sons, Ltd. Published 2014 by John Wiley & Sons, Ltd. Companion website: www.wileynursingpractice.com

Competencies (*Continued*)

5. Use up-to-date knowledge and evidence to assess, plan, deliver and evaluate care, communicate findings, influence change and promote health and best practice. They must make person-centred, evidence-based judgements and decisions, in partnership with others involved in the care process, to ensure high quality care. They must be able to recognise when the complexity of clinical decisions requires specialist knowledge and expertise, and consult or refer accordingly

6. Carry out comprehensive, systematic nursing assessments that take account of relevant physical, social, cultural, psychological, spiritual, genetic and environmental factors, in partnership with service users and others through interaction, observation and measurement.

Introduction

On nursing…A distinct profession, providing direct assistance to individuals in whatever setting they are found for the purpose of avoiding, relieving, diminishing, or curing the individual's sense of helplessness.

> (Ida Jean Orlando first described the four stages of the Nursing Process in 1958)

If you were admitted to hospital or in need of nursing care in any setting, you would expect the nurses caring for you to be gentle, considerate, compassionate and concerned for your well-being. The care you receive should be personal and centred around you as an individual. The Nursing Process has been advocated by many nurses as a means of moving nursing from a depersonalised, task-focussed, traditional style of nursing towards an individualised, patient-centred philosophy of care (Ford & Walsh 1994, p. 181). In any caring environment, this should be a given; however, it is worth remembering that for nurses to practise their art, they require a number of tools to allow this. The Nursing Process is one such tool that assists nurses to plan care; it is a framework that helps the nurse to focus on the 'person' and will help set a pathway leading to a world of patient comfort, rehabilitation and recovery depending on the observable conditions.

Defining Nursing

Before introducing the concept of the Nursing Process and how we utilise the framework, it is important to first define what nursing is. There are many definitions of nursing. The Royal College of Nursing (RCN 2003, pp. 5–7) highlights many of these, including the classic description by Florence Nightingale and that of the World Health Organization (WHO). However, the most often quoted and widely used definition comes from Virginia Henderson and was taken up by the International Council of Nurses (ICN) in 1960. In it, she describes the 'unique function of the nurse' as:

> *…to assist the individual, sick or well, in the performance of those activities contributing to the health or its recovery (or to peaceful death) that he would perform unaided if he had the necessary strength, will or knowledge…*

> (Henderson 1966, quoted in Aggleton & Chalmers 1986, p. 18)

The RCN (2003, p. 6) quite rightly points out that this is only the first part of Henderson's definition and only one part of nursing, and it is unfortunate that it is often used as if it were the full definition. It stresses the continuation:

In addition she helps the patient to carry out the therapeutic plan as initiated by the physician, and she also, as a member of a team, helps others as they in turn help her, to plan and carry out the total programme whether it be for the improvement of health, or recovery from illness, or support in death.

Hall and Ritchie (2009, pp. 6–7) put forward a number of reasons for a clear definition of what nursing is. It enables nurses to describe nursing to people who do not understand it; it helps to clarify the role within the multidisciplinary (MDT) team; it will influence the policy agenda at both a local and national level and it will develop educational curricula and identify areas where research is needed to strengthen the knowledge base of the profession. It will also inform decisions about whether and how nursing work should be delegated to others and support negotiations at local and national level on issues such as nurse staffing, skill mix and nurses' pay.

The Evidence

Experience shows that as far as the patient is concerned, they are basically unaccustomed to the way we organise our work. Christine Beasley, the then Chief Nursing Officer (CNO) for England, rightly pointed out:

Nursing may not be easy to describe but patients know when they get good nursing and when they do not. Nursing requires a high level set of skills and understanding which taken separately may seem commonplace and undemanding but combined as a whole is far more complex and powerful.

(Christine Beasley, CNO for England, DH 2006, p. 4)

It is crucial that nurses utilise the structure the Nursing Process offers in order to continue to deliver the appropriate nursing interventions based on a sound assessment and plan of care. Your patient may not be aware of the systems we use but they will certainly garner the benefits of the arrangements we put in place.

Jot This Down

- Take some time to think about your personal definition of nursing
- Discuss this with your colleagues and maybe ask your patient what nursing means to them

  How do perceptions differ?

  What have you learned from the patient's description of nursing?

No doubt, you will find from completing the 'Jot This Down' exercise above, that each individual will come up with a different definition of nursing. This obviously depends on where the person is placed at that time.

Long before the inception of the Nursing and Midwifery Council (NMC) in April 2002, guidance was provided to registrants by the United Kingdom Central Council for Nursing, Midwifery and Health Visiting (UKCC). This was set up in 1983 and like the NMC, its primary function was to underscore the principles required for nurse registration and thus present a method through which the organisation would employ its main purpose of protecting the public. It is hard to believe that in 1999, the UKCC remained uncertain about the value of trying to come up with a definition of nursing, and concluded that:

A definition of nursing would be too restrictive for the profession.

In nursing practice, however, some measurement is necessary for the intention of formulating guidelines, the design of nursing services and the advancement of programmes of nurse education. As Clark and Lang (1992) have pointed out:

If we cannot name it, we cannot control it, finance it, research it, teach it, or put it into public policy.

Nursing is:

the use of clinical judgement in the provision of care to enable people to improve, maintain, or recover health, to cope with health problems, and to achieve the best possible quality of life, whatever their disease or disability, until death.

(RCN 2003, p. 3)

The RCN (2003, p. 3) points out six defining characteristics of nursing; the list features the promotion of health, healing and growth, modes of intervention, people's physiological/psychological/social/cultural or spiritual response to health and illness and the commitment to the nurse–patient partnership. Point 4 describes the focus of nursing on the whole person and the human response, rather than a particular aspect of the person or a particular pathological condition. While all the characteristics are connected in some way to the overall concept of the Nursing Process, it is Point 4 that stands from the rest in terms of the holistic approach to care and the nursing judgement and interventions that follow a medical diagnosis.

The (RCN 2003, p. 4) continued to highlight the difficulties associated with grading the work of nurses and nursing. There will come a point in our lives where we will all experience nursing in some shape or form, and yet, it is still very complicated to explain; even nurses find it difficult to articulate an adequate definition when asked to do so.

In 1859, Florence Nightingale wrote:

The elements of nursing are all but unknown.

(Skretkowicz 1992)

Even today, this declaration rings true. Nursing can be allied to the physical tasks we deliver at the bedside, ensuring that the patient is treated as an individual in an environment that is clean, safe, and comfortable.

Jot This Down

- Think about the public's awareness of nursing and the role nurses play
- What do *you* think is the public perception of our work as nurses?

As you did in the previous 'Jot This Down' exercise, you may find that from completing this exercise, each individual will have common perceptions of the profession but there will be many variations among the group. This may depend on the person's experiences of health care and nursing.

Nursing is seen by some as supporting medicine and the physicians by carrying out work coupled to the medical management of patients. Of course, these are fundamental aspects and are part of our practice, but the idea that nursing consists of these elements alone ignores the wider contribution of professional nursing to health care, and will result in a service which does not offer its full potential (RCN 2003, p. 4). Ford *et al.* (2004, p. 3–6) have examined much of the sound research evidence that there is to demonstrate that skilled nursing makes a difference. Jane Cummings, the Chief Nursing Officer for England, and Viv Bennett, the Department of Health Nursing Director (DH & NHS 2012, pp. 4–5) acknowledged this by saying how constantly impressed they are by the dedication shown by nurses to improving the quality of care; they also point to the significant difference made by nurses. As the RCN (2003) have said, part of the paradox is that the more skilful a nurse is in what they do, the less likely it is that the observer, or even the patient, will recognise exactly what has been done.

We know that not all nursing is done by qualified nurses; anymore than all law enforcement work is done by trained police officers. A patient's relatives, unofficial carers and a variety of support workers and healthcare assistants will also carry out this work. Their involvement is precious for the patient, but it does differ from that of the registered nurse. The RCN (2003) highlights the distinction between professional nursing and the nursing undertaken by other people, stating that it does not lie in the type of task performed, nor in the level of skill that is required to perform a particular task. As for all professional practice, the difference lies in:

- *The clinical judgement inherent in the processes of assessment, diagnosis, prescription and evaluation*
- *The knowledge that is the basis of the assessment of need and the determination of action to meet the need*
- *The personal accountability for all decisions and actions, including the decision to delegate to others*
- *The structured relationship between the nurse and the patient which incorporates professional regulation and a code of ethics within a statutory framework.*

(RCN 2003, p. 4)

You will no doubt observe in practice that qualified nurses do work in a different way from support workers when caring for their patients. While assisting a patient to the toilet, the support worker will deal with the task. This will be done in the appropriate manner, with care and consideration for the patient. However, while the qualified practitioner will carry out the same task, they will also be mindful of many other aspects associated with that individual; a constant assessment and re-assessment often takes place, sometimes without the nurse really thinking about it. For instance, the nurse may be assessing her patient's mobility, asking about their diet, whether they have pain or breathlessness, as well as assessing their psychological status and asking about their home circumstances and how their family will manage when it is time for discharge. This is all done with the steps of the Nursing Process in mind. What is a fundamental aspect of care now becomes a holistic approach to the actual and potential needs of the patient. Clearly, the qualified nurse has been prepared for this through her/his education and development, and appreciative of the underlying principles and evidence base for the care she/he delivers. With the task completed and with the new information gathered, the nurse will now revisit the care plan and update it accordingly.

What the Experts Say

> Ann-Marie is a student nurse in her 2nd year; she is currently working on an acute medical ward. Her mentor tells her that the Nursing Process is 'a complete waste of time and it's just a lot of unnecessary paperwork'.
>
> Ann-Marie is currently working on a patient-centred essay that requests that she use a Nursing Process approach. Her mentor's statement is the last thing she wants to hear if she is to remain motivated to complete the essay.
>
> (Ann-Marie, 2nd year student nurse, University of Salford)

In the scenario in the 'What the Experts Say' above, Ann-Marie is faced with a dilemma; she has completed a lot of reading, including numerous analyses of the Nursing Process, and she is shocked by her mentor's sweeping statement and is disheartened by the opinion put forward.

Jot This Down

- What do you think Ann-Marie should do?
- How should she approach the issue with her mentor?

In the 'Jot This Down' exercise above, you may have highlighted Ann-Marie's need to speak to her mentor (in a professional manner) to establish exactly what she meant by the comments. This may be an opportunity for both practitioners to discuss their own views and explain their judgements to each other. This makes for a healthy debate and gives them both an opening for reflection. This can be done in an informal manner – over the coffee break perhaps?

Florence Nightingale's focus on the promotion of health and healing, as distinct from the cure of illness and the harmony of the person, health and the environment, remains central to modern definitions of nursing (Skretkowicz 1992). This too, can be linked to the process of nursing. Person-centred nursing allows for recovery, rehabilitation or comfort of people who present with any illness or condition. Planning the care for these people helps them to deal with the situations, needs or requirements associated with the circumstances.

The RCN (2003, p. 7) refers to the same key concepts found in the definition of nursing developed by the World Health Organization (WHO 1991) in response to the Strategy of Health for All by the year 2000.

The Evidence

The mission of nursing in society is to help individuals, families and groups to determine and achieve their physical, mental and social potential, and to do so within the challenging context of the environment in which they live and work. This requires nurses to develop and perform functions that relate to the promotion and maintenance of health as well as to the prevention of ill health. Nursing also includes the planning and implementation of care during illness and rehabilitation, and encompasses the physical, mental and social aspects of life as they affect health, illness, disability and dying. Nursing is the provision of care for individuals, families and groups throughout the entire life-span – from conception to death. Nursing is both an art and a science that requires the understanding and application of the knowledge and skills specific to the discipline. It also draws on knowledge and techniques derived from the humanities and the physical, social, medical and biological sciences.

(RCN 2003, p.7)

Organisational Models of Care

Lintern (2012) reported on the workforce research carried out for the Royal College of Nursing, which concluded that patient care in the NHS could suffer because of a future shortage of nurses. Many hospitals will face difficult times in attempting to maintain nursing staff numbers and optimum skill-mix. We need to adjust the way we organise nursing care accordingly; to help us do this, it must be a guarantee that each area of practice makes best use of the available staff and utilises their skills and experience. Ford and Walsh (1994, p. 186) highlight the many criticisms of the Nursing Process and the notion that it is a waste of nursing time, with endless paperwork and a ritualistic, task-centred process. However, it can be argued that a model underpins the delivery of care via the Nursing Process and can be fully implemented within a primary nursing system. It gives structure to the assessment and guides the nurse away from irrelevant areas (Ford & Walsh 1994, p. 206). This is clearly one of the key advantages of the Nursing Process; using the documentation appropriately will help the nurse to see that from a robust assessment comes the identification of key patient-centred goals. This in turn will lead to important nursing interventions ensuring that valuable nursing time is administered accordingly, without the distractions of the more extraneous issues. What we see here is true patient-centred care and when the Nursing Process is used in combination with an appropriate organisational model of care, it results in an empowered workforce that can prioritise care, manage time, problem-solve and make decisions about patients and ultimately influence the quality of care in practice. The remainder of this section aims to give an overview of the organisational models of care and help you to appreciate how the Nursing Process could compliment the most appropriate system.

 Link To/Go To

http://currentnursing.com/nursing_theory/models_of_nursing_care_delivery.html

This page shows the models of nursing care delivery; it also links to some of the important nursing theories developed worldwide.

In their seminal work, Walsh and Ford (1990) demonstrated the rituals of clinical practice, examining the patient's day and comparing it to the nurse's day. They made recommendations for good practice, including an evaluation of the routine tasks we carry out and the need to ask patients what they want in order to improve their hospital stay and develop patient-centred care further. It was argued that many of the rituals that take place are staff-centred; getting the job done within a specific window of time was more important than dealing with patients' needs on an individual basis. Completing all the work before the staff on the late shift arrived seemed more important than addressing any wishes that the patient may have had. Not all people want to be awoken at 6.30a.m. to be given their medication; the patient may not want to be bathed first thing in the morning, opting instead for a bath during the afternoon or early evening.

Jot This Down

- What rituals have you noticed in practice?
- How should we deal with these issues for the benefit of the patient?
- Is the care on your ward/area patient-centred or staff-centred?

In the 'Jot This Down' exercise above, you have been asked a number of key questions in relation to the way nursing work is organised. You may have thought about the habitual practice we experience at handover; a group of nurses sat huddled in the office for up to 60 minutes! In this time, we are expected to write down the important facts associated with the mass of information given to us. If you have four nurses in the office during handover, 60 minutes becomes 240 minutes (4 hours) of nursing time. Think about it!

Is it any wonder that when the nurses on the late shift finally emerge from the report that they spend the next few hours playing 'catch up', possibly missing a much needed break later due to the obligation to recover that lost time? Walsh and Ford (1990, p. 119) declared that a much more efficient use of time would be to have a bedside report, during which the nurse is responsible for a group of patients. That way you have three or four reports going on at the same time, but in the process you cut the time down to 10–15 minutes, thus saving several nursing hours. This is also an opportunity to involve the patient in the process; patients will become part of the handover, contributing to the dialogue that takes place at the bedside. This is true patient-centred care, and much more resourceful, thus giving nurses the time to get on with other work.

The Evidence

Think about the two situations below:

- I was admitted to a Dermatology Unit, because I required daily PUVA (ultraviolet) treatment. The ward staff insisted that I changed immediately into my pyjamas because they say that 'all patients have to remove their outdoor wear on admission'.
(Male, aged 23 years)
- I was admitted on to a rheumatology ward for treatment of my osteoporosis. I have managed to monitor and take my medication with no problems for the past 2 years. However, on arrival to the ward the staff insist on taking all my medication from me, telling me that from now on the staff will administer my tablets at the stipulated times on my medication sheet. I was not happy about this and I asked to speak to the nurse in charge. From their reaction to me I think the staff are beginning to think I'm going to be a 'difficult' patient.
(Female, aged 57 years)

What do you think about these two scenarios? Both scenarios are based in fact and you may want to reflect on them before you come to a reasonable conclusion. You could possibly think that this is perfectly reasonable. You may have witnessed this in practice. However, we need to ask ourselves a couple of questions here. Why does a young man need for ultraviolet in his pyjamas all day when, other than his need to take a patient, he is perfectly fit and well? Why do we are admitted to the ward medication from them as soon as they deprive the person of patient need to be in control and thus in control of her medication care? If the patient has been any problems, why shred them that length of time without What right have we to strip people of individual responsibility? independence? We must ensure that uniqueness, dignity and intact and that they have the freedom to determination is left their lives.

The Organisation of Care: A History

A lot of the organisation previously mentioned nursing, where nurses are ordered according to task task-allocated work. This structure has a long history profession and was used during the 1970s and the early when student nurses made up the bulk of the workforce. Each jobs were allocated to staff, such as washing patients, carrying observations and dressing wounds. This was done according each practitioner's level of proficiency and, in a student's case, according to their educational preparation and competence. The tasks were distributed in a hierarchical manner. Third-year students would be elevated to dealing with the more complex wounds or would be allowed to complete the 'medicines round', whereas a first-year student would be serving the morning coffee/tea or doing 2-hourly 'turns' dealing with those patients most at risk of pressure sores. It was efficient and very useful when staffing levels were low; it was easy to manage and organise and it was a way of making sure that all patients got the basic care required. In this author's experience, when involved in task allocation, his patients were clean, comfortable, safe, well-fed and adequately hydrated. It is a pity that the nurse had little or no time to form a truly therapeutic relationship or even communicate for any length of time with the patient. It was almost impossible to sit and talk to your patient at this time. Aspects of care, such as counselling, listening, health education, were virtually non-existent. Whenever nurses did get time for this, the ward sister always found something for them to do; sitting at the bedside talking to the patient was seen as 'idle time' and there was always work to be done. It was simply not seen as important at the time. You could liken it to a factory assembly line and although it clearly affected the job satisfaction of many, it got the job done!

Task allocation has consistently been shown to give low job satisfaction rate (Gullick *et al.* (2004, p. 36); again, something that this author was aware of during this period. The observation trolley, laden with the required equipment for the 'obs' round, was approached with consternation; the thought of recording the temperature, pulse and respirations of all 30 patients on the ward did not really inspire or motivate. In fact, by the time the round was well under way, it was the norm just to make an approximate calculation of the respiratory rates or to compare them with the previous recording. If a patient did not look distressed or was showing no signs of change, then a detailed individual assessment was not completed. Walsh and Ford (1990, p. 56) highlighted this and stated that respiratory rate is one of the most dreadfully neglected vital signs and it was intimated that estimation was at work here.

115

In today's healthcare environment, you would not expect ...s to happen, especially with the introduction of the Early Warning Score (EWS) for all patients. That said, nurses ne.of breathing, of the importance of a patient's depth and rh.they are to avoid as well as any pain associated with breathi.ring the task alloca- a similar situation to that which transpi. tion period.

Jot This Down

During the 197... .sual for wards to have a 'bath book' and '... .s'. Staff would be allocated to the task of ... .patients were bathed and in some elder... .en every day. Without any thought, th... .had not opened their bowels that day would ...a small enema, a laxative or suppositories to ...hem.

...nat do you think of the 'Jot This Down' scenario above?

It is hard to believe that this was the case back then. There never seemed to be any thought about the individual needs of the patients; care seemed to be centred on the staff completing their daily work. Looking back, surely it would have been more appropriate to ensure that the elderly patients be given meals that had higher roughage content, that the nurses ensured sufficient hydration and that the patient was correctly mobilised. It was this thoughtless practice that led nurses to lose sight of the patient as a holistic being and not just a body of separate parts.

Other forms of organising care included patient allocation, team nursing and primary nursing.

Patient allocation is distinguished by its ability to achieve a more holistic approach to the delivery of nursing; it could meet the requirements of the individual and demonstrated that the patient was the chief focus of our care.

Team nursing allowed for a small group of nurses to be separated into different teams often over a six- or eight-bedded area, where they would provide care for that specific cluster of patients.

Primary nursing (the author was introduced to this model during the early 1980s) aimed to develop organisation further, and link nursing care through the allocation of a single, 'named nurse' who would have 24-hour responsibility and accountability for the patient's care for the period of their hospital stay. An Australian study by Gullick et al. (2004, p. 36) was undertaken to ascertain which organisational models were used in a Sydney hospital, and how well these enabled nurses to provide a high standard of care. The findings did suggest that the patient-allocation model should be maintained where practical, and that team nursing should be trialled where poor numbers and skill-mix demand a greater degree of supervision and support. Task nursing was seen as no better or worse that any of the other organisational models. Nurses clearly knew all the people on the ward and seemed to have a broader overview of their patients, rather than knowing a lot of information about a few people. However, it did not allow nurses to develop relationships with patient or family, and more importantly, there was less staff satisfaction associated with this approach to nursing. Primary nursing seemed to harvest little in the way of appraisal in Gullick et al's (2004) study; however a number of authors have viewed the design positively, including Pearson (1988), Walsh and Ford (1990, p. 132), Manthey (1992), and Jonsdottir (1999, p. 235).

It has been reported that there are many benefits of primary nursing:

- *The provision of high quality care is facilitated*
- *Authority is decentralised*
- *Continuity of care is increased*
- *Nurses work in a professional way with responsibility for individual patients*
- *Nursing is more visible and it is easier to see one's responsibility*
- *Nursing care plans are better used*
- *Nursing care is based on individual needs.*

(Jonsdottir 1999, p. 236)

In the author's experience, it seemed an appropriate combination to participate in the delivery of primary nursing and to continue to develop the key skills associated with the Nursing Process and care planning. It allowed for high quality care that helped nurses to establish a connection with the patient. It was both challenging and rewarding; it demanded nurses have a higher degree of accountability and independence as practitioners, but the rewards were fulfilling and meant that much of the nurses' everyday work fully complimented the expectations of their patients. Therapeutic relationships were formally developed; the nurse would sit down and join forces with the patient to plan their care together. Fragmented care was becoming a thing of the past. The requirements of patient-centred care were beginning to prevail over the self-interest previously observed through staff-centred care.

Jot This Down Organisational Models of Care

Take a look at the five organisational models illustrated (Figure 6.1, Figure 6.2, Figure 6.3, Figure 6.4 and Figure 6.5) and think about what you have been exposed to in practice. Which do you think is the most appropriate, and how does this link to the way nurses make use of the Nursing Process and care planning?

You may have seen one way, all of the above or a combination. What you need to think about is which was the most effective in your experience and were you and your colleagues utilising your time and the nursing documentation accurately? If the answer is no, then why do you think this is? Low staffing levels, different shift patterns, staff detached from the Nursing Process and care plans, the ward culture and ritualistic practice may have come to mind. Clearly, what we need to do is to look for solutions to such barriers

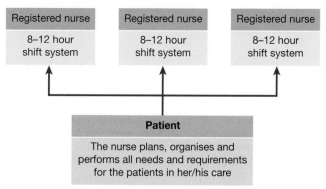

Figure 6.1 Patient allocation.

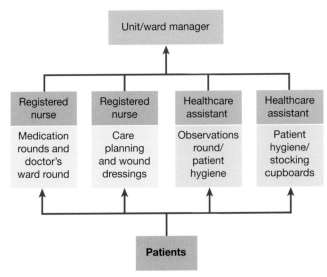

Figure 6.2 **Task allocation.**

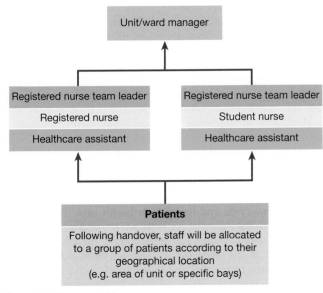

Figure 6.3 **Team nursing.**

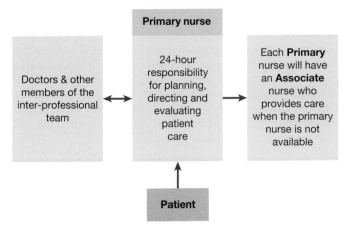

Figure 6.4 **Primary nursing.**

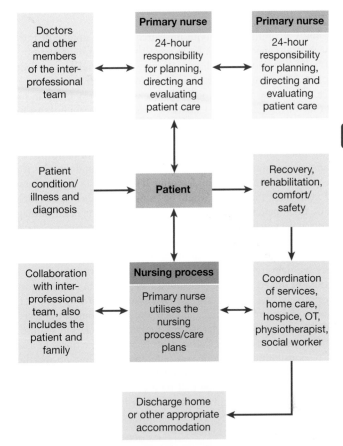

Figure 6.5 **Primary nursing and the Nursing Process.**

to ensure that personalised care is upheld and sustained, so that our patients will do well in our care.

The Nursing Process

The Influence from the USA

During the early part of the 1960s, we began to witness the nursing profession pressing forward in the education of its workforce, stressing the need to further develop the knowledge base and competencies of nursing students and those already in practice. This was especially the case in the USA, leading to new explanations and theories. Nurse lecturers and researchers were finding ways of explaining the nature of nursing to new entrants on the programmes offered. The aim of such theories was to make the work of nurses understandable and guide nursing education and training. Theorists, such as Peplau, Orem, Henderson, Neuman and, in the UK, Roper, Logan and Tierney (as cited in Aggleton & Chalmers 1986), highlighted different features of the patient, which included their biological, social and psychological needs. From the 1950s onwards, the development of the 'Nursing Process', and the concept of nursing diagnosis, focussed attention on the identification of those patient problems that nurses know about and treat. As nursing began to develop in the universities in countries such as the USA, Canada, Australia and the Netherlands, the development of nursing science (the discipline-specific knowledge base of nursing) in these countries rapidly accelerated and came to be incorporated into definitions of nursing (RCN 2003, p. 8).

The UK Picture

In the UK, things were more measured and the uptake of these theoretical concepts was a lot slower. The development of a body of 'nursing science' was disappointingly underdeveloped and the notion of the 'nursing diagnosis' was rarely (if ever) used in practice. In fact, the medical model of care was still very much in use at this time. Aggleton and Chalmers (1986, p. 11) point out that for many years, the medical model formed the basis not only of medical training but of most nurse training as well. The model focusses on anatomical, physiological and biochemical causes of ill health. On commencing nurse training in 1976, the author found that this was very much at the heart of his learning. It is difficult to imagine now, 37 years later, that nurses would be using this model. As a student back then, patients were nursed according to their medical diagnosis; what you had was a set of guidelines and strategies associated with each diagnosis and it was not unusual for patients to be referred to as the 'appendix in bed 6' or 'the coronary in bed 2'. The way we delivered nursing care for surgical patients for instance, would be linked to where the patient was situated in the days post-operatively. The initial guidelines were carried out preoperatively, with some common features applied; but there would be a degree of uniqueness associated with the individual operation planned. The first day post-surgery (Day 1) would direct the nurse to a set of responsibilities; each one was different, depending on whether the patient had returned from theatre having had a cholecystectomy, a gastrectomy or toe nail removal. To some extent, this is where some individuality of the care delivered was evident but overall it was this set of rigid guidelines that stifled the nurse–patient relationship.

The Evidence Definition: the 'Medical Model' of Care

The traditional approach to the diagnosis and treatment of illness as practiced by physicians in the Western world since the time of Koch and Pasteur. The physician focuses on the defect, or dysfunction, within the patient, using a problem-solving approach. The medical history, physical examination, and diagnostic tests provide the basis for the identification and treatment of a specific illness. The medical model is thus focused on the physical and biologic aspects of specific diseases and conditions. Nursing differs from the medical model in that the patient is perceived primarily as a person relating to the environment holistically; nursing care is formulated on the basis of a holistic nursing assessment of all dimensions of the person (physical, emotional, mental, and spiritual) that assumes multiple causes for the problems experienced by the patient. Nursing care then focuses on all dimensions, not just physical.

(*Mosby's Medical Dictionary* 2009)

Definition

A shift away from the medical model was not too far away, and it was the introduction of the Nursing Process that helped to achieve this movement. However, the Nursing Process alone does not provide nurses with a set of understandings about people and their health-related needs around which to plan and deliver care. This stems from the fact that, while the Nursing Process suggests that nurses should assess, plan, intervene and evaluate, it does not indicate what should be the focus of such activities (Aggleton & Chalmers 1986, p. 15). When used alongside nursing models (explored in Chapter 7), the Nursing Process helps us to focus on the individual, their specific characteristics and their health-related requirements.

Jot This Down

Take a look at the definition of the 'medical model' and how nursing differs from it.

Imagine using the medical model in practice, where the patient is referred to by his medical diagnosis and his bed number. Individualised nursing care was virtually non-existent and the nursing contribution to patient care was directed by this method. Nurses at the time were often regarded as 'physicians' assistants' and there needed to be a clear move towards enhancing the nursing profession's contribution to health care.

Take some time to discuss this 'Jot This Down' exercise with your mentor and peers. You may like to think about how valuable the Nursing Process and care planning is and how it contributes to the quality of your nursing practice. Miller (1985, p. 63) found a reduction in length of stay in hospital, patient dependency and a better chance of surviving the hospital stay after the implementation of the Nursing Process. This individualising of patient care led to less dependent patients who could be discharged earlier. Walsh and Ford (1990, p. 147) pointed out that any statement refuting the merits of the Nursing Process is therefore a myth.

Barrett and Richardson's (1996) **Le**arning **Ma**terial **O**n **N**ursing (LEMON) highlighted that nursing was becoming functional and task-oriented rather than person-centred. It was believed at the time that the knowledge base for practice within nursing was developing at an unhurried pace and even where it existed, it was often not utilised to inform nursing practice. Society's view of nursing was increasingly that it was about supporting and complimenting medicine. It became evident, through consultation with various nursing organisations, that only through the study of the practice of nursing would nursing be able to define, develop and fulfil its unique role and function in health care. The LEMON manuscript defines nursing as both an art and a science that requires the understanding and application of the knowledge and skills specific to the discipline. It draws on knowledge and techniques from the humanities and the physical, social, medical and biological sciences.

Meleis (1995, p. 111) remarked that, while the Nursing Process addresses patterns in assessing, diagnosing and intervening, nursing therapeutics considers the content of nursing interventions and the goals of intervention. The ultimate goal of theory development in nursing is to develop theories that guide the care that nurses give to patients. Nursing was beginning to move away from the medical model, which could be argued as reductionist. Rather than nursing a specific condition against a background of guidelines and medical orders, nursing was now looking at the individual. **Holism** was now a key word in the nursing vocabulary, referring to an approach that underlines the whole person rather than their component parts and systems. Plainly speaking, 'the whole is greater than the sum of its parts'.

A Systematic Approach

Hall and Ritchie (2009, p. 67) comment that the Nursing Process offers a systematic approach to planning and delivering nursing care using a problem-solving cycle in which the needs of the individual patient are taken into account. Howatson-Jones *et al.* (2012, p. 55) highlighted that this systematic way integrates assessment information with decisions made about care. It includes critical thinking about potential nursing interventions to develop a care strategy and then evaluating the outcomes of the care provided.

> ### Jot This Down
>
> Think about the care plans you have observed and used in practice. What sort of information do you look for when assessing your patient?
>
> What information is important?
>
> As you collect the data, are you already beginning to think about a plan for this individual?
>
> Are you thinking about nursing interventions and the evaluation of your actions?

For the 'Jot This Down' exercise above, you may have thought about objective data, such as the symptoms associated with the patient's condition. If a patient is admitted to your ward with pyrexia or a swollen calf muscle or nausea and diarrhoea, this can be seen immediately and is quite clearly a symptom of an underlying condition. On the other hand, there is subjective data to be collected; this data is personal to the patient and it is necessary to question the patient (at the appropriate point) about their experiences to assemble a more complete picture of the individual. Both sets of data complement each other and the assessment is also a time for establishing a meaningful nurse–patient relationship, although this may not be the most immediate action possible if the patient's health problem is critical (Holland *et al.* 2008, p. 14).

> ### Nursing Fields Adult Health
>
> A 45-year-old male patient presents with a history of palpitations, light-headedness and a feeling of weakness and low energy for the past 4 weeks. His pulse is irregular and you can feel 'missed beats' when recording his pulse. When determining his apex beat, it always sounds louder when an ectopic impulse is evident. The patient seems to get more breathless at night when he lies down to sleep.
>
> He admits to a 'fluttering' in his chest. It radiates to his throat and he's feeling more breathless when mobilising. This has increased his anxiety levels and he's afraid that he may collapse and die at any minute. He is normally an outgoing person but the situation is now beginning to affect his mood and he feels depressed. He stopped socialising with his friends because of the way this makes him feel and he is concerned that it may be serious; he is now very frightened of what may happen. He has not wanted to talk about it to anyone.
>
> Although it has been difficult, he has continued to go to work. He is troubled that it may have had an effect on his productivity. If his boss notices this and given the current climate, he fears the company may sack him or look at making him redundant.

You can see from the above scenario that (**a**) draws attention to the patient's symptoms, the 'objective data', whereas (**b**) the 'subjective data' expands on the information and adds greatly to the information already assembled. The symptoms (**a**) described here, provide us with the physiological response to what sounds like a cardiac arrhythmia. The individual's experience (**b**) also describes symptoms but tells us much more. You not only have physiological data, you now have a measurement of the patient's psychological well-being and the effect this condition is having on his work and social life. You can see how the two sets of data broaden the overall assessment and can help the nurse to lay down a suitable plan of action for the patient.

The four key steps of the Nursing Process have been illustrated in many texts over the years (Yura & Walsh 1978; Roper *et al.* 1985, p. 14; Holland *et al.* 2008, p. 12; Howatson-Jones *et al.* 2012, p. 56). The main stages of this process are APIE:

- **A**ssessment
- **P**lanning
- **I**mplementation
- **E**valuation.

Holland *et al.* (2008, p. 12) refer to an expansion of the four phases:

- Collecting the information and assessing the patient
- Planning the care and defining the relevant objectives for nursing care
- Implementing actual interventions
- Evaluating the results.

They also considered that in some areas, further stages are added to these, one of which is 'making a diagnosis', and that all the stages 'guide the production of nursing care plans and documentation of care in all fields of nursing'. Matthews (2010, p. 5) also points to the steps of the Nursing Process but includes the 'nursing diagnosis', placing it between assessment and planning. **A**ssessment, **P**lanning, **I**mplementation and **E**valuation (APIE, see Figure 6.6) now becomes **A**ssessment, **D**iagnosis, **P**lanning, **I**mplementation and **E**valuation (ADPIE, see Figure 6.7).

Figure 6.7 represents the continuous loop and is a progression of actions that continually recycle as patient problems and priorities change or resolve (Matthews 2010, p. 7).

Myra Estrin Levine was said to be the first person to question the idea of the 'nursing diagnosis'. Marriner-Tomey and Alligood (1998) pay tribute to her work as a nursing theorist, while Bullough and Sentz (2000, p. 179) go further, pointing to where she began her scholarly activities and her contribution to the concept of the Nursing Process. As an author and principal investigator of a surgical dressing project at the University of Chicago (1952–1953),

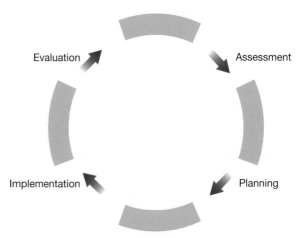

Figure 6.6 The four phases of the Nursing Process.

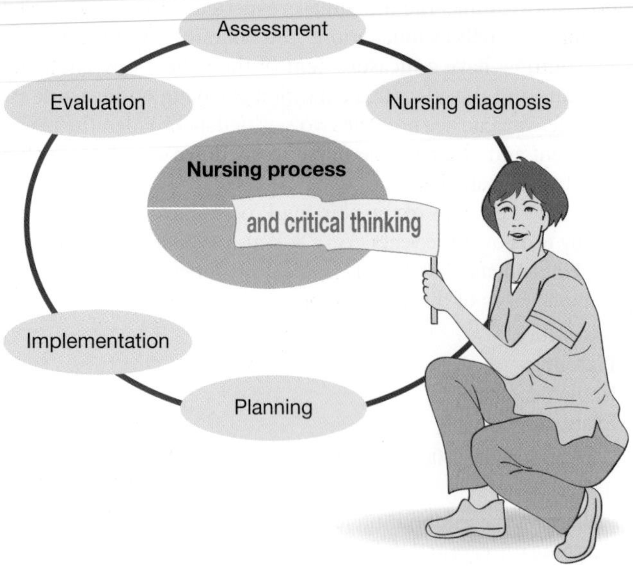

Figure 6.7 The four phases plus the nursing diagnosis.

Levine went on to contribute in 1966 the concept of 'trophicognosis', a term she coined to replace 'diagnosis' which she felt to be incorrect and legally unsound when applied to nursing. She defined 'trophicognosis' as a nursing care judgement arrived at by the scientific method. 'Trophico' is derived from the Greek words *trophikos techne* and translates as the 'art of nursing', while *gnosis* literally means 'knowledge'. Trophicognosis is seen then, as the application of science to resolve an individual's nursing care needs, and is suggested as an alternative to the term 'diagnosis'. Whether you want to call it a nursing diagnosis (ADPIE) or trophicognosis (ATPIE) is not a major issue: what Levine has highlighted is the importance and significance of the art and science of nursing. It is the nurse's task to bring a body of scientific principles on which decisions depend to the precise situation that she shares with the patient. Sensitive observation and the selection of relevant data form the basis for her assessment of nursing requirements. The essence of Levine's theory is that:

When nursing intervention influences adaptation favourably, or toward renewed social well-being, then the nurse is acting in a therapeutic sense; when the response is unfavourable, the nurse provides supportive care. The goal of nursing is to promote adaptation and maintain wholeness.

(Levine, quoted in Marriner-Tomey and Alligood 1998, p. 199)

At the beginning of the 1990s Walsh and Ford (1990, p. 144) commented that experience shows that many nurses still do not understand how to devise a care plan. The theory of care-planning is simply not practised they said.

Jot This Down

- Do you think this is still the case today?
- If so, why do you think this is?
- When using a care plan, do you tend to include and document information that is not relevant?
- Do you think it has all become a ritual?

For this 'Jot This Down' exercise, you may have thought about the documentation you have used, and that you have felt obliged to robotically complete all sections on the care plan. You may have become frustrated at the fact that you did not have the time or opportunity to sit down with the patient to identify patient problems, whether they were actual or potential. For a lot of nurses, this becomes a source of irritation, and switches the attention from the patient. The nurse wants to sit with the patient and discuss 'patient' problems so that they can collaborate and work in partnership and the patient can see from this, that you place a value on his well-being and recovery.

What the Experts Say

> A 75-year-old gentleman with a known history of ischaemic heart disease but no history of a previous myocardial infarction (MI) was admitted to the ward suffering from a sudden onset of severe angina; this was the worst pain he had ever suffered. On admission, he was very anxious with slight breathlessness. He was pain-free, having had a dose of nitrate (GTN) therapy while in the A&E department. The patient lives alone, his wife having died some years ago and his only child, a daughter, now lives in Canada.
>
> Once I had settled him into bed and had given him a cup of tea, I asked him if he had any worries. Thinking that he would share his fear that this time it may be a heart attack and the impact this may have on him being able to get back home and live a 'normal' life, I was surprised at his response to my question.
>
> 'My only worry at the moment', he said was 'who is going to look after my dog? He is on his own in the house and will need feeding and taking out for his walk this evening'.
>
> I immediately called his next door neighbour (who he was very friendly with and holds a spare key to his house). She had already taken his dog to her house and wanted me to pass on the message that everything was fine and that the dog would be staying with her until he was discharged and well enough once more.
>
> I passed on the message; he was extremely grateful and then said, 'I have no more worries, just do what you need to do and I can get home as soon as possible'.

(Registered Nurse, care of the elderly ward)

Think about the 'Expert' comments – the registered nurse had presumed that the patient would share thoughts and feelings related to his medical condition and the symptoms he had been admitted with. However, the patient's anxieties were completely different in terms of priority; this is unmistakably a patient-centred problem and is of no less concern.

Patient Goals

Failure to state clear and realistic goals will lead to planning failure as the care implemented rarely resembles the plan (Ford & Walsh 1994, p. 211). What we have seen in the goals section in the past are phrases such as 'to observe' and 'to avoid' or 'to ensure'. What will nurses observe? What will they ensure will happen and what will they avoid? Such goals are not patient-centred and are very ambiguous, especially for the student nurse, newly qualified nurse and those new to the ward. The evaluation paperwork is no better; you often read 'slept well', 'no complaints', 'up to the toilet', 'eating and drinking' and 'on a fluid balance'. These expressions mean absolutely nothing when analysed closely. The term 'eating and drinking' can mean the patient has had only one spoonful of porridge all day or that he enjoyed three whole meals throughout the day. What does 'slept well' mean to the night nurse? The patient may have settled down at 10p.m. and slept undisturbed until 6a.m. the next morning. On the other hand, it may be that the night staff felt he slept well because he did not request anything during the night and that his bedside light was off all night. Think about this situation – he may have been lying there all night feeling anxious at the thought of his forthcoming surgical procedure tomorrow afternoon. The nucleus of the Nursing Process should always be linked to your patient; nurses need to get away from the thought that it is only about completing the documentation.

Matthews (2010, p. 71) states that all outcomes must be patient-orientated and expressed in the form of a statement. This is the outcome statement or goal and can be pigeonholed into four components:

1. A specific behaviour that shows the patient has reached his goal
2. Criteria for measuring that behaviour
3. The condition under which the behaviour should occur
4. A time frame for when the behaviour should occur.

An example of this would be a patient with a nursing diagnosis of headache and photophobia with vomiting and nausea secondary to a severe migraine. The expected outcome may be that the patient's pain will be less severe within 2 hours following medication and that he will be pain free within 6 hours. Thinking about and documenting a realistic time frame for completion of the desired behaviour are vital and must be constantly appraised to ensure that a new outcome statement is written if required. The goal should clearly stipulate what the patient will be able to do once a nursing intervention takes place. Howatson-Jones *et al.* (2012, p. 70) comment that a goal should be formulated in a way that is **S**pecific, **M**easurable, **A**chievable, **R**elevant and **T**ime-limited (SMART). If the goal is unclear to the nurse, it becomes very difficult to assess patient progress or to encourage the patient towards the desired outcome. Nurses need to set goals that are both short and long term.

Nursing Fields Children's Health

Children's nursing concerns a parent–nurse partnership. Nursing goals are:

· To promote a therapeutic relationship between parent and child
· Accomplished by family-centered care
· To promote continued growth and development.

Jot This Down

· Do you think that goal setting has become a lost art?
· If so, why do you think this is?
· When setting goals do you always think about the three important components set out above?

For the 'Jot This Down' exercise above, you may have thought about the way you document patient goals and discussed this with

your mentor and other colleagues. It is a commonsense approach and you may already be doing this. However, if you are not, then you need to think about whether your care is truly patient-centred. Walsh and Ford (1990, p. 146) point out that documenting care actually saves time: it saves the nurse 15 minutes trying to find the nurse who looked after the patient yesterday, to clarify issues. A patient-centred goal using the SMART principles will give the nurse a clear signal as to what exactly needs to be done and this will lead to a number of beneficial factors. It is an appropriate use of the resources available, allowing the nurse to use her skills in the proper manner and in a timely fashion; the nurse becomes more productive, patients will see the improvement and gain more confidence, which will lead to a more rapid recovery, rehabilitation and quicker discharge. Think about it – if your work is more fruitful and reduces the length of a patient's stay in hospital, the organisation will reap the benefits. It makes financial sense and while giving value for money, more importantly it boosts the quality of care for your patients.

Nursing Fields Mental Health Nursing

Mental health nursing practice should establish goals in relation to the health, educational, employment, social and recreational needs of the client.

The 'Nursing Fields' examples above express plainly how to set out a patient goal. The nurse who reads this will be in no doubt as to, exactly what is required in terms of the behaviour and outcome for her patient. If you get this part of the Nursing Process correct, you will have set up the perfect starting point for the rest of your care plan.

 Link To/Go To

For more information linked to SMART and ADPIE goals go to:

1. SMART = **http://www.youtube.com/watch?v=k9TuE4 —IuY**
2. ADPIE = **http://www.youtube.com/watch?v=fILK28z3rPA**

These 'YouTube' presentations demonstrate a brief overview of: (1) How to recognise and write SMART goals and (2) the Nursing Process.

Writing the Care Plan

Following the previous discussion, you can now appreciate just how important the Nursing Process is and how the care plan becomes central to the method. The five steps of the Nursing Process have been highlighted and you can see the relationship between each stage. Matthews (2010, p. 119) points out that the nursing care plan is the core of your nursing practice – a vital source of information about your patient's problems, needs and goals and the quintessential blueprint to direct your treatment and care. If you perform this with accuracy, it will lead you systematically through your everyday practice and assist your patient to recover in a more timely fashion.

Putting your patient at the centre of everything you do is of paramount importance and especially in view of what is a significant year for the NHS (2013/2014). The 'Putting Patients First' document (NHS England 2013, p. 4) comments that, the Francis report demonstrated the tragic consequences when standards of care fall woefully short. This is why we in the NHS must, and will, put patients at the heart of everything we do. The overarching theme of the Francis report is clear: a fundamental cultural change is needed in order to put patients at the centre of the NHS.

The principles and philosophy of the Nursing Process facilitates this, making it possible for nurses to see their patient as the single most important person when delivering care. Add to this, a robust nursing care plan and you have a situation that is person-centred, allowing for a therapeutic relationship. The nurse now begins to see the individual in the patient and can focus on the appropriate approach to care in partnership with the person.

Take a look at the following 'Jot This Down' exercise and think about the nursing interventions that may be required when caring for Mr Simpson.

Jot This Down

Mr Simpson, a 70-year-old gentleman, is admitted with an exacerbation of chronic obstructive pulmonary disease (COPD). He is extremely breathless on admission and is very anxious.

1. Using the stages of the Nursing Process, think about his immediate needs and produce an appropriate care plan for him
2. Now think about his potential needs and plan his care accordingly.

You may have thought about a number of acute needs (Box 6.1) associated with his medical condition; some of these are emphasised below. He will also have potential needs that need to be planned for and you can see these in the next box (Box 6.2).

Box 6.1 Mr Simpson's Immediate Needs

Thinking about his immediate problems/needs you may have highlighted:

1. Assistance with breathing
2. Maintaining patient safety (internal and external)
3. Difficulties with communication
4. Problems mobilising.

Box 6.2 Mr Simpson's Potential Problems/Needs

Thinking about his potential problems/needs you may have highlighted:

1. Potential deterioration due to pneumonia (think about a possible hospital acquired infection on top of his chest condition – think patient safety!)
2. The potential for pressure sore development and deep vein thrombosis (DVT), given his mobility problems
3. Potential dehydration and weight loss due to poor appetite and fluid intake

Remember, patients who are extremely breathless burn a lot of calories (think about the overload to his intercostal muscles and vital fluid loss due to excess expiration).

An example of Mr Simpson's care plan follows. You will see the actual and potential problems, and the associated activity of living based on the model of nursing developed by Roper *et al.* (1985).

Implementation Stage

The implementation stage of the Nursing Process allows the nurse to set aside a plan of action for the patient. Once again, this plan is specific to each individual and centres on a feasible and measurable end-product. The actions taken by the nurse at this point will include the constant monitoring and examination of the patient for signs of change or improvement, the continuous delivery of direct care, carrying out necessary medical tasks, communicating with the patient, coaching and teaching the patient about further health management, and referring the patient to other members of the interprofessional team for specialised treatment.

When implementation takes place, the nursing care can be maintained over hours, days, weeks or even months. Hogston (2011, p. 13) observed that, implementation is the 'doing' phase of the Nursing Process. This is where the nurse puts into action the nursing care that will be delivered and addresses each of the diagnoses and their goals. The nurse will undertake the instructions written in the care plan in order to assist the client in reaching these goal(s). This will involve a process of teaching and helping clients to make decisions about their health. In an ideal situation, the nurse should sit with the patient, taking the time to talk about the needs and requirements based on the individual problems identified. This will depend on the condition and symptoms of the patient given their medical diagnosis. The nurse will then discuss with the patient, the most suitable method for providing nursing care with further discourse to stress the importance of involving other healthcare professionals in an attempt to develop the most appropriate patient outcome.

Jot This Down

As a nurse, you are in a unique position when caring for patients (see Figure 6.3), constantly working at the bedside.

Thinking about all members of the interprofessional team:

· Do you know their principal roles and tasks?
· Do you know when it may be appropriate to liaise with the different members of the team?
· What issues will you discuss with your patient when considering any communication with a member of the interprofessional team?

From the 'Jot This Down' exercise above, you may already have a general idea of the functions attributed to each member of the healthcare team. A good nursing assessment will help you to grade the essential needs of your patient and from this, you may be aware of the additional input required. A physiotherapist for instance, can be employed to assist a patient with mobility problems or one who has breathing difficulties. The speech therapist may be required to assist the stroke patient with communication. Similarly, the community nurse, podiatrist, dietician, psychologist and pharmacist among others, can be contacted when a specialist opinion is required (Figure 6.8).

Matthews (2010, p. 59) points out that not all nursing diagnoses can be managed solely by the nurse. The nurse must be aware that

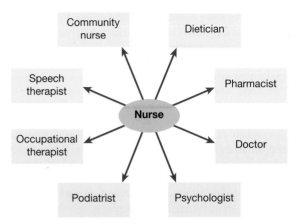

Figure 6.8 The pivotal role of the nurse when communicating with the interprofessional team.

to meet the best outcome for the patient, some findings will necessitate collaboration with others as the management of care will be based on a partnership. A truly good relationship with your patients will help them to understand that what you are planning is in their best interests. Keeping the patients informed and raising their awareness of the role each person takes, will help them to appreciate the care delivered. It also encourages the person's participation in his or her own care (Barrett & Richardson 1996, p. 23).

Evaluation Stage

Once all nursing interventions have been carried out, the nurse should then complete an evaluation of the care administered. This will help the nurse to establish whether the goals set for the patient have been successful.

The outcomes of your nursing care are commonly expressed in three ways: this relates to (a) the improvement of his/her condition; (b) whether the patient's condition has become stable or (c) his/her condition has deteriorated/the patient has died/been discharged. If a patient's condition has shown no progress, or if the goals are not achieved in the time frame set, the nurse will have to return to the first step of the Nursing Process and a reassessment of the situation will be considered with a new set of realistic objectives planned.

When evaluating, it is necessary to revisit the problem definitions and goals statements in order to identify any changes that have occurred and also any modifications that need to be made (Howatson-Jones *et al.* 2012, p. 70). As you work through the care plan, it will become apparent that not all problems you have identified will be resolved totally; this means that the nurse will have to adjust her care accordingly and fine-tune the original goals set on the patient's admission. Matthews (2010, p. 104) declares that evaluation is an on-going practice that occurs with every patient encounter. *Remember* that this incorporates many factors:

- Continuous reassessment of your patient
- Measure your findings against your outcome standard or the goals you have set
- Establish whether your patient's condition has improved, have they met the goals you set, met them to some degree or not at all?
- Documentation must be completed continually
- Amendments to the care plan must also include changes to the nursing diagnoses as required.

After discussion with your colleagues, you may have thought about many patient related issues and questions to ask when delivering care. Physiological measurements such as blood pressure, temperature, pulse and respiration allow the nurse to constantly appraise the patient's health status.

The appropriate use of assessment tools, such as pain scales, the Malnutrition Universal Screening Tool (MUST) and the falls risk assessment, helps the nurse to ascertain a strongly balanced assessment leading to a robust plan of care to meet the individual needs of the patient. The nurse may ask herself 'what changes have taken place and has there been any sign of progress since I activated the care plan?' The key issue here is whether the nurse can document that the original purpose and objective have been achieved. This process would appear to be time consuming and relies on the nurse being ever vigilant in her observations. This is even more difficult in a busy healthcare setting where staffing levels are low, patient turnover is rapid and the care is becoming ever more complex. However, as Howatson-Jones *et al.* (2012, p. 76) succinctly put it, taking time with people may be difficult but is also extremely rewarding in terms of achieving nursing outcomes and quality nursing care.

The use of care planning can improve the continuity of care and save time if carried out in a rational manner. Ritualistic filling in of forms however, will waste time and be of no benefit to the patient (Walsh & Ford 1990, p. 146). In fact, the same authors go to some length in their argument to dispel the myth that the Nursing Process does not work. They refer to the work of Miller (1985), as cited in Walsh and Ford (1990, p. 147), who measured the length of stay in hospital and patient dependency. The study showed a reduction in both after the implementation of the Nursing Process. Individualising patient care led to less dependent patients who could be discharged earlier.

Nurses need to be aware of the value of using the Nursing Process approach to care; they must appreciate that the documentation is an instrument to be used for the effective delivery of practice; it must be seen as an accessory to the many other mechanisms and resources we use and not detached from them.

With regard to the 'Jot This Down' exercise above, you may have thought about a number of reasons why the Nursing Process is beneficial to patient care. It is quite clear that if care planning is done correctly, then the patient will be treated as an individual, valued by the nurse and allowed to become a partner in the care process. This patient-centred approach means that they will work in collaboration with the nurse and the patient places their trust in her; this ultimately leads to a therapeutic relationship. The nurse encourages patient involvement at every level, allowing them to be a part of all the decisions made about their care – the result of which is patient empowerment. Ryder and Wiltshire (2001) point out that empowerment has implications for the relationship between nurse and patient.

Nurses wishing to 'empower' clients must understand the complexity of this approach because failure to do so could result in the nurse not recognising the need for an individual approach, which takes into account patients' differing circumstances. This could result in patients being overloaded with information, creating unnecessary anxiety, rather than the nurse using his/her skills to assess and address individual needs.

The care plan is outcome driven; it calls for individual goal setting, which means that the main focus is on the 'person' who should remain independent from everything else that is going on around them. Nurses need to think 'smarter not harder' when using the Nursing Process. In other words, the nurse needs to use the care plan to her and the patient's advantage and not regard it as another chore, inconveniently adding another burden to her busy day.

How Does 'Intentional Rounding' Fit in?

Nurses today continue to be taught about holistic care, treating their patients as individuals and as we can see, the Nursing Process is a way of providing this. It can be pondered whether the application of the Nursing Process when combined with primary nursing (see Figure 6.4 and Figure 6.5) is an impressive design that provides holistic care. The idea that each patient has a 'named' nurse who is responsible for their care would seem very patient-focussed and can lead to job satisfaction for the nurse. In fact, recommendation 15 of the Francis Report (2013) embraces this vision for nurses and healthcare support workers, making the point:

Each patient should be allocated a named key nurse for each shift who would be responsible for coordinating the provision of the care needs of that patient.

(quoted in Harrison 2013, p. 13)

What the Experts Say

> ...the evidence for 'intentional rounding' consists almost exclusively of weak studies and that nurse managers appear to have so readily adopted the interventions in the absence of robust justifying evidence and it speaks loudly of nursing's insecurity as an autonomous profession.

(quoted in Duffin 2013, p. 5)

Duffin (2013, p. 5) points to David Cameron, the Prime Minister's flagship policy on 'Intentional Rounding' (IR) – an arrangement involving systematic checks to see that patients are pain free

and comfortable, and assisted to eat and drink or to mobilise to the toilet if necessary. Chinn (2012) sparked an interesting online discussion, questioning whether 'intentional rounding' actually provides holistic care. Some of the discourse pointed out that it lacked 'personalisation' and, although it meant that observations and fluids got done, it was going back to ritualistic practice. The debate is set to continue for some time yet. Duffin (2013, p. 5) refers to Paul Snelling, a programme leader in health and life sciences at the University of the West of England, who has scrutinised evidence on the 'rounding' system and questions whether it makes any difference to patient outcomes. Snelling regards it as nothing more than a tick-box exercise. The health think tank The King's Fund (2012) has analysed 'intentional rounding' as part of its Point of Care policy. It seems to argue that, while it does have its merits, there is not a wealth of evidence to support the idea. A DH spokesperson stated that it has reduced the number of patient complaints and significantly improved patient satisfaction levels. That said, *it would appear that what is required here is a robust, peer reviewed study to support some of the statements we hear.*

Jot This Down

Think about 'intentional rounding (IR)' and the Nursing Process

- What are your views?
- Discuss this with your mentor/colleagues
- Jot down the strengths and weaknesses of IR

There is a fine line between the concept of individualised care and holism and the safety of our patients. The question is: Do we need both? – The Nursing Process for holistic care and IR bringing us the elements of patient safety. Surely, the 'named nurse', using a Nursing Process approach to care on each shift covers the very aspects of safety currently advocated by IR. The Nursing Process allows the nurse these moments at the bedside as much as IR does.

 ### Link To/Go To

http://www.youtube.com/watch?v=s5FKx22-gc4

This short 'YouTube' video from Cape Cod Hospital, Hyannis, Massachusetts, USA, explains what IR is and gives some indication of the benefits of the idea.

You can see from the Cape Cod video clip that the concept is based on regular practice to meet patient needs, improve their safety and comfort and reduce the number of call bells, leading to improved patient satisfaction levels. You can also see that the nurse completes any programmed procedures, such as administration of analgesia or wound checks. The environment is also assessed and equipment is positioned within easy reach of the patient. The questions we may want to ask here are: Is this a new practice and does it stand independently from the Nursing Process approach?

The National Nursing Research Unit (NNRU 2012) policy paper states that IR can help 'organise workload and can provide more systematic reliable care'. It was also reported that patients liked IR because they felt less isolated and know that they will be checked on regularly. In contrast, the policy document also highlighted that further evaluation of IR is needed to determine the evidence of its effectiveness and cost implications within the UK. Once again, it could be argued that the Nursing Process advocates all these things – it is a systematic approach to individual care that allows for a therapeutic nurse–patient relationship where patients take an active part in their plan of care; a plan that nurse and patient constantly review together during the course of the 'named' nurse's shift.

Compassion

Compassion is the new buzzword. It has appeared at the top of the healthcare agenda for some time now, and similarly within education circles (Willis 2012, p. 2). Dewar (2013, p. 48) states that while increased value is placed on compassion and caring, there is little understanding about how it can be promoted in the healthcare setting. Compassion has been defined (Chochinov 2007) as 'a deep awareness of the suffering of another coupled with a wish to relieve it'. Dewar (2013, p. 49) continues by saying, to be compassionate towards a patient requires you to relate with that person. It is not so much about what people choose to do for each other but about what they choose to do together. Compassion implies a level of reciprocity and interdependence. Some of the key dimensions of compassionate care include:

- It is a subjective experience
- It is about the quality of the relationship between individuals
- It requires that individuals acknowledge the person with the illness
- It requires emotional connection and interpersonal skills.

Nearly 20 years ago, the Tresolini and Pew-Fetzer Task Force (1994, p. 26) recommended that clinicians embrace patient-centred care, which involves communicating openly with patients and practising with a healing and caring ethic. If we are meant to develop a good relationship with our patients, connect with the individual, value their needs and requirements and involve them in the decision-making process (see Box 6.3), then clearly, we need a process that is robust, not a 'questionable' system such as IR, a tick-box system that so far has not demonstrated any real quality outcomes of note.

Consider the questions in Box 6.3 – they can help you to deliver compassionate care. Dewar (2013, p. 51) observes that it is through engaging with people in this way that practitioners can find out what matters to them and understand how they feel. This in turn can help healthcare professionals to work with people in a way that minimises vulnerability. IR may be safe practice in some ways, but it can be argued that it still leaves your patient vulnerable in other ways. Simply asking the patient if they have had a drink in the past hour is not the same as asking: 'tell me what I can do for you that could make your stay on the ward much better?' The latter question is linked to quality, while the former merely allows the nurse to add to her ever-growing quantitative measurements during her working day. If we continue to adhere to a hierarchical way of working, fearing punishment for not conforming to what could be argued to be ritualistic practice, then we are less likely to give a high quality of care showing the compassion that organisations see as essential. A revisit to the Nursing Process approach may well be the answer for nurses.

Jot This Down

- Some of the literature suggests that we use IR and that it does have a place in health care
- The idea of a compassionate workforce is also important
- The Nursing Process is a systematic approach to individualised patient care

  What is your impression of the ideas discussed here? Discuss these with your mentor and think about their place in practice.

Having thought about the questions in the 'Jot This Down' exercise above, you may have reflected and believe that, as nurses, we need to be more measured in what we use. You may have seen the benefits of both systems.

Conclusion

What we require is a questioning attitude and not a time where nursing staff simply conform to every new-fangled thing that is introduced and sold as the next piece of the jigsaw or innovative to practice. We must be cautious of these novel ideas, requesting the evidence and the appropriate evaluations of their origins and thus avoid their introduction based on individual anecdotal substantiation. Checking whether a patient has been to the toilet in the last hour somehow oversimplifies things, and if your drive is to tick the box at the patient's bedside, why not use the hourly rounding opportunity to take the patient's care plan with you and develop it and update it in a similar fashion.

Key Points

- This chapter offers insight into the various definitions of nursing.
- An introduction to the history of the Nursing Process and understanding of the concept (philosophy/principles) of the Nursing Process is provided.
- Consideration is given to the practice of nursing and various organisational models of care.
- Having an understanding of the stages of the Nursing Process; assessment, diagnosis, planning, implementation and evaluation (ADPIE) can help the nurse use a systematic approach to care provision.
- An understanding of how 'intentional rounding' and compassion impact on the concept of individualised care is provided.

Box 6.3 Do You Really Know Your Patient?

Questions to help you to get to know the person:

- What matters to you most while you are in hospital?
- Tell me something that will help us to care for you here?
- How do you feel about your experience?
- What helps you to feel upbeat (positive) and well?
- How would you like us to respond if you are feeling low?
- Who are the most important people to you?
- What worries or concerns do you have?
- What things have worked well for you here?

(Dewar & Nolan 2013, p. 8)

Glossary

Art of nursing: the intentional creative use of oneself, based upon skill and expertise, to transmit emotion and meaning to another. It is a process that is subjective and requires interpretation, sensitivity, imagination and active participation

Care plan: a design to direct nurses and other healthcare professionals involved with patient care. Such plans are patient specific and are meant to address the individual and the best possible outcomes for patients

Health promotion: the process of enabling people to increase control over their health and its determinants, and thereby improve their health

Holism: the conception of man as a functioning whole

Integrated care pathway: an interprofessional plan for delivering health and social care to patients with a specific condition or set of symptoms

Nursing model: a set of theoretical and wide-ranging statements about the concepts that serve to provide a framework for organising ideas about patients, their environment, health and nursing

Nursing process: a method that provides an organisational structure for nursing practice

Positivism: a philosophy of science, based on the view that information derived from logical and mathematical treatments and reports of sensory experience is the exclusive source of all authoritative knowledge, and that there is valid knowledge (truth) only in scientific knowledge

World Health Organization: A global administration concerned with world health and welfare

References

Aggleton, P. & Chalmers, H. (1986) *Nursing Models and the Nursing Process.* Macmillan, London.

Barrett, K. & Richardson, J. (1996) The nursing process and documentation. In: R. Rogers (ed.) *LEMON Package*, Ch. 4. R. World Health Organization, Copenhagen, Denmark.

Bullough, V.L. & Sentz, L. (eds) (2000) *American Nursing: a biographical dictionary*, Vol. 3. Springer, New York.

Chinn, T. (2012) #WeNurses – Didn't we stop rounding years ago? *NursingTimes.net.* http://www.nursingtimes.net/nursing-practice/clinical-zones/educators/wenurses-didnt-we-stop-rounding-years-ago/5049670.article (accessed 25 February 2013).

Chochinov, H. (2007) Dignity and the essence of medicine: the A, B, C, and D of dignity conserving care. *British Medical Journal*, 335, 185–187.

Clark, J. & Lang, N. (1992) Nursing's next advance: an international classification for nursing practice. *International Nursing Review*, 38(4), 109–112.

DH (2006) *Modernising Nursing Careers: setting the direction.* Department of Health, London. http://webarchive.nationalarchives.gov.uk/20130107105354/http://www.dh.gov.uk/prod_consum_dh/groups/dh_digitalassets/@dh/@en/documents/digitalasset/dh_4138757.pdf (accessed 25 March 2013).

DH & NHS (2012) *Developing the culture of compassionate care: creating a new vision for nurses, midwives and care-givers.* Department of Health & NHS Commissioning Board, Leeds. http://www.england.nhs.uk/wp-content/uploads/2012/10/nursing-vision.pdf (accessed 2 April 2013).

Dewar, B. (2013) Cultivating compassionate care. *Nursing Standard*, 27(34), 48–55.

Dewar, B. & Nolan, M. (2013) Caring about caring: developing a model to implement compassionate relationship centred care in an older care setting. *International Journal of Nursing Studies.* www.researchgate.net/.../9c96051927afed8f0e.pdf.

Duffin, C. (2013) Evidence for intentional rounding said to be 'flimsy and questionable'. *Nursing Standard*, 27(32), 5.

Ford, P., Heath, H., McCormack, B. & Phair, L. (2004) *What a Difference a Nurse Makes: an RCN Report on the Benefits of Expert Nursing to the Clinical Outcomes in the Continuing Care of Older People.* Royal College of Nursing, London. Publications code: 000 632. https://www.rcn.org.uk/__data/assets/pdf_file/0009/78489/000632.pdf (accessed 2 April 2013).

Ford, P. & Walsh, M. (1994) *New Rituals for Old: nursing through the looking glass.* Butterworth & Heinemann, Oxford.

Francis, R. (2013) *Report of the Mid Staffordshire Foundation Trust Public Enquiry.* The Stationery Office, London.

Gullick, J., Shepherd, M. & Ronald, T. (2004) The effect of an organisational model on the standard of care. *Nursing Times*, 100, 36–39.

Hall, C. & Ritchie, D. (2009) *What is Nursing? Exploring Theory & Practice.* Learning Matters, Exeter.

Harrison, S. (2013) The caring, committed majority of nurses need better support. *Nursing Standard*, 27(24), 12–13.

Hogston, R. (2011) Managing nursing care. In: R. Hogston & B. Marjoram (eds) *Foundations of Nursing Practice: themes, concepts and frameworks*, 4th edn. Palgrave Macmillan, Hampshire.

Holland, K., Jenkins, J., Solomon, J. & Whittam, S. (2008) *Applying the Roper, Logan and Tierney Model in Practice*, 2nd edn. Churchill Livingstone, Edinburgh.

Howatson-Jones, L., Standing, M. & Roberts, S. (2012) *Patient Assessment and Care Planning in Nursing Learning Matters.* Sage, London.

Jonsdottir, H. (1999) Outcomes of implementing primary nursing in the care of people with chronic lung diseases: the nurse's experience. *Journal of Nursing Management*, 7, 235–242.

King's Fund (2012) *Will Hourly Rounds Help Nurses to Concentrate More on Caring?* Paper by Jocelyn Cornwell. http://www.kingsfund.org.uk/blog/2012/01/will-hourly-rounds-help-nurses-concentrate-more-caring (accessed 12 February 2014).

Lintern, S. (2012) NHS faces a nursing shortage, review for RCN warns *NursingTimes.net.* http://www.nursingtimes.net/nhs-faces-a-nursing-shortage-review-for-rcn-warns/5050873.article (accessed 5 April 2013).

Manthey, M. (1992) *The Practice of Primary Nursing.* King's Fund Centre, London.

Marriner-Tomey, A. & Alligood, M.R. (1998) *Nursing Theorists and their Work*, 4th edn. Mosby, St Louis.

Matthews, E. (2010) *Nursing Care Planning Made Incredibly Easy!* First UK edn. Wolters Kluwer/Lippincott, Williams and Wilkins, London.

Meleis, A.I. (1995) *Theoretical Nursing: development and progress*, 2nd edn. Lippincott, Philadelphia.

Miller, A. (1985) Nurse patient dependency; is it iatrogenic? *Journal of Advanced Nursing*, 10(1), 63–69.

Mosby's Medical Dictionary (2009) 8th edn. Elsevier. http://medical-dictionary.thefreedictionary.com/medical+model (accessed 15 April 2013).

NHS England (2013) NHS England Business Plan 2013/14–2015/16 *Putting Patients First* NHS Constitution, NHSE041302. http://www.england.nhs.uk/wp-content/uploads/2014/04/ppf-1415-1617-wa.pdf (accessed 29 April 2013).

NNRU (2012) *Policy+ 35: Intentional Rounding: what is the evidence?* National Nursing Research Unit, Policy+Review, King's College, London, p. 69. http://www.kcl.ac.uk/nursing/research/nnru/publications/Policy-plus-Review.pdf (accessed 12 June 2013).

Pearson, A. (ed.) (1988) *Primary Nursing.* Chapman & Hall, London.

RCN (2003) *Defining Nursing.* Royal College of Nursing, London. Publications code: 001 998. http://www.rcn.org.uk/__data/assets/pdf_file/0003/78564/001983.pdf (accessed 26 March 2013).

Roper, N., Logan, W.W. & Tierney, A.J. (1985) *The Elements of Nursing*, 2nd edn. Churchill Livingstone, Edinburgh.

Ryder, E. & Wiltshire, S. (2001) Understanding empowerment. *Nursing-Times*.net. http://www.nursingtimes.net/nursing-practice/leadership/understanding-empowerment/200691.article (accessed 19 May 2013).

Skretkowicz, V. (ed.) (1992) *Florence Nightingale's Notes on Nursing (Revised with additions)*. Scutari Press, Middlesex.

Tresolini, C.P. & The Pew-Fetzer Task Force (1994) *Health Professions Education & Relationship–Centred Care*: report of the Pew-Fetzer Task Force on advancing psychosocial health education. http://rccswmi.org/uploads/PewFetzerRCCreport.pdf (accessed 1 July 2013).

Walsh, M. & Ford, P. (1990) *Nursing Rituals: research and rational action*. Heinemann Nursing, Oxford.

WHO (1991) *Nursing in action project. Health for All Nursing Series No 2: mission and functions of the nurses*. WHO, Copenhagen.

Willis, P. (2012) *Quality with Compassion: the future of nursing education*. Report of the Willis Commission 2012. Executive Summary. http://www.williscommission.org.uk/__data/assets/pdf_file/0008/485009/Willis_Commission_executive_summary.pdf (accessed 13 June 2013).

Yura, D. & Walsh, M.B. (1978) *The Nursing Process: assessing, planning, implementing and evaluating*. Appleton Century Crofts, New York.

Test Yourself

1. The Nursing Process is:
   (a) Task-focussed care
   (b) A traditional style of care
   (c) Individualised patient-centred care
   (d) All of the above

2. There is only one true definition of nursing.
   (a) True
   (b) False

3. The NMC was preceded by the:
   (a) General Medical Council
   (b) Allied Health Professionals Council
   (c) United Kingdom Central Council
   (d) Health and Care Professional Council

4. Which organisational model of care was considered to give a low job satisfaction rate when used by nurses in practice?
   (a) Primary nursing
   (b) Team nursing
   (c) Patient allocation
   (d) Task allocation

5. Planning is the doing phase of the Nursing Process.
   (a) True
   (b) False

6. Documenting care in a care plan:
   (a) Takes up valuable nursing time
   (b) Is a waste of time
   (c) Saves time
   (d) Is redundant information

7. Which report recommended that each patient should be allocated a 'named nurse' for each shift?
   (a) The Keogh Report
   (b) The Francis Report
   (c) The Griffiths Report
   (d) The McKinsey Report

8. The evidence illustrating the benefits of 'intentional rounding' is comprehensive.
   (a) True
   (b) False

9. It has been reported that nursing care plans are better used and the continuity of care is increased when using the following patient care delivery system:
   (a) Primary nursing
   (b) Team nursing
   (c) Patient allocation
   (d) Task allocation

10. Which nurse theorist was said to be the first person to question the idea of the 'nursing diagnosis'?
    (a) Hildegard Peplau
    (b) Dorothea Orem
    (c) Myra Estrin Levine
    (d) Ida Jean Orlando

Answers

1. c
2. b
3. c
4. d

5. b
6. c
7. b
8. b
9. a
10. c

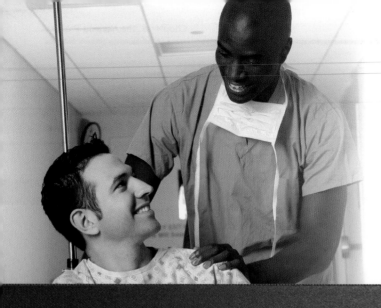

7

Models of Nursing

Mike Lappin

University of Salford, UK

Learning Outcomes

On completion of this chapter you will be able to:

- Be aware of the history and principles of nursing models
- Have an insight into the concept (philosophy/principles) of nursing models
- Provide an overview of nursing models and how a nursing model links to patient-centred care and safety
- Understand the stages of the Roper, Logan and Tierney activities of living model of nursing
- Demonstrate a knowledge of the dimensions of Roper, Logan and Tierney's model, Orem's model, a chosen model related to the Child and Young Person and a Mental Health model
- Have an insight into the Art and Science of Nursing

Competencies

All nurses must:

1. Work in partnership with service users, carers, families, groups, communities and organisations. They must manage risk, and promote health and well-being, while aiming to empower choices that promote self-care and safety.
2. Build partnerships and therapeutic relationships through safe, effective and non-discriminatory communication. They must take account of individual differences, capabilities and needs
3. Use a range of communication skills and technologies to support person-centred care and enhance quality and safety. They must ensure people receive all the information they need in a language and manner that allows them to make informed choices and share decision-making. They must recognise when language interpretation or other communication support is needed and know how to obtain it.
4. Maintain accurate, clear and complete records, including the use of electronic formats, using appropriate and plain language

(Continued)

Nursing Practice: Knowledge and Care, First Edition. Edited by Ian Peate, Karen Wild and Muralitharan Nair.
© 2014 John Wiley & Sons, Ltd. Published 2014 by John Wiley & Sons, Ltd. Companion website: www.wileynursingpractice.com

5. Use up-to-date knowledge and evidence to assess, plan, deliver and evaluate care, communicate findings, influence change and promote health and best practice. They must make person-centred, evidence-based judgements and decisions, in partnership with others involved in the care process, to ensure high quality care. They must be able to recognise when the complexity of clinical decisions requires specialist knowledge and expertise, and consult or refer accordingly.

6. Carry out comprehensive, systematic nursing assessments that take account of relevant physical, social, cultural, psychological, spiritual, genetic and environmental factors, in partnership with service users and others through interaction, observation and measurement

Introduction

It seems appropriate that Chapter 6, relating to the nursing process, should be followed by a chapter on nursing models. There are countless volumes, articles, book chapters and presentations covering both aspects within the nursing literature. In fact, it can be argued that you could fill a library alone with the information available. This author, like many nurses, has read numerous pieces of the available work; various narratives go back to before the author entered the nursing profession in the late 1970s. What we have is an arsenal of information written by many renowned theorists, including: Virginia Henderson, Hildegard Peplau, Betty Neuman, Martha Rogers, Sister Callista Roy, Patricia Benner and probably the most famous of all, Florence Nightingale. In general, the texts often go on to consider the nursing process and highlight some of the key models developed by these nursing philosophers, exploring the main differences between them and how they link to care planning.

The purpose of this chapter is not to completely follow this pattern; in fact the author would doubt whether he can improve upon that which has gone before, and it would be extremely difficult to follow in such esteemed footsteps. The plan, therefore, is to structure the discussion around many of the key issues related to nursing today. It is the intention of this chapter to link factors such as patient safety, risk management and the effect of organisational culture on patient well-being to nursing models.

Realistic patient-centred care, individualism, holistic care and the systematic approach to nursing is the order of the day, and in view of the recent failings at the Stafford Hospital and the call for sweeping changes to end the perceived disregard for patient safety (Francis 2013), perhaps what we need to do is to re-focus our attention on the care plans and the correct use of the frameworks we have at our fingertips in an attempt to deliver the elementary aspects of care.

…models were devised to move nursing away from task-oriented and ritualistic care towards more thoughtful practice…

(Jones 1989)

Nursing Theory

Theofanidis and Fountouki (2008) observe that, in order to practice competent nursing, nurses have to combine knowledge already generated from many other disciplines, as well as solid and rigorous facts from the nursing profession. As professionals, we are aware of the fact that when working in the clinical setting, it is not just the practical aspects of our work that are important; the theoretical knowledge that strengthens our actions is equally vital. Theories enable us to distinguish facts from fallacies (Roberts 1985). In addition to this, Colley (2003, p. 33) highlights that Nursing Theory should provide the principles that underpin practice and help to generate further nursing knowledge. However, a lack of agreement in the professional literature on Nursing Theory confuses nurses and has caused many to dismiss Nursing Theory as irrelevant to practice.

As you work through your nursing programme, you will become increasingly more aware of this situation and you will come across the many opinions of authors, educators, researchers and practitioners. In fact, Colley (2003, p. 33) comments that:

Lack of agreement in the professional literature serves to confuse nurses and has caused many to dismiss nursing theory as long-winded and irrelevant to everyday practice.

Marriner-Tomey (1998, p. 3) distinguishes theory as helping nurses to provide knowledge to improve practice by describing, explaining, predicting and controlling phenomena. Nurses' power is increased through theoretical knowledge because systematically developed methods are more likely to be successful. Nurses will also be able to explain why they are doing what they are doing if confronted by their patients or members of the interprofessional team. Theory presents nurses with a sense of professional autonomy, by steering their clinical practice, their learning and their research function. Torres (1990, p. 6) sets out the seven basic characteristics of a theory, the first of which is that it can interrelate concepts in such a way as to create a different way of looking at a particular phenomenon.

Torres uses the following example:

What the Experts Say

A theory might identify the two concepts 'need' and 'nursing'. The concept of *need* may be described in terms of actual experiences that the person might encounter that interfere with an optimal health state.

The concept of *nursing* may be defined in terms of actions that can be taken to reach an optimal health state such as touch, listening, or teaching.

The theory, in turn, may connect the two concepts of *need* and *nursing* in such a way that nursing actions can be deliberately viewed as meeting needs, and in so doing reach a goal of optimal health.

(Torres 1990, p. 7)

You may be able to see from this that without the theory, we may not perceive the relationship between a need and a nursing action: the theory should provide a unique way of viewing nursing actions as meeting a particular goal; a specific relationship (Torres

1990, p. 7). Interestingly, the same author highlights that theories should be relatively simple but generalisable. The effusive and extraneous descriptions of nursing theories highlighted by Colley (2003, p. 33) seem like a world away from the thought of a 'good theory' stated in the most simple of terms.

132

> ### Jot This Down
>
> Mrs Ireson, a 35-year-old woman, has attended her local gastroenterology clinic for bowel problems for some years now. She has suffered long-term Crohn's disease, which has failed to respond to medical treatment and as a consequence, a section of her colon was surgically removed and a permanent colostomy was formed. She keeps herself fit by attending her local gym twice weekly. The only time she does not attend is when she has an exacerbation of the disease. She is married with two children, both at school during the day. She works part-time as a secretary in a solicitor's office, and it is an ideal situation for her as her office hours allow her to pick up the children after school. Her husband is an architect and works away quite a lot, having to travel across the country to meet new clients and manage new building projects.
>
> - When reviewing the circumstances here, reflect upon a number of the key theories that will illustrate the need for specialist knowledge in order to deliver a better quality of care for Mrs Ireson.

A small sample of the theories you identified may include:

Body Image Theory

Cash (2004, p. 1) points out that body image is a multifaceted psychological experience of embodiment that profoundly influences the quality of human life. The nurse needs to establish how the patient is going to deal with this new set of circumstances; this will be done through a robust assessment. The theory should give you some indication as to how she will deal with both the physiological and psychological aspects of her condition.

Adaptation Theories

An assessment of Mrs Ireson's capability to adjust to her colostomy (physical needs) and the way she perceives her new look (psychological needs) will be established. What follows should be a comprehensive explanation by the nurse, who will utilise this theoretical concept to inform her practice and advice to her patient.

Teaching Theories (Patient-Centred)

The nursing literature is awash with information related to patient teaching; it is a fundamental part of your role and the Nursing and Midwifery Council makes this quite clear in its Code:

> *You must act as an advocate for those in your care, helping them to access relevant health and social care, information and support.*
> *You must support people in caring for themselves to improve and maintain their health.*

(NMC 2008, p. 3)

An awareness of teaching theories will ensure that you appreciate what exactly an adult learner requires, that the skills you employ in this situation will help the person to take some or more control of matters and that you can make a difference to their life when maximising the information available.

Family Theories

Torres (1990, p. 10) points out that the structure and function of the family unit and the interrelationships of a family group are reflected in theories related to the family. Although you may have never met Mr Ireson, you will be able to assess the relationship of the two as she perceives it and the possible impact this may have on their sexual relationship for example. As a relatively young woman, Mrs Ireson will be aware of the changes to her body; the formation of a stoma may lead to embarrassment and psychological discomfort. It may make her feel undesirable and this feeling of being less attractive could well influence the relationship she has with her husband. Theories concerning family structure and needs will assist the professional nurse in health teaching and nursing diagnoses (Torres 1990, p. 10).

> ### Link To/Go To
>
> If you go to the link below you will find a very useful power point (ppt) presentation that relates to Theories of Nursing Practice. Admittedly, it is rather a long entry, but worth the time taken to read it:
>
> **http://intranet.tdmu.edu.ua/data/kafedra/internal/socmedic/ presentations/en/nurse/ptn/bsn/RN-BSN%20(2%20year%20 program)/Current%20Topics%20in%20Nursing/2/12.%20 Theories%20of%20nursing%20practice.ppt**
>
> (Delmar Learning 2004)

The presentation itself explores the role of theory and highlights three main qualities, stating that:

- Theory is the representation of reality in a way that seeks to make explicit underlying factors, connections and outcomes
- Theory helps us explore reality and identify changes we might seek to make
- Theory identifies the range of possible interventions and their ramifications, as well as factors that might impede progress.

Looking back at the circumstances surrounding Mrs Ireson, you can begin to see how this fits with the theories identified when dealing with her individual needs. The nurse will use her knowledge of each theory, link this to her patient's position and work on a plan of care to meet each of her patient's needs; using a recognised model of nursing, her requirements will be identified and a deliberate plan of nursing action will be prepared.

> ### Jot This Down
>
> At this point, you may want to think about the purpose of *Nursing Theory*.
> Discuss this with your colleagues and your mentor in practice.
>
> - What is the function of Nursing Theory?
> - Why do nurses need to learn about this supposition?
> - How do we make use of Nursing Theory in our daily practice?

You may have thought about how Nursing Theory helps us to channel our practice and the new knowledge it creates. It could be that you thought about how theory helps us to explain nursing to people both within and outside of the profession. When coming into the profession and beginning a programme of education and development, the study of such theories may change the views and ideas we have about nursing. It may help us to think in different ways and understand the gaps that exist between theory, research and our practice. It may have helped you to think 'smarter' not 'harder', using new ideas, skills and methods of performance to enhance practice further. It may be seen as empowering practitioners, enabling them to plan and carry out work with a level of accountability and responsibility that benefits the patient, themselves and their organisation.

When put into practice, Nursing Theory helps us to organise our care and to understand and question patient information, and it allows us to make clinical decisions, which gives us an idea about what we actually do for the patient. Nursing Theory aids our planning, so that we can go on to anticipate and calculate potential outcomes for our patients. Finally it will help us to measure and evaluate the care delivered.

Colley (2003, p. 34) declares that, broadly speaking, nursing theories can be divided into different categories according to function.

Theories can also be classified according to the extent their principles can be generalised.

They can also be categorised as:

- Needs theories
- Interaction theories
- Outcome theories
- Humanistic theories.

The categories above signify the fundamental philosophical underpinnings of the theories.

Needs Theories

These theories are based around helping individuals to fulfil their physical and mental needs. The basis of these theories is well-illustrated in Roper, Logan and Tierney's model of nursing (1985).

Interaction Theories

As described by Peplau (cited in George 1990, p. 51; Marriner-Tomey & Alligood 1998, p. 337), these theories revolve around the relationships nurses form with patients. Riehl's model (Aggleton & Chalmers 1986, p. 75) declares that part of the nurse's role involves an attempt to enter into the subjective world of patients in order to see things as they do. Only by doing this can a nurse make an accurate assessment of an individual's needs and plan an appropriate series of nursing interventions.

Outcome Theories

Roy (1980) sees the nurse as the changing force, enabling individuals to adapt to or cope with ill health (cited in Aggleton & Chalmers 1986, p. 48). In fact, Roy suggests that, while doctors focus on biological systems and disease processes, the nurse's specific role is to promote adaptation in health and illness (Aggleton & Chalmers 1986, p. 53).

History and Principles

Ford and Walsh (1994, p. 205) stated that much has been written about conceptual models of nursing, ranging from outright rejection as just another North American import we can do without, through to total slavish acceptance of a one-model-only approach. However, nursing models have been seen as a set of frameworks based on the environment of care, the people involved in nursing activity, the health status of the patient or service user and the nursing capabilities and knowledge of the practitioner (Hinchcliff et al. 2008). Howatson-Jones (2012, p. 80) argue that the nursing approach to care must vary accordingly to the specialty of practice – nursing a patient with intensive care unit (ICU) needs is different from nursing a patient in an ambulatory care environment or in the community.

> **Jot This Down**
>
> Think about the model(s) of nursing you have used and been exposed to in practice
> - Did the model fit well within that specialty?
> - Did you find it easy to use or understand?
> - If you had no framework to help you focus, how would this affect your practice?

Chapter 6 asserts that the patient is a unique individual with a series of differing healthcare needs. If this is regarded to be a truly accurate declaration, the use of a 'one-size-fits-all' model is neither desirable nor practical. Fawcett (1992) observed that many nursing models lack a clear linkage to the clinical practice they seek to guide. As a model is tried in practice, staff should be reflecting on its strengths and weaknesses, changing and adapting the model, perhaps grafting and attaching sections of another model if it is philosophically consistent. Models would then be seen as more vibrant and forever evolving in reaction to the real world of nursing.

You may have used the most familiar framework here in the UK, the Roper, Logan and Tierney (1980, 1981, 1983) model of nursing. You may possibly have applied Orem's self-care model (1980, 1985) or perhaps Roy's adaptation model (1980, 1984) or a combination of models (all cited in Aggleton & Chalmers, 1986). Thinking back, if you used Roper, Logan and Tierney's model for example, it may well have helped you to understand each of the 12 Activities of Living (see Box 7.1) – assisting patients to return to an independent state using the dependence to independence continuum (Roper et al. 1985; Holland et al. 2008).

The Roper, Logan and Tierney Model

The use of the Roper, Logan and Tierney activities of living model helped this author to both appreciate and focus on the individual patient. When using the model in everyday practice, it became clear that no matter what the patient's medical condition, it was the nursing model that helped to shape the nursing practice. It allowed for true patient-centred care and when applied, the 12 activities of living meant that the patient's requirements and needs were dealt with in an efficient manner.

To illustrate this, think about the 12 activities (see Figure 7.1) as they relate to *you* as an individual.

> **Jot This Down**
>
> Imagine you are getting up for work. From the moment your alarm clock rings, the 12 activities of living will become noticeable, but they will not enter your consciousness, as these things have become a part of your everyday life.
>
> If you were to think (consciously) about the 12 activities as you wake up and get ready for work, what would you discover about them and how much they influence everything we do?

Box 7.1 The 12 Activities of Living

1. Maintaining a safe environment
2. Communication
3. Breathing
4. Eating and drinking
5. Controlling body temperature
6. Working and playing
7. Expressing sexuality
8. Elimination
9. Personal cleansing and dressing
10. Mobilising
11. Sleeping
12. Dying/fears for the future.

(Roper *et al.* 1985)

NOTE: The final activity of living is dying; this is not always relevant when dealing with the individual. However, when assessing patients against the 12 activities, it will always be relevant to gauge and consider any fears that the patient may have. It is true s/he may fear death or s/he may be apprehensive about an impending operation or medical condition. In any event, the nurse must ascertain any angst the patient presents with. As was discussed in Chapter 6, it may be the smallest of issues that have the most profound effect on the patient. More often than not, the nurse can easily deal with such issues and alleviate the worries and so minimise the patient's fears.

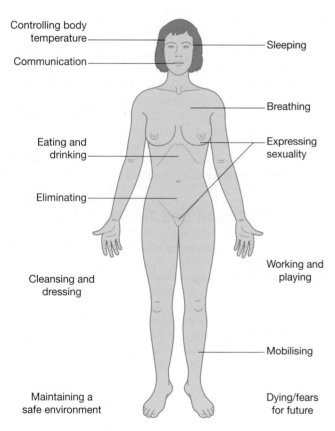

Figure 7.1 The 12 activities of living.

The 'Jot This Down' exercise above may seem pointless, but its purpose should become clearer once you start it. To put the activities into context may help you appreciate your patient's needs in both health and illness:

*You wake (**sleeping**); you'll take your first (conscious) breath of the day (**breathing**); you may say good morning to a loved one (**communication**); you'll get out of bed (**mobilising**); and go to the bathroom (**elimination and personal cleansing and dressing**). After this, you may go back to the bedroom to put on your uniform (**personal cleansing and dressing**); you may put some make-up on and brush your hair, or if you're a male, you may have shaved in advance (**expressing sexuality**). Once ready, you'll go to the kitchen to prepare some breakfast and make a hot drink (**eating and drinking**). You may be thinking about the day ahead and the visit to the gym after work (**working and playing**). Breakfast over, it's time to get your coat on; the weather outside will dictate your choice of clothing, as you will want to be comfortable for the journey to work (**controlling body temperature**). Depending on your mode of transport, you will be mindful of a safe trip and what is required when driving, cycling or simply crossing the road (**maintaining a safe environment**). Finally, you may be thinking about certain anxieties related to specific issues in your social life, family relationships or work (**fears for the future**).*

It could be argued that nursing models, when used correctly, can assist nurses, allowing a sound structure and as Ford and Walsh (1994, p. 206) point out, they guide the nurse away from irrelevant areas, while directing their attention to the way problems are understood and goals are set. It should also influence how interventions are carried out and evaluated.

Orem's Model

According to Orem:

> *… nursing has as its special concern for the individual's need for self-care action and provision and management of it on a continuous basis in order to sustain life and health, recover from disease and injury, and cope with their effects.*
>
> (cited in George 1990, p. 92)

Self-care is the 'practice of activities that individuals initiate and perform on their own behalf in maintaining life, health, and well-being' (Foster & Janssens 1990, p. 92). This model expresses awareness that the patient has the capacity and restrictions to self-care. Howatson-Jones (2012, p. 85) highlights a number of features related to self-care:

- **Self-care agency** – this can be aligned to the patient taking purposeful action to meet his desired goals. An example of this may be sitting himself up in bed without assistance prior to lunch
- **Universal self-care requisites** – this links to what the patient requires in order to maintain life: water, nourishment and air to breathe
- **Development self-care requisites** – this relates to the physical, psychological and functional across the various stages of life
- **Health deviation self-care requisites** – this relates to the patient's condition and how it can impede with attaining what is essential for the individual
- **Helping methods and nursing systems** – the actions taken by nurses to help balance the patient's health and well-being in pursuit of self-care
- **Self-care deficit** – individual patients may require help to complete tasks that they would otherwise do for themselves if well enough. Their current limitations require nursing support at this point, for example assistance with drinking or maintaining oral hygiene.

As a model that values personal responsibility for health, it is also a framework that recognises prevention and health education as key aspects of nursing actions. Aggleton and Chalmers (1986, p. 60) examined the work of Orem who suggested that western society expects adults to be self-reliant and to take a degree of personal responsibility for their dependants. Such a view concurs with those expressed by Ivan Illich (b.1926) during the 1960s and 1970s, in his assessment of the increasing 'medicalisation' of everyday life and in consideration of the patient's growing trend to a dependence on the interventions of the doctor, nurse or local hospital. Porter (1997, p. 687) refers to Illich who maintained that:

> …the medical establishment has become a major threat to health.

In laying bare what he styled as 'iatrogenesis' (doctor-caused illness), Illich exposed many facets of modern medicine as positively counter-productive: pharmaceutical products made you ill; hospitals were hotbeds of infection; surgery was often carried out inappropriately and mistakes made; tests were lacking or misleading, or they created maladies of their own. Not least, argued critics of for-profit, free-market, fee-for-service medicine, among others, there were too many unnecessary procedures (Porter 1997, p. 687).

While it is not the intention of this author to critique these circumstances any further, what he is attempting to point out is that, by placing an emphasis on self-care where it is appropriate, may free patients from the shackles of the clinical setting and thus allow the patient more control of his environment and ultimately his existence.

For those working with the Orem model of nursing, nursing intervention is indicated only when individuals (or their relatives and significant others) are unable to achieve or maintain a balance between their 'self-care abilities' and the demands made on these. Such a situation will occur when 'self-care demands' exceed the self-care abilities of a particular person.

Self-care demands > self-care abilities = nursing intervention

According to Orem, the need for nursing arises from health-related experiences. In other words, adults will not normally require nursing to meet their 'universal self-care needs' unless there are also 'health deviation self-care needs' affecting them. Thus, nursing interventions aim to restore a balance between 'self-care abilities' and the demands made on them (Aggleton & Chalmers 1986, p. 62).

From a 'universal self-care' perspective, it has become quite clear that the patient's standard of living leaves him at risk for impaired cardiovascular functioning and perhaps this is related to a lack of knowledge about the connection between his current lifestyle and the potential threat of a myocardial infarction or stroke. He may also have little understanding of his increased vulnerability caused by the onset of diabetes. The 'self-care deficit' is the difference between his knowledge base and the life choices, all of which increase the undoubted risk to his cardiovascular health. The plan of care must include interventions that will help him to reduce the risks to his well-being. The nurse will aim to develop an agreement with him to help reduce his cholesterol level.

Asking the patient to keep a food diary, teaching him about foods high in fats and the effect that these have on the cardiovascular system will allow him to think about foods on offer that have a lower cholesterol content. The importance of gentle exercise and reducing his smoking habit will be discussed and he will be given the opportunity to think about what he can do to achieve his goals. Strategies will be considered and examined together; the nurse assisting the patient in his decision-making and allowing him to manage the situation. You can see from this that the nurse directs and guides her patient, teaching him along the way, providing psychological support and ensuring that it is done in a sympathetic environment.

What the Experts Say

My name is Richard, I'm an 18-year-old male who was recently diagnosed with end-stage renal failure (ESRF) – I have had a history of renal problems since my early childhood.

Following consultation with my renal physician and the specialist nurses I have decided to go onto peritoneal dialysis (PD) which is a self-care management therapy. Once discharged, I am keen to go home and maintain an independent life. Don't get me wrong, I realise my condition is long term but I wish to remain self-sufficient, as this is very important to me as a person. I have never liked to rely on people too much; I want to be as free as possible from the restraints of the hospital environment.

- Using Orem's self-care model, what questions might you ask Richard when assessing him prior to discharge from the ward?
- What will the nurse be looking for when assessing his self-care abilities?
- What nursing interventions may be required?

There are many other settings where the Orem self-care model would be appropriate; on a renal ward for instance, where patients with long-term conditions require support. For many student nurses and those new to the profession for example, the very thought of using and understanding such complex models can be a daunting prospect. However, you may have found the framework very useful, helping to guide you in your assessment of the patient.

In Richard's scenario, you may have thought of asking him about his home environment, for example whether his PD supplies and equipment could be adequately stored in his house. You would have to assess his knowledge of the procedures required when caring for his dialysis. From a mobility point of view, he will require assessment in terms of his dexterity and any visual problems would have to be taken into consideration. No matter what the patient's

Jot This Down

Imagine you are caring for a 38-year-old man in the community, who has recently been diagnosed with diabetes, and is a heavy smoker, overweight and eats a lot of convenient/fast foods. He lives alone, is unemployed, and has a family history of heart disease. His blood pressure is within a normal range at 130/78 mmHg, however his cholesterol is above the normal level. He does very little exercise due to a previous back injury sustained in his last job when working on a building site as a hod carrier.

Given this short history, using Orem's self-care model, what are the key factors to consider from a nursing perspective?

Discuss this with your colleagues and with your mentor in practice.

age, he will be called upon to manage his dialysis alone throughout the day. Nursing interventions will include teaching the necessary procedures to Richard; he will have to care for and maintain his PD exit site, monitor his own blood pressure, maintain fluid control and weight, together with problem-solving his dialysis regimen.

Aggleton and Chalmers (1986, p. 59) cite Orem, who defined self-care as:

> …the practice of activities that an individual initiates and performs on their own behalf in maintaining health and well-being…

Thus, self-care is a concept applicable to individuals when they are in a state of health and well-being, rather than when they are in a state of ill health or sickness. For Richard, the Orem framework places a value on his desire to take personal responsibility for his life after discharge, while the nurse commits to this through a series of strategies related to communication, education and motivation of her patient.

Jot This Down

Think about how this nursing model helps you deliver consistent care:

- What evidence do you think about and use to inform your practice when writing down the nursing interventions section of your care plan?

You may have thought about the importance of communicating with your patient, educating and informing him and understanding the importance of building a nurse–patient relationship.

The NHS Plan (DH 2000b) emphasises the importance of patient-centred care and service-user involvement. Crawford et al. (2002) highlight that in England and Wales, the involvement of patients is central to current efforts to improve the quality of health care. The belief generally is that putting patients at the centre of care will lead to more services that are available and will help to develop the health and quality of life of patients. Ward (2011) comments that:

> We as nurses have a responsibility to tend to our patients' needs, but we have an equal responsibility to teach. Providing 'care' means ensuring that patients are fully educated about their condition and their proposed treatments. Through education, patients can be made aware of their disease process and potential treatment options…

Furthermore, she highlights that through teaching and empowering our patients, we are giving them the tools they need to manage their disease process and this will result in fewer hospitalisations and in an improved quality of life. The positive results of effective communication are well documented and are essential in achieving, among other things, increased recovery rates, a sense of safety and protection, improved levels of patient satisfaction and greater adherence to treatment options. Aside from these, successful communication through a patient-centred approach also serves to reassure relatives that their loved ones are receiving the necessary treatment. Within the nursing field, such skills are considered indicative of best practice (McCabe & Timmins 2006).

Orem's model allows the nurse to focus on exactly what skills the patient possesses and what he actually knows to care for himself. Once the nurse uses her expertise in assessment, she can then put into place the appropriate approach to supporting and leading patients down an avenue to self-care.

A Framework for Children's Nursing

It has been 25 years since Anne MacDonald (1988) and her colleagues devised their own paediatric nursing model. At the time, she was the Director of Nursing at the Royal Manchester Children's Hospital. Being frustrated at the limited success of the nursing process, MacDonald felt that a unique structure for their practice was required. Well-versed in many of the models in use at the time, she remained unconvinced that any of them suited the nursing needs of the children in their care. Uncertain of their reaction, she mentioned to her colleagues how good it would be to devise their own model, using their experience, knowledge, enthusiasm and commitment, to create a stout paediatric model of care. The work of Wright (1986) inspired the team to action; his work became the chosen text because it described an inductive approach. It was a logical transcript that helped them to guide and influence this working group in the production of a philosophy that would then lead to the creation of a model to suit the philosophy. Wimpenny (2002, p. 347) also referred to the work of Wright, highlighting the implementation of a model by building it from the ground. At this point, MacDonald worked closely with Dawn Clarke (1988) and from the model's inception, it became quite clear that there was a need to link the developmental stages of the child to the activities of living, an adaptation of the model defined by Roper et al. (1985). Four main developmental stages were identified:

- Birth to 1 year
- 1 year to 5 years
- 6 years to 12 years
- Adolescence.

It was thought by both authors that this would act as a learning tool, providing nurses with an instant reference to the developmental stage which could be expected and helping them to consider the child's development/behaviour when identifying individual problems and planning care.

Clarke (1988, p. 33) recognised that the child and his parents were fundamental to paediatric nursing practice. The individual child, within the family unit, is viewed as a unique and dynamically developing human being, vulnerable because of his age, and in certain conditions, at risk of physical and psychological trauma from others around him. The child is also seen as a character who has physical, psychological, socio/environmental and spiritual needs, which must be met so he can develop his full potential, according to the attitudes, values and beliefs of his own family traditions.

Jot This Down

Think about how the adapted model (MacDonald 1988; Clarke 1988) described above will assist you to carry out reliable care for your young patient, mindful of his/her developmental/behavioural stage.

You may have thought about all the activities of living and considered how each is associated with the healthy developmental stage of that particular patient. This will then be followed by thoughts related to the altered state, caused by an illness or a disability.

Some of the examples that you may have thought about here will have included:

- **Maintaining a safe environment** – you will have considered the child's age, condition and incapacity. Is the child in his own bed at this stage or does he sleep in a cot? Does he require protection from excessive temperature levels in his room during the day/night? Does he have any mobility problems that could severely restrict his movement and cause pressure sore development, chest infection and/or pneumonia?
- **Personal cleansing and dressing** – consider the patient's hygiene on admission; depending on his level of development, he will display different phases of independence. Can he dress and wash alone without any help? Is he allergic to any materials worn? Can he manage to brush his own teeth?
- **Expressing sexuality** – does the patient get embarrassed or anxious at the thought of intimate procedures? Depending on his age, he may have different levels of self-image. Girls particularly, may be more conscious of using special toiletries, make-up and costume jewellery.
- **Working and playing** – you will probably have considered the type of school he attends (nursery, play group, secondary school or special needs). Are there any learning difficulties? What toys and games does he play with or does he have any hobbies/pastimes? A teenager may have a Saturday job or a paper round for example.

Casey (1988, p. 8) described her model as one that lends itself to adaptation. From birth, the healthy child is able to meet some of his own fundamental needs – he breathes, expresses discomfort, digests food, eliminates waste, sleeps and moves. All other needs are met by his family in the early stages. As he grows and develops he becomes more independent and thus, from complete dependence he learns to care for himself until he reaches maturity. The care of children in sickness and in health is best carried out by their families, with varying degrees of assistance from members of the healthcare team, whenever it is required (Casey 1988, p. 8).

Shields (2011, p. 1) observed that 'family-centred care' in now widely regarded as a way to care for children in hospitals, and it has become almost universal in the world of paediatrics. It is a way of caring for children and their families; it centres on a plan for the whole family, not just the individual admitted to your ward; each one of them is regarded as a receiver of health care. Casey's model (1988) ensured that parents work in partnership with nurses to provide care for their child; in fact the parent is encouraged to give the so-called 'basic' care, while the nurse educates and supports the parent to do so.

Jot This Down

At this point, you may want to revisit Orem's self-care model and think about how this framework could assist you as you plan the care. Remember Orem's model allows the nurse to focus on the abilities of the patient in pursuit of self-care. In this situation, a family member, parent, sibling or significant other would also be involved to help the nurse recognise exactly what is required to help their loved one make progress.

It may be a worthwhile exercise if you were to share this with a fellow student and you both attempted to write a series of care plans based on the Royal Manchester Children's (1988) model (Clarke 1988). As Orem (cited in George 1990, p. 358) pointed out, the focus of the assessment is on appraising the situation: determining why a person needs care; considering his life history and lifestyle. When planning care for the child, an agreement has to be made with the individual and with their parents and significant others about the role each will play in the overall process.

The Tidal Model in Mental Health Nursing

Stevenson and Fletcher (2002, p. 29) point to the work of Barker and Barker (2005) who developed the 'Tidal Model' following a comprehensive study into a need for psychiatric nursing. The 'Tidal' heading relates to the flowing, ever-changing nature of the experiences of people, and echoes the words used by those who are suffering, uneasy, and in pain – 'washed up', 'swimming against the tide', 'drowning', 'all at sea' and so on.

The model represents a multidimensional approach to the provision of quality psychiatric and mental health care. From the very beginning, the Tidal Model generated attention and enthused many. Inspired by Barker's theory, the passion for this framework has spread rapidly across many parts of the world, including Ireland, Canada, Japan, Australia and New Zealand.

 Link To/Go To

Click onto the following link: **http://www.tidal-model.com/**
Here you can learn more about the Tidal Model from Dr Phil Barker and Poppy Buchanan-Barker. This site provides introductory information about the Tidal Model and how different groups of people might use the Tidal Model to further develop or enhance their efforts to help others.

You will see from the link that the beginner's guide to using the model is quite clear and that Barker has developed a specific theory of personhood, based on people sharing their stories with themselves (**Self-domain**); they also allocate some of the story of their existence with others (**World Domain**) and act out the living of their lives, influence others and are, in turn, influenced by them (**Others' Domain**).

The three domains provide the academic foundation for the person and group-based methods of the Tidal Model:

- The holistic assessment
- One-to-one sessions
- The personal security plan.

    And the three forms of group work:

- Discovery
- Solutions
- Information-sharing.

Stevenson and Fletcher (2002, p. 29) go on to suggest that people, their families and those close to them need to conceptualise psychiatric situations, e.g. admission, as resulting from the problems of living they have encountered and not as a mysterious illness, which is within the patient. This down-to-earth approach respects the lived experience of psychiatric distress as meaningful to the patient and his significant others. As a consequence of placing the person at the centre of care, a mutually satisfying definition of the individual's circumstances and his proposed treatment is developed within the Tidal Model, where the duty for change remains with the person.

Link To/Go To

Click on the following link: **http://www.youtube.com/watch?v=LAp9SKp1DEc**

This YouTube video presentation is based on a real case study and features 'Jack's story: the holistic initial assessment'. The interview is led by Phil Barker and is intended for students who are currently studying mental health nursing. Hopefully, this will be a helpful tool for you.

Jot This Down

Looking back at 'Jack's story: the holistic assessment', think about the interpersonal relationship between Phil, the nurse and Jack, the patient.

- What did you notice about the scene?
- What did Phil do to ensure that the situation remained patient-centred?

It may help to discuss this with your colleagues and mentor to explore the key issues.

The National Service Framework (NSF) for Mental Health (DH 1999) set out to illustrate and direct the provision of future mental health services. Its focus is on guiding the practitioner in the overall development and delivery of their work, highlighting the need for appraisal of their performance and telling them exactly what needs to be accomplished to ensure a high quality service. Some of the key principles are:

- Involve service users and their carers in planning and delivery of care
- Deliver high quality treatment and care, which is known to be effective and appropriate
- Promote the safety of service users and that of their wider family, carers and staff
- Offer choices and promote independence
- Deliver continuity of care for as long as this is needed.

Stevenson and Fletcher (2002, p. 30) imply that the Tidal Model is a means of addressing the key issues within these proposals. Relating to Barker's work, it is clear that both professionals and people as patients are keen for nurses to be able to relate in an ordinary everyday way. The special nature of the interpersonal relationship between the nurse and service user was universally accepted, echoing the work of Peplau (b.1909).

In fact, Peplau's (1952) orientation phase makes it quite clear that the nurse and her patient come together as strangers; in a meeting initiated by the patient who expresses a 'felt need', they then work together to recognise, clarify and define facts related to the need (George 1990, p. 52). Peplau believes that the counselling role has the greatest emphasis in psychiatric nursing. In the nurse–patient relationship counselling is reflected in the way nurses respond to patients' demands. She continues by saying:

The purpose of interpersonal techniques is to help the patient remember and understand fully what is happening to him in the present situation, so that the experience can be integrated rather than dissociated from other experiences in life.

(cited in Marriner-Tomey & Alligood 1998, p. 338)

The Tidal Model also advocates: being respectful of the person's knowledge and expertise about his own life; putting the person in the driving seat in relation to the interaction; seeking permission to explore the person's experience and valuing the person's contribution; being curious as a way of validating the person's experience; finding a common language to describe the person's situation; taking stock and reviewing collaboratively; inspiring hope through designing a realistic future together (Stevenson & Fletcher 2002).

Following your discussions, you may have identified a number of themes. You will see from the video of Jack's story that the relationship between Phil and the patient, Jack, is one of collaboration. It is set in an environment where they are both working together to remedy the health concerns discussed. Phil is using the therapeutic relationship with his patient as a means of identifying, assessing and planning individual goals. With a good communication strategy and a cooperative partnership, Jack begins to understand that change is inevitable in him as a person. The Tidal Model focusses on the patient's strengths and the nurse teaches the person to live independently. The way Phil facilitates the meetings will allow Jack to use his own knowledge and skills to solve his own problems. Phil listens to the story offered, because the patient is living the experience and so knows it better than anyone else. The nurse can then focus on the patient's strengths to make best use of the effectiveness of the healthcare system available.

Many patients feel a loss of power when entering the healthcare system; the Tidal Model conveys the idea that nurses promote power of freedom to patients. By allowing the patient to use his own words and by writing this down in his plan of care, he is not baffled by healthcare jargon. The nurse will approve of the patient making his own decisions, so that he is not solely dependent on the medical professionals he meets.

Des (2012, p. 20) highlights the work of Travelbee (1971) who emphasised the importance of human-to-human relationships stating that:

Every interaction, every encounter, with the ill patient supplies an opportunity for the nurse to meet the patient on his or her premises; allowing her to assess his needs and to build a "human-to-human relationship". An encounter entails all interactions between the two; where all treatment, all conversation and all actions take place.

Travelbee's (1971) human-to-human relationship includes four phases:

- The original encounter
- Emerging identities
- Empathy
- Sympathy.

Des (2012) chose not to use the four phases but rather to use the idea that lay behind the phases. Des believes that Travelbee's concept is that both the nurse and patient come into an encounter as **people** not as 'patient' and 'nurse'; and that the relationship is built through them, realising each other's uniqueness, giving reciprocal equality to each other.

She suggests that in order for this to take place, the nurse needs to be able to meet the patient where he is, as he is. The nurse must obtain an understanding of the patient, where he comes from, what his experiences are and what his needs are. In order to be able to observe and find out these things, the patient should be met with understanding, acceptance and a non-judgemental attitude. You can see from 'Jack's story', that Phil displays all of these characteristics in order to get the best outcome for his patient. For this to be able to take place, the nurse needs to view humans as unique individuals and not as patients; encouraging the patient to view the nurse as a human being allows the two to build a relationship on reciprocal understanding of each other (Travelbee 1971). Phil also attempts to build trust between them; this is a vital factor for building their partnership, allowing him to involve his patient in all aspects of the assessment. Finding a common ground of compassion and illness utilises one's humanity; allowing the nurse and patient to meet as equal human beings (Travelbee 1971).

Jones *et al.* (n.d.) refers to the inpatient psychiatric case management model; a case management model involving the use of a managed care agent (MCA) to perform the initial assessment and develop an initial treatment plan. It is quite clear from the video presentation that Phil Barker is an MCA but in using the Tidal Model, he collaborates with the individual to plan the delivery of his care. He is attempting to empower Jack by making certain that 'his sequence of events' is at the heart of his care plan.

What the Experts Say

The nurse is responsible for helping the patient avoid and alleviate the distress of unmet needs.

(Joyce Travelbee 1926–1973)

Link To/Go To

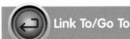

http://currentnursing.com/nursing_theory/Joyce_Travelbee.html

This web page will take you to a companion to nursing theories and models. Travelbee, a psychiatric nurse, educator and writer regarded the interpersonal relationship between the nurse and her patient as paramount in the nurse's role to help the patient to maintain hope and avoid hopelessness.

The Tidal Model encourages a full assessment and innovative plans of care for your patients. It aims to boost and protect the patient's physical and psychological well-being. Working effectively and efficiently with people in mental distress is demanding and requires the investment of both time and emotional commitment (Stevenson & Fletcher 2002, p. 37). This section of the chapter has presented a straightforward introduction to how psychiatric nurses can work in partnership with people in their care, helping to support the individual to influence their healthcare journey. Like all models, this framework is there to guide you through certain circumstances with your patient and not dictate the way you ought to practice.

Many models and theories have an alliance to a mnemonic in an attempt to aid a student's learning and as a way of allowing the retention of information. Surprisingly, for this author, the Tidal Model does not. However, if it were to be associated to a mnemonic* it could well be something like this:

Therapeutic, **I**ndividualised, **D**irects care,

Active participation, **L**ucrative

*My apologies to Professor Phil Barker for taking the liberty of introducing and using a mnemonic as a personal prompt.

In essence, the Tidal Model teaches the importance of the person as an individual, supporting both the nurse and patient to plan a course of action leading to a successful outcome. Working in unison, the pair will generate a healing bond that will give support to the therapeutic process and will ultimately lead to the excellence of care desired by both.

The Art and Science of Nursing

Colley (2003, p. 34) comments that coupled with the confusion surrounding Nursing Theory is the question of whether nursing is an 'art' or a 'science'. For many years, there have been countless deliberations by the nursing profession with regard to this concept. You may even be reading this chapter as part of your degree (BSc) in nursing studies at university and relating it to your nursing practice (Art). Since the move to higher education institutions, it could be argued that nursing has had to align with one of these main schools of learning and knowledge. The two schools – art and science – were traditionally, and to some extent still are, seen as mutually exclusive (Colley 2003, p. 35).

Colley continues:

As nursing shares common ground with both schools, it is stuck between them.

In the past, it was common practice for nursing to follow in the footsteps of medicine, a much more scientific advance to patient care. This more precise knowledge is considered to be more candid and substantial; which in turn, has led scholars to the conclusion that it is more academically sound than the subject matter (nursing), whose concepts cannot be measured.

However, the wider agreement is that nursing is both an art and a science. Carper (1978) encompasses both schools of knowledge through the identification of four ways of knowing in nursing: empirical, ethical, personal and aesthetical.

The Evidence

Carper's contribution to the debate was to encourage nurses to move away from the empirical knowledge and address their discipline in terms of artistry. This offered the nursing profession the opportunity to move away from a world dominated by medicine and allowed nurses to describe their unique role within the healthcare environment.

(Carper 1978)

Link To/Go To

To read more of the work of Barbara Carper, click on the link below:

http://samples.jbpub.com/9780763765705/65705_CH03_V1xx.pdf

While it may appear more complicated to categorise the art over the science of nursing in practice, it is an extremely important aspect to address. Some of the ways of knowing are difficult to validate, as nurses often follow these ways without being aware of them, for example intuition and the therapeutic use of self. This might not be such a problem if nursing in particular and health care as a whole, stopped trying to validate their existence through scientific outcomes (Colley 2003 p. 35).

There has been a counterattack against the traditional view of science as an absolute; Clifton (1991, cited in Colley 2003, p. 35) condemned it as presenting a narrow picture of humans. This positivist observation is a philosophy of science, based on the view that information derived from logical and mathematical treatments and accounts of sensory experience is the exclusive source of all authoritative knowledge and that there is valid data only in facts that are scientific in nature.

Nurses were now being driven to produce a unique body of knowledge specific to their line of work; however, nurse education is based on theory loaned from other disciplines. This has included physiology, sociology and psychology. Colley (2003) has regarded the application of this knowledge from other professions as further diluting nursing practice. Castledine (1994, p. 180) and Crossan and Robb (1998, p. 608) dispute this by declaring that as the occupation of nursing is focussed on humans, perhaps it is inevitable that nursing uses knowledge from other social sciences. They argue that no knowledge is exclusive and because of the diverse nature of our work, it is impossible to have a unique body of knowledge and one unified body of theory.

> ### Jot This Down
>
> Imagine you have fractured your clavicle (collar bone) after a fall:
>
> 1. The doctor will make a diagnosis using his skills of interpretation when viewing your X-ray
> 2. The doctor will prescribe analgesics for your pain and discomfort
> 3. The next phase will involve a nursing intervention: you will require someone who recognises your mobility/agility and dexterity problems; she will also recommend and order further treatment through a number of ways: ordering physiotherapy and requesting specialist advice on exercises, arranging a visiting nurse, making plans for an occupational therapist and equipment to be available.
>
> Is this an example of nursing as a science, the art of nursing or a combination of both?
>
> Discuss this with your mentor and colleagues and together explore whether you think it is one or other of the current schools of knowledge or a blend of both.

You may have thought about the skills and knowledge required to make an accurate nursing assessment in this situation. It could be argued that this will take a degree of scientific expertise; the nurse will also need to be aware of the best evidence to help support the decisions she makes and to plan the subsequent interventions for you as the patient. The medical model might consider the nursing intervention here as a 'soft science' but which one is going to make your life better, not just your collar bone?

Without the medical diagnosis, the nurse cannot start a plan of care, but once this has been established, the nurse can then use her scientific knowledge and skills to actively move things forward. Using this specialist knowledge and combining it with compassion, consideration for the patient's plight and the care required, she can then introduce the art of nursing into the equation. You may have also thought about both the quantitative and qualitative features of the care for the patients we come across on a daily basis.

An example of this could be: **Quantitative** data will show the number of hip operations done per year and if targets are met, then this will be commended; however, getting your patient back on his feet without any complications and in a timely manner and fittingly is **qualitative** data, not often as celebrated as the numerical evidence. It is the qualitative data in such cases that means more to the patient; it is this measure of quality, which in the long term saves the patient from avoidable discomfort (resulting in a shorter hospital stay), the NHS money and enhances the satisfaction of the staff caring for the individual. A win–win situation!

When patients cannot attend to their own personal hygiene needs or they are unable to move up the bed to eat a meal or welcome their visitors to the bedside, it can be very distressing. Things that we take for granted, even the most uncomplicated tasks, can become such a burden for the patient that it frustrates, upsets and causes unthinkable emotional distress. In hospital, the nurses provide almost all of the care the patient receives; armed with their new found knowledge of medical and nursing language, biochemistry, human anatomy and physiology (the science), they now practise the art of nursing. This practice progresses and the skills become more advanced with time in the healthcare environment. Technically, the nurse becomes adept at assessing, diagnosing, planning and implementing care before finally evaluating their actions. Using these technical skills, they complement this with proficiencies in communication, listening, attending to the physical, emotional and spiritual needs, while demonstrating a devotion to their duty of care. In view of the most talked about and newsworthy reports to be published in recent years (Francis 2013), nursing remains one of the most honourable professions in our society.

The nurse needs to explain the plan of care to each individual, using a language they understand. She has to be truthful, having the confidence to admit that she does not have all the answers, but that she will make sure that she will do everything in her power to find the answers when required. The art in nursing is the quality you bring to the bedside, presenting your personality to the patient, showing empathy, demonstrating an attention to detail and offering kindness and thoughtfulness. Science leaves an empty space if the patient lacks trust in you as a person or your nursing practice. Your conduct in practice will be noticed and measured very quickly by the patient and their relatives. Granted, it is subjective data, but it is a dimension that seems to be much less credible in academic terms, although it could be argued it is of equal measure.

In delivering a quality service, it is the nurse who takes on the responsibility to organise and plan care; she is the one who is responsive to the individual needs and requirements of people, therefore the skills of planning care are not to be underestimated and the use of a robust nursing model throughout this period will help to develop a safe and caring culture.

Patient-Centred Care and Safety

Murphy (2011) studied a US report comparing the quality and cost-effectiveness of healthcare systems in seven major countries (Figure 7.2).

A summary of the data demonstrates that the UK ranks second overall. Of the key indicators, it ranked in the top 3 on eight of them. An interesting finding was that it finds itself rock bottom where patient-centred care is concerned.

> ### Jot This Down
>
> Think about why the UK might be in this position when we hear so much about the importance of patient-centred care.
>
> · Discuss this with your colleagues and explore the possible explanation for this.

Country Rankings
1.00–2.33
2.34–4.66
4.67–7.00

Exhibit ES-1. Overall Ranking

	AUS	CAN	GER	NETH	NZ	UK	US
OVERALL RANKING (2010)	3	6	4	1	5	2	7
Quality Care	4	7	5	2	1	3	6
Effective Care	2	7	6	3	5	1	4
Safe Care	6	5	3	1	4	2	7
Coordinated Care	4	5	7	2	1	3	6
Patient-Centered Care	2	5	3	6	1	7	4
Access	6.5	5	3	1	4	2	6.5
Cost-Related Problem	6	3.5	3.5	2	5	1	7
Timeliness of Care	6	7	2	1	3	4	5
Efficiency	2	6	5	3	4	1	7
Equity	4	5	3	1	6	2	7
Long, Healthy, Productive Lives	1	2	3	4	5	6	7
Health Expenditures/Capita, 2007	$3,357	$3,895	$3,588	$3,837*	$2,454	$2,992	$7,290

Figure 7.2 **The quality and cost-effectiveness of healthcare systems. Note: 1 is top rank; 7 is lowest.** *Source*: Davis, K., Schoen, K. & Stremikis, K. (2010) Reproduced with permission of The Commonwealth Fund.

You may have thought about staff shortages, the ward skill-mix or the ever increasing responsibilities placed upon nursing staff in the healthcare environment. Murphy (2011) feels that in clinical practice, we trade something important here: price for patient focus. Of course patients should be at the heart of the NHS, but we seriously increase the cost of care if we double the time seeing our patients. Labour is expensive and in an environment with a vast workforce you can see the need to reduce payments. We have seen this with the number of nursing redundancies and reconfigurations that have taken place since the coalition government came to power in May, 2010.

The choice is a straightforward one: you can have a patient focused NHS so long as you're willing to pay for it.

(Murphy 2011)

What can we conclude from this?

Many nurses would argue that they are finding it progressively more difficult to deliver patient-centred care and it is one indicator that is related to a large amount of nursing effort. Employing lots of nurses is expensive for the NHS; any further increase in numbers will be seen as unattainable. It could be argued that in the ever-present, target driven clinical environments, the excessive use of assessment tools and the need to constantly 'tick the boxes' actually highlights an organisational-centred situation. As Chinn (2012) quite succinctly pointed out, this sort of practice lacks the personal touch and it is heading back to ritualistic practice.

McCaughan and Kaufman (2013, p. 48) highlight that many of the harms associated with health care are preventable. They relate to a report from the Institute of Medicine in the USA, from 1999. At that time, it was estimated that as many as 1 million people were injured and 98 000 individuals died annually as a result of medical error. A similar report in the UK found that around 10% (equating to approximately 850 000) of UK hospital admissions were associated with some form of patient safety incident, which could have or did lead to harm for one or more patients (DH 2000a). The report goes further, indicating that such incidents cost the NHS approximately £2 billion in additional hospital days per year, alongside human costs, such as unnecessary suffering for patients and feelings of self-blame on the part of clinicians.

Jot This Down

From a nursing perspective, can you think about any situations and examples were patient safety may be compromised, leading to any potential risks to their well-being and comfort?

Explore these conditions with your mentor and colleagues in practice.

Following your discussions, you may have highlighted situations, such as the potential development of pressure sores in people who have very limited mobility or who are so incapacitated that they cannot get out of bed. You may have identified the risk of falls in the elderly population or the consequences of a poor nursing assessment and how it may lead to a practitioner missing key indicators linked to patient deterioration. You may have recognised the importance of maintaining good hand washing technique and the appropriate hygiene practices required in the challenges we face with hospital acquired infections, such as those related to indwelling urinary catheters, intravenous cannulation and surgical wounds. Other aspects that may have been debated, are the importance of maintaining adequate nutrition and hydration for all patients in your care. You may also have thought about a robust psychological assessment in an attempt to gauge a patient's thoughts and frame of mind. McCaughan and Kaufman (2013, p. 49) comment that it is important to be mindful that the notion of harm encompasses psychological as well as physical harm. Patients who feel their concerns are rebuffed or dismissed by healthcare professionals can experience mental anguish.

Florence Nightingale noted in the 1860s that 'the first requirement of a hospital is to do the sick no harm' (Skretkowicz 1992). This famous quote will be forever allied to her name. However, it is as relevant today as it was back in the 19th century; patient safety remains a dominant force in health care and is considered to be the most important test facing health care in the early decades of the 21st century (National Patient Safety Agency, NPSA 2011). Clearly, nurses and other healthcare professionals need to understand that a major reduction in unnecessary harm to our patients is essential.

Kaufman and McCaughan (2013, p. 52) highlighted that record-keeping was one of the most important components ensuring patient safety and quality of care. Interestingly, when investigating the Mid Staffordshire NHS Foundation Trust, Francis (2013) reported that record-keeping and handover were not carried out appropriately on many occasions, resulting in poor standards of care. We now know that when patients move through the healthcare system they are entitled to be treated with compassion and are to be valued as a partner in their care, involving them in the decision-making process throughout their passage – it is a truly patient-centred approach. Maintaining 'open communication' channels and documenting care in the correct manner will go some way to dealing with the failings exposed by both Francis (2013) and the Keogh review (2013).

McSherry (2013, p. 15) commented that it is imperative that the core principles of caring, compassion and patient-centred care underpin all aspects of nursing practice in the future. Sharing and learning from the Francis Report (2013) is undoubtedly everyone's business and responsibility. If we fail to communicate appropriately with our patients and do not allow them to share in the decision-making process, it will ultimately influence our nursing actions and we will fall short of following a planned pathway of care using the nursing process and current nursing model(s) within our sphere of practice.

From a legal and professional point of view, it is compulsory for nurses to accurately record plans of care (NMC 2010) for all individuals to provide a legitimate document that demonstrates care has been carried out. The nursing process and the employment of nursing models assist in the organisation and prioritising of nursing care. Cardwell *et al.* (2011, p. 1378) point out that in systematically assessing, planning and documenting care to meet the individual's needs, models of nursing like that of Roper *et al.* (1985) must be reinforced and their application practised. In fact, Cardwell (2011, p. 1382) and her colleagues (all of whom are children's nurses) stress that care planning skills are fundamental to safeguarding vulnerable children, their families and indeed the nursing profession in this current challenging socioeconomic climate.

From this author's observation, the belief is that the nursing process, care plans, models of nursing and other frameworks such as integrated care pathways (ICPs) are all useful instruments in our pursuit of safeguarding and protecting patients whichever field of nursing we practice.

Conclusion

What becomes clear from the discussion throughout this chapter (and Chapter 6) is that when using a nursing process approach to care, all nurses can benefit from using the framework and when combining a nursing model with this method, it helps support the delivery of care that is of a high quality. It is true to say that there are many critics who have judged nursing models to be excessively abstract and that they have little place in modern nursing.

What the Experts Say

 Peter Wimpenny (2002) examines many of the criticisms of nursing models. His article highlights features such as their complexity of language, inflexibility and lack of rigorous testing. Others add that nursing models as promoted by theorists and educators have made little or no positive impact on clinical practice.

Wimpenny points to the suggestion that theoretical models may be more valuable as tools for thought rather than tools for use. He comments on the fact that nursing models are often presented as some final truth and defended as such with the result that they attract pros and cons without examination of their worth or limitations.

The article is a **must read** and can be accessed at the address below:

http://asheehan.brinkster.net/nursing/downloads/articles/The%20meaning%20of%20models%20of%20nursing.pdf (accessed 8 September 2013).

The numerous criticisms in the media and from the general public have declared, on many occasions, that nurses are spending too much valuable time away from the bedside and placing too much emphasis on the input of data into ward computers. Add to this is the feeling that nursing students spend a lot of their time studying and would be better placed with their patients.

It is easy to criticise the design of the way we organise care; perhaps the answer to this lies in the way we apply nursing models and the nursing process in practice. The framework helps to support our nursing practice and what we need to do is make sure we use it to our advantage. Nurses need to be more confident when using care plans and models; the framework is like a skeleton, it provides an outline. The essential action for nurses is to build the muscle, sinew and exterior around the frame in an attempt to enhance our assessment of patients and deliver excellence in health care. For student nurses, a model provides a comprehensive guide to each stage of care planning. The more experienced you become the more you will be able to develop your own ideas based on the theoretical concepts, freeing you from the limitations that some authors so often highlight.

When beginning his nurse education and training in the 1970s this author experienced a system that was largely based on directives from such things as the procedure manual, the bath book and the dressing's book. During his time, as both a student nurse and then a newly qualified practitioner, it was quite clear that nursing was considered as supplementary to the medical team, rather than an independent profession. The introduction of the nursing process and nursing models seemed to emancipate a lot of nurses at the time (including this author) and although many colleagues regarded them as vague and unclear, the benefits seemed to be clear to many.

As nurses began to appreciate the whole process, the benefits shone through. The introduction of the nursing process and nursing models:

- Helped to support communication between the nurse and her patients
- Allowed patients to participate in the decisions made about them and their on-going care
- Allowed the nurse and patient to spend valuable time together
- Improved safety of care through open communication channels
- It was a very useful education tool especially for student nurses

- It enhanced information and the nurses had better access to information about patients
- Patients felt staff valued them and dealt with their individual needs
- The time spent with patients was used appropriately helped nurses to understand the patient's condition and the preparation required to give them the best care available.

If we are to use models and the nursing process appropriately, assessing the person against his individual needs and requirements, then why are we using so many risk assessment questions and an increasing number of risk assessment tools when the model of nursing should envelop all of these factors? The key is to develop staff awareness and for them to extend their skills in care planning. A comprehensive ongoing assessment linked to patient activities of living for instance, should help the nurse to identify the potential dangers to patient safety and in doing this, can take the opportunity to involve the patient fully in the process to avoid the potential for harm. Regular, active patient involvement in identifying care that meets their needs should cover all aspects, including risk to patient safety, comfort, health and well-being.

Sitting at the bedside with the patient's care plan and engaging more frequently with your patient, will result in meaningful dialogue. A therapeutic partnership, one that is supportive and compassionate, putting the patient at the centre of everything we do, is a measure of quality.

Key Points

- This chapter has provided an introduction to the history and principles underpinning nursing models.
- Undertaking a comprehensive, systematic nursing assessment that takes account of relevant physical, social, cultural, psychological, spiritual, genetic and environmental factors, in partnership with service users and others through interaction, observation and measurement ensures that care provision is patient-centred.
- Various nursing models have been discussed, demonstrating how a nursing model links closely to patient-centred care and safety.
- The Roper, Logan and Tierney activities of living model of nursing (or derivatives thereof) is most the most widely used nursing model in the UK.
- The chapter provides insight into the dimensions of Roper, Logan and Tierney's model, Orem's model, a model related to the child and young person and a nursing model used in mental healthcare settings.
- Nursing models allow nurses to articulate the art and science of nursing.
- Nurses are required to work in partnership with service users, carers, families, groups, communities and organisations, managing risk and promoting health and well-being, empowering people to make choices that promote self-care and safety.
- All nurses must build partnerships and therapeutic relationships through safe, effective and non-discriminatory communication. This can enable the nurse to take account of individual differences, capabilities and needs.
- When assessing, planning, delivering and evaluating care, nurses must use up-to-date knowledge and evidence.

Glossary

Art of nursing: the intentional creative use of oneself, based upon skill and expertise, to transmit emotion and meaning to another. It is a process that is subjective and requires interpretation, sensitivity, imagination and active participation (Jenner 1997)

Care plan: a design to direct nurses and other healthcare professionals involved with patient care. Such plans are patient specific and are meant to address the individual and the best possible outcomes for patients

Health promotion: the process of enabling people to increase control over their health and its determinants, and thereby improve their health

Holism: the conception of man as a functioning whole

Integrated care pathway: an inter-professional plan for delivering health and social care to patients with a specific condition or set of symptoms

Nursing model: a set of theoretical and wide-ranging statements about the concepts that serve to provide a framework for organising ideas about patients, their environment, health and nursing

Nursing process: a method that provides an organisational structure for nursing practice

Positivism: a philosophy of science, based on the view that information derived from logical and mathematical treatments and reports of sensory experience is the exclusive source of all authoritative knowledge, and that there is valid knowledge (truth) only in scientific knowledge

World Health Organization: a global administration concerned with world health and welfare

References

Aggleton, P. & Chalmers, H. (1986) *Nursing Models and the Nursing Process.* Macmillan, London.

Barker, P. & Barker, P.B. (2005) The Tidal Model: A guide for mental health professionals. Brunner-Routledge, London.

Cardwell, P., Corkin, D., McCartan, R., McCulloch, A. & Mullan, C. (2011) Is care planning still relevant in the 21st century? *British Journal of Nursing*, 20(21), 1378–1382.

Carper, B.A. (1978) Fundamental patterns of knowing in nursing. *Advances in Nursing Science*, 1(1), 13–24. http://samples.jbpub.com/9780763765705/65705_CH03_V1xx.pdf (accessed 3 September 2013).

Casey, A. (1988) A partnership with child and family. *Senior Nurse*, 4, 8–9.

Cash, T.F. (2004) Body image: past, present and future. *Body Image: An International Journal of Research Body Image* 1:1–5. http://www.ufjf.br/labesc/files/2012/03/Body-Image_2004_Body-Image-past-present-and-future.pdf (accessed 21 February 2014).

Castledine, G. (1994) Nursing can never have a unified theory. *British Journal of Nursing*, 3(4), 180–181.

Chinn, T. (2012) #WeNurses – Didn't We Stop Rounding Years Ago? *NursingTimes*.net. http://www.nursingtimes.net/nursing-practice/clinical-zones/educators/wenurses-didnt-we-stop-rounding-years-ago/5049670.article (accessed 25 February 2013).

Clarke, D. (1988) Framework for care. *Nursing Times*, 84(35), 33–35.

Colley, S. (2003) Nursing Theory: its importance to practice. *Nursing Standard*, 17(46), 33–37.

Crawford, M.J., Rutter, D., Manley, C., *et al.* (2002) Systematic review of involving patients in the planning and development of health care. *British Medical Journal* 325:1263. http://www.bmj.com/content/325/7375/1263 (accessed 22 August 2013).

Crossan, F. & Robb, A. (1998) Role of the nurse: introducing theories and concepts. *British Journal of Nursing*, 7(10), 608–612. http://www.hadassah.org.il/media/2469999/RoleoftheNurse.pdf (accessed 3 September 2013).

Delmar Learning (2004) *Theories of Nursing Practice* (ppt presentation, 42 slides). A Division of Thomson Learning Inc. https://www.google.co.uk/#q=++%22Theories+of+nursing+practice.ppt%22 (accessed 13 February 2014).

Des, J.D. (2012) *Encountering isolation: can the nurse through use of her encounter with the patient, help patients with tuberculosis to avoid the negative psychological effects of isolation?* Publiseringsavtale bacheloroppgave Haraldsplass diakonale høgskole, Bergen. http://brage.bibsys.no/dhh/bitstream/URN:NBN:no-bibsys_brage_35938/1/Janelle%20Nes.pdf (accessed 26 August 2013).

DH (1999) *A National Service Framework for Mental Health*. Department of Health, London. https://www.gov.uk/government/uploads/system/uploads/attachment_data/file/198051/National_Service_Framework_for_Mental_Health.pdf (accessed 29 August 2013).

DH (2000a) *An Organisation with a Memory*. Department of Health, London. http://webarchive.nationalarchives.gov.uk/20130107105354/http://www.dh.gov.uk/prod_consum_dh/groups/dh_digitalassets/@dh/@en/documents/digitalasset/dh_4065086.pdf (accessed 4 September 2013).

DH (2000b) *The NHS Plan: a plan for investment, a plan for reform*. Department of Health, London. http://webarchive.nationalarchives.gov.uk/20130107105354/http://www.dh.gov.uk/prod_consum_dh/groups/dh_digitalassets/@dh/@en/@ps/documents/digitalasset/dh_118522.pdf (accessed 4 September 2013).

Fawcett, J. (1992) Conceptual models and nursing practice: the reciprocal relationship. *Journal of Advanced Nursing*, 17(2), 224–228.

Ford, P. & Walsh, M (1994) New Rituals for Old: nursing through the looking glass Butterworth & Heinemann, Oxford.

Foster, P.C. & Janssens, N.P. (1990) Dorothea E. Orem. In: J.B. George (ed.) *Nursing Theories: the base for professional nursing practice*, Ch. 7, 3rd edn. Prentice-Hall, New Jersey.

Francis, R. (2013) *Report of the Mid Staffordshire Foundation Trust Public Enquiry*. The Stationery Office, London.

George, J.B. (ed.) (1990) *Nursing Theories: the base for professional nursing practice*, 3rd edn. Prentice-Hall, New Jersey.

Hinchcliff, S., Norma, S. & Schober, J. (eds) (2008) *Nursing Practice and Healthcare*, 5th edn. Hodder Arnold, London.

Holland, K., Jenkins, J., Solomon, J. & Whittam, S. (2008) *Applying the Roper, Logan and Tierney Model in Practice*, 2nd edn. Churchill Livingstone, Edinburgh.

Howatson-Jones, L. (2012) Relationship of nursing models to care planning. In: L. Howatson-Jones, M. Standing & S. Roberts (eds). *Patient Assessment and Care Planning in Nursing*, Ch. 6. Learning Matters, Sage, London.

Jenner, C.A. (1997) The art of nursing: a concept analysis. *Nursing Forum*, 32(4), 5–11. http://onlinelibrary.wiley.com/doi/10.1111/j.1744-6198.1997.tb00970.x/pdf (accessed 21 February 2014).

Jones, J.S., Fitzpatrick, J.J. & Rogers, V.L. (n.d.) An Interpersonal Approach: student guide. Springer, New York. http://www.springerpub.com/content/downloads/Jones_Student_Guide.pdf (accessed 26 August 2013).

Jones, S. (1989) Is unity possible? *Nursing Standard*, 3(1), 22–23.

Kaufman, G. & McCaughan, D. (2013) The effect of organisational culture on patient safety. *Nursing Standard*, 27(43), 50–56.

Keogh, B. (2013) Review into the quality of care and treatment provided by 14 hospitals in England: overview report. http://www.nhs.uk/NHSEngland/bruce-keogh-review/Documents/outcomes/keogh-review-final-report.pdf (accessed 4 September 2013).

MacDonald, A. (1988) A model for children's nursing. *Nursing Times*, 84(34), 52–55.

Marriner-Tomey, A. (1998) Introduction to analysis of nursing theories. In: Marriner-Tomey, A. & Alligood, MR. (eds) *Nursing Theorists and their Work*, Ch. 1, 4th edn. Mosby, St Louis.

Marriner-Tomey, A. & Alligood, M.R. (eds) (1998) *Nursing Theorists and their Work*, 4th edn. Mosby, St. Louis.

McCabe, C. & Timmins, F. (2006) *Communication Skills for Nursing Practice*. Palgrave Macmillan, Basingstoke.

McCaughan, D. & Kaufman, G. (2013) Patient safety: threats and solutions. *Nursing Standard*, 27(44), 48–55.

McSherry, R. (2013) Can clinical governance act as a cultural barometer? *Nursing Times*, 109(19), 12–15.

Murphy, R. (2011) *The NHS – a Stunningly Cost Effective Supplier of High Quality Healthcare* Tax Research UK. http://www.taxresearch.org.uk/Blog/2011/06/06/the-nhs-a-stunningly-cost-effective-supplier-of-high-quality-healthcare/ (accessed 6 August 2013).

NMC (2008) *The Code: Standards for Conduct, Performance and Ethics for Nurses and Midwives*. Nursing and Midwifery Council, London. www.nmc-uk.org

NMC (2010) *Standards for pre-registration nursing education*. Nursing and Midwifery Council, London. http://standards.nmc-uk.org/PreRegNursing/statutory/competencies/Pages/Competencies.aspx (accessed 4 September 2013).

NPSA (2011) *Patient Safety First: 2008–2010. The Campaign Review*. National Patient Safety Agency, London. http://www.patientsafetyfirst.nhs.uk/ashx/Asset.ashx?path=/Patient%20Safety%20First%20-%20the%20campaign%20review.pdf (accessed 4 September 2013).

Porter, R. (1997) *The Greatest Benefit to Mankind: a medical history of humanity from antiquity to the present*. Harper Collins, London.

Roberts, K.L. (1985) Theory of nursing as curriculum content. *Journal of Advanced Nursing*, 10(3), 209–215.

Roper, N., Logan, W.W. & Tierney, A.J. (1985) *The Elements of Nursing 2nd Edition*. Churchill Livingstone, Edinburgh.

Shields, L. (2011) Family-centred care: effective care delivery or sacred cow? *Forum of Public Policy*, pp. 1–10. http://forumonpublicpolicy.com/vol2011.no1/archive2011.no1/shields.pdf (accessed 27 August 2013).

Skretkowicz, V. (ed.) (1992) *Florence Nightingale's Notes on Nursing (Revised with additions)*. Scutari Press, Middlesex.

Stevenson, C. & Fletcher, E. (2002) The Tidal Model: the questions answered. *Mental Health Practice*, 5(8), 29–38.

Theofanidis, D. & Fountouki, A. (2008) Nursing Theory: A discussion on an ambiguous concept. *International Journal of Caring Sciences*, 1(1), 15–20.

Torres, G. (1990) The place of concepts and theories within nursing. In: J.B. George (ed.) *Nursing Theories: the base for professional nursing practice*, Ch. 1, 3rd edn. Prentice-Hall, New Jersey.

Travelbee, J. (1971) *Interpersonal Aspects of Nursing*, 2nd edn. F.A. Davis Company, Philadelphia.

Ward, J. (2011) How to educate patients. *NursingTimes*.net. http://www.nursingtimes.net/nursing-practice/clinical-zones/educators/how-to-educate-patients/5030180.article (accessed 22 August 2013).

Wimpenny, P. (2002) The meaning of models of nursing to practising nurses. *Journal of Advanced Nursing*, 40(3), 346–354. http://asheehan.brinkster.net/nursing/downloads/articles/The%20meaning%20of%20models%20of%20nursing.pdf (accessed 27 August 2013).

Wright, S.G. (1986) *Building and Using a Model of Nursing*. Edward Arnold, London.

144

Test Yourself

1. Nursing models allow the nurse to plan:
   (a) Realistic patient-centred care
   (b) Holistic care
   (c) Individualistic care
   (d) All of these

2. Nursing Theory has many definitions.
   (a) True
   (b) False

3. Which theorist introduced nurses to the idea of the individual's need for self-care action?
   (a) Virginia Henderson
   (b) Patricia Benner
   (c) Dorothea Orem
   (d) Martha Rogers

4. Who discussed 'iatrogenesis'?
   (a) Aggleton & Chalmers
   (b) Ivan Illich
   (c) Roy Porter
   (d) Ford and Walsh

5. Who declared: 'it is the nurse's specific role to promote adaptation in health and illness'?
   (a) Betty Neuman
   (b) Sister Callista Roy
   (c) Florence Nightingale
   (d) Joyce Travelbee

6. In which year did Anne MacDonald and her colleagues devise their own paediatric nursing model?
   (a) 2003
   (b) 1978
   (c) 1990
   (d) 1988

7. When using the Tidal Model (mental health) the duty for change remains with …
   (a) The family
   (b) The person
   (c) The nurse
   (d) The patient's consultant

8. The positivist philosophy is considered a 'soft science'.
   (a) True
   (b) False

9. Nursing has been regarded as:
   (a) A science
   (b) An art
   (c) A combination of both
   (d) Neither

10. The approximate cost to the NHS annually as a result of patient safety incidents is:
    (a) £20 million
    (b) £2 billion
    (c) £12 million
    (d) £20 billion

Answers

1. d
2. a
3. c
4. b
5. b
6. d
7. b
8. b
9. c
10. b

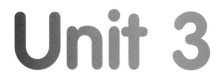

Unit 3

The Principles of Care

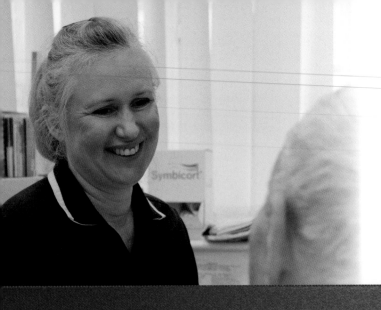

8

The Principles of Safeguarding and Dignity

Iain McGregor

Millington Springs Care Home, Elder Homes Group, UK

Learning Outcomes

On completion of this chapter you will be able to:

- Define what is meant by the terms 'safeguarding' and 'dignity'
- Consider how safeguarding and dignity can directly affect an individual that you care for and support
- Demonstrate an understanding of the legislative frameworks around safeguarding and dignity
- Gain an insight into the application of the principles relating to safeguarding and dignity
- Demonstrate an awareness of the dignity challenges and framework
- Have an insight into dignity action planning and influencing

Competencies

All nurses must:

1. Support and promote the principles of safeguarding and dignity in care
2. Apply the principles of the Mental Capacity Act in a capacity assessment
3. Encourage and advocate the application of the dignity challenges and practice framework
4. Participate in the delivery of safe and dignified care and support to individuals in a health or social care setting
5. Practice within the Nursing and Midwifery Council's Code (Nursing and Midwifery Council, NMC 2008), when caring for and supporting individuals
6. Complete a dignity action plan, relating to one influence or change within your practice area

Visit the companion website at **www.wileynursingpractice.com** where you can test yourself using flashcards, multiple-choice questions and more.

Unit 3 image source: Science Photo Library
Nursing Practice: Knowledge and Care, First Edition. Edited by Ian Peate, Karen Wild and Muralitharan Nair.
© 2014 John Wiley & Sons, Ltd. Published 2014 by John Wiley & Sons, Ltd. Companion website: www.wileynursingpractice.com

Introduction

Within this chapter, you will learn the key principles of 'safeguarding adults at risk' and of 'dignity in care', and be able examine how these can and do directly relate to your practice and practice setting. There will be many situations where you will be required to gain informed consent. Because of this, it is imperative that you understand the legal considerations required for gaining valid consent from individuals and how the capacity assessment might be utilised within situations where the individual is not able to give valid consent at that time.

The important issue of human rights are discussed and how specific articles of the Human Rights Act relate to all aspects of health and social care practice. You will be required, when practicing as a Registered Nurse, to understand how these important rights could be potentially breached and always be aware that you must act, at all times, in the best interests of the people you care for.

Dignity in Care forms part of everyday practice within nursing care and application of the dignity challenges and framework allows you, as a practitioner, to ensure that all aspects of care delivery are completed in a just and dignified manner. An understanding of how to influence dignity in care practices is also be introduced through the use of 'SMARTIES' objective development, and the opportunity to create and apply your own dignity action plan and objectives.

All knowledge and learning that takes place after reading this chapter directly supports practice in line with the NMC's: The Code (NMC 2008), and will allow you to practice with confidence with respect to accountability and responsibility for your actions and omissions.

With the media coverage of poor care and practices within the Winterbourne and Mid-Staffordshire enquiries, safeguarding and dignity of individuals is even more widely recognised than ever before. These cases have proven why it is vital for everyone within health and social care to have a sound knowledge and understanding of safeguarding and dignity, and practice conscientiously and professionally in-line with the professional and legislative frameworks.

What Is Safeguarding?

'Safeguarding' is considered to be an umbrella term that includes the concepts of promoting the welfare and well-being of an individual, as well as protecting from harm (SCIE 2012).

The key point to remember when thinking about safeguarding is to ensure that the individual you are supporting is the highest priority and that they are cared for and supported in a way that is dignified and respectful. This means making sure that they have an active involvement in any planning, decisions and implementation of care and support they are receiving.

Safeguarding should not be seen as a negative or restrictive option, but as a positive way of promoting individualised care and support to individuals. Often, it can be viewed as this, because of the requirement of organisations having policies and procedures in place, highlighting the roles and responsibilities of individual practitioners, and the actual act of safeguarding an individual.

Safeguarding of adults aims to ensure that each individual maintains (to the best of their abilities):

- Dignity and respect
- Quality of life
- Health
- Choice
- Control
- Safety.

Who Is Responsible for Safeguarding?

Safeguarding is ultimately everyone's business, whether they are directly involved in the care and support of an individual or not. We all have a duty to watch out for people in society who have difficulty in protecting themselves and their interests from harm or exploitation.

To Whom Does Safeguarding Apply?

Safeguarding could and may apply to any 'adult at risk'. This term itself could apply to a wide range of people, some for a short period of time and some for a substantial period of time or indefinitely.

Anyone with a condition or illness that affects their ability to maintain their own safety, well-being or interests and express their views could be included in safeguarding principles and procedures. A young gentleman, for example, who has been involved in a motorbike accident and is temporarily incapacitated both physically and mentally due to his injuries and condition, or a person who has a dementia, learning disability or mental health condition that can fluctuate in mental capacity, could require the principles of safeguarding applied to their care.

Principles of Safeguarding

The Department of Health (DH 2011) issued a Statement of Government Policy on Adult Safeguarding, which outlined six principles of safeguarding adults; these are detailed in Box 8.1.

Box 8.1 Principles of Safeguarding Adults	
Empowerment	This includes a belief that the individual has been involved in person-led decisions and informed consent
Protection	This includes the support and interpretation of those in utmost need
Prevention	This includes the anticipation and avoidance of situations before harm could occur
Proportionality	This includes a balanced and least restrictive option and response, which is fitting to the risk identified
Partnership	This includes working within the local communities, to prevent, identify and report any signs of neglect or harm to an individual
Accountability	This includes the need to be accountable for all actions, transparent with care and support for individuals and while taking part in safeguarding

(*Source*: DH 2011)

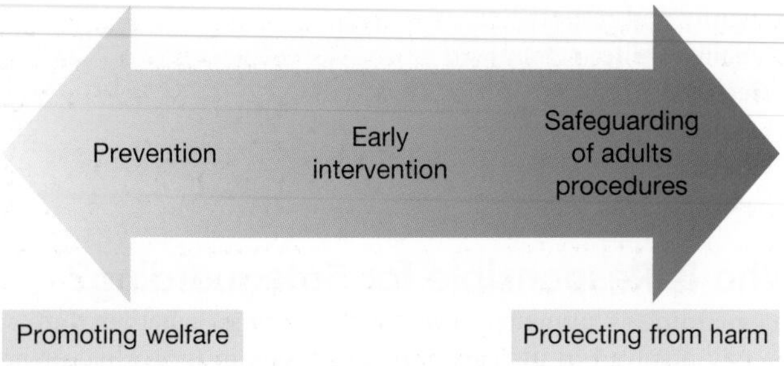

Figure 8.1 Safeguarding continuum. *Source:* SCIE 2013c.

Safeguarding Continuum

Safeguarding of adults should never be viewed in isolation or as a single act once safeguarding procedures have commenced. It should be viewed as a two-way continuum that travels from promoting welfare and well-being to protecting from harm. Figure 8.1 highlights how the continuum of safeguarding is envisaged by multiple local authorities and safeguarding boards (SCIE 2013c).

Safeguarding in Action

The six principles of safeguarding (see Box 8.1) can be applied in practice with some practical guidelines, which will ensure that you deliver the best care and support to the individuals for whom you are responsible.

These guidelines may vary in styling or phrasing from one organisation to the next and it is always recommended to acquaint yourself with the guidelines and policies for your local practice area, although they will include similar guidelines to those listed below:

- Service provision should be suitable and fitting to the individual, and non-discriminatory
- Allow individuals to make their own decisions, as far as possible and support or offer advocacy support to make choices
- Presume that adults do have the mental capacity to make informed decisions about their lives, unless they have been assessed as not having capacity at that point in time
- Provide information, advice and support to any identified adult at risk, in a format that they can understand, and that their wishes and chosen outcomes are central to any safeguarding decision made about them and their lives
- Ensure that any decision taken by health or social care professionals about an individual's life should be done in a timely fashion, be reasonable, justified and proportionate to the risks identified.

As well as the six principles of safeguarding being included in the organisational policy, there are some other inclusions which you will be able to locate within the opening statement or throughout the document. These are:

- A statement on the fact that the individuals you care for and support are kept safe and lead lives that are rewarding
- Information on the staff's responsibilities
- Evidence that your organisation is taking its responsibilities about safeguarding seriously
- Legal disclaimers to protect staff members and the organisation
- Identify routes of which referral to a professional body or safeguarding authority may take, and the circumstances associated with these

- Compliance with legislation and regulations, including good practice guidance and evidence-based support.

Who is an adult at risk?

The 'No Secrets' guidance from the Department of Health (DH & HO 2000) offers definitions on who might be an adult at risk and exists to protect and support some of the most vulnerable adults in society. Adults at risk are defined as:

Any adult over the age of 18, who is or may be in need of community care services by reason of mental or other disability, age or illness; and who is or maybe unable to take care of him or herself, or unable to protect him or herself against significant harm or exploitation.

(DH & HO 2000)

> **Jot This Down**
> - Think of some of the **characteristics** that might make someone more at risk of harm.
> - Think of some of the **factors** that might make someone more at risk of harm.

What does 'mental capacity' mean?

In a safeguarding situation, mental capacity is the ability of an individual to:

- Understand the potential implications of their situation and the risks to themselves
- Take appropriate measures to protect themselves against abuse
- Take part in any decision-making process involving them as individuals, to the fullest extent, regardless of it relating to everyday matters or significant life events.

The Mental Capacity Act 2005 and the Adults with Incapacity (Scotland) Act 2000 are both based on five principles. These principles are detailed in Table 8.1.

You will see from Table 8.1 that there are some differences between both elements of law relating to mental capacity, although ultimately they are both in place to ensure the safety and well-being of individuals and prevent the likelihood of harm or exploitation.

For the purposes of this chapter, we will explore the five principles of the Mental Capacity Act (MCA) 2005 in greater depth.

Table 8.1 Principles of the Mental Capacity Act and Adults with Incapacity (Scotland) Act.

MENTAL CAPACITY ACT 2005	ADULTS WITH INCAPACITY (SCOTLAND) ACT 2000
Principle 1 – Assumption of capacity	**Principle 1 –** Benefit
Principle 2 – Support to make decisions	**Principle 2 –** Least restrictive option
Principle 3 – Right to make unwise decisions	**Principle 3 –** Take account of the wishes of the person
Principle 4 – Best interests	**Principle 4 –** Consultation with relevant others
Principle 5 – Least restrictive option	**Principle 5 –** Encourage the person to use existing skills and develop new skills

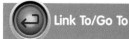

Link To/Go To

Further information on the Adults with Incapacity (Scotland) Act 2000 can be found at: http://www.scotland.gov.uk/Resource/Doc/217194/0058194.pdf

Principle 1 – Assumption of Capacity

Everyone, even those with a diagnosis of an illness or condition, have the right to make their own decisions and must be assumed to have capacity, unless it is proved otherwise.

This requires a 'balance of probability' test initially, where we need to ensure that 'a reasonable person' would think that there is evidence of an individual understanding the required decision and its consequences.

Following this, a two-stage functional test of capacity is required to decide if an individual has capacity to make a decision.

The two stages are:

Stage 1 – Is there an impairment of or disturbance in the functioning of a person's mind or brain? If so,

Stage 2 – Is the impairment or disturbance sufficient that the person lacks the capacity to make a particular decision?

(SCIE 2010)

Following this functional test of capacity, the MCA states that an individual is not able to make their own decision if they cannot achieve one or more of the following:

- Understand and retain the information given to them to be able to make a decision
- Process the information that has been made available to them to make the decision
- Communicate their decision.

After the assessment has been completed using the above criteria and the balance of probabilities (and your findings) have shown it is more likely than not that the individual lacks capacity, it is essential to document all findings and how you have come to the conclusion that their capacity is lacking for the particular decision.

When considering how an individual can communicate their decision, health and social care professionals can not solely consider verbal communication as a valid communication method and every effort should be made to establish ways of communicating with someone before the decision that they lack capacity is made.

Alternative communication methods that may need to be considered including: use of sign language, written word or a slight movement of a muscle within given parameters.

Who should assess mental capacity?

Jot This Down

Take time to list some of the members of the multiprofessional team, and think who would be the best person from your list to assess mental capacity on individuals.

The answer to the question in the 'Jot This Down' exercise above, about who should assess mental capacity, is dependent on who is directly involved in the care delivery and who is immediately involved in the outcome from that decision. This means that everyone in the list you have made above, including yourself, will be involved in assessing an individual's capacity at different times and for different decisions.

Jot This Down

- Consider your practice, and identify some decisions that an individual might be asked to make, while you are present, and where you may be involved in assessing the capacity of the individual.

151

Principle 2 – Support to Make Decisions

Some individuals are able to make decisions when supported in doing so. Any adult at risk must receive all the help and support possible to make decisions before anyone presumes that they cannot do so.

The Department of Constitutional Affairs (DCA 2007) in the Mental Capacity 2005 Code of Practice identifies several items to be taken into consideration to ensure that a person has been supported to make a decision and these should be followed as part of the overall assessment of the individual's abilities.

- Has the individual received all of the significant information to make a decision?
- If there are alternatives available, has the individual been given the information on all of the alternatives?
- Would the individual be able to understand or process the information better if it was presented differently?
- Does the individual demonstrate a better understanding at different times of the day?
- Does the individual feel more comfortable in different places, and therefore able to make decisions better?
- Does the decision have to be made at this point in time or can it be delayed until the conditions are different, allowing the individual to make the decision.
- Does the individual need anyone else to help them to make their choices or views known?

Principle 3 – Right to Make Unwise Decisions

Any adult has the right to make decisions that others might consider as being unwise or eccentric. This also applies to adults at risk, and the person cannot be treated as lacking capacity because of these reasons.

However, if someone repeatedly makes unwise decisions that place them at significant risk, this might be grounds to question and assess their capacity.

Throughout the considerations within Principle 3, it is important to remember that everyone has their own values, beliefs and preferences, which may not be the same as yours. People cannot be treated as lacking in capacity because they hold different values, beliefs or preferences from those we hold.

As members of the health and social care team, it is essential to try and understand, to the best of our abilities, the beliefs and values of the person whose capacity to make decisions is under question. This is done by seeking evidence of a person's beliefs and values, which can be found in things such as:

- Cultural background
- Religious beliefs

- Political convictions
- Past behaviour or habits.

Some people set out their beliefs and values in a written statement while they still have capacity.

Principle 4 – Best Interests

If it is essential to make a decision on behalf of someone who has been assessed as lacking capacity, then whatever the decision made needs to ensure that it is in the person's best interests.

The term 'best interest' is not actually defined within the Mental Capacity Act 2005 because the Act deals with so many different types of decisions and actions.

The Mental Capacity Act Code of Practice (DCA 2007) does, however, provide a checklist of common factors that must always be considered by anyone who needs to decide what is in the best interests of a person who lacks capacity in any particular situation. It is only the starting point; in many cases, extra factors will need to be considered.

Link To/Go To

The aforementioned checklist can be accessed via:

http://www.justice.gov.uk/downloads/protecting-the
-vulnerable/mca/mca-code-practice-0509.pdf

Principles governing 'best interest' decisions

When working out what is in the best interests of the person who lacks capacity to make a decision or act for themselves, decision-makers must take into account all relevant factors that it would be reasonable to consider, not just those that they think are important.

They must not act or make a decision based on what they would want to do if they were the person who lacked capacity rather what the person themselves would do if they did not lack capacity.

The following principles should be applied while making a 'best interest' decision on behalf of a person who is lacking capacity:

- Do not discriminate. Do not make assumptions about someone's best interests merely on the basis of the person's age or appearance, condition or any aspect of their behaviour
- Take into account all relevant circumstances
- If faced with a particularly difficult or contentious decision, it is recommended that practitioners adopt a 'balance sheet' approach (weighing up the advantages and disadvantages of each option in turn).
- Will the person regain capacity? If so, can the decision wait?
- Involve the individual as fully as possible
- Take into account the individual's past and present wishes and feelings, and any beliefs and values likely to have a bearing on the decision
- Consult as far and as widely as possible.

Principle 5 – Least Restrictive Option

If a best interest decision is made on behalf of someone who is judged to be lacking capacity, it is important that you make the choice that least restricts the person's liberty.

This means, before you make a decision or act on behalf of a person who lacks capacity to make that decision or consent to the act, you must always question whether you can do something else that would interfere less with the person's basic rights and freedoms

(and would not close down or reduce the future choices available to them). This includes considering whether there is a need to act or make a decision at all.

It is also essential that you record your decision given the evidence-based approach required by the Mental Capacity Act, so that you have an objective record should your decision or decision-making process later be challenged. This should be in-line with the Nursing and Midwifery Council's *Record Keeping: Guidance for nurses and midwives* (NMC 2009).

What Is Meant by Deprivation of Liberty Safeguards?

The Deprivation of Liberty Safeguards (DoLS) is an amendment to the Mental Capacity Act 2005. It applies to England and Wales only. The Mental Capacity Act allows restraint and restrictions to be used – but only if they are in the person's best interests. Extra safeguards are needed if the restraint and restrictions will deprive a person of their liberty and they do not have the capacity to consent – these are called the Deprivation of Liberty Safeguards.

The DoLS can only be used if the person will be deprived of their liberty within a care home or hospital setting. In other settings, the Court of Protection can be asked if a person can be deprived of their liberty.

The ways in which a person's freedoms can be curtailed include:

- Using locks or key pads, which stop a person going out or into different areas of a building
- The use of some medication, for example to calm a person
- Close supervision in the clinical setting
- Requiring a person to be supervised when out
- Restricting contact with family, friends and acquaintances, including if they could cause the person harm
- Physically stopping a person from doing something that could cause them harm
- Removing items from a person that could cause them harm
- Holding a person so that they can be given care or treatment
- The use of bedrails, wheelchair straps or splints
- The person having to stay somewhere against their wishes
- The person having to stay somewhere against the wishes of a family member.

Members of the health and social care teams need to ensure that they are using the least restrictive alternative and have sought the permission of the correct supervisory body.

From April 2013, the supervisory bodies for care homes and hospitals are the local authorities where the person is ordinarily resident. Usually, this will be the local authority where the care home or hospital is located unless the person's care is funded by a different local authority.

What Is Abuse or Harm?

The term 'abuse' or 'harm' is often interchangeable and, dependant on the location of your studies, may be included in the Country's laws and legislation. The Adult Support and Protection (Scotland) Act 2007, for example uses the term 'harm' to adults at risk, rather than abuse. For the purposes of this text, the term 'abuse' will be utilised.

'Abuse' in its broadest term relates to the misuse or application of power and control over one individual from another, and can take place in virtually any environment within society, regardless of circumstance.

The Department of Health (DH & HO 2000) 'No Secrets' document formally defines abuse as:

the violation of an individual's human or civil rights by any other person or persons.

To reiterate, there are several groups of adults that could potentially be at higher risk of being abused because of their vulnerabilities, and additional considerations need to be paid when caring and supporting these individuals.

Abuse does not always require motive or be intended, and can be considered on the harm caused or the impact of the harm caused on the individual. Examples of this will be explored when looking at the types of abuse.

The Social Care Institute for Excellence (SCIE 2011) states that early legal or police involvement in any suspected or alleged abuse is vital and should be a key consideration with any circumstances, although not all cases of reported abuse escalate to legal or criminal proceedings.

The Nature of Abuse

Abuse however, is not as straight forward in practice, as the misuse of power or control over an individual, and several complexities come into play within this arena. There are four main themes to consider when identifying the nature of the abuse taking place, as well as the type. Table 8.2 highlights the nature in which abuse can take place.

Consent

When considering abusive acts and the reporting and dealing with such, consent from the individual must be a consideration within the process. The application of the Principles of the Mental Capacity Act and the Adults with Incapacity (Scotland) Act, which have already been described, would need to be a consideration at these times.

While also considering if consent was given, thought should be paid to if consent was given under duress, such as fear, intimidation and for potential outcomes for other family members. If consent was given in any of these circumstances, it is likely to be regarded as non-consensual and action can be taken against the perpetrator.

Types of Adult Abuse

Legislation within England outlines seven different types of abuse, while the Adult Support and Protection (Scotland) Act (2007) details eight, i.e. with the inclusion of 'any conduct which causes self-harm'. In essence, this means that any conduct performed by a health or social care professional which leads to the individual self-harming, will be considered abusive and could potentially lead to criminal prosecution being made against them.

The other seven types of abuse are comparable across the legislation and are detailed in Figure 8.2.

While each of these types will be explored individually, there are often overlapping aspects of each. Sexual abuse, for example, is unlikely to take place without some form of emotional or psychological abuse also taking place.

Physical abuse

Physical abuse can be comprised of several actions, both deliberate and unintentional, including: punching, kicking, shaking, hitting, scalding, pinching, over or under use of medication and the misuse of restraint.

The SCIE (2011b) defines physical abuse in one of two ways:

The use of force which results in pain or injury or a change in the person's natural physical state.

The non-accidental infliction of physical force that results in bodily injury, pain or impairment.

Although the second definition offered by SCIE states 'non-accidental', there are times when 'accidental' physical abuse may take place, although it would be potentially considered as neglect or an act of omission. Failing to check the temperature of a bath, for example and submersing the individual into it, causing scalding to legs and torso could be considered as accidental physical abuse.

Table 8.2 The nature of abuse. (*Source*: SCIE 2011)

NATURE OF ABUSE	DESCRIPTION
A single act or repeated acts	Abuse may take place in a single act or a series of acts, both large and small, that could have abusive consequences for the individual in question
Unintentional	Causing harm may have been unintentional and not wilful, but harm has been caused and abuse has taken place. Regardless of intent, a response under the safeguarding procedures is required
An act of neglect or a failure to act	Neglect or failing to act may still cause harm to an individual and would require a response under the safeguarding procedures, to identify and deal with the contributing factors that are often associated with this abusive nature
Multiple acts	The individual receiving care and support may be experiencing several forms of abuse at the same time; some more discreet than others

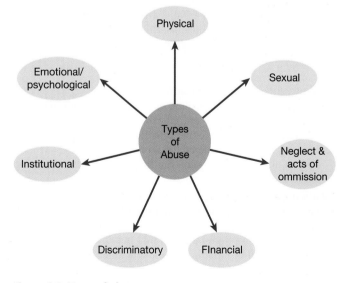

Figure 8.2 Types of abuse. *Source*: Department of Health and Home Office 2000.

> **Box 8.2 Emotional Abuse**
> - Undermining self-esteem or belittling an individual
> - Humiliation
> - Ignoring
> - Removal of the right for an individual to make choice
> - Threatening behaviour
> - Bullying
> - Coercion
> - Withdrawal of contact with others
>
> (*Source*: SCIE 2012a)

Emotional or psychological abuse

'Emotional abuse' or 'psychological abuse' are terms that can often be interchangeable. They ultimately mean any act or deed that could be harmful to the well-being, health or growth of an individual who is at risk (SCIE 2012b). For the purposes of this text, the term 'emotional abuse' will be used, although reference should be made to organisational policies and procedures for use of the correct terminology within practice.

Emotional abuse can include any of the issues identified in Box 8.2.

Sexual abuse

Sexual abuse can be both direct and indirect in nature, involving an individual in sexual activity or relationship, who:

- does not want to take part or has not given valid consent to
- does not understand and lacks the mental capacity to give consent
- has been coerced into taking part because the perpetrator is in a position of power and trust.

Sexual abuse can also take into account the viewing or being included in the making of pornographic materials, against the individual's wishes, this can either be through video materials or through imagery.

Sexual abuse is often under reported and the figures published in the NHS Information Centre's report (NHS 2012) suggest that sexual abuse only forms 6% of all referrals made.

The risk of sexual abuse from a stranger is significantly lower than those known to the individual, although the ever growing use of the internet for social media and online dating is posing more of a threat within modern society.

Neglect and acts of omission

This is often known as the failing or failure of a person who has responsibility for the safe and effective care and support of an individual. Neglect can be either intentional or unintentional and acts of omission are considered the same.

Neglect and acts of omission can include any of the following in isolation or as multiple failings:

- Lack of social or educational provision
- Withholding or lack of provision for basic needs such as food, water and warmth
- Lack of protection from other hazards and adverse risk-taking
- Lack of medical or nursing care and attention.

The development of a pressure ulcer in any care setting could be considered an act of neglect, due the lack of essential care being provided to the individual. The same could be considered for any individual who becomes dehydrated or malnourished while receiving care and support from health or social care staff.

Financial abuse

Financial abuse is often considered one of the less obvious forms of abuse that can take place until the matter has developed so considerably that it becomes apparent to others.

Forms of financial abuse can include: theft or fraudulent behaviour; exploitation; misappropriation of property; possessions or financial income; excessive pressure on the individual in relation to property, inheritance, wills and other financial transactions.

Financial abuse could also be considered as the financial gain from an individual who is not able to give valid consent. An example of this is collecting a supermarket's loyalty points from shopping, which you have undertaken for an individual who you are caring for and supporting and they have paid for.

Discriminatory abuse

This can take place when there is a difference in values, beliefs or culture and an exploitation of power takes place over a group or individual. It has the potential to be a characteristic in other types of abuse, but can also be performed in isolation.

It has been found that discriminatory abuse can be motivated by age, gender, disability, religion, class, culture, sexuality, language and race or ethnic origin (SCIE 2011c).

It often results in situations where the group or individual feels vulnerable and excluded from aspects of life that are open to others, such as accessing health or social care services.

The Equality Act 2010 was developed and established as a vital piece of legislation to minimise and reduce the likelihood of any discriminatory practices.

> **Jot This Down**
>
> Before accessing further information on The Equality Act 2010, detailed in this chapter, can you list some of the aspects of equality and diversity that you may already be aware of?

 Link To/Go To

Further information on The Equality Act 2010 can be found at:
https://www.gov.uk/equality-act-2010-guidance

Institutional abuse

Institutional abuse violates an individual's dignity, right to make choices and basic human rights. It is the maltreatment and restrictive practices of some care providers that still makes institutional abuse apparent today.

It is often associated with the lack of flexibility in service delivery, systems and regimes that brings this type of abuse to the forefront. It is often connected with organisations that fail to respond to the poor and inadequate practices taking place and addressing these matters when brought to their attention.

It can take place in any establishment or organisation where care and support on any level is offered, and can be difficult to differentiate between a poor service and institutional abuse.

Identifying Abuse

Depending on your level of contact and support with an individual can affect how abuse can be identified. If you are supporting the individual with personal care, you might be able to notice signs more readily than someone who is providing support in a social capacity.

The identification of abuse can be split into three potential indicator groups, which may make it easier to formulate into a firmer suspicion or confirmation of abuse taking place.

The three indicator groups are:

- **Physical signs** – Does the individual have any or show any physical changes or signs that may indicate abuse taking place?
- **Behavioural signs** – Are there any changes in the individual's behaviours that may lessen or increase your concerns? Are the behaviours significantly different from usual?
- **Other factors** – Are there any historical influences that need to be considered at this time, and do they increase your concern or reduce it?

 Link To/Go To

Further information on the potential signs of abuse can be accessed as follows:

Types and Signs of Abuse:

http://www.hertsdirect.org/infobase/docs/pdfstore/app2signs.pdf

Identifying the Signs of Abuse:

http://www.scie.org.uk/publications/elearning/adultsafeguarding/resource/documents/Identifying%20the%20signs%20of%20abuse.pdf

Jot This Down

From the information that has been accessed on the signs of abuse – can you list three potential signs of abuse for each of the following types?

Physical abuse

Emotional/psychological abuse

Sexual abuse

Institutional abuse

Discriminatory abuse

Financial abuse

Neglect and acts of omission

Safeguarding Is Everybody's Business

Safeguarding is everybody's business. However, your responsibilities may vary depending on your role, which may include being: a family member, friend, volunteer, health and social care worker, professional, safeguarding professional or manager.

There are six key principles of safeguarding that are applicable to all roles, and require everyone to be aware of:

1. **Empowerment** – presumption of person-led activities and informed consent
2. **Protection** – support and representation for those in greatest need
3. **Prevention** – it is better to take action before harm occurs
4. **Proportionality** – proportionate and least intrusive response appropriate to the risk presented

5. **Partnership** – local solutions through services working with their communities (communities have a part to play in prevention, detection and reporting neglect and abuse)
6. **Accountability** – accountability and transparency in delivering safeguarding.

Policy Framework for Safeguarding Adults

Adult safeguarding is framed in terms of the responsibilities of the local authorities and its partners in the National Health Service, Police forces and other emergency services, with the Safeguarding Adults Boards managing the delivery of services across all agencies.

The Centre for Public Scrutiny and the Improvement and Development Agency (CPS & I&DeA 2010) published an 'Adult Safeguarding Scrutiny Guide', recognising the need for safeguarding to be everybody's business, and identified four main work streams involved in adult safeguarding, with varying responsibilities depending on your role and relationship to the adult at risk.

Prevention and awareness raising

These incorporate ways to improve the general well-being of everyone, to support communities to look out for each other and to help the public know what to do if they think that someone may be being harmed or abused.

Inclusion

This is where people who are vulnerable to poor life circumstances, and have been identified as an 'adult at risk', are actively engaged in activity provided services and they may be alerted to the people at risk, and concerns from other organisations.

Personalise management of benefits and risks

This involves specific actions taken by those who are responsible for the commissioning, design and delivery of services to people at risk. Personalised management ensures the identification and support of people to help them to protect themselves and make informed decisions about action.

Specialist safeguarding services

These are the people responsible for providing the specific responses to those who have or may have experienced harm or abuse and include their involvement in decision-making as far as possible. This will involve specific action to ensure that people who lack capacity are supported through advocates and processes to ensure that their best interests are pursued. It also includes ensuring that justice is facilitated where people at risk are the victims of crime (CPS & I&DeA 2010).

Jot This Down

List some of the emotions that you think a person might be feeling when considering whether to talk about abuse

- Make a separate list of what they might be looking for or wanting from the person they are disclosing to

If someone chooses to disclose abuse to you, it is because they trust you. If someone confides in you, no matter what position you hold or your relationship to the person making the disclosure, you must act. Your responsibility is not to decide whether they are being abused, that is the responsibility of the relevant social work and safeguarding teams.

From the two activities completed concerning abuse and disclosure, you may have identified that a person who is disclosing abuse to you, could potentially be feeling:

- Sad
- Lonely
- Angry
- Frightened
- Guilty
- Confused
- Worried
- Anxious
- Worthless.

They may be looking for any of the following from the person they are disclosing to:

- To be listened to
- To be believed
- Reassurances
- Help
- Support
- Empathy
- Privacy
- Understanding
- Kindness
- To make it stop.

Responding to Disclosures

If an individual chooses to disclose harm or abuse to you, you will need to have an awareness of the feelings they could be experiencing and what they may be looking for, by disclosing to you – which can be identified from the lists above.

Other guidelines, which are listed below should be followed when responding to an adult at risk, who is disclosing to you.

- Assure the individual that you are taking them seriously
- Listen carefully to what they are telling you, stay calm, get as clear a picture as you can, but avoid asking too many questions at this stage
- Do not give promises of being completely confidential
- Explain that you have a duty to tell your manager or other designated person, and that their concerns may be shared with others who could have a part to play in protecting them
- Reassure the individual that they will be involved in decisions about what will happen
- Explain that you will try to take steps to protect them from further abuse or neglect
- If they have specific communication needs, provide support and information in a way that is most appropriate to them
- Do not be judgemental or jump to conclusions.

These guidelines may be presented slightly differently within your local practice areas, although the underlying principles will remain the same. Regardless of the guidelines that you are utilising, it is essential that you consider the guidelines, and react and behave appropriately to the individual needs of the person.

Immediate Action

Everyone who witnesses abuse or has abuse disclosed to them needs to know what immediate action to take. It is vital to become familiar with the local organisations policies and procedures, so responses are made in-line with these documents.

If no policy or procedure is in place or available, the following steps should be utilised as a framework for response in an emergency:

- Make an immediate evaluation of the risk and take steps to ensure that the adult is not in immediate danger
- If there is need for emergency medical treatment, dial 999 (or the emergency response number in your location) for an ambulance. If you suspect that the injury is non-accidental, alert the ambulance staff, so that appropriate measures are taken to preserve possible forensic evidence. Wherever possible, establish with the adult at risk the action they wish you to take
- Consider contacting the police if a crime has been or may have been committed. Professional staff should alert their safeguarding lead or deputy, as they will be the ones to involve the police
- Do not disturb or move articles that could be used in evidence, and secure the scene, for example by locking the door to a room
- Contact the children and families' department if there is also or is suspected that there is also a child at risk
- As far as is possible, make sure that others are not at risk.

What to Do If a Criminal Offence Is Suspected

The first concern of everyone must be to ensure the safety and well-being of the alleged victim.

It is the responsibility of the police to gather and preserve evidence in order to pursue criminal allegations against people causing harm and they should be contacted immediately.

However, the victims themselves and other people and organisations play a vital role in the preservation of evidence to ensure that vital information or forensics is not lost.

In some situations, it is important that you do not touch anything, so resist the natural inclinations to tidy up or wash away blood or other forensic materials. It may also contaminate evidence if the victim eats drinks or smokes a cigarette – so think carefully about what the individual is doing.

Resist the temptation to take pictures of the scene with your phone. Your pictures are unlikely to be of sufficient quality to be submitted to court as part of a prosecution case, as they are unlikely to be used in court; the police will also confiscate your phone. The preferable option is to leave the scene undisturbed and allow a police photographer to capture the evidence.

Do not question the alleged victim any more than you need to in order to clarify that possible abuse has taken place. Police are required to obtain oral (spoken) evidence in specific ways. Questioning the alleged victim at this stage runs the risk of contaminating their oral evidence and a defence lawyer may be able to allege that the victim was coached by you.

Red Flag

Preventing abuse means doing three things:

- Listening to people and their caregivers
- Intervening when you suspect abuse
- Educating others about how to recognise and report abuse

Making a Record

Anybody who is witness to or alerted to a situation of abuse should make a written record of any incident or allegation of crime as soon as possible, and keep a signed, dated and timed copy.

The record must reflect as accurately as possible, what was said and done by the people initially involved in the incident (the victim, suspect and potential witnesses). Use the words actually spoken and not a sanitised version of them – this is important.

This does not mean that the alleged victims or suspects should be questioned in any detail. This record is an account of what was observed, disclosed or witnessed at the time and not an investigation. Investigation is the responsibility of the safeguarding professionals.

The notes must be kept safe, as it may be necessary to make records available as evidence and to disclose them in court.

Key Stages of the Safeguarding Adult's Process

There are seven key stages in the safeguarding adult's process, brief information will be given on all of the stages but this chapter will focus on the first two stages, as the later ones require further specialist training.

- Stage 1 – Raising an alert
- Stage 2 – Making a referral
- Stage 3 – Strategy discussion or meeting
- Stage 4 – Investigation
- Stage 5 – Case conference and protection plan
- Stage 6 – Review of the protection plan
- Stage 7 – Closing the safeguarding adult's process.

Stage 1 – Raising an alert
Everyone has a responsibility for safeguarding adults. If you are raising a concern within an organisation, then the concern should be passed immediately to the person responsible for dealing with safeguarding adults.

If there is no organisation involved, the person raising the alert should contact the local Social Services Department directly.

Stage 2 – Making a referral
The decision to make a referral will normally be made by the person responsible for dealing with safeguarding.

If there is no organisation providing service to the adult at risk, the person who is concerned can make a referral directly to the local Social Services Department.

Stage 3 – Strategy discussion or meeting
This is a multiagency meeting convened and coordinated by the Safeguarding Adults Manager (SAM) in the local authority, who will discuss the allegations with a range of professionals (usually including the police, where appropriate) to:

- Consider the wishes of the adult at risk
- Agree whether an investigation will take place, and if so, how it should be conducted and by whom
- Undertake risk assessment
- Agree an interim protection plan
- Make a clear record of the decisions
- Record what information is shared
- Agree an investigation plan with timescales
- Agree a communication strategy
- Consider whether a child (under 18 years) may also be at risk
- Circulate decisions to all invitees within 5 days, using the appropriate pro forma.

Stage 4 – Investigation
The nature of the investigation is decided by those at the strategy meeting, who will also appoint an investigating officer. The purpose of the investigation is to:

- Establish the facts and contributing factors leading up to the referral
- Identify and manage risk and ensure the safety of the individuals and others.

If a mental capacity assessment is indicated, the meeting should also consider instructing an Independent Mental Capacity Advocate (IMCA). This may be appropriate where the person lacks other appropriate support to represent their interests.

Stage 5 – Case conference and protection plan
The aim of a case conference is to:

- Consider the information contained in the investigating officer's report(s)
- Consider the evidence and, if substantiated, plan what action is indicated, or alternatively:
  - Plan further action if the allegation is not substantiated
  - Plan further action if the investigation is inconclusive
- Consider what legal or statutory action or redress is indicated
- Make a decision about the levels of current risks and a judgement about any likely future plans
- Agree a protection plan
  - Agree how the protection plan will be reviewed and monitored.

The protection plan, which will be overseen by a designated protection plan coordinator, focusses on minimising the risk of harm to the person at risk and developing strategies to enhance their resilience. This does not include actions taken against the person causing harm.

Stage 6 – Review of the protection plan
The purpose of the review is to ensure that the actions agreed in the protection plan have been implemented and to decide whether further action is needed, including any service improvements.

Stage 7 – Closing the safeguarding adult's process
The safeguarding adults process may be closed at any stage, if it is agreed that an ongoing investigation is not needed or if the investigation has been completed and a protection plan has been agreed and put in place.

In most cases, a decision to close the safeguarding adult's process is taken at the case conference or at a protection plan review.

Jot This Down

More in-depth details on the seven stages of the safeguarding adults process can be accessed and read in the following document: Social Care Institute for Excellence (SCIE 2011a) *Adult Services Report 39. Protecting adults at risk: London multi-agency policy and procedure to safeguard adults from abuse.* SCIE, London.

When reading this, think about your role as a student nurse, how you can work with other professionals to promote safeguarding, and which of the seven stages you may be potentially involved in. Make notes.

Timescales of the Key Stages of the Adult Safeguarding Process

It is vital that each of the stages of the adult safeguarding process takes place within the stipulated timescale and with certain tasks and responsibilities being completed at each of the stages, allowing the correct systems to be in place and utilised, also ensuring the safety and welfare of the individual who might be subject to the safeguarding process.

Link To/Go To

These timescales and further information can be downloaded from the Social Care Institute for Excellence website:

http://www.scie.org.uk/publications/elearning/
adultsafeguarding/resource/documents/Key%20stages%20
of%20adult%20safeguarding.pdf

Stage 1 – Raising an Alert

Raising an alert means passing on a concern. Everyone has a responsibility for safeguarding adults. If you are raising a concern within an organisation, then the concern should be passed immediately to the person responsible for dealing with safeguarding alerts (the 'alerting manager').

If an adult is on the receiving end of abuse... An adult at risk, may find it difficult to identify their vulnerabilities and to respond to neglect or ill-treatment by others.

You must contact your local Social Services Department. If it is difficult for you to do this directly, speak to someone you trust – a family member, friend or professional not involved in the abuse – and ask them to do this for you.

You should expect a response from Social Services within 24 hours. If the situation is an emergency, ring 999 and the police will ensure that your concerns are passed onto Social Services and that you get an immediate response.

If you are a friend or family member... Discuss with the adult concerned the need to involve Social Services. As adults, we have the right to make our own decisions, even unwise ones, so always try to obtain consent of the person involved before contacting the local Social Services Department.

However, you may contact them without gaining their consent if:

- You doubt their capacity to understand the consequences of their decision to take no action
- You fear for the safety of others
- You feel there is an immediate danger.

When contacting Social Services, explain your fears and the fact that the adult concerned did not want you to involve them. They will decide how best to take matters forward.

If you are a professional (including all healthcare students), care worker or volunteer... If you are concerned that a member of staff has abused an adult at risk, you have a duty to report these concerns. You must inform your line manager immediately; as a student nurse, it can be difficult to identify who your line manager is – while on practice placements, this would be your link lecturer or university tutor.

If you are concerned that your line manager has abused an adult at risk, you must inform a senior manager in your organisation, or another designated manager for safeguarding adults, without delay.

If you are concerned that an adult at risk may have abused another adult at risk, inform your line manager immediately.

Responsibilities of the 'alerting manager'

An 'alerting manager' is the person within an organisation designated to make safeguarding adult referrals. The alert may be made to them by the adult at risk, their family or friends, care workers, volunteers or other professionals.

They must decide without delay on the most appropriate course of action.

If you are a staff member or a volunteer it is your responsibility to find out who is the designated person within your organisation to make a safeguarding referral.

Jot This Down

What areas do you think, as a student nurse, you may need to consider at the point that you are making someone aware of a safeguarding matter? List your thoughts.

Depending on the circumstances, the alerting manager needs to consider the adults immediate:

- **Health needs** – have they sustained an injury or does the neglect they have experienced warrant medical attention?
- **Forensic needs** – if they need to see a doctor, should it be someone competent to collect forensic evidence? If the matter is to be referred to the police, the alerting manager should discuss any potential forensic considerations, particularly if the abuse is thought to be of a sexual nature
- **Legal needs** – has a crime been committed? In which case, immediate consultation with the police is necessary
- **Safety needs** – are they at continued risk in their current home? What additional supports are necessary? Do they need to be provided with alternative services or accommodation?

They may need to make a referral to the relevant adult care services or Community Mental Health Team (CMHT), or the relevant adult care services Emergency Duty Team (EDT) if out of hours.

If the person causing the harm is also an adult at risk, they should arrange for a member of staff to attend to their needs and make a parallel referral to Social Services to address their needs.

If a staff member is suspected of causing the abuse, their manager should consider suspending the staff member (or otherwise removing them from the person at risk) in-line with their organisation's safeguarding policy.

Responsibilities to the alleged abuser The alerting manager should also consider the action they need to take in relation to the person alleged to have caused harm. It is always worth considering liaison with the police regarding the management of any risks.

Where the allegation is against a staff member, the first consideration should be whether to separate them from the person at risk. This may involve suspending them, without prejudice, pending further investigation, while the staff member has a right to know that allegations have been made against them (the details of the allegation should not be shared at this stage). The strategy meeting (identified in Stage 3 of the seven stage adult safeguarding process) will decide on what will be shared and when. Consideration must also be given to the risks, if any, to other service users and staff members, particularly if the conduct of the staff member came to light as the result of whistle-blowing.

If the person alleged to have caused harm might also be considered an adult at risk, the alerting manager needs to arrange for a professional in Social Services or another involved agency to ensure that any immediate needs they have in relation to the health and safety are met, and that they understand the need for legal representation and the possibility that they may need to provide forensic evidence.

Speaking to the adult at risk The alerting manager may feel that it is appropriate to speak to the adult at risk before contacting Social Services. They should consider their communication needs and their capacity to understand the information they are being provided with and their ability to make decisions. Specifically, they should:

- Speak to them in a private and safe place to inform them of the concerns
- Obtain their views on what has happened and what they want done about it
- Provide information about the safeguarding adults process and how it could help to make them safer
- Ensure that they understand the parameters of confidentiality
- Explain how they will be kept informed, particularly if they have communication needs
- Consider how the abusive experience might impact on the ongoing delivery of services, particularly personal care arrangements and access arrangements
- Explore their immediate protection needs.

They should not conduct an investigation – that is the responsibility of the safeguarding professionals in Social Services and the police. An organisation may need to conduct a disciplinary investigation, coordinated at the strategy meeting.

In the event that the adult at risk does not have capacity to make decisions for themselves, any action taken or decisions made on their behalf must be made in their 'best interests'.

Stage 2 – Making a Referral

The consent of the adult at risk is a significant factor in deciding what action to take in response to an allegation but this in turn will depend on the capacity of the adult to make a decision.

When considering whether to *refer* or not and assessing their capacity, the following questions need to be included as part of the overall assessment:

- What do they understand about the abuse they have experienced?
- What do they think will be the consequence of making or not making a referral, both in terms of their immediate safety and in the longer term?
- What outcome do they want?
- What action do they think will be taken and by whom?
- What is their ability to protect themselves from future harm?

What if the adult at risk decides not to refer?

The safeguarding processes are based on an assumption of capacity and the right of the individual to make their own choices, even unwise ones. In situations where the adult alleging abuse decides they do not want action taken:

- They should be given information about where to get help if they change their mind or if the abuse or neglect continues and they subsequently want support to promote their own safety
- The referrer/alerting manager must assure themselves that the decision to withhold consent is not made under undue influence, coercion or intimidation
- A record must be made of the concern, the adult at risk's decision and of the decision not to refer, along with both your and their reasons
- A record should also be made of what information/advice they were given in a separate part of the individual's file or record that is clearly labelled 'safeguarding'.

If the referrer/alerting manager feels uncomfortable making this decision alone, they should seek a consultation with their local adult safeguarding team to discuss the situation, without naming the individual, and document any advice they are given.

Overriding the adult at risk's decision

Where the referrer/alerting manager believes that there is an overriding public interest or vital interest if gaining consent would put the individual at further risk, a referral must be made and the views of the individual overridden.

The key issue in deciding whether to make a referral is the harm or risk of harm to the adult at risk and any other individual who may have contact with the person who could have caused harm. Be especially vigilant where the person who could have caused harm remains in contact with the same organisation, service or care setting.

This would include situations where:

- Other people or children could be at risk from the person causing harm
- It is necessary to prevent crime
- There is a high risk to the health and safety of the adult at risk
- The person lacks capacity to consent.

If the alerting manager is unsure whether to refer, they should contact the relevant local safeguarding adult's organisation for advice.

Preventing the Abuse of Adults at Risk

In recent years, the debate about prevention in safeguarding has been assisted and developed further with the introduction of the personalisation agenda and the self-directed care initiatives and schemes that have been running. It is important to achieve a balance between the individual's rights to make choices for themselves and the duty of those caring and supporting the individual to keep them free from harm.

In practice, this means not being overprotective or risk adverse, but rather promoting empowerment and positive risk taking within any care setting.

The prevention of the abuse or neglect of the vulnerable in our society requires a multidimensional approach. Figure 8.3 represents the people and services that any individual may reasonably expect to 'look out' for them.

The Right to be Free from Abuse

Everyone needs to know that they have the right to be free from abuse. Some adults need support in exercising this right. This might mean ensuring they have access to advocacy services.

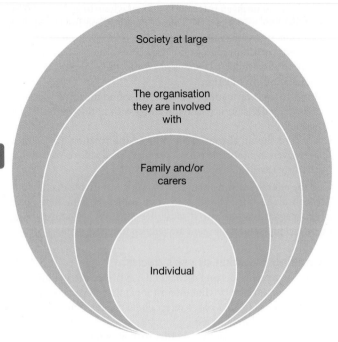

Figure 8.3 Multidimensional approach to preventing abuse or neglect. *Source:* SCIE 2011.

In order for adults at risk to be able to exercise their rights, those around them need to be made aware that these rights exist and the reasons for them.

Empowerment and Choice

Many people at risk have reported wanting help to deal with situations in their own way, specifically, they want to do their own safeguarding. People want help with information, options, alternatives, suggestions, mediation, talking to others in a way that helps them get what they want, and so on.

What they do not want is decisions being made for them.

To facilitate this, adults at risk should have regular practice in making independent decisions.

The 'personalisation' police agenda provides one such environment within which to exercise choice and, despite the potential for the financial exploitation of vulnerable adults, there is a range of strategies identified, which can help empower adults to make their own decisions (Carr 2010).

Person-Centred Practice

Limited resources are a reality, but there is a range of very simple steps we can all take to demonstrate that we acknowledge the individuality of the person we are caring for and supporting.

These steps can be summarised as 'person-centred practice'. There is much written about person-centred practice throughout nursing and care literature but the main features can be summarised as talking to and about the person to build up a picture of:

- How the individual sees themselves
- How others see them
- Their routines
- Their hopes for the future.

The aim is to identify with them (or their advocate) how best to support them. The outcome of these discussions can then be written as a care or support plan.

Person-Centred Planning

Person-centred planning can be defined as a way of assisting people to work out what they want and the support they require, and helping them to get it. A range of planning tools ensures that the adult being supported is centre stage at all times and that the services they receive are the ones they both want and need.

This approach was initially used in work with people with learning disabilities and their networks. Person-centred planning is now used with older people, those with mental health issues and those with substance misuse problems. It has become key to the implementation of self-directed support and personal budgets.

There are several different approaches or styles of person-centred planning. They differ in the way in which information is gathered and whether emphasis is on the detail of the day-to-day life or on longer-term plans for the future. However, all start with who the person is and end with specific actions to be taken.

A range of techniques are employed in person-centred practice, many of which use graphic or pictorial approaches.

Some practitioners favour 'maps' as assessment and engagement tools. Some of the different ways in which 'maps' can be used are outlined in the Box 8.3.

Prevention and Families

Where the adult at risk has a family or social network, efforts should be made to involve them in the planning and support, assuming that this is what the person concerned actually wants. There may be some difficulties faced when thinking about involving the family of an adult at risk. Each of these is listed below with how it can be potentially problematic for those involved.

There is no involved family – In the absence of an involved family, the person may be isolated and benefit from increased involvement with their local community

The family may be intentionally or unintentionally harming the individual – Getting to know the family helps to understand the problem, the risks and how best to intervene

The person may not want their family involved – The person has the right not to involve others but an exploration of the reasons will give a better understanding of their perspective and occasionally may assist reconciliation

The family may not understand that the person has a right to make choices so long as they have capacity and should be supported to do so – Getting involved with the family is the best way to help them understand that the person has the right to make choices

Involving the family takes time – Involving the family does take time but it can be time well spent in the longer term, if it has the effect of empowering them and their relatives, making them more independent of services. It is likely to improve the quality of the provision being made. It can also have the benefit of revealing important information needed to achieve an appropriate balance, avoiding conflicts and the possibility of strategies being undermined because their perspective is not understood or valued.

More often than not, the family are concerned about the welfare of the adult at risk and have a meaningful contribution to make. However, in some situations, their actions contribute to risk or harm to the individual. Even then, it is important to have a dialogue with them in order to understand how best to intervene, particularly because carers who feel isolated may be more likely to be abusive. Wherever possible, involving the family should be done with the consent of the person at risk.

Box 8.3 Maps Assessment Tools

Relationship map	Identifies who is important to the person and could contribute to the planning process or identify the balance of family, friends and paid workers in the person's life to help maintain the person at the centre
Places map	Shows where the person goes and how they spend their time, so as to identify time spent in segregated and community places and illustrate opportunities for increasing the time spent in the community
Background map	Can be useful in understanding the experiences in a person's life that should be celebrated and those which need to be avoided, enabling the identification of positive experiences to build on
Preferences map	Describes what the person likes and dislikes. This map can show what the person enjoys and is good at, and can contribute to identifying things that the person may want to do more often or to show what situations and experiences should be avoided
Dreams, hopes and fears map	Helps to identify future goals and the barriers to achieving them. This map is useful to get a sense of how someone would like their life to be and to identify what the person is most afraid of happening, and can help to set the agenda for the planning meeting
Choices map	Shows what decisions the person makes and which are made by others. This map can help to establish what autonomy the person has, so as to indicate the areas in which the person could have more control
Health map	Describes what helps and what damages the person's health. This map can help to specify aspects of the person's health that need attention or to show what makes the person healthier and needs to be continued or developed

(*Source*: McCormack & McCance 2011)

Promoting Resilience

The consequences of experiencing abuse or neglect can vary from person to person, depending on their resilience. Resilience is that quality in us all which helps us withstand adversity better. It has been described as 'the ability to cope with life's knocks', or 'the ability to pick yourself up and dust yourself off and start all over again' (SCIE 2013d).

How resilient we are depends on a number of factors; the personal attributes we were born with, the sort of parenting we received and the amount and nature of the supports available to us. However, these are things we can do for ourselves.

Box 8.4 Core Components of Promoting Resilience

- Multiple social roles
- Positive leisure pursuits
- Taking care of others
- Making the most of educational opportunities
- Stability
- Spirituality
- Involvement in the creative or expressive arts

(*Source*: SCIE 2013d)

The principles on what helps to promote resilience agree on the core components, which are listed in Box 8.4.

What Is Dignity?

Over recent years, there has been a considerable amount of literature produced about the subject of dignity in care, both in professional reading, as well as in the media and on the internet.

Despite the coverage that has been given to this subject, there has been no formal decision on the definition of what 'dignity' is.

It can often be easier to describe what dignified care is not, as there are examples highlighted within the media on a regular basis, for example the recently published Francis report and the Winterbourne inquiry published in 2012 – which actually detracts from the quality of dignified care that is being delivered in many of the health and social care settings across the UK.

The Royal College of Nursing (RCN) (2008) offer a definition of dignity being related to how individuals might think, feel or behave as to their own worth and value, as well as that of others. It also offers insight into treating someone in a respectful manner.

There are two main perspectives that are evident, despite the term being used in overlapping ways, depending on the groups of individuals being discussed at the time.

These two main perspectives are:

- *Dignity is a quality of the way we treat others*
- *Dignity is a quality of a person's 'inner-self'*.

(HASCAS 2010)

Dignity is a quality of the way we treat others – Dignity is one **quality** of our behaviour and actions towards others (e.g. the person was treated with dignity). You will find that when discussing care of vulnerable adults, dignity seems to be most often considered from this perspective.

Dignity is a quality of a person's 'inner-self' – Everyone has psychological needs and these are related to feelings of self-respect, self-esteem and self-worth.

The term 'dignity' can be used in more complex ways, for example:

- **Expectations of being treated with dignity** – People want to be treated with dignity and most people have a very individual finely tuned sense of whether or not they are being treated with the dignity they believe they deserve. Some vulnerable adults have considerable expectations with feelings of self-worth associated with previous achievements or status
- **Appearing and acting dignified** – Dignity can be used to describe how a person can appear or behave (e.g. looking or acting dignified). First, the outward appearance or behaviour of a person may be a direct indication of how they feel about themselves (self-esteem). Second, maintaining a dignified appearance

may be a major contribution to whether a person is treated with dignity by others. It takes training and experience to see past how a person looks or acts and to treat them with dignity and even then, they themselves do not look or act in a dignified way.

The European Commission (EC 2004) through their Dignity and Older Europeans Project Study, fashioned four 'types of dignity' using the perspectives and evidence collected through the study. Although the study focussed on older people, the findings can be related to any group of adults at risk.

- **Dignity of the Human Being** – This type of dignity is based on the principles of humanity and the universal worth of human beings and their inalienable rights – which can never be taken away. This is a moral approach, which considers that we all have a moral obligation to treat other human beings with dignity because of the belief that all human beings have 'nobility' and 'worth' and people need to be treated with dignity as part of fulfilling their human lives. Various international conventions and legal instruments define this in terms of human rights and how all human beings ought to be treated. This brings with it other ideas such as equality, where, for example, it is expected that all people merit treatment as human beings on an equal basis, whoever they are, whatever their age, whatever their background, how they are behaving or whatever they may be suffering from.
- **Dignity of Personal Identify** – This form of dignity is related to personal feelings of self-respect and personal identity, which also provides the basis for relationships with other people. Most people have a self-image and wish to be treated by others in the manner they believe they deserve. Most people, even those who may have learning disabilities or mental health issues, have a sense of self and whether or not they are being treated in a dignified and respectful matter. They may not be able to put it into words, but respect can be sensed. On the other hand, it is relatively easy to damage a person's perception of their self-esteem and self-worth with a few harsh words or with physical mistreatment.
- **Dignity of Merit** – This form of dignity is related to a vulnerable adult's status. Many vulnerable adults may have held positions in society, been awarded honours and had significant achievements in their lifetime. Uniforms, awards, badges and titles all bring to the owner a level of respect and dignity in society. People have a reasonable expectation of continued recognition for their achievements and can be very disappointed when this does not happen.
- **Dignity of Moral Stature** – This is a variation of dignity of merit, where people had status as they stand out because of the way they lead their lives according to their principles. This form of dignity is very difficult to appreciate because the meaning and value of 'stature' will vary, and unlike awards or honours, 'moral stature' is not something everyone recognises. For example, an unelected 'community leader' may well carry considerable moral stature and be treated with the dignity the role demands by members of the community. Yet to others, this unelected individual may seem to have no legitimate right to represent anyone and just be ignored. In this sense 'dignity of moral stature' will be very much in the 'eye of the beholder'. What is seen by one individual as being vitally important and deserving of respect, may be unimportant to another person. This has many implications for the care of adults at risk with dignity and the maintenance of their perceptions of themselves.

What Is Respect?

'Respect' is a term which is intimately related to dignity. 'Respect' is a verb and is probably the most important action word used to describe how dignity works in practice.

Respect can be defined by the dictionary as:

- Paying attention to
- Honouring
- Avoid damaging – insulting – injuring
- Not interfering with or interrupting
- Treating with consideration
- Not offending.

The Nursing and Midwifery Council (NMC) supports this through the Code of Conduct (NMC 2009) as well as their publication *Care and Respect: what you can expect from nurses* (NMC 2012).

Dignity is brought to life by the level of *respect* given to people's:

- Rights and freedoms
- Capabilities and limits
- Privacy, personal space and modesty
- Culture
- Habits and values
- Freedoms
- Individual beliefs of self-worth
- Personal merits
- Reputation
- Personal beliefs.

Thinking about and Understanding Dignity

When thinking about dignity in practice and trying to understand how dignity in care can be applied to practice, it can create emotions and reflections on situations we have already been in, both personally and professionally.

This is where a clear framework is useful when thinking about and understanding the subject of dignity in care, and it is recommended that the idea of dignity is considered from two linked points of view:

- Human rights
- Human needs.

Human Rights

The framework for human rights has been present within society for a number of years, although it is only more recently that it has had a larger presence within everyday practice and life in general.

Figure 8.4 demonstrates how human rights along with the relevant laws and legislation within the UK have been developed from wider declarations.

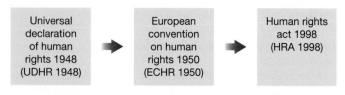

Figure 8.4 Universal Declaration of Human Rights 1948. *Source:* **HASCAS 2010.**

The Universal Declaration of Human Rights, which was adopted by the United Nations General Assembly in 1948, was the result of the experience of the Second World War. With the end of that war, and the creation of the United Nations, the international community vowed never again to allow atrocities such as those in that conflict happen again.

European Convention on Human Rights (ECHR) 1950

Following on from the United Nations' work on Human Rights, the European Court of Human Rights was established and the publication of the European Convention on Human Rights 1950 followed, with its full implementation being by 1953.

Human Rights Act 1998

The Human Rights Act 1998 was formulated as a 1997 White Paper by the UK Government 'Rights Brought Home', which stipulated the need for UK domestic law on maintaining and overseeing the application of the European Convention of Human Rights a little closer to home.

Part of the reasons for its introduction was to reduce the time and the costs involved in applying to the European Court of Human Rights for review and application of the articles to specific cases from the UK.

There is a direct correlation between the Universal Declaration of Human Rights, the European Convention on Human Rights and the Human Rights Act, with the 16 human rights in UK law being taken from the ECHR (Box 8.5).

Some of the articles in Box 8.5 are more applicable than others within a health and social care setting. Examples of some of the potential breaches to the articles are displayed in Box 8.6.

Other UK legislation relating to human rights

There are a number of other key pieces of UK legislation that can and do directly relate to the protection of Human Rights, some have already been discussed within this chapter, others will require you to undertake some additional reading to develop your knowledge and understanding of them:

- Mental Capacity Act 2005
- Adults with Incapacity (Scotland) Act
- Equality Act 2010
- Safeguarding Vulnerable Groups Act 2006
- Mental Health Act 2007
- Mental Health (Care and Treatment) (Scotland) Act
- Health and Social Care Act 2012.

Human Needs

All people have complex overlapping personal needs, each of them relating to dignity and respect as part of normal life. Maslow's hierarchy of needs, which was published in 1954 explores the needs of a human being in five sections, each of them having relevance and direct connections to providing dignified care to individuals, his theory originally stems from his initial work in 1943, where his developmental psychology theory focussed on the successful growth of humans (Maslow 1943).

Figure 8.5 illustrates the hierarchy of needs as established for every individual. It is often represented as a pyramid, with the most fundamental needs at the bottom and the greater needs at the top (Simons *et al.* 1987; Steere 1988).

The hierarchy of needs is based on the successful fulfilment of the lower levels initially leading to rising up the framework to reach self-actualisation.

Box 8.5 Summary of the Human Rights Act 1998

Article 1	Introduction
Article 2	Right to Life
Article 3	Prohibition of torture, and inhuman, degrading or humiliating treatment (Abuse)
Article 4	Prohibition of slavery and forced labour
Article 5	Right to liberty and security
Article 6	Right to a fair trial
Article 7	No punishment without law
Article 8	Right to respect for private and family life
Article 9	Freedom of thought, conscience and religion
Article 10	Freedom of expression
Article 11	Freedom of assembly and association
Article 12	Right to marry
Article 14	Prohibition of discrimination
Article 16	Restrictions on political activity of aliens
Article 17	Prohibition of abuse of rights (unless objective reasons)
Article 18	Limitation on use of restrictions on rights
Protocol	Protection of property
Additional protocols	Right to education Right to free elections Abolition of the death penalty

(*Source*: HASCAS 2010)

Jot This Down

List three aspects of each need, and how these can be supported within health and social care practice: physiological needs; safety needs; love/belonging; esteem; self-actualisation

Physiological needs

These are the most basic of human needs and requirements. They are essential for human survival, and if these are not met, the human body will not function properly, and will ultimately lead to illness, disease or death. These needs should be met first, as they are considered the most important.

Physiological needs will include the need for air, water and food along with clothing, shelter and protection from the elements.

Safety needs

With an individual's physical needs being met or relatively satisfied, the individual safety needs take priority. Safety and security needs, could be potentially inclusive of: personal safety; financial safety; health and well-being; safety net against accidents/illness and its impact.

Love and belonging needs

Once the physiological and safety needs have been met, there is a requirement for a sense of belonging and acceptance within an individual's social groups. The term 'social groups' can be used to cover a wide range of circumstances, including family members, loved ones, friends, as well as the wider communities like social groups or clubs.

Box 8.6 Examples of Potential Article Breaches

Article 2	Right to Life	No proper assessment of needs
Article 3	Prohibition of torture or degrading treatment (abuse)	Not being given enough diet or fluids
Article 5	Right to liberty and security	Individuals being given sedatives, tranquillisers and being physically restrained
Article 8	Right to respect for private and family life	Going through someone's belongings without permission
Article 9	Freedom of thought, conscience and religion	Restricting access to place of worship
Article 10	Freedom of expression	An individual being too frightened to complain
Article 14	Prohibition of discrimination	Restricted access to health or social care services because of discrimination
Protocol	Protection of property	Disposal of personal property without proper consent or permission

(*Source*: HASCAS 2010)

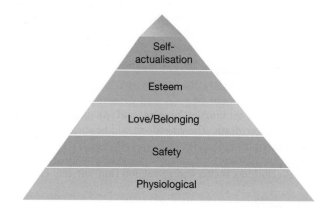

Figure 8.5 Maslow's hierarchy of needs. *Source*: Maslow 1943.

Every human has the need to be loved and to love, both in a sexual and non-sexual way and many people may become prone to loneliness, social isolation and potentially depression if there is an absence of this love or belonging need.

Esteem

All humans have a need to feel respected; this includes the need to have self-esteem. The overall need within this section is to be accepted and valued by others. Maslow did identify that the relationship between this and the lower levels of the hierarchy are not completed separated, but more a gently blended from one to the other.

Self-actualisation

This is the final level of the hierarchy; this is where the individual realises what their full potential is and achieves this. Maslow believes that for this to be achieved the previous levels have to be mastered rather than just met.

This level of the hierarchy can often be described as:

the desire to accomplish everything that one can, to become the most that one can be.

(Maslow 1954)

When relating the hierarchy of needs to dignity and respect within a health and social care setting, there are five main needs that can be drawn from all of the levels to compliment already existing thoughts and practices:

- The need to have personal identity, self-respect, self-esteem self-worth and resilience
- The need to feel respected by others
- The need to be treated as an individual
- The need to have independence, choice and control in personal lives
- The need to develop and maintain interpersonal relationships.

The concept of personal needs remaining unfulfilled, can lead to unhappiness and frustration and a poor quality of life. Adults at risk can potentially have more complicated personal needs than others.

Dignity from a human needs perspective is difficult to define, but the term which is often used in this way is to describe the *quality* of the way people:

- treat other people with 'dignity', which affects a person's feelings of self-esteem and self-worth
- Behave and look, and so deserve to be treated with dignity.

The 'human rights' and 'human needs' points of view can provide a clear framework to:

- understand the current problems, and wider challenges associated with dignity
- consider the dignity challenges that face you in day-to-day practice
- deliver care practices with a deeper awareness of dignity
- identify local dignity in care problems and make action plans to resolve them.

Medicines Management

Insomnia often affects the quality of life of the older person and acute episodes are often treated with drugs such as a benzodiazepine or a benzodiazepine receptor agonist (zolpidem, zopiclone, zaleplon) for sleep problems.

There are adverse events that are associated with sedative use, such as ataxia, falls, memory impairment or the inability to consent to treatment and these are particularly detrimental for older people. The nurse needs to be aware of these potential adverse events.

Types of Dignity

The study completed by the European Commission and University of Cardiff (EC 2004) merges the human rights and needs of individuals along with the types of dignity into one framework, allow-

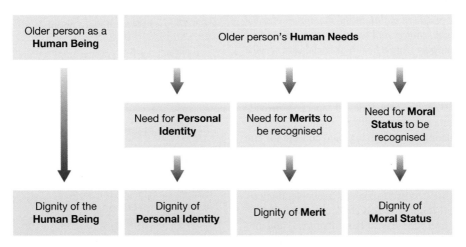

Figure 8.6 **Combined Framework of Human Rights and Needs.** *Source:* HASCAS 2010.

Table 8.3 **Concepts and considerations towards application to practice.** (*Source:* HASCAS 2010)

DIGNITY OF HUMAN BEING	DIGNITY OF PERSONAL IDENTITY	DIGNITY OF MERIT	DIGNITY OF MORAL STATUS
Conventions and Laws	Personal Identity	Achievements	People's Moral Principles
Right to Life	Self-respect	Rank and Seniority	Religious Faith
No Abuse	Self-esteem	Place in Society	Community Membership
Justice	Resilience	Honours and Awards	Leadership
Privacy	Personal Relationships	Employment	Recognised Roles
No Discrimination		Knowledge and Skills	
Freedoms/Respect		Experience	
		Qualifications	
		Financial Worth	
		Success in Life	
		Independence	

ing easier application of theory into practice, regardless of the setting or client group that is being provided with care and support. Figure 8.6 demonstrates the merged concepts of human rights and needs.

Following on from the combination of the human rights and human needs approach, further exploration can be made into each of the types of dignity, with some concepts of application and consideration being introduced. Table 8.3 demonstrates this.

Dignity in Care Campaign

The Dignity in Care campaign was launched in November 2006, following a number of consultations, and frameworks being produced. A number of factors were identified during this time, establishing the absence of the focus of dignity in care before this time, such as poor management, absence of training and education and the rapid turnover of staff within some health and social care settings (SCIE 2013a).

The National Dignity Council leads on the campaign, maintaining the focus of having 'dignity in our hearts, minds and actions' (SCIE 2013b). Part of the Dignity in Care campaign, was the creation, launch and embedding of 10 dignity challenges, which will be discussed later in the chapter.

The other parts of the Dignity in Care campaign were to recruit and register health and social care practitioners, who are passionate and committed to delivering quality dignified care to all of the individuals, they care and support for. The campaign now has over 40 000 registered dignity champions who work both locally and nationally on raising the profile of the campaign and improving the outcomes for individual's receiving care and support. Education

and sharing of best practice was also another theme to the campaign, with the creation of key learning materials and messages for all to utilise and access.

The 10 dignity challenges

The Dignity in Care campaign created and launched 10 challenges for all health and social care organisations and practitioners, to meet and exceed, each having their own rationale, definitions and requirements. The requirements of each of the challenges have been called dignity tests and are key markers on the standard and quality of the service delivery.

1. **Abuse** – *have a zero tolerance of all forms of abuse.* Respect for dignity is highlighted as a priority for most health and social care organisations. To meet this challenge, services should provide care and support in a safe and harm-free environment.

2. **Respect** – *support people with the same respect you would want for yourself or a member of your family.* Individuals should receive care in a courteous and considerate manner, allowing time to get to know the individual. Individuals should be encouraged and supported within this challenge to manage their care as independently as possible.

3. **Person-centred care** – *treat each person as an individual by offering a personalised service.* This is seen as an essential behaviour and attitude to have at all levels of service provision. Although each service will have standards to meet in relation to their regulatory requirements, the care delivery for each of the individuals should not be standardised and customised to each of their care needs.

4. **Autonomy** – *enable people to maintain the maximum possible level of independence, choice and control.* Any individual receiving care and support from a health or social care service should be encouraged to participate in daily life and be involved in decisions about their care and support.

5. **Communication** – *listen and support people to express their needs and wants.* This challenge includes all aspects of providing information relating to care delivery, including seeking agreement in care planning, and seeking valid consent for any care and support taking place.

6. **Privacy** – *respect people's right to privacy.* People's personal space is essential for the provision of dignified care and support. Ensuring that it is accessible and available, demonstrates a commitment to dignity. This challenge also incorporates the right that everyone has to basic manners, and not feeling embarrassed or humiliated while receiving any care and support.

7. **Complaints** – *ensure people feel able to complain without fear of retribution.* Any individual receiving care and support from a health and social care organisation should be provided with information and advice that they need to pass comment on the service provision as well as the quality markers and standards that each service is regulated on. The provision or access to advocacy services would be inclusive within this challenge. Health and social care practitioners should also feel comfortable to raise concerns and complaints to the appropriate person as needed, without the fear of retribution or concern for their job security.

8. **Care partners** – *engage with family members and carers as care partners.* Family members, informal carers and significant others should be kept fully informed on care needs of their loved one and this should be given in a timely fashion. Engagement with everyone involved in the care and support for an individual should feel engaged and listened to when accessing health and social care services.

9. **Self-esteem** – *assist people to maintain confidence and positive self-esteem.* Individuals should be supported in a manner that promotes confidence and self-esteem, which in turn would support and promote health and well-being. Any active support relating to care needs can be included within this challenge.

10. **Loneliness and isolation** – *act to alleviate people's loneliness and isolation.* Any individual receiving care and support should be offered to engage in age appropriate, enjoyable and stimulating activities that hold personal meaning to them. This provision should be commensurate with the needs, abilities and interests of the individual, and engagement with the wider community is seen as a key part of this 10th challenge.

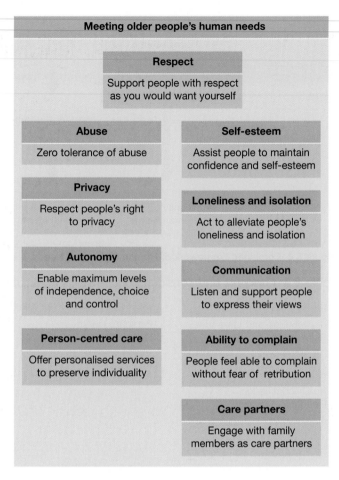

Figure 8.7 Dignity Challenges Framework. *Source:* HASCAS 2010.

Dignity Challenges Framework

The majority of these 10 challenges can be 'fitted' into one of two headings: either treating individuals as human beings or meeting individual's human needs.

Figure 8.7 demonstrates how the 10 challenges can be fitted into the framework model.

What the Experts Say

> Loneliness and social isolation can affect everyone but older people are particularly vulnerable after the loss of friends and family, reduced mobility or limited income.

Services that aim to reduce loneliness and social isolation can be divided into one-to-one interventions, group services and wider community engagement. The number of services and the different ways of measuring their success make it difficult to be certain what works for whom. Those services that look most promising include befriending schemes, social group schemes and community navigators.

Jot This Down

Identify from your practice experiences so far, examples of where you have been able to demonstrate aspects of meeting each of these 10 dignity challenges

- Respect
- Zero tolerance of abuse
- Privacy
- Autonomy
- Person-centred care
- Confidence and positive self-esteem
- Communication
- Complaints
- Engage with family and carers

What To Do If ...

Think about the 'Jot This Down' exercise above. What would you do if a relative makes a complaint about the care home manager saying the manager speaks to her mother in an uncivil way? What do you do next?

Essence of Care 2010

As well as the dignity challenges and framework being made available, the Department of Health have published the *Essence of Care 2010: benchmarks for respect and dignity* (DH 2010), which identifies seven factors associated with dignity in care. Each of these factors outlines indicators of best practice, which can be applied on an individual or organisational basis.

The seven factors that have been identified within this document are:

Factor 1 – Attitudes and behaviours
Factor 2 – Personal world and personal identity
Factor 3 – Personal boundaries and space
Factor 4 – Communication
Factor 5 – Privacy, confidentiality
Factor 6 – Privacy, dignity and modesty
Factor 7 – Privacy, private area.

(DH 2010)

Influencing Dignity in Care Practice

Every member of the health and social care workforce should hold dignity at the heart of everything that they do, regardless of practice setting, job role or discipline, thus being in the optimal position to be influencing dignity in care. You do not have to be 'a person of influence' to be influential.

Dignity can be influenced by a number of factors, but ultimately can be placed into three themes: **place, people and process** (RCN 2009).

The RCN elaborate on each point a little further in their guide to state what is meant:

Place – relates to the physical environment where the services are delivered
People – relates to the behaviours and attitudes of others and the organisational culture in which you are practicing
Process – relates to the way the care and support is actually delivered.

Influencing dignity in care does not have to need considerable changes in practice or organisational policy but can be done on a singular basis, which relates to a specific area of practice.

When considering what (if any) influences or change is needed in relation to dignified care practice, the following points might be useful to consider:

- Who is affected?
- Why are they affected?
- How do you know they are affected?
- What effects are being experienced by the individual?

Once you have established the answers to these, you will be in a position to discuss the matter with colleagues and other practitioners within your practice setting. It will also allow you to establish some dignity action plans and goals relating to the influences or changes that you have identified.

Any goal or influence that you establish should be able to demonstrate the main required characteristics for action plans or objectives. The main characteristics that are looked for allow for **SMART** action plans or objectives:

Specific – including clear statements of what is to be achieved, using terms and phrasing relating to the individual or organisation in which it relates
Measurable – this is probably the most important consideration, as being able to measure the response or influence will be allow you to evidence the effects that it is having, both positive and negative
Achievable – the influence that you are planning, must be achievable – there is little point in starting a change if it is not likely to be completed
Realistic – is the influence or change that you have identified as realistic, both within your scope of practice and organisation
Timed – any influence or change that has been identified should be timed, providing a focus for the tasks in hand, along with allowing for a balance of optimism and pessimism.

Along with these required characteristics, there are some additional ones that can be considered when looking at influencing practice or completing dignity action plans – resulting in the objectives being SMART**IES**

Inspiring – will the action plan or objective encourage and inspire other people to change their practice, attitudes or behaviours relating to dignity in care?
Enthusiastic – will the action plan or objective excite and enthuse other people?
Sustainable – will the objective be maintained in the long term?

Jot This Down

Can you identify one aspect of the dignity challenges that you are able to complete an action plan on? Try using the SMARTIES approach to objectives.

S	Specific
M	Measurable
A	Achievable
R	Realistic
T	Timed
I	Inspiring
E	Enthusiastic
S	Sustainable

Conclusion

This chapter has provided you with an understanding of the principles of safeguarding 'adults at risk' and the different types of abuse that could be presented within a health or social care setting. The application of the knowledge to nursing practice will be essential when recognising the potential physical and behavioural signs of abuse, and what to do if abuse is suspected.

As a nursing student, you play an essential and vital part of the health and social care team, providing direct care and support to a number of vulnerable adults within all of your practice placement settings.

Not only will your practice placements give you the practical skills required to register as a nurse, they will also develop your knowledge and understanding of working in partnership with families, friends and other professionals, which is fundamental when protecting and safeguarding vulnerable adults.

Abuse can take place in a number of environments, including health and social care settings, and you may at times be required to recognise these situations and report these to the appropriate managers and organisations. This chapter has identified how to respond to a disclosure of abuse, and some of the general processes that are in place to assist you to do this, regardless of setting or role.

Key Points

- In all aspects of society, there are vulnerable individuals who should be afforded dignity, protection and safeguarding against abuse or inequality.
- This chapter has focussed on the older person, however the principles discussed here can be applied to all fields of nursing.
- Key terms have been defined and discussed in this chapter, with consideration on how safeguarding and dignity can directly affect care and support.
- There are a number of legislative frameworks concerning safeguarding and dignity and these have been outlined.
- The chapter has offered insight into the application of the principles relating to safeguarding and dignity.
- Supporting and promoting the principles of safeguarding and dignity in care, among other things, requires the nurse to apply the principles of the Mental Capacity Act in a capacity assessment, encourage and to advocate the application of the dignity challenges and practice framework.
- When nurses participate in the delivery of safe and dignified care, offering support to individuals in any care setting, they must practice within the Nursing and Midwifery Council's (NMC 2008) 'Code of Conduct'.

Glossary

Bullying: the use of force, threat or coercion to abuse, intimidate or aggressively impose domination over another person or others. This behaviour is often repeated and habitual

Dignity: the quality or state of being worthy of esteem or respect

Compassion: compassion is associated with the feeling of empathy for others. Compassion is the emotion that is felt in response to the suffering of other people, motivating us to help

Discrimination: the unfair or prejudicial treatment of different categories of people, particularly on the grounds of ethnicity, age, ability, socioeconomic status or sex

Empowerment: in respect to health and social care, empowerment refers to the balancing of rights and responsibilities of an individual, community, health promoting agencies and the nation (the state). Empowerment can enhance the spiritual, political, social, educational, gender or economic strength of individuals and communities

Human Rights Act: the Human Rights Act 1998 came into force in the UK in October 2000. All public bodies (such as courts, police, local governments, hospitals, publicly funded schools and others) and other bodies carrying out public functions have to comply with the convention rights. The act sets out the fundamental rights and freedoms that individuals in the UK have access to.

Humiliation: the act of humiliating degradation. This is the belittlement of a person, the abasement of pride and can create or lead to a state of being humbled or reduced to lowliness or submission. It is an emotion that a person feels, whose social status has decreased. It can be brought about through intimidation, physical or mental mistreatment or trickery or by embarrassment.

Informed consent: agreement to permit an occurrence, for example the provision of an aspect of care, based on a complete disclosure of facts that is needed to make the decision intelligently, such as knowledge of the risks entailed or alternatives available

Principle: a moral rule or belief that can assist you in knowing what is right and wrong and this then influences your actions

Resilience: the capacity to withstand stress and catastrophe. The ability to recover quickly from illness, change or misfortune; buoyancy

Spirituality: broadly, this is an individual's search for understanding the true meaning of life and the desire to integrate with the transcendent or sacred. Spirituality is that which gives meaning to one's life drawing one to transcend oneself. Spirituality is a broader concept than religion, although that is one manifestation of spirituality

References

Carr, S. (2010) *Enabling Risk, Ensuring Safety: self-directed support and personal budgets.* Social Care Institute for Excellence, London.

CPS & I&DeA (2010) *Adult Safeguarding Scrutiny Guide.* Centre for Public Scrutiny and Improvement and Development Agency, London.

DCA (2007) *Mental Capacity Act 2005 Code of Practice.* Department of Constitutional Affairs, London.

DH & HO (2000) *No Secrets: guidance on developing and implementing multi-agency policies and procedures to protect vulnerable adults from abuse.* Department of Health, London.

DH (2010) *Essence of Care 2010: benchmarks for respect and dignity.* Department of Health, London.

DH (2011) *Statement of Government Policy on Adult Safeguarding.* Department of Health, London.

EC (2004) *Educating for Dignity: The Dignity and Older Europeans Project.* European Commission, University of Cardiff, Cardiff.

HASCAS (2010) *Dignity through Action (Vulnerable Adults) Resource 2: Dignity Workshop Pack.* Health and Social Care Advisory Service, London.

Maslow, A. (1943) A theory of human motivation. *Psychological Review,* 50(4), 370–396.

Maslow, A. (1954) *Motivation and Personality.* Harper, New York.

McCormack, B. & McCance, T. (2011) *Person-centred Nursing: theory and practice.* Wiley, London.

NHS Information Centre, Social Care Team (2012) *Abuse of Vulnerable Adults in England 2010–2011: experimental statistics.* The NHS Information Centre, London.

NMC (2008) *The Code: Standards of Conduct, Performance and Ethics for Nurses and Midwives.* Nursing and Midwifery Council, London.

NMC (2009) *Record Keeping: guidance for nurses and midwives.* Nursing and Midwifery Council, London.

NMC (2012) *Care and Respect: what you can expect from nurses.* Nursing and Midwifery Council, London.

RCN (2008) *The RCN's definition of dignity.* Royal College of Nursing, London.

RCN (2009) *Small Changes Make a Big Difference: how you can influence to deliver dignified care.* Royal College of Nursing, London.

SCIE (2010) *At a Glance 05: Mental Capacity Act 2005.* Social Care Institute for Excellence, London.

SCIE (2011a) *Adult Services Report 39. Protecting adults at risk: London multi-agency policy and procedure to safeguard adults from abuse.* Social Care Institute for Excellence, London.

SCIE (2011b) *At a Glance 44: Protecting adults at risk: London multi-agency policy and procedure to safeguard adults from abuse.* Social Care Institute for Excellence, London.

SCIE (2011c) *Adult Services Report 41. Prevention in adult safeguarding.* Social Care Institute for Excellence, London.

SCIE (2012a) *Guide 45: Safeguarding and quality in commissioning care homes.* Social Care Institute for Excellence, London.

SCIE (2012b) *Adult Services Report 60: Safeguarding adults: multi-agency policy and procedures for the West Midlands.* Social Care Institute for Excellence, London.

SCIE (2013a) *Adult Services Guide 15: Dignity in care.* Social Care Institute for Excellence, London.

SCIE (2013b) *The Dignity in Care Campaign.* Social Care Institute for Excellence, London. http://www.dignityincare.org/Dignity_in_Care_Campaign (accessed 14 February 2014).

SCIE (2013c) *1.3 Safeguarding Continuum.* Social Care Institute for Excellence, London. http://www.scie.org.uk/publications/elearning/adultsafeguarding/resource/2_study_area_1_3.html (accessed 14 February 2014).

SCIE (2013d) *5.1.1 Promoting Resilience.* Social Care Institute for Excellence, London. http://www.scie.org.uk/publications/elearning/adultsafeguarding/resource/2_study_area_5_11.html (accessed 14 February 2014).

Simons, J.A., Irwin, D.B. & Drinnien, B.A. (1987) *Psychology – The Search for Understanding.* West Publishing Company, New York.

Steere B.F. (1988) *Becoming an Effective Classroom Manager: a resource for teachers.* SUNY Press, New York.

Further Reading

SCIE (2012) *Guide 46: Commissioning Care Homes: common safeguarding challenges.* Social Care Institute for Excellence, London.

SCIE (2011) *Guide 42: Good Practice Guidance on Accessing the Court of Protection.* Social Care Institute for Excellence, London.

169

Test Yourself

1. Who is responsible for the safeguarding of adults at risk of harm? (Choose all that are applicable)
   (a) Adult Social Care
   (b) The police
   (c) Government
   (d) The public
   (e) The adult at risk
   (f) All of the above

2. Which of these sentences best describes 'safeguarding' in practice?
   (a) Safeguarding is an umbrella term for 'protecting from harm' and 'dealing with complaints of abuse'
   (b) Safeguarding is about responding appropriately and quickly to allegations of abuse or neglect
   (c) Safeguarding can be described as a continuum with 'promoting welfare' at one end and 'protecting from harm' at the other
   (d) Safeguarding is about promoting resilience in adults at risk

3. The Mental Capacity Act is in place to stop adults at risk of harm from making unwise decisions?
   (a) True
   (b) False

4. An adult you are supporting has dementia with fluctuating mental capacity. They have previously stated a desire to move into a care home, but now, faced with the reality of that decision they want to change their mind. They seem to have forgotten all the reasons they had for wanting to move, and the information you provided that helped them come to this decision. What should you do?
   (a) Talk it through with them again, at a time when you believe they have the mental capacity to make an informed decision
   (b) Say nothing to the person, but go ahead with the plans made. You are confident they made the right decision when they had the mental capacity to do so. It is in their best interests
   (c) Tell them it's too late to change their mind, and remind them of their reasons for making the decision
   (d) Respect their wishes, and cancel the arrangements made

5. You support an adult with learning disabilities, who retains mental capacity. The woman discloses to you that her 'uncle' (a family friend who helps her with odd jobs) has been touching her in a way that makes her feel uncomfortable. She is very clear that she had told you this in secret and does not want anyone else to know about it. She doesn't want any trouble. You are concerned that she is being abused. What do you do?
   (a) Explain that you can't promise not to tell anyone else (because you might not be the best person to help). Reassure her that you won't do anything without her knowl-

edge. Support her and provide information that can help her make an informed decision on whether to take the matter forward herself
   (b) Respect her wishes to keep this disclosure secret, but try to persuade her to talk to her social worker or the police
   (c) Inform the appropriate authority, this is acting in her best interests
   (d) Ask lots of questions, take photographs and get as much evidence as possible so that you can go to the police with a complaint
   (e) Confront the alleged perpetrator so that he will back-off

6. Dignity of the Human Being, Dignity of Merit, Dignity of Moral Status have all been identified as types of dignity, can you identify the 4th from the list below?
   (a) Dignity of Personal Hygiene
   (b) Dignity of Personal Integrity
   (c) Dignity of Personal Identity
   (d) Dignity of Personal Honour

7. The Dignity in Care campaign identifies 10 challenges within it, and two halves of the dignity framework – which one of the challenges though overlaps both parts of the framework?
   (a) Care partners
   (b) Autonomy
   (c) Person-centred care
   (d) Respect
   (e) Loneliness and isolation

8. When considering who can influence dignity in care practices, who can be involved?
   (a) Only Senior Managers – they have the experience behind them
   (b) Only Registered Practitioners – they have the professional knowledge to support their decisions
   (c) Only service users – they are the ones receiving the care and support
   (d) Only members of the public – as they love to get involved in scandals
   (e) Everyone – dignity in care is everyone's business, so all should be involved in it

9. When considering creating objectives for dignity action plans, SMART objectives are required – what do we need to do to make them SMART**IES**?
   (a) Inquire, Enthuse, Sustain
   (b) Inspire, Encourage, Sustain
   (c) Inspire, Enthuse, Sustain
   (d) Inspire, Enthuse, Suspend
   (e) Inquire, Encourage, Suspend

10. A vulnerable adult can be abused by:
   (a) Another patient/service user
   (b) A health or social care professional
   (c) A family member
   (d) All of the above

Answers

1. f
2. c
3. b
4. a

5. a
6. c
7. d
8. e
9. c
10. d

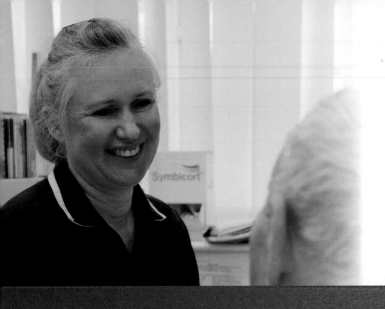

9

The Principles of Older People's Care

Helen Paterson

Royal Berkshire NHS Foundation Trust, Reading, UK

Learning Outcomes

On completion of this chapter you will be able to:

- Define communication and appreciate why effective communication is essential when offering care to older people
- Understand the importance of maintaining and respecting dignity when providing care to older people
- Understand the importance of effective and timely assessment of an older person's nutritional needs
- Demonstrate an insight concerning the critical role of the nurse in the assessment of risk and the reduction of falls in the older person
- Gain an understanding of the discharge and transfer process

Competencies

All nurses must:

1. Communicate effectively so that appropriate information is shared in a timely manner
2. Provide individual, evidence-based care to older people
3. Carry out competent assessment of an older person's nutritional needs
4. Identify factors associated with the potential development of pressure ulcers
5. Perform a timely falls-risk assessment in order to identify those at risk of falls
6. Identify different types of communication
7. Ensure that the older person has a structured discharge plan tailored to their individual needs

 Visit the companion website at **www.wileynursingpractice.com** where you can test yourself using flashcards, multiple-choice questions and more.

Nursing Practice: Knowledge and Care, First Edition. Edited by Ian Peate, Karen Wild and Muralitharan Nair.
© 2014 John Wiley & Sons, Ltd. Published 2014 by John Wiley & Sons, Ltd. Companion website: www.wileynursingpractice.com

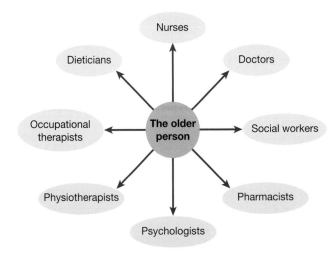

Figure 9.1 Some members of the multidisciplinary team.

Introduction

Caring for the older person requires a skilled competent and confident practitioner. Nurses are required to use clinical judgement in order to enable the older person to improve, support, or recover health, to manage their health problems, and to achieve the best possible quality of life, regardless of their disease or disability, or until death.

In order to offer care that is safe, effective and person-centred, nurses are required to work in partnership with the person, their relatives and other care providers in the statutory, independent and voluntary sectors. A multidisciplinary approach is advocated with the nurse at the centre of care provision leading, prescribing, delegating and supervising the work of others. At all times, the nurse remains personally and professionally accountable for his or her own decisions, actions and omissions. Some members in a multidisciplinary team (MDT) are outlined in Figure 9.1.

This chapter provides you with an insight into the ways in which the nurse can excel at care provision for this group of people. Communicating effectively is an absolute pre-requisite.

Attitudes and Stereotyping

With the global trend towards an increasingly ageing population, Doherty *et al.* (2011) put forward that nurses need to be more equipped with the knowledge and skills to fulfill significant roles in responding to older people's future health and supportive needs. Conversely, Nay (1993) (cited in Nay & Garratt 2004) found that many nurses in the acute care setting have had little if any, specialist education in the care of older people and therefore do not understand the extent of their needs. Higgins *et al.* (2007) imply that this may be due to many nurses preferring to care for younger patients with acute illnesses, who are curable, supporting Pursey and Luker's (1995) suggestion that the high dependency levels of older people and the structure of nursing work with older people in hospitals means that fewer nurses make this area a positive career choice. However, McKinlay and Cowan (2003) point out that due to the ageing population, it means that care of older people will become an increasingly important part of nurses' remit, despite employment statistics, suggesting that this is an unpopular nursing special-

ism. This, they say, constitutes a potential problem, especially if such attitudes have an impact on the quality of care provided (McKinlay & Cowan 2003).

Familiar stereotyping of older people can result in older patients deemed to be unpopular because of their perceived personality, attitudes or communication, and because their needs fit poorly with the service available to the them; along with poor staffing levels, length of stay and the older person's expectations (Price 2013). An increasing number of older people utilise the acute setting and attitudes of registered nurses caring for older people could affect the quality of care provided (Courtney & Tong 2000). Complaints contain many themes within the acute settings, such as older patients experiencing reduced independence; limited decision-making opportunities; increased probability of developing complications; little consideration of their ageing related needs; limited health education and social isolation (Courtney & Tong 2000). Interestingly, a study by McLafferty and Morrison (2004) showed that student nurses who worked with older adults were very positive about their work and the nursing opportunities they offer student nurses. However, there was criticism of the nurses who worked in the acute setting, and the pre-registration curriculum attributing to negativity towards nursing older people. A large proportion of healthcare professionals portray negative views about the older person, reflected in their attitudes and stereotyping, potentially resulting in a 'lack of time to care' of older people and risks thus becoming problematic (Higgins *et al.* 2007). All healthcare professionals need to be aware of their influence on the attitudes of student nurses towards older people; good practice includes the ability to demonstrate that older people in hospital settings are valued. Moreover, nurse tutors need to review the way they prepare students for this specialist work, in order to avoid inadvertently conveying negative attitudes (McLafferty & Morrison 2004). The care a nurse provides should reflect the needs and preferences of the older people. In order to do this, you need not only to talk to them but also listen to what they expect from you in terms of the care they receive (NMC 2009a,b).

Effective Communication

Effective communication is critical during the countless interactions that occur among healthcare workers on a daily basis. Staff must know how to communicate effectively and work collaboratively in teams, so that appropriate information is shared in a timely manner. When effective communication is absent, patient care is compromised (Henry *et al.* 2009). Yet, despite the emphasis on teaching communication skills over the past two decades, good communication is often curtailed by structural factors, an overwhelming emphasis on increased patient throughput, together with the greater use of bank and agency staff, placing further limits on nurses' ability to develop a substantial rapport with patients (Naish 1996). The art of effective communication is a skill that is learned with time and exposure to different situations (Magee 2013). The Department of Health (DH 2010b) defines communication as a process that involves a meaningful exchange between at least two people, to convey facts, needs, opinions, thoughts, feelings or other information, through both verbal and non-verbal means, including face-to-face exchanges and the written word.

Communication in the nursing profession can be a complicated process, and the possibility of sending or receiving incorrect messages frequently exists. It is essential that we know the key components of the communication process, how to improve our skills, and the potential problems that exist with errors in communication (Anderson 2012).

The *Essence of Care* (DH 2010a) consultation paper suggests a number of best-practice benchmarks for communication. Most importantly, it is essential that professionals ensure communication takes place in an environment that is acceptable to all parties; that staff have effective interpersonal skills; that communication needs are assessed and information effectively shared Francis (2013). Furthermore, if staff communicate more effectively with the older person, recognise their individual identity and involve them in shared decision-making, it may result in more positive experiences for that older person (Bridges *et al.* 2010). Conversely, the Commission for Healthcare Audit and Inspection (CHAI 2007) found that older patients are least likely to be critical of any particular hospital situation, so it is particularly worrying that these same people are less likely than those in middle age and early old age to describe their hospital care as '*excellent*' and most likely to feel talked over '*as though they were not there*' by staff. The introduction of a new national friends and family test from 1 April 2013, asks patients if they would recommend their ward or A&E department to friends and family if they needed similar care or treatment (DH 2013a). This has financial implications for acute Trusts; they are tasked with ensuring that they receive 15% 'highly recommended' returns of this test. If this is achieved, the Trust is rewarded by the DH financially. However, if they do not achieve this, the Trusts are not only unable to get the financial incentive to achieve the targets, but also the results are made public, which could potentially affect the reputation of the Trust. Therefore, it is essential nurses promote a person-centred approach to care of the older person, to ensure they have a positive experience during their journey from admission to discharge.

What the Experts Say

Admission to and treatment in hospital is almost invariably a time of great anxiety, not only for the patient but also for those closest to him or her.
Patients and those closest to them naturally require to be kept informed of developments and will be worried if they are denied this or if they have to make great efforts to find out what they want to know. It is of the very essence of modern medical care that it is provided in partnership with the patient and always subject to the consent of the patient or authorised representative, following the provision of the information needed to make decisions. This requires a continual professional conversation with the patient and those authorised by him or her to receive treatment information, so that those involved are thoroughly informed of the current position and enabled to play their full part in the process. Communication in a hospital setting is not a one-way process. It is as vital that patients and their relatives are listened to – for in many ways they are the experts on the patient and his or her needs – as it is for hospital staff to provide information

(Francis 2013)

The Nursing and Midwifery Council (NMC 2008) make it clear that nurses should communicate effectively and share knowledge, skills and expertise with other members of the team, as required for the benefit of patients and clients. To achieve this, acute Trusts must ensure appropriate clinical supervision of student nurse–older person communication by preceptors, increasing theoretical input in relation to interpersonal skills and communication theory, facilitating reflective practice whilst students are on clinical placement and regular auditing of clinical placements as suitable learning environments (Tuohy 2003).

Indicators to support best practice for communication have been produced by the DH (2010b):

- Communication is managed effectively and sensitively, including potentially difficult communication, such as conveying bad news, dealing with complaints and resolving disputes and hostile situations
- All staff are courteous, especially when faced with challenging situations
- Staff are aware of the importance of body language and effectively use non-verbal communication to facilitate communication
- Communication is adapted to meet the needs of *people*, carers and groups. This includes consideration of their emotional state, hearing, vision and other physical and cognitive abilities and developmental needs, as well as their preferred language and possible need for an interpreter and translator
- Communication is open, honest and transparent
- Staff are able to establish rapport, undertake active and empathic listening, and are non-judgemental
- Straightforward language is used when communicating with *people* and carers
- Initiatives are in place to assess and provide feedback on the interpersonal skills of staff, such as through the use of audits on the views of *people* and carers.

Effective communication between nurses and other caregivers is critical to patient safety, yet numerous challenges contribute to poor communication and an unhealthy reliance on individual action (Henry *et al.* 2009). Effective communication is the way to ensure that your knowledge and clinical skills are used to best effect. Use language and terminology that are familiar to the patient and are culturally sensitive and always check their understanding (DH 2010b).

Jot This Down

Identify specific communicate strategies and the obstacles that can prevent effective communication particularly when working with older people.

Types of Communication

Verbal and non-verbal: Language is both verbal and non-verbal, our body language can confirm or contradict the words we are actually saying (RCN 2008b).

Facial expression: Ekman *et al.* (1987) identified seven main facial expressions:

1. Happiness
2. Surprise
3. Fear
4. Sadness
5. Anger
6. Disgust
7. Interest.

However, interpreting them may be hindered, as the older person may have injury to the face, facial nerves or muscle weakness or a disease, such as people with Parkinson's, who often exhibit an expressionless, mask-like facial expression (Ekman *et al.* 1987).

Gestures: Often closely coordinated with speech, and form an important part of the communication process, however, a physical condition, which may affect movement such as stroke or Parkinson's, may impinge on an older persons ability to use gestures or body movement (Fook & Morgan 2000).

Body language and posture: These again can enhance and expand communication, particularly when communicating with someone with a visual or hearing impairment (Fook & Morgan 2000).

Barriers to effective communication

Poor listening skills: Communication can become difficult if a listener does not appear to be interested in what the older person is saying, or provides them with adequate time to say what they want to say. Some older people may have memory problems, so it may take them a little longer to process what it is they are trying to communicate.

Environmental: Noise, poor lighting and telephones can make communicating with the older person difficult. On a busy ward or clinic, it is can be too easy for the older person to become distracted.

Staffing: A high throughput of patients, together with poor staffing or skill mix, can restrict the time nurses spend *with* patients (DH 2010b). A study by Agewell's (2005) suggests the following strategies to assist when communicating with the older person face-to-face:

- Places where you give face-to-face information should have low levels of background noise. Remember a hearing aid amplifies the background noise, as well as speech. Some florescent strip lighting may emit a humming noise, which can be distracting to hearing aid wearers
- When talking to older people, staff should try to keep their faces visible and not obscure their mouths, as some older people rely on lip reading to supplement their hearing. Try not to turn your back on someone while talking to them
- Places where you give face-to-face information should be well lit and ideally, your seating arrangements should place the older person with their back to windows or lighting sources. This ensures that shadows do not fall on the staff member's face, which can obscure their mouth and therefore prevent the older person from reading their lips
- It is important to speak clearly and not too fast but shouting or over-mouthing will alter the lip pattern and may not be helpful
- When you initiate any conversation with the older person, do not assume that the person to whom you are talking wishes to be called by their first name; ask how they would like to be addressed.

What the Experts Say

> I am 78 years of age, I still have all of my faculties, my left leg is a bit dodgy but, I'm all there. To be addressed by the nurses as love, dear, sweetie really irks me. For me, this is a lack of respect. I think they should ask me what is I want to be called, this way I am still being seen as an individual.

(Miss Mary O'Leary)

Therefore, it is important that staff communicate effectively with older people, recognise their individual identity and involve them in shared decision-making, thus ensuring a more positive experience for patients (Bridges *et al.* 2010).

Handover

The nursing change of shift report or handover is a communication process that occurs between groups of nurses and carers, whereby the specific purpose is to communicate information about patients under the care of nurses (Lamond 2000). Problems typically arise at shift or patient handovers and/or involve ambiguous or poorly recorded information in patient files (JCR 2007).

The explicit function of handover according to Evans *et al.* (2008) is to communicate information from one nurse or group of nurses to the next group of nurses, to formally hand over responsibility for patients.

Furthermore, effective communication at clinical handover is important for improving patient safety and reducing adverse outcomes (Porteous *et al.* 2009). By the same token, information is often poorly communicated and inaccurate due to the omission of important detail (Currie 2000). When information is missed in patient handovers, people could potentially die (Wilson 2007).

Higgins *et al.* (2007) found that prejudiced beliefs about patients are transferred from one nurse to another during handover and colleague's attitudes towards patients were influenced through informal communication and the use of stereotypical labels. This would suggest that negative behaviour reduces the older person's ability to maintain autonomy over healthcare choices (Baillie 2007).

The NMC (2008) state, 'that you must not discriminate in any way against those in your care'.

Jot This Down

Perform a literature review of clinical handover. Compare the methods described and compare those with what you have experienced on your placements. Would a change in practice enhance the quality of information provided during handover? If yes, consider discussing this with the ward manager with rationale for the need for change.

Briefing tools such as SBAR (**S**ituation, **B**ackground, **A**ssessment and **R**ecommendation) give opportunities for team members to share information effectively (NHS Institute for Innovation and Improvement 2008; Risky Business 2012; WHO 2009).

Failure of Communication between Staff
Documentation to communicate care provision

Purpose: Communication is central to human interaction. Without it, people cannot relate to those around them, make their needs and concerns known, to make sense of what is happening to them. One of the most basic goals for nursing staff is that their patients and clients and those who care for them experience effective communication (DH 2010a).

Legal concerns: Keeping accurate up-to-date documentation is an essential part of a nurse's role; remember that documentation is essential for legal purposes to demonstrate clarity of decision-making, advice and follow-up plans, if appropriate (RCN 2006). You are at risk of being suspended from the Nursing and

Midwifery Council's (NMC) register if you are found to repeatedly fail in keeping accurate records of the care you provide to your patients. It has to be assumed if it is not documented, then it did not happen. Good record-keeping helps to improve accountability and shows how decisions related to patient care were made (NMC 2009b). Furthermore, effective documentation provides evidence of the assessment, plan of care, nursing interventions (care, teaching, safety measures), outcome of care, change in status, healthcare team communication, and how the nurse left the patient (RCN 2008b).

What the Experts Say

'All nurses must ensure that the healthcare record for the patient is an accurate account of treatment, care planning and delivery'. The record should provide clear evidence of the care planned, the decisions made, the care delivered and the information shared within the team.

(NMC 2009)

The communication process in health and social care settings can be complicated. As Anderson (2012) points out, the possibility of sending or receiving incorrect messages frequently exists. It is essential that you understand the key components of the communication process, how to improve your skills, and the potential problems that exist with errors (Anderson 2012). Furthermore, effective communication is the way to ensure that your knowledge and clinical skills are used to empower older people to become partners or participants in the care they receive (DH 2010b). Highlighting the importance of effective communication should ensure that nurses working with older people, regardless of health or social care setting, focus on the individualised needs of the older person when communicating with other professionals, the patient and significant others.

Patient-Centred Care

The needs of the patients and communities that nurses serve must be at the heart of all we do. Responding to the individual needs and respecting individual choices can help to demonstrate that nurses respect the needs of the older person and their families.

Preetinder (2013) defines patient-centred care as care that leads to higher level of patient engagement. The five constituent dimensions of patient engagement include:

Communication

1. Provider effectiveness
2. Alignment of objective
3. Information and encouragement
4. Patient incentive.

Jot This Down

Describe what person-centred care means to you.

When asked what patient-centred care is, it is usually referred to as 'individualised care' or some say 'it's all about the person'. Many struggle to be more specific (Butterworth 2012).

The phrase 'person-centred care' is often encountered when reading about how older people should be supported. The essential standards of Quality and Safety (Care Quality Commission, CQC 2010), which sets out how adults receiving health and social care in England should be supported, make little reference to this phrase. But the outcomes support a person-centred approach, resulting in patient satisfaction due to an enhanced environment that ensures older people are fully involved with any decision-making relating to their care (Pope 2011).

Older people are often addressed using terms of endearment, such as darling or sweetheart, which is not appropriate. It is good practice for staff to ask and record what a person likes to be called; if they like the terms of endearment (Butterworth 2012). The NMC (2009a) guidance for the care of older people reinforces this approach. Older people occupy two-thirds of general and acute hospital beds in the UK (DH 2010c). Although nurses spend most of their time caring of older people, the needs of this patient group are not being met (CQC 2011a,b). How to tackle the challenges is addressed in the 'Silver Book' which provides quality standards for older people (Conroy 2012).The focus of this guide is on care standards for older people over the first 24 hours of an urgent care episode, with the specific remit to:

- *Help decrease variations in practice*
- *Influence the development of appropriate services across the urgent care system*
- *Identify and disseminate best practice*
- *Influence policy development.*

(Silver Book 2012)

Older people are admitted to hospital more frequently, have a longer length of stay and occupy more bed days in acute hospitals compared with other patient groups (Cooke *et al.* 2012). In addition, older people admitted to hospital, find it difficult to get discharged and have the highest risk of readmission to hospital than any other group (Triggle 2012). There is a pressing need to change how older people are cared for with urgent care needs to improve care quality, outcomes and efficiency.

Lloyd (2010) suggests that practitioners must think of as many ways as possible to involve the person in planning their care. An important aspect of person-centred approach is that people have choices and can make decisions about their care and support. Respect for the autonomy and dignity of the older person must underpin our approach and practice at all times (Cooke *et al.* 2012).

What the Experts Say

High quality care is care where patients are in control, have effective access to treatment, are safe and where illnesses are not just treated, but prevented.

(DH 2008)

Pope (2011) explored nurses' attitudes towards older people in hospital and how they can impact on patient outcomes. She argues that moving towards a patient-centred culture can improve nurses' attitudes and enhance the nurse–patient relationship. The principles of person-centred care are outlined in Box 9.1.

The importance of person-centred care is acknowledged in standards of conduct and national guidance (DH 2001; NMC 2008). The Royal College of Nursing (RCN) launched the *Principles of Nursing Practice* (RCN 2010). Developed in partnership with patient and user organisations, the Department of Health and The

---

Box 9.1 Principles of Person-Centred Care

· Listen to patients
· Treat patients as individuals
· Understand patients rights and values
· Respect dignity and confidentiality
· Empower individuals and encourage autonomy
· Build mutual trust and understanding.

(*Source*: Adapted from DH 2001 and McCormack & McCance 2010)

Nursing and Midwifery Council describe what people and service users can expect from nursing services (in any setting) and from those providing their nursing care – be it from a Registrant, Healthcare Assistant or a Nursing Student (RCN 2010). The principles underpin practice with peoples' expectations and rights to be autonomous, treated equally and fairly and treated with dignity and respect. To put it simply, the *Principles of Nursing Practice* describe what everyone can expect from nursing (Cooke *et al.* 2012).

The NHS Constitution emphasises patients' right to be involved in decisions and this is reinforced in standards set by professional regulators. Compassion and respect have always been enshrined in the value statements of the health professions (NMC 2009). However, 'compassion' has recently gained a higher profile with policy-makers. The NHS Constitution sets out certain NHS values, including respect, dignity and compassion (DH 2009).

McCormack and McCance (2010) developed a person-centred framework, which they suggest has the potential to improve care by encouraging nurses to appreciate patients as significant and autonomous individuals in healthcare settings. They state that the framework can be used to evaluate quality of care and enable practice development that results in the most effective individualised care pre-requisites of the nurse, care environment, care processes and person-centred outcomes (McCormack & McCance 2010). In summary, the framework comprises four constructs. Pre-requisites focus on the attributes of the nurses and include: being professionally competent; having developed interpersonal skills; being committed to the job; being able to demonstrate clarity of beliefs and values; and knowing self (McCormack & McCance 2006).

Jot This Down

Undertake a literature search on McCormack and McCance's (2010) framework. Would you find it a useful tool to implement in order to improve care provision?

When dignity is present, people feel in control, valued, confident, comfortable and able to make decisions for them. When dignity is absent, people feel devalued, lacking control and comfort. They may lack confidence and be unable to make decisions for themselves. They may feel humiliated, embarrassed or ashamed (RCN 2008c).

What the Experts Say

While the dignity of a patient who survives can doubtless usually be recovered, even if the experience remains an unpleasant and distressing memory, the memory of the undignified circumstances in which their loved one died will be the last that those left behind have.

(Francis 2013)

The Essential Standards of Quality and Safety (CQC 2010) set out 28 outcomes of what a person receiving care can expect in a range of health and social care settings. The first is 'respecting and involving people who use the service, by ensuring personalised care, treatment and support through involvement'.

Personalisation

Standard Two of the *National Service Framework for Older People* (DH 2001) aims to ensure that older people are treated as individuals and that they receive appropriate and timely packages of care, which meet their needs as individuals, regardless of health and social services boundaries. Lord Darzi (DH 2008) set out a vision for improving quality in the NHS in which the personalisation of services is central. Personalisation means different things to different people but the following 'What the Experts Say' definition may be useful:

What the Experts Say

Personalisation reinforces the idea the individual is best placed to know what they need and how those needs can be best met. It means that people can be responsible for themselves and can make their own decisions about what they require, but that they should also have information and support to enable them to do so. In this way services should respond to the individual instead of the person having to fit with the service.

(DH 2008)

Older people want to be treated as individuals and receive care that is tailored around their needs. They want to be offered treatment choices, backed up with information, and recognition of their preferences (Help the Aged/Age Concern 2009). The NMC (2008) require nurses to uphold people's rights to be fully involved in decisions about their care.

Link To/Go To

http://www.ageuk.org.uk

Age UK aims to improve later life for everyone through the provision of information and advice, services, campaigns, products, training and research.

Capacity

For people to have the capacity to make a particular decision, they must be able to comprehend and retain information material to the decision, especially as to the consequences of having or not having the intervention in question (Butterworth 2012). Chapter 8 of this text discusses capacity in more detail, along with the principles of safeguarding and dignity. If the older person is not involved in their care it may be due to the fact they may lack the mental capacity to do so. If this is the case, it must be documented as to why they were not involved (DH 2001). The RCN (2010) discusses dignity in care centres based on three integral aspects:

- **Respecting** patients' and clients' diversity and cultural needs; their privacy – including protecting it as much as possible in large, open-plan hospital wards; and the decisions being made

- Being **Compassionate** when a patient or client and /or their relatives need emotional support, rather than just delivering technical nursing care
- Demonstrating **Sensitivity** to patients' and clients' needs, ensuring their comfort.

Dementia

In the UK, there are an estimated 8 000 000 people with dementia (Alzheimer's Society 2012). Up to one-quarter of hospital beds are occupied by people over the age of 65 years with dementia, who may have other age-related conditions that require hospital admission (Alzheimer's Society 2009; Health Foundation 2011).

Link To/Go To

http://www.alzheimersresearchuk.org

Alzheimer's Research UK is the UK's leading dementia research charity. The organisation's science and innovation hold the key to defeating dementia and they invest in the scientists discovering more about the condition and its causes.

The National Dementia Strategy (DH 2009) aims to raise awareness, facilitate assessment and improve service provision for those diagnosed with dementia. Although this strategy is unquestionably correct, the assumptions, emphases and economic predictions are questionable (Greaves & Jolly 2010). While supporting the aims of the Strategy, Greaves and Jolly (2010) suggest from their experience, that many patients and families will be better provided with affordable assessment and continued support, by strengthening the activities of primary care, rather than referral of everyone to secondary care centres.

Students' experiences of caring for people with dementia are important, as these experiences can influence their future as registered nurses (Baillie *et al.* 2009). Embracing every opportunity to spend more time with patients with dementia will provide student nurses with valuable learning experiences (Nolan 2006).

The Alzheimer's Society (2010) produced a leaflet 'This is Me' with spaces and photographs and information to support people with dementia going into hospital. The Royal College of Psychiatrists (RCP 2011) recommended that personal information such as the 'This is Me' booklet should be implemented in hospital. As a result, many acute Trusts have implemented the usage of this or similar booklets, as it enables significant others knowledge of the older person to be acknowledged, as well as enabling more effective care provision for the older person with dementia. Despite this, valuable information is being utilised in acute sectors. Douglas-Dunbar and Gardiner's (2007) findings suggest that carers of people with dementia admitted to hospital report their knowledge was often ignored.

Dignity

Dignity in patients' care include maintaining privacy of the body, providing spatial privacy, giving sufficient time, treating patients as a whole person and allowing patients to have autonomy (Lin & Tsai 2011). To explore how older people view human dignity in their lives, three major themes were identified: respect and recognition; participation and involvement; and dignity in care (Bayer *et al.*

2005). Patients are vulnerable to loss of dignity in hospital, staff behaviour and the hospital environment can influence whether patients' dignity is lost or upheld. Reports have highlighted cases of undignified care of older people in our hospitals and care homes; in too many instances, people have been let down when they were vulnerable and most needed help (Berry 2012). Therefore, it is essential a conducive physical care environment, and individual nurse's actions promote the dignity of older people while they are undergoing health care (Baillie *et al.* 2009). For dignity of older people to be enhanced, communication issues, privacy, personal identity and feelings of vulnerability need to be addressed (Bayer *et al.* 2005).

The *National Service Framework Next Steps* report (DH 2006b) aimed to ensure that, within 5 years, all older people receiving care services will be treated with respect and dignity. The report acknowledges the need for wide-reaching culture change and zero tolerance of negative attitudes towards older people. Seven years later, the shocking finding from the Francis Inquiry (2013) sadly indicates vital components of care are being lost. While the case at Mid Staffordshire NHS Foundation Trust was unique in its severity and duration, pockets of poor care do exist elsewhere, and some of the features that contributed to the tragedy – patients and families ignored, staff disengaged or unable to speak up – point to wider problems (DH 2013b).

RCN *Defending Dignity* (RCN 2008a) suggests nurses reflect on their practice to ensure they embed the following practices when caring for the older person:

- Respect privacy by pulling curtains (ensuring there are no gaps)
- Shutting doors
- Provide assistance to older people to walk to the toilet or bathroom when possible
- Checking or knocking before entering curtains and rooms
- Not exposing patients unnecessarily during procedures.

Delivering Dignity is the final report of the Commission on Dignity in Care for Older People and sets out the Commission's work and recommendations. It focusses on how to tackle the underlying causes of poor care. Some hospitals and care homes are already providing dignified care for older people; this report and the follow-up programme of activities are intended to build on existing good practice, so that we get it right for every person, every time (Local Government Association, NHS Confederation, Age UK 2012).

Jot This Down

The Commission on Improving Dignity in Care released its draft report and recommendations on 29 February 2012. Review the 10 recommendations of 'The Commission on Improving Dignity in Care'. Compare these to the hospital settings you are familiar with. Have they improved the care provided for older people in hospital? If not what improvements are needed to meet those recommended?

Disappointingly, fewer hospitals are respecting people's privacy and dignity, with 82% meeting people's need. CQC inspectors saw call bells left unanswered, older people being left without help to get to the toilet and without support for other needs (CQC 2010).

Box 9.2 outlines a number of principles that may be applied to improve the care of older people with an emphasis on dignity and respect.

Box 9.2 Principles of Care

- All patients are individuals with their own backgrounds, needs, interests and wishes for which they are entitled to recognition and respect.
- No patient should ever be referred to by a name other than that which he or she wishes to be called.
- Staff should be readily identifiable by name and grade.
- If for whatever reason, a patient has received less than acceptable care, every effort must be made to recognise the effects on the patient, remedy them, and explain to the patient the reason for what has happened.
- Sensitive information, particularly concerning diagnosis and prognosis, must be given to patients in privacy, and in earshot only of those people the patient agrees to being present.
- The patient's right to physical privacy should be respected wherever possible, and in no circumstances should a patient be left in an undressed state visible to those passing by the bed.

(*Source*: Adapted from Francis 2013)

What the Experts Say

 It is a national scandal that six out of 10 older people are at risk of becoming malnourished, or their situation getting worse, in hospital. Malnourished patients stay in hospital for longer, are three times more likely to develop complications during surgery, and have a higher mortality rate than well-fed patients. Ending the scandal of malnourished older people in hospitals will save lives.

(Age Concern 2006)

There is no universally accepted definition of malnutrition, however, Elia (2003) defines it as:

…a state of nutrition in which a deficiency or excess (or imbalance) of energy, protein, and other nutrients causes measurable adverse effects on tissue/body form (body shape, size and composition) and function, and clinical outcome.

Jot This Down

Identify why it is so important to ensure older people are assessed within 4 hours of being admitted to hospital of their nutritional status and what are the aims of nutritional interventions in older patients?

Being aware of and identifying the key principles of person-centred care can help to improve care provision, as well as the perception of caring for older people, regardless of the care setting. This should effectively ensure that nurses deliver quality care, which promotes dignity by nurturing and supporting the older person's self-respect and self-worth (NMC 2009).

The Older Person's Nutritional Needs

Older people have specific nutritional requirements that are different from other groups. In older people, the nutritional status of many is poor with regards of some key nutrients. Older people are at higher risk of malnutrition if they are ill, live alone or have difficulty eating. Older patients should have their nutritional status assessed and nutritional intake monitored regularly, to ensure they are receiving adequate nutrition. Failure to do this is tantamount to professional misconduct.

Chapter 17 of this text discusses nutrition in more detail. In this section of the chapter, nutritional needs are related to the older person, with a focus upon their specific needs.

Prevention and management of malnutrition surveys have shown that older people in both community and institutional settings are either malnourished or at risk of becoming so (McLafferty & Morrison 2004). Following admission to hospital, many older people are known to lose weight and sustain a further deterioration in their nutritional status, with associated risk of an increasing morbidity and mortality (BAPEN 1992). The incidence of under-nutrition among people admitted to hospitals in the UK is 23% for those aged less than 65 years but 32% for those aged 65 (Cooke *et al.* 2012). The cost of malnutrition in the UK is estimated to be over £7.3 billion a year; over half of this cost is expended on people aged 65 years and over (NICE 2006). Plausibly, patients over the age of 80 admitted to hospital have a five times higher prevalence of malnutrition than those under the age of 50 (Elia 2003; Age Concern 2006).

Having enough to eat and drink is one of the most basic human needs (*Dignity in Care Campaign*, DH 2006a), yet some vulnerable people are not having this fundamental need met (DH 2007b). Indefensibly, five years later, Cooke *et al.* (2012) found that under-nutrition remains poorly detected by nursing and medical staff.

The Age Concern (2006) report prompted key policy initiatives to highlight the importance of creating the right environment to support eating and drinking (Cooke *et al.* 2012). The risk of under-nutrition is increased in elderly patients due to their decreased lean body mass and too many other factors that may compromise nutrient and fluid intake. Consequently, an adequate intake of energy, protein and micronutrients has to be ensured in each patient independently of his/her previous nutritional status. Since restoration of body cell mass (BCM) is more difficult than younger persons, preventive nutritional support has to be considered (Volkert *et al.* 2006). Moreover, nutritional interventions in malnourished hospital patients can reduce complications, lengths of stay and mortality (National institute of Clinical Excellence, NICE 2006) this reinforces Edington *et al.*'s (2000) findings that patients who are malnourished stay in hospital for a longer time, require more medications, and are more likely to suffer from infections.

The NICE (2006) guidance recommends that:

- All hospital inpatients on admission should be screened (weighed, measured and have their body mass index (BMI) calculated).
- Screening should be repeated weekly.
- A clear process should be established for documenting the outcomes of screening and the subsequent actions taken if the patient is recognised as malnourished or at risk of malnutrition.

In addition to these guidelines, Volkert *et al.* (2006) suggest that the assessment should take into account a nutritional programme that reflects ethical as well as clinical considerations. Furthermore (the authors recommend when designing a programme), it should be remembered that the majority of sick, elderly patients require at least 1 g protein/kg per day and around 30 kcal/kg per day of energy, depending on their activity, as many elderly people also suffer from specific micronutrient deficiencies, such as folic acid,

179

vitamin B12, vitamin B6, niacin, vitamin C, vitamin E, iron, or zinc, which should be corrected by supplementation (Volkert *et al.* 2006). Remedying micronutrient deficiencies should lead to a major improvement in health and an increase in longevity, at low cost (Ames 2001).

The number of malnourished people leaving NHS hospitals in England has risen by 85% over the past 10 years; surveys elsewhere consistently find that about 20% of patients in general hospitals are malnourished (Lean & Wiseman 2008). Signifying that malnutrition is currently under-recognised and therefore under-treated (The Malnutrition Universal Screening Tool, MUST report, Elia 2003). Malnutrition affects the function and recovery of every organ system, increases the risk of infection, extends hospital stay, and makes readmission more likely. Clinicians need to be able to identify patients who have malnutrition or are at risk of malnutrition and then to refer them to dietitians or multidisciplinary nutrition support teams as appropriate, and provide an action plan for those at risk, as this can greatly improve outcomes (Lean & Wiseman 2008). Assessments should be reviewed regularly, either weekly or if the patient's condition changes, and any risks addressed, including making timely referrals for nutritional advice or treatment (CQC 2012). However, it must be emphasised that this tool must support not replace clinical judgement.

Jot This Down

When you are next on practice placement, note if there are adequate systems in place that enable staff to identify those at risk of malnutrition but, more importantly, what interventions are initiated?

What the Experts Say

My examination of the medical records of many patients suggested that proper records of fluid balance and nutritional intake were not maintained. In many cases, charts would be started but not continued, or filled in for some days but not others, allowing no picture to be built up of patients' progress. I very much doubt that such incomplete records would be of any significant assistance in assessing patients' continuing nutrition and hydration needs. This deficiency was remedied in a striking way by one patient's family. The mother of the patient in Ward 11 in September 2007, who saw her tray being taken away untouched, resorted to self-help in this regard.

Francis (2013)

Despite malnutrition being high on the professional, political and media agenda, the Care Quality Care (2013) review of various hospitals supported the findings from the Francis (2013) report. Unacceptably, they found some hospital staff are not giving patients the help they need to eat and drink, accurately recording what they eat and drink or not always providing patients a suitable choice of menu. This underpins the concerns raised by older people and their relatives who worry about not knowing whether they will be given appropriate food or help with eating it (RCN 2007).

Red Flag

Consider allocating staff members to patients who require assistance. This way there is some accountability in ensuring the patient has been fed. Especially if the ward is very busy.

Do not complete the menu care for the patient just because it is quicker to do so; encourage the patient to make choices, ask relatives to complete the menu card with the patient, to increase the likelihood of the patient eating what is served at meal times.

Ensure the amount they eat is documented correctly, and note previous day's intake, if they are not eating adequately they should be referred to the dietician.

Ensure the MUST score is reviewed weekly or when there has been a change in the patient's condition.

Evaluate the patient's dexterity when using cutlery; they may find specialised cutlery easier to eat with.

Specific common themes that emerged from the Francis (2013) report and the CQC (2012) inspections were:

- Lack of choice in the menus
- Inappropriate food given to patients in light of their condition
- Patients not provided with a meal
- Patients' meals placed out of reach and taken away even though they have not been touched
- No assistance provided to patients to unwrap a meal or cutlery
- No encouragement to patients to eat
- Relatives and other visitors denied access to wards during meal times
- Visitors having to assist other patients with their meals
- Visitors prevented from helping patients with feeding
- No water available at the bedside
- Water intake not monitored or encouraged
- Problems with drips not addressed adequately
- Lack of monitoring and appropriate records of fluid balance and nutritional intake.

The acuity and dependency of older people being admitted to hospital are increasing, due to the ageing population. Despite this, the staffing levels on elderly care wards in many acute hospitals have not been increased accordingly. As a result, this can impact on the staff's ability to provide the amount of time required per patient, especially if that older person has dementia, to ensure they eat adequately. Furthermore, *The Scottish Inpatient Patient Experience Survey* (Scottish Government 2010) found that interruptions to patients' meal times impacted on the problem of ensuring adequate nutrition and hydration in hospital. They identified that these interruptions occur for different reasons including: ward rounds, drug rounds and tests and investigations that may involve taking the patient away from the ward. As a result, meals became cold, missed, food wasted, patients losing their appetite and those requiring help and encouragement with feeding not receiving the support they need.

Red Flag

Ensure patients are not interrupted during meal times. Encourage doctors to stop ward rounds during for the hour food is being served.

Ensure no staff go on breaks during meal times. All staff should be available to assist with feeding.

Encourage the use of volunteers to assist patients at meal times.

Some Trusts have started up social dining. This not only encourages the patient to eat more, but the time after meals can be utilised to do activities such as reminiscence sessions or discussion around world events using the daily paper.

It is also important to remember that older people with a diagnosis of dementia may develop a loss of interest in food or overeat. The Alzheimer's Society (2009) explain in their literature, that if a person with dementia appears to have a poor appetite, this may develop for numerous reasons, for example a change in food preferences, difficulties chewing and swallowing, coordination problems affecting eating and drinking or depression. Conversely, while some lose their appetite, others may start to eat far more food than they normally would. This may be down to increased activity levels and genuine hunger, eating out of boredom or loneliness or developing a fondness for higher calorie sweet flavoured foods (Alzheimer's Society 2009).

Red Flag

 Ensure patients have their dentures cleaned and put in their mouth and not left on the side in the denture pot. Ask relatives to bring in snacks they know the patient likes.

Encourage the patient to have their meals in the dining room, if one is available.

As the dementia progresses, some patients lose the ability to use cutlery; in this case, ensure that more finger food is available to them.

Volunteers or student nurses could sit down with the patient and do some activities with them to reduce boredom. Biography not only lets you get to know the patient, it allows them to time to talk about events in their lives which makes them happy.

There are many initiatives around the country aiming to improve the way that older people are provided food in hospitals (DH 2010b). One is the 'red tray system' for identifying patients who require assistance at meal times. Serving their food on red – or any different colour – trays allows all staff to easily recognise who needs help at meal times, and does not compromise the dignity of the patient (Age Concern 2006). A red tray is also a simple reminder to staff to check the patient's notes for guidance on any specific help or nutritional needs (DH 2010). Over the years. staff have sought innovative ways to improve the provision of food to older people, which include:

- Protected meal times for all non-urgent activity. Ward and drug rounds or tests should not be allowed to happen during meal times. This allows patients to eat their meals without being interrupted by other activity and gives ward staff the time needed to help those who need help with eating (Age Concern 2006)
- More Trusts are training volunteers and other Trust staff members to assist at meal times, on elderly care wards. Key players in the area of patient care, such as Age UK, the National Patient Safety Agency and the Royal College of Nursing support the use of trained volunteers at meal times, as one way to assist patients who require help with eating and drinking. Volunteers can be especially useful in helping patients who have visual impairments or those who may have difficulty in cutting food and lifting food to their mouths. They can also offer encouragement to those who do not feel like eating (RCN 2007)
- Verbal prompting by nursing staff to encourage patients to eat and drink can have a significant impact on increasing oral intake
- Use of the MUST and personalised dietary care plans (NHS 2010).

When some older people decline food, this must be recorded by nurses as the patient's choice. However, some older people,

What To Do If …

 You are working with a community nurse caring for an older person who has been diagnosed with Alzheimer's disease. The partner of the person tells you he has noticed his partner has not been eating very much in the last 2 days; he says, 'I have noticed he has not been so keen on the food I have been giving him. I have tried coaxing him, giving him treats'. What would you do in this situation?

including those with mental health needs such as dementia need encouragement to eat – especially in the strange environment of a hospital ward (Age Concern 2006). This highlights a need to ensure that the older patient's food intake is recorded and acted upon if concerns are raised, indicating a referral to a dietician, nurse swallow assessment or just simply asking the relatives to assist the patient to fill in their menu card.

Box 9.3 outlines some examples of records and nutrition which are accurate and fit for purpose.

Box 9.4 provides examples of records that are not accurate or fit for purpose.

Being aware of the nutritional needs of older people and their individual preferences is an essential nursing duty that requires

---

Box 9.3 Examples Where Records Concerning Nutrition Are Both Accurate and Fit for Purpose

- Multidisciplinary records demonstrate that patients have had their nutritional risk assessed on admission and this was reviewed on a regular basis. Appropriate referrals were made to other healthcare professionals (e.g. dietitians)
- Patients' weights are recorded and monitored if required
- Records of patients' food intake and fluid balance are accurately completed
- Working records, for example, fluid balance charts, are kept near to the patient, and other nursing and medical notes holding confidential information being held securely but within easy reach of staff.

(*Source*: Adapted CQC 2011a,b)

Box 9.4 Examples Where Records Concerning Nutrition Are Not Fit for Purpose

- Staff concentrate on delivering the food in a timely manner, but patients are not always positioned in a way that helped them to eat without assistance
- Food is left for patients who are lying in bed, by the bedside table
- Person is slumped in bed and the table is not near enough to the patient
- Care assistants remove trays without asking if the patient has finished
- The food charts are not always completed for evening meals
- Food charts are not reviewed to ensure that people's nutritional needs are regularly updated
- Insufficient evidence to inform clinical decisions about treatments and interventions in order to ensure people are protected from inadequate nutrition and hydration.

(*Source*: Adapted CQC 2011a,b)

skill in order to act competently and confidently and above all, in the person's best interests. Nurses working with older people regardless of care setting, must focus on the individualised needs of the older person, in order to prevent malnutrition, strategies must be in place to identify those at risk of malnutrition and care plans must reflect the care that is required.

Best practice by the Council of European Alliance (UK) highlighted the key principles in effective nutritional care in hospitals:

- All patients are screened on admission to identify the patients who are malnourished or at risk of becoming malnourished
- All patients are re-screened weekly
- All patients have a care plan which identifies their nutritional care needs and how they are to be met
- The hospital includes specific guidance on food services and nutritional care in its Clinical Governance arrangements
- Patients are involved in the planning and monitoring arrangements for food service provision
- The ward implements 'protected meal times' to provide an environment conducive to patients enjoying and being able to eat their food
- All staff have the appropriate skills and competencies needed to ensure that patient's nutritional needs are met. All staff receive regular training on nutritional care and management
- The hospital supports a multidisciplinary approach to nutritional care and values the contribution of all staff groups working in partnership with patients and users.

Pressure Ulcer Prevention

Chapter 18 of this text considers skin integrity and the reader is advised to access that chapter in order to learn more. In this section, a brief consideration of pressure ulcer prevention in the older person is discussed.

Around 1 in 20 people who are admitted to hospital with an acute illness will develop a pressure ulcer, arising from many inter-related factors, and people over 70 years old are particularly vulnerable to pressure ulcers due to a combination of factors (NHS 2012). Failure in assessing the appropriate care could be detrimental to the well-being of the patient; therefore it is imperative that nurse understand and implement the latest evidence-based knowledge associated with wound care management.

Pressure Ulcers

Pressure ulcers are also referred to as pressure sores, decubitus ulcers and bedsores (Beldon 2006). Direct pressure is the major causative factor in the development of pressure ulcers. This occurs when the soft tissue of the body compressed between a bony prominence and a hard surface. This occludes the blood supply, leading to ischemia and tissue death (JWC 2013).

In some situations, deep tissue damage may have occurred in the day's prior admission to hospital, which is why it is an essential reason for inspecting the skin within 6 hours following admission (Butcher 2001).

Shear forces in combination with pressure can also contribute to pressure ulcer development, as this twisting and dragging effect occludes blood vessels, causing ischaemia and usually leads to the development of more extensive tissue damage (European Pressure Ulcer Advisory Panel and National Pressure Ulcer Advisory Panel; EPUAP & NPUAP 2009). Furthermore, shear forces can be exac-

erbated by the presence of surface moisture through incontinence or sweating and by friction when the skin slides over the surface with which it is in contact (JWC 2013).

> **Jot This Down**
>
> With regards to an older person, what do you think are the main causes of a developing pressure ulcer?
> What are the pressure ulcer points on the body?

Those most at risk

The list of those who are at risk of developing a pressure ulcer is extensive. Some examples of those at risk have been highlighted in the NHS Choices (2012) guidelines, as those:

- Who have problems moving
- Who cannot change position by themselves without help
- Who cannot feel pain over part or all of their body
- Are incontinent
- Are seriously ill
- Undergoing surgery
- Have had pressure ulcers in the past
- Have a poor diet and do not drink enough water
- Have damaged their spinal cord and can neither move nor feel their bottom and legs
- Are older people who are ill or have suffered injury.

Areas at risk of developing a pressure ulcer

NICE (2005) suggest that the most common places for pressure ulcers to occur are over bony prominences (bones close to the skin), such as the sacrum, heel and elbow, ankle, shoulder, back (bony prominences) and the back of the head (occipital).

In order to prevent the occurrence of pressure sores, those most at risk of developing them require early identification of their level of vulnerability, thus reducing unnecessary distress to the patient. To enable this, it is necessary to have a reliable evidence-based method of assessing pressure sore risk (see Chapter 18). The RCN (2005) suggest that prevention is key and older people accessing urgent care should be routinely screened for their risk of developing pressure sores, for example using the Waterlow score.

Pressure Ulcers Avoidable versus Unavoidable

An avoidable pressure ulcers is one that developed when the care provider did not do one of the following:

- Evaluate (assess) the person's clinical condition and pressure ulcer risk factors
- Plan and implement interventions that are consistent with the person's needs and goals, and recognised standards of practice
- Monitor and evaluate the impact of the interventions or revise them as appropriate.

An unavoidable pressure ulcer is one that has developed, even though the care provider did all three actions (DH 2011).

Pressure Ulcer Assessment Tools

Accurate assessment of pressure ulcer risk must be carried out as part of the holistic assessment of the patient, this enables the nurse to identify risk factors associated with the potential development of pressure ulcers in order to minimise cost, protect against litigation and improve standards of care (Phair & Heath 2010).

Red Flag

 It is essential to ensure any risk assessment tool is used in conjunction with professional judgement and not solely on the assessment score.

Pressure ulcer risk assessment and prevention should be seen as an interdisciplinary issue not just a nursing one (RCN 2001). The European Pressure Ulcer Advisory Panel (EPUAP & NPUAP 2009) guidelines endorse that risk assessments should be used in adjunct to clinical judgement and not as a tool in isolation from other clinical features. They suggest assessment tools can lean to rigid and over prescriptive approaches to patient care.

Jot This Down

Review the assessment scores on a patient who has developed a pressure ulcer in the care environment you are currently allocated to. Is there evidence to support that there is continued assessment being carried out?

Jot This Down

The two most commonly used tools to predict pressure ulcer risk are the Braden scale and the Waterlow scale. Perform a review of the assessment tools used in your area of work and perform a literature review. What are the advantages and/or disadvantages of either tool? Do you think the right one is being utilised in your work area?

Using a system which makes it easy for staff to identify quickly who is at risk of developing a pressure ulcer, will assist staff to focus their efforts on who needs pressure ulcer prevention care (NHS Choices 2012).

Preventive Measures
Pressure relieving devices

When an assessment has been carried out and the needs of the person have been determined, there may be need to order appropriate pressure relieving aids, such as an alternating pressure device that mechanically varies the pressure beneath the individual, thus reducing the duration of applied pressure. This must be based in the unique individual needs and preferences of the older person.

Positional changes

Making regular and frequent changes to the person's position is one of the most effective ways of preventing pressure ulcers. If a pressure ulcer has already developed, regularly changing position will help to avoid putting further pressure on it, and give the wound the best chance of healing (NHS Choices 2012). The use of 'Turn charts' is becoming embedded practice in many care environments. It not only provides guidance and prompts to the person providing care but is also useful evidence.

Nutrition

Nutrition status is an essential aspect of care provision. The section earlier in this chapter emphasised the importance of nutrition in the older person.

Ensuring an older person eats a healthy, balanced diet that contains an adequate amount of protein and a good variety of vitamins and minerals can help to prevent skin damage and enhance the healing process.

Incident forms

If an older person develops a pressure ulcer in a care environment, the nurse (or other healthcare professional) must complete an incident form, and if it is graded 3 or more this should be investigated as per hospital policy, for a route cause analysis (RCA):

- Look for learning points and improvements
- Establish how recurrence may effectively be reduced or eliminated
- Formulate realistic recommendations which address root causes and learning points to improve care delivery systems
- Provide a consistent means of sharing learning from the incident.

The aim of this brief overview of the prevention of pressure sore formation in the older person was to raise awareness and make the prevention of pressure ulcers a fundamental concern for nurses working with older people, regardless of the care setting. It is imperative that nurses provide a structured approach to skin assessment, care provision and evaluation of needs relevant to the setting.

Falls Prevention

There are approximately 2 000 000 falls reported in acute hospitals across England and Wales every year (PSF 2007). A Significant number of these falls result in death or severe/moderate injury. In an average 880 bed acute hospital, there will be around 1260 falls every year, resulting in estimated costs of about £92 000 for an average acute Trust (Patient Safety Observatory 2007).

The NPSA's (2007) definition:

A fall is defined as "an event whereby an individual comes to rest on the ground or another lower level, with or without loss of consciousness".

This definition includes a fall from height, which would include an environmental risk assessment. In relation to falls, this is defined as: "a process that seeks to identify hazards in the environment that could contribute to falls so that action can be taken to reduce the risk of harm".

There is significant underestimation of the overall burden from falls once the costs of rehabilitation and social care are taken into account, as up to 90% of older patients who fracture their neck of femur fail to recover their previous level of mobility or independence (Murray *et al.* 2007).

Preventing patient falls and related injuries in acute care settings has been an elusive goal for many hospitals. Falls are a high-risk and high-cost problem (human and fiscal) for all healthcare facilities. An estimated 30% of hospital-based falls result in serious injury (Stevens 2004). An ageing population, rising patient acuity, nurse shortages and an inefficient work environment for caregivers, can make any process improvement a challenge (Hendrich 2006).

Falls are also the commonest single reason for older people to present to urgent care. It is a misconception that falls are an inevitable part of ageing; they are often due to underlying disease or impairment that may be amenable to treatment or modification (Cooke *et al.* 2012). The Royal College of Physicians National Falls Audit (RCP 2009) suggests that older people often do not receive optimum care and preventative advice when they are admitted to hospital following a fall in the community. Falls prevention has become increasingly challenging, and more patients are in fact at risk for falling (Hendrich 2006). While it is important to prevent further falls in hospital, it is also important to ensure that older people are enabled to move around safely, in order that they can get the best from rehabilitation programmes (NHS 2010).

All areas of acute care hospitals are now required to assess for fall risk if their goal is to eliminate harm and injuries from falls. The number of emergency department (ED) hospital admissions is very high; as a result, the number of ED falls is increasing in many hospitals, these are the same patients who will be assessed as high risk for falling, once they go to their hospital beds (Hendrich 2006).

Those most vulnerable to falls include people with dementia or delirium; key components of falls prevention training are how to provide good care for patients with short-term memory problems or agitation, and how to prevent, detect and manage delirium (IHI [Institute for Health Care Improvement] 2009).

The Impact of a Fall for an Older Person

Falls and fractures (the majority of which result from a fall) are significant public health issues. Although not an inevitable consequence of old age, around one in three people over the age of 65 will fall each year, increasing to one in two of those over 80 (DH 2009). The psychological impact of falling can be devastating, with lower levels of confidence and independence, and increased isolation and depression inhibiting prompt recovery. Those who fall may also have to contend with a range of physical injuries, such as fractures. Half of those with hip fractures never regain their former level of function and one in five die within three months (Age UK 2012). Although the *National Service Framework for Older People* (DH 2001) set out 'to reduce the number of falls which result in serious injury and ensure effective treatment and rehabilitation for those who have fallen' and the NICE (2004) guidance has been published, there has been little significant impact.

The after-effects of even the most minor fall can be catastrophic for an older person's physical and mental health. Fear of falling again among older people and those who care for them, reduces their quality of life and well-being, even if a fall does not result in serious consequences (Age UK 2012).

> ### Jot This Down
>
> Falls in hospital are the most commonly reported patient accident in the country (Patient Safety Observatory 2007). People may fall in hospital for a variety of reasons. What do you think they are? Review the notes of some older patients who have fallen. What are the main contributing factors causing them to fall?

Causes of Falls

Oliver *et al.* (2007) note that the causes of falls are complex and hospital patients are particularly likely to be vulnerable because of the following conditions:

- Confusion related to delirium
- Cardiac
- Neurological
- Musculoskeletal
- Side-effects from medication
- Problems with balance, strength or mobility.

However, patient safety has to be balanced with independence, rehabilitation, privacy and dignity. A patient who is *not allowed* to walk alone will quickly become a patient who is *unable* to walk alone (Healey 2010). Boushon *et al.*'s (2012) findings propose that, regarding all patients who want to walk alone, although unsafe to do so, training needs to provide an overview of legislation, including the Mental Capacity Act (2005) and professional guidance, including the Royal College of Nursing's *Let's Talk about Restraint* (RCN 2007).

Red Flag

Some examples of medicines that may contribute to a fall:

Drugs that cause sedation: Any drug which causes sedation can worsen a pre-existing or create a new state of confusion in the elderly and is one of the most common causes of drug-induced falls. However, almost any of the commonly used sedating drugs can cause confusion in the elderly who then tend to present with confusion as the main symptom of an adverse effect.

Drugs which affect the central nervous system: These include antipsychotics, antidepressants and sleeping tablets (including benzodiazepines). They can cause confusion, sedation, impaired balance and low blood pressure, especially on standing. Some drugs can also cause symptoms of Parkinson's disease, such as tremor and abnormal body movements. It should be remembered that these drugs are often prescribed for conditions which in themselves can cause confusion, such as depression.

Every nurse should be aware there is no such thing as a simple fall. Even a fall where there is no injury can cause a level of psychological damage to the patient, often resulting in a loss of confidence and independence. Older people in hospital settings or care homes are more at risk of falling than non-hospitalised people, due to the increased incidence of confusion, confounding medical conditions and environmental factors (Fonda *et al.* 2006). It is predictable that an elderly, confused patient who is mobile, will fall if left unsupervised and out of bed (Francis 2013). It is essential that a 'falls prevention care plan' is initiated, and preventable measures put in place, such as: to ensure the patient is being nursed in an observable area or nursed on a bed that goes right to the floor (high-low bed); falls sensor alarms, which are placed under the patient, if they move off the sensor pad an alarm sounds alerting the staff the patient is at risk of falling so they attend straight away. If the patient is very confused, it may necessitate the usage of 1:1 (one nurse to one patient) nursing to ensure the patient's safety is maximised. Given the many different causes of falls in hospital patients, engagement of all the multidisciplinary team is needed and will be most effective if they engage nurses, doctors, therapists, pharmacists, housekeeping staff and relevant others to work together to develop key aspects to reduce older people falling in hospital (Boushon *et al.* 2012).

Assessment of Falls Risk

Undertaking and documenting a risk assessment for patient falls for each patient within 4 hours of admission is a necessity. Reassessing and documenting falls risk factors on should be done on a regular basis, at least weekly or if the condition of the patient changes or if the patient falls. Oliver *et al.* (2007) suggests that even with the most validated tool such as the fall risk assessment tool (FRAT), there is a risk they will miss patients who are likely to fall or conclude a patient that is likely to fall, when they are not. Even if the tools were more effective at predicting falls, there is a risk that the recording of the score is where the action ends (Healey 2010).

Treating a fall risk assessment as an integrated component of an individual care plan is the first best step for proactive prevention of falls; too often, fall prevention strategies begin after a fall occurrence, not before (Hendrich 2006). While it is important there is a trigger mechanism in place, it is far more important to ensure interventions have been implemented to prevent a fall/further falls. Equally, after any fall, the interventions put in place should be reviewed and further interventions initiated. It is important to remember that there are some older people who will fall, regardless of what interventions are put in place. However, it is important to provide documented evidence to support that there are interventions in place.

Jot This Down

Review and compare different falls risk assessment tools. How accurate did you think the numerical fall risk assessment tools are at predicting those at risk of falls? What actions were taken as a result of the risk assessment? In areas you have worked/working what mechanisms are in place to ensure a falls prevention care plan is initiated in an effort to prevent the person falling/falling again?

Recent reviews of the reliability of numerical falls risk assessments suggest there is a risk of such tools missing patients who are likely to fall or identifying a patient as a likely faller when in fact they are not (Oliver *et al.* 2007).

Older people are concerned about asking for nursing help, given how 'busy' they perceive nursing staff to be. Regularly scheduled patient contact to high-risk patients with impaired gait and mobility due to functional deficits or medication side-effects, will reduce falls in most acute care hospitals between 50% and 70%, yet this intervention is inconsistently applied (Hendrich 2006).

Jot This Down

Following the completion of a falls risk assessment, it identifies an older person at a high risk of falls. As part of a falls prevention care plan, what measures can be initiated to prevent a further fall?

Initiatives to Prevent an Older Person Falling

- Ensure environment is free from clutter
- Ensure they have adequate footwear
- Ensure walking aids are near them
- Ensure the call bell is within reach
- Ensure a medication review has occurred to reduce any unnecessary hypnotics or sedatives
- Ensure they have been assessed by the physiotherapist for an appropriate walking aid and assessment of their balance and gait
- Consider the use of equipment, such a falls prevention sensor alarms
- Consider the usage of high-low bed
- Ensure those high at risk of falls are in observable bays
- Ensure one to one monitoring/observation is in place if an older person is unsafe to be left unsupervised.

After a Fall

Immediate Checks Post-Fall

After a fall has occurred, the initial focus has to be on rapidly identifying and treating any resultant injury (Boushon *et al.* 2012). The nurse finding any patient who has fallen must check for signs and symptoms of fracture or potential for spinal injury before the patient is moved. If there is any suspicion that the patient has sustained a head/spinal injury, the patient should **NOT** be moved unless their airway is compromised (Patient Safety Observatory 2007). If a patient is suspected of having sustained a head/neck injury, they should be transferred to bed following the 'stabilisation and transfer of patients with a suspected or confirmed spinal injury' and will require the use of equipment such as a hover jack, however, this specialised equipment should only be used by those who have the competencies to do so.

Timescale for Medical Examination

If an adult patient has had an un-witnessed fall it is important to ensure that neurological observations are performed as per the National Institute for Clinical Excellence (NICE) guidance and the instructions given by the attending doctor. A medical examination should take place immediately if the patient displays an altered Glasgow Coma Scale score, possible signs of fracture/spinal/head injury or new pain, confusion or distress (NICE 2013).

Informing Significant Others

It is essential that the identified main contact for the patient is informed of any fall, even if no injury has been incurred. This is good practice and is usually in most acute Trusts 'Falls Prevention Policy' and on the clinical incident form that has to be completed by the staff member who found/witnessed a patient who had a fall.

Incident Form

Ensure an incident form has been completed, providing details, such as: was the fall witnessed/un-witnessed; immediate actions taken post-fall (assessment of the patient's condition, any concerns of a neck/head injury); how the patient was transferred back into bed; and what observations and preventative measures were initiated to prevent further falls.

Patients Who Sustain Serious Harm

Any patient who sustains severe harm must have a full Root Cause Analysis (RCA) completed with 24 hours of the incident (Patient Safety Observatory 2007).

The Evidence

Route cause analysis (RCA)

The report should explain:

- What happened (i.e. chronology of events)
- When it happened
- Where it happened
- How it happened (i.e. what went wrong)
- Why it happened (i.e. what underlying, contributory factors caused things to go wrong).

The 'How it happened' and 'Why it happened' form the most valuable parts of the investigating process in order to try to get to the root causes of the incident. It is necessary to establish whether any failings had occurred.

The RCA investigation process should:

- Look for learning points and improvements
- Establish how recurrence may be effectively **reduced** or **eliminated**
- Formulate realistic recommendations, which address root causes and learning points to improve care delivery systems
- Provide a consistent means of sharing learning from the incident.

The identification and assessment of the older person at risk of falls; the management of care of those at risk of falling in hospital; the minimising of risk of injury as a result of falling and the process of managing the care of the patient who has fallen to minimise the risk of further injury, are key aspects of the role and function of the nurse.

Discharge Planning

The aim of discharge planning is to reduce the length of time an older person has to stay in hospital, prevent unnecessary readmission to hospital and improve the coordination of services following discharge from hospital (Shepperd *et al.* 2013). On admission to an acute hospital, planning for discharge or transfer of care should begin as soon as possible (DH 2010). Older people may require complex support networks, both formal and informal, to support them in their own homes, therefore comprehensive discharge planning is crucial to ensure individual's problems have been addressed, so they can return safely to their own home (Shepperd *et al.* 2013; Heath *et al.* 2010). Therefore, a well-ordered system of discharge management is an essential part of the hospital service (Francis 2013). It is important to remember that discharge involves coordinating many services the patient may require, from the pharmacy and transport to care packages provided by agencies outside the trust. The involvement of additional people makes coordination and planning even more critical to discharge (DH 2010). It is important to ensure adequate and timely information is shared between services whenever there is a transfer of care between individuals or services (Cooke *et al.* 2012).

Discharge planning concerns the facilitation of a person's discharge from one healthcare setting to another or back to the person's own home. This is a multidisciplinary process involving, for example, nurses, doctors, social workers and if appropriate, other health professionals. The goal is to enhance continuity of care. The process begins on admission.

The pressure on a busy hospital to discharge patients is considerable. It is possible that even a small reduction in length of stay or readmission rate could free-up capacity for subsequent admissions in a healthcare system where there is a shortage of acute hospital

beds (DH 2008). However, it is essential that the older person should only be discharged from hospital with adequate support and with respect for their preferences (Cooke *et al.* 2012). The nurse acting as advocate has a key role to play here.

Older people may be especially vulnerable and will require a holistic assessment of their home circumstances before discharge. The evidence suggests that a structured discharge plan tailored to the individual patient probably brings about a reduction in hospital length of stay and readmission rates and an increase in patient satisfaction and ultimately, the need for long-term care (Cooke *et al.* 2012; Shepperd *et al.* 2013). Furthermore, discharge planning should ensure that older people are discharged from hospital at an appropriate time in their care, with adequate notice, and the provision of other services organised (DH 2010).

A crucial part of effective discharge planning is to ensure the older person, and where appropriate their carers and families, are involved in the decision-making process around assessment and management of ongoing and future care, and self-care (Cooke *et al.* 2012). The NMC (2008) stipulate that 'You must be aware of the legislation regarding mental capacity, ensuring that people who lack capacity remain at the centre of decision-making and are fully safeguarded'. This is a key element in working with the older person and their family when considering discharge planning.

Francis (2013) found that patients and their families had raised some principal matters for concern with regards to discharge:

- Premature discharge from wards resulting in readmission to hospital
- Protracted process of discharge
- Failure to communicate discharge arrangements to patients and their families
- Discharge at an inappropriate time or in an inappropriate condition
- Failure to ensure appropriate support
- Lack of communication about changes in discharge plans.

Jot This Down

What is your experience of the discharge process? As a nurse, how can you influence the discharge process and what are your responsibilities to ensure a safe and effective discharge is achieved?

Discharge planning commences the day the older person is admitted to hospital and this entails seeking collateral history from the patient and/or family and/or carers within 24 hours of admission (DH 2010). This will enable MDT to collaboratively, with the patient and significant others, plan care, agree on who is responsible for specific actions and make decisions on the process and timing of discharges and transfers to plan (Lees & Delpino 2007).

What the Experts Say Nurses Responsibilities

- Listen to people in their care and respond to their needs and preferences
- Share with people in a way they understand the information they want and need to know about their health and care
- Share information with colleagues and keep them informed
- Work effectively as part of a team
- Ensure that patient consent is gained before intervention
- Act as advocate for patients

(NMC 2008)

The MDT need to develop an understanding of how the patient managed prior to admission, for example with regard to activities of living, mobility, issues concerning continence, nutrition and any concerns the older person or significant others may have with regard to discharge planning. Nurses and doctors can often predict when a patient is likely to respond to treatment and an estimated discharge date (EDD) can be set. This date should be communicated to the patient and family, so that they can make any necessary preparations. This is usually the time when the older person and/or relatives will voice any concerns that they may have. Setting an EDD is important, as the older person needs to know how long they are likely to be in hospital, so they can plan for their return home (DH 2001). It is important to remember that older people must be treated as individuals with dignity and respect; their wishes and those of their significant others must be acknowledged, with shared decision-making based on clinical considerations (Cooke *et al.* 2012). Adopting this approach will enable discharge and transfer planning to anticipate or pre-empt potential problems, arrange for appropriate support to be put in place and agree an expected discharge date.

It is essential that the nurse establishes a trusting relationship with the older person and family. This will enable the older person and the nurse to identify specific concerns which may affect how the person is going to continue living independently or how much assistance is going to be required for a safe discharge. Effective discharge planning can only occur if individualised needs are assessed appropriately (Heath *et al.* 2010).

> ### Jot This Down
> Effective interpersonal skills are not always sufficient themselves in creating the right environment. What other factors may undermine attempts for the older person to express a need?

Carers/Significant Others' Involvement

Nurses should not make an assumption that a person's carer will necessarily be able to, or want to, continue in a caring role. Older people and their carers may have different needs and aspirations. Check the accuracy of any information that has been provided from the patient about their relative's willingness and ability to care (Lees & Delpino 2007).

Assessment Notification – Section 2

When a patient is deemed fit for discharge and there has been an identified need for community support, with the patients consent or, in the patient's best interest, a Social Services referral is required. Following this notification, social care departments have a minimum period of 3 days to carry out an assessment and arrange services.

> ### Primary Care
> It is important to ensure the GP receives a full summary of the admission to hospital to ensure continuity of care.
>
> If the older person has complex needs or a long-term condition, consider a referral to the community matron to assess the patient post–discharge.
>
> District nurses will require a referral if the patient requires medication to be administered by them, catheter care or dressings to wounds (ensure they have at least 3 days supply of dressings on discharge, as it takes time for the district nurse to get a prescription from the GP for the appropriate dressing, especially if it is a newly acquired wound).

Discharge Notification – Section 5

Discharge notification – Section 5 gives notice of the day on which it is proposed that the patient is discharged. Reimbursement liability commences on the day after the minimum 3-day period (Section 2) or the day after the proposed discharge date (Section 5), whichever is the later (Lees & Delpino 2007).

It is important to remember that older people and their carers must be involved at all stages of discharge planning, provided with adequate information and assisted to make care planning decisions and choices. Remember that patients and their carers are the experts in how they feel and what it is like to live with, or care for someone with, a particular condition or disability. Listen to their concerns and give consideration to their past and present circumstances and aspirations. Pay attention to their frame of mind, how they are feeling and who else might be involved (DH 2010). To have the ability and skill to manage patient and carer expectations by involving them at all stages of decision-making, ensures fewer problems and surprises at the end of an episode of care. A mismatch of expectations between the patient, carer and MDT is the result of inconsistent or poor communication earlier in the process (Lees & Delpino 2007).

What To Do If …

 An older person is due to be discharged – he is excited and very keen to be going back home with his wife. His wife has called you aside to say that she no longer feels able or willing to care for her husband at home. She feels the burden is too great, as she herself has a number of health issues that restrict her physically.
What will your next steps be?

If discharge planning is not coordinated, the older person has not been involved in the discharge process, this can result in potential problems. The DH (2010) suggests that premature discharge can leave the patient:

- with some unmet needs
- poorly prepared for home
- with the likelihood of readmission
- inappropriate move to residential or nursing home care.

A protracted length of stay increases the risk of:

- infection
- depression/low mood
- boredom
- frustration
- loss of independence and confidence
- NHS resources being used inappropriately.

There are occasions when an older person will decide against the identified need for a care package by the MDT and want to be discharged accordingly. As long as they have the mental capacity to make that decision, the nurse and other members MDT must respect their decision, despite how unsafe that decision may appear to them.

Those older people who do not have the capacity to make decisions are given their rights and obligations under the Mental Capacity Act. Where the patient cannot represent themselves, the next of kin, carer, relative or an independent mental capacity advocate (IMCA) must be involved. Their role is to represent the patient's interests, and to challenge any decision that does not appear to be in the best interest of the patient.

NHS continuing healthcare patients who do have complex health needs are eligible to have their needs considered against the criteria (DH 2009). Eligibility for NHS Continuing Healthcare is based on an individual's assessed health needs. In order to inform consistent decision-making on a person's eligibility, the *National Framework for NHS Continuing Healthcare* was introduced in October 2007 and revised in July 2009 (DH 2007a).

Decision Support Tool (DST)

This tool is designed to ensure that the full range of factors that have a bearing on the person's eligibility are taken into account in making a decision. This should be completed following a full assessment of need and risk by the MDT. The older person's needs should be evaluated and a level of need apportioned. Completion of the DST should be coordinated by a clinician (e.g. a consultant nurse or nurse specialist) who has specialist knowledge of the NHS eligibility criteria and with the agreement of the MDT. A recommendation should then be made on the person's eligibility for NHS Continuing Healthcare. Patients who are not eligible for NHS Continuing Healthcare and who enter a nursing home, are eligible for an assessment for NHS-funded nursing care. This is a standard weekly payment made directly to the nursing home to meet the cost of the care from a registered nurse.

The following ten steps to an effective and timely discharge has been produced by the DH (2010):

1. Start planning for discharge or transfer before or on admission
2. Identify whether the patient has simple or complex discharge and transfer planning needs, involving the patient and the carer in your decision
3. Develop a clinical management plan for every patient within 24 hours of admission
4. Coordinate the discharge or transfer of care process through effective leadership and handover of responsibilities at ward level
5. Set an expected date of discharge or transfer within 24–48 hours of admission, and discuss with the patient and carer
6. Review the clinical management plan with the patient each day, take any necessary action and update progress towards the discharge or transfer date
7. Involve patients and carers so that they can make informed decisions and choices that deliver a personalised care pathway and maximise their independence
8. Plan discharges and transfers to take place over seven days to deliver continuity of care for the patient
9. Use a discharge checklist 24–48 hours prior to transfer
10. Make decisions to discharge and transfer patients each day.

Understanding how the discharge process works and all of the issues associated with it can help to ensure that the care package is seamless – from hospital to home. This should effectively ensure that nurses working with older people regardless of the care setting will focus their attention on the individualised needs of the older person when planning discharge. The need for timely discharge and care transfer requires nurses and others to plan, communicate, negotiate and ensure a smooth transition for individuals and their families (DH 2010). Underpinning this is the need for:

- Effective communication with individuals and across settings
- Alignment of services to ensure continuity of care
- Clear clinical management plans

The discharge process is an essential part of care management in any setting; it is equally essential in settings where older people are being cared for. It ensures that health and social care systems are proactive in supporting older people and their families and carers to either return home or transfer to another setting. It also ensures that systems are using resources efficiently (DH 2010). Assessment is about putting together information concerning an older person's needs and circumstances, making sense of that information in order to identify needs and agreeing what advice, support or treatment to provide (Lees & Delpino 2007). Approximately 20% of patients have more complex needs and may need additional input from other professionals such as social workers, therapists. The involvement of additional people makes coordination and planning even more critical to discharge (DH 2010).

Key Points

- The chapter has emphasised the importance of communication in the older person setting and also when communicating with older people and their families.
- Key issues associated with all aspects of care have been discussed; these included dignity and respect. The need to ensure that people are treated as individuals has been highlighted.
- It is imperative that care planning is (when possible) done with patients reflecting and respecting their individual needs.
- When undertaking an assessment of individual needs, a holistic approach must be adopted. The person undertaking the assessment of needs must be deemed competent and confident in this important aspect of care. Assessment tools must be used judiciously, be fit for purpose and be relevant.
- There are a number of tools available to assess the needs of the person's nutritional needs. Assessment of need concerning nutrition has ben discussed.
- Falls are a major cause of morbidity and mortality in the ageing population. Undertaking a detailed and patient-centred assessment can identify those at risk and help to prevent a fall occurring.
- Caring for people in their own homes in a safe and effective manner will require the nurse to plan the discharge in such a way that the patient is at the centre of any decisions being made. A multidisciplinary team approach has been advocated.

Glossary

Advocate: a person, group or organisation supporting and championing individuals or groups, making sure that their views are considered and their rights defended

Assessment notification – section 2: issued for patients who are considered likely to require social services involvement in order to expedite their discharge; it is a notification of need of care to the relevant social services authority

Autonomy (nursing): the freedom of a person to make binding decisions, within the scope of their practice, based on professional ethics, expertise and clinical knowledge

Care pathways: a system of care delivery that organises a service user's care from their first contact with health services to the end of their journey. Care pathways aim to improve continuity and coordination across different professions and sectors. Other types include integrated care pathways, clinical pathways, multidisciplinary pathways, care maps and collaborative care pathways

Clinical governance: a systematic approach to maintaining and improving the quality of patient care within health and social systems

Comorbidity: the presence of more than one health problem in one person at the same time

Competence: refers to the overarching set of knowledge, skills and attitudes required to practise safely

Diversity: valuing people, recognising them for their skills, their talents and experiences, acknowledging that everyone is different

Malnutrition: a condition caused by an imbalance between what a person eats and the nutrients that they need to maintain good health

Nursing: the use of clinical judgement in the delivery of care to assist people to improve, maintain or recover health, to cope with health problems, and to attain the best possible quality of life, regardless of their disease or disability until their death (Royal College of Nursing, RCN 2008b)

Recovery: a person's ability to live what they believe is a meaningful and satisfying life, with or without symptoms. Recovery means having control over and input into your own life

Root cause analysis (RCA): this practice (approach) tries to solve problems by endeavouring to identify and correct the root causes of events, instead of simply addressing their symptoms

Safeguarding: associated with acting in the best interests of people when they are using or requiring the services of healthcare providers; it relates to protecting children, young people and vulnerable adults from abuse and neglect, as well as explicitly promoting their welfare

References

Age Concern (2006) *Hungry to be Heard, the Scandal of Malnourished Older People.* http://www.ageuk.org.uk/health-wellbeing/doctors-hospitals/campaign-against-malnutrition-in-hospital/ (accessed October 2013).

Age UK (2012) *Stop Falling: Saving Lives and Money.* http://www.ageuk.org.uk/documents/en-gb/campaigns/stop_falling_report_web.pdf?dtrk=true (accessed October 2013).

Agewell's (2005) *A Good Practice Guide to Communicating with Older People.* Agewell's Working Group, West Bromwich.

Alzheimer's Society (2009) *Counting the Cost: caring for people with dementia in hospital wards.* Alzheimer's Society, London.

Alzheimer's Society (2010) *This is Me.* Alzheimer's Society, London.

Alzheimer's Society (2012) *Dementia 2012: a national challenge.* Alzheimer's Society, London.

Ames, B.N. (2001) DNA damage from micronutrient deficiencies is likely to be a major cause of cancer. *Micronutrients and Genomic Stability*, 475(1–2), 1–188.

Anderson, L. (2012) *Why Communication in the Nursing Profession is Important.* http://www.nursetogether.com/why-communication-in-the-nursing-profession-is-important (accessed 12 April 2013.)

Baillie, L. (2007) The impact of staff behavior on patients dignity in acute hospitals. *Nursing Times*, 103(34), 30–31.

Baillie, L., Ford, P., Gallagher, A. & Wainwright, P. (2009) Nurses' views on dignity in care. *Nursing Older People*, 21(8), 22–29.

BAPEN (1992) *A Positive Approach to Nutrition as Treatment.* British Association for Parenteral and Enteral Nutrition, Kings Fund Central Report.

Bayer, T., Tadd, W. & Krajcik, S. (2005) Dignity: the voice of older people. *Quality in Ageing and Older Adults*, 6(1), 22–29.

Beldon, P. (2006) Pressure Ulcers: prevention and management. *Wound Essentials*, 1, 68–81.

Berry, L. (2012) University courses should stress the value of dignity. *Nursing Older People*, 24(6), 5.

Boushon, B., Nielsen, G., Quigley, P. et al. (2012) *How-to Guide: reducing patient injuries from falls.* Institute for Healthcare Improvement, Cambridge, MA. www.IHI.org (accessed 18 April 2013).

Bridges, J., Flatley, M. & Meyer, J. (2010) Older people's and relatives' experiences in acute care settings: systematic review and synthesis of qualitative studies. *International Journal of Nursing Studies* 47(January), 89–107.

Butcher, M. (2001) NICE Clinical Guidelines: pressure ulcer risk assessment and prevention – a review.

Butterworth, C. (2012) How to achieve a person-centred writing style in care plans. *Nursing Older People*, 24(8), 21–26.

CHAI (2007) *Ageism and age discrimination in secondary health care in the United Kingdom.* Commission for Healthcare Audit and Inspection, Centre for Policy.

Conroy, S. (2012). *Quality Care for Older People with Urgent and Emergency Care Needs.* (The Silver Book). Age UK, London. Association of Directors of Adult Social Services (ADASS); British Geriatrics Society (BGS), June 2012.

Cooke, M., Oliver, D. & Burns, A. (2012) *Quality Care for Older People with Urgent and Emergency Care Needs.* Silver Book. http://tinyurl.com/cebaqz3 (accessed 17 February 2013).

Courtney, M. & Tong, S. (2000) Acute-care nurses attitudes towards older people: at literature review. *International Journal of Nursing Practice*, 6(2), 62–69.

CQC (Care Quality Commission) (2010) *Guidance about Compliance: Essential Standards of Quality and Safety.* Care Quality Commission, London.

CQC (2011a) *Dignity and Nutrition Inspection Programme: National Overview, October 2011.* Care Quality Commission, London.

CQC (2011b) *Publish First of Detailed Reports in to Dignity and Nutrition for Older People.* Care Quality Commission, London.

CQC (2012) The state of health care and adult social care in England in 2011–2012.

CQC (2013) *Time to Listen in NHS Hospitals Dignity and Nutrition Inspection Programme 2012 Summary.* Care Quality Commission, London.

Currie, J. (2000) Audit of nursing handover. *Nursing Times* 9(6), 42–44.

DH (2001) *National Service Framework (NSF) for Older People.* Department of Health, London.

DH (2006a) *Dignity in Care Campaign.* Department of Health, London.

DH (2006b) *National Service Framework Next Steps.* Department of Health, London.

DH (2007a) *The National Framework for NHS Continuing Healthcare and NHS-funded Nursing Care* (revised July 2009). Department of Health, London.

DH (2007b) *Valuing People Now.* Department of Health, London.

DH (2008) *High Quality Care For All. NHS next stage review final report, Lord Darzi.* Department of Health, London.

DH (2009) *Living Well with Dementia: a national dementia strategy.* Department of Health, London.

DH (2010a) *Essence of Care 2010: benchmarks for communication.* Department of Health, London. http://bit.ly/hloYIx (accessed 23 July 2013).

DH (2010b) *Essence of Care Communication, Promoting Health and Care Environment.* Department of Health, London.

DH (2010c) *Ready to Go? Planning the discharge and the transfer of patients from hospital and intermediate care.* Department of Health, London.

DH (2011) *Defining Avoidable and Unavoidable Pressure Ulcers*, Department of Health, London. www.patientsafetyfirst.nhs.uk_ashx_Asset.ashx_path=_PressureUlcers_Defining%20avoidable%20and%20unavoidable%20pressure%20ulcers (accessed 19 April 2013).

DH (2013a) *Treating Patients and Service Users with Respect, Dignity and Compassion.* Department of Health, London.

DH (2013b) *Patients First and Foremost:* The initial government response to the Report of the Mid Staffordshire Foundation Trust Public Enquiry. Department of Health, London.

Doherty, M., Mitchell, E.A. & O'Neill, S. (2011) Attitudes of healthcare workers towards older people in a rural population: a survey using the Kogan Scale. *Nursing Research and Practice*, 2011, 352627. http://dx.doi.org/10.1155/2011/352627 (accessed 13 September 2013).

Douglas-Dunbar, M. & Gardiner, P. (2007) Support for carers of people with dementia during hospital admission. *Nursing Older People*, 19(8), 27–30.

Edington, J., Boorman, J., Durrant E.J. *et al.* (2000) Prevalence of malnutrition on admission to four hospitals in England. The Malnutrition Prevalence Group. *Clinical Nutrition*, 19(3), 191–195.

Ekman, P., Friesen, W.V., O'Sullivan, M. *et al.* (1987). Universals and cultural differences in the judgments of facial expressions of emotion. *Journal of Personality and Social Psychology*, 53(4), 712–717.

Elia, M. (2003) *Screening for Malnutrition: a multidisciplinary responsibility.* Development and use of the 'Malnutrition Universal Screening Tool' ('MUST') for adults. BAPEN, Redditch.

EPUAP & NPUAP (2009) *Prevention and Treatment of Pressure Ulcers: Quick Reference Guide.* European Pressure Ulcer Advisory Panel, London and National Pressure Ulcer Advisory Panel, Washington DC.

Evans, A., Pereira, D. & Parker, J. (2008) Discourses of anxiety in nursing practice: a psychoanalytic case study of the change of shift handover ritual. *Nursing Inquiry*, 15(1), 40–48.

Fonda, D., Cook, J., Sandler, V. *et al.* (2006) Sustained reduction in serious fall-related injuries in older people in hospital. *Medical Journal of Australia*, 184(8), 379–82.

Fook, L. & Morgan, R. (2000) Hearing in Older People: a review. *Postgraduate Medical Journal*, 76, 537–541.

Francis, R. (2013) Independent Inquiry Into Care Provided by Mid Staffordshire NHS Foundation Trust: January 2005–March 2009.

Greaves, I. & Jolly, D. (2010) National Dementia Strategy: well intentioned – but how well founded and how well directed? *British Journal of General Practice*, 60(572), 193–198.

Healey, F. (2010) A guide on how to prevent falls and injury in hospital. *Nursing Older People*, 22(9), 16–22.

Health Foundation (2011) *Spotlight on Dementia Care: a health foundation improvement report.* The Health Foundation. London.

Heath, H., Sturdy D. & Cheesly, A. (2010) A. Discharge planning: A summary of the Department of Health's guidance, Ready to go? Planning the discharge and the transfer of patients from hospital and intermediate care. RCN Publishing, Harrow.

Help the Aged/Age Concern (2009) *Waiting for Change: how the NHS is responding to the needs of older people.* Age UK, London.

Hendrich, A. (2006) *Inpatient Falls: Lessons from the Field.* Lionheart Publishing, Inc., Holywood.

Henry, L.N., Martin, L., Hunt, S. & Crippen, P. (2009) A quality improvement project to optimise patient outcomes following the maze procedure. *Journal Nursing Care Quality*, 24(2), 160–165.

Higgins, I., Van Der Reit, P., Slater, L. & Peek, C. (2007) The negative attitudes of nurses towards older patients in the acute setting: A qualitative descriptive study. *Contemporary Nurse*, 26(2), 225–237.

IHI (Institute for Healthcare Improvement) (2009) Pursuing perfection in health care: involving patients in redesigning care (healthcare workforce).

JCR (2007) *Improving Hands-Off Communication.* Joint Commission Resources, Illinois (Made available by Google eBooks). (accessed 13 March 2013).

JWC (2013) Wound Assessment Supplement. *Journal of Wound Care*, MA Healthcare. http://info.journalofwoundcare.com/features/wound_assessment/ (accessed 12 February 2013).

Lamond, D. (2000) The information content of the nurse change of shift report: a comparative study. *Journal of Advanced Nursing*, 31(4), 794–804.

Lean, M. & Wiseman, M. (2008) Malnutrition in hospitals. *British Medical Journal*, 336(7639), 290.

Lees, L. & Delpino, R. (2007) Facilitating an effective discharge from hospital. *Nursing Times*, 103(29), 30–31.

Lin, Y.P. & Tsai, Y.F. (2011) Maintaining patients' dignity during clinical care: a qualitative interview study. *Journal of Advanced Nursing*, 67(2), 340–348.

Lloyd, M. (2010) *A Practical Guide to Care Planning In Health and Social Care.* Open University Press, Maidenhead.

Local Government Association, NHS Confederation & Age UK (2012) *Delivering Dignity: Securing dignity in care for older people in hospitals and care.* http://www.nhsconfed.org/priorities/Quality/Partnership-on-dignity/Pages/Draftreportrecommendations.aspx (accessed May 2013)

McCormack, B. & McCance, T. (2010) *Person-centred Nursing Theory and Practice.* Wiley-Blackwell, Oxford.

McCormack, B. & McCance, T.V. (2006). Developing a conceptual framework for person-centred nursing. *Journal of Advanced Nursing*, 56(5), 472–479.

Magee, M.B. (2013) *Barriers to Effective Communication in Nursing.* eHow.com http://www.ehow.com/list_6797926_barriers-effective-communication-nursing.html/ixzz2ReYx2xYA (accessed April 2013).

McKinlay, A. & Cowan, S (2003) Students attitudes towards working with older patients. *Journal of Advanced Nursing*, 43(3), 298–309.

McLafferty, I. & Morrison, F. (2004) Attitudes towards hospitalised older adults. *Journal of Advanced Nursing*, 47(4), 446–53.

Murray, G.R., Cameron, R.D. & Cumming, R.G. (2007) The consequences of falls in acute and subacute hospitals in Australia that cause proximal femoral fractures. *Journal of the American Geriatrics Society*, 55(4), 577–582.

Naish, J. (1996) The route to effective nurse-patient communication. *Nursing Times*, 92(17), 27–30.

Nay, R. & Garratt, S. (2004) *Nursing Older People: Issues and innovation*, 2nd edn. Churchill Livingstone, Sydney.

NHS Choices (2012) *Pressure Ulcers.* http://www.nhs.uk/Conditions/Pressure-ulcers/Pages/Treatment.aspx (accessed 13 November 2012).

NHS Institute for Innovation and Improvement (2008) *SBAR Situation – Background – Assessment – Recommendation.* http://www.nice.nhs.uk (accessed 15 February 2013).

NHS Practice Guide (2010) *Achieving age equality in health and social care* –29, Ch. 5. *High Quality Care for All.* www.southwest.nhs.uk/age-equality.html (accessed 10 March 2013).

NICE (2004) Clinical Guidelines. *The Assessment and Prevention of Falls in Older People.* National Institute for Health and Clinical Excellence, London.

NICE (2005) *Clinical Guideline 29: pressure ulcer management.* National Institute for Health and Clinical Excellence, London.

NICE (2006) *Clinical Guideline 32: nutrition support for adults: oral nutrition support, enteral tube feeding and parenteral nutrition.* National Institute for Health and Clinical Excellence, London.

NICE (2013) *Falls: Assessment and Prevention of Falls in Older People.* NICE Clinical Guideline 161. National Institute for Health and Care Excellence, London.

NMC (2008) *Performance and Ethics for Nurses and Midwives.* Nursing and Midwifery Council, London.

NMC (2009a) *Guidance for the Care of Older People.* Nursing and Midwifery Council, London.

NMC (2009b) *Record Keeping – Guidance for Nurses and Midwives.* Nursing and Midwifery Council, London.

Nolan, L. (2006) Observations of the experiences of people with dementia on general hospital wards. *Journal of Research in Nursing*, 11(5), 453–465.

NPSA (National Patient Safety Agency) (2007) *Slips, Trips and Falls in Hospitals.* NPSA, London.

Oliver, D., Connelly, J., Victor, C. *et al.* (2007) Strategies to prevent falls and fractures in hospital and care homes and the effect of cognitive impairment: systematic review and meta-analyses. *British Medical Journal*, 334(7584), 82.

190

Patient Safety Observatory (2007) *Slips, Trips and Falls in Hospital*. National Patient Safety Agency, London.

Phair, L. & Heath, H. (2010) Neglect of older people in formal care settings part two: new perspectives on investigation and factors determining whether neglect has taken place. Peer reviewed policy and practice paper. *Journal of Adult Protection*, 12(4), 6–15.

Pope, T. (2011) How person-centred care can improve nurses attitudes to hospitalised older patients. *Nursing Older People*, 24(1), 32–36.

Porteous, J., Stewart-Wynne, E., Connolly, M. & Crommelin, P. (2009). ISOBAR-a concept and handover checklist: The National clinical handover initiative. *Medical Journal of Australia*, 190(11), S152–S156.

Preetinder, S. Gill (2013) Patient engagement: an investigation at a primary care clinic. *International Journal of General Medicine*, 6, 85–98.

Price, B. (2013) Countering the stereotype of the unpopular patient. *Nursing Older People*, 25(6), 27–23.

PSF (2007) *The How to Guide for Reducing Harm from Falls*. Patient Safety First, London.

Pursey, A. & Luker, K. (1995) Attitudes and stereotypes: nurses' work with older people. *Journal of Advanced Nursing*, 22(3), 547–555.

RCN (2001) *Pressure Ulcer Risk Assessment and Prevention*, Royal College of Nursing, London.

RCN (2005) *The Management of Pressure Ulcers in Primary and Secondary Care*: A clinical practice guideline. Royal College of Nursing, London.

RCN (2006) *Telephone Advice Lines for People with Long Term Conditions: guidance for nurse practitioners*. Royal College Of Nursing, London.

RCN (2007) *Nutrition Now Campaign*. Royal College of Nursing, London. http://nursingstandard.rcnpublishing.co.uk/campaigns/nutrition-now, (accessed 13 February 2013).

RCN (2008a) *Defending Dignity: challenges and opportunities for nurses*. Royal College of Nursing, London.

RCN (2008b) *Delivering Dignified Care: a practice support pack for workshop facilitators*. Royal College of Nursing, London.

RCN (2008c) *Small Changes Make a Big Difference: How You can Influence to Deliver Dignified Care*. Royal College of Nursing, London.

RCN (2010) *Discharge Planning: a summary of the department of health's guidance ready to go? Planning the Discharge and the Transfer of Patients from Hospital and Intermediate Care*. Royal College of Nursing, London.

RCP (2009) *National Audit of the Organisation of Services for Falls and Bone Health of Older People*. Royal College of Physicians, London.

RCP (2011) *Report of the National Audit of Dementia Care in General Hospitals*. Royal College of Psychiatrists, Healthcare Quality Improvement Partnership, London.

Risky Business (2012) SBAR acute handover. An example video of how to do an acute handover using the SBAR technique. http://www.powershow.com/view/505e8-NGYzM/SBAR_powerpoint_ppt_presentation (accessed 20 January 2013).

Scottish Government. (2010) *Scottish Inpatient Patient Experience Survey 2010*, Vol. 1: National results. Scottish Government, Edinburgh.

Shepperd, S., Lannin, N.A., Clemson, L.M., McCluskey, A., Cameron, I.D. & Barras, S.L. (2013) Discharge planning from hospital to home. *Cochrane Database of Systematic Reviews*, (1):CD000313.

Silver Book (2012) *Quality Care of Older People with Urgent and Emergency Care Needs* University of Leicester, Leicester.

Stevens, J.A. (2004). Falls among older adults-risk factors and prevention strategies. In: *Falls Free: promoting a national falls prevention action plan*, pp.3–18. National Council on Aging, Washington, DC.

Triggle, N. (2012) Standards aim to boost care, *Nursing Older People*, 24(7), 6–7.

Tuohy, D. (2003) Student nurse-older person communication. *Nursing Education Today*, 23(1), 19–26.

Volkert, D., Berner, Y.N., Berry, E. *et al.* (2006) ESPEN guidelines on enteral nutrition: geriatrics. *Clinical Nutrition*, 25(2), 330–360.

WHO (2009) *Human Factors in Patient Safety. Review of Topics and Tools. Report for Methods and Measures Working*. World Health Organization, Geneva.

Wilson, M. (2007) A template for safe and concise handovers. *Medical Surgical Nursing*, 16(3), 201–206.

191

Test Yourself

1. Grimacing, raised eyebrows and shrugs are all examples of:
   - (a) Culture
   - (b) Verbal communication
   - (c) Good communication
   - (d) Body language

2. Which the following are barriers to effective communication:
   - (a) Invasion of personal space
   - (b) Noise
   - (c) Inappropriate body language
   - (d) All of these

3. What should nurses do to promote dignity in care:
   - (a) Speak clearly
   - (b) Understand, offer support and reassure patients
   - (c) Write clearly
   - (d) Be knowledgeable

4. Out the following groups, to whom does abuse usually happen:
   - (a) The elderly
   - (b) The child
   - (c) The person with a mental health problem
   - (d) All of them

5. The Waterlow Assessment Tool assesses:
   - (a) Risk of developing a stomach ulcer
   - (b) Risk of developing a pressure sore
   - (c) Risk of being under-nourished
   - (d) Risk of developing a deep vein thrombosis

6. The acronym MUST means:
   - (a) Microscopic utilisation of skills in treatment
   - (b) Malnutrition Universal Screening Tool
   - (c) Malnutrition Universal Scoping Tool
   - (d) None of the above

7. When a patient is admitted they should have falls assessment undertaken:
   - (a) Only if they fall
   - (b) When being discharged
   - (c) On admission
   - (d) On a daily basis

8. Risk factors contributing to a fall include:
   - (a) Culture
   - (b) Some medications
   - (c) The type of ward
   - (d) The height of the person

9. The majority of older people have dementia:
   - (a) True
   - (b) False

10. Physical strength declines in old age
    - (a) True
    - (b) False

Answers

1. d
2. d
3. b
4. d
5. b
6. b
7. c
8. b
9. b
10. a

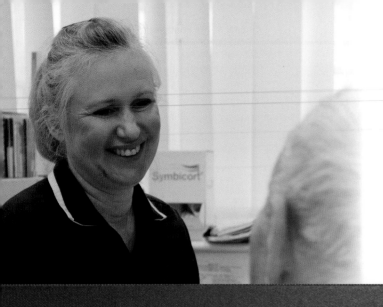

10

The Principles of Caring for People with Learning Disabilities and Autism

Paul Maloret and Jo Welch

The Centre for Learning Disability Studies, University of Hertfordshire, UK

Learning Outcomes

On completion of this chapter you will be able to:

- Understand the nature of learning disabilities, causes and prevalence
- Have a greater understanding of why people with learning disabilities are more susceptible to inequalities in health care
- Gain an insight into the role of the learning disability nurse
- Consider how enhanced communication awareness can improve the care of people with learning disabilities and autism
- Understand how services can be *reasonably adjusted* to meet needs
- Be aware of contemporary legislation impacting upon the care delivery

Competencies

All nurses must:

1. Support and promote the health, well-being and rights of people with learning disabilities and autism
2. Work in partnership with specialist learning disability services to address needs in all healthcare settings
3. Assess physical and psychological needs in a user friendly manner
4. Encourage person-centred planning to empower choices in health care
5. Secure equal access to health screening, health promotion and healthcare
6. Ensure people receive all the information they need in a language and manner that allows them to make informed choices and share decision-making
7. Recognise and respond to the major causes and social determinants of health, illness and health inequalities

 Visit the companion website at **www.wileynursingpractice.com** where you can test yourself using flashcards, multiple-choice questions and more.

Nursing Practice: Knowledge and Care, First Edition. Edited by Ian Peate, Karen Wild and Muralitharan Nair.
© 2014 John Wiley & Sons, Ltd. Published 2014 by John Wiley & Sons, Ltd. Companion website: www.wileynursingpractice.com

Introduction

This chapter is designed to meet the learning needs of healthcare professionals working within a nursing environment in which they would come in direct contact with patients with learning disabilities and autism. An estimated 26% of people with learning disabilities are admitted to hospital each year, compared with 14% of the general public (NHS Health Scotland 2004). The reputation of general hospitals and the way in which they care for adults with learning disabilities was considerably tarnished in 2007, when *Death by Indifference* (Mencap 2007) explained the circumstances of very poor practice surrounding the deaths of six people with learning disabilities while they were in the care of the NHS. Some of the material from this report is shocking and would be more suited to Victorian Britain when society held people with disabilities in far lower regard and segregation, and institutional care was a way of life for the majority. While many positive changes have occurred in the care of people with learning disabilities, it would appear that there is still a long way to go and far more progress to be made. *Death by Indifference* (Mencap 2007) suggested that people with learning disabilities, their families and carers were facing institutional discrimination in healthcare services; the subsequent report of the independent inquiry called *Healthcare for All*, which was led by Sir Jonathon Michael (DH 2008a) exposed the unequal health care that people with learning disabilities often receive within the NHS (DH 2006).

Link To/Go To

www.mencap.org.uk/campaigns/take-action/
death-indifference

This link will provide you with the full *Death by Indifference* report.

The access to mainstream services is unquestionably the way forward and people who have a learning disability will be accessing these services now and in the future. It is worth noting that the Department of Health (DH) estimates there will be a 1% increase in the population of people who have a learning disability by 2015 (DH 2001). There are an estimated 1.2 million people in Great Britain with a learning disability. A further 200 babies with learning disabilities are born each week. Emerson and Hatton (2008) also estimate that the total number of adults with a learning disability (aged 20 or over) will increase by 8% to 868 000 in 2011 and by 14% to 908 000 by 2021. Whereas people with a learning disability are 58 times more likely to die before the age of 50 than the rest of the population (DRC 2006; RCN 2011; Heslop & Marriott 2011), this highlights the need for change in health profile of these individuals. Often, these individuals have additional health needs. It is known that people with learning disabilities carry a disproportionate health burden when compared with the general population (Emerson & Baines 2011) and therefore, as a result an increase in admissions to acute care, but many healthcare professionals do not feel effectively prepared (Sowney & Barr 2006). As a result, there is a need for improvements in the education across all fields of nursing in meeting the needs of people with learning disabilities and autism, which must become an education priority at both pre- and post-registration levels.

'The Evidence' box below shows key reports contributing to a call for further Inquiry into the deaths of people with learning disabilities. This chapter highlights some of the reasons for these shortcomings and acknowledges that having a greater knowledge and understanding of this different kind of patient can go a long way to being able to provide a level of care that is acceptable to those with intellectual disabilities.

Additionally, this chapter will give you an overview of the different types of people with learning disabilities and the particular health needs for which they may require a service and why they find it so difficult accessing those services. Some of the issues facing adult nurses are of an ethical nature; some examples of previous dilemmas will be discussed with guidance. There will be times when the level of your knowledge is not enough and you will require support from specialist learning disability services and an outline of what they are and how they can help is available in this chapter (DH 2007).

This chapter also explores patients with learning disabilities whose nature is potentially of a greater complexity due to an associated mental health problem, autistic spectrum condition or the inability to communicate pain, etc. Communication is very often at the heart of good nursing and there is no better example of when a practitioner is faced with the challenge of a patient whose communication skills are significantly impaired. Some quick and easy skills will be identified that can have an impact upon the success of your care and interventions. The legalities of working with people who find it difficult to communicate their needs and desires can be complicated and this chapter will assist in making lawful and beneficial decisions regarding their care.

195

The Evidence Key Reports Contributing to a Call for Further Inquiry into the Inequalities of Health Care for People with Learning Disabilities and Autism

Valuing People (DH 2001) – This is the first White Paper on learning disability for 30 years and sets out an ambitious and challenging programme of action for improving services.

Treat Me Right (Mencap 2004) exposes inequalities in health care for people with learning disabilities.

Disability Rights Commission report (DRC 2006) considered it 'alarming' that little or nothing had been done to implement the recommendations of Mencap's 'Treat Me Right' report by those with the power to do so, i.e. the government.

Disability Rights Commission report (DRC 2006) criticised the lack of strategic change and prioritisation that had taken place following its report the previous year, calling it 'quite literally a matter of life and death'.

***Death by Indifference* (Mencap 2007)** defined the circumstances surrounding the deaths of six adults with learning disabilities while they were in the responsibility of the NHS. It is suggested that people with learning disabilities, their families and carers were facing institutional discrimination in healthcare services (Mencap 2007).

***Healthcare for All* (2008)** is the report of the 'Michael Inquiry' which was established to learn lessons from the six cases highlighted in the Mencap report (*Death by Indifference*). It reported evidence of 'a significant level of avoidable suffering and a high likelihood that there are deaths occurring which could be avoided' (DH 2008a).

High Quality Care for All (2008) – Lord Darzi sets out a 10-year plan to provide the highest quality of care, including improvements to those patients with disabilities (DH 2008b).

Valuing People Now (2009) acknowledges that learning disability services have so far struggled to deliver real change on the ground and hopes to address this issue. The strategy covers all areas of a person's life and has set some ambitious targets (DH 2009).

The Autism Act (2009) – building on the success of the 'I Exist Campaign', The Act made two key provisions: that the government produce an adult autism strategy by 1 April 2010 and that the Secretary of State for Health issues statutory guidance for local authorities and local health bodies on supporting the needs of adults with autism by 31 December 2010.

Definitions of Learning Disabilities

Defining learning disabilities can be tricky, as the tendency is to explain it in a very clinical way that would suggest that it is an illness, which it is not. It is however a lifelong condition, with its beginning before, during or after birth, or as a result of a brain injury, which can affect a person's ability to learn and communicate effectively. While the condition cannot be 'cured', it is possible for someone with a learning disability to lead an independent life or, with support, develop new skills and progress.

Too often, the terminology used confuses people as to the specific group we are discussing. For example the media, television in particular, use the term 'learning difficulty' when reporting on a person with a learning disability. In actual fact, a person with learning difficulties is normally considered to have educational needs, such as dyslexia, dyspraxia or hyperactive disorders. Additionally, learning disabilities is not a mental illness, although the general consensus is that around 40% of people with learning disabilities will experience an associated mental illness in their lifetime (Priest & Gibbs 2004).

Mackenzie (2005), cited in Grant *et al.* (2005, p. 49), outlines the two similar diagnostic classifications in the following way:

ICD-10 defines "mental retardation" (WHO terminology for learning disabilities) as a condition of arrested or incomplete development of mind, which is characterised by impairment of skill manifested during the development period, which contribute to the overall level of intelligence, i.e. cognitive, language, motor and social abilities.

DSM-IV defines as a significantly sub average intellectual functioning: an intelligence quotient (IQ) of approximately 70 or below. Concurrent deficits or impairments in present adaptive functioning in at least two of the following areas: communication, self-care, home living, social/interpersonal skills, use of community resources, self-direction, functional academic skills, work, leisure, health and safety.

Additionally, it is important to think about groups of people within the wider learning disability context, for example 75–80% of people with Autistic Spectrum Conditions will have a measured IQ of below 70 and therefore, diagnosed as learning disabled. Some of their needs would be similar to other people with learning disabilities; however, they could have further needs around communication, flexibility of thought and emotional detachments (NAS 2012).

The Evidence Defining Learning Disability According to Mencap (2012):

- A learning disability is a reduced intellectual ability and difficulty with everyday activities – for example household tasks, socialising or managing money – which affects someone for their whole life
- People with a learning disability tend to take longer to learn and may need support to develop new skills, understand complex information and interact with other people
- The level of support someone needs depends on individual factors, including the severity of their learning disability. For example, someone with a mild learning disability may only need support with things like getting a job. However, someone with a severe or profound learning disability may need full-time care and support with every aspect of their life – they may also have physical disabilities
- People with certain specific conditions can have a learning disability too. For example, people with Down's syndrome and some people with autism have a learning disability
- Learning disability is often confused with dyslexia and mental health problems. Mencap describes dyslexia as a 'learning difficulty' because, unlike a learning disability, it does not affect intellect. Mental health problems can affect anyone at any time and may be overcome with treatment, which is not true of learning disability
- It is important to remember that with the right support, most people with a learning disability in the UK can lead independent lives.

Over the years, different terms to describe this group of people are now deemed inappropriate, mostly because they have been taken out of context and used as a way of insulting another.

Jot This Down

Think about the terms you may have heard used to describe people with learning disabilities. Note them down and consider how they would sound to a person with learning disabilities?

In the 'Jot This Down' exercise above, you might have identified a number of negative labels that have been associated with people with learning disabilities. In 'What the Experts Say' below, you can see how this kind of behaviour affects the emotional and social health of a person with autism and learning disabilities.

What the Experts Say

David is a man in his 30s who has learning disabilities and autism; he has struggled to cope with day-to-day living all his life, but now attends college regularly. David explains below the impact of some of the name calling he experiences from the teenagers in the college.

When I am at college, some of the people would call me names, and laugh at me because I am different. They have called me freak, geek, monster and a few more that I wouldn't want to repeat. I feel very vulnerable and I am not able to stop it; instead I try and act as "normal" as possible so I can fit in and not stand out from the crowd. However, I am rubbish at this and it causes me a lot of stress when I can't do it. I don't want to involve the staff at college, because then I would be a grass as well as odd!

Autistic Spectrum Conditions Defined

The variation in presentation of autistic spectrum conditions (ASC) is wide; therefore the intervention and support required are clearly varied and can be very different from patient to patient. However, there are three consistent traits with all people with an ASC diagnosis. All people with ASC will to some degree experience impairments in the following three key areas:

1. Social interaction
2. Communication
3. Lack of flexibility in thinking and behaviour.

This is often referred to as the 'Triad of Impairment', 'The Evidence' box below outlines the more definitive diagnostic tool of the 5th edition of the *Diagnostic and Statistical Manual of Mental Disorders* (DSM), DSM-IV, which uses a very similar 'Triad of Impairment' (APA 1994).

The Evidence Outline of the Autistic Spectrum Criteria Belonging to the DSM-IV

The DSM-IV autistic spectrum conditions criteria:

· Onset before 3 years old
· At least six from the following (at least two from category 1):
  1. Qualitative impairment in social interaction
     · Marked impairment in the use of non-verbal behaviours such as eye contact, facial expression, body posture, etc.
     · Failure to develop peer relationships appropriate to developmental level
     · Lack of spontaneity in seeking to share enjoyment, interests with others
     · Lack of social reciprocity
  2. Qualitative impairments in communication
     · Delay or lack of spoken language with no compensatory non-verbal communication
     · In people with speech impairment in the ability to initiate or sustain conversation
     · Stereotypical/receptive/idiosyncratic language
     · Lack of spontaneous and varied pretend play
  3. Restricted, repetitive and stereotyped patterns of behaviour, interests and activities.
     · Preoccupation with one or more restricted interest that is unusual in intensity or focus
     · Inflexible adherence to routines or rituals
     · Stereotyped and repetitive movements
     · Preoccupation with parts of objects
     · Social play

In children's services, this checklist will often be completed by the health visitor or a GP. In adult services, very often a learning disability nurse would use this while in liaison with a clinical psychologist. Regardless of who is using this, it is important that it used as a discourse of information gathered via interviews and observations. However, within the changes made in the DSM-V, the 'Triad of Impairment' will be reduced to two main areas:

1. *Social communication and interaction*
2. *Restricted, repetitive patterns of behaviour, interests or activities.*

(NAS 2012)

Additionally, sensory behaviours will be included in the criteria for the first time, under restricted, repetitive patterns of behaviours

descriptors. There is an ever-growing body of research analysing the hypersensitivities that people with ASC experience to some sounds, smells and visuals, which can impact upon their behaviour. Knowing this is crucial to the care of someone with ASC in a hospital setting, later in this chapter 'reasonable adjustments' are discussed and challenge services to consider if any alterations can be made to existing services to help people with different needs. In this instance, awareness of hypersensitivities for people with ASC can make a huge impact upon their general anxiety levels, while they are in hospital and out of their usual, more controlled, environment. Reports of strobe lighting, the smell of cleaning products and constant noises from machines, all of which can be seen, heard and smelt in a very magnified way, are very common. Some of these can be easily addressed, while others present greater challenges and it is very difficult to eradicate these completely.

Another change is that the DSM will no longer give a specific diagnosis, i.e. the current terms used in the DSM-4, which are autistic disorder, Asperger's disorder, childhood disintegrative disorder and PDD-NOS (pervasive developmental disorder - not otherwise specified). The proposals mean that when people go for a diagnosis in the future, instead of receiving a diagnosis of one of these disorders, they would be given a diagnosis of 'autism spectrum disorder'. The National Autistic Society (NAS 2012) have collated information from those people with Asperger's in particular, as they appear to be unhappy that this term will no longer be used in the DSM. They are very proud to have Asperger's and often refer to themselves as 'Aspies'.

What the Experts Say

Malcolm is a man who was diagnosed with Asperger's syndrome 20 years ago – now in his 40s, he feels that his diagnosis is an essential part of his identity...

The term Aspie or Asperger's is who I am, I do not want to be called anything else and they are suggesting changing it to autistic something or other. Firstly I am autistic, but I don't like to use the terminology, because people are ignorant and automatically think I have a learning disability and treat me very differently. I don't have a learning disability, not there is anything wrong with that, it's just not me, I have an above average IQ and many people know this about Aspies and respect us for it. Besides, people on the spectrum hate change, so please don't change our identities!

Prevalence and Causes of Learning Disabilities

The causes of learning disability are multifaceted and can be complex. The causative factors can be divided into two parts: first, *heredity*, i.e. the transmission of genetic characters from parents to offspring, and second, *environmental*, for example childhood infections that could cause brain injury and consequentially a learning disability. Additionally, we can consider these two causative factors within periods of time: **Pre-conceptual**, **Prenatal**, **Perinatal** and **Postnatal**.

The main causes of learning disability can be considered as follows:

- Pre-conceptual
  - Heredity – parental genotype
  - Environmentally – maternal health
- Prenatal
  - Heredity – genetic conditions such as Down's syndrome
  - Environmentally – infection, maternal health, nutrition and toxic agents
- Perinatal
  - Environmentally – prematurity and injury during birth
- Postnatal
  - Environmentally – infection, trauma, toxic agents, sensory and social deprivation, brain injury and nutrition.

Genetic abnormalities are estimated to be the cause of 50% of learning disabilities. Michael (DH 2008a) explains that the numbers of people with learning disabilities in the UK is expected to increase by around 1% per annum for the next 10 years. This is largely attributable to improvements in prenatal and perinatal care. Additionally, the increasing use of alcohol and consequential fetal alcohol syndrome will also have an impact upon these figures.

However, estimating the prevalence of learning disability within the UK population is difficult, it is clear that severe or profound people (see 'The Evidence' box below), are more easily recognised, diagnosed and recorded as requiring service interventions. Accurate reporting of mild to moderate learning disabilities (again refer to 'The Evidence' box below), is more difficult, with a number of people not being diagnosed until much later in their lives or not at all. The Department of Health (DH 2001) reported that approximately 1.5 million people have mild to moderate learning disability and an estimated 210 000 individuals with severe or profound learning disabilities are in the UK.

Classification of Learning Disability

It can be true that by understanding more about the classification of a person with learning disabilities it can help you to potentially know more about their abilities and perhaps their limitations. However, great care must be taken not to make assumptions based upon their classification of learning disabilities. 'The Evidence' box below shows how, according to a person's IQ, they are classified in the severity of their learning disability. As a novice worker in the field, it is easy to make assumptions of their ability according to their classification, for example the majority of people with mild learning disabilities have the potential to communicate well, be able to address their own personal care needs and, to a degree, be independent. As the IQ diminishes, usually the ability to communicate and be independent does as well. But great care must be taken here not to make assumptions that people can or equally cannot achieve certain tasks due to their classification or even their learning disability label. This chapter later explains how the correct information regarding the person's needs can be obtained efficiently and how this can help you care for the individual.

An intelligence quotient or 'IQ' is a score derived from one of several tests standardised designed to assess intelligence. The abbreviation 'IQ' comes from the German term *Intelligenz-Quotien*. The average of the test's scores for the vast majority of us (95%) will score between 70 and 130. Below 70 will indicate significant intellectual/learning disability. For the small 5% that can reach scores of above 130, they would be considered to have an above average IQ and intelligence. Interestingly, a number of these extremely intelligent people would have an autistic spectrum condition, normally people with Asperger's syndrome, which is positioned on the higher end of the autistic spectrum.

> **The Evidence** Disease Classifications ICD 10 and DSM IV Divide Learning Disability into Four Categories:
>
> 1. Mild – IQ 50–70
> 2. Moderate – IQ 35–49
> 3. Severe – IQ 20–34
> 4. Profound – IQ below 20

Inequalities in Health Care

The learning disability population have poorer health than the general population and are more likely to suffer from mental illness, epilepsy, physical and sensory problems, as well as chronic health problems. Yet, they are less likely to access health care in a way that the rest of us take for granted. These health inequalities have been highlighted in a number of formal inquiries. Already in this chapter, we have discussed Mencap's report 'Death by Indifference' (Mencap 2007) and its significant impact upon service delivery in general hospitals, along with the findings of the Independent Inquiry into the health inequalities of people with learning disabilities (Michael & Richardson 2008). Others are worth looking into:

- **Closing the Gap** – a report from the Disability Rights Commission (DRC 2006)
- **Six Lives**: the provision of public services to people with learning disabilities (Parliamentary and Health Service Ombudsman 2009)
- **Health Inequalities & People with Learning Disabilities in the UK: 2010**. The Public Health Learning Disabilities Observatory (Emerson *et al.* 2012).

A range of barriers to accessing health care and other services have been identified in 'The Evidence' box below.

> **The Evidence**
>
> These include:
>
> - Scarcity of appropriate services
> - Physical and informational barriers to access
> - Unhelpful, inexperienced or discriminatory healthcare staff
> - Increasingly stringent eligibility criteria for accessing social care services
> - Failure of healthcare providers to make 'reasonable adjustments' in light of the literacy and communication difficulties experienced by many people with learning disabilities
> - 'Diagnostic overshadowing' (e.g. symptoms of physical ill health being mistakenly attributed to either a mental health/ behavioural problem or as being inherent in the person's learning disabilities)

People with learning disabilities have a shorter life expectancy compared with the general population. While life expectancy is increasing with people with mild learning disabilities approaching that of the general population, the mortality rates among people with moderate to severe learning disabilities are three times higher than in the general population; despite this, people with learning disabilities are less likely to receive regular health checks and access screening opportunities, which again are routine and taken for granted by many of us (Tyrer & McGrother 2009).

Some people with a learning disability and additional complex or profound physical disabilities will require health professionals from mainstream and specialist learning disability services to work in partnership, in order to use medical technology and to access essential therapeutic assessments and interventions from nurses, physiotherapists, psychiatrists, psychologists, occupational therapists, speech therapists and dieticians. Similar partnership arrangements are also needed to ensure that people with more complex needs gain access to the best care and treatment in the full range of health services, from maternity services through to end of life care (DH 2009).

Their health needs can be perceived as complex, which can add to the accessibility problem. Very often, these complexities are too intricate to address within a regular appointment with the GP. The interactions of behavioural, physical and mental health issues can appear to be difficult to interpret and may cause illness to be overlooked, so that serious conditions can present too late for prevention or cure. This is called 'diagnostic overshadowing' and may lead to some healthcare professionals not investigating early enough. Very often, a person with significant communication problems will express pain in different ways; this can often be changes in their behaviour and commonly, aggression will increase. To exemplify these complexities, read the 'What the Experts Say' scenario, below.

What the Experts Say A Community Learning Disability Nurse's Account as She Attempts to Gain Equitable Mental Health Care for a Service User in Her Care.

" Esme is a 53-year-old woman with Down's syndrome and moderate learning disability, who for the past five years has lived in supported-living accommodation.

Esme's support mechanisms have consisted of a 24-hour call-out support network, provided by an outreach team, and two hours a week support with her weekly budgeting and shopping provided by a social support worker.

Esme works in a charity shop two days a week, though her time in the shop is mostly spent sorting and tidying in the back, as her speech is considered to be both too quiet and unclear to communicate effectively with customers.

Until recently, Esme has always appeared a quiet and contented lady, preferring to keep herself to herself, but in the last few weeks, Esme has been seen exhibiting some strange behaviours. One neighbour, Tom, said he saw a very 'red faced' Esme talking loudly and aggressively to herself while fiddling with her door key and when he approached her, she spat at him. Her colleagues in the shop have also reported Esme to be vague and disinterested in her work and far from being her normal punctual self, she has been arriving late for work and inappropriately dressed for the cold weather.

Her social support worker, Susan has also noticed Esme's flat to be uncharacteristically untidy and Esme still in her nightwear, complaining of being too hot, in the afternoon. Susan was concerned and contacted her GP and made an appointment. Esme was seen by a doctor who she had never met before and despite Susan explaining that Esme is normally able to communicate her feelings in a more coherent manner, the doctor had read her notes and appeared to have made up her mind that all these behaviours were due to her learning disability. The GP asked them to refer her to social services if she needed more support.

Unsatisfied with the GP's assessment, Susan contacted the local Community Learning Disability Team. A nurse in the team carried out their own assessment and found clear evidence that Esme was beginning to show signs of dementia and knowing that there is a direct link between Alzheimer's and Down's syndrome, the psychiatrist in the team agreed that a formal diagnostic assessment should follow. Within weeks, a formal diagnosis was in place and Esme's care package was reviewed in the likelihood that her condition could deteriorate further.

Jot This Down

1. The GP clearly found this case to be complex, why?
2. What would you have done differently if you were the nurse?

In the 'Jot This Down' exercise above, you may have considered the complexity of the case by thinking about the similarities that can exist between the two conditions of dementia and moderate learning disability. Both can manifest themselves in a variety of ways and a baseline of Esme's intellectual abilities needs to be assessed, in order for differences to be more easily noted and ensure they are documented, so the nurse can show evidence when engaging with a GP or a psychiatrist.

The Royal College of General Practitioners (2010) have published a step by step guide on annual health checks for people with learning disabilities. It is a clear step in the right direction and an indication that GPs are willing to listen to changes within their practice to meet the needs of people with learning disabilities. The introduction of annual health checks is important for improvements to health outcomes: to help identify and treat medical conditions early; to screen for health issues particular to people with learning disabilities and specific conditions; to improve access to generic health promotion in people with learning disabilities; and lastly to develop relationships with GPs, practice nurses and primary care staff, particularly after the comprehensive paediatric care finishes at the age of 18. The evaluations in 2012 of these annual checks are very good and have had an impact upon many people and their general health (Hoghton et al. 2010).

Over many years of research, our understanding of the increased prevalence of physical health issues for those with learning disabilities and in particular those with genetic or chromosomal abnormalities have increased. The annual health check assessments used by GPs will assess for those particular health needs, which are very common to those with specific chromosomal syndromes. For example there is an increase in the prevalence of *ophthalmic problems* (cataract, glaucoma, keratoconus and refractive errors) with people with Down's syndrome, therefore part of the annual health checks would include an eye test. However, it would be true to say that many healthcare practitioners would not be aware of the health issues pertinent to those with specific chromosomal abnormalities and this information is important to assist with the assessment and diagnosis of the patient as well as their experience as a patient.

Attitudes Towards People with Learning Disabilities

According the Chief Nursing Officer, Jane Cummings (2012), there is a lack of 'basic values' in way that the nursing profession is caring for its patients. Her 3-year strategy 'Compassion in Practice' will see senior nurses being sent on training courses to learn how to promote care and compassion among their teams of nurses and support workers (DH 2012a). This strategy involving the Royal College of Nursing and the Department of Health has emerged from repeated complaints from patients and those close to them, regarding issues of neglect and people being stripped of their dignity. The strategy cites the abuse of the residents with learning disability at Winterbourne View, which has become infamous after the BBC 'Panorama' programme in 2012 (BBC 2012).

BBC One's 'Panorama' showed patients at a residential care home near Bristol being slapped and restrained under chairs, having their hair pulled and being held down as medication was forced into their mouths. The victims, who had severe learning disabilities, were visibly upset and were shown screaming and shaking. One victim was showered while fully clothed and had mouthwash poured into her eyes.

Undercover recordings showed one senior care worker at Winterbourne View asking a patient whether they wanted him to get a 'cheese grater and grate your face off?'. The abuse was so bad that one patient, who had tried to jump out of a second floor window, was then mocked by staff members. Dr Peter Carter, head of the Royal College of Nursing, said: 'The sickening abuse revealed in this programme is more shocking than anything we could have imagined' (BBC News Website, BBC 2012).

'Health Care for All' (DH 2008a) states that: 'The health and strength of a society can be measured by how well it cares for its most vulnerable members. For a variety of reasons, including the way society behaves towards them, adults and children with learning disabilities, especially those with severe disability and the most complex needs are some of the most vulnerable members of our society today'.

Health Liaison

The Learning Disability Nurse has a unique and pivotal role in supporting individuals to develop their specialist skills and champion the needs of people with learning disabilities in health care (Gates 2011a,b). The Liaison Nurse role exists: to ensure the needs of the person with a learning disability are met on admission to an acute hospital setting; to facilitate open and easy access to the various wards and departments by ensuring the provision of appropriate environments of care; to enable access to care through arrangement and adjustment of appointments; ensure pre-hospital preparation; ensure accessible information. This will involve a range of communication with an array of clinicians and services in both hospital and community settings; identifying and offering training (formal and informal) and where appropriate, providing training support alongside specialist nursing advice. It will also warrant and require extensive close communication and involvement with individuals, family, carers and others during the pre-admission, admission and discharge; actively engaging with hospital staff to assist, support and empower them to provide care that meets the needs of people with learning disabilities and those

that support them. This is the opportunity to 'mind the gap' which is today present for those with a learning disability.

Care, Dignity and Compassion The Role of the Liaison Nurse Is Summarised as Follows:

Advocate
- *An ambassador for people with a learning disability, fostering equal care through recommending reasonable and achievable adjustments*
- *Representing the views of patients and carers to hospital staff*
- *Ensuring recognition of and adherence to specific legislation and sensitive policies such as 'do not resuscitate' orders*

Collaborator
- *Often the connection between services, families and individuals*

Communicator
- *Enabling information flow across healthcare sectors, professionals and between health staff and carers*
- *Advising hospital staff on specific communication issues and methods*

Educator
- *Through induction, updates, CPD programmes and skill development (formal)*
- *Opportunistic learning opportunities and role modelling; sharing information (informal)*
- *Educating across professional groups, including input for medical staff*
- *Offering advice and support in Mental Capacity Act and Safeguarding*
- *Contribution and development of accessible healthcare resources*

Mediator
- *Networking with key individuals, departments, services and agencies*
- *Translating information between the person with a learning disability and hospital staff*
- *Removing barriers to appropriate health care. Forming effective working relationships with clinicians and ward teams*

Facilitator
- *Creating and using accessible information*
- *Supporting reasonable and achievable adjustments; reasonable adjustments may mean a greater use of accessible information*
- *Demonstrating new ideas and explicitly explaining what is required*
- *To actively engage with hospital staff to assist and empower them to provide care, which meets the needs of people with learning disabilities and their carers.*

A key to all of this is the working together to achieve the outcome for people with a learning disability. Better health is a key priority and working together enables everyone to meet the 10 key recommendations in *Health Care for All* (DH 2008).

The responsibility of the liaison nurse is to raise the profile of the healthcare needs of people with a learning disability across secondary care provision, bridging the gap between acute clinical care areas to enable better communication and access to healthcare. The liaison nurses should make themselves visible to healthcare staff in order to be able to continue to support them in the role they have in the provision of such care. In this way, they will have to be creative in the work they undertake; minimising constraints and challenges to ensure a successful outcome for all involved, specifically the person with a learning disability. As part of the wider team, the nurse aims to ensure people with a learning disability receive the health care required to live a healthy life and importantly, have equity with others in society (DH 2001; DH 2009). This is also essential to meeting the collaboration and other elements of the 6Cs (DH 2012a).

Health Action Plans

Health action planning (DH 2002) is a requirement for all healthcare providers to ensure each person with a learning disability was offered a plan that outlined their needs, to use as a baseline of information for any health professional when this person presents for an appointment, consultation or assessment. This contains an information passport, which enables the health staff to see a snapshot picture and use this in helping formulate outcomes with the individual, providing an increasingly cohesive picture. Everyone with a learning disability has the opportunity to access a health action plan, which draws together aspects of their 'health picture' into a useable framework and informs the healthcare staff they come into contact with (DH 2002).

Jot This Down
Consider you are being asked for information about your childhood health by a healthcare practitioner. What is your history of immunisation – did you have chicken pox as a child? More than likely you will have something to inform you of when these were or you can refer back to your family, medical history or others for such information. Often, the challenge to someone who has led a life where the information is not so joined up, this is missing or non-existent. The Health Action Plan enables all this to be bought together in one place.

The Hospital Passport

This is different from the Health Action Plan, in that it also informs the local partnership boards as to the extent of the individual's health needs. The passport presents the healthcare professional with a picture of the 'whole person'. It contains information not only relevant to health but also about the individual. By owning the passport, this individual is empowered to participate further in the care they may require and will bring this with them to appointments and consultations. They vary from area to area and additionally, people often add their own personalised touches. This provides the healthcare practitioners with additional information about how they will focus care and about choices in healthcare opportunities, rather than denying opportunity to the individual or trial and error. They can base decisions on this information and be far more confident of the outcome. The increased information (present and historical) can enable the individual to be more involved in the decisions and this provides for a safer environment for everyone. It can enable services to be flexible and responsive to individual needs and this can educate the healthcare professional by default (Blair 2011). These also enable the staff to make reasonable adjustments with the person to enable better adherence to treatment planning, admission and discharge.

Care, Dignity and Compassion
Reasonable Adjustments

The *Healthcare for All* (DH 2008a) report also highlights the need for nurses and other healthcare practitioners to show these very vulnerable people our upmost compassion, but also identifies insufficient attention to making *'reasonable adjustments'* to support the delivery of equal treatment, as required by the Disability Discrimination Act 2005. Adjustments are not always made to allow for communication problems, difficulty in understanding (cognitive impairment) or the anxieties and preferences of individuals concerning their treatment.

Under the *Disability Equality Duty*, cited in the Equality Act (2010), all public sector organisations are required to make 'reasonable adjustments' to services to ensure they are accessible for disabled people. This includes making adjustments for people with learning disabilities. The NHS Standard Contracts for 2012/13 (NHS 2011) requires service providers within the NHS to demonstrate how reasonable adjustments are made. The law says that all health services must think about people with disabilities. They have to ask 'what extra things do we need to do, so people with learning disabilities can get health services that are equitable to other people?' If the organisation fails to make these reasonable adjustments, it is considered discrimination (Blair 2012) This might be:

- Making sure that information on health services is accessible to people with learning disabilities
- Nurses with special skills to look out for people with learning disabilities
- Giving people more time with doctors and nurses, so they have a chance to explain what is wrong or they can be assessed comprehensibly.

The 'Improving Health and Lives: Learning Disabilities Observatory' was set up in April 2010, as a 3-year programme following one of the recommendations of the 'Report of the Independent Inquiry into Access to Healthcare for People with Learning Disabilities' (The Michael report, DH 2008a). The 'Improving Health and Lives: Learning Disabilities Observatory' in 2012 contacted the 400 NHS Trusts in the UK and asked them what they were considering reasonable adjustments; 119 replied and a database has been produced so examples of the adjustments can be accessed by other organisations outside of the NHS (IHL 2012). 'The Evidence' box below shows the key actions that all NHS Trusts and health services need to consider when implementing reasonable adjustments.

The Evidence Key Actions that All NHS Trusts and Health Services Need to Consider When Implementing Reasonable Adjustments

1. Ensure that people with learning disabilities are easily identified in records systems
2. Foster a culture in which everyone understands reasonable adjustments and how they can help everyone when applied in a timely and appropriate manner
3. Have a policy on accessible information and review coverage and use on a regular basis
4. Promote the involvement of family carers in the healthcare of people with learning disabilities
5. Continuously monitor how well the Mental Capacity Act is being implemented

6. Develop clear and widely used protocols for service delivery and where applicable, discharge arrangements that take account of the additional support needs of people with learning disabilities
7. Ensure that people with learning disabilities and their family carers can influence what happens within the organisation at all levels.

(The Improving Health and Lives: Learning Disabilities Observatory, IHL 2012)

The example in Box 10.1 is of reasonable adjustments made by the Mid Yorkshire NHS Trust in 2012, when caring for a person with learning disabilities on a ward in their hospital (Gibb 2012).

Jot This Down

Think about people with learning disabilities in general hospitals that you have worked with. Use the example of the reasonable adjustments from the Mid Yorkshire NHS Trust and jot down any adjustments you have witnessed and consider if those made above would have improved the patient experience?

In the 'Jot This Down' exercise above, you may have considered the experiences of those with learning disabilities in hospitals; it is important to keep in mind that it can very often be the small things that really matter and that can play a significant part in the overall experience.

Person-Centred Planning (PCP)

Person-centred planning discovers and acts on what is important to a person. It is a process for continual listening and learning, focussing on what are important to someone now and in the future, and acting on this in alliance with their family and their friends (Thompson *et al.* 2008).

Put simply, PCP is a means of ascertaining what people want, the support they need and how they can achieve it. This is empowering and is useful to create change with people, as it shifts the balance of power from people who work in services to those that use or participate within them to lead an independent and inclusive life. There are many different approaches to achieving the goal of PCP. One you may come across is 'Essential Lifestyle Planning' (ELP), there are also 'PATH MAPs'. These tools are there to support the formulation of plans which reflect the individual. PCP aims to consider aspirations and capacities, rather than needs and

---

Box 10.1 'Reasonable Adjustments' Made by the Mid Yorkshire NHS Trust in 2012, When Caring for a Person with Learning Disabilities on a Ward in Their Hospital.

Orientation to the ward

Patients with learning disabilities can often feel isolated on busy wards. Please consider the following actions where appropriate to the patient:

- Orientate the patient to the ward
- Introduce them to other patients in their ward area
- Ensure that toilets and bathrooms have appropriate signage and the patient understands where they can find them if able to carry out their own personal care
- Remember that you might need to repeat information on where they can find the toilet/bathroom/rest room during their stay
- Make sure the patient and their carer, if appropriate, knows who their named nurse on duty is.

Environment

- Assess the patient's clinical and individual need for a single cubicle or a ward bay
- Some patients with a learning disability will be more comfortable cared for alongside other people, and may feel isolated and frightened in a single cubicle. Others with complex needs, autism or challenging behaviour will benefit from the quieter environment of a cubicle, where there are less distractions from the general activity of a busy ward
- Involve the patient with a learning disability and their carer/support worker in decisions regarding individual requirements
- Ensure lighting is not too bright or intrusive, as this can be stressful for a person with a learning disability and for people who have autistic spectrum disorder
- Reduce distracting noise if possible, as this can be stressful for a person with a learning disability and for people who have autistic spectrum disorder
- Reduce general clutter and objects which are not required in the provision of care, as these can distract a patient with a learning disability and make it difficult for them to visually focus on you and may become a general hazard

- Make sure that the environment is physically accessible and safe
- Use the **Health Action Plan** to determine individual needs.

General nursing care

- Patients with severe learning disabilities may be very dependent on ward staff. They might have difficulty expressing their needs, such as hunger, thirst, pain, distress, toilet and washing requirements, so staff should anticipate these needs and involve the carer/support workers if there are any indications or non-verbal signals the patient with learning disabilities uses to communicate their needs
- Please refer to the patient's **Health Action Plan**.

Ward routine

- Predictability and routine are often important to patients with a learning disability: develop a routine as soon as possible to reduce anxiety. Ask the patient's carer/support worker to help write an accessible timetable that includes meal times, ward rounds and other activities.

Discharge planning

- Consider the need to hold a discharge planning meeting, this is particularly relevant to patients with severe learning disabilities, complex health care needs and patients who are vulnerable. Discharge planning meetings offer the opportunity to share important information, amend care plans and adjust support required in community.
- Inform the discharge coordinator, as soon as possible, whenever a patient with a learning disability is admitted to your ward. Patients with learning disabilities often experience severe delays in the discharge process if potential problems are not considered on admission.
- Provide a discharge sheet with accessible 'Easy Read' information, covering diagnosis, treatment, when to return for follow-up appointments, any possible side-effects of medication and details of someone on the ward to contact if necessary.

deficiencies. At its core, it attempts to include the individual's family and wider social network, emphasising the provision of support to achieve goals, rather than limiting goals to what services can manage to achieve (Mansell & Beade-Brown, cited in Cambridge & Carnaby 2005, p. 20). Planning is not just about one aspect of an individual's life, it is about every aspect, including health and how health needs will be met (DH 2012b).

PCP should have at the heart of it, the individual, not the services. It should take account of wishes and aspirations. PCP is a mechanism for reflecting the needs and preferences of a person with a learning disability and covers such issues as housing, education, employment and leisure (DH 2001). This is something that takes time and understanding of the individual, although it is imperative the important people in life are involved, including healthcare workers. The health liaison nurse is part of the commitment to develop healthcare practices and therefore the quality of care for people with a learning disability. The work undertaken by these nurses is paramount in ensuring that people with a learning disability receive the health care in a person-centred manner. To enable us to best understand the aspirations of people with a learning disability regarding their health, we must, together, encourage and facilitate complete engagement with individuals at all levels of healthcare delivery and inclusion of service design and delivery, as we do for other members of the population. To include someone in their future will help determine the outcomes for them and as such, it is vital that individuals are involved (Scottish Government 2012).

Communication

Many of the reports and additional evidence suggests that communication is one of the most significant issues for people with learning disability when admitted to hospital. Of all the people with learning disabilities admitted to general hospitals, it is estimated that 40% of them will have hearing deficiencies, while 50% will have serious communication problems and around 80% will have some level of communication problem (Hannon & Clift 2011). Generally speaking, nurses are good communicators; they pride themselves on having good interpersonal skills, which aid their need to bond well with people and communicate effectively. However, even those of us who are highly skilled communicators will be challenged when working with people with learning disabilities. As a two-way process, it can be affected by a person's ability to express themselves, i.e. explain their symptoms and the capability to receive messages and understand what is being said. It is important to note that communication may also be non-verbal and alternative methods of communication such as sign language, symbols, photographs and objects of reference are all commonplace when with people with learning disability.

Many people with learning disabilities and especially those with autism, have difficulty with abstract language; they have a more literal understanding of what is being said to them. Our language is full of idioms and expressions, which when analysed literally, make very little sense. Examples of this could be *'pull your socks up'* or *'step up to the plate'* and unless you have experience of using these expressions and understand their meaning, they are difficult to comprehend.

Simple guidelines on face-to-face communication can help, such as the following, suggested by the National Development Team for Inclusion (2012):

- Maintain a quiet, calm, low voice with people who dislike too much expression
- Replace gesticulation, facial expression, body language and metaphor with clear literal statements
- Do not demand eye contact
- Avoid an angry or aggressive tone as the person may fear that they will be harmed by you
- Allow longer for the person to establish trust
- Provide simple explanations of complex treatment interventions
- Be confident in approaching and speaking to the patient.

An individual's level of comprehension should always be clarified; often, people who accompany the patient with learning disabilities may make statements such as, 'he understand what you say to him'. A person's level of comprehension can also be altered if they are anxious and being in hospital is likely to cause some level of anxiety, additionally if a medical procedure is being discussed, this is likely to increase anxiety further. It is always important to check that someone has listened and understood what you have said before carrying out a healthcare intervention. Very often, people with learning disabilities will be accompanied in hospital by a carer from the residential home, a family member or perhaps a health liaison nurse from the local learning disability team. It is easy to make the mistake of talking to them instead of the patient. It is however, important to include them in the discussion and often if they are trusted by the patient, then they can help to keep a person's anxiety at a level which assists in clear and concise communication. Consider the 'What the Experts Say' scenario, below.

What the Experts Say Kevin's Mum

Kevin is autistic and has a moderate learning disability, although he has some verbal communication skills, he uses Makaton for the majority of his communication. However, consistent with many people with autistic spectrum conditions, he uses communication in a very minimalistic manner, i.e. he does tend to engage in 'small talk' and only initiates a conversation if he needs someone to help him. Therefore, he has a few Makaton signs (Figure 10.1) which he uses regularly; some of these are shown in Figure 10.1 (Bailey 2012).

Kevin was visiting outpatients to have an endoscopy as part of a gastrointestinal investigation. Kevin had been suffering from severe chest pains, which are thought to be associated with a suspected hiatus hernia. As part of a desensitisation process, on a previous visit, Kevin and his mum were given pictures of the procedure, showing how and where the camera will be inserted and what it will show. Kevin and his mum had spent time talking about the procedure and attempting to alleviate Kevin's understandable anxiety.

However, the difficult part was trying to explain the discomfort as the camera passed into his stomach. When this happened, Kevin reacted by standing up, pulling the camera from his throat and attacking the very shocked medical team.

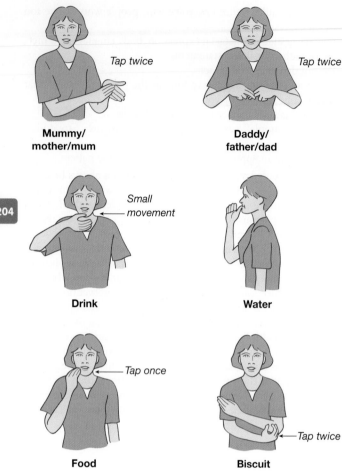

Figure 10.1 Examples of Makaton signs.

people and the world around them. Many people who work with adults and children with learning disabilities have undertaken Makaton training. As well as signs, the training incorporates a range of symbols, which are used widely. In some hospitals, the use of Makaton is prevalent, as part of the reasonable adjustments made to enhance equality, healthcare workers have taken advice from speech and language therapists on which signs and symbols to learn. One example of its use by the nursing staff on a children's ward has been very well evaluated as a great time-saving adjustment for staff and patients alike.

Communication with people with learning disabilities is always easier if you develop a relationship with the patient, it is only then that it is possible to understand what a person's learning disability means to them. Additionally, a rapport with your patient helps them to feel understood, valued and supported; it is of great importance for the person to be considered an equal partner in the healthcare process. Involving the patient as far as possible in their care is central to its success and can assist in reducing potential conflict. It is important to display a respectful and accepting attitude towards people with learning disabilities; too often nurses and doctors speak to the person with them, rather than directly to them. Try to change your posture and voice tone to appear more relaxed and this will help them to relax more. However, it is also true to say that some people with learning disabilities will try to be overly friendly and overstep what is considered to be appropriate in a nurse–patient relationship. If there are behaviours such as attempting to hug or kiss which are uncomfortable, it is important to provide boundaries; very often such boundaries are perceived as positive and actually enhances the relationship.

Jot This Down

Do you feel you can be assertive with a patient with learning disabilities who attempts to give you a hug? How do you feel about giving physical contact to a patient? Is there a time when this is OK?

In the 'Jot This Down' exercise above, you may have considered the vulnerability of people with learning disabilities and how physical contact in the correct context can help to significantly reassure patients. However, as a practitioner, you also need to be aware of your own vulnerabilities; physical contact can very often be misunderstood. Be aware of how this could be perceived by a patient who may be in particular need of emotional support, which they are seeking via an embrace. You can over-analyse such scenarios but be sure to be aware of any potential risks.

Mental Capacity Act 2005 (MCA)

Death by Indifference (Mencap 2007) demonstrated clearly that there was a void in the understanding of people's rights in hospital and significant confusion around the MCA and its implications for decision-making for those who do not have capacity.

The MCA is intended to provide protection to people who cannot make a particular decision at a particular time because their mind or brain is affected. That could be because of mental illness, injury or learning disability. The MCA affects everyone working with or caring for adults who lack capacity and applies to everyday

---

Jot This Down

Consider if you would have done anything better to manage this intervention and support his mum with explaining the procedure? Kevin was only mildly sedated, could more have been done, and should more have been done? Would you expect Kevin to be able to consent to his treatment?

In the 'Jot This Down' exercise above, you may have considered the experiences of those with learning disabilities and an intrusive intervention, such as the endoscopy described. There are often no right or wrong answers in these scenarios, however, it is important to exhaust all avenues and in using a community learning disability nurse or a health liaison nurse to help Kevin, he may have been better prepared for the very frightening insertion of the camera into his stomach.

Makaton is the most widely used sign language for people with learning disabilities. Today, over 100 000 in the UK are users. For those who have experienced the frustration of being unable to communicate meaningfully or effectively, Makaton alleviates some of that frustration and enables individuals to connect with other

matters or life altering events. The MCA looks at how decisions are made concerning adults. It applies to all people who are 16 and over in England and Wales (different rules apply to children).

We all have a responsibility to enable people to make their own decisions wherever possible (House of Lords *et al.* 2008). In the situation where an individual is unable at that time to make a decision others will need to step in on their behalf. When a person cannot make their own decision, other people will need to decide what is in their best interests. Frequently, the family, carers and other important people get involved but sometimes other people must make the decision. If it is a medical decision, this will be made by the doctor but not independently from others involved. Sometimes the local authority will be involved in making decisions. Anybody making 'best interests' decisions on behalf of a person with profound and multiple learning disabilities must consult with the person's family and others who know the person well.

The Evidence The Five Principles of the MCA

1. Assume a person has capacity unless proved otherwise
2. Do not treat someone as incapable of making decisions before everything practicable has been done to help them decide for themselves
3. A person should not be treated as unable to make a decision merely because their decision may seem unwise
4. Always do things, or take decisions, for a person without capacity in their best interests
5. Before doing something to someone, or making a decision on their behalf, consider how the outcome could be achieved in a way which is least restrictive of their basic rights and freedoms

---

The responsibility lies with the person requiring the decision, to determine if the individual has capacity, i.e. if a patient needs surgery, then the surgeon must be satisfied that they have capacity to consent.

Professional and Legal Issues

Lacking capacity – someone lacks capacity to make a particular decision if they cannot do one or more of the following:

- Understand information given to them
- Retain that information long enough to be able to make the decision
- Weigh up the information available to make the decision
- Communicate their decision.

Note: someone can lack capacity on one area of life and not in another.

If a person cannot make one particular decision, this does not mean that they are not able to make any decisions at all. Also, if they are not able to make a decision at one point in time, this does not mean they are able to make a similar decision at another time. It is time- and topic-dependant (Blair 2012).

Best Interests

If and when a person lacks capacity, then actions subsequently taken or decisions made on behalf of the individual must be done in their best interests. The person who has to take the decision about what is in someone's best interest must:

- Involve, as much as possible, the individual who is lacking capacity in deciding what actions will be taken
- Explore the views and feelings of the individual, including anything they may have said or written at a time when they did have capacity, e.g. lasting power of attorney, advanced decisions, discussions and conversations with relatives or friends
- Sometimes it is appropriate to consult other people involved in the care of the person, such as relatives and friends, and take their views into account.

If decisions are being made about serious medical treatment or significant changes of residence, and the patient is 'without friends', i.e. they have no one at all involved in their life apart from paid carers, a referral must be made to the local Independent Mental Capacity Advocate (IMCA) service. The IMCA service can be accessed via the Local Authority.

The MCA now points out that it is a criminal offence to ill-treat or wilfully neglect a person who lacks capacity. 'Before the act is done, or the decision is made, regard must be had to whether the purpose for which it is needed can be as effectively achieved in a way that is less restrictive of the person's rights and freedom of action' (Mental Capacity Act 2005). They must prove that they have made every effort to enable the person to be able to make a decision. All this evidence must be documented and dependent on the nature of the decision, the assessment may need to be repeated at different times of the day, so you can see when they are functioning at their optimum level.

Lasting Power of Attorneys (LPAs)

LPAs now replace Enduring Power of Attorneys (EPAs). This is a legal document and has to be registered with the Office of the Public Guardian. The main difference to an EPA is that the appointed person can be 'authorised to make decisions on behalf of the individual in relation to personal welfare which includes health' (DH 2007). Thus, an individual could have a relative or friend who is willing to make decisions about their health care once that individual no longer has capacity. Day-to-day care, as well as consenting or refusal of medical treatment/examination, could be included. The appointed person is not able to consent or refuse life-sustaining treatment unless the LPA expressly states and authorises this.

Advanced Decisions

Someone over 18 is able to specify, while they still have capacity, to refuse specific medical treatment for a time in the future when they may lack capacity to consent or refuse that treatment. This includes people with a learning disability, although often they are not given the opportunity. This has to be valid and applicable to the current circumstances to be effective and is treated as a decision made by that individual when they had capacity. An advanced decision can be written or verbal. However, the exception is where there is life-sustaining treatment, then the advanced decision must be in writing and witnessed.

Court of Protection (CP)

The CP is intended to deal with decision-making for individuals who may lack capacity to make specific decisions for themselves. This deals with property and affairs and now deals with serious decisions affecting health care and personal welfare matters.

Deprivation of Liberties Safeguards (DoLS)

This became part of the MCA in April 2009, as a result of the Bournewood Inquiry and applies to people over 18 who lack capacity. The premise here is that all care must be carried out in the 'Best Interest' and in the 'Least Restrictive' approach.

This sets out the criteria for when a person may be deprived of their liberty:

- If you are acting in their Best Interest to protect them from harm
- Proportionate action/response in the event of likelihood of serious harm

The only less restrictive alternative:

This is so the person is free from harm and must not be used:

- As a form of punishment
- Staff/Carer's/Organisation's convenience
- Without the appropriate DoLS assessment carried out by a Best Interest assessor
- Indefinitely.

Consent

Consent is an individual's agreement for a health professional to provide care. In the case with someone who has a learning disability, this is exactly the same, however the person may indicate consent in a different way from other people. People often indicate consent in a variety of ways. They may indicate consent non-verbally (e.g. by presenting their arm for their pulse to be taken), orally or in writing.

For the consent to be valid, the patient must:

- Be competent to take the particular decision
- Have received sufficient information to take it
- Be able to weigh up and communicate a decision
- Not be acting under duress.

Where an adult patient lacks the mental capacity (either temporarily or permanently) to give or withhold consent for themselves, a decision may be made on behalf of a person who lacks capacity – a Lasting Power of Attorney (LPA), as discussed above. If there is no LPA, treatment can be given if it is in the patient's best interests, as long as it has not been refused in advance in a valid and applicable manner.

Individuals being supported to make their own decisions:

- A person must be given all practicable help (e.g. use of simple language, photographs, drawings, sign language, interpreters) before anyone treats them as not being able to make their own decisions
- An individual may choose to make what might seem an unwise decision: just because they make a decision that others may think is unwise, it should not be assumed that they lack capacity.

Safeguarding

Each and every person in health services has a responsibility for the safety and well-being of patients and colleagues. Safeguarding adults is a fundamental part of all aspects of safety and well-being and the outcomes expected within the NHS. Safeguarding adults is also fundamental to complying with legislation, regulations and delivering effective care. These notes should be used by you as a guide to form the principles. If you have a safeguarding concern they should always be used alongside your organisation's safeguarding policy and procedures.

The Evidence

- Living a life that is free from harm and abuse is a fundamental human right of every person and an essential requirement for health and well-being
- Safeguarding adults is about the safety and well-being of all patients but providing additional measures for those least able to protect themselves from harm or abuse.

(*No Secrets*, DH 2000)

Definition of a vulnerable adult

Aged 18 years or over –

who may be in need of community care services by reason of mental or other disability, age or illness; and who is or may be unable to take care of him or herself, or unable to protect him or herself against significant harm or exploitation.

(*No Secrets*, DH 2000)

You have a responsibility to follow the six Safeguarding principles:

1. *Promotion of empowerment and well-being* – presumption of person-led decisions and consent
2. *Protection* – support the rights of the individual to lead an independent life based on self-determination and personal choice
3. *Prevention* – from harm or abuse and reducing unacceptable risks
4. *Proportionality* – the least intrusive response to harm or abuse rights and take account of the person's age, culture, wishes, lifestyle and beliefs. Managing concerns in the most effective and efficient manner
5. *Partnerships* – working to implement local solutions, with communities working together collaboratively to prevent, identify and respond accordingly
6. *Accountability* – be accountable and transparent in the delivery of services ensuring all those involved are aware of safeguarding and accountable to those the service is for patients, public and to their governing bodies. Working in partnerships also entails being open and transparent with the partner.

Significant harm

'Harm should be taken to include not only ill treatment but also the impairment of, or avoidable deterioration in, physical or mental health; and the impairment of physical, intellectual, emotional, social, or behavioural development' (Law Commission 1995).

Whistle-blowing

You must always take action whenever abuse is suspected, including when your legitimate concern is not acted upon. Whistle-blowers are given protection under the Public Interest Disclosure Act 1998. If in doubt, contact your nominated lead for adult safeguarding.

Categories of abuse

- *Physical abuse*, including hitting, slapping, pushing, kicking, misuse of medication, restraint or inappropriate sanctions
- *Sexual abuse*, including rape and sexual assault or sexual acts to which the vulnerable adult has not consented, or could not consent or was pressured into consenting

- *Psychological abuse*, including emotional abuse, threats of harm or abandonment, deprivation of contact, humiliation, blaming, controlling, intimidation, coercion, harassment, verbal abuse, isolation or withdrawal from services or supportive networks
- *Financial or material abuse*, including theft, fraud, exploitation, pressure in connection with wills, property or inheritance or financial transactions, or the misuse or misappropriation of property, possessions or benefits
- *Neglect and acts of omission*, including ignoring medical or physical care needs, failure to provide access to appropriate health, social care or educational services, the withholding of the necessities of life, such as medication, adequate nutrition and heating
- *Discriminatory abuse*, including racist, sexist, that based on a person's disability, and other forms of harassment, slurs or similar treatment
- *Institutional abuse* can happen in residential homes, nursing homes or hospitals, when people are mistreated with poor or inadequate care, neglect and poor practice.

Death by Indifference (Mencap 2007) and *Healthcare for All* (DH 2008a) both highlight the need for good commissioning to address the quality of health care. Acute services have issues in ensuring they have effective care pathways and communication strategies. Knowledge of staff within these services have the opportunity to work with the liaison nurses to support in identifying and implementing reasonable adjustments, systems of support are instigated and there is provision of training to meet the need of those involved (DH 2009).

'Getting it Right' (Mencap 2008) identifies the need for health professionals, healthcare authorities and others involved in the lives of people with a learning disability, need to work together to ensure the health needs of individuals with a learning disability are being met in a timely and equitable manner. Learning from other services, opportunities of best practice and reasonable adjustments can assist in the provision of a unified service, where we are able to share ideas thoughts and protocols to the benefit of everyone and thus see a change in the future in the health status of people with a learning disability. This is not the responsibility of one agency but one that affects everyone and each have a part to play.

Conclusion

This chapter has provided you with insight and understanding concerning the care of adults with learning disabilities and autism. Working with any patient is very individual and this chapter provides a guide to thinking holistically about the person and their experience in health care. It is fair to say that the more time you have to understand the patient, the more time can be saved making mistakes; however, it is acknowledged that the vast majority of healthcare practitioners are providing the best care possible in sometimes very difficult situations. The implementation of some of the simple points in this chapter can help clarify some of those difficulties and increase confidence where needed. The access to mainstream services is unquestionably the way forward and people who have a learning disability will be increasing their access to these services now and in the future, therefore awareness of how to work with this group of people is crucial to the continued growth in their quality of their care.

Key Points

- This chapter has provided the reader with an understanding of the nature of learning disabilities, causes and prevalence. Gaining insight into these issues can help the nurse provide person-centred care.
- People with learning disabilities are more susceptible to inequalities in health and social care when compared with other people in society.
- Enhanced communication awareness and the use of effective communication skills has the potential to improve the health and well-being of people with learning disabilities.
- When service provision has been reasonably adjusted, the needs of the person with learning disabilities can be met more effectively.
- Legislation has the ability to impact positively on care delivery for people (and their families) with learning disabilities.
- The key role of the nurse is to support and promote the health, well-being and rights of people with learning disabilities.
- Partnership with specialist learning disability services is essential when offering health and social care services to those with leaning disabilities.
- The nurse is required to assess the person's physical and psychological needs using communication strategies that are appropriate and effective.
- When encouraging person-centred planning, the nurse empowers the person with regards to choices in health and social care.

Glossary

Brain injury: the physical damage to brain tissue or structure that occurs before, during or after birth that is verified by EEG, MRI, CAT or a similar examination, rather than by observation of performance. When caused by an accident, the damage may be called traumatic brain injury (TBI)

British sign language: a form of sign language developed in the UK for the use of deaf people, the fourth most widely used indigenous language in Britain

Court of Protection: makes decisions and appoints deputies to act on behalf of those people who are unable to make decisions about their personal health, finance or welfare

Diagnostic and Statistical Manual of Mental Disorders: used by clinicians and psychiatrists to diagnose psychiatric illnesses; published by the American Psychiatric Association, it covers all categories of mental health disorders for both adults and children. Focusses mostly on describing symptoms, as well as statistics concerning which gender is most affected by the illness, the typical age of onset, the effects of treatment and common treatment approaches

Dyslexia: a difficulty in understanding or using one or more areas of language, including listening, speaking, reading, writing and spelling

Dyspraxia: a difficulty in performing drawing, writing, buttoning, and other tasks requiring fine motor skill, or in sequencing the necessary movements

Health inequalities: these are preventable and unjust differences in health status experienced by certain population groups

(Continued)

Inclusion: a term used by people with disabilities and other disability rights advocates for the idea that all people should freely, openly and without pity, accommodate any person with a disability without restrictions or limitations of any kind

Intelligence quotient (IQ): an estimate of intelligence level. The IQ is usually calculated by dividing the mental age, derived through psychological testing, by the chronologic age and multiplying the result by 100. The average IQ is considered to be 100.

Social skills: any skill facilitating interaction and communication with others. Social rules and relations are created, communicated and changed in verbal and non-verbal ways. The process of learning such skills is called socialisation.

Makaton: this is a language programme using signs and symbols to help people to communicate; designed to support spoken language, the signs and symbols are used with speech, in spoken word order

Whistle-blowing: this occurs when a worker reports suspected wrongdoing at work. Formally this is called 'making a disclosure in the public interest'.

References

APA (1994) *The Diagnostic and Statistical Manual of Mental Disorders,* 4th edn. American Psychiatric Association, Washington DC.

Bailey, J. (2012) Makaton. http://www.jacobbailey.com/2012/04/makaton. (accessed 23 November 2012).

BBC (2012) *Winterbourne View: abuse footage shocked nation.* BBC Panorama. http://www.bbc.co.uk/news/uk-england-bristol-20084254.

Blair, J. (2011) Care adjustments for people with learning disabilities in hospitals. *Nursing Management,* 18(8), 21–24.

Blair, J. (2012) Caring for people who have intellectual disabilities. *Emergency Nurse,* 20(6), 15–19.

Cambridge, P. & Carnaby, S. (2005) *Person Centred Planning and Care Management with People with Learning Disabilities.* Kingsley, London.

Cummings, J., Chief Nursing Officer for England (2012) Compassion in practice: nursing has to change if patients are going to be treated well. *The Times,* London, 4 December 2012.

DH (2000) No Secrets: guidance on developing and implementing multi-agency policies and procedures to protect vulnerable adults from abuse. Department of Health, London.

DH (2001) Valuing People: a new strategy for learning disability for the 21st century. Department of Health, London.

DH (2002) Action for Health: health action plans and health facilitation; detailed good practice guidance for learning disability partnership boards. Department of Health, London.

DH (2006) *Our Health, Our Care, Our Say.* Department of Health, London.

DH (2007) *Putting People First: a shared vision and commitment to the transformation of adult social care.* Department of Health, London.

DH (2008a) *Healthcare for All.* Report of the independent inquiry into Access to Healthcare for People with Learning Disabilities, Sir Jonathan Michael. Department of Health, London.

DH (2008b) *High Quality Care for All: NHS next stage review final report* (CM 7432) Lord Dazi report. Department of Health, London.

DH (2009) *Valuing People Now.* Department of Health, London. https://www.gov.uk/government/uploads/system/uploads/attachment_data/file/215891/dh_122387.pdf (accessed 24 February 2014).

DH (2012a) *Compassion in Practice: nursing, midwifery and care staff our vision and strategy.* Department of Health, London.

DH (2012b) *Improving the Health and Well-being of People with Learning Disabilities: a commissioning guide for clinical commissioning groups (CCGs).* Department of Health, London. http://www.improvinghealthandlives.org.uk/event.php?eid=2267 (accessed 12 March 2014).

DRC (2006) *Equal Treatment: closing the gap,* Part one. Disability Rights Commission, Stratford Upon Avon.

Emerson, E. & Baines, S. (2011) Health inequalities and people with learning disabilities in the UK. *Tizard Review,* 16(1), 42–48.

Emerson, E. & Hatton, C. (2008) *Estimating Future Need/Demand for Supports for Adults with Learning Disabilities in England.* Institute for Health Research at Lancaster University Centre for Disability Research, Lancaster.

Emerson, E., Vick, B., Graham, H., Hatton, C., Llewellyn, G. & Madden, R. (2012) Disablement and health In: N. Watson, C. Thomas, A. Roulstone (eds), *Companion to Disability Studies.* Routledge, London.

Gates, B. (2011a) Envisioning a workforce fit for the 21st century. *Learning Disability Practice,* 14(1), 12–18.

Gates, B. (2011b) Learning Disability Nursing: Task and Finish Group: Report for the Professional and Advisory Board for Nursing and Midwifery – Department of Health, England. https://uhra.herts.ac.uk/dspace/bitstream/2299/6289/1/Gates3.pdf

Gibb, M. (2012) *Guide to Caring for an Adult Patient with a Learning Disability.* Mid Yorkshire Hospitals NHS Trust, Wakefield.

Grant, G., Goward, P., Richardson, M. & Ramcharan, P. (2005) *Learning Disability – A Life Cycle Approach to Valuing People.* Open University Press, London.

Hannon, L. & Clift, J. (2011) *General Hospital Care for People with Learning Disabilities.* Blackwell, London.

Heslop, P. & Marriott, A. (2011) The Confidential Inquiry into the deaths of people with learning disabilities – the story so far. *Tizard Learning Disability Review,* 16(5), 18–25.

Hoghton, M. & the RCGP Learning Disabilities Group (2010) *A Step by Step Guide for GP Practices: annual health checks for people with a learning disability.* The Royal College of General Practitioners, London.

House of Lords, House of Commons, Joint Committee on Human Rights (2008) *A Life Like Any Other? Human Rights of Adults with Learning Disabilities,* 2008 HL Paper 40–1 HC 73–1.

IHL (2012) *Improving Health and Lives.* http://www.improvinghealthandlives.org.uk/projects/reasonableadjustments

Law Commission for England and Wales (1995) *Mental Incapacity,* Report No. 231. HMSO, London.

Mencap (2004) *Treat Me Right!* Mencap, London.

Mencap (2007) *Death by Indifference.* Mencap, London.

Mencap (2008) *Getting It Right.* Mencap, London.

Mencap (2012) *What is a Learning Disability?* http://www.mencap.org.uk/all-about-learning-disability/about-learning-disability (accessed 13 March 2014).

Michael, J. & Richardson, A. (2008) Healthcare for all: the independent inquiry into access to healthcare for people with learning disabilities. *Tizard Learning Disability Review,* 13(4), 28–34.

NAS (2012) *What is Autism?* National Autistic Society. http://www.autism.org.uk/about-autism/autism-and-asperger-syndrome-an-introduction/what-is-autism.aspx

National Development Team for Inclusion (2012) http://www.ndti.org.uk/publications/ndti-articles/ (accessed 12 March 2014)

NHS Health Scotland (2004) *Health Needs Assessment Report – Summary. People with Learning Disabilities in Scotland.* http://www.healthscotland.com/documents/1040.aspx (accessed 6 January 2013).

NHS (2011) *NHS Standard Contracts 2012/13.* Department of Health, London.

Parliamentary and Health Service Ombudsman (2009) *Six Lives: the provision of public services to people with learning disabilities.* The Stationery Office, London.

Priest, H. & Gibbs, M. (2004) *Mental Health Care for People with Learning Disabilities.* Churchill Livingstone, London.

Royal College of General Practitioners (2010) http://www.rcgp.org.uk (accessed 21 February 2014).

RCN (2011) *Learning from the Past – Setting Out the Future. Developing Learning Disability Nursing in the United Kingdom*. An RCN position statement on the role of the learning disability nurse. Royal College of Nursing, London. http://www.rcn.org.uk/__data/assets/pdf_file/0007/359359/PosState_Disability_170314b_2.pdf (accessed 11 January 2013).

Scottish Government (2012) *Strengthening the Commitment: The report of the UK modernising learning disability nursing review*. Scottish Government, Edinburgh http://www.scotland.gov.uk/Publications/2012/04/6465/downloads (accessed 6 January 2013).

Sowney, M. & Barr, O. (2006) Caring for adults with intellectual disabilities: perceived challenges for nurses in accident and emergency units. *Journal of Advanced Nursing*, 55(1), 36–45.

Thompson, J., Kilbane, J. & Sanderson, H. (2008) *Person Centred Practice for Professionals*. Open University Press, Berkshire.

Tyrer, F. & McGrother, C. (2009) Cause-specific mortality and death certificate reporting in adults with moderate to profound intellectual disability. *Journal of Intellectual Disability Research*, 53(11), 898–904.

Test Yourself

1. Which of the following was NOT used in government policy to describe people with learning disabilities?
   (a) Idiots
   (b) Imbeciles
   (c) Feeble minded persons
   (d) Lunatic

2. Which of the following is the first and second priority when asked to triage a person with a learning disability?
   (a) Pain relief
   (b) Diagnosis
   (c) Determining their method of communication
   (d) Discharge

3. Does a person with learning disabilities lack capacity?
   (a) Yes it is presumed to be so under the Mental Capacity Act 2005
   (b) There is no presumption that a person with learning disabilities automatically lacks capacity. If capacity is in doubt a proper assessment under the Mental Capacity Act 2005 must be made
   (c) Yes, pursuant to the Mental Health Act 2007
   (d) Yes, in accordance with the Bournewood principles

4. Some people with learning disabilities may have difficulties with communication which can impact on their health. There are a number of techniques which have been developed to help support people for whom speech is difficult. Which of the following have been developed specifically for people with a learning disability?
   (a) Widget, Makaton BSL
   (b) Makaton, BSL, Easy Read Symbols
   (c) Speech and Language Therapy, BSL, Widget
   (d) Widget, Makaton, PECS, Easy Read Symbols

5. The Directed Enhanced Service (DES) requires GPs to provide people with learning disabilities with annual health checks from what age?
   (a) Birth
   (b) 5 years of age
   (c) 16 years of age
   (d) 18

6. All of us experience challenges to our emotional well-being at some stage in our lives, and children and adults with learning disabilities are not exempt from this. What does the research tell us about the number of people with learning disabilities who also have mental health problems?
   (a) An estimated 25–40% of people with learning disabilities have mental health problems
   (b) An estimated 10–15% of people with learning disabilities have mental health problems
   (c) An estimated 20–30% of people with learning disabilities have mental health problems
   (d) An estimated 5–10% of people with learning disabilities have mental health problems

7. Under the *Disability Equality Duty* cited in the Equality Act (2010), all public sector organisations are required to do which of the following?
   (a) Make reasonable adjustments to services to ensure they are accessible for disabled people and people with learning disabilities
   (b) Not have to make any adjustments to services to ensure they are accessible for disabled people and people with learning disabilities
   (c) Make any adjustments to services to ensure they are accessible for learning disabilities groups only
   (d) None of the above

8. Many people with learning disabilities and especially those with autism, have difficulty with which one of the following?
   (a) Abstract language
   (b) Written language
   (c) Smell
   (d) All of the above

9. Materials used in verbal learning are:
   (a) Unfamiliar words
   (b) Familiar words
   (c) Nonsense syllabus
   (d) All of the above

10. Consent is an individual's agreement for a health professional to provide care. In the case of someone who has a learning disability, which of the following statements is true?
    (a) You do not have to get their consent
    (b) You need to get their consent
    (c) Ignore the consent form
    (d) Two nurses can consent for the patient

Answers

1. d.

   Feedback: 'idiots', 'imbeciles' and 'feeble-minded persons' were used in The Mental Deficiency Act (1913); lunatic was used to describe people with chronic mental illness.

2. a, b.

   Explanation: It is of course imperative that pain is controlled as quickly as possible and that should always be the number one priority; however, despite determining the presenting condition and formulating a diagnosis being the primary function of the triage nurse, this relies heavily on reporting the history of the condition and the symptoms. It also relies on the ability to describe the nature and the intensity of the pain. Therefore, determining their method of communication would be the second priority.

3. b

4. d

5. d

   Feedback: The 2011 Government Green Paper 'Support and aspiration: A new approach to special educational needs and disability' (PDF) proposes that annual health checks should start from the age of 16.

6. a

7. a

8. a

9. d

10. b

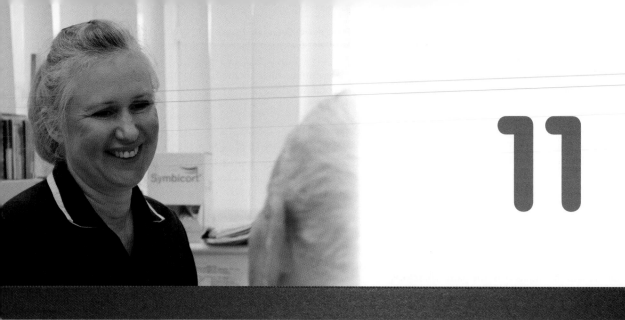

11

The Principles of Caring for Children and Families

Ann Foley and Linda Sanderson

University of Central Lancashire, UK

Learning Outcomes

On completion of this chapter you will be able to:

- Recognise the key stages in relation to the development of infants, children and young people
- Utilise a range of communication strategies, which will help to establish a caring relationship with infants, children, young people and their families
- Have an awareness of the common physical and mental health problems associated with infants, children and young people
- Understand the basic care requirements of infants, children and young people, in order to meet their essential needs
- Recognise the importance of acting to protect infants, children and young people, where there is a risk of harm to their well-being
- Identify signs of deterioration in the general health of infants, children and young people and be aware of best practice relating to end of life care

Competencies

All nurses must:

1. Work in a professional manner with children and their families, demonstrating integrity and respect for dignity at all times
2. Care and safeguard the child in all clinical environments
3. Utilise excellent and appropriate communication skills when working with children and young people of all ages and abilities and their families
4. Assess the physical and emotional needs of children and young people in a variety of clinical settings
5. Attend appropriately to the fundamental care needs of children and young people, adapting to their age and abilities
6. Work with a team of healthcare professionals and the child's family to offer safe, effective and compassionate care

 Visit the companion website at **www.wileynursingpractice.com** where you can test yourself using flashcards, multiple-choice questions and more.

Nursing Practice: Knowledge and Care, First Edition. Edited by Ian Peate, Karen Wild and Muralitharan Nair.
© 2014 John Wiley & Sons, Ltd. Published 2014 by John Wiley & Sons, Ltd. Companion website: www.wileynursingpractice.com

Introduction

Children attend the healthcare services in a variety of clinical areas. No matter in which field of nursing you are working, you will come into contact with children and their families. It is essential that you care for children and their families compassionately, appropriately and confidently. In this chapter there is a lot of information offering guidance for when you are caring for children. Caring for children of different age groups is fascinating, challenging and rewarding. It is hoped that this chapter will stimulate your interest and encourage you to explore the care of children, so that you enjoy working alongside them in your future career.

The Key Stages in Relation to the Development of Infants, Children and Young People

Jot This Down

Write down what you think is meant by Development.
What would you think the key stages are?

Child health professionals working with children find early childhood fascinating, as it is a period of major growth and development. The child explores a world where opportunities abound! Parents, guardians and carers of children also have much to offer in this process. Growth and development is affected by a myriad of factors, e.g. nutrition, sleep and maintaining safety. In addition, there are inherited attributes and the social, economic, geographic and political factors cannot be forgotten. All of these factors interact and affect the overall child's development into adulthood. Within this chapter, development will be considered in the following age ranges: the baby 0–18 months, the pre-school child, the school-age child and the adolescent.

Childhood is a period of rapid growth and development and children of varying ages from birth through to adolescence have very different needs (Bee & Boyd 2010). The information contained herein will not make you an expert in child development – there are books entirely given over to the subject matter (e.g. Lightfoot *et al.* 2009) – but it is important for student nurses to know about child development, so that they are able to:

- Teach and advise parents
- Have reasonable expectations of what the child can and cannot do
- Be able to undertake suitable play activities with the child
- Be able to identify their limits
- Be able to recognise where there are changes from the normal and be able to recognise disabilities and irregularities.

The Evidence

Growth and development occur throughout the lifespan. Growth implies an increase in size . . . Development refers to the acquisition of skills and abilities that take place throughout life.
(Devitt & Thain 2011, p. 15)

As a baby develops, the increase in the complexity of their development involves their learning, physical growth and maturation. Maturation in the main is considered to centre on an increase in competence and adaptability to the child's experiences and surroundings (Bee & Boyd 2010). There continues to be differing schools of thought about what development actually is and what it is affected by. An important debate relevant to child development is the extent to which 'nature' and nurture' influence the child (Lightfoot *et al.* 2009). Professionals supporting the influence of 'nature' argue that behaviour and development are affected and guided by inborn factors and hereditary factors. Professionals supporting the influence of 'nurture' suggest that individual human differences are down to life experiences. However, these two 'camps' are polarised and child development is mainly considered to be a combination of both nature and nurture (Lightfoot *et al.* 2009). Child development is an amazing, complex process and nurses need to look at each child and family unit on an individual basis to consider their stage of development.

Baby 0–18 Months

Development is generally assessed by the utilisation of developmental scales in the following distinct areas.

1. Physical – which includes growth, vision, hearing, gross motor development and coordination
2. Cognitive – this is language and understanding
3. Psychosocial – which involves adapting to the society and culture to which the child belongs
4. Emotional – where we consider the control of feelings and emotions.

Jot This Down

Think back to when you were growing up; were there any differences in how you and your friends were growing?
Think about motor skills and fine skills and jot down some notes.
Think about when you were growing up . . .

Within the health professional realm, it is the responsibility of the Health Visitor (HV) and General Practitioner (GP) to undertake developmental assessments. Occasionally, a paediatrician may also undertake this assessment.

The assessments are aimed at underpinning observations as they relate to the above four areas. Generally, the HV would be looking for:

- Gross motor development by referring to large muscle skills
- Fine motor skills by referring to small muscle skills
- Hearing and speech
- Vision
- Social development – feeding dressing and social behavioural traits.

The development of a child between the ages of 0–18 months is an incredible complex and sometimes mind-blowing experience but to aid your knowledge of this, below is an overview of major milestones. You also need to realise that there may be individual differences in the rate and timing of specific developmental progress

Box 11.1 Major health milestones

- Smile – 1–2 months
- Laugh – 6 months
- Sits (with support) – 6 months
- Sits (without support) – 8–9 months
- Crawls – 8–9 months
- Stands/walks – 12 months
- Pincer grip – 12 months
- Delicate pincer – 18 months
- Walks backwards – 18 months

– e.g. three perfectly normal infants may sit unaided at 5, 6 or 9 months. However, the sequence will always be the same.

Box 11.1 gives an indication of some of the major milestones that healthcare professionals will look for, with an approximate age that these milestones can usually be seen.

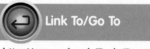

Link To/Go To

http://www.nhs.uk/Tools/Pages/birthtofive.aspx#close
Information about expected development of the baby.

What needs to be considered in relation to development is that all aspects of it are interlinked. Developmental skills of babies are always achieved chronologically. In this respect, head control is always developed before the baby is able to sit independently – crawling follows on from this and then the control of the lower limbs facilitates standing and walking.

The Pre-school Child

When observing the pre-school child, it can be noted that their growth rates relating to the body and brain are considerably slower than when they were a baby.

Jot This Down

Spend some time watching children in a playground – this will show you the remarkable differences in physical and motor development that separate the baby and the pre-school child – look at the Table 11.1 and see if you can pick out some of these developmental traits

At the same time, the ability that children have to control what their body can do grows enormously.

Table 11.1 identifies a vast array of skills, motor and fine, that the pre-school child masters developmentally – but what is also awe-inspiring, is the liveliness with which they practise them. Watch a child in the supermarket or waiting for a bus hopping around just for the sheer joy of it because it is a new skill!

Table 11.1 Milestones in the pre-school child. (Sheridan 2008)

AGE (IN YEARS)	GROSS MOTOR SKILLS	FINE MOTOR SKILLS
2	Walks well	Uses a spoon and fork
	Runs	Turns pages in a book
	Up and down stairs alone	Imitates a circle stroke
	Kicks a ball	Builds a tower of 6 cubes
3	Runs well	Feeds themselves well
	Marches	Puts on socks and shoes
	Rides a tricycle	Buttons and unbuttons
	Stands in one foot	Builds a tower of 10 cubes
4	Skips	Draws a person
	Can do a broad jump	Cuts with scissors (not expertly)
	Throws a ball over hand	Dresses self well
	High motor drive	Washes and dries face
5	Hops and skips	Dresses without help
	Good balance	Prints simple letters
	Rides scooter	

Jot This Down

Consider the link of sleep to development and also consider the impact of malnutrition and under-stimulation of a young child – what might you see?

This vast increase in developmental skills strikingly increases the child's ability to explore – and provides them with abundant occasions for the development of new ways to think and do.

School-Age Child

Within this age range, the physical changes are much less obvious than in the baby and pre-schooler. However, children are growing taller, they are changing in their body shape and still adding to their toolbox of skills. Broadly speaking, by the time the child reaches school age, their height and weight are increasing gradually at the rate of 5 cm and 2–3 kg per year up until adolescence. Generally speaking, boys are on average 2.5 cm taller and 1 kg heavier than girls in the early school years but by around 12 years of age, girls are both taller and heavier than boys in their peer group.

Look for the following in age groups:

5 year olds can:

- Write their own name, draw a person or/and a house
- Hop, skip, swing jump, balance, climb, dance and throw a ball
- Choose their friends and be very clear who they will play with
- Undress and dress – although not able to tie laces
- Undertake play activities alone or in groups – like imaginative play.

6 year olds can:

- Swing by the arms on monkey poles in playgrounds
- Skip with a rope

7 year olds can:
- Be proficient with a bat and ball.

8–10 year olds can:
- Play hopscotch
- Team games.

Jot This Down

When in a placement area, undertake some or all of the following activities to underpin your knowledge around child development.

Look at the age and gender of the child initially and the context of where you are observing them.

Look at their:
- Social behaviour and how they play
- Hearing and speech
- Fine motor skills and their vision
- Gross motor skills
- Feeding
- Physical appearance
- Personality and interactions with others

Adolescence

As a range of complex factors affect development in the 0–18-month-old baby, so adolescence is triggered by a range of hormonal effects that bring on a further set of very visible physical changes. These hormonal changes are controlled by the anterior pituitary, in response to a stimulus from the hypothalamus (Figure 11.1).

Puberty can begin in boys as early as 10.5 years and as late as 16 years, with the average onset at 12 years. In girls, puberty can begin as early as 7.5 years and as late 11.5 years, with the average onset at 10 years.

During adolescence, there is a rapid growth spurt. The internal organs grow and this includes the lungs and the heart, which in turn increases physical endurance. At this time, the lymphoid system, which includes the tonsils and adenoids, decreases in size, which for some teenagers leads to improvements in asthma. Boy's longer skeletal growth is reflected in their greater height, with longer legs and arms. Muscle mass increases in boys and girls – for girls it peaks at menarche and then slows down – for boys it continues with the resultant leaner body mass (Coleman 2011).

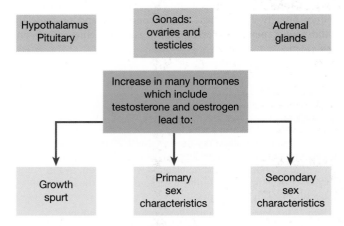

Figure 11.1 Hormones produced in adolescence.

The brain also continues to grow during adolescence. There is no increase in the number of neurones but the myelin sheath does continue to grow at least until puberty, which ensures faster neural processing with the resultant development of cognitive abilities.

 Link To/Go To

The following websites is an excellent reference guide for highlighting pubertal processes:

http://www.nhs.uk/Conditions/Puberty/Pages/ Introduction.aspx

---

Student nurses may have a variety of experiences in placement areas. These should be utilised to gain valuable learning. Children across their developmental age range are an amazing subject from whom a vast amount of information can be gathered. By watching and recording data, talking to the child and parents, student nurses can begin to understand child development. There follows a list (not exhaustive) of where student nurses can begin their knowledge journey.

- Child health clinics
- Home visits with the Health Visitor
- School health checks with the school nurse
- Placement at a children's centre
- Mother and toddler groups
- Playgroups
- Nurseries
- Youth centres
- Voluntary sector child focussed organisations – play centres, youth centres.

What To Do If ...

 Student nurse, Gemma, was attending a baby clinic with her mentor, an HV. Gemma noticed a mum and baby at the clinic who were sat quietly on their own, so she went to talk to them. The conversation moved to the baby, who was 6 months old. The mum told Gemma that she was very worried about her baby as he was not taking notice of his environment like other babies were and also not smiling much.

In this situation, it would be very important to report the mum's concerns to the HV. A developmental assessment could be undertaken to see if the baby was reaching expected milestones or not. If the baby is reaching the milestones mum can be reassured and given suggestions about interacting with her baby to promote his interest in the environment, for example reading to the baby, explaining and describing everything happening around him, helping to establish a regular sleep and rest pattern.

If the baby is not reaching the expected milestones, then the HV could refer the mum and baby to the community paediatrician for a more thorough assessment of vision, hearing and neurological system.

A Range of Communication Strategies

Children, young people and their families often come into contact with health services: health centres, neonatal units, accident and emergency departments, outpatient clinics, acute ward areas, community nurses, school nurses. Whatever the situation, the child/young person will be uncertain/anxious or openly distressed and fearful. The likelihood is that the child or young person will be asked to cooperate with the care that is thought to be in their best interests, but which may appear to be unacceptable to the child, e.g. taking a medicine, passing urine into a bedpan, holding a position for an X-ray. It is essential that the nurse uses appropriate and genuine communication to support the child or young person to undergo the procedures that they would really rather not undergo.

Alongside the child or young person is often a parent or carer. The communication between parent/carer and nurse is understandably focussed on the child or young person. The parent/carer may be feeling anxious and protective of their child in a situation where the nurse is perceived to be the expert and powerful. The nurse must enable the parent/carer to support the child or young person in a way which ensures they feel involved and contributing positively to their child's care.

Communication with the child, young person and family is not just about passing on information. It is about building caring relationships, which promote rapport, trust and openness. In such circumstances, the child, young person and family are afforded their best opportunity to experience health care in a positive way, even in the face of difficult, even tragic circumstances. This approach to communication is not an optional extra; it is embedded in the value set of nursing.

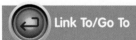

Link To/Go To

Read *Compassion in Practice: the implementation plans.* Excellent communication is considered central to compassionate nursing care.

http://www.england.nhs.uk/2013/04/15/cip-implementation/

In this chapter, aspects of communication will be considered, particularly in relation to children of different ages and abilities, and their families. The reader will be encouraged to think about their own practice and some tips will be offered to develop their approach to communicating with children, young people and their families.

Using Communication to Build Relationships

Jot This Down

Think about your experiences with children, young people and their families.

Think of a situation where you felt you had a 'good' and a 'not so good' relationship with them.

What aspects of communication between you and the child, young person or family contributed to the different relationships?

At a basic level, communication is the passage of a message from a 'sender' to a 'receiver', and possibly a reply (Figure 11.2).

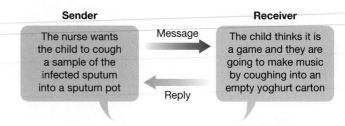

Figure 11.2 Communication from the sender to the receiver.

Box 11.2 Barriers to Effective Communication

Physical: Visual or hearing impairment, speech impediment, neurological impairment or other factors causing poor health status, e.g. diarrhoea and vomiting

Cognitive: The age of the child, learning difficulties, stress, anxiety, mental health problems, e.g. depression, anorexia nervosa

Environmental: Noise level, temperature, seating arrangements, privacy, interruptions, time available

Personal: Confidence, experience and skills in communication, perception of the power relationship between health professionals, children, young people and their families, perception of hierarchy in a relationship, culture, language.

The ideal scenario is for the sender and receiver of the message to have the same mental image of the message and the same understanding of what is required, e.g. 'Please cough into this pot'. Even at this simplistic level, it is possible to see that there may be barriers to the sending and receiving of the message.

The potential barriers to conveying information between nurses, children, young people and their families are many and varied (Box 11.2) but establishing a caring relationship is not just about conveying information.

Effective verbal communication is one aspect of establishing a caring, trusting relationship with children, young people and their families. Verbal communication, non-verbal communication, listening skills and valuing the child, young person and family as fellow human beings are all vital components of effective relationship building between the nurse, child and family. With this genuine approach to communication, rapport can be established and trust built between the child, young person, family and the nurse, which is likely to facilitate cooperation during procedures, reduce anxiety and distress for all concerned and promote the child/young person's developing sense of achievement and self-worth.

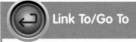

Link To/Go To

The Nursing and Midwifery Council (NMC 2010) have clear expectations of the knowledge, skills and behaviours of all nurses, in relation to communication with children, at the point of registration. You may want to consider these before continuing with the chapter.

http://standards.nmc-uk.org/PreRegNursing/statutory/competencies/Pages/Specific-knowledge-and-skills.aspx

Communication and relationship formation with children of different ages and abilities, and their families will now be considered.

Babies and infants

Babies and infants are reliant upon those around them to provide food, security, warmth and social interaction, in order for them to achieve their full potential (Bee & Boyd 2010). Social interaction with consistent caring adults is essential for the baby to learn about all aspects of communication: verbal communication and the development of language; body language, particularly facial expressions; experiencing love, security and the emotions associated with communication. The quality of early social experiences is linked to the child's mental health and well-being, particularly their resilience and ability to cope with stressors as they grow and develop.

Link To/Go To

You may want to explore the importance of early social interaction:

http://www.educationscotland.gov.uk/video/p/video_tcm4637473.asp

http://www.developingchild.net/about/history.htm

Jot This Down

Baby Joe is 3 months old. He has been admitted to a children's ward, with diarrhoea. He is likely to be on the ward for 1 or 2 days. Joe's mum and dad visit between 10a.m. and 2p.m. each day but then have to leave Joe to care for their other three children who attend nursery and school.

How would you promote communication and social interaction with baby Joe?

In the 'Jot This Down' exercise above, which introduces you to baby Joe, you might have thought about sitting down with Joe's parents; showing that you want to listen to them by smiling, making eye contact, and sitting in a relaxed way, so as not to appear rushed. If you only have limited time, say this in a positive way, 'It is really important for me to find out about the usual care you give Joe. I have 10 minutes now if that is convenient for you?'

The nurse should discuss Joe with his parents – What is his usual routine? When Joe's parents are there, what care would they like to give Joe, what care would they like the nurses to give Joe?

Make sure Joe's parents know who will be looking after Joe in their absence. One nurse per shift should be allocated to care for Joe to provide as much consistency as possible. When caring for Joe, make him feel special. Smile, coo and talk to him. Hold him closely and securely, so he feels safe. This all communicates the care that he will thrive on.

Listen to Joe, what are his cries like? Is he trying to tell you he is hungry, hot/cold, he has a soiled nappy or he wants comfort and security?

Even at this young age, Joe requires excellent communication.

Children

'Children' covers a large age range, from toddlers to 12 year olds; it is beyond the scope of this chapter to address communication issues related to each year group. Some aspects of child development are covered elsewhere in this chapter and it is clear to see that a child's language develops tremendously over the period of childhood, as does their ability to communicate through body language; listening becomes more purposeful and intuitive; social interaction opportunities increase; their knowledge improves as does their ability to understand new information. In healthcare settings, all of these factors, which influence the way in which messages are sent and received, must be taken into consideration to ensure the child feels involved and considered in communication about the care they are being offered. The United Nations Convention on the Rights of the Child (UNCRC 1989, ratified by the UK in 1992) emphasises this important point in article 12: 'When adults are making decisions that affect children, children have the right to say what they think should happen and have their opinions taken into account'.

The majority of children enjoy adult company and will be happy to communicate with them if the adult is genuine in the relationships they are seeking to build. Here are some tips for building relationships with children.

Minimise the size difference between yourself and the child, sit on a chair or on the floor, so that you can make eye contact with the child and hear what they are saying.

- Play is an essential part of the child's world and can be a useful way of 'breaking the ice' with a child
- Show an interest in what the child is doing; invite the child to tell you what is happening, rather than making an assumption from your perspective. 'This looks like an interesting game, can you tell me about it please?' rather than 'I used to love playing farms with my tractors, can I be the farmer?' If you make the wrong assumption this can create an unnecessary barrier to conversation (Howard & McInnes 2013).

Some children will not have the words to explain to you how they are feeling, or what hurts, or give you the details of an illness. Parents and carers will often fill in the details of their child's situation but this does not mean you cannot show a genuine interest in the child and pick up on any cues that the child may present, e.g. 'I don't like going to the toilet at school', respond to this and try to get more information – 'What are the toilets like at school?' This may help to explain why a child has severe constipation and abdominal pain.

Some children may find it easier to communicate while playing; provide toys, dolls that represent what the child is undergoing, e.g. a teddy bear with a cannula, and listen to what the child is explaining to the teddy bear. Is the child explaining the benefits of the cannula to the bear or are they telling the bear that it is horrible and painful, which may indicate that you need to try a different explanation so the child can be reassured that you are trying to make them better.

Even very young children may be able to paint or draw their feelings or the situation they perceive themselves to be in. For example some children have complex family arrangements and it may be very important to find out who the child sees as the important people around them. Ask them to draw their family and then sit down with them and ask questions about the child's picture.

Adults who work with children on a regular basis often appear to be 'natural' in their relationships with children of different ages but for others, it is a skill that needs to be developed. Watch the experienced people, e.g. children's nurses, play specialists, nursery nurses and listen to the interactions between child and adult and note some of the helpful phrases that are used. Prepare yourself with topics of conversation by watching popular TV programmes, reading children's literature, playing children's computer games. Another tip is to have something about you that might help you to begin a conversation with a child, e.g. a pen with a character on, paper and a pen to play a game or draw or a pack of cards to show your magician's skills. Take the opportunity to develop your skills with children by getting feedback from your mentor and reflect on your relationships with particular children.

What the Experts Say

> At the University of Central Lancashire, some of the student children's nurses are given an opportunity to develop their communication skills in local primary schools, when they run a 'Teddy bear clinic'. The children, aged 6 and 7, bring their teddy bear to school. The student nurses go to the school in uniform and take real equipment that the children are likely to encounter if they need acute healthcare, e.g. a stethoscope, thermometer, pen torch. This activity has been evaluated very positively by the students; many have commented on their increased confidence in talking to children.
>
> The teacher reported that the children had learnt about the equipment and talked about it for a long time afterwards. Some children thought they might want to be a nurse. Some Year 6 children reported that one of their highlights of school was the Teddy bear clinic. Ofsted visited one Teddy bear clinic and mentioned it in the school report as good practice!
>
> The student nurses also enjoyed the Teddy bear clinic. Their evaluations include the following statements:
>
> *I learnt that it is an important part of our role as student nurses to prepare children for hospital – in a way that is fun and age appropriate*
>
> *We still had to think about how to answer some of the questions we were asked, therefore it was reinforcing our knowledge base and developing our learning*
>
> *I enjoyed listening to the children's stories of their time in hospital*
>
> *A brilliant, hectic hour and a half!*

Young people

Many of the tips for forming a relationship with children, above, apply equally to 'young people', i.e. 13–18 years of age, but an important point to take into consideration is the natural, increasing, independence of the young person. A barrier to communication can be created if the young person feels that their opinions are not being heard or if they perceive the information they require is not being made available to them.

Jot This Down

Jodie (15 years) is awaiting a surgical review, following an appendectomy, to discuss discharge plans. Jodie has been up and dressed since 8a.m. and it is now lunchtime. When you come onto the late shift, it is reported that Jodie has been 'slamming' about all morning, abrupt and increasingly uncommunicative.

How would you go about establishing a caring, professional relationship with Jodie?

In the 'Jot This Down' exercise with the Jodie scenario, it may well be that Jodie is not receiving the information that she requires to stay calm. She may perceive she is being treated 'like a child'. An important step to establishing a relationship is to acknowledge her frustration but also to find an explanation. With an explanation, Jodie is more likely to appreciate the situation.

It is important to find some common ground when talking to younger people. Familiarise yourself with popular music, sport, magazines, internet sites, books, films, so that you can offer conversation rather than a string of questions – young people do not like to feel interrogated.

An increasingly popular way for young people to communicate is via social media networks. This media can be used to convey important messages about health and well-being if face-to-face communication cannot be established.

Children/Young People with Problems Affecting Communication

It is important to consider children/young people who may have problems which affect their ability to communicate as would be anticipated for their age, for example children with hearing or visual impairments; children with developmental disorders affecting communication, e.g. autism, and children with global developmental delay. These children require creativity when communicating with them. If a verbal approach is not possible, then other strategies must be used to convey your enthusiasm in establishing a relationship with the child.

Jot This Down

Hassan (aged 8 years of age) has profound developmental delay. He is dependent on his carers to meet all of his needs. Hassan cannot talk but he smiles and hears well.

When you meet Hassan for the first time, what can you do to communicate with him?

In relation to the 'Jot down box' concerning Hassan, before approaching Hassan take the time to get some information about him by talking to his parents or other carers who have known him for a long time, to find out about him. What makes him happy? What makes him sad? How does he communicate that information to you? What does Hassan like to do?

Approach Hassan confidently, as you would with any child, sit down, smile and talk to Hassan. Use play as a way of communicating, e.g. sensory toys, music, books. Listen to Hassan and respond to his communication with you. Is he making sounds which are conveying happiness or unhappiness?

Some children may have particular aids to assist with their communication, e.g. picture boards (Vaz 2013). Other children may use a form of sign language, such as Makaton or British sign language. It is useful to learn some of the signs, such as 'Hello', 'Goodbye', 'Where does it hurt?', in case you meet a child who uses sign language. However, if you intend to work with children who use sign language, a more detailed course would be valuable.

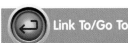

Link To/Go To

For further information about communication aids go to:

http://acecentre.org.uk/

http://www.makaton.org/

Jot This Down

When meeting a parent/carer for the first time, what steps can you take to minimise the formation of barriers and promote a rapport?

Some tips for developing a rapport with parents

Introduce yourself and your position in the team looking after the child. Sit down, make eye contact and smile. Unless it is an acute situation, make time to talk to the parents before commencing any intervention to show that you are taking a genuine interest in the family and their child.

Find out, from the parents' perspective, why the child has come into contact with the health services and what they hope to get out of the experience. Find out about the child. Explain how you may be able to support them to care for their child, or what you can offer to participate in the care of their child.

Parents/Carers

The relationship between the parent/carer and nurse can be very effective in offering the 'best' care for a child or young person but it does not 'just happen'. The professional, i.e. the 'nurse', may be perceived by the parent/carer as the expert and this can create a barrier for the parent; they may feel unsure about their role in caring for their child; unconfident about talking to a professional, particularly at initial meetings. Alternatively, the parent may be dismissive of the nurse, considering that the nurse 'does not know their child as they do', again creating a barrier to establishing a relationship.

In order to understand what it is like to care for a child who requires nursing support, there is an increasing body of research you may wish to consider, for example Williams *et al.* (2012) and Sanders *et al.* (2012) and the seminal work of Phillip Darbyshire (1994) *Living with a Sick Child in Hospital. The Experiences of Parents and Nurses.*

It is important to recognise that when communicating with a parent/carer they may have many influences on them, which can affect their communication. Great sensitivity and a professional approach are required to avoid unnecessary misunderstandings, even confrontation, in communication. Always sit down when talking to a parent/carer; show a willingness to listen and acknowledge the emotions the parent may be showing, e.g. 'You seem a bit fed up today?' This approach will encourage the parent/carer to

share their concerns with you and facilitate the open, honest communication necessary to offer the best care to the child.

Some Common Physical and Mental Health Problems

Within this part of the chapter, common physical and mental health problems for infants, children and young people will be considered. This is only a 'flavour', and signposts have been given for further information. First, the immunisation programme will be considered and then the following will be discussed:

- The febrile child
- The child with a respiratory problem
- The child with a skin problem
- The child with gastroenteritis
- Mental health and well-being of young people.

Immunisation

Significant and beneficial effects on children's health have been seen since the introduction of immunisation programmes. The World Health Organization (WHO 1981) adopted the goal of eliminating measles, poliomyelitis, neonatal tetanus, diphtheria and rubella by the year 2000. For this to be achieved in England, a primary objective of the immunisation of 90% of children had to be attained by 1995. This was met and by 1992, the target was increased to 95%. There have been challenges with the MMR immunisation due to conflicts given about the side-effects of the vaccination. In 2013, an increase of measles cases were seen in England and Wales, due to reduced uptake of the MMR immunisation. The government announced a programme to encourage older children and young people to have the vaccination (PHE 2013). Crawford (1995) found that the factors which influences parental uptake of immunisation most profoundly lies in the knowledge, confidence and overall enthusiasm of the healthcare professionals they are working with.

Jot This Down

You are working with the Health Visitor but a parent asks you about immunisations. She tells you her daughter is 6 weeks old and her other daughter is 5 years old and has just started school.

Link To/Go To

Go to the following site for information about immunisations:

https://www.gov.uk/government/collections/immunisation

You can find information to support your discussions with this parent by going to the link.

Jot This Down

Jenny asks your opinion about whether she should let her baby daughter Poppy have the MMR vaccine.

- Consider your own feelings, knowledge base beliefs and attitudes about MMR.
- Do you think that the media and other views have shaped your opinions?
- Can you give an informed opinion?

Table 11.2 Overview of childhood immunisations (UK 2013 immunisation schedule). Taken from http://www.patient.co.uk/health/immunisation-usual-uk-schedule

AGE	DISEASE TO PROTECT AGAINST	VACCINE
2 months	Diphtheria, tetanus, pertussis (whooping cough), polio and *Haemophilus influenzae* type b	DTaP/IPV(polio)/Hib all-in-one injection: Pediacel®
	Pneumococcal infection	Pneumococcal conjugate vaccine (PCV) in a separate injection: Prevenar 13®
	Rotavirus gastroenteritis	Rotavirus vaccine oral route (drops): Rotarix®
3 months	Diphtheria, tetanus, pertussis (whooping cough), polio and *Haemophilus influenzae* type b	DTaP/IPV(polio)/Hib (2nd dose: Pediacel®)
	Meningitis C	Men C in a separate injection: NeisVac-C® or Meningigate®
	Rotavirus gastroenteritis	Rotavirus vaccine oral route (drops): Rotarix®
4 months	Diphtheria, tetanus, pertussis (whooping cough), polio and *Haemophilus influenzae* type b	DTaP/IPV(polio)/Hib (3rd dose: Pediacel®)
	Pneumococcal infection	Pneumococcal conjugate vaccine (PCV) in a separate injection (2nd dose: Prevenar 13®)
Between 12 and 13 months	*Haemophilus influenzae* type b and Meningitis C	Hib/MenC combined as one injection (4th dose of Hib and 2nd dose of MenC: Menitorix®)
	Measles, mumps and rubella	MMR combined as one injection: Priorix® or MMR II®
	Pneumococcal infection	Pneumococcal conjugate vaccine (PCV) in a separate injection (3rd dose: Prevenar 13®)
3 years and 4 months to 5 years	Diphtheria, tetanus pertussis and polio	Pre-school booster of DTaP/IPV(polio) Repevax® or Infanrix-IPV®
	Measles, mumps and rubella	MMR (2nd dose: Priorix® or MMR II®)
Around 12–13 years (girls)	HPV (human papillomavirus types 16 and 18)	Three injections: Gardasil® . The second injection is given 1–2 months after the first one. The third is given about 6 months after the first one
Around 13–18 years	Tetanus, diphtheria and polio	Td/IPV(polio) booster: Revaxis®
	Meningitis C	MenC in a separate injection (booster: NeisVac® or Meningitec®)

Table 11.2 gives the normal immunisation schedule for all people in the UK – each vaccination is given as a single injection in the muscle of the thigh or the upper arm.

The Febrile Child – Febrile Convulsions

In relation to the febrile child (a child with a temperature) there are a few points to consider:

- A fever is defined as an abnormal rise in temperature usually above 37.5 degrees, although children's temperatures are higher than adult temperature
- 3% of children between 3 months and 6 years will experience a febrile convulsion – usually caused by a bacterial or viral infection
- Febrile convulsions usually occur up to the age of 7 years
- Usually last between 1–2 minutes and are generalised in nature
- If they last longer, i.e. more than 30 minutes, the child would need further investigation (Lissauer & Clayden 2011).

The Child with a Respiratory Problem

Earlier on in the chapter, the development of young children was considered. Physiologically, children aged 1–4 are more susceptible to respiratory illness due to immaturity of the respiratory system and anatomically, they have narrower airways and often enlarged adenoids and tonsils.

Upper Respiratory Tract Infections (URTI)

Around 80% of respiratory problems involve only the nose, ears and sinuses and thus cover a number of conditions such as the common cold (coryza), sore throat, acute otitis media and sinusitis (Lissauer & Clayden 2011).

The child may present with a sore throat, fever, nasal blockage and earache – these symptoms are usually accompanied by a troublesome cough. Management of these children is normally in the home environment, with possibly a visit to the GP for advice. This would usually centre upon antipyretics to bring the temperature down, such as paracetamol, rest and encouraging the intake of plenty of fluids. These symptoms can precipitate a hospital admission if the child develops a febrile convulsion (due to increasing temperature), becomes wheezy and has difficulties with breathing, activities or develops a sever upper respiratory tract infection, which may need medical and nursing interventions.

Red Flag

 Paracetamol is a commonly used medication. It is presented in many different forms, e.g. liquid, tablet, caplet, soluble tablets, and has many different proprietary names. The parents may not realise that a supermarket home brand medicine contains paracetamol. It is essential that the healthcare professional clarifies with the parents what medication they have already given to their child before giving the child further paracetamol, to avoid over-dosage.

Asthma

Asthma is a chronic inflammatory condition of the airways, and according to Kieckhefer and Ratcliffe (2000), the cause is still not completely understood. It has been described as:

An airway obstruction that is reversible with airway inflammation and an increased airway responsiveness to a variety of stimuli.

The inflammation results in a narrowing of the airway with an associated cough and wheeze. Although the cause is not completely understood, there is a variety of causative factors, which include:

- Genetic predisposition
- Environmental factors
- Parental smoking
- Exposure to allergens in infancy.

Jot This Down

Identify what types of environmental factors might increase the incidence of asthma.

 Link To/Go To

Find out how many children have been diagnosed with asthma in the UK.

http://www.asthma.org.uk

http://www.nhs.uk/Conditions/Asthma-in-children/Pages/Introduction.aspx

Diagnosis and management of asthma Diagnosis in the child under 5 is inherently difficult, mainly because wheezing and cough are really prevalent in this age group. However, generally, a diagnosis is considered if the child is being troubled by the following:

- Frequent episodes of wheezing – more than once a month
- A nocturnal cough
- Wheezing that happens in all seasons
- Symptoms persisting after the child turns 3 years of age
- Cough which is induced by activity.

 Link To/Go To

Children are introduced to the Step approach to drug management and you can find further information on this from:

http://www.sign.ac.uk/pdf/sign101.pdf

http://www.brit-thoracic.org

Management lies with focussing on controlling the underlying inflammatory response and this is achieved by using prophylactic therapy and breakthrough symptoms, which are generally treated by bronchodilators. It is really important to highlight to the child and family that asthma cannot be cured but that symptoms can be managed. The nursing aim is that symptoms are controlled well, so that the child can lead a full and active life (Kieckhefer & Ratcliffe 2000).

Jot This Down

Find out about drug therapy utilised to treat asthma:

Bronchodilators

Steroid therapy

 Link To/Go To

British Thoracic Society: http://www.brit-thoracic.org.uk

Asthma UK: http://www.asthma.org.uk

National Institute of Health and Care Excellence: http://www.nice.org.uk

Eczema

Infantile eczema is also known as 'atopic dermatitis' or 'atopic eczema'. The terms are used synonymously. *Eczema* has its origins in Greek language and it means 'to boil over'. Eczema describes itchy skin which develops into a rash of pustules, which break down and leak serous fluid. It usually appears in the first year of life but can happen to adults and children at any time in their lives. The areas most commonly affected are:

- The neck
- Flexures of the wrist and ankles
- Antecubital areas
- Popliteal areas.

Atopic eczema is an inflammation of genetically sensitive skin (National Institute for Health and Clinical Excellence, NICE 2007). Eczema is a symptom rather than a disorder. The condition in infants and children is multifactorial and indicates an over sensitivity to substances which are referred to as allergens.

The allergens gain entry into the body via the following routes:

- Digestive tract – in foods
- Inhalation of dust and pollen
- Direct contact with wool, soap, and in some cases, strong sunlight
- Injections, some insect bites, some vaccinations.

221

Jot This Down

Define the following terms in relation to the child with eczema:

Blister, erythema, excoriation, petechiae, pruritus purpura, pustule, urticarial, vesicle

Atopic eczema usually begins around 2–6 months of age and generally undergoes spontaneous remission by 3 years. This infant has a greater chance of developing dry skin and eczema in later life. Eczema can also occur in later childhood at 2–3 years and in this instance, the skin is usually healed by 5 years. Adolescent eczema can begin at about 12 years of age and continues into adulthood. Some children will develop the trio of atopic eczema, asthma and hay fever.

Signs and symptoms of atopic eczema
Signs
- Erythema
- Vesicles that weep
- Developing a dry crust
- Scaling
- Worse in winter
- The lesions are easily infected by bacteria
- Extremes of temperature, humidity and sunlight can irritate the skin.

Symptoms
- Intense itching (pruritus)
- Scratching
- Irritable
- Broken sleep patterns.
  These symptoms may worsen following immunisations.

 Link To/Go To

The National Eczema Society provide a lot information concerning incidence, triggers and treatment:

http://www.eczema.org

Principles of care in children with eczema
The main principles of care are to hydrate the child's skin, reduce the pruritus, reduce the inflammation and prevent secondary infection.

Hydrate the skin
- Give lukewarm, NOT hot baths
- Use emollient bath treatments
- Apply the emollient immediately after the bath (Spagnola & Korb 2002)
- Avoid bubble baths
- Pat the skin, DO NOT RUB.

Red Flag

 Emollients can make the bath slippery – stay with the child to prevent accidents.

Relieve pruritus
- Prevent scratching wherever possible
- Distract the child from scratching
- Keep fingernails short
- May need to put cotton gloves on the young child to stop scratching
- Avoid wool
- May use prescribed sedating antihistamines at night-time.

Reduce inflammation
- Protect skin from excessive moisture
- Avoid overheating
- Limit exposure to dust, cigarettes smoke and pollens
- Recognise and limit emotional stressors
- Flare-ups may need pharmacological intervention – topical steroids/wet wraps.

Prevent secondary infection
- Recognition of skin infections – seeking prompt treatment.

 Link To/Go To

Have a look at the systematic review of atopic eczema treatments at:

http://www.ncbi.nlm.nih.gov/pubmed/11134919

Secondary infections can be treated by systemic antibiotics.

Gastroenteritis
Acute gastroenteritis in children and young people is characterised by the sudden onset of diarrhoea and/or vomiting and also includes a variety of other symptoms, including poor appetite, general fever and abdominal cramps. The vast majority of cases are caused by rotavirus, although there can be bacterial and also parasitic causes.

The results of gastroenteritis can be very serious, particularly in infancy and early childhood because loss of fluid will affect the fluid balance of the child. This is primarily due to an increased metabolic rate and the distribution of extracellular and intracellular fluid.

Gastroenteritis should be treated with oral rehydration for around 3–4 hours with a resumption of normal feeding following this. The management of severe dehydration caused by gastroenteritis would need more intensive treatment by intravenous fluids.

Jot This Down

Undertake an internet search for causative organisms of gastroenteritis

Table 11.3 Causative organisms of gastroenteritis.

CAUSATIVE ORGANISM	SIGNS
Rotavirus	Severe diarrhoea, watery frequent stool, nausea and vomiting
Adenovirus	Diarrhoea – also linked to URTI
Hepatitis A	Fever, malaise, nausea and jaundice
Campylobacter	Pyrexia, abdominal pain, watery foul smelling diarrhoea, which may contain blood
Salmonella	Rapid onset, nausea, vomiting, pain, diarrhoea contains blood and pus
Shigella	High fever, cramping pain, watery diarrhoea with mucous and blood
Escherichia coli	Gradual or sudden onset, explosive watery green diarrhoea pyrexia and abdominal distension
Escherichia coli 157	Colitis, bloody diarrhoea and sever abdominal cramps

Organisms will spread, particularly in areas such as nurseries and schools but competent hand washing is a very effective method of reducing the incidence of gastroenteritis.

Table 11.3 highlights specific causative organisms and gives an overview of the presenting signs from the child.

Mental Health and Well-Being in Young People

Earlier the development of young people was considered and the vast physical changes the young person deals with was highlighted. There are other inherent pressures; peer pressure, examination stress and some young people may be acting in a caring role within their family unit. There is not sufficient scope within this chapter to examine, in significant depth, the health challenges which face young people but it is useful to consider specific policy documents that influence the health care of young people and provide an insight into some of their health challenges.

> **Jot This Down**
>
> Look in more depth at some of the challenges young people face, e.g. alcohol misuse, eating disorders and depressive illnesses.

The main policy documents which frame the health care of young people are:

- *Bridging the Gaps: healthcare for adolescents* (RCPCH 2003)
- *National Service Framework for Children, Young People and Maternity Services* (DH 2004)
- *Every Child Matters* (DfES 2004)
- *Youth Matters* (DfES 2005).

For young people the main factors which contribute towards health risk behaviours are closely related to factors which can contribute to emotional distress and mental health problems. Adolescence is also considered a time when patterns of health behaviour and the use of health services are developed. Mortality among young people has not fallen significantly over the last 50 years. The main causes of mortality in young people are accidents and self-harm, with a worrying rise in suicide among young men (RCPCH 2003).

> **Jot This Down**
>
> What makes us mentally healthy?
> Think back to your own adolescence and jot down any factors which affected your mental well-being.
> How did you maintain your mental health?

The list below is not exhaustive but gives a flavour of which attributes relate to young people being mentally healthy. The policy documents referred to above look to some of these factors when considering what services should look like and why the young people need skilled staff who are able to interpret their worries and concerns.

- Self-esteem
- Physical growth
- Emotional growth
- Resilience
- Ability to make good personal relationships
- A sense of right and wrong
- The motivation to face setbacks and learn from them
- A sense of belonging
- A belief in their ability to cope
- A way through solving problems.

It has been identified that certain factors increase the young persons' resilience in the face of specific stressors. It is also generally considered that the interplay of risk and protective factors determines whether the adolescent overcomes the stressors that they face. In certain situations, the stressors may be so great that they cannot be overcome.

> **The Evidence**
>
> Cooper (cited in Glasper & Richardson 2006) summarises the factors within the young person, family unit and the environment, which enhance resilience.

Factors which enhance resilience within the young person:

- Being female
- More intelligent
- A secure attachment as an infant
- Easy temperament when an infant
- Positive attitude – problem-solving approach
- Good communication skills
- Planner
- Strong faith
- Capacity to reflect.

Factors which enhance resilience within the family unit:

- At least one good parent–child relationship
- Affection
- Supervision – authoritative/discipline
- Support for education
- Supportive marriage/relationship

Factors which enhance resilience within the environment:

- Wider supportive network
- Good housing

- High standards of living
- High school/college with moral and positive attitude with policies for behaviour attitudes and bullying
- Schools/colleges with strong academic opportunities
- Schools/colleges with non-academic opportunities
- A range of sport and leisure activities
- Appropriate relationships with adults.

Within society, maintaining good mental health for the population of young people is crucial because of the strong links there are to health risk behaviours. Poor mental health can have an effect on exercise patterns, eating behaviours and sexual activities in young people. The challenges for healthcare professionals can lie with obesity/eating disorders and body image, substance misuse and sexual behaviours.

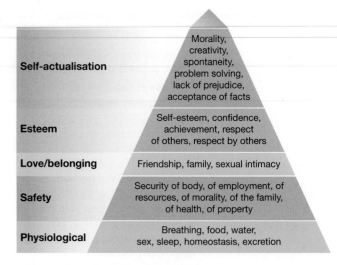

Figure 11.3 **Maslow's hierarchy of need.**

Jot This Down
Undertake an internet search in relation to the incidence of hospital admission in the under 16s for alcohol abuse

Jot This Down
Search around the use of illegal drugs and substances – note the short-term side-effects of taking them and the long-term health effects

Red Flag

Key considerations as you work with young people:
- Depressive illnesses are very common in adolescence
- In early adolescence (11–14 years), there are high rates of conduct and emotional disorders
- Mid to late adolescence is the peak time for the onset of depressive disorders
- Self-injury and self-harm – deliberate self-harm is common in adolescent girls. The peak age for presentation to services is 15–24 for females
- Eating disorders, e.g. anorexia nervosa and bulimia, which affect more females than males
- Attempted suicide – the rate is low under 14 years of age. It begins to occur around 12 years and then increases in the early and mid-teens. Young men are more at risk and are less likely than girls to show any distress before the suicide attempt.

Jot This Down
Jake is 15 and admitted to your unit. He is admitted following ingestion of alcohol and drugs.

As the admitting nurse, you are a little taken a back at the amount of alcohol he has taken and also his knowledge about illegal drugs. He has a difficult family history, in that his mum is not around and Jake acts as a carer for his dad, who suffers from a neurological disorder.

1. Consider what Jake most needs from the nurse and the health agencies at this time
2. Consider his situation and list the risk factors which may be impacting on his life at present
3. Outline short- and longer-term goals to reduce Jake's health risk behaviours and describe the role of the multi-agency team who will be working with Jake.

Basic/Fundamental Care Needs

This section discusses meeting the fundamental care needs of infants, children and young people.

Jot This Down
What do you think the fundamental care needs of infants, children and young people are?

For the purposes of this chapter, the term 'Fundamental care needs' are those needs that have to be met in order for the child to thrive. The aspects to be considered are: *physiological needs*, i.e. air, food, water, warmth; and *safety needs*, i.e. security, freedom from fear. These are loosely based on Maslow's hierarchy of need (Figure 11.3).

The fundamental care needs of a child are usually attended to by their parents or carers. As the child grows and develops, they take on more responsibility for meeting their own needs and the guidance from their parents decreases. If there is concern that a parent/carer is not attending to the fundamental needs of the child, then the child may be considered to be neglected (DfE 2013). This is a serious issue, which will be discussed in more detail later within the chapter, hence the importance of nurses attending to the fundamental needs of the infant, child or young person. For the purposes of this section, it will be assumed that the infant, child or young person is an inpatient within a ward environment, possibly without a parent/carer present.

Meeting the Fundamental Care Needs of Infants

From 0–1 year of age, the infant is totally dependent on their parent or carer to meet their fundamental care needs except, usually, for the need of air. The process of birth ensures that the baby very quickly becomes self-sufficient in inhaling air and exhaling the by-products of respiration. However, the airways of an infant are very small and if they have increased mucosal secretions for any reason, they may need assistance to meet the fundamental need for air, most specifically oxygen.

Very young babies breathe almost exclusively through the nose, so hard, crusty secretions will obstruct their tiny airways. When caring for the infant, every effort should be made to remove nasal secretions, which are clearly obstructing the baby's nasal air passage. **Note**: only remove secretions which can be removed by wiping the base of the nose with a tissue. If it appears that the nasal passages and upper airways are becoming obstructed with secretions, suctioning may be required.

Red Flag

 Nasal and upper airway suction should only be performed by individuals who have been assessed as competent to do so, as a poor technique can lead to mucosal irritation and damage and, therefore, the production of further secretions (Macqueen *et al.* 2012, p. 640).

Infants may also require oxygen therapy if they have an illness, which means they are unable to take sufficient oxygen into their body to meet their physiological needs, i.e. hypoxia. Oxygen therapy can be delivered most effectively to young infants via an incubator. Within an incubator the ambient oxygen concentration can be controlled as can the humidity of the oxygen. It is beyond the scope of this chapter to discuss the care of the infant in an incubator in detail but readers are directed to Meeks and Hallsworth (2010).

As the infant gets older, beyond 5 months, an incubator may not be appropriate. In this situation, oxygen may be delivered via nasal cannula, via a headbox (Figure 11.4) and for short periods, by holding a facial oxygen mask close to the infants face, e.g. while the infant is feeding or eating (Macqueen *et al.* 2012, p. 644).

Red Flag

 Oxygen is classed as a medicine and must be prescribed. The administration of oxygen must adhere to Trust policies and procedures.

Caring for an infant who requires oxygen demands accurate observational skills to spot signs of deterioration or distress and these will be discussed elsewhere in the chapter. Nursing assessments must be made to consider the infants other fundamental needs, while receiving the oxygen. For example feeding the infant must be considered, monitoring the infant safely, attending to hygiene needs and, very importantly, ensuring the parents/carers can continue to care for and comfort the infant. If possible, care should be organised around the parent/carer availability, to ensure they can participate in feeds, nappy changes and cuddles.

The focus of this section will now move on to the consideration of meeting the other fundamental needs that an infant may have. To facilitate this, consider the case of Maryam (Figure 11.5).

225

Jot This Down

Maryam is 8 months old. She has been in hospital for 1 day and her condition is improving; she is likely to go home later today. You have taken over her care at 7.30a.m. and Maryam's mum is due to arrive at 12 noon.

What are Maryam's fundamental care needs and how will you attend to them?

I need food!

At 8 months Maryam will be 'weaned', she will probably have cereal or toast for breakfast, mashed food for lunch and tea. Fruit snacks in between, e.g. mashed banana. Maryam will want to feed herself with assistance. She must be supervised at all times as she will not be able to recognise food that may cause her to choke. 'I love water with my meals'. Maryam will still have baby milk (breast or formula, before bed).

I need to be warm too!

Maryam will need to be dressed in clothes that will keep her warm but also enable her to move freely. No loose buttons, no tapes or cords.

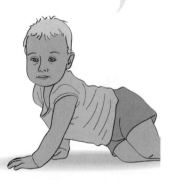

I need to feel safe and secure while my mum is away
This is a very strange place!

Ideally Maryam will have the same nurse caring for her. She needs constant supervision when out of her cot. She can crawl and will be keen to explore. When Maryam is in her cot the sides should be fully raised and securely fastened. If she is in a pushchair or highchair all of the fastenings should be in place. Maryam will enjoy sitting with her nurse, looking at books or playing, this will make her feel safe and secure. It is essential that strangers do not approach or pick up Maryam. She is totally dependent on the healthcare team to look after her while her mum is away.

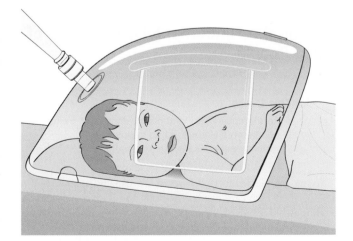

Figure 11.4 An infant receiving headbox oxygen.

Figure 11.5 Maryam's fundamental care needs.

Link To/Go To

For lots of practical advice on caring for infants go to:
http://www.nhs.uk/Tools/Pages/birthtofive.aspx
http://www.netmums.com/

Meeting the Fundamental Care Needs of Children

During childhood, 1–12 years, children begin to take a much more active role in meeting their fundamental care needs but close supervision and adult input remain an important aspect of caring for children in this age group. Whatever the age of the child, the nurse should encourage them to actively participate in meeting their fundamental needs; this is important for the child's development, as they work towards independence.

The Nursing and Midwifery Council (NMC 2010) recognise the importance of safe and competent nursing care.

Nursing Fields Nursing Practice and Decision-Making

Children's nurses must be able to care safely and effectively for children and young people in all settings, and recognise their responsibility for safeguarding them. They must be able to deliver care to meet essential and complex physical and mental health needs informed by deep understanding of biological, psychological and social factors throughout infancy, childhood and adolescence (NMC 2010).

As with infants, the child is largely independent when meeting their requirement for air. However, 1 in 11 children have asthma and one child is admitted to hospital every 18 minutes with asthma (Asthma UK 2013), so prompt, effective management of a wheeze in childhood is essential. This will include the administration of broncho-dilating inhalers or nebulisers and the appropriate administration of oxygen.

Red Flag

All medications must be prescribed and checked, according to the Trust policy and guidelines, before administering to the child.

As children get older, they are more likely to tolerate face mask oxygen but younger children, i.e. 1–4 years may find this very difficult, particularly when awake. The nurse needs to use her creative skills to encourage the young child to sit quietly and at least allow the oxygen to waft via oxygen tubing. Parents and carers can be very supportive and perhaps if they sit and cuddle the young child, the oxygen can be administered. Plenty of distractions are required to occupy the young child, e.g. books, TV, DVDs, bubble machines, light projection machines.

Other fundamental care needs to consider are similar to those of the infant, i.e. food, water, warmth, safety, security, freedom from fear, but the approach taken to meet them will differ with the age of the child.

Of course I need food and drink but I will be able to tell you what I like or if I am hungry or thirsty. I am really interested in how my body works and trying to keep healthy so if you have any information about this I would be happy to listen.

One of my friends has diabetes and she gets a bit fed up with it, she eats sweets even though she shouldn't. If she was in hospital you would really need to help her to stick to her healthy eating!

My favourite nurse is Lisa. She gives me jobs to do and just seems to know when I am not feeling well, or I am in pain. If mum's not here Lisa makes sure I get ready for bed properly and turns the lights off at a good time.

At 10 years of age Emily still likes routine to make her feel secure.

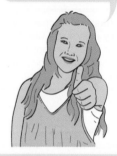

I get a bit bored in hospital if I don't have anything to do. I like it if other children are in around my own age because we can talk about school and guides and stuff. My mum lets me have my mobile so I can keep in touch with my friends.

I sometimes get nervous if there are noisy families around, that's when I really need to know where the nurses are.

Figure 11.6 Emily's fundamental care needs.

Jot This Down

You have been allocated two children to look after. Emily is 10 years old (Figure 11.6) and Josh is 3 years old (Figure 11.7). They are both well enough to be up and about out of bed. Both children have parents who are usually on the ward.

What are Emily and Josh's fundamental care needs and how will you attend to them?

Meeting the Fundamental Care Needs of Young People

Jot This Down

What are the advantages and disadvantages of caring for young people on children's wards in hospitals?

Young people from 13–18 years are usually independent at meeting their own care needs. They can find it extremely difficult to relinquish this independence, even when very unwell. The strong desire for independence should be encouraged and nurtured while receiving health care, unless this is contraindicated by the young person's health needs or illness. During this age spectrum, the

Mum or dad stay with me at night usually and then I feel safe. If they can't stay it is best if I go to sleep and have my teddies around me. If I wake up at night it is best if there is a nurse I know. They ask me to wear a bracelet so they know my name and birthday.

I am Josh and I need a little bit to eat and drink every two or three hours. I don't eat or drink much because I get fed up with it!

Mum sometimes gets a bit frustrated with me because I don't always want to eat what she gives me.

Getting dressed can be a bit of a nuisance but I always like to try and put my socks on, trouble is I get fed up and wander off to watch TV before I get my tee-shirt on!

At 3 years Josh will need guidance about what to wear but it is essential that he is offered some choice and time to try things himself.

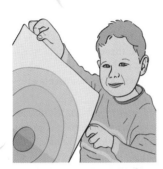

Hospital is a very strange place! I get a bit worried about some of the things I have to do such as a 'temperature' but most nurses make me giggle while they are doing it!

My favourite place is the play room because it is a bit like nursery. I get really worried if mum goes to get her tea but if she leaves her handbag and a nurse sits with me and reads me a story I can cope.

Figure 11.7 Josh's fundamental care needs.

young person is naturally decreasing their reliance on parents/carers and building strong relationships with their peers. Every effort should be made to help the young person maintain contact with their friends by allowing the use of mobile phones and internet access but the safety of all people using the healthcare services need to be considered and sometimes, an open discussion with young people is required to ensure they understand any rules that may be in place in the healthcare setting.

Young people, or adolescents, have been acknowledged as a group with particular needs. As they move through a potentially turbulent period of their life contact, with healthcare services can be an added challenge for them. Healthcare professionals can do a lot to minimise this challenge by ensuring young people have privacy, are included in all decisions about themselves and are encouraged to express their opinions. The Royal College of Nursing has produced some general guidance about caring for adolescents (RCN 2007). Some services have developed Teenage Units in recognition of the unique needs of this age group (Teenage Cancer Trust 2012) but Dodds (2010) argues that a lot can be done without major financial investment to offer good care to young people using healthcare services.

An important aspect of the fundamental care of young people, is to ensure that they are competent to make decisions about their healthcare, i.e. to consent or refuse treatment.

Jot This Down

Consider these two situations:

Paul is 16 years old, he has fractured his elbow while playing rugby. He needs prompt surgery to stabilise the fracture. His parents are away on holiday and cannot get back for 12 hours. Paul was staying with a friend and his parents are not contactable. Could consent for the surgery be taken from Paul? What will influence your thoughts about this situation?

Naeve is 14 years old, she has also sustained a fracture of her elbow, which needs prompt surgery to stabilise the fracture. Naeve has had an excessive amount of alcohol and she is refusing to tell you her parent's telephone number and insisting that she gives permission for the operation to go ahead.

Could consent for the surgery be taken from Naeve? What will influence your thoughts about this situation?

There is a legal framework which guides whether consent can be taken from a young person or not. The main considerations are:

- What is in the best interest of the child? This may require a consideration of what benefits will come from the procedure and what harm may be caused by the procedure
- Is the young person cognitively competent to consent to treatment? Does the child fully understand the potential benefits of the procedure and the potential risks?

Assessments in relation to the above questions largely rely upon a discussion between the medical and nursing staff, the young person and the parents. This can be a complex subject and dilemmas in practice can arise. The General Medical Council (GMC 2007) have produced guidance which is a useful resource.

Above the fundamental care needs of infants, children and young people have been considered. The discussion has focussed on children who are progressing as expected developmentally and who have a short-term illness. It is important to consider those children for whom chronological age does not correspond with their developmental age and those children with chronic illness.

Each infant, child or young person is of course unique and children with complex care needs are no exception. It is important to listen to the family about the fundamental care needs that the child may require, so that appropriate nursing care can be offered.

Jot This Down

Imran is 13 years old. He has global developmental delay, due to a rare genetic disorder. Imran has a poor swallow reflex and so he has gastrostomy feeds, he has occasional seizures, he moves very little and is fully dependent on his carers to meet all of his needs.

How would you ensure that Imran received excellent fundamental care?

Issues you should have considered in discussion with Imran's carers:

- Due to a poor swallowing reflex, Imran is vulnerable to obstructing his airway with secretions. He needs to have suction and oxygen available at all times
- Imran may not be able to have any foods or drinks orally, or only drinks and foods of a particular consistency. This measure is to

prevent Imran aspirating the food or drink, i.e. because of a poor swallowing reflex food and drink may enter the trachea rather than the oesophagus and lead to airway obstruction or a chest infection

- Gastrostomy feeds must be given as per the dietician's protocol. Staff must be suitably trained in caring for a child with a gastrostomy *in situ*
- Imran is dependent on carers to meet his hygiene needs. He will need washing, mouth care and frequent nappy area care to prevent excoriation of the skin. **Note:** Ensure Imran has privacy and is treated with dignity when attending to hygiene needs
- Imran is unable to move himself, so he will require frequent position changes to prevent the development of pressure ulcers, to promote circulation, prevent stiffness and to ensure comfort
- Safety must be a priority at all times. Imran must have sides on his bed to prevent him falling from bed. When moving Imran from bed to chair, an appropriate hoist must be used safely. When sat in his chair, all of the fastenings must be made to prevent falling. Care must be taken not to have the fastenings too tight and not to trap Imran's skin or clothes when securing the fasteners
- Anticonvulsant medication must be given as prescribed to minimise the risk of seizures. Rescue medication must be easily available in case Imran has prolonged seizures.

Red Flag

Oxygen is classed as a drug and must be prescribed. The administration of oxygen must adhere to Trust policies and procedures.

Nasal and upper airway suction should only be performed by individuals who have been assessed as competent to do so as a poor technique can lead to mucosal irritation and damage and, therefore, the production of further secretions (Macqueen *et al.* 2012, p. 640).

Meeting the fundamental needs of any infant, child or young person is an essential and fulfilling nursing activity. The extent to which a parent/carer, child, young person or nurse meets the child's needs must be discussed with all parties and negotiated when the child is in a healthcare setting. Nurses need to willingly learn about the fundamental care needs of each infant, child or young person, so that they can effectively participate in their care.

The Importance of Acting to Protect Infants, Children and Young People

The way in which a society treats its children is perhaps the best measure of its humanity.

(Lord Laming 2003)

Protecting infants, children and young people is everybody's responsibility. Children are the future of any society and hold the aspirations for its future. Child protection is a very sensitive area, which touches all elements of society. Hobart (2009) suggests that child maltreatment is the biggest cause of morbidity in children. Within this part of the chapter, a brief overview of the legal framework safeguarding children will be provided. Definitions of harm will be provided and the importance of parenting will be explored

to enable you to recognise the importance of protecting children across the age spectrum. Further help and support is signposted within the chapter.

Legal and Policy Framework

The legal framework relating to safeguarding sits within the legal definition of childhood which is embodied within:

- The Children Act [1989] and [2004] – England and Wales
- The Children [Scotland] Act [1995]
- The Children [Northern Ireland] Order [1995]

Moving on from the legal framework safeguarding policies, which support and guide safeguarding practices have been developed separately in England, Wales, Northern Ireland and Scotland and all these have encompassed similar principles relating to children's rights.

These key documents are:

England

Department for Education (DfE 2013). *Working Together to Safeguard Children. A Guide to Inter-Agency Working to Safeguard and Promote the Welfare of Children*, DfE, London.

Wales

All Wales area Child Protection Committees (2005). *All Wales Child Protection Procedures,* Wales Child Protection Review Group, Cardiff.

Scotland

Scottish Executive (2004) *Protecting Children and Young People: framework for standards*, Scottish Executive, Edinburgh.

Northern Ireland

Department of Health, Social Services and Public Safety (DHSSPS 2003) *Co-Operating to Safeguard Children*, DHSSPS, Belfast.

All the above policies incorporate Articles 3 and 6 of the United Nations Convention on the Rights of the Child (UNCRC 1989). Article 6 refers to every child having an inherent right to life and the article highlights that States and Governments are obliged to use every possible means within their disposal to ensure this. Article 3 concerns best interests and refers to Governments ensuring that if children's best interests are not being served by the parents or those with parental responsibility, then the authorities need to provide that care in the family unit or away from the family unit.

Jot This Down

| Undertake an internet search using Safeguarding |
| Children as your key words. |
| What concepts does your search engine unearth? |
| What are your client groups? |

In 2003, the English government commissioned a consultation of children and young people to ask what they viewed their needs were in relation to growing and developing and living fulfilled lives. From this consultation, five outcomes were adopted and these form the foundation for policies in relation to safeguarding children – they also contributed to the Children Act (2004).

Those five areas are:

1. *Be healthy*
2. *Stay safe*
3. *Enjoy and achieve through learning*

4. *Make a positive contribution to society*
5. *Achieve economic well-being.*

(Every Child Matters, DfES 2004)

Safeguarding is everyone's responsibility and the legal framework and policy underpinnings give you some insight into the enormous task that this is. It is also useful to consider that everyone approaches safeguarding based on a value set that they have developed over their lifetime, their experiences of being parented and their interactions and experiences. Some consequences from safeguarding children are very clear cut – others sometimes less so – look at the scenarios below and consider whether the behaviour described gives you concerns in relation to safeguarding activity – would you report this further?

Jot This Down

A 4-year-old in reception at school often comes to school not washed and not having had breakfast

An 8-year-old is left alone often to care for her mother who has a chronic illness

A teacher at primary school often shouts at a child in their class telling him he is useless

A 13-year-old girl is having sex with her 17 year old boyfriend

A pregnant mother is using heroin and cocaine during her pregnancy

A stressed dad caring for his children on his own hits one of his children and causes marks and bruising

A 10-year-old with hearing aids misses two of his appointments with the audiology team

As a student nurse, your interpretation of areas for concern may not always be corresponding with that of your clinical mentor but every opportunity should be taken to discuss any concerns and learn from experienced people around you. Parenting forms a central tenant of safeguarding, as parents or guardians are entrusted to provide safety for children and keep them from harm. A key part of safeguarding children is judging whether the parents are 'good enough' parents.

Deciding whether parents are 'good enough' can be challenging for all staff involved with the care of children and young people. Student nurses need to consider the concept of 'good enough parenting' but remember that the 'good enough' standard is affected by social and cultural norms. Munro (2011) points out that professionals may become accustomed to poor standards of parenting and then sometimes accept them as normal or 'good enough', with devastating consequences for children.

Categories of Abuse

There are four categories of abuse under the current legislation (DfE 2013). Below are the definitions provided by this guidance document.

Physical abuse

This may involve hitting, shaking, throwing, poisoning, burning or scalding, drowning, suffocating or otherwise causing physical harm to a child. Physical harm can also be caused when a parent/guardian fabricate the symptoms of or deliberately induces an illness in a child.

Emotional abuse

This is the persistent emotional maltreatment of the child, which causes severe and persistent adverse effects on the child's emotional development. It may involve conveying to the child that they are unloved, inadequate or worthless. It may include age or developmentally inappropriate expectations imposed upon the child. It may also involve seeing or hearing the maltreatment of somebody else. It may involve children feeling frightened or in danger.

Sexual abuse

Sexual abuse involves forcing or enticing a child or young person to take part in sexual activities including prostitution, whether or not the child knows what is happening. The activities can include physical contact, including penetrative and non-penetrative acts. They can also include non-contact acts, such as involving children looking at or be involved in the production of pornographic material or watching sexual activities.

Neglect

Neglect is defined as the persistent failure to meet a child's physical and/or psychological needs, likely to result in the serious impairment of the child's health and development. Neglect may occur in pregnancy as a result of maternal substance abuse. Once a child is born, it may involve a parent failing to provide adequate food or clothing and shelter. It may also involve failing to protect from physical harm or failure, to ensure access to appropriate medical care. It may also include neglect of a child's basic emotional needs.

Jot This Down

You are undertaking a placement with the School Nurse and attend school with the Nurse to observe the immunisations programme. Holly attends with her friend and you notice that she is very quiet but think she may be a bit nervous. You also notice that she has some bruising to her cheek and a couple of small bruises on her earlobes. She cannot have the immunisation as her consent form has not been signed. She goes back to class. The School Nurse discusses your concerns with the class teacher, who advises that Holly's mum has just started a new relationship and the man has moved into their flat.

What are your concerns?

It would be expected that a referral would be made by the School Nurse in relation to the above scenario. There are developmental pointers which relate to a withdrawn quiet child, and also physical pointers which relate to the bruises on her cheek and also on her earlobes.

Professional Advice

The following are the main organisations and individuals concerned with safeguarding and protecting children:

- Social Services
- The Police
- Health Visitors, Schools Nurses, Midwives, GPs and Practice Nurses

229

- Paediatricians, Psychologists, Nurses – Allied Health Professionals
- Addiction Services
- Named Nurses for Child Protection
- Education – Early Years workers, Teachers at primary and secondary school
- Sure Start
- Voluntary Organisations
- Probation Service
- Youth Offending Teams
- Lawyers
- Foster Carers.

As a student nurse, you will be supported with any concerns you discuss with your mentor. This entire area causes anxiety to new and also experienced healthcare practitioners alike. There have been a number of serious case reviews (Davies & Ward 2012), which have set out messages for all healthcare professionals. These key messages highlight that all healthcare professionals should be aware of the myriad of factors that could indicate a child is in need and these should always be discussed, not dismissed. The other vital key message is that all healthcare professionals should follow policies at National level and protocols at Local level, to make sure a full accurate picture is painted and that support is given for a positive outcome for the child and family unit.

Link To/Go To Child Protection Helplines and Websites

ChildLine (24 hours) 0800 1111; **http://www.childline.org.uk**

Family Rights Group 0808 801 0366; **http://www.frg.org.uk/**

Kidscape (9.30a.m.–5.30p.m. Monday–Friday) 020 7730 3300; **http://www.kidscape.org.uk**

NSPCC Child Protection Line (24 hours) 0808 800 500; e-mail: help@nspcc.org.uk; **http://www.nspcc.org.uk**

Chapter 8 of this text discusses issues concerning Safeguarding in a more general manner.

Identifying the Signs of Deterioration in General Health

Jot This Down

The discussion in this section is about identifying signs of deterioration in the general health of infants, children and young people. What kinds of illnesses may affect infants, children and young people and lead to a deterioration in their health?

Assessing the General Health of Children

In a previous section of this chapter, the fundamental health needs of children and young people were discussed. In this section, it is acknowledged that healthcare practitioners will often come into contact with children and young people when they are unwell. The spectrum of 'unwell' is vast: children with asthma, diarrhoea and vomiting, appendicitis, rashes, head injury, burns – the potential list of illness is phenomenal. The majority of children will be supported appropriately, during their illness, by their parents/carers, GPs, paramedics; acute hospitals services, and recover to full health. However, the Office of National Statistics (ONS 2013) released the Child Mortality Statistics (2011), which shows that infants, children and young people die in the UK from a variety of acute, chronic and genetic illnesses and accidents. The prevention of childhood death is not always a realistic option; however, in the majority of cases, it can be a realistic option but the infant, child and young people are reliant upon the people around them to recognise deterioration in their condition and respond accordingly and promptly to support them.

It is not possible to cover this entire topic in one section of a chapter, so the focus will be upon the nurse's role in the recognition of the deterioration of physical health in infants, children and young people with an acute onset illness. The Nursing and Midwifery Council (NMC 2010) recognise the importance of safe and competent nursing care from all nurses to all age groups. This section is concerned with the generic skills mentioned by the NMC, rather than the specialist skills of the Children's nurse.

Nursing Fields Nursing Practice and Decision-Making

All nurses must assess and meet the full range of essential physical and mental health needs of people of all ages who come into their care.

All nurses must be able to recognise and interpret signs of normal and deteriorating mental and physical health and respond promptly to maintain or improve the health and comfort of the service user, acting to keep them and others safe.

Particular skills are required from those nurses working in the Children's field of nursing.

Children's nurses must carry out comprehensive nursing assessments of children and young people, recognising the particular vulnerability of infants and young children to rapid physiological deterioration.

In order to recognise physical deterioration in an infant, child or young person, it is important to assess them at the time of admission so a 'baseline' can be recorded. From this baseline, it can be seen whether the child improves, stays the same or deteriorates. Also from this 'baseline' assessment, the nurse can begin to plan and administer appropriate care, reassessing regularly to evaluate the child's response. This cycle of assessment, planning, intervention and evaluation is commonly known as the Nursing Process and it is a useful approach to nursing, particularly if a child's condition is changing rapidly (Ellson 2008). The whole process may be done in conjunction with other healthcare professionals but it is often the nurse who spends prolonged periods with the child and family and so it is essential that the nursing assessment is thorough, systematic and reliable.

Assessment is both subjective and objective, it needs to take account of the child's physical health, mental health, developmental achievements, usual activities of living, family situation, presenting problems and any relevant past health history. To do a thorough assessment of all these aspects of the child's health requires time and the development of a trusting relationship between the nurse, child and family. However, in the acute situation, the nurse must prioritise her assessment approach. If a child is acutely unwell, then the nurse needs an assessment approach to quickly identify the child's physical status, i.e. their baseline – this is the priority. Having assessed the child's physical status, the nurse can alert other healthcare professionals to the findings and then appropriate interventions can be put into place to support the child's physical status, with the goal of preventing deterioration. Once the child is physically stable, a more detailed, general assessment can be undertaken.

A systematic approach to the assessment of an acutely ill child is suggested in Figure 11.8. This assessment is based upon the 'ABCDE' approach recommended by the Advanced Life Support Group (ALSG 2011) in the care of the seriously ill child (Figure 11.8). It is not anticipated that the readers of this chapter will have the knowledge and skills to perform the comprehensive assessments recommended by the ALSG, rather they can use this approach to make a baseline assessment and summon help quickly and appropriately if they are at all concerned by the child's physical health status.

In order to undertake a reliable assessment, it is important to use appropriate techniques to, for example, take the heart rate of an infant which requires a stethoscope, and assess the pain of a young child. The Royal College of Nursing (RCN 2011) have produced some useful standards for assessing children, and Gormley-Fleming (2010) provides a comprehensive review of the assessment of children and the expected 'normal' values of the vital signs, i.e. temperature, pulse, respiratory rate and blood pressure, for children of different ages.

 Link To/Go To

https://www.spottingthesickchild.com/

An important aspect of the assessment, is assessing the child's effort of breathing. This is about assessing whether the child is using their accessory muscles in order to breathe, i.e. intercostal and subcostal muscles. If they are, you will be able to see the child's head 'bobbing', between their ribs appearing to be 'sucked' in. These features are often most pronounced in the younger child.

 Link To/Go To

The following videos may help you when assessing the child's respiratory effort:

http://www.youtube.com/watch?v=-4OhWQ8Ppko Stridor and respiratory distress in the infant

http://www.youtube.com/watch?v=sJLHiTaXrtc Child with respiratory distress

The above approach will assist you in assessing the infant, child and young person but it is essential that you report any concerns, or difficulties with the assessment to a senior nurse or doctor. You should also document your findings and report these to the senior nurse.

In order to ensure a systematic and consistent approach to assessing infants, children and young people, and encourage the early raising of concerns, many clinical areas now use a tool known as Paediatric Early Warning Scores (PEWS). This is a chart which facilitates the recording of a variety of the observations suggested in the above assessment process, in one place. From those observations, a score is achieved. If the score increases as the observations are repeated over time, this alerts the healthcare professional to a potentially deteriorating child. As the PEWS charts have developed, there has been concern that they were not always completed thoroughly, the trigger point for seeking help was not always clear and staff did not always complete the observations correctly, therefore affecting the PEWS score. However, the NHS Institute for Innovation and Improvement have created a central repository for PEWS charts, education and guidance, to promote a consistent and effective approach to assessing infants, children and young people.

 Link To/Go To

Visit the NHS Institute for Innovation and Improvement website to find a range of resources relating to the assessment of infants, children and young people using PEWS:

http://www.institute.nhs.uk/safer_care/paediatric_safer_care/pews.html

If the child is acutely unwell, they can deteriorate quickly from the baseline observations, particularly if supportive measures are not put in place in a timely and appropriate manner, e.g. administering oxygen, fluids, medication. Having undertaken an assessment, it is important to keep reassessing the child to monitor for signs of improvement or deterioration. If the cause of the illness is known, the path of the child's illness may be anticipated but every child is individual and so the early signs of deterioration need to be identified.

Jot This Down

James is 6 months old. He has been admitted with a 2-day history of diarrhoea and vomiting. On admission, he is alert and smiling but continues to have several small vomits and two dirty nappies.

Samina is 5 years old. She has a temperature and a cough. Her voice is very husky. She is reluctant to eat and drink and she looks miserable.

Moira is 13 years old. She has abdominal pain and she is reluctant to walk about.

What would alert you to the physical deterioration of these children?

Box 11.3, Box 11.4 and Box 11.5 highlight the possible signs of deterioration in the 'Jot This Down' scenarios.

In these three scenarios, robust, systematic assessment which is on-going from the initial baseline assessment, will assist with the successful management of the children. The assessment will lead to

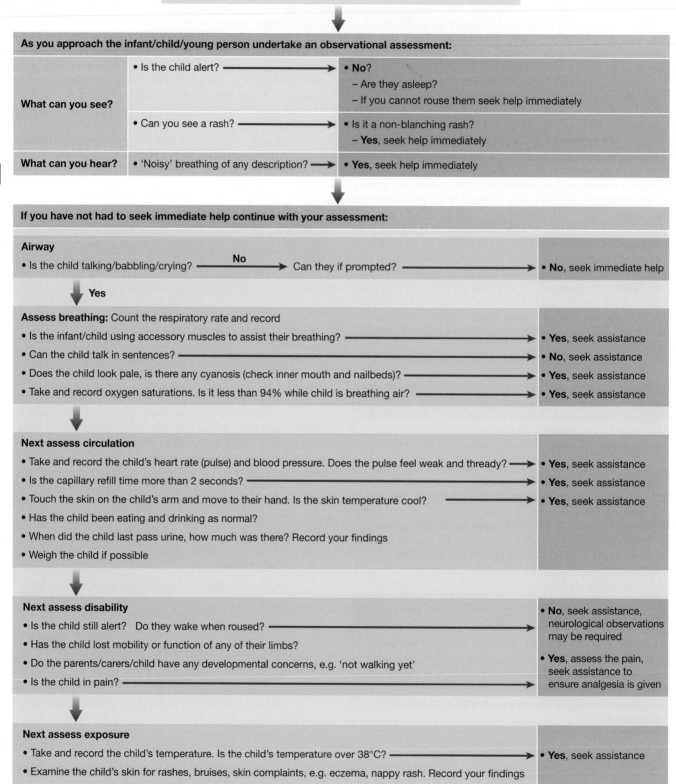

Figure 11.8 A systematic approach to assessment.

Box 11.3 James – 6 Months Old

Alert?	Will become increasingly fractious or, more worryingly, quiet and less responsive.
Airway	As James is alert and smiling, it would appear that his airway is open and stable. It is unlikely that this would deteriorate.
Breathing	There is no suggestion that James has a breathing problem. However, deterioration in any system may initially raise the respiratory rate as part of James' compensatory or 'coping' mechanism.
Circulation	As James is losing fluid and electrolyte through diarrhoea and vomiting, his circulatory system may deteriorate as he has to compensate for a decreasing fluid volume in that system. His heart rate will increase out of his normal range; his blood pressure may rise slightly initially and then begin to fall out of his normal range. His fontanel will appear sunken, his mouth dry and his urine output will decrease. He will look increasingly pale and his peripheral skin will be cooler to the touch than central skin. His capillary refill time will be more than 2 seconds.
Disability	He will become increasingly fractious or, more worryingly, quiet and less responsive. May have abdominal pain.
Exposure	Temperature may increase if there is a gastrointestinal infection. Observe for rashes with every nappy change.
Priority of management	James needs fluid and electrolyte replacement to prevent further dehydration and potential hypovolemic shock. Please refer to the NICE guidelines: http://guidance.nice.org.uk/CG84

Box 11.4 Samina – 5 Years Old

Alert?	Samina is alert but miserable.
Airway	Samina has a husky voice and a temperature, which could suggest an infection in her 'airway'. At 5 years old, it is unlikely to obstruct her airway but it is essential that this is assessed regularly.
Breathing	Samina is coughing and has a temperature which may be because of a chest infection. Her respiratory rate and effort of breathing may increase as Samina compensates to ensure adequate oxygenation of her blood. These signs and a decreasing oxygen saturation level are signs of deterioration.
Circulation	A high temperature and the increased work of breathing will raise Samina's heart rate out of her normal range. BP should remain stable. Reluctance of drinking and increased work of breathing could cause slight dehydration, urine output and fluid intake should be monitored.
Disability	May become increasingly miserable and fractious. Increasing tiredness and becoming less responsive may be due to hypoxia. A pain assessment should be undertaken, as Samina may be most miserable due to a sore throat.
Exposure	Any developing rashes should be reported.
Priority of management	If possible, the source of infection should be treated. Supportive care of respiration, e.g. oxygen therapy may be required to prevent deterioration. Adequate analgesia should be given to enable Samina to feel improved and to eat and drink.

the appropriate interventions from nurses and other members of the healthcare team. This in turn should lead to the children returning to their previous level of good health.

Best Practice Relating to End of Life Care

It is not always possible for children to recover from an acute illness. For those children who cannot recover, the goal of care becomes a dignified and pain-free death. Of course the family are central to the nursing care offered at these distressing times and another important goal of care is to assist the family to have positive memories of their child's final days until the time of death.

Jot This Down

If a child were to die in the acute care setting, e.g. a ward area or intensive care, what steps can the staff take to support the family and help them to have some positive memories from such a distressing time?

Box 11.5 Moira – 13 Years Old

Alert?	Moira is alert.
Airway	No suggestion of a problem with Moira's airway. Regular conversations with her will enable on-going assessment.
Breathing	No suggestion of a problem with Moira's breathing. Increasing pain may raise the respiratory rate above the normal range.
Circulation	Increasing pain may raise the heart rate and blood pressure, particularly if there is an infectious or inflammatory underlying cause, e.g. appendicitis.
Disability	Pain is the main problem and increasing pain will increase Moira's reluctance to move. Moira needs regular pain assessment and observation of her body posture to spot deterioration due to pain.
Exposure	Temperature may increase.
Priority of management	Pain assessment and management, referral to surgical team for assessment.

The death of a child is a significant event for the parents/carers and all their family. The minute details of the events leading up to the death of a child can be ingrained on the minds of the families forever, so it is essential that the potential for unnecessarily distressing memories are minimised. It may be that a child is brought into the resuscitation room of an accident and emergency department. There is debate and discussion about whether the parents/carers should be witnesses to the resuscitation of their child. Moore (2009) highlights the potential benefits and challenges of this scenario, for some parents they need to know that everything possible has been done for their child. Other parents may find the whole situation just too distressing to be involved in. The main issue here is to communicate openly with the family, explain the options and offer them a choice, respecting the decision made and offering the support of a caring nurse. The RCN (2002) have produced a useful guide for nurses who support relatives in the resuscitation room.

Other important aspects when caring for a dying child, is to remember to include the parents and wider family in the care that is offered the child, e.g. washing the child, changing clothes. Again choices should be given and the parent's decision respected. In the final days and hours, the family may want privacy, but the reassurance that a nurse is close by. The parents may want time alone, away from the child, but the confidence that a nurse will stay with their child so he/she is not alone. Care of the dying child requires care, compassion and a willingness to communicate openly and honestly with the parents. The nurse also needs to work closely with other health professionals to avoid offering conflicting information to the parents.

A big decision for parents concerns the environment where the child might receive their end of life care: in hospital, at home or in a hospice environment. There may not always be the opportunity to offer all of these choices if the child is so acutely ill that they die in the resuscitation room or on intensive care but if at all possible, the options should be discussed with the parents so they can make an informed choice.

Simpson and Penrose (2011) examine the issue of 'place of death' for children who are ventilated on intensive care. They advocate a consultative approach to working with parents and following their research make some useful recommendations for the care of families in this situation, showing that the choices of parents can be supported on the whole, even in the most challenging situations. Importantly, Simpson and Penrose (2011) highlight the great benefits felt by parents who had been involved in choosing their child's place of death.

There are many other important aspects to consider, such as the child's age and understanding of their imminent death, the care and support that can be offered to siblings at the end of life and the care that can be offered to the whole family following the death of their child. These are all fascinating and important topics but are beyond the scope of this chapter. There are several excellent resources which will further your understanding of these issues.

Link To/Go To

These websites bring together national care pathways, research and relevant publications for families and health professionals:

http://www.togetherforshortlives.org.uk/
http://www.childbereavement.org.uk/
http://www.winstonswish.org.uk/

Key Points

- The nurse when caring for children and their families should offer care that is safe and effective using a sound evidence base.
- Growth and development of a child is influenced by a number of factors, for example nutrition and a variety of social, economic, geographic and political aspects. These factors interact and impact on the overall child's development into adulthood.
- Childhood is a period of rapid growth and development; children of different ages from birth through to adolescence have very distinctive needs.
- During adolescence a rapid growth spurt occurs. The internal organs grow, for example the lungs and the heart, this in turn increases physical endurance.
- The nurse is required to use appropriate and effective communication skills when supporting the child or young person and their families, particularly when undergoing procedures that they would rather not undergo.
- Immunisation programmes (childhood immunisations) have provided significant and beneficial effects for the health of children since these programmes were introduced.
- Common physical and mental health problems for infants, children and young people have been considered, providing the reader with a 'flavour' and offering signposts where further information can be found.
- Protecting infants, children and young people is everybody's responsibility. Child protection is a very sensitive area, which touches all of society. A brief overview of the legal framework for safeguarding children has been provided.

Glossary

Bronchodilator: a drug causing the bronchi to widen, for example any of those taken by inhalation for the easing of asthma

Child-centred care: care that has been tailored to the individual needs and choices of the child (and family), taking into account issues such as diversity, culture, religion, spirituality, sexuality, gender, age and disability

Cognition: the mental action or process of acquiring knowledge and understanding through thought, experience and the senses

Emollient: helps to keep the skin moist by reducing water loss from the epidermis by providing a protective film

Erythema: superficial reddening of the skin, often in patches, as a result of injury or irritation resulting in dilatation of the blood capillaries

Gross motor skills: the abilities usually acquired during infancy and early childhood as part of a child's motor development. By the time the child reaches the age of two, almost all children are able to stand up, walk and run, walk up stairs

Hormones: regulatory substances produced in an organism and transported in tissue fluids such as blood to stimulate specific cells or tissues into action

Hypoxia: low circulating oxygen in the blood

Mortality: the incidence of death in a population

Personality: the particular combination of emotional, attitudinal and behavioural response patterns of an individual. Personality theorists have their own definitions based on their theoretical positions

Public health: encompasses preventing disease, prolonging life, promoting health and reducing recognised health inequalities through influencing and informing decisions by society, organisations, communities, families and individuals

Rights: rights enshrined in policy, law and values-based codes and frameworks, including human rights

Self-determination: the belief that people have the right, responsibility and ability to make their own choices about what is necessary and desirable to create a satisfying and meaningful life. In the context of nursing, this means that nurses should work with people to encourage and enable them to make informed decisions about their care and treatment and how they manage their lives.

References

ALSG (2011) *Advanced Paediatric Life Support. The Practical Approach*, 5th edn. Advanced Life Support Group. Wiley-Blackwell, Chichester.

All Wales Area Child Protection Committees (2005) *All Wales Child Protection Procedures* Child Protection Review Group, Cardiff, Wales.

Asthma UK (2013) *Facts and Frequently Asked Questions.* http://www.asthma.org.uk/Default.aspx.

Bee, H.L. & Boyd, D.R. (2010) *The Developing Child,* 12th edn. Allyn and Bacon, London.

Coleman, J. (2011) *The Nature of Adolescence,* 4th edn. Routledge, Hove.

Crawford, J. (1995) Winning the fight against disease: a review of childhood immunisation. *Child Health* 2(5), 187–191.

Darbyshire, P. (1994) *Living with a Sick Child in Hospital. The Experiences of Parents and Nurses.* Chapman and Hall, London.

Davies, C. & Ward, H. (2012) *Safeguarding Children Across Services: messages from research.* Jessica Kingsley Publishers, London.

DfE (2013) *Working Together to Safeguard Children. A Guide To Inter-Agency Working To Safeguard And Promote The Welfare Of Children.* Department for Education, London. http://www.education.gov.uk/aboutdfe/statutory/g00213160/working-together-to-safeguard-children.

DfES (2004) *Every Child Matters.* Department for Education and Skills, London.

DfES (2005) *Youth Matters.* The Stationery Office, London.

DH (2004) *National Service Framework for Children, Young People and Maternity Services*: Executive summary. Department of Health, London.

DHSSPS (2003) *Co-operating to Safeguard Children.* Department of Health, Social Services and Public Safety, Belfast.

Devitt, P. & Thain, J. (2011) *Children And Young People's Nursing Made Incredibly Easy.* Lippincott, Williams & Wilkins, London.

Dodds, H. (2010) Meeting the needs of young people in hospital. *Paediatric Nursing*, 22(9), 16–20.

Ellson, R. (2008) Assessment of patients. In: R. Richardson (ed.) *Clinical Skills for Student Nurses*, Ch. 2. Reflect Press Ltd, Exeter.

GMC (2007) *0–18 Years: Guidance for Doctors.* General Medical Council, London.

Glasper, A. & Richardson, J. (2006) *A Textbook of Children's and Young Peoples Nursing.* Churchill Livingstone, London.

Gormley-Fleming, E. (2010) Assessment and vital signs: a comprehensive review. In: A. Glasper, M. Aylott & C. Battrick (2010) *Developing Practical Skills for Nursing Children and Young People,* Ch. 9. Hodder Arnold Ltd, London.

Hobart, C. (2009) *Good Practice in Safeguarding.* Nelson Thornes Ltd., Cheltenham.

Howard, J. & McInnes, K. (2013) *The Essence of Play.* Routledge, Oxon.

Kieckhefer, G.M., Ratcliffe, M. (2000) What parents of children with asthma tell us. *Journal of Pediatric Health Care* 14(3), 122–126.

Lord Laming (2003) *The Victoria Climbie Inquiry Report.* www.education.gov.uk/publications.

Lightfoot, C., Cole, M. & Cole, S. (2009) *The Development of Children.* Worth Publishers, New York.

Lissauer, T. & Clayden, G. (2011) *Illustrated Textbook of Paediatrics,* 4th edn. Mosby, Edinburgh.

Macqueen, S., Bruce, E.A. & Gibson, F. (2012) *The Great Ormond Street Hospital Manual of Children's Nursing Practices.* Wiley-Blackwell, Oxford.

Meeks, M. & Hallsworth, M (2010) *Nursing the Neonate.* Wiley-Blackwell, Chichester.

Moore, H. (2009) Witnessed resuscitation: staff issues and benefits to parents. *Paediatric Nursing*, 21(6), 22–25.

Munro E. (2011) *The Munro Review of Child Protection: Final Report – A Child Centred System.* Department for Education, London.

NICE (2007) Atopic eczema in children: management of atopic eczema in children from birth up to the age of 12 years. *NICE Clinical Guideline 57.* http://guidance.nice.org.uk/QS44.

NMC (2010) *Standards for Pre-registration Nurse Education.* Nursing and Midwifery Council, London. www.nmc-uk.org/.

ONS (2013) *Child Mortality Statistics: Childhood, Infant and Perinatal, 2011.* Office for National Statistics, London. http://www.ons.gov.uk/ons/publications/re-reference-tables.html?edition=tcm%3A77-296223.

PHE (2013) *National MMR Vaccination Catch-up Programme Announced in Response to Increase in Measles Cases.* Public Health England, London. https://www.gov.uk/government/news/national-mmr-vaccination-catch-up-programme-announced-in-response-to-increase-in-measles-cases.

RCN (2002) *Witnessing Resuscitation. Guidance for Nursing Staff.* Royal College of Nursing, London.

RCN (2007) *Caring for Young People. Guidance for Nursing Staff.* Royal College of Nursing, London. http://www.rcn.org.uk/__data/assets/pdf_file/0004/78547/001824.pdf.

RCN (2011) *Standards for Assessing, Measuring and Monitoring Vital Signs in Infants, Children and Young People.* Royal College of Nursing, London.

RCPCH (2003) *Bridging the Gaps: healthcare for adolescents.* Royal College of Paediatrics and Child Health, London. http://www.rcpch.ac.uk/system/files/protected/page/bridging_the_gaps.pdf

Sanders, C., Carter, B. & Goodacre, L. (2012) Parents need to protect: Influences, risks and tensions for parents of prepubertal children born with ambiguous genitalia. *Journal of Clinical Nursing*, 21, 3315–3323.

Scottish Executive (2004) *Protecting Children and Young People: framework for standards.* Scottish Executive, Edinburgh.

Sheridan, M. (2008) *From Birth to Five Years: children's developmental progress,* 3rd edn. Routledge, London.

Simpson, E.C. & Penrose, C.V. (2011) Compassionate extubation in children at hospice and home. *International Journal of Palliative Nursing*, 17(4), 164–169.

Spagnola, C., Korb, J.D. (2002) Atopic dermatitis. *emedicine Journal* 3(10).

Teenage Cancer Trust (2012) *A Blueprint of Care for Teenagers and Young Adults with Cancer.* Teenage Cancer Trust, London. http://www.teenagecancertrust.org/workspace/documents/Blueprint-of-care.pdf.

UNCRC (1989) *United Nations Convention on the Rights of the Child.* http://www.education.gov.uk/childrenandyoungpeople/healthandwellbeing/b0074766/uncrc.

Vaz, I. (2013) Visual symbols in healthcare settings for children with learning disabilities and autism spectrum disorder. *British Journal of Nursing*, 22(3), 156–159.

WHO (1981) *Global Strategy for Health for all by the Year 2000.* World Health Organization. http://whqlibdoc.who.int/publications/9241800038.pdf

Williams, L., Eilers, J., Heermann, J. & Smith, K. (2012) The lived experience of parents and guardians providing care for child transplant recipients. *Progress in Transplantation*, 22(4), 393–402.

Test Yourself

1. Which of the following statements suggest that the child is developing their fine motor skills:
   (a) The child can hop on one leg
   (b) The child can pick up a pea between finger and thumb
   (c) The child can recognise her/his parent
   (d) The child can wave goodbye

2. How old is a child likely to be before they can draw a person?
   (a) 10 months
   (b) 2 years
   (c) 3 years
   (d) 4 years

3. Which of the following children may cause concern about their development?
   (a) Sarah is 18 months and is reluctant to let go of her mum's hand to walk
   (b) John is 2 years and still struggles to eat his meals without creating some 'mess'
   (c) Helen is 6 months old and she doesn't turn to the sound of her dad's voice
   (d) Sammy is 5 years old and struggles to tie his shoe laces

4. Which of the following statements is likely to promote communication with a child
   (a) The nurse always speaks to the parents rather than the child
   (b) The nurse always stands when talking to the child
   (c) The nurse asks the child about his/her drawing
   (d) The nurse writes her/his notes when the child is talking to her/him.

5. What qualities do children value in a nurse (when asked by the University of Central Lancashire)?
   (a) Smiling
   (b) Efficiency
   (c) Tidiness
   (d) Aloofness

6. Which disease would a 2-month-old be immunised against:
   (a) Measles
   (b) Mumps
   (c) Diphtheria
   (d) Rubella

7. Which of the following is unlikely to predispose the child to asthma?
   (a) If their parents smoke
   (b) The school they attend
   (c) Viral infection when a baby
   (d) Their genetic make up

8. Oxygen is NOT:
   (a) A fundamental need of the child
   (b) A drug which must be prescribed
   (c) A challenge to deliver to infants and toddlers
   (d) An essential vitamin

9. Safeguarding children is NOT:
   (a) A challenge for healthcare professionals
   (b) Guided by the law and policies
   (c) About keeping the child with their family
   (d) Something to be left to qualified professionals

10. When assessing a child you notice he has a non-blanching rash. Should you:
    (a) Chat with the mother about the child's birth
    (b) Seek help from a senior nurse immediately
    (c) Get the child a drink
    (d) Sort out the computer for the child

Answers

1. b
2. d
3. c
4. c

5. a
6. c
7. b
8. d
9. d
10. b

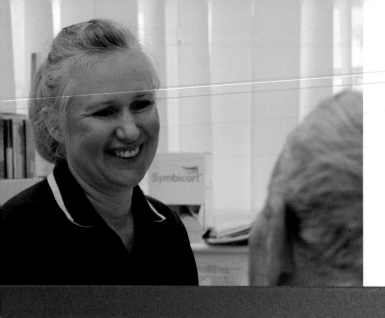

12

The Principles of Caring for People with Mental Health Problems

Steve Trenoweth,[1] Alicia Powell[2] and Wasiim Allymamod[3]

[1]University of West London, UK
[2]Hounslow Mental Health Assessment Team, West London Mental Health NHS Trust, UK
[3]Central and North West London NHS Foundation Trust, UK

Learning Outcomes

On completion of this chapter you will be able to:

- Understand the policy context for contemporary mental health nursing care and be aware of the contexts for mental health care, including settings for care and legal contexts
- Be aware of the various approaches to understanding mental disorder
- Be familiar with the principles of the 'recovery' approach
- Understand the principles of holism in the delivery of nursing care for people with mental health problems
- Appreciate how and why physical health problems may be elevated in this client group
- Understand the principles of nursing care for people experiencing mental distress and their carers, including assessment, treatment options and therapeutic nursing care

Competencies

All nurses must:

1. Practice in a holistic, non-judgemental, caring and sensitive manner; support social inclusion; recognise and respect individual choice; recognise when people are anxious or in distress and respond effectively
2. Use therapeutic principles to engage, maintain and, where appropriate, disengage from professional caring relationships; respect professional boundaries
3. Encourage health-promoting behaviour
4. Carry out systematic nursing assessments taking into account physical, social, cultural, psychological, spiritual, genetic and environmental factors, in partnership with others; respond to the physical, social and psychological needs of people
5. Recognise and interpret signs of normal and deteriorating mental and physical health and respond promptly
6. Be self-aware and recognise how your own values, principles and assumptions may affect your practice

Nursing Practice: Knowledge and Care, First Edition. Edited by Ian Peate, Karen Wild and Muralitharan Nair.
© 2014 John Wiley & Sons, Ltd. Published 2014 by John Wiley & Sons, Ltd. Companion website: www.wileynursingpractice.com

Introduction

Mental health problems are common and nurses in all fields will encounter service-users, clients and patients who experience mental distress, some of whom may warrant a psychiatric diagnosis, some of whom may not. Mental health problems, however, may not be recognised or acknowledged and as a consequence, such problems may go untreated and escalate in seriousness. This may undermine the quality of an individual's life or, worse, lead to a deterioration of a person's mental and physical condition to the point where their overall health and safety may be severely compromised. Mental health problems may also persist if untreated. It is estimated that half of all mental health problems last longer than a year (Jenkins *et al.* 2008). Left untreated, mental health problems can also lead to an 'inter-generational burden' (Jenkins *et al.* 2008), as children who grow up with a parent who has a mental health problem are at increased risk of developing a mental problem themselves, such as depression (Davies 2002; Dean & Macmillan 2002). There is also a financial cost of mental ill health to the UK economy. In 2009/10 this was estimated at £105.2 billion. This sum includes £10.4 billion or 11% of all gross NHS expenditure that is spent on mental health (DH 2010) and also other costs associated with a reduction in economic output, and the impact on people's quality of life, which may often go unacknowledged (CMH 2010).

Nurses will also encounter people who have chronic, complex and perhaps long-term needs associated with their mental health problems, who may also have co-morbid physical illnesses or learning disabilities. Some mental health problems can be persistent and are often episodic in nature. That is, such problems can vary in acuity, where at one end of a continuum (in an acute crisis) there may be the need for high-intensity care and support from nurses and other healthcare professionals and, at the other end of the continuum, low-intensity, on-going support, where independence is encouraged (i.e. when symptoms of mental distress may have abated or when the mental health problem has been resolved).

Policy Context

Service-user involvement in all aspects of their care is an important part of current mental health policy. Similarly, service-users have been increasingly involved in service development, including the ability to influence care delivery through to the commissioning of clinical services. In the UK's Coalition Government's White Paper 'Equity and Excellence: liberating the NHS' (DH 2010) service-user choice and experience was emphasised. The White Paper sought to ensure that the NHS was more accountable and responsive to the needs and wishes of service-users, including choosing treatments and providers which they feel would best meet their own needs. Similarly, the mental health strategy for England 'No Health Without Mental Health' (DH 2011) proposed to improve the mental health of people with existing mental health problems and also had a public health focus, in that it sought to prevent mental ill health wherever possible.

Link To/Go To

Mental Health Strategy for England:

https://www.gov.uk/government/publications/the-mental-health-strategy-for-england

No Health without Mental Health:

https://www.gov.uk/government/publications/no-health-without-mental-health-a-cross-government-outcomes-strategy

Mental Health Promotion and Mental Illness Prevention – The economic case:

https://www.gov.uk/government/publications/mental-health-promotion-and-mental-illness-prevention-the-economic-case

ICD-10 International Classification of Diseases

http://www.who.int/classifications/icd/en/

The Mental Health Strategy for England identified six high level priorities for mental health (Box 12.1).

> **Jot This Down**
> · Think about the implications of these mental health objectives in your field of practice
> · Considering these objectives, what contribution can you make to the health and well-being of people with mental health problems?

The strategy was '…both a public mental health strategy and a strategy for social justice' (DH 2011, p. 3), recognising that social inequalities (such as, lack of employment prospects, poor housing, social exclusion and so forth) contribute to mental distress.

In the policy 'Choosing Health: supporting the physical health needs of people with severe mental illness' (DH 2006), attention was focussed on the tendency for people with mental health problems to have an increased risk of developing serious physical disorders (Robson & Gray 2007), such as cancer, coronary heart disease, diabetes and respiratory diseases (Mentality/NIMHE 2004). In recent years, the role of medication, which has historically been the focus of mental health care (Faulkner & Layzell 2000) has been de-emphasised and there has been increasing focus on the provision of social and psychological care which is hopeful, optimistic and positive (DH 2001) and aims to support people to live a life which is meaningful to them (NIMHE 2005; Jenkins *et al.* 2008). This 'recovery approach' has found expression in mental healthcare policies which have emphasised supportive, collaborative therapeutic alliances and shared decision-making between service-users and healthcare professionals, and a recognition that people have strengths, talents and abilities as well as needs and problems.

> **Box 12.1 Six High Level Mental Health Objectives**
> 1. More people will have good mental health
> 2. More people with mental health problems will recover
> 3. More people with mental health problems will have good physical health
> 4. More people will have a positive experience of care and support
> 5. Fewer people will suffer avoidable harm
> 6. Fewer people will experience stigma and discrimination.
> (DH 2011)

239

The Evidence National Institute for Mental Health in England (NIMHE 2005) Guiding Statement on Recovery

Recovery is an experiential process, focussed on an individual's return to a state of well being. This may not necessarily mean a full restoration to the individual's prior state of health, but focusses on a change process where one achieves a state of personal satisfaction with their quality of life. Recovery involves changing one's focus about a health problem from a traumatic or difficult episode, towards restoration, self-determination and well-being.

The recovery orientated system of care for individuals with mental health difficulties, aims to empower service-users by taking a *strengths* approach to their treatment and fostering an environment of hope, optimism and enablement. Recovery-based services place value on delivering holistic care, taking into account psychological, physical, social, spiritual and emotional needs. Services aim to work collaboratively with individuals to encourage personal growth and an active role in within their own families, social groups and communities.

The Care Programme Approach (CPA) has been central to Government mental health policy since 1990 (DH 2008a). CPA aims to ensure that people with mental health problems who have been in contact with mental health services receive the ongoing care they need. It provides:

- Arrangements for health and social needs assessment
- A care plan documenting agreed mental health care and treatment and also plans to support the person enter employment; receive adequate housing; and possible entitlement to benefits
- The appointment of a key worker (care coordinator) who will provide ongoing monitoring and support, and to coordinate care
- Regular review and agreed amendments to the care plan as necessary.

Today, CPA policy has been 'refocussed', emphasising the personalisation of mental health care and active service-user involvement and engagement, along with promoting social inclusion and recovery (DH 2008a).

Jot This Down

The current unemployment rate in the UK (May 2013) is 7.8% of the economically active population (Office for National Statistics, ONS 2013). The unemployment rate of people with a mental health problem is approximately 30–45% (OECD 2012). Many people who experience long-term mental health problems are unemployed but wish to work. Consider some of the issues facing the person with mental health problems who wishes to enter the labour market.

What the Experts Say Recovery

> A young service-user worried that he would never recover from his mental health problems. He had a diagnosis of paranoid schizophrenia; the symptoms of which were not completely treated with antipsychotic medication. We worked collaboratively to determine which aspects of his life he would like to improve, focussing on his strengths. He requested help to deal with the auditory hallucinations (voices) he continued to experience. He developed some techniques to deal with the voices in a more socially acceptable way to him (including pretending he was talking on his mobile when the voices were particularly intrusive). As his confidence improved, he was encouraged to participate in voluntary work schemes. Two years later, he had gained part-time employment and was playing guitar in a band. He had developed several satisfying personal friendships. For him, this process of recovery was not about the absence of symptoms, but the integration of his condition into his life, and finding a way to feel confident, fulfil his goals, and contribute to his local community.

(Mental Health Nurse)

 Link To/Go To Recovery

Overview of recovery

http://www.mentalhealth.org.uk/help-information/mental-health-a-z/R/recovery/

Challenges to recovery

http://www.rethink.org/living-with-mental-illness/recovery/recovery-challenges

What Is Mental Disorder?

For the World Health Organization (WHO), health is '…not merely the absence of disease or infirmity' (WHO 1946). It further defines mental health as:

> …a state of well-being in which the individual realises his or her own abilities, can cope with the normal stresses of life, can work productively and fruitfully, and is able to make a contribution to his or her community.

(WHO 2007)

As such, the WHO's definition of health and mental health reflects our ability to function, cope within, and make a contribution to society. This in turn, recognises the social nature of our functioning as human beings. This definition also recognises the personal and subjective nature of one's experience of 'mental health'.

There are several models that seek to explain the development of mental health problems. For example, the biomedical model considers mental illness as a product of abnormalities or disease processes within the body, such as a genetic heritability, dysfunction with neurotransmitters, or differences in the structure of the brain amongst people with mental illnesses (Kring *et al.* 2010; Butcher *et al.* 2008). The biomedical model also seeks to establish a diagnosis, which forms the basis of clinical decision-making with respect to medical care and treatment. However, there have been many criticisms of medical diagnoses in mental health care. For example, a diagnosis may be considered as a label, which often serves to marginalise or exclude people from communities. There have also been concerns about the reliability of diagnoses as they are made on the basis of subjective data and have been found to vary according to the psychiatrist's personal bias rather than a cataloguing of objective symptoms (Boyle 2002). Here, a person's behaviour that is odd, deviant or objectionable and does not conform to prevailing 'social norms' may be considered symptomatic of a mental illness. Likewise, care must always be taken to ensure that cultural differences in communication or behaviour are not misinterpreted as signs of mental disorder. It has often been argued that psychiatric medication can be very helpful to the person in terms of their recovery and that such drugs have been the single most important development in the treatment of mental illnesses (Krauss & Slavinsky 1982). However, it must also be acknowledged that there are also sometimes significant consequences for an individual who has been prescribed medication for mental distress, including many major side-effects such as toxicity and dependence.

In 1977, Engel argued that the biomedical model may restrict our understanding of health and illness and there are other approaches which may offer a fuller explanation of mental distress (Engel 1977). The social approach, for example, sees social injustice such as inequalities, stigma and prejudice, discrimination, unemployment, chronic social adversity (such as poverty), a lack of community acceptance and tolerance and poor social support and isolation as precursors to mental ill health (Holmes & Rahe 1967; Bentall 2003). Psychological models suggest that mental distress arises from unhelpful or biased thinking or is acquired through learning unhelpful behaviours which in turn has an impact on how we think and feel about ourselves (such as our self-esteem, self-confidence and so on) and interact with others. Stress models suggest that mental ill health arises due to an inability to cope with and adjust to environmental demands (Butcher *et al.* 2008).

While the precise causes of mental health problems are not known, it is most likely that all the factors mentioned above – social, psychological, biological and environmental factors – may interact to increase the risk of developing mental disorders (Gallop & Reynolds 2004) (Figure 12.1).

There are hybrid models that seek to capture this complexity. For example, the 'Stress Vulnerability' model (Zubin & Spring 1977) recognises the complex interplay between such factors and represents a hybrid approach. This model recognises that we may become predisposed towards mental disorder (such as schizophrenia) due to biological and environmental factors (such as early upbringing) and but the risk is triggered by stressors (which may include socioeconomic issues, such as poverty or substance misuse or physical issues such as ill health) (Zubin & Spring 1977). There are further implications of the 'Stress Vulnerability' model – if one's mental health fluctuates in response to exposure to stress as

suggested by Zubin and Spring (1977), then everyone has the capacity to develop mental disorders. In this sense, there are not 'mentally ill people' as a separate or distinct group but we all exist on a continuum of people whose vulnerability varies as a function of their predispositions and exposure to stress.

To illustrate how the complex interplay between social, psychological, biological and environmental factors may lead to mental distress, let us consider 'depression'. The International Classification of Diseases (ICD-10) (WHO 2004) (the medical taxonomy developed by the World Health Organization (WHO), which catalogues medical and psychiatric disorders) describes different types of depression of varying severity – from 'mild' to 'severe' episodes (which in the latter case may be accompanied by, e.g. 'psychosis', strange beliefs and bizarre behaviour). Depression is a common mental disorder (Care Services Improvement Partnership, CSIP 2006) and typical symptoms of depression can include: feelings of sadness and despair; a loss of hope; appetite and sleep disturbances; social withdrawal; loss of interest or pleasure in activities that are normally pleasurable; decreased libido; decreased energy; and an inability to concentrate. Feelings of guilt and suicidal thoughts may be present (NICE 2009a). However, for a diagnosis to be made, the depressed mood must be persistent for a period of time (typically at least 2 weeks); be abnormal for the individual; present for most of the day (and almost every day); and largely uninfluenced by environmental circumstances (WHO 2004).

The Evidence

This study found that the majority of individuals recovering from depression attribute their recoveries to a multifaceted approach, including both intrinsic and extrinsic factors. Attributable personal and social factors include self-determination and willpower, support from friends and family, employment and leisure opportunities. The types of treatments offered, the timeliness of interventions, attitudes of healthcare practitioners and the information given by professionals, are also factors cited as important to ones experience and recovery from depression. Having ones' own role in the recovery process acknowledged, and being given choices regarding treatment options also enhances the recovery process and promotes concordance with chosen treatments. Healthcare professionals are in a key position to promote recovery by acknowledging these multiple factors involved in the recovery process, taking a 'strengths' focussed view and providing holistic care in a climate of mutual respect.

(Badger & Nolan 2007)

Adverse life events and stressors (such as financial troubles, bereavements and employment problems) are often cited as risk factors for of depression. The highest rates of depression are to be found in the most deprived neighbourhoods (Office of the Deputy Prime Minister, ODPM 2004). Brown and Harris (1978) in their seminal work on the 'social origins of depression' suggested that early maternal loss, lack of a confiding relationship, more than three children under the age of 14 at home and unemployment, can greatly increase vulnerability to depression. Women tend to have higher rates of depression than men and here, women have an approximately 30% lifetime risk of experiencing a depressive episode (Jenkins *et al.* 2008). However, it also appears that a person's biology may also be implicated. For example, depression often seems to run in families and those with the most genetic similarity

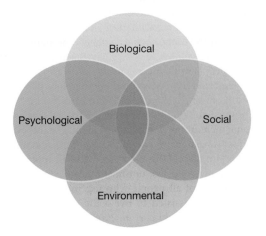

Figure 12.1 Factors affecting the development of mental disorders.

(such as monozygotic twins) seem to have higher concordance rates (Kring *et al.* 2010). Neurochemical changes in the brain may also play a part in depression (such as decreased levels of the neurotransmitter serotonin) (Martin 2006). There are also higher rates of depression among those who have suffered damage to their brain (traumatic brain injury) (Brown 2004). Depression also seems to be associated with lower volumes of grey matter in the prefrontal cortex, the part of the brain which is seen to be responsible for speech, decision-making and goal-directed behaviour, and people diagnosed with depression show elevated activity in the amygdala (the structure in the brain associated with assessing the emotional importance of a stimulus) (Kring *et al.* 2010). Poor nutrition and diet has also been linked to mental health problems (MHF 2006) and nutrients, such as folic acid, omega-3 fatty acids, selenium and tryptophan appear to reduce the symptoms of depression.

Red Flag

In 2009, the 'Adult Psychiatric Morbidity Survey' (APMS, NHSIC 2009) found that almost 17% of people reported thoughts of suicide and almost 6% said that they had made a suicide attempt. In the UK, there were 5675 suicides in 2009 (ONS 2011). Suicide is therefore a serious health issue, with depression being is a significant risk factor. It is important that the nurse is vigilant when caring for the person who is depressed and alert to any warning signs that they may be considering taking their lives. Concerns of family members and carers must be listened to and acknowledged.

Settings for Mental Health Care

Mental health care service provision in the UK is arranged in a three-tier structure comprising: primary, secondary and tertiary care. Historically, there have been many changes in how mental health care has been provided, with a current focus on maximising efficiency and reducing costs, while treating service-users in the least restrictive and socially inclusive way.

The majority of people with a mental health problem are now treated in community settings, with only the most acutely unwell and those with complex presentations being cared for in hospital settings.

Primary care refers to non-specialist care services provided through GP surgeries. GPs are often the first point of contact for anyone experiencing mental distress, and responses from these professionals depend on their skills, attitudes and experience. Therefore, it is imperative that GPs and other primary care professionals have the skills to detect mental health issues and are able to consistently instigate the most appropriate, evidence-based treatment options or refer to specialist services, where necessary (DH 1999).

Over 90% of people with mental health concerns are treated in primary care (NMHDU 2011). Common mental health problems, such as mild to moderate depression, panic and anxiety disorders, are most commonly cared for in primary care, and GPs will usually instigate treatment options based on NICE guidelines, including the use of medicines and counselling or cognitive behavioural therapy. The 'Improving Access to Psychological Therapies' (IAPT) programme has been enhancing treatment choice in primary care settings, providing increased access to trained cognitive behaviour therapists and psychologists (NMHDU 2011).

Secondary care services are specialist mental health services, based in community settings. The recent and ongoing national move to reconfigure mental health service provision towards more personalised and cost-effective care (in government policies 'Liberating the NHS' (DH 2010) and 'No Health Without Mental Health' (DH 2011), has led to changes in community mental health services. The remit of secondary care services is to assess and treat people with acute, severe and/or enduring mental health problems. Assessment services deal with referrals for persons over 18 years, excluding those with an organic condition, and provide short-term treatment and follow. Community Recovery Services provide longer-term support to service-users with enduring conditions, with the focus being on recovery, empowerment and social inclusion. Assertive Outreach Teams work with service-users who have complex presentations, are difficult to engage and who often have comorbid and dual diagnoses. Outreach working can help to reduce the number of hospital admissions for such individuals (DH 1999). Specialist services exist for older people with organic mental health problems, including dementia. Early intervention services exist for young people aged 18–35, presenting with first symptoms of psychosis. Prompt treatment within this group has shown to improve long-term mental health, reduce suicide rates and reduce hospital admissions (Singh 2010).

Services also exist for people presenting in acute crises who can be cared for outside the confines of hospital. These include psychiatric liaison teams and home treatment or crisis resolution teams. Personal benefits include enhanced control over their own mental health and the support provided by families. Cost benefits are significant with studies suggesting a saving of up to £700 per month per service-user, compared with inpatient admission (CEMH 2007).

Tertiary care mental health services refer to inpatient care usually provided in hospital-based settings. The main inpatient facilities in the UK are acute services (comprising assessment and recovery wards), psychiatric intensive care units and forensic services. Due to the increase in community-based mental health services, inpatient facilities tend to provide shorter care spells to the only the most complex, and acutely unwell service-users.

Recovery

Mental health services have often seemed to focus on medical symptomatology, and treatment has often emphasised the use of medication. In the words of Murray (2012, p. 4), in mental health care '… medication is prioritised at the expense of psychological interventions and social rehabilitation'. 'Recovery' in a biomedical sense, may be seen to have been achieved if a person is free of symptoms of mental illness or if they have been 'cured' (Matthews 2008). Many people with mental health problems, in this sense, may not be expected to 'recover' and are therefore perceived to be in need of long-term psychiatric care and medication.

As mentioned above, a new approach – the 'recovery approach' – has become increasingly important in mental health care both in terms of policy development and in mental health and nursing care (Repper & Perkins 2003). This recovery-focussed approach stresses the importance of a hopeful, optimistic positive approach to the care and treatment of all people who use mental health services (DH 2001) who are assisted to live a life of personal value and worth (NIMHE 2005; Jenkins *et al.* 2008). The recovery approach distinguishes between 'complete recovery' (in which an individual returns to their level of functioning before they experienced mental ill health accompanied by symptom relief or eradication), and 'social recovery' (which focusses on supporting the process of recovery emphasising support for the person to improve their overall quality of life, despite the presence of 'psychiatric symptoms') (Matthews 2008). 'Social recovery', then:

> ... is not about regaining a problem-free life – whose life is? It is about living life more resourcefully, living a satisfying and contributing life, in spite of limitations caused by a continuing vulnerability to disabling distress.

(Watkins 2001, p. 45)

Jot This Down
- What does the term 'recovery' mean to you?
- How is the term used in your own field?
- How does it differ in mental health care?

Mental health nurses using a (social) recovery approach stress:
- *The importance of working in partnership and shared decision-making with mental health service-users*
- *The development of a supportive and empathic professional working alliance*
- *Treatments which reflect the service-user's preference based on an informed discussion*
- *A recognition that individuals have personal strengths, abilities and assets that may be used in the recovery process*
- *Support to cope with future challenges that mental health problems may bring.*

(Trenoweth & Allymamod 2010)

Here, the emphasis is placed on the promotion of positive mental health, as well as responding to mental illness and with supporting the development of subjective well-being (Seligman 2008). Emphasis is placed on helping the person to develop satisfying social relationships and support networks, and empowering them to develop their sense of citizenship and inclusion by supporting the person's efforts to find meaningful employment or educational endeavours.

Holism

A recovery approach suggests a holistic focus in the delivery of nursing care and treatment of mental health problems (Sin & Trenoweth 2010), in that it sees beyond the psychiatric symptoms with which a person may present. It encompasses all aspects of their biological social, psychological and even spiritual being. In holism, the aetiology of mental ill health, for example is seen as being multidimensional (involving these psychological, social, emotional and spiritual dimensions of self) and not just stemming from a biological dysfunction. However, it is not just mental ill health where holism may be of importance – any healthcare problem can have a major impact on our holistic functioning and can impact upon all aspects of our world and our experiences within it, from our social life (relationships, finances, work performance for example) to our psychological health (self-esteem, confidence, and so forth) and this can affect our emotional well-being as the person may struggle with stress and uncertainty about the course their illness may take (Sin & Trenoweth 2010).

As mentioned earlier, the medical model seeks to explain mental distress in physical (biomedical) terms, stemming from a dysfunc-

tion of an individual's biology. As such, 'spirituality' as a dimension of being, which is subjective and perhaps not amenable to quantification, may be misunderstood or, worse, ignored. Spirituality is, however, an important part of our lives (Crawford *et al.* 1998) and a vital aspect of holistic nursing care (Thompson 2002).

Swinton and Pattison (2001) describe spirituality as:

> ... that aspect of human existence which relates to structures of significance that give meaning and direction to a person's life and helps them deal with the vicissitudes of existence. It is associated with the human quest for meaning, purpose, self transcending knowledge, meaningful relationships, love and a sense of the holy. It may or may not, be associated with a specific religious system.

That is, spirituality is not necessarily the same as religious affiliation. There is a clear difference – the concept of spirituality, which may be used in a religious sense to connote belief in a divine power (metaphysical) and spirituality as a reference to the philosophies, values and beliefs that helps us to make sense of our lives (existential) (Goddard 1995). There may of course be a connection between metaphysical and existential forms of spirituality in that a person's religious beliefs may help them to make sense of their lives but this cannot be assumed or expected. There are also large numbers of people in the UK who have no religious affiliation and here, it would be incorrect to say that they were not spiritual. In 2006, almost 46% of people in the UK claimed no religious affiliation (Brown 2010). Listening to the meanings that a mental health service-user places on their lives can help us to understand their frame of reference. This requires an open-mindedness and effective interpersonal skills, as we encourage people to share with us the issues that matter to them in their lives.

Ill health, particularly that which is ongoing, long term or resistant to treatment, can leave sufferers feeling helpless and hopeless – at the mercy of the symptoms they may be experiencing. This can have a major impact on the person's recovery from illness or trauma.

Jot This Down
- What does 'spirituality' mean to you?
- Many people see their 'spirituality' as being related to the meaning and purpose in their lives. Imagine for a moment that your life lacked such meaning and purpose. How would you feel?

In mental health care, there is a growing awareness that a lack of 'hope' can have a detrimental impact in the trajectory of ill health and the concept of 'hope' is central to a person's recovery (Koehn & Cutcliffe 2007). Hope, is:

> ... a process of anticipation that involves the interaction of thinking, acting, feeling and relating, and is directed toward a future fulfilment that is personally meaningful.

(Stephenson 1991, p. 1459)

It is optimism that the future will reveal a better life, as defined by the person and that the symptoms a person may be experiencing will have abated or will become manageable or less significant.

Caring for Carers

About half of all people with long-term mental health problems live with their family or with friends (DH 1999; Jenkins *et al.* 2008), who play a vital part in their treatment and care (NICE 2009a,b). Unfortunately, the needs of carers have often been overlooked and it is important to recognise the impact that such caring can have on carers who may require support themselves from mental health and social care services. In fact, the strains, responsibilities and the subsequent emotional and financial implications of caring, can lead to carers being twice as likely to have mental health problems as the general population, particularly depression (ODPM 2004). It is important to recognise that carers have specific needs, and to respond to these needs in a timely and sensitive manner. Carers may experience feelings of shame, grief, guilt or blame, may feel their views are being ignored or that they cannot participate in a meaningful way in the treatment and recovery process. A family member with a mental health problem can present a number of challenges for the wider family and times when a person is unwell can be very disruptive for a family. Parents may need to take carer's leave from work, which might have career and financial implications for the family. Other family members may be concerned that they may also develop a mental health problem. It is therefore imperative that professionals provide carers with as much up-to-date information, advice and support as they are able to, or refer them to external resources, where necessary. This may include signposting carers to support groups and voluntary agencies; providing advice regarding benefit entitlements; giving information about care and treatment options available to support recovery; and what to do, and who to contact, in the event of a crisis (DH 1999). Specialist mental health services have provisions for assessing and responding to the specific needs of carers, aiming to support the balance between the caring role, while maintaining their own health and well-being (DH 1999).

Comprehensive Assessment in Mental Health

It is clear then that nursing assessments with mental health service-users should be comprehensive and holistic, and cover a wide range of the health and social care needs, including possible physical health problems, medical/psychiatric symptoms, social functioning, psychological, occupational, economic, physical and cultural/diversity issues (NICE 2009a,b). However, this is not merely a clinical exercise where the sole aim is an interview with a service-user to extract information. Nurses who are conducting assessments in mental health care must use appropriate, supportive and empathic communication skills to encourage the individual to 'tell their personal story' (Launer 2002).

People with long-term mental health issues may also need support with their 'activities of daily living'. For example, an Office for National Statistics (ONS 2002) survey found that over a third of people with mental disorders in their sample had at least one problem in dealing with domestic affairs (including paperwork and budgeting), using public transport and household activities. A person's functional ability to lead an 'ordinary' life therefore needs also to be assessed. Assessments must also be culturally sensitive and the nurse needs to have the knowledge, skills and values required in understanding and working with diverse communities (DH 1999).

Within a recovery framework, it is important to consider the strengths and assets of the individual. Rapp (1997) and Rapp and Goscha (2006) have developed an approach which seeks to capture the strengths of individuals, which allows consideration for oppor-

---

Box 12.2 An Assessment of Strengths

A strength assessment seeks to gather information across six interrelated domains:

- The person's capacity for independent living
- Vocational and educational skills and achievements
- Social support and leisure activities
- Health resources
- Financial and legal factors
- Transportation and mobility.

---

tunities for growth and development of the individual, rather than concentrating on illness and deficits (Box 12.2). These include the individual's interests, aspirations, skills, competencies and talents (Rapp 1997).

The Physical Health of People with Mental Health Problems

Good mental and physical health is vital in maintaining our overall sense of well-being (Robson *et al.* 2008). It is important to recognise that people who experience mental health problems, such as depression, also tend to have an increased vulnerability to, and higher rates of, physical health problems (Robson & Gray 2007), such as coronary heart disease and respiratory diseases (SCMH 2003), cancers (such as breast and bowel cancers) and have increased risks of developing diabetes (Gough & Peveler 2004). Severe and chronic stress can have a detrimental impact on an individual's immunity, which increases their vulnerability to illness and disease, such as heart attacks, osteoporosis, arthritis, type 2 diabetes and some cancers (Ershler & Keller 2000; Tosevski & Milovancevic 2006). This is compounded by the fact that such people also tend to have poorer access to medical care, higher rates of hospitalisation for medical conditions, and are less likely to be offered regular physical health checks (such as blood pressure or cholesterol monitoring) or to receive advice about promoting or maintaining their health (SCMH 2003; Disability Rights Committee, DRC 2006). As a result, physical illnesses are often poorly diagnosed among people with serious mental health problems. This may be due, at least in part, to reluctance among some service-users to engage with healthcare services and accept and act upon health education advice. However, it may also be due to a possible lack of willingness of healthcare professionals to engage with people with mental health problems. There may be an over emphasis on mental health issues and such 'diagnostic overshadowing', where the focus is on a person's primary mental health diagnosis to the exclusion of other health issues (Friedli & Dardis 2002; Dean *et al.* 2001). More worryingly, physical symptoms may be dismissed as being seen to be 'all in the person's mind' (Seymour 2003).

The Evidence

It is well evidenced that individuals with serious mental illness are at greater risk of having a range of chronic diseases than the general population. This study found that the causal factors of the higher rate of morbidity and mortality this group face are multifaceted and interrelated. Significant factors include the negative side-effects of psychotropic medication, the poorer health behaviours of people with serious mental health problems (such as smoking, inadequate diets, physical inactivity and risky sexual health practices) and the lack of specific training for mental health professionals. Mental health nurses should view their role as a strategic opportunity to help improve the physical and mental health outcomes of the people they care for. Adequate training should be provided to ensure that mental health professionals feel competent to collaboratively assess, and monitor the risk of physical health issues and provide evidence-based health promoting care from the onset of treatment. Primary healthcare practitioners should be aware of the increased risks among this group and provide routine physical screenings and examinations accordingly.

(Robson & Gray 2007)

As a consequence, serious physical disorders tend to occur at a younger age among people with mental health problems, with a higher premature death rate and poorer survival rate than the general population (Harris & Barraclough 1998). Similarly, as Cohen and Rodriguez (1995) suggest, people with physical disorders also tend to have higher rates of depression. That is, depression seems to be both a cause and consequence of physical illness particularly when a person experiences chronic, long-term symptoms such as pain, breathlessness and fatigue (Care Services Improvement Partnership, CSIP 2006; Margereson 2008). Chronic pain, it appears, contributes to a higher incidence of depression, but it is important to recognise that depression also seems to affect the experience of pain (Gureje 2007). Similarly, our emotional responses can affect our experience of pain, where peace of mind appears to offer relief from pain, while fear and anger appears to amplify it (Bope *et al.* 2004). There are also increased risks of sexual health problems among people with mental health problems, particularly among younger people (Sheild *et al.* 2005) who may be at an increased risk of contracting sexually transmitted infections. They are twice as likely as their peers to be sexually active and to engage in unsafe sexual practices and are more likely to have unplanned pregnancies (DiClemente & Ponton 1993; Kessler *et al.* 1997).

It is important, therefore, to be alert to physical health problems among people with mental health problems and the possibility of mental distress among those with physical health problems. It is important to realise that people with mental health problems do care about their physical health, and would value and welcome health promotion information and advice.

What the Experts Say Physical Health

> Our community mental health team runs a monthly 'Physical Health Clinic' for service-users less likely to attend their GP surgery or recognise their own physical health issues. Service-users often feel more comfortable in familiar, relaxed environments run by health care professionals with special understanding of mental health issues. Service-users are provided an extended appointment which includes measurement of vital signs, blood sugar levels, Body Mass Index and health promotion assessment and advice. This could include information about smoking cessation, dietary advice, and referrals to in-house healthy lifestyles, cooking or sports groups. Reports are then passed onto the service-users' GP with recommendations for any follow up medical care or further investigations. Care coordinators are then able to empower and assist service-users to address any areas that require follow up and continue with health promoting support.

(Community Mental Health Nursing Team)

Red Flag

Never overlook the physical healthcare needs of people with mental health. As a nurse, you must ensure that the same advice and support is available to people with long-term mental healthcare needs as the general population. Nurses in all fields must be alert to comorbid and co-existing health issues, which can affect the holistic well-being of their patients and service-users. This may include considering and challenging one's assumptions about the overall healthcare needs of people with mental health problems (Seymour 2003).

There needs to be an assessment of lifestyle factors which may increase the risk of poor physical health among a mental health client group, such as alcohol and/or drug use; smoking, poor diet and a lack of exercise. Indeed, it is likely that these factors combine cumulatively to impact on the physical health of people with mental health problems. McCreadie (2003), for example, found that people with serious mental health problems were exposed to more risk in terms of these lifestyle factors compared with the poorest socioeconomic group within the general population.

People with mental health problems tend to smoke at higher rates, and at higher levels (i.e. smoking over a pack of 20 cigarettes per day) than the general population (McCloughen 2003). There are many possible reasons, which may account for this (including the potentially energising or conversely a relaxing effect of nicotine; boredom; habit and addiction; social reasons, and so forth). However, there is some evidence that smoking is considered to be an acceptable and positive part of the mental health culture by mental health nurses (Stubbs & Gardner 2004). If this is the case, then there may be less emphasis placed on health promotion and smoking cessation.

A good, nutritious diet contributes to good physical health, while a poor diet increases the risk of some forms of cancer (such as bowel cancer), diabetes, cardiovascular disease and hypertension. A poor diet (which is high in saturated fats and sugar and low in omega 3 fatty acids) may be predictive of poor recovery (Peet 2004). However, people with mental health problems tend to have a much poorer diet than the general population with higher intakes of saturated fat. As such, people with serious mental health problems tend to have hyperlipidaemia (raised serum cholesterol levels) (McCreadie *et al.* 2003). In one study, none of the group of people with mental health problems studied was found to be eating the recommended weekly minimum of five portions of fruit or vegetables each day and one portion of oily fish (Brown *et al.* 1999; Food Standards Agency, FSA 2001). All nurses must, therefore, be able to promote and encourage healthy eating amongst people with mental health problems.

The risks associated with smoking and unhealthy diets are compounded by a lack of regular exercise, which can increase rates of obesity and diabetes. People with mental health problems, particularly women, tend to be overweight when compared with the general population (Kendrick 1996) and this may due, at least in part, to a poorer uptake of exercise. In one study, a third of the people with mental health problems stated that they took no exercise at all (Brown *et al.* 1999). However, exercise can not only improve physical health (such as improving fitness and body strength, sleep patterns, posture and flexibility) but may also improve the symptoms of many mental health problems (Faulkner & Sparkes 1999). The National Institute for Health and Care Excellence (NICE) advise that physical activity programmes can alleviate symptoms of mild to moderate depression (NICE 2009a). There are also psychosocial benefits of exercise in terms of improving self esteem and social contacts (Daley 2002). However, encouraging and supporting the uptake of exercise is particularly challenging with this client group, due to possible symptoms of mental disorder (such as lethargy, low mood and a lack of motivation) and some medication used in psychiatry can lead to sedation, which may mean that individuals feel less able to become physically active.

People with mental health problems also have an increased risk of using drugs and alcohol. The use of such substances carry with them risks to an individual's physical health (including liver problems, and blood disorders such as Hepatitis C and HIV/AIDS), but there are other associated risks such as increases in violent behaviour, promiscuity and suicide, which can lead to a slower recovery from mental health problems (Vose 2000).

Risk Assessment and Management

There is perhaps an over-emphasis placed on the assessment and management of risk in mental health care, perhaps influenced by the perception of the general public that people with mental health problems are violent (Morgan 1998). However, the majority of people with a mental health problems are not violent. This is not to say that an assessment of the risk of violence or aggression is unwarranted –nurses need to maintain a sense of perspective. What seems to be significant is not the presence of a mental health problem when assessing the risk of violence but how acute and severe these problems may be (Davidson 2005). For example, people who are distressed by severe paranoid or persecutory ideas have an elevated risk of aggression and violence. The use of substances (such as alcohol and/or drugs) and antisocial personality traits also significantly increases the risk of violence (Paterson *et al.* 2004; Davidson 2005). Other factors which can increase the risk of violent or aggressive behaviour are:

- *Boredom and lack of environmental stimulation*
- *Too much stimulation, noise and general disruption*
- *Excessive heating, overcrowding and lack of access to external space*
- *Personal frustrations associated with being in a restricted environment*
- *Difficulties in communication*
- *Emotional distress, e.g. following bereavement*
- *Antagonism, aggression or provocation on the part of others*
- *Physical illness.*

(DH 2008b, p. 113)

Jot This Down

Why is it, do you think, that there is a perception that people who experience mental health problems are more violent that the general population?

Suicide risk assessments are also conducted regularly in mental health care. Suicide is a complex issue and any assessment of suicide risk must be undertaken compassionately and sensitively (Watkins 2001; Barker 2004). These assessments should encompass the known risk factors for suicide, which will include not only factors relating to a person's previous history and current mental state but also social and environmental factors, which may also

Box 12.3 Suicide Risk Factors

- Previous history of suicidal attempts
- Family history of suicide
- Negative view of the future – feelings of hopelessness, helplessness, perception of, and plans for the future, if any
- ental health issues – especially depression, hallucinatory voices commanding self-harm or of persecution, alcohol/drug use
- Social isolation – withdrawal, loss/lack of social support
- Behaviour warning of suicidal intent – e.g. procuring means of death, acts in anticipation of death, putting financial affairs in order, general behaviour at interview, plan to commit suicide
- Current stressors – recent bereavement (especially of partner), relationship difficulties or other stressful events, financial problems, terminal illness, accommodation issues

(*Source*: Barker 2004; Cutcliffe & Barker 2004)

increase risk. For example, 10–15% of people with major depressive disorder will eventually commit suicide (NICE 2009a). Unemployment increases the risk (ODPM 2004) and suicide rates increase with age and are higher among those who are single, widowed, divorced or separated (Box 12.3).

What the Experts Say Suicide Risk

One of the questions I am most asked by students is, 'how do you know how likely someone is to commit suicide?' I have found that therapeutic relationship and knowledge of individual clients to be the one of most valuable tools in gauging risk. A clinicians' instinct or 'gut feeling' is also an important consideration, especially when they know the service-user very well. Changes in emotional state, behaviour and social situation can be considered carefully in conjunction with knowledge of the actuarial risk factors. However, we often need to assess individuals we do not know, and it is especially important to try and establish an atmosphere of trust and openness in such situations. It can be challenging asking people sensitive questions, such as their intent to end their lives, and you may find their answers difficult to deal with. Asking key questions sensitively but directly is very important, with the aim of getting honest answers from the individual. Support should always be sought when you do not feel confident in dealing with the level of risk posed.

(Mental Health Lecturer)

However, people who experience serious, chronic, painful physical illnesses are also at heightened risk of suicide. In a recent study of suicides of people who contacted NHS Direct prior to suicide, over 50% reported physical health problems (Bessant *et al.* 2008).

There have been many strategies over the years to reduce the incidence of suicide. For example, the 'National Suicide Prevention Strategy for England' (DH 2002) sought to reduce suicide risk in high risk groups; promote well-being in the wider community; and reduce lethality and availability of suicide methods, such as by reducing the pack size of non-prescription paracetamol (DH 2002). However, consideration must be given to the particular factors which appear to underpin the person's feelings of suicide. Specialist therapy, counselling and ongoing care in an inpatient service may be required to address possible reasons underpinning the suicidal crisis and to ensure the safety of the person. There is evidence that such strategies have had a positive impact in reducing suicide rates. The latest statistics (ONS 2011) indicate that numbers of suicides are at their lowest since 1991. There were 5377 suicides in adults aged 15 and over – 940 less than in 1991 (6317), with a suicide rate for men of 16.8 per 100 000 population, and for women 5.0 per 100 000 population (ONS 2011).

People who neglect their own personal health and hygiene are relatively common in mental health care. As such, 'self-neglect' is an important risk, which needs to be assessed. It has been defined as:

> … *a form of self-care deficit in which those self-care activities that are thought to be necessary to maintain a socially accepted standard of personal and household hygiene are not undertaken.*
>
> (Lauder 2005, p. 46)

Self-neglect as a phenomenon appears to exist on a continuum (Matthews & Trenoweth 2008) with, at one end, less serious deficits (such as failure to look after diet, dental hygiene and not seeking medical attention when ill), with more extreme forms of severe self-neglect at the other (such as a failure to look after physical health problems, e.g. diabetes; the hoarding of rubbish and animals, both alive and dead; the neglect of rotting food; poor personal hygiene, which results in parasitic infestations and other infections; ignoring possible dangers from malfunctioning appliances, and so on) (Gibbons *et al.* 2006). There are many factors which must be taken into consideration when making an assessment of self-neglect. For example, self-neglect may be associated with mental health problems such as depression, dementia and stress in later life (Abrams *et al.* 2002). Self-neglect may also result from the use of prescribed medication, which is sedating and it may be exacerbated by alcohol or drug misuse (Halliday *et al.* 2000). There also may be a link between self-neglect and cognitive decline in older age (Abrams *et al.* 2002). The term 'Diogenes syndrome' is often used to describe self-neglect among older people, characterised by social withdrawal, malnutrition, the hoarding of rubbish and severe neglect of personal hygiene (Hettiaratchy & Manthorpe 1989) (Box 12.4).

Sadly, the phenomenon of self-neglect/severe self-neglect among younger people is poorly researched (Cooney & Hamid 1995) but self-neglect may be present among people who have poor social networks (few contacts with friends, rejection of help from outside agencies, often being described as being often suspicious and argumentative) (Vostanis & Dean 1992). However, any assessor of self-neglect must consider what they perceive to be socially acceptable standards of personal and household hygiene (Lauder *et al.* 2005). Perceptions of cleanliness and hygiene are likely to vary between social groups and cultures (Lauder 2001). They are, therefore, subjective. This means that nurses may have different perceptions of self-neglect than their patients, which may be, at least in part, based on their own internalisation of their own cultural values (Lauder *et al.* 2001).

There are many risks associated with mental ill health and any assessment must consider the risks that a person poses to themselves or others. But the risks to which the person is exposed also need to be considered in any risk assessment, such as the risk of abuse, being a victim of crime, social exclusion, isolation, poverty, poor access to physical health care, the risk of relapse, and so on. Social and economic factors, such as poverty, social exclusion, accommodation difficulties and overall living conditions, can carry significant risks and also have a significant impact on our physical and mental health and well-being (Mentality/NIMHE 2004). People are more likely to experience disadvantage in these areas – they are more likely to live in areas with higher rates of social deprivation, poor quality housing, high crime levels, unemployment and drug misuse. They are also more at risk of homelessness when compared with the general population (Repper 2000).

A psychiatric diagnosis itself potentially carries risks for the individual, in that it can lead to stigma, and there is evidence that people with mental health problems are discriminated against (ODPM 2004). Stigma can result from misconceptions about people with mental health problems and the level of risk that they may be deemed to pose. Discrimination may have significant consequences for the person in terms of their employment prospects. Unemployment can lead to financial problems, thereby exacerbating the feelings of frustration, low self-esteem and entrapment. This, in turn, can increase the potential for suicidal thoughts and behaviour (Mathers & Schofield 1998). This is recognised in the mental health strategy for England 'No Health Without Mental Health' (DH 2011). The strategy recognises the impact of social injustice and the risks posed by social inequalities, such as those mentioned earlier, which further compounds mental distress (DH 2011). There is also a potential danger that people with mental health problems may be vulnerable to violence or may experience sexual abuse or exploitation. Individuals, particularly at times of acute emotional or mental distress, may be especially at risk. Here, nurses must be mindful of such risks, particularly when the person has a known past history of being physically or sexually abused; when the person appears to lack boundaries in relation to sexual expression or personal space or a lack of awareness, or passivity in the face of, their own risk when exposed to people who may be wishing to exploit them.

Link To/Go To Risk Assessment and Management

Suicide prevention information:

http://www.papyrus-uk.org/

http://www.mentalhealth.org.uk/help-information/mental-health-a-z/S/suicide/

Box 12.4 Diogenes

Diogenes of Sinope (*c.* 404–323 BCE) was a 'cynic' who eschewed all material comfort and property, famously living in a barrel or jar. Unlike people who experience mental health problems, such rejection of comfort and social conventions was a political choice for Diogenes, allegedly seeking to expose corruption in his society.

Legal Context

In England and Wales, the Mental Health Act (1983 amended 2007) is the law which can be used to admit, detain and treat people against their wishes in a hospital setting who are deemed to have a mental disorder. In order for a person to be detained under the Act, there must be clear grounds that:

Box 12.5 The Guiding Principles of the Mental Health Act

The MHA is founded on a number of important guiding principles, which include:

- Keeping to a minimum restrictions which impact on a person's liberty
- Respecting a person's views, wishes and feelings as far as possible, recognising an individual's race, religion, culture, gender, age, sexual orientation or disability
- The opportunity for service-users to participate in their care, including decision-making with regards to planning and reviewing their care and the involvement of carers and family members where possible
- Providing care and treatment, which is effective and efficient in meeting identified heath care needs.

- The person is suffering from a mental disorder of a nature or degree which warrants their detention in hospital for assessment and/or to receive treatment
- The person ought to be detained in their interest of their own health and safety with a view to the protection of others.

While a person may be compulsorily detained, the Mental Health Act (MHA) emphasises the need to involve service-users in all appropriate aspects of their care and on promoting a person's overall health and well-being while supporting their recovery from mental distress (DH 2008b) (Box 12.5).

The Mental Capacity Act 2005 (MCA) differs from the MHA, in that its purpose is to ensure that adults (aged 16 or over) who lack the capacity to make decisions for themselves are protected under the law. The MCA may apply not only to people with mental health problems, dementia and learning disabilities but also to people who may have a brain injury or under the influence of substances or sedation. The Act:

> … is intended to assist and support people who may lack capacity and to discourage anyone who is involved in caring for someone who lacks capacity from being overly restrictive or controlling. But the Act also aims to balance an individual's right to make decisions for themselves with their right to be protected from harm if they lack capacity to make decisions to protect themselves.
>
> (DCA 2007, p. 15)

A person may lack capacity if they are unable to:

- *'understand information relevant to the decision,* or
- *remember the information long enough to make the decision,* or
- *weigh up information relevant to the decision,* or
- *communicate their decision – by talking, using sign language, or by any other means.*

> (Care Quality Commission, CQC 2011, p. 5)

There are two stages to making a test of capacity. First, consideration must be given to whether there is an impairment or disturbance in the functioning of a person's mind or brain. Then, if there is such impairment, is this sufficient to lead to a lack of capacity to make a particular decision?

The MCA is based on a number of important key principles: that a person has capacity unless the contrary has been established; people must be helped to make decisions; unwise decisions do not necessarily mean lack of capacity; decisions taken on behalf of the person must in the person's best interests and must be as least restrictive of freedom as possible (CQC 2011). The MCA also makes it clear that if a person lacks capacity to make **particular** decisions, this does not imply that they lack capacity to make **any** decisions about their life (CQC 2011). The MCA also provides legal protection for nurses when they offer personal care for a person who lacks capacity (such as washing, dressing or attending to personal hygiene; eating and drinking; walking and assistance with transport), providing they are working within the principles and code of practice of the MCA.

Jot This Down

What are the key differences between the Mental Health Act and the Mental Capacity Act?

Link To/Go To Legal Context

Mental Health Act Legislation
http://www.legislation.gov.uk/ukpga/2007/12/contents
Mental Capacity Act Legislation
http://www.legislation.gov.uk/ukpga/2005/9/contents

Therapeutic Nursing Care

Nursing care is, first and foremost, an interpersonal process and the relationship that nurses establish with service-users is crucial to the success of any nursing intervention. Nurses working with people with mental health problems need to be particularly aware of this and they need to develop not only excellent social and interpersonal skills but they need to be self-aware, open-minded, understanding, accepting, insightful and reflective. Sensitivity, patience, empathy, warmth and communication and listening skills are also vital qualities that are used consciously and intentionally, in order to make a positive connection with people experiencing mental distress (Heifner 1993). In so doing, the nurse communicates a genuine concern for and an interest in supporting, understanding and caring for the individual and those which care for them. This is an important part of supporting individuals on their road to recovery and is known as the 'therapeutic use of self'.

A trusting, safe and supportive relationship helps to build a therapeutic alliance between nurse and service-user, within which the person can be supported and possibly to address and resolve issues which they may be facing. The individual may be experiencing problems with their mood or may have experiences or thoughts which may be overwhelming and distressing. They may feel lonely and isolated. Whatever the particular symptoms a person may be experiencing, the nursing relationship needs to communicate sensitivity and a readiness and willingness to engage with the person in a positive, sensitive and thoughtful way (Shattell *et al.* 2006). While this is, of course, the foundation of modern professional nursing practice, there is also evidence therapeutic relationships lead to greater satisfaction with treatment and care, improved attitudes towards medication use and potentially positive clinical outcomes for service-users, such as a reduction of symptoms and admission rates and an improved quality of life for service-users in the community (Forchuk & Reynolds 2001; Nolan & Badger 2005; Hewitt & Coffey 2005).

Often the aspect of mental health nursing care most valued by service-users stems from the personal qualities that nurses bring with them. This was recognised by Carl Rogers in the 1950s, whose work on 'client-centred therapy' (Rogers 1951) has been influential in mental health nursing. Rogers identified three fundamental qualities underpinning a therapeutic relationship:

- Empathy (that is, listening to, understanding and accepting the service-user's frame of reference)
- Non-judgemental warmth or unconditional positive regard (i.e. accepting and valuing the client as a person who is entitled to respect and dignity)
- Genuineness (openness and honesty) (Sin & Trenoweth 2010).

There have been many studies which have indicated that service-users highly rate nurses who are empathic, tolerant, demonstrate personal respect and understanding (Forchuk & Reynolds 2001; Geanellos 2002; Welch 2005). For example, Nolan and Badger (2005) identified the following qualities which mental health service-users found particularly helpful in their recovery:

- Being listened to and understood
- Optimistic attitude from their healthcare workers with reference to treatment options
- Honesty from the practitioners in relation to prognosis and outlook
- Practitioners being supportive and nurturing
- Continuity of care
- Specialist knowledge
- Genuine interests and efforts to monitor the progress.

Empathy is not only a feeling of compassion for another; it is a conscious attempt to understand the frame of reference of the service-user and their experiences, perceptions and meanings that they assign to their situation. This will include an awareness of the values and belief systems arising from another's cultural, social and family backgrounds. However, empathy is also the way in which understanding about another is demonstrated and verbalised to them. We should never assume that we fully or truly 'know' another and we must have humility to recognise that our attempts to understand another person may be limited. We develop our empathy and increase the accuracy of our understanding of another's situation within the therapeutic and trusting relationship where the nurse and service-user feel safe to discuss and identify those thoughts, feelings and experiences which seem related to the person's mental health problem.

Empathy begins with an understanding our own 'self' – a connectedness to those aspects of our personality, which defines and describes us as human beings, our values and the way we experience the world (Welch 2005). An awareness of this helps us to understand how we relate to others, our own attitudes, biases, limitations and strengths and how we are likely to respond to situations and influence our thinking. Such self-awareness helps us to realise that our experiences, like the experiences of others, are subjective, and there are always different interpretations that may be placed on any given situation. Assuming that our viewpoint, and only our viewpoint, is the one which is right or correct and that we have the 'truthful' understanding will not lead to empathic understanding of others. In fact, it may lead to an assumption that our advice is in the service-user's best interests. This may be seen as coercion and limiting the service-user's choice to live their lives in the way in which they choose. Developing our own self-awareness is perhaps one of the most enriching elements of mental health nursing practice – that in the process of helping a person learn

about themselves we, in turn and through a process of self-reflection, begin to understand ourselves. This process allows us to become consciously aware of our thoughts, feelings and actions and how they may be interconnected.

Self-disclosure may form an important part of developing a therapeutic relationship with a service-user. This may also develop naturally as part of a general social conversation that may develop over time. Indeed, some nurses have consciously used self-disclosure as a therapeutic tool:

The nurses used their own experiences of living a life to: be seen as ordinary people; be credible; illustrate aspects of being-in-the-world; allow the service-users to identify with them; and to normalise the service-user's fears and difficulties.

(O'Brien 2001, p. 188)

This, of course, may be perfectly appropriate but needs to be carefully thought through in advance. It is very important to maintain professional boundaries and any aspect of the nurses' personal life must be consciously employed in furtherance of benefitting and supporting the service-user as part of a therapeutic relationship and not to use the service-user as a sounding board for one's own personal problems. This is reinforced in the NMC Code (NMC 2008), which requires nurses to maintain clear, professional boundaries by refusing any gifts, which may be seen as leading to preferential treatment; refraining from asking for loans and establishing and maintaining sexual boundaries.

A therapeutic relationship is the foundation for all nursing care, treatment and interventions in mental health nursing care. Mental health nurses often use psychosocial interventions (PSI) in their day-to-day practice, which is a collaborative approach using psychological and social principles to support service-users and their friends and families (Sin & Scully 2008). The ultimate aim of any PSI approach is to help the person to help themselves (in other words to optimise their own self-management) by empowering the service-user, their families and carers (Repper & Perkins 2003). The key features of the PSI approach include:

- Structured and systematic assessments undertaken collaboratively conducted with service-users (and their families) to explore not only needs but also strengths (such as coping abilities, knowledge, abilities, and so on)
- Educating people about mental health and mental disorders to develop understanding and knowledge and the various treatment options which may be helpful to promote and support recovery (this is often referred to as 'psychoeducation')
- Talking therapies to help the person consider how their thinking patterns may be linked to their feelings and behaviour and helping the person view a situation differently, particularly where the person feels helpless or where they feel there is no way out of their current situation) (this is often referred to as 'cognitive therapy')
- Supporting and encouraging the use of medication and to optimise the medication regimen and adherence. While medication may be important in supporting and promoting recovery (Bennett 2008), a PSI approach also seeks to help to psychologically manage their symptoms (such as helping people who hear voices to develop control of those voices and to reduce distress; supporting the management of stress by using relaxation techniques, mindfulness and meditation)
- Supporting and working with families and carers in order to develop their coping abilities and their understanding of mental health problems so that they may be better placed to help and

support people who experience mental distress. This may also include 'family therapy' (Sin & Trenoweth 2010).

Interviews are often used in PSI approaches and mental health nursing care as a forum for assessment or counselling. Successful interviews use the skills mentioned above and require skilled and thoughtful interpersonal communication and counselling skills drawn upon universally agreed approaches. Interviews should be considered a 'purposeful conversation' (Barker 2004), in which the process (i.e. the way in which the assessment is conducted) is considered as important as the outcome (the assessed information).

A typical interview involves the following.

Establishing rapport

As Rollnick *et al.* (1999, p. 57) suggest, 'If you have a good rapport with someone, you can talk about any subject' and this is an important principle, which underpins any interview with a mental health service-user. In establishing rapport, it is vital that the nurse clearly shows attention and interest in the person by using appropriate non-verbal communication (such as eye contact and body language, which emphasises calmness and interpersonal warmth, such as appropriate smiling and hand gestures) in an environment which is quiet, safe, private and relaxing.

Understanding the person's frame of reference

For Nelson-Jones (2003), understanding the person is essential to be able to most effectively offer help. Here, it is essential to understand the person's frame of reference in an interview by helping the person to talk about their experiences and their thoughts and feelings. This process is facilitated by using verbal and non-verbal prompts. One of the most common easy ways of doing this is to use open questions (which invite the person to talk freely on a subject, for example, 'How are you feeling?') and closed questions (which invite yes/no or short answers, for example, 'Are you feeling sad today?'). Closed questions should be used sparingly, as they tend to halt conversational flow and if we are interested in developing an understanding of another person it is important that they are able to do most of the talking and this is best facilitated by open questions. Other techniques which are important to encourage talk are active listening (i.e. making a conscious effort to hear what the person is saying and demonstrating you are doing this by verbal and non-verbal prompts); reflection (showing that you understand a person's point of view by reflecting back to them what they have said); and summarising (i.e. bringing together all the points that have been discussed as a conclusion to a conversation).

There are times, of course, where an interview may be quite structured, such as when you are conducting assessments to develop a clearer understanding of the nature of the person's problems. At such times, the conversation may centre on the nature of the person's current mental distress and the impact that this has on their life and holistic functioning; the broad context of the current problem, including triggers, which may have precipitated the problem; their past history and factors, which may have predisposed the person to mental distress; physical health problems; factors which are helpful and unhelpful in supporting the person; the risks that person may pose to themselves and others; and the strengths and abilities that the person may have which could be marshalled to support their recovery. In this way, the nurse can develop an understanding of what the issues might be for the service-user and what they would like to do to address their problems. The nurse is therefore able to offer suggestions and

develop a treatment or action plan which is agreeable to the service-user (Simmons & Griffiths 2009). This latter point is vital in that a service-user is not likely to be willing to work towards addressing such problems if they feel that the action plan has been imposed upon them.

Resolving problems

There are many possible ways in which the nurse and service-user (and their carers and family) may be able to address and support the current problems or difficulties of the service-user. Of course, the nurse may make constructive suggestions based on research or best-practice that might help to improve the situation. Helping the person to think about how they might manage their condition better and identify and choose a possible solution to their problems can be a significant step on the road to recovery and help the person take more control of their lives (Rollnick *et al.* 1999; Miller & Rollnick 2002). Once a course of action has been decided, the nurse must be available to offer assistance and support to the person to achieve their goals and in offering support during the change process (such as meeting regularly to review progress and offer encouragement) (Nelson-Jones 2003).

Conclusion

In this chapter, we have explored the fundamental principles of caring for people with mental health problems and the policy context, which underpins contemporary mental health care. It is important, however, to understand that while the policy context stresses a 'recovery' approach (where an emphasis is placed on social recovery and supporting people to achieve the best quality of life) contemporary mental health services are often primarily medical in nature, where medication is emphasised to the detriment of holistic and psychosocial care. An important aspect of nursing care is being able to promote and respond to the physical health care need of this group. We have explored the settings and contexts for mental health care and the principles of nursing care for people experiencing mental distress and their carers, including assessment and treatment options. Finally, we have explored how to provide therapeutic nursing care for this client group.

Key Points

- This chapter has provided you with an overview of the fundamental aspects associated with mental health nursing, the principles of care. The chapter has provided information immersed in the policy context for contemporary mental health nursing care.
- An awareness of the various approaches to understanding mental disorder have been discussed, an emphasis has been placed on the principles of the 'recovery' approach. The values of holism in the delivery of nursing care for people with mental health problems are essential if care is to be person centred.
- Understand the principles of nursing care for people experiencing mental distress and their carers, including assessment, treatment options and therapeutic nursing care have been discussed with an appreciation of why physical health problems may be elevated in this client group.
- The chapter has highlighted the need for nurses to be aware of the contexts for mental health care, including the various settings for care and the legal contexts.

- Central to the values that underpin effective mental health nursing is the need for all nurses to practise in a holistic, non-judgemental, caring and sensitive manner that avoids assumptions, supports social inclusion; recognises and respects individual choice; and acknowledges diversity. Where necessary, the nurse must challenge inequality, discrimination and exclusion from access to care.
- Emphasis has been placed on the need for all nurses to use therapeutic principles to engage, maintain and, where appropriate, disengage from professional caring relationships, respecting professional boundaries.

Glossary

Antisocial personality disorder: lack of regard for the moral or legal standards in the local culture, along with a marked inability to get along with others or abide by societal rules. Sometimes this called psychopaths or sociopaths

Anxiety disorders: chronic feelings of overwhelming anxiety and fear, unattached to any obvious source that can grow progressively worse if not treated, often accompanied by physical symptoms such as sweating, cardiac disturbances, diarrhoea or dizziness

Dementia: a condition of declining mental abilities, particularly memory. Individuals with dementia may have trouble doing things they used to do, such as driving a car safely or planning a meal. They often have trouble finding the right word and can become confused when given too many things to do at one time they may also experience changes in personality, becoming aggressive, paranoid or depressed

Depression: a disorder marked particularly by sadness, inactivity, difficulty with thinking and concentration, a significant increase or decrease in appetite and time spent sleeping, feelings of dejection and hopelessness and sometimes suicidal thoughts or attempts to commit suicide. Depression also can be experienced in other disorders such as bipolar disorder; it can range from mild to severe

Panic: an anxiety disorder whereby individuals have feelings of terror that strikes suddenly and repeatedly with no warning. Individuals cannot predict when an attack will occur. Symptoms can include palpitations, chest pain or discomfort, sweating, trembling, tingling sensations, a feeling of choking, fear of dying, fear of losing control as well as feelings of unreality

Psychiatry: the branch of medicine that deals with the science and practice of treating mental, emotional or behavioural disorders

Psychosis: a serious disorder that is characterised by defective or lost contact with reality, often with hallucinations or delusions, this may lead to a deterioration of normal social functioning

Stigma: a mark of shame or discredit. A sign of social unacceptability

Substance misuse: the inappropriate use of and possibly addiction to illegal and legal substances including alcohol and prescription and non-prescription drugs

Traumatic brain injury: traumatic brain injury (TBI) is a non-degenerative, non-congenital insult to the brain from an external mechanical force, possibly leading to permanent or temporary impairment of cognitive, physical and psychosocial functions, with an associated diminished or altered state of consciousness.

References

Abrams, R.C., Lachs, M., McAvay, G., Keohane, D.J. & Bruce, M.L. (2002) Predictors of self neglect in community-dwelling elders. *American Journal of Psychiatry*, 159(10), 1724–1730.

Badger, F. & Nolan, P. (2007) Attributing recovery from depression. Perceptions of people cared for in primary care. *Journal of Clinical Nursing*, 16(3a), 25–34.

Barker, P. (2004) *Assessment in Psychiatric and Mental Health Nursing: in search of the whole person.* Nelson Thornes, Cheltenham.

Bennett, J. (2008) Supporting recovery: medication management in mental health care. In: J. Lynch & S. Trenoweth (eds) *Contemporary Issues in Mental Health Nursing.* Wiley, Chichester.

Bentall, R. (2003) *Madness Explained: psychosis and human nature.* Penguin, London.

Bessant, M., King, E.A. & Peveler, R. (2008) Characteristics of suicides in recent contact with NHS Direct. *Psychiatric Bulletin*, 32, 92–95.

Butcher, J., Mineka, S. & Hooley, J. (2008) *Abnormal Psychology: core concepts.* Pearson, Boston.

Bope, E.T., Douglass, A.B. & Gibovsky, A. (2004) Pain management by the family physician: the Family Practice Pain Education Project. *Journal of the American Board of Family Medicine*, 17, S1–S12.

Boyle, M. (2002) *Schizophrenia. A scientific delusion?*, 2nd edn. Routledge, London.

Brown, A. (2010) Caring for the spirit. In: C. Margereson & S. Trenoweth (eds) *Developing Holistic Care for Long Term Conditions.* Routledge, London.

Brown, M. (2004) *Coping With Depression after Traumatic Brain Injury.* http://www.biausa.org/_literature_43189/depression_and_brain_injury.

Brown, G. & Harris, T. (1978) *The Social Origins of Depression: a Study of Psychiatric Disorder in Women.* Tavistock, London.

Brown, S., Birtwistle, J., Roe, L. & Thompson, C. (1999) The unhealthy lifestyle of people with schizophrenia. *Psychological Medicine*, 29(3), 697–701.

CQC (2011) *The Mental Capacity Act 2005.* Care Quality Commission. http://www.cqc.org.uk/sites/default/files/media/documents/rp_poc1b2b_100563_20111223_v4_00_guidance_for_providers_mca_for_external_publication.pdf.

CEMH (2007) *Model to Assess the Economic Impact of Integrating CRHT and Inpatient Services.* Centre for the Economics of Mental Health, Health Service and Population Research Department King's College, London.

CMH (2010) *The Economic and Social Costs of Mental Health Problems in 2009/10.* Centre for Mental Health. http://www.centreformentalhealth.org.uk/pdfs/Economic_and_social_costs_2010.pdf.

Cohen, S. & Rodriguez, M.S. (1995) Pathways linking affective disturbances and physical disorders. *Health Psychology*, 14(5), 374–380.

Cooney, C. & Hamid, W. (1995) Review: Diogenes syndrome. *Age and Aging*, 24(5), 451–453.

Crawford P., Nolan P. & Brown, B. (1998) Ministering to madness: the narratives of people who have left religious orders to work in the caring professions. *Journal of Advanced Nursing*, 28(1), 212–220.

CSIP (2006) *Crisis Resolution and Home Treatment: report from a conference linking research, policy and practice for service development*, 5 October. Care Services Improvement Partnership, York.

Cutcliffe, J. & Barker, P. (2004) The nurses' global assessment of suicide risk (NGASR): developing a tool for clinical practice. *Journal of Psychiatric and Mental Health Nursing*, 11, 393–400.

Daley, A.J. (2002) Exercise therapy and mental health in clinical populations: is exercise therapy a worthwhile intervention? *Advances in Psychiatric Treatment*, 8, 262–270.

Davidson, S. (2005) The management of violence in general psychiatry. *Advances in Psychiatric Treatment*, 11(5), 362–370.

Davies, J-A. (2002) *Trapped in the Hell of Their Parents' Suffering. National network of adult and adolescent children who have a mentally ill parent/s,*

251

Vic. Inc., Australia. http://www.nnaami.org/index.php?option=com_content&view=article&id=64:trapped-in-the-hell-of-their-parents-suffering&catid=6:featured-articles&Itemid=8.

Dean J., Todd G., Morrow, H. & Sheldon, K. (2001) Mum, I used to be good looking. Look at me now: the physical health needs of adults with mental health problems: the perspectives of users, carers and front-line staff. *International Journal of Mental Health Promotion*, 3(4), 16–24.

Dean, C. & Macmillan, C. (2002) *Serving the Children of Parents with a Mental Illness: barriers, breakthroughs and benefits.* Australian Infant, Child, Adolescent and Family mental health Association Ltd. http://www.aicafmha.net.au/conferences/brisbane2001/papers/dean_c.htm.

DCA (2007) *Mental Capacity Act 2005 Code of Practice.* Department for Constitutional Affairs. http://webarchive.nationalarchives.gov.uk/ and http://www.dca.gov.uk/legal-policy/mental-capacity/mca-cp.pdf.

DH (1999) *National Service Framework for Mental Health: modern standards and service models.* Department of Health, London. http://www.nmhdu.org.uk/silo/files/nsf-for-mental-health.pdf.

DH (2001) *The Mental Health Policy Implementation Guide.* Department of Health, London.

DH (2002) *National Suicide Prevention Strategy for England.* Department of Health, London. http://www.nmhdu.org.uk/silo/files/national-suicide-prevention-strategy-for-england.pdf.

DH (2006) *Choosing Health: supporting the physical needs of people with severe mental illness commissioning framework.* Department of Health, London.

DH (2008a) *Refocusing Care Programme Approach.* Department of Health, London. http://www.nmhdu.org.uk/silo/files/dh-2008-refocusing-the-care-programme-approach-policy-and-positive-practice-guidance.pdf.

DH (2008b) *Code of Practice: Mental Health Act 1983.* Department of Health, London. http://www.lbhf.gov.uk/Images/Code%20of%20practice%201983%20rev%202008%20dh_087073[1]_tcm21–145032.pdf.

DH (2010) *Equity and Excellence: liberating the NHS.* Department of Health, London. http://www.dh.gov.uk/en/Publicationsandstatistics/Publications/PublicationsPolicyAndGuidance/DH_117353.

DH (2011) *No Health Without Mental Health.* Department of Health, London. https://www.gov.uk/government/uploads/system/uploads/attachment_data/file/135457/dh_124058.pdf.

DiClemente, R. & Ponton, L. (1993) HIV related risk behaviours among psychiatrically hospitalised adolescents and school based adolescents. *American Journal of Psychiatry,* 150: 324–325.

DRC (Disability Rights Commission) (2006) *Equal Treatment, Closing the Gap: background evidence for the DRC's formal investigation into health inequalities experienced by people with learning disabilities and/or mental health problems.* University of Leeds, Leeds.

Engel, G. (1977) The need for a new medical model. *Science,* 196, 129–136.

Ershler, W. & Keller, E. (2000) Age-associated increased Interleukin-6 gene expression, late life diseases and frailty. *Annual Review of Medicine,* 51, 245–270.

Faulkner, A. & Layzell, S. (2000) *Strategies for Living: the research report.* Mental Health Foundation, London

Faulkner, G. & Sparkes, A. (1999) Exercise therapy for schizophrenia: an ethnographic study. *Journal of Sport and Exercise,* 21, 39–51.

Forchuk, C. & Reynolds, W. (2001) Clients' reflections on relationships with nurses: comparisons from Canada and Scotland. *Journal of Psychiatric and Mental Health Nursing,* 8, 45–51.

Friedli, L. & Dardis, C. (2002) Smoke gets in their eyes. *Mental Health Today,* Jan, 18–21.

FSA (2001) *The Balance of Good Health.* Food Standards Agency. http://www.food.gov.uk/multimedia/pdfs/bghbooklet.pdf.

Gallop, R. & Reynolds, W. (2004) Putting it all together: dealing with complexity in the understanding of the human condition. *Journal of Psychiatric and Mental Health Nursing,* 11, 357–364.

Geanellos R 2002 Transformative change of self: the unique focus of (adolescent) mental health nursing? *International Journal of Mental Health Nursing,* 11, 174–185.

Gibbons, S., Lauder, W. & Ludwick, R. (2006) Self-neglect: a proposed new NANDA diagnosis. *International Journal of Nursing Terminologies and Classifications,* 17(1), 10–18.

Goddard, N. (1995) Spirituality as integrative energy: a philosophical analysis as requisite precursor to holistic nursing practice. *Journal of Advanced Nursing,* 22(4), 808–815.

Gough, S. & Peveler, R. (2004) Diabetes and its prevention: pragmatic solutions for people with schizophrenia. *British Journal of Psychiatry,* 184(Suppl 47), S106–S111.

Gureje, O. (2007) Psychiatric aspects of pain. *Current Opinion in Psychiatry,* 20, 42–46.

Halliday, G., Banerjee, S., Philpot, M. & Macdonald, A. (2000) Community study of people who live in squalor. *The Lancet* 355, 882–886.

Harris, E. & Barraclough, B. (1998) Excess mortality of mental disorder. *British Journal of Psychiatry,* 173, 11–53.

Heifner, C. (1993) Positive connectedness in the psychiatric nurse–patient relationship. *Archives of Psychiatric Nursing,* 7(1), 11–15.

Hettiaratchy, P. & Manthorpe, J. (1989) The 'hidden' nature of self-neglect. *Care of the Elderly,* 1(1), 14–15.

Hewitt, J. & Coffey, M. (2005) Therapeutic working relationships with people with schizophrenia: literature review. *Journal of Advanced Nursing,* 52(5), 561–570.

Holmes, T. & Rahe, R. (1967) The Social Readjustment Rating Scale. *Journal of Psychosomatic Research,* 11(2), 213–218.

Jenkins, R., Meltzer, H., Jones, P. *et al.* (2008) *Foresight Mental Capital and Well-being Project. Mental Health: future challenges.* The Government Office for Science, London.

Kendrick, T. (1996) Cardiovascular and respiratory risk factors and symptoms among general practice patients with long term mental illness. *British Journal of Psychiatry,* 169, 733–739.

Kessler, R., Berglund, P., Foster, C., Saunders, W., Stang, P.E. & Walters, E.E. (1997) Social consequences, psychiatric disorders, 11: Teenage parenthood. *American Journal of Psychiatry,* 154, 1405–1411.

Koehn, C. & Cutcliffe, J. (2007) Hope and interpersonal psychiatric/mental health nursing: a systematic review of the literature, Part 1. *Journal of Psychiatric and Mental Health Nursing,* 14, 134–140.

Krauss J. & Slavinsky, A. (1982) *The Chronically Ill Psychiatric Patient and the Community.* Blackwell, Boston.

Kring, A., Johnson, S., Davison, G. & Neale, J. (2010) *Abnormal psychology,* 11th edn. Wiley, Hoboken.

Lauder, W. (2001) The utility of self-care theory as a theoretical basis for self-neglect. *Journal of Advanced Nursing,* 34(4), 545–551.

Lauder, W., Anderson, I. & Barclay, A. (2005) A framework for good practice in interagency interventions with cases of self-neglect. *Journal of Psychiatric and Mental Health Nursing,* 12, 192–198.

Lauder, W., Scott, P. & Whyte, A. (2001) Nurses' judgements of self-neglect: a factorial survey. *International Journal of Nursing Studies,* 38(5), 601–608.

Launer, J. (2002) *Narrative-based Primary Care: a practical guide.* Radcliffe Medical Press, Abingdon.

Margereson, C. (2008) Physical illness: promoting effective coping in clients with co-morbidity. In: J. Lynch & S. Trenoweth (eds) *Contemporary Issues in Mental Health Nursing.* Wiley, Chichester.

Martin, G. (2006) *Human Neuropsychology,* 2nd edn. Pearson, Harlow.

Mathers, C. & Schofield, D. (1998) The health consequences of unemployment: the evidence. *Medical Journal of Australia,* 168(4), 178–182.

Matthews, J. (2008) The meaning of recovery. In: J. Lynch & S. Trenoweth (eds). *Contemporary Issues in Mental Health Nursing.* Wiley, Chichester.

Matthews, J. & Trenoweth, S. (2008) Some considerations for mental health nurses working with patients who self-neglect. In: J. Lynch & S. Trenoweth (eds). *Contemporary Issues in Mental Health Nursing.* Wiley, Chichester.

McCloughen, A. (2003) The association between schizophrenia and cigarette smoking: a review of the literature and implications for mental health nursing practice. *International Journal of Mental Health Nursing*, 12, 119–129.

McCreadie, R. (2003) Diet, smoking and cardiovascular risk in people with schizophrenia. *British Journal of Psychiatry*, 183, 534–539.

MHF. (2006) *Feeding Minds: the impact of food on mental health*. Mental Health Foundation. http://www.mentalhealth.org.uk/campaigns/food-and-mental-health/.

Miller, W.R. & Rollnick, S. (2002) *Motivational Interviewing: Preparing People for Change*, 2nd edn. Guildford Press, New York.

Morgan, S. (1998) The assessment and management of risk. In: C. Brooker & J. Repper (eds) *Serious Mental Health Problems in the Community: Policy, Practice and Research*. Baillière Tindall, London.

Murray, R. (2012) *The Abandoned Illness: A report by the Schizophrenia Commission*. https://www.sussex.ac.uk/webteam/gateway/file.php?name=tsc-executive-summary1.pdf&site=75.

NHSIC (2009) *Adult Psychiatric Morbidity in England, 2007: results of a household survey*. The NHS Information Centre. http://www.ic.nhs.uk/webfiles/publications/mental%20health/other%20mental%20health%20publications/Adult%20psychiatric%20morbidity%2007/APMS%2007%20(FINAL)%20Standard.pdf.

NIMHE (2005) *NIMHE Guiding Statement on Recovery*. National Institute for Mental Health in England. http://www.psychminded.co.uk/news/news2005/feb05/nimherecovstatement.pdf.

NIMHE (2004) *Healthy Body and Mind: Promoting Healthy Living for People who Experience Mental Distress. A Guide for People Working in Primary Health Care Teams Supporting People with Severe and Enduring Mental Illness*. National Institute for Mental Health in England & Mentality.

NMHDU (2011). *Improving Access to Psychological Therapies*. National Mental Health Development Unit, England.

Nelson-Jones, R. (2003) *Basic Counselling Skills: A Helpers' Manual*. Sage, London.

NICE (2009a) *The Treatment and Management of Depression in Adults with Chronic Physical Health Problems*. National Institute for Health and Care Excellence. http://guidance.nice.org.uk/CG91.

NICE (2009b) *Schizophrenia: core interventions in the treatment and management of schizophrenia in adults in primary and secondary care*. National Institute for Health and Care Excellence. http://www.nice.org.uk/CG82.

Nolan, P. & Badger, F. (2005) Aspects of the relationship between doctors and depressed patients that enhance satisfaction with primary care. *Journal of Psychiatric and Mental Health Nursing*, 12, 146–153.

NMC (2008) *The Code: Standards of Conduct, Performance and Ethics for Nurses and Midwives*. Nursing and Midwifery Council. http://www.nmc-uk.org/Documents/Standards/The-code-A4-20100406.pdf

O'Brien, A.J. (2001) The therapeutic relationship: historical development and contemporary significance. *Journal of Psychiatric and Mental Health Nursing*, 8(2), 129–137.

ODPM. (2004) *Mental Health and Social Exclusion: Social Exclusion Unit Report*. Office of the Deputy Prime Minister, Wetherby.

OECD (2012) *Sick on the Job?* Organisation for Economic Co-operation and Development. http://www.oecd.org/els/emp/49227189.pdf.

ONS (2002) *The Social and Economic Circumstances of Adults with Mental Disorders*. Office for National Statistics, London.

ONS (2011) *Suicide Rates in the United Kingdom, 2000–2009*. Office for National Statistics. http://www.ons.gov.uk/ons/rel/subnational-health4/suicides-in-the-united-kingdom/2009/suicide-rates-in-the-united-kingdom-2000-2009.pdf

ONS (2013) *Labour Market Statistics, May 2013*. Office for National Statistics. http://www.ons.gov.uk/ons/dcp171778_307508.pdf.

Paterson, B., Claughan P. & McComish, S. 2004 New evidence or changing population? Reviewing the evidence of a link between mental illness and violence. *International Journal of Mental Health Nursing*, 13(1), 39–52.

Peet, M. (2004) Diet, diabetes and schizophrenia: review and hypothesis. *British Journal of Psychiatry*, 184(Suppl 47), S102–S105.

Rapp, C. (1997) *The Strengths Model: Case Management with People Suffering from Severe and Persistent Mental Illness*. Oxford University Press, New York.

Rapp, C. & Goscha, R.J. (2006) A beginning theory of strengths. In: C.A. Rapp & R.J. Goscha (eds) *The Strengths Model: Case Management with People with a Psychiatric Disability*, 2nd edn. Oxford University Press, New York.

Repper, J. (2000b) Social inclusion. In: T. Thompson & P. Mathias (eds) *Lyttle's Mental Health and Disorder*. Elsevier, London.

Repper, J. & Perkins, R. (2003) *Social Inclusion and Recovery: a Model for Mental Health Practice*. Bailliere Tindall, Edinburgh.

Robson, D. & Gray, R. (2007) Serious mental illness and physical health problems: a discussion paper. *International Journal of Nursing Studies*, 44, 457–466.

Robson, H., Margereson, C. & Trenoweth, S. (2008) Comorbidity in physical and mental ill health. In: J. Lynch & S. Trenoweth (eds) *Contemporary Issues in Mental Health Nursing*. Wiley, Chichester.

Rogers, C. (1951) *Client-centred Therapy: Its Current Practice, Implications and Theory*. Houghton Mifflin, Boston.

Rollnick, S., Mason, P. & Butler, C. (1999) *Health Behaviour Change: A Guide for Practitioners*. Churchill Livingstone, Edinburgh.

SCMH (2003) *Economic and Social Costs of Mental Illness in England*. Sainsbury Centre for Mental Health, London.

Seligman, M. (2008) Positive health. *Applied Psychology: An International Review*, 57, 3–18.

Seymour, L. (2003) *Not All in the Mind: the physical health of mental health service-users*. Briefing paper 2. Radical Mentalities, London.

Shattell, M.M., McAllister, S., Hogan, B. *et al*. (2006) She took the time to make sure she understood': mental health patients' experiences of being understood. *Archives of Psychiatric Nursing*, 20(5), 234–241.

Sheild, H., Fairbrother, G. & Obmann, H. (2005) Sexual health knowledge and risk behaviour in young people with first episode psychosis. *International Journal of Mental Health Nursing*, 14, 149–154.

Simmons, J. & Griffiths, R. (2009) *CBT for Beginners*. Sage, London.

Sin, J. & Scully, E. (2008) An evaluation of education and implementation of psychosocial interventions within one UK Mental Healthcare Trust. *Journal of Psychiatric and Mental Health Nursing*, 15, 161–169.

Sin, J. & Trenoweth, S. (2010) Caring for the mind. In: C. Margereson & S. Trenoweth (eds) *Developing Holistic Care for Long Term Conditions*. Routledge, London.

Singh, S. (2010) Early intervention in psychosis. *British Journal of Psychiatry*, 196, 343–345.

Stephenson, C. (1991) The concept of hope revisited for nursing. *Journal of Advanced Nursing*, 16, 1456–1461.

Stubbs, J. & Gardner, L. (2004) Survey of staff attitudes to smoking in a large psychiatric hospital. *Psychiatric Bulletin*, 28, 204–207.

Swinton, J. & Pattison, S. (2001) Spirituality. Come all ye faithful. *Health Service Journal*, 111(5786), 24–25.

Thompson, I. (2002) Mental health and spiritual care. *Nursing standard*, 17(9), 33–38.

Tosevski, D.L. & Milovancevic, M.P. (2006) Stressful life events and physical health. *Current Opinion in Psychiatry*, 19, 184–189.

Trenoweth, S. & Allymamod, W. (2010) Mental health. In: C. Margereson & S. Trenoweth (eds) *Developing Holistic Care for Long Term Conditions*. Routledge, London.

Vose, C.P. (2000) Drug abuse and mental illness: psychiatry's next challenge! In: P.L. Thompson & P. Mathias (eds) *Lyttle's Mental Health and Disorder*. Elsevier, London.

Vostanis, P. & Dean, C. (1992) Self-neglect in adult life. *British Journal of Psychiatry*, 161, 265–267.

Watkins, P. (2001) *Mental Health Nursing: the Art of Compassionate Care*. Butterworth Heinemann, Edinburgh.

Welch, M. (2005) Pivotal moments in the therapeutic relationship. *International Journal of Mental Health Nursing*, 14, 161–165.

253

WHO (1946) International Health Conference, New York, 19 June–22 July. *Official Records of the World Health Organization*, No. 2, p. 100. World Health Organization, Geneva.

WHO (2004) *International Statistical Classification of Diseases and Related Health Problems,* 10th revision (ICD-10), Vol. 2. World Health Organization, Geneva.

WHO (2007) Mental health: strengthening our response. *Fact sheet N°220.* WHO Media Centre, World Health Organization, Geneva. http://www.who.int/mediacentre/factsheets/fs220/en/index.html.

Zubin, J. & Spring, B. (1977) Vulnerability: a new view of schizophrenia. *Journal of Abnormal Psychology*, 86(2), 103–124.

Test Yourself

1. Which of the following is NOT a high level priority for mental health?
   (a) More people will have good mental health
   (b) More people with mental health problems will have good physical health
   (c) More people will be cared for in hospital
   (d) Fewer people will suffer avoidable harm

2. Recovery is:
   (a) focussed on an individuals' return to a state of well-being
   (b) achieved when a person no longer experiences symptoms of mental illness
   (c) achieved when a person returns to work
   (d) best facilitated by service-user's listening to and being compliant with healthcare treatment

3. Which of the following is NOT usually a symptom of depression?
   (a) Feelings of sadness and despair
   (b) A loss of hope
   (c) Appetite and sleep disturbances
   (d) Increased energy

4. In 2013, the unemployment rate was 7.8% of the economically active population (Office for National Statistics, ONS 2013). What was the unemployment rate of people with mental health problems?
   (a) 7.8%
   (b) 15–20%
   (c) 30–45%
   (d) 60–70%

5. What does the National Institute for Health and Clinical Excellence (NICE) advise may alleviate symptoms of mild to moderate depression (NICE 2009a)?
   (a) Physical activity
   (b) Homeopathy
   (c) Anti-psychotic medication
   (d) A holiday

6. How many people with a major depressive disorder will eventually commit suicide (NICE 2009a)?
   (a) 0–10%
   (b) 10–15%
   (c) 20–25%
   (d) 40–50%

7. Which of the following are guiding principles of the Mental Health Act?
   (a) Keeping to a minimum restrictions which impact on a person's liberty
   (b) Respecting a person's views, wishes and feelings as far as possible, recognising an individual's race, religion, culture, gender, age, sexual orientation or disability
   (c) The opportunity for service-users to participate in their care, including decision-making with regards to planning and reviewing their care and the involvement of carers and family members where possible
   (d) Providing care and treatment, which is effective and efficient in meeting identified heath care needs
   (e) All of the above

8. Which of the following is NOT one of three fundamental qualities underpinning a therapeutic relationship, as identified by Rogers (1951)?
   (a) Empathy
   (b) Non-judgemental warmth or unconditional positive regard
   (c) Sympathy
   (d) Genuineness

9. According to the Mental Capacity Act, a person may lack capacity if they are unable to:
   (a) Understand information relevant to the decision
   (b) Remember the information long enough to make the decision
   (c) Weigh up information relevant to the decision
   (d) Communicate their decision by talking, using sign language, or other means
   (e) All of the above

10. Which of the following are NOT typically key features of the PSI approach?
    (a) Structured and systematic assessments undertaken collaboratively conducted with service-users (and their families) to explore not only needs but also strengths (such as coping abilities, knowledge, abilities and so on)
    (b) Telling people what is wrong with them and what they must do to recover
    (c) Talking therapies
    (d) Supporting and encouraging the use of medication and to optimise the medication regimen and adherence
    (e) Supporting and working with families and carers in order to develop their coping abilities and their understanding of mental health problems

255

Answers

1. c
2. a
3. d
4. c
5. a
6. b
7. e
8. c
9. e
10. b

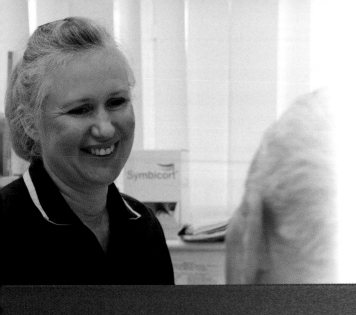

13

The Principles of Maternity Care

Rosemary McCarthy and Jean Mason Mitchell

University of Salford, UK

Learning Outcomes

On completion of this chapter you will be able to:

- Have an understanding of the role of the midwife in maternity care
- Identify the options available for maternity care and birth
- Gain an insight into the physiology of pregnancy
- Be aware of the screening offered during pregnancy
- Have an understanding of the common minor disorders of pregnancy and appropriate management
- Understand the care a woman receives in the antenatal, intranatal and postnatal period and gain insight into the care of the neonate
- Have an awareness of some of the complications of pregnancy and childbirth

Competencies

All nurses must:

1. Support and promote the health, well-being, rights and dignity of people, groups, communities and populations
2. Work in partnership with service-users, carers, families, groups, communities and organisations
3. Manage risk, and promote health and well-being, while aiming to empower choices that promote self-care and safety
4. Understand the roles and responsibilities of other health and social care professionals, and seek to work collaboratively for the benefit of all who need care
5. Practise independently, recognising the limits of competence and knowledge
6. Reflect on these limits and seek advice from, or refer to, other professionals where necessary

 Visit the companion website at **www.wileynursingpractice.com** where you can test yourself using flashcards, multiple-choice questions and more.

Nursing Practice: Knowledge and Care, First Edition. Edited by Ian Peate, Karen Wild and Muralitharan Nair.
© 2014 John Wiley & Sons, Ltd. Published 2014 by John Wiley & Sons, Ltd. Companion website: www.wileynursingpractice.com

Introduction

Maternal health is incorporated into the pre-registration nursing curriculum and although most normal maternity care is provided by midwives, nurses will meet pregnant women in a variety of situations. Nurses need to have an awareness of pregnancy as a normal physiological event and have an understanding of the implications of pregnancy and childbearing on women's health.

There were almost 730,000 live births in England and Wales in 2012 (Office of National Statistics 2013) and most of these births follow on from healthy, uncomplicated pregnancies that are considered to be low in risk. In low risk, normal pregnancies the midwife is the lead health professional who delivers and coordinates maternity care. The midwife may share this care with other health professionals, depending on the woman's specific and unique needs. If complications or risk factors are identified, midwives refer to obstetricians who manage clinically complex pregnancies.

The Role of the Midwife in Maternity Care

A midwife is a person who has been educated and trained and successfully completed a course of studies in midwifery (see the NMC website for a full definition of the midwives role) (NMC 2012). The midwife is a health professional who works in partnership with women to give support, care and advice during pregnancy, labour and the postpartum period.

> ### Jot This Down
>
> From your experience, what would you say are the principal roles that the midwife has in pregnancy and after care?
>
> **http://www.nmc-uk.org/Publications/Standards/**

In the 'Jot This Down' exercise above, you will have thought about the midwife's role in preparing women for motherhood and maintaining safety.

The midwife assists the woman birthing and is the lead professional during normal labour and birth and she also provides care for the newborn and the infant. Midwifery care includes preventative measures, the promotion of normal birth, the detection of complications in mother and child, the accessing of medical care or other appropriate assistance and the carrying out of emergency measures. The midwife also has a vital role in antenatal education, preparation for parenthood, health counselling and education for the women and their families (ICM 2011).

All midwives in the UK must be registered with the Nursing and Midwifery Council (NMC 2010) who regulate their practice. In addition to the 'Code of Conduct' (NMC 2008), which all nurses and midwives must adhere to, midwives must also adhere to the 'Midwives Rules' (NMC 2012).

All midwives registered in the UK have to be supported by a Supervisor of Midwives (NMC 2006). A supervisor of midwives is an experienced midwife who has undertaken additional training and her role is to protect women and babies from poor practice and to support midwives in clinical practice.

 Link To/Go To

The NMC website for midwifery-related content and documents will provide you with further information:

http://www.nmc-uk.org/Nurses-and-midwives/Midwifery-New/

Overview of the Physiology of Pregnancy

Pregnancy is a normal physiological event and is not pathological; however, pathological processes can occur in pregnancy as they can in any individual at any time. Thus, nurses need to be aware of the pregnant woman and the potential changes to her physiology and the care she may require.

 Link To/Go To

You can read about the physiological changes that occur during pregnancy at:

http://www.patient.co.uk/doctor/physiological-changes-in-pregnancy

The duration of pregnancy is 40 weeks or 280 days; this is described in three parts called 'trimesters', each lasting three calendar months. The first trimester is from conception to 12 weeks; the second (mid)-trimester is from 12 weeks to 24 weeks; and the third is from 24 weeks to delivery of the fetus. The estimated date of delivery (EDD) is calculated by adding 7 days to the first day of the last menstrual period (LMP) and counting back 3 months. Ultrasound scans (USS) are commonly used to confirm gestation; the earlier these are undertaken the more accurate they are.

> ### Jot This Down
>
> **Naegele's Rule** is a standard way of calculating the due date for a pregnancy. The rule estimates the expected date of delivery (EDD) by adding one year, subtracting 3 months, and adding seven days to the first day of a woman's last menstrual period (LMP). The result is approximately 280 days (40 weeks) from the LMP. See example of Naegle's rule calculation in Box 13.1.

Box 13.1 Example Calculation to Estimate Date of Delivery (Naegele's Rule)

LMP = 8 May 2012
+1 year = 8 May 2013
−3 months = 8 February 2013
　+7 days = 15 February 2013 is estimated delivery date (EDD)

The calculation method does not always result in 280 days because not all calendar months are the same length; it does not account for leap years. Naegele's Rule assumes an average menstrual cycle length of 28 days. In modern practice, calculators, reference cards, or sliding wheel calculators are used to add 280 days to LMP.

Calculate the EDD if the LMP is 25 July 2013.

The signs and symptoms of pregnancy are largely due to hormonal changes and the increasing size of the gravid uterus.

Signs and Symptoms – First Trimester

These are not diagnostic tests and do not confirm pregnancy.

1. Amenorrhoea (absence of menstruation) – in women with a previously predictable cycle
2. Positive pregnancy test
3. Breast changes – they may become larger, tender and veins may appear more prominent and the pigmentation of the areolar may become darker
4. Skin pigmentation
   - **Chloasma** – also known as the 'mask of pregnancy'. This is a brownish pigmentation that appears on the face of approximately 50–70% of women in a butterfly-like pattern. This exacerbates as the pregnancy develops
   - **Linea nigra** – a dark line may be noted on the abdomen between the sternum and the symphysis pubis
   - **Striae gravidarum** – reddish/purple stretch marks that may be noted on the thighs, buttocks, abdomen and breasts.
5. Nausea and vomiting (morning sickness) can occur from as early as 2 weeks but usually subsides by 12 weeks
6. Fatigue
7. Frequency of micturition
8. Pica (cravings).

Additional Signs and Symptoms – Second and Third Trimester

1. Enlargement of the abdomen and the uterus can be felt through the abdominal wall.
2. Fetal movements are felt and heart sounds may be heard from approximately 20–22 weeks in a primigravid woman and 16–18 weeks in a multigravid woman. Many things can affect this, such as the mothers' weight, muscle tone and position of the placenta and the fetus.
3. Changes may be seen in the cervix and vagina on speculum examination. The colour of the vagina, cervix and labia may appear to be darker purple in colour (**Jacquemier's/Chadwick's** sign). Stronger pulses may be palpated on vaginal examination (**Osiander's** sign).
4. Increase in normal vaginal discharge (leucorrhoea)
5. Braxton Hicks contractions – intermittent contractions of the uterus may be felt from the second trimester.

What the Experts Say A Mother to Be

I think it's (Braxton Hicks contractions) different for everyone, for sure. Mine don't hurt. I can just feel the tightness. It's definitely not comfortable, but not painful at all for me.

(Julie's experience in her first pregnancy.)

Diagnostic Tests that Confirm Pregnancy

- Fetal parts palpable abdominally
- Fetal movements felt by examiner
- Fetal heart heard
- Ultrasound scan that confirms the presence of a fetal heart.

Overview of Antenatal Care

Pregnancy, birth and motherhood affect women physically, psychologically and socially and the role of the midwife is to support women during this process. Pregnant women often seek out information from a number of sources, including books, websites and health professionals. It is important for nurses to understand the aims of antenatal care, however they should refer to the midwife who is the lead professional in normal childbirth.

Antenatal Appointments

NICE (2010) advocate a schedule of antenatal appointments but contact with women during pregnancy should be based on their individual needs. This is commonly ascertained during the booking appointment. This is often the first contact between the mother and maternity services. The appointment is longer than subsequent appointments so that information can be gathered regarding the woman's obstetric, medical, family and social history. The midwife gives the woman information about the pregnancy, screening, options for care and lifestyle choices. This appointment is considered pivotal for assessing risk and identifying the woman's needs.

Care should be sensitive to the needs of the woman and take place at venues that are easily accessible for her; this may be the woman's home or a local medical/family centre. Women with complicated pregnancies or specific medical conditions will be offered consultant-led appointments at the hospital or appointments shared between the consultant and midwife at hospital and community-based venues.

Clinical Care, Assessment and Advice

The clinical care, observations, assessment and advice offered to the woman and her family during the antenatal period are fully explored in NICE's (2010) *Routine Care for the Healthy Pregnant Woman*.

 Link To/Go To

To access the full range of NICE recommendations and advice for antenatal care, go to:

http://www.nice.org.uk/nicemedia/live/11947/40110/40110.pdf

Abdominal Examination

At each antenatal appointment from the second trimester, the midwife will examine the mother's abdomen to confirm fetal growth and well-being. A full abdominal examination consists of:

- **Inspection** – the midwife observes the abdomen for skin changes, scars, shape and size
- **Palpation** – the midwife palpates the abdomen using the palmar surfaces of her hands. Palpation is also broken down into three elements:
  - *Fundal* – the uppermost border of the uterus is palpated. This reflects growth and assists the midwife in determining the presentation of the fetus
  - *Lateral* – the sides of the uterus are palpated. This assists the midwife in determining the position of the fetus
  - *Pelvic* – the lower aspect of the uterus is palpated to assist the midwife in determining the presentation of the fetus. This is

259

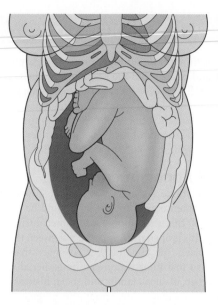

Figure 13.1 Terminology used during abdominal palpation. In this case, the presentation is cephalic. The position is left occiptio anterior (the fetal occiput is anterior and is on the left of the maternal pelvis). The lie is longitudinal. The attitude is one of flexion and the head is not engaged.

assessed from 36 weeks of gestation, as the presentation will be variable when the fetus is less mature and has more room to move.

Terminology used during the abdominal examination
(Figure 13.1)

- **Presentation** – this is the part of the fetus lying lowest in the maternal uterus, i.e. directly above the cervix. Most commonly, this is the head and is called a cephalic presentation
- **Position** – this most commonly reflects the position of the head in the maternal pelvis
- **Lie** – this refers to the long axis of the fetus in relation to the long axis of the maternal uterus, i.e. longitudinal (length ways), transverse (across), oblique (diagonally)
- **Attitude** – this means the degree to which the fetus has its limbs, body and head flexed. The most common attitude is one of flexion, i.e. the fetal position (curled up)
- **Engagement** – this is how much of the presenting part, usually the head, has passed through the narrowest part of the maternal pelvis.

The assessment of fetal growth is a vital aspect of role of the midwife as fetal growth correlates with fetal well-being. If growth is less than or more than would be expected for the gestational age of the fetus, the midwife will refer the woman to an obstetrician. Growth is initially assessed by measuring the fundal height of the mother's uterus, as discussed in NICE (2010). Fetal growth is demonstrated pictorially in Figure 13.2. At weeks 1–4, the approximate size is 0.6 cm. By weeks 13–16, the estimated measurement is 18 cm and the uterus containing the pregnancy can be palpated abdominally. The approximate measurement at weeks 26–29 is 32–42 cm and by 36 weeks to the end of pregnancy it is 50 cm.

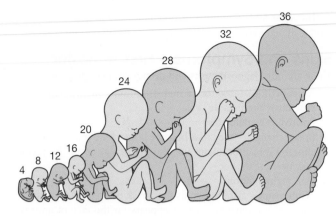

Figure 13.2 Fetal growth from week 4 to week 36.

During the antenatal period women will be offered a range of screening tests.

Antenatal Screening
Tests are offered usually early in pregnancy to check for potential problems. Blood tests and ultrasound scans can be offered to woman, who should be given enough information to make an informed choice about the test. You can see the schedule of screening tests for mothers in Figure 13.3.

Common Blood Tests and Investigations
Maternal
Haemoglobin (Hb) – there is an increase in the number of red blood cells in pregnancy but this is not equal to the increase in plasma volume. Consequently, there appears to be a drop in the haemoglobin level. This is called haemodilution of pregnancy. Tests to confirm anaemia may need to be carried out if the haemoglobin level falls significantly

Blood group and antibodies – these are taken to check for antibodies that may cause a problem in this or subsequent pregnancies

Infection screen – blood is taken to check for rubella, hepatitis, HIV, syphilis

Haemoglobinopathies such as sickle cell anaemia and thalassemia – are inherited blood disorders

Chlamydia screening is offered to women under 25 years.

Fetal
Early pregnancy ultrasound scan – confirms the pregnancy and due date and may detect abnormalities

20-week detailed scan – this does not detect all abnormalities and may also lead to problems being suspected in healthy babies. Subsequent scans may be undertaken to assess fetal growth and well-being

Down's syndrome (Trisomy 21) – a chromosomal abnormality detected using a combination of blood tests, and sonography at approximately 16 weeks of gestation. An invasive diagnostic test would be offered following a positive screening test, e.g. amniocentesis.

Women may feel anxious during pregnancy and need information to reassure them that their pregnancy is progressing normally.

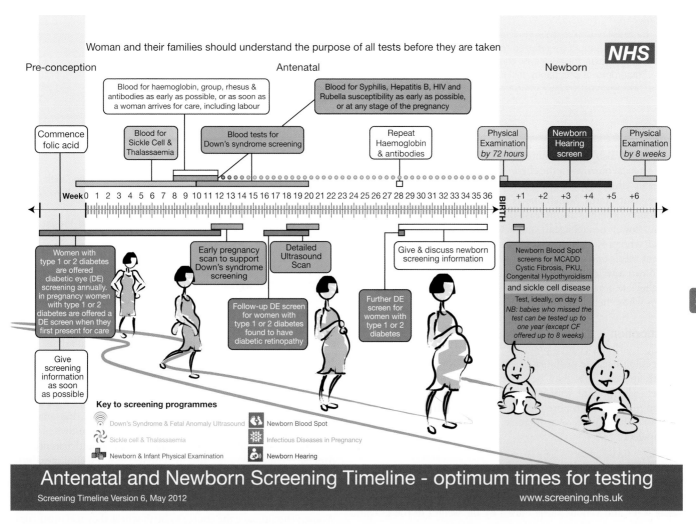

Woman and their families should understand the purpose of all tests before they are taken

NHS

Pre-conception   Antenatal   Newborn

Blood for haemoglobin, group, rhesus & antibodies as early as possible, or as soon as a woman arrives for care, including labour

Blood for Syphilis, Hepatitis B, HIV and Rubella susceptibility as early as possible, or at any stage of the pregnancy

Commence folic acid

Blood for Sickle Cell & Thalassaemia

Blood tests for Down's syndrome screening

Repeat Haemoglobin & antibodies

Physical Examination *by 72 hours*

Newborn Hearing screen

Physical Examination *by 8 weeks*

Week 0 1 2 3 4 5 6 7 8 9 10 11 12 13 14 15 16 17 18 19 20 21 22 23 24 25 26 27 28 29 30 31 32 33 34 35 36   +1 +2 +3 +4 +5 +6

BIRTH

Women with type 1 or 2 diabetes are offered diabetic eye (DE) screening annually. in pregnancy women with type 1 or 2 diabetes are offered a DE screen when they first present for care

Early pregnancy scan to support Down's syndrome screening

Detailed Ultrasound Scan

Give & discuss newborn screening information

Newborn Blood Spot screens for MCADD Cystic Fibrosis, PKU, Congenital Hypothyroidism and sickle cell disease
Test, ideally, on day 5
NB: babies who missed the test can be tested up to one year (except CF offered up to 8 weeks)

Follow-up DE screen for women with type 1 or 2 diabetes found to have diabetic retinopathy

Further DE screen for women with type 1 or 2 diabetes

Give screening information as soon as possible

Key to screening programmes

Down's Syndrome & Fetal Anomaly Ultrasound

Sickle cell & Thalassaemia

Newborn & Infant Physical Examination

Newborn Blood Spot

Infectious Diseases in Pregnancy

Newborn Hearing

Antenatal and Newborn Screening Timeline - optimum times for testing

Screening Timeline Version 6, May 2012   www.screening.nhs.uk

Figure 13.3 Antenatal and neonatal screening test schedule. This information was originally developed by the UK National Screening Committee/NHS Screening Programmes (www.screening.nhs.uk) and is used under the Open Government Licence v1.0.

261

This may include information about screening tests and also about the physical changes the woman is experiencing, which can result in minor symptoms of pregnancy. Nurses need to have an awareness of common minor disorders and their treatments but it is important for nurses to refer pregnant women to a midwife for on-going advice and support. It is important to differentiate between minor symptoms and pathological disorders.

Care, Dignity and Compassion

In order show compassion we need to understand the impact of what we say and do. Not all women are comfortable exposing their bodies or bumps, even when they are pregnant. It is important to maintain privacy and dignity for women at all times. Always ask permission to expose any parts of their bodies. Examination room doors should be locked or privacy signs and screens used. Sheets should be used to prevent women from being overexposed during examinations. These considerations demonstrate to women that their privacy and dignity is respected.

Minor Disorders of Pregnancy and Their Management
Nausea and vomiting

This is very common and affects over 50% of pregnant women. It is usually worse in the first trimester and often occurs in the morning, hence its colloquial name 'morning sickness'. Women should be reassured that this usually resolves by 20 weeks of gestation. The exact cause is unknown but it is thought that high levels of the circulating hormone hCG contribute to the condition.

What to Do If...A Pregnant Woman Complains of Morning Sickness

There are several ways to manage morning sickness; these may be broken into pharmacological and non-pharmacological.

Non-pharmacological methods used are ginger and P6 (wrist) acupressure

Pharmacological treatments include prescribed antihistamines.

Red Flag

Women should be referred to a midwife, GP, pharmacist or obstetrician for advice on the management of minor disorders of pregnancy, including morning sickness.

Heartburn

Heartburn is also very common in pregnancy. Women complain of retrosternal burning in the chest or discomfort that can be more noticeable when they are lying down. It is caused by the weight of the pregnant uterus, which affects the emptying of the stomach. Additionally, there is an increase in progesterone that relaxes the cardiac (lower oesophageal) sphincter leading to gastric reflux. Women who present with symptoms should be advised to eat small frequent meals and avoid fatty foods. An upright position and not lying down after meals may help, and sleeping with extra pillows may alleviate nocturnal heartburn. Antacids may be offered to women whose heartburn remains troublesome.

Constipation

Constipation can occur in pregnancy due to decreased peristalsis in the colon because of the effects of progesterone, which relaxes smooth muscle. This may be exacerbated by oral iron tablets. Women who present with constipation in pregnancy should be advised to take a high fibre diet with extra fresh fruit, vegetables, bran or wheat fibre. An increase in fluid intake should be encouraged.

Varicosities

Varicosities may develop in pregnancy in the legs, anal area and also the vulva, due to the relaxing effect of progesterone on the vessel walls and venous stasis caused by the weight of the gravid uterus.

Women should be informed that varicose veins are a common symptom of pregnancy that will not cause harm and that compression stockings can improve the symptoms but will not prevent varicose veins from emerging.

In the absence of evidence of the effectiveness of treatments for haemorrhoids in pregnancy, women should be offered information concerning dietary modification to avoid constipation. If clinical symptoms remain troublesome, standard haemorrhoid creams may be considered.

Women may be distressed or concerned especially about vulval varicosities and should be reassured they will subside after delivery of the baby.

Vaginal discharge

An increase in vaginal discharge is a common physiological change that occurs during pregnancy, however women should be advised that if it is associated with itching, soreness or has an offensive smell or pain on passing urine, there may be an infection present and this should be investigated. Common infections can include *candida albicans* (thrush) and urinary tract infections (UTIs).

Backache

This is caused by softening and relaxation of the ligaments in the pelvis. The gravid uterus results in an exaggerated curvature of the spine that increases back strain and can lead to pain. Exercising in water, massage therapy and back care classes might help to ease the symptoms.

Link To/Go To

Advice about backache can be obtained from:

http://www.nhs.uk/conditions/pregnancy-and-baby/pages/backache-pregnant.aspx#close

An obstetric physiotherapist may be useful in dealing with specific problems associated with pregnancy. Find out more from *Physiopedia* at:

http://www.physio-pedia.com/Low_Back_Pain_and_Pregnancy

Carpal tunnel syndrome

This is caused by soft tissue swelling resulting from increases in the circulating volume that may cause compression of the median nerve in the wrist. The woman may experience weakness and tingling in the thumb and forefinger and pain, particularly at night. The symptoms usually resolve following delivery of the baby. A light splint may support the wrist and alleviate the symptoms along with simple analgesia.

Discussing the physiological changes of pregnancy is an important part of antenatal care. This can take place during antenatal appointments or during sessions delivered by the midwife to help prepare the woman and her partner for birth and parenthood. Antenatal education may also include relaxation techniques, birth choices, infant care and feeding.

Options Available for Birth

Women should have the choice to birth where they feel most comfortable. The birth environment can affect a woman's chances of having a normal birth. Options for birthing currently include home birth, midwifery-led birth centres and obstetric units. Birth centres offer the comforts of a home environment, with a team of midwives available. Birthing in an obstetric unit provides direct access to obstetricians, anaesthetists, neonatologists and other specialist care, including epidural analgesia and it is important that women are aware of this to enable them to make an informed choice about the place they birth their babies (NICE 2007b, 2010).

If women give birth at home or in a midwife-led unit, there is a higher likelihood of a normal birth, with less intervention however, some women require additional care and may be advised to birth in an obstetric unit. For example if the woman has any pre-existing medical conditions, develops complications during the pregnancy or has had a previous complicated birth.

In 2011/2012 over half (51.4%, 299 528) of NHS deliveries took place in designated consultant wards; 35.9% (208 937) in wards associated with a consultant, GP or midwife and 12.3% (71 590) in midwife or non-maternity wards. The percentage of deliveries in midwife or non-maternity wards has seen the most change in recent years, indicating a trend towards midwifery-led care. This has increased by 4.9% since 2005–2006 (HSCIC 2012; **http://www.hscic.gov.uk/hes**).

Most women in the UK birth their babies in obstetric units, however, this has not always been the case and it is important that women understand all the available options for birth.

Link To/Go To

To find out more about places where women birth, go to:

http://www.nhs.uk/conditions/pregnancy-and-baby/pages/where-can-i-give-birth.aspx

http://www.nct.org.uk/birth/choosing-where-have-your-baby

http://www.nct.org.uk/birth/faqs-home-birth

Overview of Intranatal Care

Normal birth occurs spontaneously between 37 and 42 completed weeks of a singleton (one fetus) pregnancy, without induction, without the use of instruments and without general, spinal or epidural anaesthetic before or during delivery. It is generally accepted that the head delivers first in normal birth (cephalic).

Giving birth is generally very safe in the UK and over 60% of women will have a normal vaginal birth (**http://www.hscic.gov.uk/hes**). This is not the case throughout the rest of the world, particularly in parts of SE Asia and sub-Saharan Africa, where women birth without professional help. The consequences of this are illustrated in the high maternal mortality rates in those countries.

The Evidence

Some 90% of these deaths occur in the developing world where most women's lives are restricted by illiteracy, poor education and poverty.

For every woman who dies in childbirth, around 20 more suffer injury, infection or disease – a total of some 10 million women each year.

Fewer than 50% of all births in developing countries take place with the help of a skilled birth attendant.

 Link To/Go To

For more information, go to:

http://www.womenandchildrenfirst.org.uk/what-we-do/key-issues/maternal-health-maternal-mortality/maternal-mortality-statistics?utm_source=google&utm_medium=cpc&utm_campaign=maternal_mortality_statistics

Labour

Labour is the process by which the fetus, placenta and membranes are born.

The onset of labour is not fully understood but it is thought to be due a combination of factors, including the influence of maternal and fetal hormones. Labour is confirmed by the presence of regular, rhythmical contractions, which dilate the cervix. Contractions may also be accompanied by a clear or lightly blood stained plug of mucus per vagina. This is called a 'show'. Rupture of the membranes may or may not accompany labour. Labour is not predictable and is experienced by different women in different ways. Women may also find differences in each of their own pregnancies.

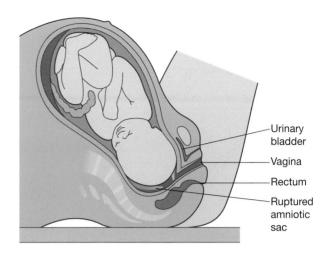

Figure 13.4 **The cervix is effaced and dilated.**

The Stages of Labour

Labour is often divided into three stages:

First stage: the onset of labour from the onset of regular rhythmical contractions that result in the dilatation (opening) and effacement (shortening) of the cervix. The dilatation of the cervix is estimated digitally from 1 cm to 10 cm (full dilatation), as shown in Figure 13.4.

Second stage: from full dilatation of the cervix to the complete expulsion of the fetus. Figure 13.5 demonstrates the expulsion of the fetal head during the second stage of labour.

Third stage: from the birth of the baby to the complete expulsion of the placenta and membranes. Figure 13.6 shows the placenta prior to separation after delivery of the baby. This stage of labour also includes the control and management of bleeding.

Normal Labour and Birth

This is considered to occur at term (37–42 weeks); it is spontaneous in onset and the head of the fetus presents. This is called a *cephalic presentation*. The process is completed within 24 hours of its onset and there are no complications or interventions (RCM 2012).

Other Types of Labour and Birth

Multiple births – 1 in 80 births following natural conception in the UK are multiples, i.e. twins, triplets, quadruplets, quintuplets, sextuplets.

The Evidence

In 2009, 16 women per 1000 giving birth in England and Wales had multiple births. This compares with 10 per 1000 in 1980.

This is due to increasing use of assisted reproduction techniques, including in-vitro fertilisation (IVF).

Up to 24% of successful IVF procedures result in multiple pregnancies.

Multiple births currently account for 3% of live births.

(NICE 2011)

Induced labour – this is when the onset of labour is started artificially and occurs in 12% of all births (**http://www.hscic.gov.uk/hes**). The method of choice depends on each individual woman and her preferences, as well as the clinical presentation. The cervix may be manually stretched to stimulate labour; this is

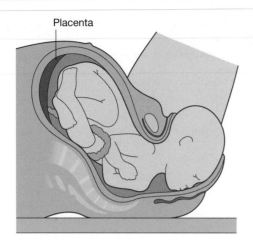

Figure 13.5 **Expulsion of the fetal head during the second stage of labour.**

264

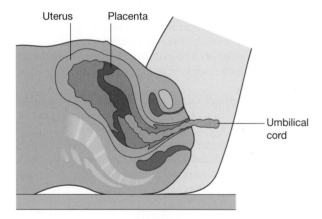

Figure 13.6 **The placenta after delivery of the baby and prior to separation from the wall of the uterus.**

known as a cervical sweep. Drugs can be administered directly into the vagina or can be given via an intravenous infusion. Finally, a procedure called amniotomy or artificially rupturing the membranes can be undertaken. This is often called 'breaking the waters'.

What To Do If ...

 You are asked about some old wives tales and their supposed rationale. Always refer the woman to a midwife for further discussion. Some of these examples may be harmful and professional advice is essential:

Sex – prostaglandins in the semen ripen the cervix and stimulate labour onset

Castor-oil – increases peristaltic action, which can stimulate the uterus to contract

Walking – upright position and the effects of gravity may help to stimulate the onset of labour

Raspberry leaf tea – stimulates effective contractions and shorter second stage of labour

Nipple stimulation – stimulates the release of hormones associated with the onset of labour

Eating fresh pineapple – meant to help you release the enzyme bromelain that in turn softens the cervix

Breech birth – this happens when the fetus presents by the breech (or buttocks). When this occurs women are advised to discuss their options with a midwife and obstetrician, as there are concerns about the safety of breech vaginal birth.

Caesarean section – the baby is delivered through an incision made into the abdomen and the uterus. Usually in the UK, this will be a small transverse incision low down on the abdomen and the uterus. Occasionally in an emergency or premature caesarean birth, it is necessary to incise both the abdomen and the uterus lengthways; this is called a classical incision.

Instrumental deliveries

Forceps – these are spoon-shaped instruments that are applied to the fetal head to allow traction to be applied to aid delivery. This is undertaken by a specially trained practitioner or obstetrician.

Ventouse – this is a suction cup that is applied to the fetal head and allows traction to be applied to aid delivery. This is undertaken by a specially trained practitioner or obstetrician.

Midwifery Care in Normal Labour

The midwife will diagnose the onset and monitor the progress of normal labour, referring to the multidisciplinary team when necessary. During labour, a fundamental role of the midwife is to work with women and their partners to support their choices and facilitate their needs. Evidence has shown that continuous support in labour improves outcomes for mothers in terms of less analgesia, shorter labours, reduced instrumental intervention and fewer caesarean sections (Hodnett *et al.* 2013). The midwife should advise women how to promote normality in birth. This will include advice about positions and movement during labour and hydration and nutrition. Women should consider these things before going into labour and are advised to write a birth plan.

 Link To/Go To

Consider the things a woman may wish to include in a birth plan:

http://www.nhs.uk/conditions/pregnancy-and-baby/pages/birth-plan.aspx#close

Assessing Progress and Well-Being

There are many ways of assessing progress in labour and the midwife needs to be aware of both subtle and obvious changes. These may include changes in the woman's behaviour, such as breathing patterns, movements, mood and the noises she makes. There are also anatomical changes, which the midwife is trained to measure.

These include:

Abdominal examination – the midwife can palpate the strength, length and frequency of the uterine contractions and can assess the descent of the fetus through the maternal pelvis. Contractions need to be strong enough to cause effacement and dilatation of the cervix. These are counted over a 10-minute period and up to five contractions in 10 minutes are considered normal. Contractions may last up to 90 seconds. The frequency and length of the contractions may depend on the stage of the labour, with increasing intensity and frequency as labour progresses.

Vaginal examination – this is a procedure during which the midwife feels the dilatation and effacement of the cervix. She can also determine the position and descent of the fetal head. This is an extremely intimate examination and women may feel uncomfortable physically and/or psychologically during the procedure. The midwife needs to be sensitive and should explain the procedure fully and gain the woman's consent. It is essential to maintain the woman's privacy and dignity and at all times, the midwife should be aware of the invasive nature of the examination.

The midwife will assess the woman and her unborn baby's well-being throughout the labour. She will undertake recordings of blood pressure, temperature, pulse, respiration rate, urinalysis and these are all recorded on a labour observation chart called a partogram. This is a graphic record of a woman's well-being and progress in labour and is used by all midwives caring for labouring woman.

Fetal well-being is also recorded on the partogram and is assessed by regularly listening to the fetal heart (auscultation) and if the membranes have ruptured the colour of the liquor is observed, this should be clear.

Methods of fetal heart rate auscultation

Intermittent auscultation is when the midwife listens to the fetal heart at intervals during labour, using either of the following:

- Pinard stethoscope – this is a simple trumpet-shaped instrument that amplifies fetal heart sounds
- Sonicaid Doppler - this is an electronic handled device that amplifies the fetal heart sounds through a speaker so that both mother and midwife can hear.

Continuous electronic fetal heart rate monitoring is sometimes required in more complex labours. This is undertaken using a cardiotocograph (CTG), which is a form of electronic fetal heart rate monitoring that amplifies the heart sounds and makes a recording on graph paper similar to an electrocardiograph (ECG).

Working with Labour Pain

There are two main beliefs about pain in labour. First, that experiencing labour pain is an important part of the labour process and fundamental to normal birth. Second, that pain is unnecessary and can be alleviated. Healthcare professionals should consider how their own values and beliefs inform their attitude to coping with pain in labour and ensure their care supports the woman's choice (NICE 2007b). Women are told about various options open to them in labour. These can be broadly separated into non-pharmacological and pharmacological methods, as identified in Table 13.1.

Care Specific to the Second Stage of Labour

During the second stage of labour, uterine contractions may become expulsive and women may feel an urge to bear down and to change to a different position. The midwife continues to monitor maternal and fetal well-being throughout. She also supports the

Table 13.1 Methods of pain relief in labour.

NON-PHARMACOLOGICAL METHODS	PHARMACOLOGICAL METHODS
Breathing and relaxation techniques Water, e.g. birthing pool/bath Massage techniques Transcutaneous electrical nerve stimulation (TENS)	Inhalational analgesia, e.g. Entonox Intramuscular opioids, e.g. pethidine/diamorphine Regional analgesia

woman in adopting positions and behaviours to facilitate a normal delivery for example encouraging the woman to push when she has the urge to bear down. Women should be encouraged to combine spontaneous pushing with upright positions. Episiotomy is a surgical incision into the perineum to enlarge the introitus. This should not be routine during spontaneous vaginal birth.

Care Specific to the Third Stage of Labour

This stage has been described as the most hazardous for the mother, due to the risk of haemorrhage and other complications (Stables & Rankin 2010). After the birth, the placenta continues to supply the baby with blood until it separates from the uterine wall or the umbilical cord is clamped and cut by the midwife. Natural separation and birth of the placenta is appropriate if the woman has experienced a physiological normal labour and birth (Fahy *et al.* 2010). NICE (2007b) advocate an active approach involving the use of a drug that stimulates a contraction of the uterus. The midwife then clamps and cuts the umbilical cord and delivers the placenta manually.

> **The Evidence**
>
> In 1801, Darwin considered the tying and cutting of the navel string too soon to be injurious to the child, as a portion of blood is left in the placenta.
> (Edwards & Wickham 2011)
> Find out more about contemporary views using the following references on the third stage:
> Weeks, A. (2007) Umbilical cord clamping after birth. *British Medical Journal*, 335(7615), 312–313.
> Fahy, K., Hastie, C., Bisits, A., Marsh, C., Smith, L. & Saxton, A. (2010) Holistic physiological care compared with active management of the third stage of labour for women at low risk of postpartum haemorrhage: a cohort study. *Women and Birth*, 23(4), 146–152.
> Was Darwin right?

The placenta needs to be examined after birth to check it appears to be healthy and complete. The maternal surface is dark red in colour. Figure 13.7 demonstrates the appearance of the fetal surface of the placenta.

The midwife may take a sample of blood from the vessels in the umbilical cord to confirm the baby's blood group and Rhesus status. If the maternal and fetal blood group and Rhesus status are not compatible, then there a risk of the mother developing antibodies. This may affect future pregnancies and result in fetal morbidity and mortality.

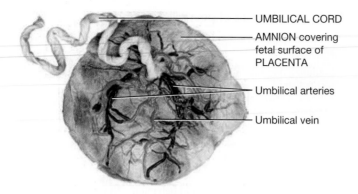

Figure 13.7 The fetal surface of the placenta. Source: Jenkins & Tortora (2013) Reproduced with permission of John Wiley & Sons Singapore Pte. Ltd.

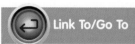

Link To/Go To

To understand about more about the Rhesus factor and how it affects pregnancy visit the NHS Blood and transplant site, go to:

http://www.blood.co.uk/the-donor/winter2011/am-i-rhesus-positive-or-rhesus-negative.asp

Unexpected and Rapid Deliveries

Occasionally, women will deliver their baby's unexpectedly or rapidly. If a woman appears to be birthing her baby without a midwife or doctor in attendance, the nurse should:

- Call for help/ambulance
- Provide reassurance that help is on the way
- Consider the woman's privacy and dignity
- Ensure the area is as warm and draught free as possible
- Hands off! Let events proceed naturally. Do not cut the cord or attempt to deliver the placenta
- If the baby delivers, place on mother's abdomen directly on her skin and, if possible, provide a warm cover
- Do not separate mother and baby.

Initial Care of the Mother and Baby after Birth

This is an important time for the mother and her birth partner to meet the baby and ideally, the mother and baby should be left undisturbed. It is thought this can help with bonding and breast-feeding (UNICEF 2010). Following delivery, the baby should be dried and placed on the mother's chest. Skin-to-skin contact should be encouraged but it is vital that the baby is not allowed to get cold. The mother's skin temperature will help to keep the baby warm but towels and blankets should cover the baby.

The mother and baby are discreetly observed during this time for signs of normality. The mother will be observed for any signs of bleeding from the genital tract and vital signs will be recorded. Each mother will be assessed individually and will be cared for according to her needs and wishes. It is important to ensure the mothers comfort and dignity during this time (NMC 2008).

Table 13.2 Apgar score.

SIGN	SCORE – 0	SCORE – 1	SCORE – 2
Heart rate	Absent	Below 100 beats/minute	Above 100 beats/minute
Respiratory effort	Absent	Weak irregular or gasping	Good, crying
Muscle tone	Flaccid	Some flexion of arms or legs	Well flexed, or active movements of extremities
Reflex irritability	No response	Grimace or weak cry	Good cry
Colour	Blue or pale all over	Body pink, hands and feet blue	Pink all over

Approximately 70% of women will sustain some trauma to the genital tract during birth (NICE 2007b). This can range from minor skin grazes to tears that require suturing. This should be assessed after birth and repairs need to be performed as soon as it is possible. Urinary incontinence, haematoma, infection and fistulas are rare but possible complications of perineal injury. If these are not identified and treated, they could impact on the quality of the mother's future physical and psychological well-being.

The baby will be assessed at approximately one minute after delivery using a scale called the 'Apgar score', see Table 13.2. This score assesses a baby's general well-being at birth and identifies if there is a need for resuscitation. A baby that does not require any intervention will achieve a score of ≥ 7.

Overview of Postnatal Care – Mother

The transition to parenthood is considered one of the greatest and most challenging responsibilities most people will ever face (Wilkins 2006). The postnatal period marks the establishment of a new phase of family life for most women and their partners.

Jot This Down

Consider what 'family' means to you and what it means to other people. How have families changed over the years.

Do most families still consist of mother, father and their children? Think about the needs of different types of families – will they be the same?

Sadly, some women may experience the loss of their baby or babies may be born with disabilities. Social services may be involved with support plans or the removal of a child from the mother in extreme circumstances. It is vital that all health professionals caring for these women and their families adopt a sensitive approach to care and incorporate the 6Cs (Care, Compassion, Competence, Communication, Courage and Commitment) of professional practice (Cummings 2013).

The puerperium or postnatal period lasts between 6 and 8 weeks following birth. During this time, the woman's body reverts to its pre-pregnant state. Ischaemic changes lead to the breakdown of uterine muscle fibres and the uterus returns to its pre-pregnant size, shape and position. This is called *involution*. Lactation will commence and breast-feeding may become established if the mother chooses to breast-feed. Multiple physiological changes to the body that have occurred throughout pregnancy are reversed.

If the woman has birthed at home, then her initial care and on-going postnatal care will be continued in the home. Women who birth in hospital are generally transferred to a postnatal ward that specialises in the care of new mothers and their babies within a few hours of delivery. The length of the hospital stay will depend on the mother's unique circumstances. However, it is thought to be in the mother and baby's best interests to return home as soon as possible, to establish normal family life and to reduce the risks associated with hospitalisation.

Traditionally on-going postnatal care has been offered within the mother's home, but current practice has seen the introduction of postnatal clinics and telephone support (RCM 2010).

Jot This Down

List the advantages and disadvantages of postnatal visiting and newer methods of postnatal support for woman.

Which do you think will provide the most effective support?

The midwife's role in the postnatal period is to support the woman and her family, to detect any problems and to refer to an appropriate professional when required. Although midwifery care should be based on individual circumstances, CMACE (2011) recommend that routine postnatal observations will lead to better recognition and management of potentially life-threatening conditions.

A range of clinical examinations and observations to assess the mother and confirm normal progress may be undertaken.

- Blood pressure, pulse, temperature and respirations within 6 hours after birth (NICE 2006)
- The lochia – these are the vaginal losses following delivery. They are heavily blood stained immediately post-delivery but become less so as the postnatal period advance
- Uterine involution – abdominal palpation of the uterus is thought to be unnecessary to assess the progress of involution unless the lochia becomes abnormal
- The midwife should check if the woman has passed urine within 6 hours of birth (NICE 2006) and assess if micturition continues to be normal.

Following a discussion with the mother, the midwife will determine if additional examinations are necessary, for example if the mother complains of discomfort. The midwife will also ascertain the return of normal bowel function.

It is also important to consider the woman's emotions, as this is a time of immense change. Many women will experience 'baby blues' soon after delivery, usually on the second or third day. Following the initial euphoria post-delivery, mothers may feel tired, tearful and low in mood. This is a normal transient occurrence and should resolve spontaneously. It is not fully understood why the baby blues occur, however suggestions include a rapid fall in hormones following delivery and the realisation of the responsibility of motherhood. If the symptoms of baby blues have not resolved within 14 days, the mother should be assessed for postnatal depression (NICE 2006).

Postnatal depression (PND) is a much more serious mental illness that affects 10–15% of mothers (NICE 2007a). The onset of postnatal depression is usually later. If the midwife, mother or her family have concerns about the mothers emotional well-being, the 'Edinburgh postnatal depression scale' can be used to assess for depression. Appropriate referrals must be made to specialist health professionals to ensure the mother receives adequate support and treatment. This is particularly important, as recent evidence suggests that in addition to the effect on women and their families, PND can also lead to cognitive and emotional impairment in the baby (NICE 2006). Suitable support and care that is accessed early is crucial to achieving optimum health for both the parents and those of their future children (DCSF 2009).

Jot This Down

Social isolation is a known risk factor for postnatal depression

What support services are available in your area?

Contact local family centres or health visitors for information.

How will mothers access these services?

Health and Advice in the Postnatal Period

Mothers will require advice and information about a variety of subjects, depending on their particular circumstances, ranging from baby care to the legal registration of the baby's birth (Box 13.2). The midwife will tailor information to meet the needs of the mother, baby and wider family but advice should enable mothers to make choices about her own health and the health and well-being of their babies.

The midwife should ensure that the woman and her family are given information about serious complications that may occur in pregnancy and the postnatal period so they are aware when to access urgent medical attention. Women may present for example at GP clinics or Accident and Emergency departments with complications that may be potentially life-threatening. The signs and symptoms of life-threatening conditions are identified in Table 13.3. Nurses need to be aware of these complications and ensure that women who are pregnant or have recently given birth are identified and receive the appropriate and timely treatment. It is also important that nurses are aware of the potential response to infections during pregnancy, particularly community acquired Group A streptococcal (GAS) infections. Young children are often carriers of GAS, which is a common causative organism in sore throats. GAS can have devastating effects on pregnant and newly delivered women. CMACE (2011) identified a rise in the number of maternal deaths due to GAS. Nurses should be aware of the need to advise pregnant or newly delivered women about the prevention of transmission. Women should be advised to wash their hands before and after using the toilet. This is because transmission occurs from contaminated hands to the genital tract when wiping following toilet use. Hands can be easily contaminated when caring for young children. This is an important message health professionals should share during all interactions with pregnant or newly delivered women. This simple advice could save lives. Urgent liaison with an obstetrician is required if there are any concerns about the health of a pregnant or newly delivered woman.

267

Table 13.3 Signs and symptoms of potentially life-threatening conditions. (*Source*: NICE 2006)

POSSIBLE SIGNS AND SYMPTOMS	SIGNS MOTHER NEEDS TO BE AWARE OF	EVALUATE FOR:	ACTION
Sudden or profuse blood loss or blood loss and signs and symptoms of shock, including tachycardia, hypotension, hypoperfusion, change in consciousness	Persistent increased blood loss, faintness, dizziness, palpitations or racing pulse	Postpartum haemorrhage	Emergency action
Offensive excessive vaginal loss, tender abdomen or pyrexia. If no obstetric cause, consider other causes	'Smelly' vaginal loss, abdominal pain, shivering and/or fever	Postpartum haemorrhage, sepsis or other pathology	Urgent action
Pyrexia, shivering, abdominal pain and/or offensive vaginal loss. If temperature exceeds 38°C, repeat in 4–6 hours. If temperature still high or there are other symptoms and measurable signs, evaluate further	Fever, 'smelly' vaginal loss, abdominal pain and/or shivering	Infection/genital tract sepsis	Emergency action
Severe or persistent headache	Unusual, severe or persistent headache	Pre-eclampsia, eclampsia	Emergency action
Diastolic BP is >90 mmHg and accompanied by another sign/symptom of pre-eclampsia, e.g. visual disturbance, oedema, proteinuria, seizures, headache, epigastric pain	Unusual, severe or persistent headache, visual disturbance, excessive swelling, upper abdominal pain, fits	Pre-eclampsia, Eclampsia	Emergency action
Diastolic BP is >90 mmHg and no other symptom. Repeat BP within 4 hours. If it remains above 90 mmHg after 4 hours, evaluate	N/A	Pre-eclampsia, eclampsia	Emergency action
Shortness of breath or chest pain	Shortness of breath or chest pain	Pulmonary embolism	Emergency action
Unilateral calf pain, redness or swelling	Calf pain in one leg, redness or swelling	Deep vein thrombosis	Emergency action

---

Box 13.2 Advice and Guidance for Postnatal Well-Being

· Infant feeding and baby care
· Sudden infant death syndrome
· Emotional well-being
· Contraception and resuming sexual intercourse
· Diet and exercise
· Common health problems
· Life-threatening conditions
· Breast care
· Cervical screening
· Postnatal examination and appointment at 6/52
· Postnatal examination and appointment at 6/52

Information about all of these issues can be found at:

   http://www.nice.org.uk/nicemedia/live/10988/30143/30143.pdf

---

Jot This Down

The new born baby can lose heat through four mechanisms:
Evaporation, conduction, radiation, convection.

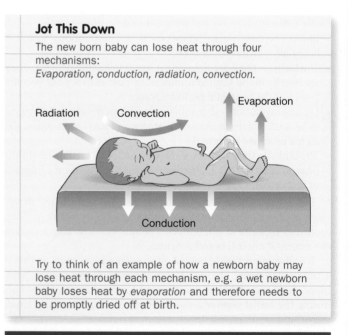

Try to think of an example of how a newborn baby may lose heat through each mechanism, e.g. a wet newborn baby loses heat by *evaporation* and therefore needs to be promptly dried off at birth.

Postnatal midwifery care continues for as long as the midwife feels it is necessary (NMC 2012). Often this will be between 10 and 28 days but will depend on the mother's individual circumstances. Visits should be flexible and arranged to meet the needs of the mother, baby and family. The midwife should liaise with the health visitor and GP to ensure care is provided after discharge from midwifery services.

Care of the Neonate after Birth

The role of the midwife in the early postnatal period is to give the mother the confidence to care for her baby and to confirm normal progress and well-being.

Following birth, the baby should be immediately dried with a warm towel. Parents should be given time to look at and be with their baby soon after birth. Women should be encouraged/offered to have skin-to-skin contact with their baby as soon as possible following birth. Physical contact encourages attachment and initiation of breast-feeding. The baby should be covered with a warm, dry towel and a hat applied while maintaining skin-to-skin contact. Initiation of breast-feeding should be encouraged within one hour of birth. A woman and her baby should not be separated within the first hour, unless it is necessary for immediate care of the woman or baby. The babies temperature should be recorded soon after birth, as the effects of cold stress on a new born baby can include breathing problems and hypoglycaemia. These could result in serious consequences for the baby.

Following the birth of the baby, a thorough examination will be undertaken by the midwife. This examination is to confirm gross normality and to detect any problems that need referral.

An important aspect of this examination is to reassure the parents that their baby appears normal. The baby will be weighed to provide a baseline for future measurement. If birth takes place in a hospital, it is important that name bands and security tags are applied to the baby. Parents should check that the information is correct. Mothers and babies should stay together as one unit throughout their stay in hospital if possible. Vitamin K will be offered to prevent a condition called vitamin K-deficiency bleeding (VKNB).

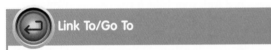

Link To/Go To

To find out more about vitamin K deficiency in the new-born:

http://www.patient.co.uk/doctor/Haemorrhagic-Disease-of-Newborn.htm

Despite the potentially catastrophic consequences of VKNB, some parents choose not to give their baby additional vitamin K. Why do you think this may be?

The examination of the baby in the early postnatal period monitors the progress and assesses on going well-being. The midwife in conjunction with feedback from the mother will confirm that the baby is thriving.

Signs of a thriving baby are:

- Alert when awake and asks for feeds
- Good colour and muscle tone
- Calm and relaxed during feeding
- Satisfied after feeds
- Regular wet and soiled nappies
- When feeding established, gaining weight.

The midwife teaches the parents skills, such as bathing, dressing and nappy changing and by example and discussion, will demonstrate good habits such as hand washing. The midwife will teach and advise the parents about how to care for the umbilical cord. The cord will separate by a process of necrosis between day 7 and day 10. Some parents are anxious about care of the umbilical cord but should be advised to keep the cord clean with water and as dry as possible. The midwife will show parents how to put on a nappy leaving the cord exposed. Creams and lotions should not be applied to the cord. Parents should be observant for signs of infection such as redness around the base of the cord, offensive odour or the presence of pus. This should be reported to the GP for appropriate treatment. A healthy baby should have regular wet and soiled nappies, increasing in frequency. By 7 days, parents should anticipate up to six or more heavy wet nappies with at least two being soiled. Parents should be made aware of the changing stool pattern. The colour and consistency will change from the first stool, which is called *meconium*. This is the sterile content of the baby's bowel and is black and has a sticky tar like consistency. As the baby starts to breast-feed and milk is absorbed by the bowel, the colour and consistency of the stools change and by 5 days, they have a yellow, watery appearance (Figure 13.8). The stools of artificially-fed babies appear more formed and may also have a seedy appearance.

The midwife also needs to ensure parents know when to seek advice on other common health problems in babies (Table 13.4).

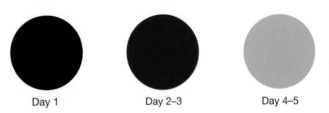

| Day 1 | Day 2–3 | Day 4–5 |

Figure 13.8 Stool colour chart. Approximate colour guide for the first few days of a baby's life. This should be used as a guide only.

Table 13.4 Common health problems in babies. (*Source*: NICE 2006)

HEALTH PROBLEM	SIGNS AND SYMPTOMS	ACTION
Jaundice in the first 24 hours	Yellow discolouration of the skin and eyes	Emergency action
Jaundice after the first 24 hours		Monitor overall well-being, hydration and alertness – *refer urgently* if concerned
Jaundice which starts after 7 days and persists after 14 days		Urgent referral
Thrush	Nappy rash and/or white patches on the babies tongue	Offer information and advice on hygiene; refer for possible anti-fungal treatment
Nappy rash	Redness, spots, excoriation	Offer information and advice on hygiene; refer for possible treatment
Constipation in formula-fed babies	Reduction in the number of soiled nappies <1 in 24 hours	Evaluate feed preparation and refer to GP/HV
Diarrhoea	Persistent watery stools	Refer to GP
Excessive, persistent crying		Reassure parents and assess the general health of the baby. Refer to HV and support groups

269

The early postnatal period is a time for guiding and advising parents and also supporting and encouraging them in their new role. Parents will need information in order to make decisions about neonatal screening tests. (Refer to Figure 13.3 for the Antenatal and neonatal screening schedule.)

What the Experts Say Caela's Story

Caela's daughter was born with medium-chain acyl-CoA dehydrogenase deficiency (MCADD), which was detected through newborn screening. Caela sits as a parent representative on the MCADD-PKU board, and contributes greatly to the information and resources available for parents.

I have a 5-year-old daughter, J, who was diagnosed with MCADD at 9 days old. I was asked by our clinical nurse specialist if I would become a parent representative on the MCADD board.

The screening for MCADD was initially part of a trial, which we were lucky enough to be a part of, although oblivious of at the time. J's heel-prick test was taken and I vaguely remember being told not to worry as nothing ever shows up.

A few days later, our world was shattered by a phone-call from our GP who asked me to call the hospital as something called MCADD had showed up from J's heel-prick test. The next few hours were a whirlwind, as we learned the basics of this condition and prepared to be at the hospital the next morning.

The team that now manage J's MCADD have given us the confidence to meet this condition head on, ensuring J maintains a completely normal life.

We have had our ups and downs with this condition, a few hospital trips with a few days here and there on a glucose drip for J, but it does not consume our lives.

(http://newbornbloodspot.screening.nhs.uk/cms
.php?folder=2697)

Infant Feeding

There has been a great deal of published research over the last two decades that demonstrates that breast-feeding is a significant factor in improving public health (UNICEF 2010).

Breast-fed babies may have better development, cholesterol, blood and dental health. They may also have less cardiovascular disease in later life and a lower incidence of childhood cancers. There is evidence to suggest women who breast-fed are at lower risk of breast and ovarian cancer, hip fractures and poor bone density. Artificially-fed babies may be at higher risk of gastrointestinal, respiratory and urinary tract infections, ear infections, eczema, asthma and wheezing, type 1 and type 2 diabetes, obesity, childhood leukaemia and sudden infant death syndrome (SIDS) (UNICEF 2010).

Infant feeding choices should be made by the parents. It is the midwife's role to give clear, factual information and to support the mother in the feeding method of her choice. Currently in the UK, by the age of 6 weeks, most babies are bottle-fed.

In 2010, the initial breast-feeding rate was 83% and at 6 weeks was 24% in England. The breast-feeding rates were lower in the rest of the UK (HSCIC 2012).

Link To/Go To

To read about the UNICEF baby friendly initiative, which identifies 10 steps for HCPs to follow, go to:

http://www.unicef.org.uk/BabyFriendly/Health-Professionals/
Going-Baby-Friendly/Maternity/
Ten-Steps-to-Successful-Breastfeeding/

Mothers who choose to bottle-feed should be shown how to prepare bottles and infant formula, to make sure the principles of hygiene are maintained and to ensure the correct nutritional balance of the feed (UNICEF 2010). It is important to remember that feeding a baby is not just a time for providing nutrients, it is also a time for biological nurturing. Breast feeding is believed to reduce the risk of sudden infant death syndrome (SIDS). It is important that parents know about the risk of SIDS and all parents should be given advice about safe sleeping. In addition to promoting breast-feeding to reduce risk, other advice includes:

- Place your baby on their back to sleep in a cot in a room with you
- Use a firm waterproof mattress in good condition
- Never fall asleep with your baby on a sofa or armchair
- Do not share a bed with your baby if you or your partner:
  - Smoke
  - Have recently drunk any alcohol
  - Have taken legal or illegal medication that could make you sleepy/drowsy
- Keep your baby smoke-free before and after birth
- Make sure your baby does not get too hot and keep your baby's head uncovered when sleeping.

Link To/Go To

For more advice and information about cot death and keeping babies safe, go to:

http://www.lullabytrust.org.uk/

Conclusion

The role of the midwife in maternity care is to work as part of the larger multidisciplinary team, to provide mothers and babies with high quality evidence-based care centred around the woman. Much of maternity care is about working in partnership with women to empower them to make decisions about their bodies, their pregnancies and their babies. As nurses, you may come across pregnant women and mothers in a variety of situations. Mothers may ask for your advice and opinions, however it is your responsibility to refer mothers to the health professional who can provide appropriate care (NMC 2008). In most cases, this will be the midwife.

Key Points

- This chapter has explored the role of the midwife in maternity care and the options available for maternity care and birth.
- It has provided an insight into the physiology of pregnancy and links for further reading.
- There is an overview of the important screening tests offered to woman during pregnancy and there are recommended links for further reading.
- Discussed some of the common minor disorders of pregnancy and their appropriate management.
- The importance of the care a woman receives in the antenatal, intranatal and postnatal period and the initial care of the neonate has been emphasised.
- Highlighted some of the complications of pregnancy and childbirth and the actions required by health professionals.
- There are many opportunities where nurses can impact on maternal and child health.

Glossary

Amniotomy: also known as 'artificial rupture of membranes'. The membranes may be ruptured using a specialised tool, such as an amnihook or amnicot

Apgar score: a score designed to quickly evaluate a newborn's physical condition and to determine any immediate need for extra care or emergency care

Auscultation: the act of listening for sounds made by internal organs, e.g. the heart and lungs, to aid in the diagnosis of certain disorders

Autonomy: self-governing, self-regulating; taking responsibility for one's decisions and actions

Braxton Hicks contractions: intermittent contractions of the uterus occurring during pregnancy

Chlamydia: a sexually transmitted infection

Haemoglobinopathy: an hereditary condition involving an abnormality in the structure of haemoglobin

Multigravid: a woman who is or has been pregnant before

Neonatologist: a clinician dedicated specifically to the care of newborn infants faced with critical illness or premature birth

Opioid: one of the main functions of opioids is to produce sedation and pain relief, for example, pethidine and diamorphine

Partogram: a graphical representation of the progress of labour

Peristalsis: a series of muscular contractions

Primigravid: a woman who is pregnant for the first time

Sudden infant death syndrome: the sudden unexpected death during sleep of infants, usually between the ages of two weeks and one year. The causes are not fully understood, they are believed to involve failure of automatic respiratory control

Transcutaneous electrical nerve stimulation: a non-invasive pain relieving aid that uses low-voltage electrical current for pain relief

Varicosity: a vein that has become distended

References

CMACE (2011) *Saving Mothers' Lives: reviewing maternal deaths to make motherhood safer: 2006–2008*. The Eighth Report on Confidential Enquiries into Maternal Deaths in the United Kingdom. Centre for Maternal and Child Enquiries, London.

Cummings, J. (2013) *Compassion In Practice*. Department of Health, London.

DCSF (2009) *Getting Maternity Services Right for Pregnant Teenagers and Young Fathers*. Department for Children, Schools and Families, London.

Edwards, N.P. & Wickham, S. (2011) *Birthing Your Placenta*. Association for Improvements in Maternity Services, p. 19.

Fahy, K., Hastie, C., Bisits, A., Marsh, C., Smith, L. & Saxton, A. (2010) Holistic physiological care compared with active management of the third stage of labour for women at low risk of postpartum haemorrhage: a cohort study. *Women and Birth*, 23(4), 146–152.

Hodnett, E.D., Gates, S., Hofmeyr, G.J. & Sakala, C. (2013) Continuous support for women during childbirth. *Cochrane Database of Systematic Reviews*, (7):CD003766.

HSCIC (2012) *Infant Feeding Survey 2010: Summary*. Health and Social Care Information Centre. https://catalogue.ic.nhs.uk/publications/public-health/surveys/infant-feed-surv-2010/ifs-uk-2010-sum.pdf.

ICM (2011) *Definition of a Midwife*. International Confederation of Midwives. http://www.internationalmidwives.org/who-we-are/policy-and-practice/icm-international-definition-of-the-midwife/.

NICE (2006) *Routine Post Natal Care of Women and their Babies*. National Institute for Health and Clinical Excellence, London.

NICE (2007a) *Antenatal and Postnatal Mental Health*. National Institute for Health and Clinical Excellence, London.

NICE (2007b) *Care of Healthy Women and their Babies during Childbirth*. National Institute for Health and Clinical Excellence, London.

NICE (2010) *Routine Care for the Healthy Pregnant Woman*. National Institute for Health and Clinical Excellence, London.

NICE (2011) *Multiple Pregnancy: the management of twin and triplet pregnancy in the antenatal period*. National Institute for Health and Clinical Excellence, London.

NMC (2006) *Standards for the Preparation and Practice of Supervisors of Midwives*. Nursing and Midwifery Council, London.

NMC (2008) *The Code: Standards of Conduct, Performance and Ethics for Nurses and Midwives*. Nursing and Midwifery Council, London.

NMC (2010) *Standards for Pre-Registration Nursing Education*. Nursing and Midwifery Council, London.

NMC (2012) *Midwives Rules and Standards*. Nursing and Midwifery Council, London.

Office of National Statistics (2013) http://www.ons.gov.uk/ons/rel/vsob1/birth-summary-tables--england-and-wales/2012/stb-births-in-england-and-wales-2012.html.

RCM (2010) *Audit of Midwifery Practice*. Royal College of Midwives, London.

RCM (2012) *Evidence Based Guidelines*. Introduction. http://www.rcm.org.uk/college/policy-practice/evidence-based-guidelines/ (accessed 12 December 2013).

Stables, D. & Rankin, J. (2010) *Physiology in Childbearing*. Bailliere Tindall, London.

UNICEF (2010) *The Baby Friendly Initiative*. http://www.unicef.org.uk/babyfriendly/.

Weeks, A. (2007) Umbilical cord clamping after birth. *British Medical Journal*, 335(7615), 312–313.

Wilkins, C. (2006). A qualitative study exploring the support needs of first-time mother on their journey towards intuitive parenting. *Midwifery*, 22(2), 169–180.

271

Test Yourself

1. The lead professional caring for a healthy pregnant woman is:
   (a) The obstetrician
   (b) The GP
   (c) The midwife
   (d) The health visitor

2. Who are midwives accountable to?
   (a) The mother
   (b) The NMC
   (c) Their employer
   (d) All of the above

3. A common minor disorder of pregnancy is:
   (a) Headache
   (b) Abdominal pain
   (c) Heartburn
   (d) Hair loss

4. Uterine contractions in labour will cause the cervix to:
   (a) Efface and dilate
   (b) Constrict and efface
   (c) Dilate and palpate
   (d) Contract and stretch

5. During a ventouse delivery:
   (a) An incision is made into the abdomen
   (b) Spoon-like instruments are applied to the baby's head
   (c) An incision is made into the perineum
   (d) A suction cup is applied to the baby's head

6. A reduction in caesarean sections may be achieved by:
   (a) Writing a birth plan
   (b) Birthing in a hospital
   (c) Continuity of midwifery care
   (d) Using epidural anaesthesia

7. What is the ratio of multiple births in the UK?
   (a) 1 in 20
   (b) 1 in 40
   (c) 1 in 60
   (d) 1 in 80

8. How can new born babies lose heat?
   (a) Convection, conduction, condensation and evaporation
   (b) Evaporation, condensation, radiation and conduction
   (c) Evaporation, conduction, radiation and convection
   (d) Condensation, radiation, evaporation and compensation

9. Vitamin K is given to newborn babies to prevent the risk of:
   (a) Haemolytic disease of the newborn
   (b) Hepatitis infection
   (c) Vitamin K deficiency bleeding
   (d) none of the above.

10. Breast-feeding can reduce the risk of:
    (a) Sudden infant death syndrome
    (b) Acne
    (c) All infections
    (d) Anorexia

Answers

1. c
2. d
3. c
4. a

5. d
6. c
7. d
8. c
9. c
10. a

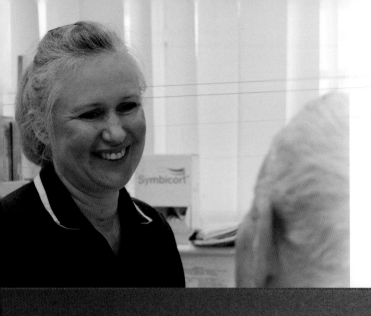

The Principles of Surgical Care

Carl Clare

University of Hertfordshire, UK

Learning Outcomes

On completion of this chapter you will be able to:

- Differentiate between the different classifications of surgery
- Discuss the potential reasons for preoperative anxiety and ways of relieving it
- Understand preoperative risks that must be identified on admission
- Understand the ASA grading system
- Explain the importance of early mobilisation in the postoperative period
- Explore the value of PCA in postoperative pain relief

Competencies

All nurses must:

1. Communicate a simple relaxation technique
2. Teach postoperative exercises for breathing and circulation
3. Carry out a systematic postoperative assessment
4. Safely remove simple sutures
5. Assess a patient for the potential suitability for day surgery
6. Safely discharge the surgical patient

  Visit the companion website at **www.wileynursingpractice.com** where you can test yourself using flashcards, multiple-choice questions and more.

Nursing Practice: Knowledge and Care, First Edition. Edited by Ian Peate, Karen Wild and Muralitharan Nair.
© 2014 John Wiley & Sons, Ltd. Published 2014 by John Wiley & Sons, Ltd. Companion website: www.wileynursingpractice.com

Introduction

We often think of surgery as a 'modern' procedure, however evidence suggests it is one of the earliest forms of medicine. The earliest known evidence of a surgical procedure is from the remains of Neolithic skeletons, which show signs of 'trepanning' (the creation of a hole in the skull) and cave paintings recording the procedure (Porter 1997). Since that time, surgery has been a mainstay of curative treatment throughout history, with ancient Egyptian texts detailing surgical procedures dating to 2700BC. The word 'surgery' is derived from the Ancient Greek work *cheirourgia*, which roughly translates as 'hand work.' While continuing technological advances have introduced forms of robotics into the operating theatre, the control, decision-making and knowledge still remain with the surgeon (Lanfranco *et al.* 2004) and many surgical procedures are still performed by direct contact by the surgeon.

Surgical nursing in the UK is the care of the patient on the ward/unit before and after surgery, as opposed to *Theatre* nursing, which is the care of the patient within the operating department. It is the unique role of the surgical nurse to support patients through a procedure that is, for many, a major life event. To the nursing and medical staff, surgery is routine and 'nothing to be scared of,' however for the patient, the prospect of surgery can be one of the most novel and alien experiences they will ever undergo. Even if the patient has undergone surgery before, any new operation (or repeat procedure) remains an unnerving episode that creates anxiety and stress. The whole process of becoming a patient is debilitating and both the anxiety about the forthcoming surgical procedure and the surgery itself have physical, psychological and social effects. The on-going care of the patient by the surgical nurse requires that the nurse both recognises and attempts to alleviate or prevent these effects. It is almost unique in the hospital setting that the patient may come into the ward 'well' and then be subjected to procedures that can leave them acutely ill.

The Classification of Surgery and Risk

Surgery is primarily classified according to purpose:
- *Diagnostic*: surgery to confirm or establish a diagnosis
- *Palliative*: surgery intended to relieve pain or reduce symptoms of a disease
- *Ablative*: surgery to remove diseased body parts
- *Constructive*: restores function or appearance that has been lost or reduced
- *Transplant*: replaces malfunctioning structures.

Jot This Down
Try to place as many surgical procedures as you can think of into the categories defined above.
For instance, hip replacement is a form of *transplant* surgery.

Surgery is further classified by the degree of urgency and the degree of risk. The degree of urgency is often defined by the necessity to preserve the patient's life, body part or bodily function. Thus, it is usual to talk of emergency (or immediate) surgery, urgent surgery, expedited surgery and elective surgery (NCEPOD 2004).

- *Emergency surgery* is performed immediately to preserve life, limb or function (for instance to stop bleeding after a trauma)
- *Urgent surgery* is normally carried out within hours of the decision to operate for events that potentially threaten life, limb or function or for the relief of pain (for instance the fixation of fractures)
- *Expedited surgery* is surgery that is normally carried out within days of the decision to operate and where the condition is not an immediate threat to life, limb or function
- *Elective surgery* is surgery that is performed when surgery is the preferred treatment to achieve the required outcome for the patient and is planned and booked in advance.

Surgery can also be categorised according to the degree of risk:
- *Major surgery*: involves a high degree of risk in that it may be a complex and/or prolonged operation. Large losses of blood may occur and vital organs may be affected
- *Minor surgery*: surgery with little risk, few potential complications are expected. Often performed as day surgery or short stay surgery.

Box 14.1 Example Surgery Grades

Grade 1 (minor): excision of lesion of skin; drainage of breast abscess

Grade 2 (intermediate): Primary repair of inguinal hernia; excision of varicose vein(s) of leg; tonsillectomy/adenotonsillectomy; knee arthroscopy

Grade 3 (major): Total abdominal hysterectomy; endoscopic resection of prostate; lumbar discectomy; thyroidectomy

Grade 4 (major +): Total joint replacement; lung operations; colonic resection; radical neck dissection.

(NICE 2003)

Needless to say, all operations are 'major' to the patient and while these classifications are useful for healthcare staff, there should be consideration in their use around patients and relatives. Furthermore, the degree of risk of surgery is affected by several other factors, independent of the nature of the operation and these will be discussed later in the chapter.

Box 14.2 Minimally Invasive Surgery

It is worthwhile at this juncture to mention the concept of *minimally invasive surgery* (often referred to as 'keyhole' surgery by patients), for instance laparoscopic procedures. Minimally invasive surgery has been used in all surgical specialities (Kehlet & Wilmore 2008) and its use continues to expand. The use of this technique reduces wound size and thus decreases the unwanted inflammatory responses and pain leading to shortened recovery times and earlier discharge. However, not every patient is suitable for minimally invasive surgery (for instance, obese patients or patients who have undergone previous surgery to the proposed operative site), furthermore minimally invasive surgery requires specialist expertise and equipment and thus, many procedures may not be available outside of specialist centres (for instance, minimally invasive cardiac surgery), whereas other procedures (such as arthroscopy) are commonly performed.

The Phases of Surgery

Surgery is comprised of three distinct phases:

1. *Preoperative*: This phase begins when the patient makes the decision to undergo the recommended surgical procedure

and ends when the patient is transferred into the operating theatre

2. *Intraoperative phase*: Begins on admission to the operating theatre and ends on transfer to the recovery area

3. *Postoperative phase*: Begins on admission to the recovery area and ends when healing is complete.

It is the intention of this chapter to discuss the nursing care of the patient on their journey through the pre- and postoperative phases of their journey. However, as the recovery area is considered to be a critical care area, the postoperative discussion will begin with the transfer of care from the recovery nurse to the collecting (ward) nurse.

The Preoperative Surgical Phase

The decision to offer surgery is that of the surgeon but the decision to agree to undergo surgery remains with the patient, unless the patient is deemed incompetent to make the decision (see Chapter 5). From that moment on, the patient enters into the preoperative phase of their surgical journey. The effect the decision will have on the patient will vary from patient to patient but in the majority of patients, there will be an element of trepidation and anxiety. While much of the nursing care undertaken during the surgical journey of the patient will be based around physical care (the biological care), it is imperative that the nurse does not lose sight of the fact that a major role of the surgical nurse is to educate, reassure and alleviate anxiety.

What the Experts Say

...to understand and respond adequately to patients suffering – and to give them a sense of being understood – clinicians must attend simultaneously to the biological, psychological and social dimensions of illness.

(George Engel, creator of the 'Biopsychosocial model.')

It has long been established that patients are anxious about their anaesthetic and surgery and anxiety can focus on many factors:

- Fear of the unknown
- Fear of the treatment
- Concerns about pain
- Concerns about safety
- Concerns about recovery and the effect on daily life
- Loss of control
- Fear of death and dying.

It is suggested that the patients' experiences of anxiety begin at the point that surgery is planned and agreed to and reaches its peak on the day of the operation (Pritchard 2009). Anxiety causes a wide range of physical responses:

- Tachycardia
- Increased blood pressure
- Increased temperature
- Sweating
- Nausea
- Heightened awareness.

In addition, the psychological responses can be varied and include changes in behaviour, such as increased tension, apprehension, aggression, nervousness and withdrawal. Often, surgery is carried out on patients who already have a long-term condition (which may or may not be the reason for surgery) and it is recog-

nised that patients with long-term conditions have a higher rate of psychological distress and rates of depression are double those found in the 'healthy' population (National Institute for Health and Clinical Excellence, NICE 2009). Furthermore, anxiety is a subjective experience and may be affected by factors such as age, gender and previous hospital experiences (Boker *et al.* 2002).

There is a growing body of evidence that addressing the psychological needs of the patient can reduce the risk of complications and improve postoperative outcomes. For instance, anxiety can increase experiences of pain (Carr *et al.* 2005), nausea, fatigue and discomfort (Montgomery & Bovbjerg 2004) and reduce the patient's immune response, potentially leading to delayed healing and thus longer hospital stays (Kiecolt-Glaser *et al.* 1998). The obvious need of the patient is information, and the traditional approach to anxiety reduction is that information giving and allowing the patient to ask questions will reduce preoperative anxiety. However, this is not universally agreed to be the most effective method, as the psychological changes noted earlier may make it more difficult for the patient to attend to information giving and to understand and retain information. With some patients, information giving may have no benefit at all, even with the use of written information the patient can take away and revisit as often as they like (Ivarsson *et al.* 2005). Thus, the suggestion has been made that the use of a validated assessment tool such as the Amsterdam Preoperative Anxiety and Information Scale (APAIS), developed by Moerman *et al.* (1996) to assess anxiety may be valuable in allowing the nurse to stratify the needs of the patient and target anxiety reduction interventions and information. The APAIS has six questions that are related to the anaesthetic and to the procedure and was further developed by Boker *et al.* (2002) to create subscales. This led to a modified scale that assesses both the anxiety levels (anaesthetic and procedure related) individually and also gives an indication of the amount of information the patient wishes to know.

As well as information giving, it is worthwhile suggesting other anxiety reduction strategies that the patient may wish to try:

- *Medication*: the use of medication in the reduction of preoperative anxiety is gradually decreasing, as it is recognised that it increases postoperative sedation. Furthermore, its use other than in the immediate preoperative period is not considered to be desirable due to the risks of dependence
- *Distraction techniques*: the use of distraction techniques has long been recommended, however while self-reported anxiety is reduced, there appears to be no effect on physiological parameters in the immediate preoperative period (Ni *et al.* 2011)
- *Relaxation techniques*: such as visualisation or deep breathing.

Box 14.3 A Simple Relaxation Technique

Sit in a comfortable chair that supports your head or lie on the floor or bed. Place your arms on the chair arms, or flat on the floor or bed, a little bit away from the side of your body with the palms up. If you are lying down, stretch out your legs, keeping them hip-width apart or slightly wider. If you are sitting in a chair, do not cross your legs.

Good relaxation always starts with focussing on your breathing. The way to do that is to breathe in and out slowly and in a regular rhythm, as this will help you to calm down.

- Fill up the whole of your lungs with air, without forcing. Imagine you are filling up a bottle, so that your lungs fill from the bottom

· Breathe in through your nose and out through your mouth
· Breathe in slowly and regularly, counting from one to five (do not worry if you cannot reach five at first)
· Then let the breath escape slowly, counting from one to five
· Keep doing this until you feel calm. Breathe without pausing or holding your breath.

Practise this relaxed breathing for three to five minutes, two to three times a day (or whenever you feel stressed).

(NHS Choices 2013)

Box 14.4 Breathing Exercise

1. Put yourself in a comfortable position – ideally sitting up straight with your back supported.
2. Take a deep breath in and hold your breath for approximately 3 seconds, then breathe out slowly and relax.
3. Repeat step 2.
4. Take a 3rd deep breath in and hold your breath for approximately 3 seconds. Open your mouth wide and force the air out in a short sharp breath as if you are steaming up a glass window (this is called a huff).
5. Finally, take a deep breath in and perform a strong cough, clearing any secretions/mucous that may be present.

Once the patient's preoperative information requirements have been ascertained, then the nurse can focus on the delivery of tailored teaching to help with the reduction of anxiety and to aid postoperative recovery. As noted, for the majority of patients, surgery will be a novel experience and even for those who have undergone surgery before, there may be incomplete memories/recollection. In educating patients it is always best practice to ascertain what the patient already knows. Assuming the patient is familiar with the processes and procedures of the operative admission is almost always going to be a mistake. Even if the patient appears to be reasonably certain of their knowledge, there is always the possibility that they are mistaken in some of their beliefs and thus identifying and rectifying incorrect information may avoid problems for both patient and staff. Increasingly, patients are being given preoperative information leaflets and many are also now asked to watch a video presentation in pre-admission clinics. Regardless of the method of information delivery, it is essential that patients and relatives are allowed the time to question staff on matters that have not been addressed or the patient did not understand. Often, information delivery is based on what the staff think the patient should be told not the patient priority (Mordiffi *et al.* 2003) and therefore allowing patients to explore their own information needs ensures that those needs can be addressed.

The information provided to patients preoperatively will vary from institution to institution and according to the surgical procedure to be undertaken however as a guide it can be categorised into five main areas:

• Details of the procedure
• Preoperative preparation
• The theatre environment
• Postoperative expectations (including length of stay)
• Details of the anaesthesia.

Other information of value will include visiting times, meal times and where possible, orientation to the ward environment. It has been a popular model of pre-admission care for patients also to be offered a chance to visit the operating theatre or for those who will be admitted electively to a critical care area postoperatively to be able to visit the critical care unit (Daykin 2003).

Jot This Down

Think about the preoperative information needs of different types of clients. How would you tailor the information giving and teaching for:

· Children
· Clients with learning disabilities
· Older patients
· Patients with communication difficulties (such as the deaf patient).

Preoperative teaching

Alongside information giving, the preoperative phase is also used for the delivery of teaching to aid the patient with their postoperative recovery, such as deep breathing exercises, leg exercises and splinting/supporting incisions when coughing.

Deep breathing exercises are encouraged, as the postoperative incidence of chest infections is increased when the patient has reduced mobility and thus is not taking breaths deep enough to expand the lungs. Teaching the patient to deep breathe before surgery means they are more likely to undertake the exercise post-surgery, encouraging lung expansion and also aiding in the clearance of inhaled anaesthetic gases that may be trapped in the lung bases. An example of a breathing exercise is detailed in Box 14.4. Alternatively, patients may be supplied with a device, known as an incentive spirometer, to aid deep breathing exercises.

Teaching patients to splint or support incisions when they are going to cough, is vitally important in several types of surgery. Patients who have undergone abdominal or thoracic surgery are less likely to cough post-surgery, as they are both frightened that the sudden pressure will 'split the scar' and also because it either will hurt or there is at least a fear that it will hurt. Thus, the patient will often suppress the cough reflex and thus are less likely to clear sputum leading to an increased risk of chest infection. Advise the patient to have a pillow or cushion available when they wish to cough. They can then hold the pillow over the wound site and 'hug it' into the wound just before they cough, this splinting reduces the pain experienced and also reassures patients. Patients who have undergone hernia repair surgery are often taught to support the incision when coughing, as there is the worry that the sudden increase in intra-abdominal pressure may lead to the repair being breached and the hernia reappearing (though this in fact is uncommon).

Leg exercises are taught to patients in an attempt to mitigate the effects of reduced mobility on the circulation. Generally, it is preferable for the patient to mobilise as soon as possible after an operation, as this increases lung expansion and also improves circulation. However, depending on the operation the patient has undergone, early mobilisation may not be possible or may only be limited. The reduced mobility leads to pooling of the blood in the veins of the legs (venous stasis) and this in turn can lead to the development of thrombi in the veins (especially the veins in the calf), known as a deep vein thrombosis. If this thrombus then breaks free and enters the circulation as an embolus, it can travel to the lungs and lead to a pulmonary embolus and potentially the death of the patient. An example of a passive leg exercise is detailed in Box 14.5.

Box 14.5 An Example of a Passive Leg Exercise

1. With your legs straight, first point your toes, then bring your toes up toward your head. Do this exercise 10 times every hour with one foot and then the other.
2. With your legs straight, rotate your ankles one at a time, as if you were drawing little circles with your toes. Do this exercise 10 times with one foot and then the other.

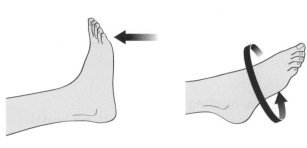

Figure 14.1 Leg exercises post-surgery.

Pre-admission clinics

Patients who are to undergo a planned (elective) surgical procedure are often asked to attend a pre-admission clinic, which is often nurse-led. A preoperative assessment of the patient is carried out as well as preoperative information giving and teaching. The nurse will often carry out a brief physical examination to generate baseline information that can be used to evaluate the patient postoperatively but also to assess for potential risks during the operative period.

Physical assessment and tests: suitably trained nurses may carry out a physical assessment, including listening to breath sounds and heart sounds. Depending on the local policies, nurses may also be able to carry out or order preoperative tests and investigations if required (otherwise, this will be done by the medical staff):

- *Electrocardiogram (ECG)* to assess the patient for pre-existing cardiac conditions (though it must be noted that a normal ECG does not guarantee the absence of heart disease)
- *Full blood count*: red blood cell count, haemoglobin level and haematocrit are important indicators of the oxygen-carrying capacity of the blood. Reduced capacity will affect recovery postoperatively. Raised white blood cell counts can help to identify infections
- *Blood grouping and cross-matching*: in case of the need for blood transfusion
- *Serum electrolytes*: to evaluate fluid and electrolyte status
- *Fasting blood glucose*: to screen for diabetes mellitus. Diabetes mellitus is a major potential cause of postoperative complications and poor wound healing
- *Blood urea nitrogen (BUN)*: to evaluate renal function
- *Alanine aminotransferase (ALT), aspartate aminotransferase (AST) and bilirubin*: to evaluate liver function
- *Urinalysis*: to assess for potential problems, such as diabetes mellitus, urinary tract infection or renal disease
- *Chest X-ray (CXR)*: to help evaluate respiratory function and heart size.

The Evidence

NICE Clinical Guideline 3 *Preoperative tests* (2003) gives a series of 'traffic lights' (red, amber and green), indicating when a certain preoperative test is required.

For instance, a patient with pre-existing heart disease undergoing a minor operation requires an ECG (green traffic light) but not a blood glucose test (red traffic light).

Risk assessment

Risk assessment prior to a surgical procedure is a vital element of ensuring patient safety. In general, the degree of risk of an operation begins with a baseline of the grade of the surgery (see Box 14.1). Surgical risk is also increased by the urgency of the operation, in that the more urgent the surgery is, the less time there is to both assess the patient and to attempt to alleviate any operative risks inherent to the patient. When reviewing patients for surgery, the anaesthetist will usually grade the patient according to the American Society of Anesthesiologists (ASA) grade (Box 14.6). The ASA grade has been shown to be correlated to the mortality (death) risk of the patient undergoing surgery independently of the operation to be carried out. For instance, a patient with an ASA grade of I has an independent risk of 0.05%, whereas a patient with an ASA grade of IV has a mortality risk of 25%. However, the ASA grade is not the only risk factor and must not be taken alone as the sole indicator of risk. Operative risk is a combination of several factors (Fitz-Henry 2011):

- The physical status of the patient
- The physiological derangement that the operation will cause
- The skill and experience of the surgeon
- The skill and experience of the anaesthetist
- The physiological support service in the perioperative period (including preoperative optimisation and postoperative care).

Optimising the patient's physical condition and health prior to surgery will help to reduce the risk the operation poses to that particular patient. Several factors cannot be altered (such as age)

Box 14.6 ASA Grades

Though the term 'ASA grade' is in common use, the actual classification system is known as the 'ASA physical status grade' (ASA PS grade) and it is acceptable to use either Roman numerals (I, II, III, etc.) or standard numbers (1, 2, 3, etc.).

ASA Grade Definition

I. Normal healthy individual
II. Mild systemic disease that does not limit activity
III. Severe systemic disease that limits activity but is not incapacitating
IV. Incapacitating systemic disease which is constantly life-threatening
V. Moribund, not expected to survive 24 hours with or without surgery.

The grading system takes into account the nature of the disease and the impact that it has on the patients' life. For instance a patient with well-controlled diabetes mellitus and no complications would be classed as ASA grade II, whereas a patient with poorly-controlled diabetes mellitus, or complications of diabetes mellitus, would be classed as grade III.

but the control of disease processes and the alteration of other factors can make a significant difference to operative risk and the speed of recovery.

- *Malnutrition* – can lead to delayed wound healing, increased rates of infection and reduced energy. The body requires a variety of nutrients for recovery, such as protein and vitamins for wound healing and vitamin K for clotting.
- *Obesity* – leads to hypertension, impaired cardiac function and impaired respiratory function. Obese patients are more likely to have impaired wound healing and have an increased risk for wound infections as adipose tissue impedes blood circulation and this reduces the delivery of the nutrients, antibodies and enzymes necessary for wound healing (Doyle *et al.* 2010).
- *Smoking* – smoking increases the risks of some postoperative complications, such as pulmonary complications, cardiovascular complications and wound-related complications (such as infection). Even a brief period of not smoking may reduce the risk of postoperative complications (Warner 2005). The use of nicotine replacement therapy (NRT) is certainly recommended in helping patients to stop smoking but there is a theoretical risk of delays in wound healing if this is carried on through the surgical period. Yet, it is currently thought that the proven benefits of NRT in helping people to quit smoking and remain non-smokers and thus reduce actual postoperative complications, far outweigh any theoretical risk to wound healing (Thomsen *et al.* 2009).

Admission to the ward

On admission to the ward, the patient will understandably feel anxious and disorientated. It is essential for the patient to feel as though they are welcome and expected. There can be little more disturbing to a patient on the day of their operation than to attend the ward only to be ignored or placed in the day room, with little information or even with such phrases as 'We don't know if we have a bed yet.' This is the point where a ward clerk can be an invaluable member of the ward team. A welcome from a member of staff who is clearly expecting the patient can make all the difference to their early impressions of the hospital and ward. If the patient's bed space is not ready and available for them to occupy, then the patient should be informed of the delay and reassurance given. Regardless of whether the patient has a bed to go to or is asked to wait in the day room, there should be an immediate orientation to the ward environment (such as the location of the toilets). Once the nurse has been made aware of the presence of the patient, then she should endeavour to at least introduce herself to the patient and any relatives that may be present. This way, the patient is reassured that they have not been abandoned or forgotten and has the name of a member of staff to whom they can turn if required. If not already done, a full nursing history should be taken from the patient. Even if a set of baseline vital signs were taken in the pre-admission clinic, it is important that the patient's blood pressure, pulse, respiration rate and temperature are recorded on the ward documentation. Full nursing documentation should be recorded on the relevant paperwork in conjunction with the patient and/or relatives:

- *Breathing* – including baseline respiration rate and smoking status. Any history of respiratory diseases, such as asthma, COPD, history of shortness of breath or frequent chest infections. Take this time to teach, or revise, breathing exercises
- *Cardiovascular system* – baseline observations. History of cardiac disease, arrhythmias, chest pain or shortness of breath on exertion. Any history of claudication or other peripheral vascular

disease – peripheral vascular diseases are linked with an increased risk of deep vein thrombosis (Libertiny & Hands 1999) and any patient with known or suspected peripheral vascular problems should also be considered high risk for pressure sores including those caused by compression stockings (NICE 2005). A history of hypertension should be recorded, as it is associated with increased risk of cardiovascular complications in surgery and anaesthesia (Foëx & Sear 2004)

- *Maintaining body temperature* – a raised temperature may be an indication of an infection
- *Hygiene (washing and dressing)* – building a picture of what the patient was able to do before surgery is a valuable aid in the postoperative goal setting ready for discharge and also helps with discharge planning. At the same time, the nurse should be aware of the actual physical state of the patient at the time of admission. Many patients will not be willing to admit that they are struggling with day-to-day tasks or may not be aware of the possibility of aids to washing and dressing or home adaptations. Oral hygiene should be discussed, including the presence of dentures, caps, crowns and loose teeth. A labelled denture pot should be made available where necessary and any loose teeth or implants should be recorded.

Jot This Down

You are admitting 80-year-old Mrs Jones to the ward prior to hip replacement surgery. Despite denying any difficulty with washing and dressing at home, Mrs Jones has long dirty toe nails, unwashed hair and her clothes are stained and dirty.

What do you think may be the reasons for the difference between what she is saying and her physical state? What may be some of the potential reasons for her inability to maintain her own hygiene?

- *Eating and Nutrition* – as well as recording patient dietary preferences and normal intake, the nurse should take the time to commence patient education in the benefits of healthy eating and review the patient's normal diet with them. Height and weight should be recorded and the body mass index (BMI) calculated. An accurate weight aids the anaesthetist in calculating the correct anaesthetic dose. Enquiring about any significant weight loss in recent times can be a valuable discussion, as if the weight loss was not deliberate (due to patient dieting) it may be an indication of an underlying disease process. Weight loss of greater than 10% in the preceding 6 months is associated with a greater risk of surgical morbidity and mortality and should be addressed with the multidisciplinary team. Fluid intake (including alcohol consumption) should be discussed and recorded.

Red Flag

Patients who are underweight should have their score calculated on the Malnutrition Universal Screening Tool (MUST) to help direct suitable interventions to improve the patient's nutritional status.

The most recent version of the tool is always available to download from the British Association of Parenteral and Enteral Nutrition website (**http://bapen.org.uk**).

- *Elimination* – record the patient's normal patterns. Are they often constipated? Do they rely on laxatives? If so have the patient's normal laxatives been prescribed? Do they have regular bowel movements? A large proportion of patients will find it difficult to have their bowels open during a hospital stay and patients with regular bowel habits should be reassured that this is normal but if they wish, laxatives can be made available. Patterns of micturition should also be recorded. For instance a patient who routinely wakes in the night to use the toilet may try to get up in the night on a darkened ward and fall.

- *Communication* – note should be made of the patient's native language and any need for a translator. Any difficulties with communication must be noted clearly on patient documentation and handed over effectively to all members of the healthcare team who come into contact with the patient. Hearing aids should be labelled if the patient is going to wear it until the point of anaesthetic, otherwise it should be stored carefully with the patient's belongings and available for the postoperative period. The use of glasses and contact lenses should be noted and storage made available.

- *Mobility* – what is the patient's usual mobility? If the patient has reduced mobility, what is the cause? Being aware of the patient's normal abilities allows for realistic goal setting for postoperative mobilising and also allows the nurse to refer to any appropriate services, such as physiotherapy or occupational therapy for assessment. A 'slips, trips and falls' assessment may be required to help maintain patient safety, as well as a pressure sore risk assessment such as a Waterlow score. Finally, the patient should be assessed for the risk of venothromboembolism (VTE) using a recognised scoring system (NICE 2010)

- *Expressing sexuality/gender* – this is a section of the nursing admission that is often ignored but sexuality and gender are important aspects of care delivery. Patients may wish to discuss when they will be able to resume sexual activities and/or if there will be any restrictions? Some patients may have express wishes about wearing make-up until the last possible moment and having make-up available as soon as they are orientated after surgery. Muslim women may have preferences as to who should nurse them and may wish to wear their *hijab* until they are in the theatre environment. Homosexual patients may be concerned about whether they can record their partner as their next of kin (Fish 2010). The use of the contraceptive pill should be noted and the date it was stopped checked with the patient, as there may be an increased risk of deep vein thrombosis. The possibility of pregnancy should be considered in all menstruating female patients. If, in discussion, they cannot be certain they are not pregnant, then a pregnancy test should be undertaken (National Patient Safety Agency, NPSA 2010a)

- *Dying/plans for the future* – it has already been noted that admission to the ward prior to surgery will be a point of great anxiety for the patient. While it may be inappropriate to discuss death and dying with some patients at this point, other patients may wish to address their feelings or to be directed to a place where they can spend some time praying/in contemplation. Some patients may look for reassurance about the risks they are about to undertake. This is an issue that should be approached with sensitivity and the discussion tailored to the wishes of the patient. Depending on the surgical procedure to be undertaken, the patient may wish to discuss possible changes in body image that will occur as a result of the surgery

- *Work and leisure* – many patients will wish to know when they can return to work and any limitations on the activities they can undertake at work or for leisure and for how long. For instance, a patient who swims regularly may need advice on how long it will be before they can expose their wound to immersion in water.

- *Support systems* – will the patient be having visitors? Do they know which ward and what the visiting times are? It is worthwhile allocating one family member who will contact the ward and then update other members of the family. This avoids having multiple phone calls enquiring after one patient but also reduces the possibility of breaching patient confidentiality over the phone. Who is looking after any pets or dependents that are usually reliant on the patient? Who will be available on discharge and what support mechanisms will be available for activities, such as shopping?

Preparation for surgery

On the day of surgery, the patient will be required to be nil by mouth (NBM) for a set period. Traditionally, patients have been asked to be nil by mouth from midnight, however it is now recognised that keeping patients nil by mouth for potentially prolonged periods is not necessary and may even be detrimental. Patients who are starved for several hours before surgery will often enter the operating theatre with a reduced blood volume due to poor hydration, thus increasing the chances of some perioperative and postoperative complications, such as shock and the development of thrombi (NCEPOD 2011). Recent recommendations are that patients can drink clear fluids up to 2 hours prior to surgery and eat food up to 6 hours prior to surgery (RCN 2005). However, the nature of surgical theatre lists are such that the patient will often be NBM for longer, due to delays or reorganisation of the running order in theatre. Therefore, patients who are NBM should be offered mouth care packs or mouth care should be given to those who cannot perform it themselves. Good communication is necessary between ward and theatres, as when operations are cancelled a patient's NBM status may be prolonged unnecessarily (National Patient Safety Agency, NPSA 2011). Prescribed medication should be reviewed and only those deemed medically necessary should be administered but nurses must be sure that medicines that are critical are administered (NPSA 2010b). Premedication may be prescribed for a variety of reasons and these may be taken with up to 60 mL of water. Care should be taken to ensure that time-critical premedication (such as antibiotics) is given as prescribed.

Unless directed otherwise by the surgeon, the patient should wash or shower the night before surgery using soap and water; antibacterial washes are not normally required (NICE 2008). For certain types of surgery (such as orthopaedic surgery), more rigorous skin decolonisation may be required. Nail-polish and make-up should be removed before surgery, as otherwise the effects of cyanosis or shock may not be as evident, as the changes in colour are masked.

If hair removal is required, it should be done on the day of surgery using depilatory cream or electric clippers with a single use disposable head. Shaving hair from surgical sites before theatre has been shown to increase the rate of surgical site infection. If shaving is undertaken, then it should be done in the theatre environment as close to the point in time of surgical skin preparation as possible but outside of the theatre itself.

Jewellery should be removed if possible, as rings can harbour bacteria; loose items of jewellery could become snagged while

Box 14.7 Some of the Contraindications to Anti-embolism Stockings

· Severe peripheral artery disease
· Severe peripheral neuropathy
· Gangrene
· Oedema of the legs
· Certain types of skin diseases, e.g. dermatitis
· Cellulitis
· Pressure sore of the heels.

transferring the patient onto and off the operating table; and all metal jewellery increase the risk of burns where diathermy is used during the procedure. Local policy may allow difficult to remove rings to be covered with tape. Transdermal patches should also be removed, as they carry a risk of burns or explosion with the use of diathermy or the need for defibrillation in the event advanced life support is required.

Menstruating females should be advised of the risk of toxic shock syndrome if they use tampons during the operative period. If a tampon is left in place for more than six hours, the risk of toxic shock is increased and therefore patients are best advised to use sanitary towels until after the operation. If a tampon is left in place, then this must be documented and handed over, thus in the case of an unexpected transfer to critical care areas postoperatively, staff are aware of the presence of the tampon.

Antiembolic stockings and/or low molecular weight heparin (LMWH) injections may be required. This will depend on surgeon choice, the results of a venous thrombosis risk assessment and the existence of any contraindications to antiembolic stockings (Box 14.7). Stockings must be measured and applied appropriately, ensuring a wrinkle-free result to avoid areas of high pressure on the skin. The nurse should ensure that prescribed anticoagulants are administered prior to surgery.

The details on the patient's wrist band must be checked with the patient and against the medical notes, X-rays, test results and nursing documentation. Patient allergies should be documented and recorded on a suitable allergy wrist band. As well as medication allergies, food allergies should be recorded, as certain food allergies give an indication of the potential for allergies to certain drugs or substances. For instance a seafood allergy indicates a high risk of potential allergy to the iodine-based dyes used in some procedures.

The site of the surgery should be marked by the operating surgeon using an indelible marker before the patient receives any medication that may cause drowsiness (NPSA 2003).

Red Flag – Wrong Site Surgery

Wrong site surgery is an adverse event whereby a surgical procedure is performed on the wrong site (for instance organ, limb, eye or wrong patient). The effects of wrong site surgery can be devastating to the patient and the use of a preoperative marking checklist is strongly recommended (NPSA 2003).

The consent form must be placed on the front of the patient notes (or other prominent place according to local policy) and confirmed with the patient. While a formal, written consent is gained for the surgical procedure, it should be noted that patients should also be consented for any anaesthetic they are to receive (Association of Anaesthetists of Great Britain and Ireland, AAGBI 2006), though this is not normally recorded on a formal consent form but in the patient's notes. (For further details of the ethical and legal aspects of consent, please refer to Chapter 5.)

Ensure the patient's bed is prepared for transfer to theatre, with canvas and bedding, and the patient is wearing a surgical gown.

Care, Dignity and Compassion

Maintaining patient dignity while they are wearing a surgical gown is difficult – as they are worn backwards (with the opening to the patient's rear) and patients often complain that the gowns do not keep them covered. Wherever possible, the patient may keep on their underwear until the moment they are to be transferred. Patients who have a dressing gown should be encouraged to wear it and those who do not have a dressing gown with them should be given a second surgical gown to wear in the place of a dressing gown.

Waiting on the ward on the day of surgery is the time when patient's anxiety is most likely to peak and thus the availability of distractions, such as reading materials, televisions or radios may be useful. Patients with learning disabilities, or paediatric patients, will benefit from the presence of a family member or familiar carer and this should be encouraged, regardless of standard visiting times.

Surgical safety checklist

The use of a surgical checklist for use in the preoperative period is now standard practice in the UK (NPSA 2009). The checklist is used to ensure that certain mandatory items are not forgotten. It is intended to give teams a simple, efficient, set of checks that have been shown to improve patient safety. The use of the checklist has undoubtedly had a significant effect on surgical morbidity and mortality, with one study noting an overall drop in surgical complications of 36% following the introduction of the World Health Organization (WHO) checklist in a number of hospitals.

Link To/Go To

The NPSA has a video showing how to use the surgical checklist at:

http://www.nrls.npsa.nhs.uk/resources/?entryid45=59860

Transfer to theatres

Once the theatre staff have asked for the patient to be transferred to theatre, the patient should be accompanied by a staff nurse who remains with the patient until handover to the theatre staff (using the checklist and patient notes) has been completed.

The Postoperative Surgical Phase

Collection of the patient from the recovery area must be carried out by a suitably qualified member of staff (normally a registered nurse). The patient is considered safe for discharge from recovery to the ward when the patient is:

- Awake with their eyes open
- Extubated
- Maintaining satisfactory blood pressure and pulse
- Is able to lift their head from the pillow on command
- Not hypoxic
- Breathing quietly and comfortably
- Not persistently bleeding from wound sites or into drains
- Appropriate analgesia has been prescribed and is safely established.

Handover from the recovery nurse to the ward nurse must include comprehensive orders for:

- Vital signs
- Pain control
- Rate and type of IV fluids
- Urine and gastrointestinal fluid output
- Other medications
- Laboratory investigations.

The handover must incorporate information on:

- The procedure undertaken
- Any complications
- Any changes in treatment from that planned
- A comment on medical and nursing observations.

Red Flag

If the patient is restless, then something is wrong, look out for:

- · Airway obstruction
- · Hypoxia
- · Uncontrolled pain
- · Shivering/hypothermia
- · Bleeding (external or internal)
- · Vomiting

If you are unhappy with the state of the patient, then you should refuse to transfer them and request a medical review.

The immediate postoperative period

On return to the ward, postoperative patients must be monitored and assessed for any deterioration. Vital signs should be assessed and recorded in-line with local policy and guidance and compared with baseline levels (preoperative and immediately postoperatively).

When reviewing vital signs, take into account both the current observations and the trend the vital signs have followed over an appropriate period of time (e.g. the last few hours). Increasingly, hospital Trusts in the UK are adopting the use of 'early warning scores,' such as the National Early Warning Score (NEWS) (RCP 2012). The NEWS is an at-risk scoring system that helps in the identification of patients who are clinically deteriorating and measures six parameters:

- Respiratory rate
- Oxygen saturations
- Temperature
- Systolic blood pressure
- Pulse rate
- Level of consciousness.

Link To/Go To

A web-based e-training module on the use of the NEWS is available at:

http://tfinews.ocbmedia.com/

While the use of the NEWS system has undoubtedly improved the clinical recognition of the deteriorating patient, it is preferable that the score is used as part of an A–E assessment of the patient, to enable a holistic assessment and gain a complete clinical picture.

When assessing the patient, ensure that you use all the appropriate senses. Touch your patient to feel the skin temperature and assess for clammy skin; listen to the sound of the patient's breathing; look at their colour and be aware of any smells (such as the smell of faeces, melena or acetone breath).

Airway

A disordered airway may be the result of several potential causes:

- Direct trauma to the airway from intubation leading to inflammation and oedema
- Reduced conscious level leading to a loss of the ability to maintain a patent airway
- Foreign body aspiration.

Assessing the airway requires the nurse to look, listen and feel. Look at the patient's chest for movement, while at the same time, listening and or feeling for breath being expired from the mouth. Complete airway obstruction will be identified by the lack of air movement from the patient, although the chest may be moving in the early stages of obstruction. Partial airway obstruction is often associated with an increased effort to breathe and added noises to the breathing. Listen for:

- Snoring noises
- Crowing noises (stridor)
- Gurgling noises (indicating fluid in the upper airway).

Left untreated, partial airway obstruction will often lead to complete airway obstruction and cardiopulmonary arrest. The treatment of airway obstruction depends on the cause but may include:

- Placing the patient in the recovery position
- The use of suction
- Removal of foreign bodies
- Head tilt-chin lift
- Advanced airway manoeuvres (such as intubation or the use of a laryngeal mask airway).

In the instance of a patient with a disordered airway, constant monitoring is advised until the situation is resolved. In many cases, it is recommended that the nurse asks for an urgent medical review of the patient.

Breathing

Causes of disorder in breathing in the surgical patient include:

- Increased bronchial secretions following the use of anaesthetic gases
- Decreased respiratory rate or work of breathing due to opiate analgesia

- Pain
- Pneumothorax
- Respiratory diseases such as asthma or COPD
- Increasing respiratory rates are often the earliest sign of shock (NCEPOD 2005).

To assess breathing:

- Look, listen and feel for signs of respiratory distress:
  - sweating
  - central cyanosis
  - the use of the accessory muscles of respiration
- Assess the respiratory rate. The normal rate is 12–20 breaths/minute. A high (or increasing) respiratory rate is a sign that the patient is potentially severely ill and may deteriorate suddenly
- Assess the depth of each breath, the rhythm of breathing and whether the chest is expanding equally on both sides
- Note the amount of oxygen being delivered and the oxygen saturations
- Listen for noisy breathing. For example rattling or wheezing.

Red Flag

When using oxygen saturation monitoring, remember to change the position of the probe regularly to prevent the development of pressure sores.

Treatment of respiratory problems will almost always require medical help to treat the underlying cause but where possible, consider:

- Commencing oxygen as prescribed (if not already being administered)
- Positioning the patient in a semi-recumbent position to allow for increased lung expansion.

Circulation

Disturbances of blood pressure and pulse are often late signs of an underlying problem. To assess circulation:

- Look to see if the patient's hands are mottled, pale or blue
- Assess the limb temperature by touching the patient's hands
- Measure the capillary refill time
- Monitor the heart rate
- Take a pulse – is it regular or irregular? Weak or strong? A weak pulse may indicate shock. A bounding pulse may indicate sepsis
- Take the blood pressure
- Consider the patient's conscious level (poor cerebral perfusion will lead to a reduced conscious level)
- Measure and record the hourly urine output (less than 0.5ml/kg per hour can be a sign of poor renal perfusion due to a low blood pressure)
- Measure and record the patient's temperature.

Post-anaesthetic, many patients will show a transient drop in blood pressure that will rectify itself quite rapidly. However, a continuing trend of decreasing blood pressure or patients showing other signs of haemodynamic instability should be assumed to be deteriorating and appropriate help should be sought. In almost all patients with signs of circulatory shock, consider hypovolaemia as the potential cause. Assess the wound site for signs of bleeding and check any drains for output. If the fluid balance is not already being recorded, then this should be commenced.

If haemodynamic compromise is suspected, then consider the following actions:

- Asking for a review by the surgical team
- Tilting the patient's bed to a head down position to improve venous return. Be aware that this may be inappropriate in patients with a compromised airway. Do not tilt the bed of patients post-gynaecological surgery, as this masks vaginal bleeding.

If the patient's temperature is reduced, then consider the use of extra blankets or a warm air blanket. In the event of a raised temperature, consider the potential onset of sepsis. Nursing interventions for pyrexia include prescribed antipyretics and indirect fan therapy. Direct fan therapy and tepid sponging should not be used, as they are fundamentally illogical and based on ritual. Direct therapies only lead to vasoconstriction of the skin blood vessels, thus reducing heat loss and raising core temperature (Woodrow 2011).

Disability

- This refers to the point where the patient's conscious level is assessed
- Measurement of the Glasgow Coma Score is very effective but a quicker method is to use the **AVPU** score:
  - The **A** stands for **A**lert (a patient who is awake and talking to you)
  - **V** refers to voice, i.e. the patient is only responding to **V**oice, such as direct questions or commands
  - **P** refers to **P**ain, i.e. the patient is only responding to painful stimuli
  - **U** is the **U**nresponsive patient, who does not even respond to pain.

A patient found to score **P** or **U** on the scale is considered to have a Glasgow Coma Score of less than 8 and therefore the airway is in danger – this patient needs to be seen by an anaesthetist as a matter of urgency.

Following on from this review the patient's drug chart for causes of a change in conscious level (for instance opiate drugs), check the blood sugar by taking a BM and consider nursing the patient in the recovery position if appropriate.

Exposure

This refers to exposing the patient in order to carry out a primary survey of the patient to assess for bleeding, rashes, early signs of pressure sores, etc. Ensure that you expose and assess the whole of the patient from the top of the patient to their toes. Remember to maintain dignity and prevent heat loss at all times. Pay particular attention to wound sites and drains to assess for signs of bleeding.

Depending on the operation, as the patient's blood pressure stabilises they may be able to sit up. The patient may need to be reminded that the operation is over and where they are, as disorientation can occur. Children and patients with learning disabilities will benefit from the presence of a relative or carer at the bedside, while they are recovering from the immediate effects of an anaesthetic.

Complications of Surgery

While each different surgical procedure will carry its own potential complications, there are several potential complications that are common to all surgical patients:

283

Basal Consolidation Leading to Chest Infection

Signs to look for include:

- A raised temperature
- Rapid shallow respirations
- Decreased chest expansion
- Potential chest pain
- A productive cough (though this is less likely in the elderly patient)
- Oxygen saturations may or may not be reduced.

Patients with increased risk of basal consolidation are smokers; patients who have undergone chest or abdominal surgery; and patients who are dehydrated. Prevention requires the encouragement of breathing and coughing exercises, early mobilisation and maintaining appropriate hydration. Patients suspected of basal consolidation should be referred to the physiotherapist and, if possible, a sputum sample should be obtained and sent for microbiological culture and sensitivity testing.

Renal Failure or Urinary Retention

In patients who are not being monitored on a fluid balance chart, this can be missed in the early stages. Patients most at risk of renal failure are those who have had a period or hypovolaemia/hypotension (see Chapter 29 for more details). Renal failure must be distinguished from urinary retention, as renal failure is a medical emergency. Patients with urinary retention will have a full bladder that may also be painful and will be unable to urinate, despite having the urge. It is expected that all patients will pass urine within 24 hours after their operation and when they do, this should be documented in the notes. No patient should be discharged from hospital without documented evidence that they have passed urine. Anaesthesia can affect the bladder, which may make it difficult for the patient to pass urine. Retention may be prevented by ensuring that the patient is appropriately hydrated, providing privacy and encouraging the patient to sit up to urinate. Where appropriate, male patients can be encouraged to sit on the side of the bed to use the bottle and female patients should be provided with commodes. Until the nurse is confident of patient safety, they should remain with any patient who gets out of bed in case of fainting or collapse. The use of bed pans and urinals in bed should be avoided if at all possible, as the patient will find it difficult and will also not be able to empty their bladder entirely. Mobilising the patient out to the toilet once it is safe to do so, will often encourage patients to pass urine.

Deep Vein Thrombosis (DVT)

The most common site for deep vein thrombosis are the calf veins. The cause is often a mix of dehydration, venous stasis and reduced venous return.

Jot This Down

Consider the causes of deep vein thrombosis. How would you help to prevent a DVT occurring in your patient?

The signs and symptoms of DVT are a swollen, painful calf that is hot to the touch. If a DVT is suspected, the medical staff must be informed immediately. Treatment involves bed rest and anticoagulation. The peak incidence for DVT is 5 days' postoperatively, however some patients can be vulnerable up to 12 weeks' postoperatively.

Nausea and Vomiting

Postoperative nausea and vomiting (PONV) may be a reaction to opiates, anaesthetics or other drugs. Other potential causes include pain, abdominal distension and electrolyte imbalances in the blood. Those most at risk of PONV are:

- *Patients under 3 or over 70 years of age*
- *Menstrual age females*
- *Obese patients*
- *Patients who were excessively starved preoperatively*
- *Patients with a history of motion sickness*
- *Patients with a previous history of PONV*
- *Patients who are highly anxious.*

(Gan *et al.* 2003)

The treatment for PONV is:

- If able, find and remove the cause
- Recovery position for patients at risk of aspiration
- Suction if required
- Withhold food and fluids
- Once the PONV subsides, start the patient on sips of fluids and small amounts of dry solid food (such as biscuits)
- Acupressure wrist bands may be of use in some patients
- If prescribed, antiemetics can be administered.

Haemorrhage

There are three main types of post-surgical haemorrhage:

- *Primary haemorrhage* – occurs at the time of the operation
- *Reactionary haemorrhage* – occurs within a few hours of surgery and is a reaction to a rising blood pressure
- *Secondary haemorrhage* – occurs days later, often as a result of infection.

First aid response to haemorrhage is to apply pressure either manually or by applying pads to the dressing. If bleeding persists, then surgical review is required.

Acute Confusion

Acute confusion may affect the elderly patient with no previous history of dementia. The key features of acute confusion are:

- Sudden in onset
- Impaired attention
- Apathy or hyperactivity
- Thought, perception and short-term memory impairment
- Mood fluctuation – especially at night
- Disorientation in time, place and person
- Disturbed sleep/wake patterns
- Hallucinations and delusions.

Acute confusion tends to last less than a month and is often followed by a full recovery.

Constipation

Often patients reason that, as there has been no food intake, there will be no faeces produced and thus tend not to report altered bowel habits to the nurse. Gastrointestinal peristalsis will be decreased for at least 24 hours in patients who have undergone gastrointestinal surgery. Furthermore, immobility, dehydration and opiate analgesia will also contribute to constipation. Nurses must also take into account the psychological effect of using

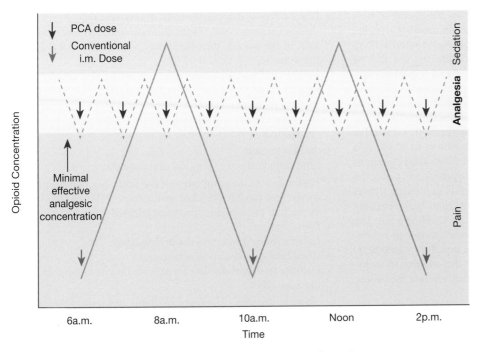

Figure 14.2 Serum levels of analgesia using PCA and intramuscular regimes. Source: Grass (2005). Reproduced with permission of LWW.

commodes on a busy ward. Where possible, patients should be mobilised out to the toilet. For many patients, normal bowel habits will return relatively quickly but without questioning, the nurse may not be aware of patients who have become constipated. Encouraging a high fibre diet and adequate hydration, as well as encouraging mobility will help to prevent constipation.

Pressure Sores

Pressure sores often begin in the operating theatre and it is worthwhile ascertaining the positioning the patient was placed in on the operating table, as pressure sores can develop in unusual places. The longer the patient is in the operating theatre the greater the risk of developing a pressure sore. When assessing patients for pressure sores, the nurse must ensure she inspects areas that are at risk due to equipment use, such as oxygen saturation probes, nasal specs, the elastic straps from oxygen masks and nasogastric tubes.

Pain

For full details of pain assessment and pain relief, please refer to Chapter 23. One aspect of pain control that is specific to surgical patients, is the use of patient-controlled analgesia (PCA). PCA is any method that allows the patient to control and administer their own pain relief and so can include all methods of drug administration. There are two main systems used for PCA post-surgery:

- *Disposable PCA* – this is a system that uses a non-electric pump based on the elastic properties of certain materials, a spring-based mechanism or pressure generated by patient action. Disposable systems have the advantage of not requiring an external power source (useful in transport situations) and eliminating programming errors. However, these systems have been shown to be generally inaccurate with variations in flow rates being affected by temperature, length of storage, atmospheric pressure and the volume of the remaining solution in the reservoir (Skryabina & Dunn 2006).

- *Non-disposable PCA* – this is the system most commonly used in the hospital setting. Based on a computerised system with disposable giving sets, these are considered to have much greater accuracy and have the advantage over disposable systems, in that they are programmable and thus rates of infusion and delivery can be changed.

Regardless of the choice of delivery system, the principle of intravenous PCA remains the same. Occasionally, the pump device will deliver a pre-set 'background' infusion rate of analgesia and nurses should be aware of this and be vigilant for the effects of over-sedation. Using a hand-held button, the patient can activate the delivery of small doses of bolus analgesia. Once activated, the button is then subject to a timed delay (lock-out), during which the delivery of another bolus dose cannot be activated, thus avoiding potential overdose. The benefits of the patient-controlled system are that the patient can have control of when analgesia is delivered, thus avoiding waits for nursing staff to be available and evidence suggests that patient control improves their perception of pain relief (Chumbley & Mountford 2010). Overall, the PCA system has been shown to provide a relatively steady serum concentration of analgesia, avoiding the peaks and troughs of traditional intramuscular regimes (Figure 14.2) and also avoiding excessive pain or sedation (Grass 2005).

Not all patients are suitable for PCA, as there is a requirement for baseline levels of dexterity to activate the button and an ability to understand the concept of PCA and its use. If a patient chooses to use PCA, then part of the preoperative teaching should include the use of PCA, including an opportunity for the patient to handle the device.

PCA analgesia does not guarantee that the patient will be pain-free and thus nurses should be aware of the need to administer further analgesia if required and to refer to the pain control team for the PCA regimen to be altered if it is providing inadequate analgesia for patient comfort.

Further Care of the Surgical Patient

Early Mobilisation

Even short-term immobility and bed rest are associated with:

- Increased risk of DVT
- Muscle wasting
- Increased insulin resistance in the muscle tissues
- Decreased pulmonary function and tissue oxygenation
- Increased risk of chest infection
- Loss of appetite
- An inability to effectively empty the bladder, leading to an increased risk of urinary tract infections
- Constipation.

Thus, early mobilisation is a vital part of the recovery of any surgical patient. Canes and other walking aids should be available to patients who require them. Depending on the operation performed, there may be particular restrictions on mobility and this should be clearly detailed in postoperative plans and in the nursing documentation. Patients who cannot mobilise on the day of surgery should be encouraged to perform leg and breathing exercises. On the first day after surgery, the patient should be aiming to spend two hours out of bed and on subsequent days, the goal should be six hours a day up to the day of discharge. When the patient is to mobilise for the first time, it is essential that the nurse (or other staff member) is present. Have the patient sit on the side of the bed for a few minutes to allow the cardiovascular system to compensate for the effect of any postural hypotension (a drop in blood pressure when the patient sits or stands up). Furthermore, if the patient does subsequently feel faint, then it is relatively simple for them to lie back onto the bed thus avoiding a fall. The patient may then stand while the nurse remains in close proximity in order to guide the patient back onto the bed if they feel dizzy. The nurse will then stay with the patient as they attempt to mobilise, to offer support and reassurance until they are sure the patient is safe to mobilise alone.

Patients are often understandably concerned that mobilising will place pressure on their wound and it will then 'split open.' Adequate pain relief and reassurance will be required. The wound will have developed most of its tensile strength immediately after the operation and thus the patient can be reassured that it is safe to mobilise. Mobility can also be restricted by the use of monitoring equipment and intravenous giving sets, and thus it is necessary to ensure that patients are disconnected from any monitoring equipment or intravenous sets as soon as they are no longer required.

Eating and Drinking

As soon as the patient is able, they should be encouraged to take sips of water and the amount taken increased as tolerated. Patients should also be encouraged to eat as they feel able (unless there are medical orders to the contrary). Small, frequent snacks may be better tolerated than full meals in the first days after surgery. In the case of abdominal surgery, appetite may not return for some time and medical orders should be followed as to when eating and drinking may be attempted.

Intravenous Infusions

Many patients return to the ward with an intravenous infusion in progress. The reasons for infusions vary from the replacement of fluid volume (rehydration), replacing blood loss (transfusion) or to return serum electrolyte levels to a normal range. Discontinuation of fluids is normally on medical orders and in terms of rehydration, this often occurs when eating and drinking are established. (Further information on intravenous infusions can be found in Chapter 19.)

Surgical Drains

Wound drains are used to remove body fluids and/or air from the area of the operation. Unless removed from the tissues, collections of body fluids can become a focus for infection. A tube is placed in the area where fluid is likely to collect and this tube exits the skin via a puncture wound. The tube is stitched to the skin to prevent the tube being accidentally dislodged and the exit site is then dressed to prevent infection of the wound. Normally, the drain is attached to a closed system to prevent the entry of pathogens and air into the body via the drainage system. There are two main types of closed system:

- *Gravity drainage*: a passive collection system that is kept below the level of the wound. If the collection container rises above the level of the wound, then there may be a backflow of fluid into the wound
- *Suction drainage*: an active collection system that usually uses a vacuum created in the collection container. Occasionally, a vacuum pump may be used. The other form of suction drainage is the underwater seal chest drain (see Chapter 27).

Regardless of the drain type, it is essential that strict aseptic technique is used.

The complications of surgical drain use are:

- Failure to function properly – if the drain has not been placed correctly or has been blocked with tissues or clotted blood or the vacuum in the container has been released
- Pain
- Inflammatory reaction to the drainage tube
- Accidental disconnection or removal
- Damage to tissues due to excessive suction or movement of the drainage tube.

Patients are often frightened of drains and restrict their movement. Adequate analgesia, education on drain handling and reassurance will help to alleviate this.

Removal of drains is dependent on the decrease in drainage and is often very painful. Removal will almost always require the administration of adequate analgesia – allow an appropriate amount of time for it to act. Patients often appreciate being given control of the speed of removal of drainage tubes through the use of previously agreed verbal or hand signals.

Wound Care and Surgical Site Infections

The patient will return from theatre with a dressing *in situ* and this should be left in place for at least 48 hours to help reduce the chance of surgical site infection (SSI). The principles of wound healing and wound care are discussed in Chapter 18. Surgical site infections (SSI) represent about a fifth of all hospital acquired infections and about 5% of patients develop an SSI after surgery (Leaper 2010). An SSI is defined as an infection manifesting within 30 days of a surgical procedure (or within one year if a prosthesis is left in place during the procedure) and affecting either the incision or the deep tissue at the operation site (Public Health England 2013). Symptoms include pus, inflammation, swelling and pain. Fever may or may not be present. The majority of infections will not manifest until after the patient has been discharged from hospital.

The risk of SSI is normally related to the class of surgical procedure undertaken:

- *Clean* – no microbial contamination has been encountered and none of the body spaces are entered
- *Clean-contaminated* – gastrointestinal, respiratory or urinary tracts are entered under controlled conditions and without contamination occurring
- *Contaminated* – contamination does occur following entry of the gastrointestinal, respiratory or urinary tract. Recent acute trauma wounds are also classed as contaminated
- *Dirty* – dead or infected tissue is present at the site of surgery.

Actions to prevent SSIs include:

- The administration of prescribed antibiotic prophylaxis in the 60 minutes before surgery starts for patients undergoing high-risk surgery
- Ensuring the preoperative, perioperative and postoperative core temperature of the patient remains above 36.5°C (NICE 2008)

- Leaving the wound covered with an interactive dressing for at least 48 hours postoperatively to ensure the wound seals
- Ensuring the free drainage of exudates and discharge
- Removing wound drains at the earliest possible opportunity
- Dressing changes are undertaken using strict aseptic technique.

Skin closure methods

There are two commonly used skin closure methods:

Skin clips (staples) These are used when there is little tension on the wound and a good general blood supply. This means they can be removed earlier than sutures (around 4–5 days postoperatively). Each of the different types of clip has an associated removal device, all of which work by deforming the clip, thus freeing the barbs of the clip from the skin. If a clip is proving difficult to remove, it can help to gently rock the clip using the device after the clip has been deformed and then gently pulling the clip away.

Sutures (stitches) Two commonly used forms of suture are the subcutaneous continuous suture and intermittent skin sutures:

- *Subcutaneous continuous sutures* are used to improve the cosmetic end-result of surgery. They can be recognised by the presence at each end of the wound of a retaining bead attached to the end of the suture (Figure 14.3). Removal of the suture is performed by cutting one end of the suture close to the skin (therefore beneath one of the retaining beads) and then applying traction to the opposite end of the suture lateral (along the same axis as) to the wound. The patient will often report that this procedure 'stings' but they should be reassured that the acute sensation will subside quickly to an ache, for which simple analgesics are perfectly suitable.
- *Intermittent skin sutures* take longer to remove and the patient may wish to have analgesia for this procedure. Each suture will have a knot, which must be identified (Figure 14.4) and lifted slightly away from the skin. Each suture is cut once just below the knot; it is important not to cut both sides of the suture, as otherwise the suture could retract under the skin (the knot will prevent this). The suture is then grasped with forceps under

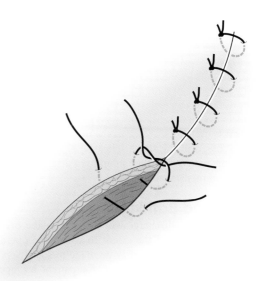

Figure 14.4 Intermittent skin sutures.

the knot (the knot helps prevent the suture slipping through the forceps) and traction put on the suture by pulling across the wound to prevent excessive traction on the wound edges.

In many cases dissolvable sutures may be used, in which case the sutures do not need to be removed but trimmed close to the skin as the suture under the skin will dissolve over a period of time.

Red Flag

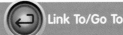

Always be sure of the type of suture you are dealing with. Trimming non-dissolvable sutures on both sides will result in a painful process for the patient when the sutures have to be dug out from under the skin.

Once sutures or clips have been removed, if there is any doubt as to the wound edges (such as the wound edges gaping open), then adhesive skin closure strips can be applied.

Discharge

Wound Infection

Patients should be educated to watch out for:

- Redness and soreness that does not appear to be part of the normal wound healing
- Hot and swollen skin around the wound
- Green or yellow coloured discharge (pus) from the wound
- If they feel unwell, feverish or have a temperature.

If any of these symptoms occur, they should contact their GP.

Link To/Go To

For more information on advising patients about monitoring for wound infections go to the patient guide on the Health Protection Agency website at:

http://www.hpa.org.uk/Publications/InfectiousDiseases/SurgicalSiteInfectionReports/1307Monitoringsurgical woundsforinfection/

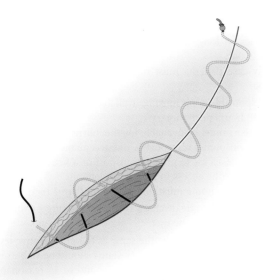

Figure 14.3 Subcutaneous continuous suture showing one of the retaining beads.

Bowels

The patient may find that their bowel habit is altered in the days following surgery. There are several potential reasons for this, including the constipating effects of some analgesics and diarrhoea caused by antibiotic use. Encouraging a healthy balanced diet with plenty of fruit and vegetables and ensuring a good fluid intake will encourage bowel action. Patients with antibiotic-related diarrhoea may benefit from the use of one of the many probiotic drinks that can be purchased in the shops (Hickson *et al.* 2007). It must be stressed to the patient that they should not discontinue the antibiotics except on medical advice.

Dressing and Bathing

The advice given on discharge will depend on the preoperative ability of the patient and the extent to which the operation has affected this ability. Referrals may be made to social services and occupational therapy, to ensure that the patient has appropriate equipment and support. In the days following surgery (and definitely while clips or sutures are in place), the wound may be exposed to water (such as a shower) but prolonged immersion (such as a bath) should be avoided.

Driving

Generally, patients should not drive for 7–10 days after an operation. While driving is not illegal, the patient's insurance may not be valid and if the patient intends to drive, then they should be encouraged to contact their insurer. After some operations, there may be medical advice not to drive for longer than 10 days; the patient will be advised of this by their surgical team.

Drugs

The patient must be given verbal and written instructions or any drugs they are to take home. Any changes to the drugs the patient used to take before the operation should be discussed and patient understanding checked.

Exercise

Specific exercises may be prescribed after surgery and these will be taught to the patient by the physiotherapy staff. The patient should be informed that it is essential that they mobilise regularly to avoid complications and aid recovery. Patients can slowly increase daily exercise until they have returned to normal levels.

Rest and Fatigue

The period after surgery often involves a period of fatigue and this will vary from patient to patient. The patient should be informed that this is normal and that they may need to take afternoon naps for a week or so.

Sexuality

Many patients will wish to know when they can resume sexual activities. It is difficult to give definite timescales on this and the patient is often the best judge of this. For menstruating females, there may be the need to discuss the appropriate timescales to resume taking the contraceptive pill.

Work

Returning to work will depend on the nature of the surgery and the nature of the work. The surgical team will be able to advise the patient about this. Patients should be issued with a certificate for the period of their hospital stay and advised to see their GP for a medical note if required.

Wound Care

An appointment must be made to have sutures or clips removed by the community nurses or the GP practice nurse.

The appearance of the wound will vary as healing takes place. It will start out red and swollen (densely black in the skin of patients of Afro-Caribbean heritage) and gradually become flat and silvery white (or black). This process may take up to 2 years. Sensations around the wound site will be altered due to the trauma of the incision. Pain and soreness will be related to the incision but also due to bruising and the inflammatory process. Wounds may become itchy but patients should be discouraged from scratching it. If the itching must be relieved, then patients are best advised to 'slap' the wound rather than scratching it.

The best results for a scar may be achieved by lightly moisturising the wound but this must not start until 24 hours after any sutures or clips are removed and the wound edges are healed. After a few weeks, thicker creams may be applied and the wound gently massaged to discourage adhesions and to encourage a flatter scar. If the scar is to be exposed to sunlight, then it is best to apply sunblock to the scar for the first year after operation.

Overgrowth of the scar occasionally occurs, which leads to a raised itchy scar (a keloid). The chest and shoulders are the areas that seem to be most at risk of keloid development and they also seem to be more common in patients of Afro-Caribbean heritage. The only treatment option for a keloid scar (if the patient wishes) is referral to a plastic surgeon.

Day-Case Surgery

Day-case surgery is becoming increasingly common and the types of operations undertaken as day cases is expanding rapidly. However, the choice of patients for day-case surgery is not just based on the type of operation to be undertaken. Traditionally, only patients with ASA grade I or II were considered for day-case surgery but now patients with ASA grade III are being treated as day cases so long as their disease processes are well-controlled (RCN 2004).

Day-case patients must be able to meet the following social criteria:

- A responsible adult must be available to stay with the patient for 24–48 hours post-surgery
- An escort must be available for the journey home
- Travel on public transport is not acceptable and so the patient must have access to private transport or a taxi
- There must be access to a private telephone
- The journey home must not take more than 1 to 1.5 hours.

For a patient to be discharged from a day surgery unit, the following criteria must be met:

- Conscious level must be the same as the preoperative level
- Cardiovascular and respiratory status should be stable
- The patient must have passed urine and be in reasonable fluid balance
- Pain, nausea and vomiting must be minimal and controlled
- Bleeding should be minimal
- Mobility should be at the preoperative level.

Conclusion

This chapter has discussed the role of the surgical nurse in the patient's journey. It has reviewed the preoperative and postoperative periods, discussing the role of the nurse. The primary role of the nurse in a patient's surgical journey is to maintain safety through information giving, appropriate assessment and intervention. While different surgical procedures carry their individual risks and complications, there are a number of risks and complications common to all operations.

Key Points

- The effect of surgery on patients is not restricted to the physical.
- Preoperative teaching is vital to both patient safety and patient satisfaction.
- Preoperative checklists are an essential tool in ensuring patient safety.
- Collecting patients from the recovery area involves a complete handover and patients should not be transferred unless the nurse is sure it is safe to do so.
- Immediately on return to the ward, the nurse should undertake a complete assessment of the patient including vital signs.
- The trends of vital signs are just as important as any single result and are often more useful to the nurse.
- Mobilising patients early after surgery has the potential to reduce the incidence of several postoperative complications.

Glossary

Adipose tissue: a form of connective tissue often referred to as 'body fat' or 'fat'
Anaesthesia: making the patient unaware of sensations (such as pain) by using pharmacological means
Analgesia: pain killers
Antiemetic: drug to take away the sensation of nausea and prevent vomiting
Arthroscopy: form of minimally invasive surgery for joints
Blood grouping: ascertaining the blood group of a patient
Body mass index (BMI): measure of body fat based on height and weight
Cellulitis: infection of the deeper layers of the skin
Complication: unfavourable development after treatment
Cross matching: determining the compatibility of blood from a donor with a recipient
Cyanosis: blue discolouration of the skin or mucosa suggestive of hypoxia
Defibrillation: delivery of an electric shock to the heart to treat a life threatening heart rhythm
Dermatitis: inflammation of the skin often in response to an allergen
Diathermy: use of a high frequency electric current to generate heat with the intention to coagulate bleeding, cut or destroy bodily tissues
Embolus: a mass (often a blood clot) travelling freely in the circulation
Electrocardiogram (ECG): a test to record the heart's electrical activity

Electrolytes: a group of chemical elements or compounds that includes sodium, potassium, calcium, chloride and bicarbonate
Endoscopy: looking inside the body using a flexible optical instrument
Excision: removal by cutting
Extubate: removal of a tube (often refers to removal of endotracheal tube used in mechanical respiratory ventilation)
Fracture: a break of a bone
Gangrene: death of bodily tissue with decomposition
Haemorrhage: bleeding
Hernia: the protrusion of an organ through the wall of the cavity that it is usually contained in
Hydration: the process of ensuring adequate water for bodily needs
Hypertension: high blood pressure
Hypoxia: lack of oxygen
Intra-abdominal: within the abdominal cavity
Laparoscopic: minimally invasive surgery involving the abdomen or the pelvis
Malnutrition: condition where a person's diet does not contain the correct levels of nutrients
Micturition: passing urine
Mucous: slippery secretion covering the mucous membranes or respiratory system
Nausea: unpleasant sensation in stomach and head with urge to vomit
Nicotine replacement therapy (NRT): providing nicotine to the body without smoking to aid smoking cessation
Obesity: overweight with a high degree of body fat (BMI greater than 30)
Occupational therapy: treatment to maintain, develop or recover the skills for the activities of daily living
Oedema: accumulation of fluid beneath the skin or in a bodily cavity
Pneumothorax: abnormal collection of gas or air in the pleural space around the lung
Pus: liquid formed at the point of infection containing dead cells, white blood cells and debris
Pyrexia: high body temperature
Physiotherapy: treatment using physical methods to maximise movement and function
Renal: relating to the kidneys
Sepsis: a potentially lethal condition of whole body inflammation in response to infection. Characterised by pyrexia, high heart rate, high respiratory rate and low blood pressure
Sputum: mucus that is coughed up from the respiratory system
Stasis: a slowing or stoppage of the normal flow of a bodily fluid
Tachycardia: a high heart rate (over 100 beats/minute)
Thrombus: a blood clot
Transdermal: a route where drugs are delivered across the skin (for instance from a patch)
Venothromboembolism: a blood clot that forms within a vein

References

AAGBI (2006) *Consent for anaesthesia.* Revised edn. Association of Anaesthetists of Great Britain and Ireland, London.

Boker, A., Brownell, L. & Donen, N. (2002) The Amsterdam preoperative anxiety and information scale provides a simple and reliable measure of preoperative anxiety. *Canadian Journal of Anaesthesia*, 49(8), 792–798.

Carr, E.C., Nicky Thomas, V. & Wilson-Barnet, J. (2005) Patient experiences of anxiety, depression and acute pain after surgery: a longitudinal perspective. *International Journal of Nursing Studies*, 42(5), 521–530.

Chumbley, G. & Mountford, L. (2010) Patient-controlled analgesia infusion pumps for adults. *Nursing Standard*, 25(8), 35–40.

Daykin, S. (2003) Implementation of pre-operative visiting for critical care patients. *Nursing Times*, 99(41), 26–28.

Doyle, S.L., Lysaght, J. & Reynolds, J.V. (2010). Obesity and postoperative complications in patients undergoing non-bariatric surgery. *Obesity Reviews*, 11(12), 875–886.

Fish, J. (2010). Promoting equality and valuing diversity for lesbian, gay, bisexual and trans patients. *InnovAiT: The RCGP Journal for Associates in Training*, 3(6), 333–338.

Fitz-Henry, J (2011) The ASA classification and peri-operative risk. *Annals of the Royal College of Surgeons of England*, 93(3), 185–187.

Foëx, P. & Sear, J.W. (2004) The surgical hypertensive patient. *Continuing Education in Anaesthesia Critical Care and Pain*, 4(5), 139–143.

Gan, T.J., Meyer, T., Apfel, C.C. et al. (2003) Consensus guidelines for managing postoperative nausea and vomiting. *Anesthesia and Analgesia*, 97(1), 62–71.

Grass, J.A. (2005) Patient-controlled analgesia. *Anesthesia and Analgesia*, 101(55), S44–S61.

Hickson, M., D'Souza, A.L., Muthu, N. et al. (2007). Use of probiotic Lactobacillus preparation to prevent diarrhoea associated with antibiotics: randomised double blind placebo controlled trial. *British Medical Journal*, 335(7610), 80–83.

Ivarsson, B., Larsson, S., Lührs, C. & Sjöberg, T. (2005) Extended written preoperative information about possible complications at cardiac surgery: do the patients want to know? *European Journal of Cardiothoracic Surgery*, 28(3), 407–414.

Kehlet, H. & Wilmore, D.W. (2008) Evidence based surgical care and the evolution of fast track surgery. *Annals of Surgery*, 248(2), 189–198.

Kiecolt-Glaser, J.K., Page, G.G., Marucha, P.T., MacCallum, R.C. & Glaser, R. (1998) Psychological influences on surgical recovery. Perspectives from psychoneuroimmunology. *American Psychologist*, 53(11), 1209–1218.

Lanfranco, A.R., Castellanos, A.E., Desai, J.P. & Meyers, W.C. (2004) Robotic surgery. A current perspective. *Annals of Surgery*, 239(1), 14–21.

Libertiny, G. & Hands, L. (1999) Deep venous thrombosis in peripheral vascular disease. *British Journal of Surgery*, 86(7), 907–910.

Leaper, D.J. (2010) Surgical site infection. *British Journal of Surgery*, 97, 1601–1602.

Moerman, N., van Dam, F.S., Muller, M.J. & Oosting, H. (1996) The Amsterdam preoperative anxiety and information scale (APAIS). *Anaesthesia and Analgesia*, 82(3), 445–451.

Montgomery, G.H. & Bovbjerg, D.H. (2004). Presurgery distress and specific response expectancies predict postsurgery outcomes in surgery patients confronting breast cancer. *Health Psychology*, 23(4), 381.

Mordiffi, S.Z., Tan, S.P. & Wong, M.K. (2003) Information provided to surgical patients versus information needed. *AORN Journal*, 77(3), 546–562.

NCEPOD. (2004) *The NCEPOD Classification of Intervention*. National Confidential Enquiry into Patient Outcome and Death, London.

NHS Choices. (2013) *Relaxation Tips to Relieve Stress*. National Health Service. http://www.nhs.uk/Conditions/stress-anxiety-depression/Pages/ways-relieve-stress.aspx. (accessed 9 August 2013).

NICE (2003) *Preoperative Tests. The use of preoperative tests for elective surgery (CG3)*. National Institute for Clinical Excellence, London.

NICE (2005) *Clinical Guideline 29: the management of pressure ulcers in primary and secondary care*. National Institute for Health and Clinical Excellence, London.

NICE (2008) *Clinical Guideline 74: surgical site infection prevention and treatment of surgical site infection*. National Institute for Health and Clinical Excellence, London.

NICE (2009) *Depression With a Chronic Physical Health Problem (CG91)*. National Institute for Health and Clinical Excellence, London.

NICE (2010) *Clinical Guideline 92: venous thromboembolism: reducing the risk of venous thromboembolism (deep vein thrombosis and pulmonary embolism) in patients admitted to hospital*. National Institute for Health and Clinical Excellence, London.

NCEPOD. (2005) *An Acute Problem?* National Confidential Enquiry into Patient Outcomes and Death, London.

NCEPOD. (2011) *Knowing The Risk: a review of the peri-operative care of surgical patients*. National Confidential Enquiry into Patient Outcomes and Death, London.

NPSA. (2003) *Patient Safety Alert 6: preoperative marking recommendations*. National Patient Safety Agency, London.

NPSA (2009) *Patient Safety Alert 2: WHO Surgical Safety Checklist*. National Patient Safety Agency, London.

NPSA (2010a) *Rapid Response Report. NPSA/2010/RRR011. Checking Pregnancy Before Surgery*. National Patient Safety Agency, London.

NPSA (2010b) *Rapid Response Report. NPSA/2010/RRR009. Reducing Harm from Omitted and Delayed Medicines in Hospital. Supporting Information*. National Patient Safety Agency, London.

NPSA (2011) *Risk Of Harm to Patients Who are Nil by Mouth: Signal 1309*. National Patient Safety Agency, London.

Ni, C., Tsai, W., Lee, L., Kao, C. & Chen, Y. (2011) Minimising preoperative anxiety with music for day surgery patients – a randomised clinical trial. *Journal of Clinical Nursing*, 21, 621–625.

Porter, R. (1997) *The Greatest Benefit to Mankind. a Medical History of Humanity from Antiquity to the Present*. Harper Collins, London.

Pritchard, M.J. (2009) Identifying and assessing anxiety in preoperative patients. *Nursing Standard*, 23(51), 35–40.

Public Health England (2013) *Protocol for the Surveillance of Surgical Site Infection. Surgical Site Infection Surveillance Service*. Public Health England, London.

RCN (2004) *Sheet 1: Day Surgery Information*. Royal College of Nursing, London.

RCN (2005) *Clinical Practice Guidelines. Perioperative Fasting in Adults and Children*. Royal College of Nursing, London.

RCP (2012) *National Early Warning Score (NEWS): standardising the assessment of acute-illness severity in the NHS*. Royal College of Physicians, London.

Skryabina, E.A. & Dunn, T.S. (2006) Disposable infusion pumps. *American Journal of Health-System Pharmacy*, 63(13), 1260–1268.

Thomsen, T., Tonnesen, H. & Muller, A.M. (2009) Effect of preoperative smoking cessation interventions on postoperative complications and smoking cessation. *British Journal of Surgery*, 96, 451–461.

Warner, D.O. (2005) Helping surgical patients quit smoking: Why, when and how. *Anesthesia and Analgesia*, 101, 481–487.

Woodrow, P. (2011) *Intensive Care Nursing: a framework for practice*, 3rd edn. Routledge, London.

Test Yourself

1. Surgery to remove a diseased body part is known as:
   (a) Diagnostic
   (b) Transplant
   (c) Palliative
   (d) Ablative

2. Patients should stop drinking clear fluids:
   (a) 2 hours before surgery
   (b) when they leave the ward for the operation
   (c) 12 midnight
   (d) 6 hours before surgery

3. After an uncomplicated anaesthetic, patients can usually return to driving:
   (a) The same day
   (b) 1 day after
   (c) 1 week after
   (d) 2 weeks after

4. Preoperative skin preparation includes:
   (a) Shaving on the morning of the operation
   (b) Using iodine wash the morning of the operation
   (c) Using chlorhexidine wash the night before surgery
   (d) Showering the night before surgery

5. Toxic shock syndrome is caused by:
   (a) A sanitary towel left in place
   (b) A tampon left in place
   (c) A contraceptive coil left in place
   (d) An operation swab left in place

6. If a patient cannot remove a ring before surgery, then:
   (a) It should be cut off using a ring cutter
   (b) It should be taped over
   (c) It should be washed in iodine solution
   (d) The operation should be cancelled

7. Gurgling noises from the airway may indicate:
   (a) Fluid in the upper airway
   (b) Fluid in the lower airway
   (c) Constriction of the upper airway
   (d) Constriction of the lower airway

8. In the event of hypotension post-surgery do not tilt the bed of patients who have undergone:
   (a) Leg surgery
   (b) Gynaecological surgery
   (c) Abdominal surgery
   (d) Chest surgery

9. Day surgery patients can be discharged home if a responsible adult will be with them for:
   (a) 1–12 hours
   (b) 12–24 hours
   (c) 24–48 hours
   (d) 48–72 hours

10. An allergy to seafood indicates the potential for an allergy to:
    (a) Latex
    (b) Heparin
    (c) Anaesthetic drugs
    (d) Iodine-based dye.

291

Answers

1. d
2. a
3. c
4. d
5. b
6. b
7. a
8. b
9. c
10. d

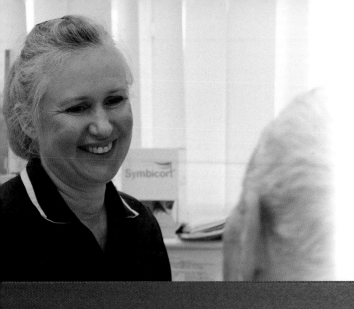

15

The Principles of Cancer Care

Laureen Hemming

University of Hertfordshire, UK

Learning Outcomes

On completion of this chapter you will be able to:

- Describe the environment in which cancers develop and the factors that contribute to cancers spreading throughout the body
- Consider the impact of lifestyle choices on the development of and recovery from cancers
- Outline the investigative procedures used to determine the presence of cancer
- Explain the rationale for the various options used to treat cancers and the role guidelines and protocols have in standardising treatment
- Examine the care required for the person with cancer throughout their cancer experience and their survivorship issues once treatment has been completed
- Explore the support available for people with cancer that is provided by charitable funded organisations

Competencies

All nurses must:

1. Explain investigative and treatment procedures to the person with cancer in a succinct manner in-keeping with their role in providing care
2. Assess, plan and deliver appropriate care for the person with cancer within their level of competency
3. Monitor the progress of a person with cancer who is in receipt of treatment, whether it is curative of palliative in intent
4. Evaluate the effectiveness of the care provided
5. Provide sensitive support to those closest to the person with cancer while maintaining confidentiality at all times
6. Relate sensitively to spiritual and cultural needs of the person with cancer

 Visit the companion website at **www.wileynursingpractice.com** where you can test yourself using flashcards, multiple-choice questions and more.

Nursing Practice: Knowledge and Care, First Edition. Edited by Ian Peate, Karen Wild and Muralitharan Nair.
© 2014 John Wiley & Sons, Ltd. Published 2014 by John Wiley & Sons, Ltd. Companion website: www.wileynursingpractice.com

Introduction

Cancer is a generic term used to cover over 200 different diseases and it is beyond the remit of this chapter to explore them all fully. The chapter takes a holistic overview of cancers because the various different cancers have a many similarities and evoke similar responses in people. It is said that Hippocrates (460–370BC), a Greek doctor, first used the word *karkinos* because cancer seemed to spread sideways with long finger-like projections, like a crab (Fayed 2009). It is believed that cancer cases were reported from as early as 3000BC on papyrus in Egypt, where they treated breast cancer by cauterising the tumours, so it is not a disease of the modern age. The first links between lifestyle choices and cancer date back to 1761, when John Hill, a London doctor and botanist, wrote a thesis on the relationship between the use of tobacco in the form of snuff and the development of nasal cancer. While cancer has a long history, it is a particularly exciting field of nursing because of the many advances being made and the cutting edge research being used to treat it. Good nursing care makes a real difference to the person's experience of their cancer journey. Despite the success rates and improved survival times for some cancers, it is still largely perceived as a fatal illness and people dread receiving a cancer diagnosis; however, with the use of combination therapies and newer targeted treatments, it is now considered a chronic illness because over half of the people diagnosed with cancer live for five years or more. It is largely a disease of 'older' age; three out of five cancers are diagnosed in those over 65 years of age, as a result, in part, of lifestyle choices and behaviours, and the reasons for this will be explored later. Having said that, younger people also develop cancer: children develop leukaemias (cancer of the blood cells), and young adults develop melanomas (skin cancers), however, they only represent 1% of the cancer cases (Cancer Research UK 2012).

Despite improvements in cancer care, England still lags behind Europe. If we were to achieve the average survival rate in Europe, 5000 lives would be saved, and if we matched Europe's best results, 10 000 lives would be saved each year. Unfortunately, most cancers are diagnosed as the result of an emergency admission to health care and there is thus a need for improved health screening to detect cancers earlier, which enables better recovery rates and this is reflected in the increase of health awareness advertising in the media.

Factors that Increase the Risk of Developing Cancer

Smoking

The link between tobacco and cancer, as stated above, was first made in 1761. The evidence is now indisputable and one in four cancer deaths in the UK occur in smokers. While lung cancer is the most common cancer from smoking, people who smoke could develop cancer of the mouth, oesophagus, stomach, pancreas, liver, kidney, bowel, ovaries, bladder, cervix or leukaemia.

Alcohol

Each year, 4% of diagnosed cancers are as a result of drinking alcohol, the main ones being mouth, throat, oesophagus, stomach, liver, bowel and breast. While a small glass of red wine (2 units) a day may reduce the incidence of heart disease, it contributes a significant risk to developing cancer, especially if consumption is greater than 2 units a day.

Obesity

Scientists have sought to find a link between what we eat and the potential to develop cancer as a result of this. Colorectal cancers are associated with a diet lacking in fibre and high in animal fats. Obesity combined with a sedentary lifestyle seems a predictive factor for other cancers such as breast and renal cancers. Hamilton-West (2011) talks of a 'global obesity epidemic' that has resulted in other diseases as well as cancer and points out that these illnesses are related to human behaviour rather than biological malfunctions.

Infections

Certain infections are also associated with a greater risk of developing cancer. For example the human papilloma virus is implicated in cervical cancers, and girls are now vaccinated at the age of 13 to decrease their risk of getting the disease.

Stress and the immune response

Cells in the body are under constant bombardment from carcinogenic (cancer causing) substances but they do not all succumb and become cancerous because the immune system detects abnormalities developing and removes these cells through apoptosis (cell death). The effectiveness of the immune system is determined by the person's ability to cope and manage with the stressors it encounters, whether these are physical or psychological (Hamilton-West 2011). How this works will be described in the section considering the pathophysiology of cancer.

> **Jot This Down**
>
> Can you think of any occupations that could put the person more at risk of developing cancer?
> What risks do the following workers face that make them potentially liable to develop cancer?
> - Builders
> - Carpenters
> - Chefs
> - Corporate bankers
> - Farmers
> - Gardeners
> - Taxi drivers

Occupational risks

In 1775, Percival Pott, a doctor at St Bartholomew's Hospital in London, made the connection between skin cancer and soot, from caring for chimney sweeps who presented with sores around the scrotum. Today, employment law sets out to protect workers from hazardous substances, but people working outside are more susceptible to skin cancers from exposure to the sun. Healthcare workers are exposed to radiation from X-rays and are routinely monitored for exposure levels.

Pathophysiology

The cell is the basic single unit from which the body develops. The first embryonic cells divide and develop to take on specific functions, thus they become differentiated, that is they become different tissues and the embryo develops skin, nervous tissue, bone, etc. and take on different roles within the body, develop at different rates, secrete different enzymes and chemicals and work in their own unique way for the benefit of the whole organism or person. Cancer starts in a single cell; it is this mutation of a cell arising from a genetic malfunction that leads to the development of further cell mutations and the development of the growth referred to as cancer. The many different cancers that exist are because different tissues become cancerous, thus carcinomas are growths arising from epithelial tissue in the body and sarcomas are cancers from supporting tissue such as bone, muscle, cartilage and fat. Lymphomas are cancers of the white blood cells and leukaemias are cancers of the cells in the blood system. Cancers are further classified according to the tissue in which they are growing, thus an osteosarcoma is growing in the bone and adenocarcinoma is growing in a gland.

Cell Division and Replication

Each cell in the body has a determined lifespan, for some cells, such as those that line the mouth, the lifespan is short; while others, such as those that make up bone have a much longer lifespan. When cancers develop in slow growing cells, the cancer develops at a slow rate, however, in a rapidly changing tissue, the cancer development may be quite aggressive and this will also affect the rate in which the cancer spreads through the body. Whether the cell is slow growing or fast, the cycle through which the cell proceeds remains the same (Figure 15.1).

Taking the starting point as G_0, where the cell is in a resting phase, chemicals signal to the nucleus within the cell the need to replicate. Under this influence, changes occur within the cell and it moves from the G_0 to the G_1 phase where it doubles the organelles within it and the cell prepares for duplication. Certain chemical enzymes, called *kinases,* check that the preparation is in order and if all is well, the cell proceeds to the next phase, called the *S phase*; however, if all is not detected to be in order, cell death (or apoptosis) is triggered. It is believed that an enzyme called p53 is responsible and although it is absent in some cancers, it is not absent in all.

The S phase sees the cell preparing further for replication and the DNA in the cell doubles. Proto-oncogenes within the cell cause the DNA helix to unwind and split into two. There is another check before the cell proceeds to the G_2 phase, where the cell expands and becomes ready for the mitotic phase where it splits in two (Figure 15.2).

The time taken for each phase varies according to the type of cell undergoing replication and this knowledge is used when timing cycles of chemotherapy treatment, so that the greatest 'cell kill' can occur.

Thus, in normal conditions, as cells reach maturity, they prepare to replicate, thus replacing themselves at regular intervals. Fortunately, cells do not all undergo this process at the same time, if they did, we would then shed layers of tissue at a specific point in time.

It is believed that cancer cells develop when the normal regulatory processes are damaged; either through the defects of ageing, which is why most cancers develop in older people, or as a result of exposure to agents, which cause the cells to mutate. Some agents are initiators, that is, exposure to them cause cancer; certain viruses are initiators; while other substances are promoters, that is prolonged exposure is required before cancer develops. Nicotine and other chemicals in cigarettes are promoters. The squamous epithelial cells lining the bronchus change after repeated exposure to cigarette smoke; however, if the person stops smoking, these cells can repair themselves. Sunburn damages cells in the skin and results in the development of skin cancers.

The UK Department of Health (DH 2007) believe that over half of all cancers are preventable and invest in national campaigns to raise public awareness, with the aim of developing a healthier nation. The main areas that the government target are:

- Smoking
- Diet and exercise
- Alcohol consumption.

In addition, the government promotes screening programmes with a view to recognising disease early enough to treat effectively. Routine screening is undertaken for:

- Cervical cancer, women aged between 25 and 64 years can have smear tests taken to check for any abnormal cells
- Breast cancer, women aged between 45 and 74 years, can attend for mammography; 73.4% of women targeted attended for screening in 2012
- Colorectal cancer, everyone over the age of 60 years is sent test-kits to collect stool samples every two years.

Publicity campaigns include advice on tanning, with the use of sun beds prohibited to those less than 18 years of age. Sunburn in childhood increases the risk of acquiring skin cancer later in life. Other campaigns have focussed on improving diet by increasing the amount of fruit and vegetables eaten and reducing red meat consumption and at the same time increasing the amount of exercise taken.

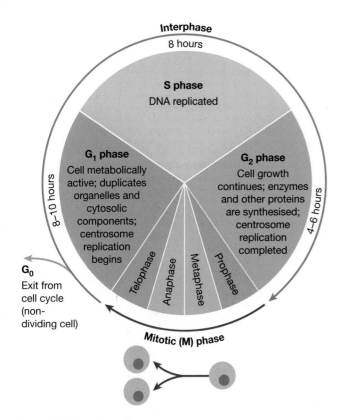

Figure 15.1 The cell cycle.

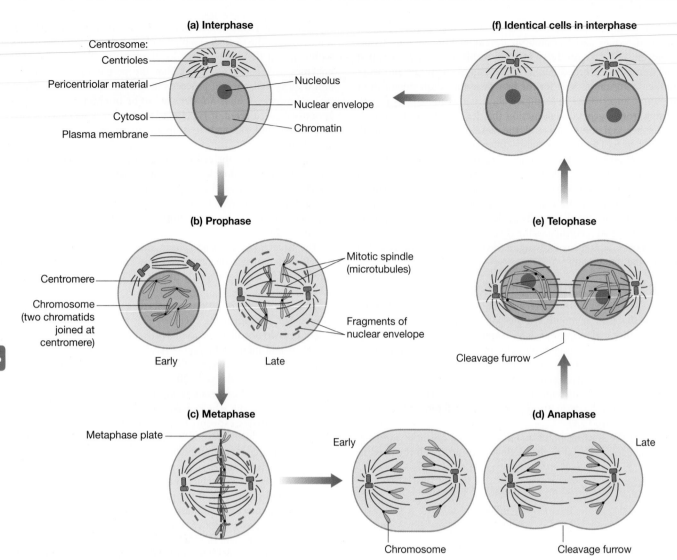

(a) Interphase

Centrosome:
Centrioles
Pericentriolar material
Nucleolus
Nuclear envelope
Cytosol
Plasma membrane
Chromatin

(f) Identical cells in interphase

(b) Prophase

Centromere
Chromosome
(two chromatids
joined at
centromere)

Mitotic spindle
(microtubules)

Fragments of
nuclear envelope

Early   Late

(e) Telophase

Cleavage furrow

(c) Metaphase

Metaphase plate

(d) Anaphase

Early   Late

Chromosome   Cleavage furrow

Figure 15.2 **Cell division – mitosis.**

296

Signs and Symptoms

As there are over 200 different cancers, it is impossible to describe all the signs and symptoms that people may experience and that may prompt them to seek medical advice. Some cancers are discovered through screening programmes, where a risk is known and measures can be taken to discover the cancer in its early stages. While mammography screening enables some breast lumps to be seen on the X-ray at an early stage, many people (it affects men and women) discover a lump in their breast tissue and this drives them to seek medical opinion. Lumps can be felt in the testes and men are advised to examine their genitalia regularly, just as women are encouraged to examine their breasts.

Changes in bowel habit could indicate colorectal cancers, especially if accompanied by bleeding. Abnormal bleeding and discharge is also an indicator that help should be sought from the medical profession as soon as possible.

However, some cancers are difficult to detect until the disease is quite advanced. People who smoke may well have a morning cough, so dismiss a persistent cough as a 'normal' state of affairs. It is also difficult to detect lung cancer on a chest X-ray, as some of the lung is not visible; some of the tissue is obscured by the heart and diaphragm.

Unexplained weight loss is a key symptom; this is referred to as cancer cachexia.

Cancer Cachexia

There is some debate as to whether people develop anorexia (loss of appetite) first and then become cachectic or whether the cachexia develops first. It would seem that cachexia precedes the anorexia because the weight loss occurs while the person is still eating normally. In advanced disease, or where the cancer grows quickly, the person can lose one-fifth of their body weight in less than 3 months, which significantly impacts on their prognosis and their response to treatment.

Cachexia develops from altered metabolism within the cells prompted by the secretion of certain cytokines (chemical messengers) that affects the metabolism of glucose. Cancer cells require amino acids obtained from proteins to grow and develop and obtains these through the breakdown of skeletal muscle. As cells usually utilise glucose for energy before using proteins, the cytokines place a block on this process by blocking the action of insulin in the liver so glycogen is not used and this leads to a raised insulin and sugar level in the blood. The cells in the hypothalamus recognise the raised serum blood sugar levels and excrete a neuropeptide, leptin, which depresses the appetite resulting in a state of anorexia.

It is believed that approximately 30% of people die from muscle wasting as the cachexia depletes muscle from the heart and the intercostal muscles, making respiration difficult.

Various interventions have been tried to help people eat more and reverse the decline, such as supplementing the diet with high protein feeds rich in omega-3 fish oils. The supplements can be unpalatable and result in pale offensive stools and 'fishy' burps. Research into this field has not yielded any encouraging results and these supplements can be expensive.

Pain

Pain is one of the most feared symptoms associated with cancer; approximately 70% of people with cancer experience pain. Unfortunately, the heightened stress that accompanies fear of a prospective cancer diagnosis can intensify the pain. Pain also arises physically as the cancer grows and infiltrates nerves or presses on nociceptors (nerve endings that sense pain). Thus, pain has psychological and physical dimensions; Hamilton-West (2011) explains that the endocrines produced in response to stress affect the nociceptor, which is why pain is not merely experienced following physical trauma.

People still associate cancer with being a fatal illness rather than a chronic illness, so a cancer diagnosis may lead them to question the meaning of life, whether they have achieved their life ambitions or not and to question the issue of mortality, and this may cause spiritual angst and pain.

Pain is always an individual experience that has physical, psychological and spiritual origins, making it a complex symptom to manage and control effectively. It is the main symptom that will drive people to seek medical help and may denote a problem. If acute pain is ignored or managed ineffectually, it will develop into chronic pain. (For more information on pain, please refer to Chapter 23.)

Investigations and Diagnosis

In the UK, a 2-week rule applies, which means if a GP suspects a person has cancer, that person needs to be seen by a specialist consultant within 2 weeks. It is a legal requirement that the person gets treated for cancer within 18 weeks of being seen by the consultant. This is part of the government strategy regarding people with cancer, as it aims to improve outcomes for people with cancer (DH 2013; NHS Choices 2013).

Link To/Go To

Department of Health (DH 2013) *The Handbook to the NHS Constitution* for England:

http://www.nhs.uk/choiceintheNHS/Rightsandpledges/ NHSConstitution/Documents/2013/handbook-to-the-nhs -constitution.pdf

The most important assessment is to glean the person's history, what has prompted them to seek medical help. This is followed by a physical examination, as cancer tumours can be palpated and felt. Cancers can be seen through:

- Bronchoscopy – used to detect cancer in the lung
- Cystoscopy – used to detect cancers in the bladder
- Endoscopy – used to detect cancer in the oesophagus and stomach
- Sigmoidoscopy – used to detect colorectal cancers.

However, cancers can grow in areas that are difficult to palpate and are not so obvious, necessitating further investigation.

Diagnostic investigations, depending on the type of cancer suspected, will include a range of imaging procedures:

- Angiography
- Computed tomography (CT scans)
- Magnetic resonance imaging (MRI)
- Nuclear imaging
- Ultrasonography
- X-rays.

These procedures site the cancer and give an indication of its size.

Cytological screening, which is viewing a sample of tissue using an electron microscope, will determine the morphological features of the cells; that is their size shape and degree to which they have changed. Tissue may be gleaned from taking a scraping of cells as in cervical smear tests, or taking a sample by needle aspiration or by looking at fluid or a blood sample.

Blood samples are also viewed for the presence of tumour markers, for example PSA (prostate specific antigen) levels are raised in cancer of the prostate and this would indicate the need for further investigations.

Nursing Care While the Person Is Undergoing Investigations

People undergoing investigations for cancer are very frightened and therefore require psychological support. It is important that they are not given false reassurance, as this can lead to a lack of trust in hospital staff, which may affect the way they respond to treatment.

Being supportive means the nurse should:

- Always refer to the person by their name
- Engage in eye contact when speaking to them
- Always listen patiently to the person's concerns
- Where possible, be honest BUT if you have insufficient information for this, say so and tell them you will find out and return with an answer.

It is not possible to have all the answers and you may not have sufficient knowledge to deal with their queries, so it is important that this is conveyed to the person.

Treatment of Cancer

As far back as 3000BC, physicians have been attempting to treat cancers, initially with cauterising the tumour, which is applying a burning iron; then surgery became the treatment of choice but the real breakthrough in treatment came in the early 20th century, following the development of radiotherapy and chemotherapy.

Decisions on the Course of Treatment

Treatment choices are largely dependent on the stage at which the cancer is discovered. Staging and grading of cancers is dependent on the **TNM** (tumour, node, metastases) status:

- *Tumour size* (**T**) – tumours are graded as T_1, T_2 or T_3. This is determined following a biopsy of the tumour. When tumour samples are examined under the microscope, it is possible to see the extent to which the cells have changed from how they should look. Cells in the body 'differentiate'; that is the embryonic cells in the fetus change from the original 'stem' cell to become specialist cells. Therefore, from the original stem cells, skin, nerve, muscle, blood, bone cells develop and take on their specific characteristics. When the cells become cancerous, they lose their specific characteristics and no longer look like the tissue they are in.
  - In T_1, only a quarter of the cells no longer look like the tissue. these cells are referred to as 'undifferentiated'
  - T_2 means that between a quarter and half of the tissue sample contains undifferentiated cells
  - T_3 means that over three-quarters of the tissue is undifferentiated, that is, the cancer has taken over most of the tissue and the tissue no longer functions as expected
- The **N** refers to the lymph nodes near the site of the cancer. Cancer spreads through the lymphatic and blood system and can seed in adjacent nodes. N_0 refers to no nodal involvement, suggesting the cancer is still relatively new and contained within the tissue where it is found. N_1 means one node near the cancer site has been altered, N_2 means more nodes are involved and N_3 means that nodes distant to the tumour are involved.
- Finally **M**, refers to the number of different sites in which the cancer has metastasised. Again, it could be M_1 or M_2 or M_3.

If the person's cancer is graded as T_1, N_0, M_0, then the cancer is in its early stages and may be easily removed by surgery. Surgery could be followed-up with either chemotherapy or radiotherapy, to ensure that any 'seeds' of cancer are eradicated. However, if the person's cancer is graded as T_3, N_3, M_3, the cancer is advanced and may be beyond removal by surgery. Surgery will be undertaken to provide symptom relief by removing blockages or to insert a stent to keep an opening patent. It may be possible to slow down its growth using chemotherapy or radiotherapy, but the prospects of curing the person are not realistic. Treatment is 'palliative' and focusses on controlling symptoms and keeping the person comfortable. The palliative phase can last a long time, particularly if symptom management is effective and the cancer is slow growing, however aggressive cancers reduce the time the person has left.

Treatment decisions are now made at multidisciplinary team (MDT) meetings, where a group of healthcare professionals meet and discuss each individual case.

Jot This Down

List the healthcare professionals you would expect to attend an MDT meeting for a person with a cancer diagnosis.

Surgery

Surgical procedures are used to diagnose and stage 90% of all cancers and surgery is used to treat 60% of cancers. As a primary treatment, the aim is to remove the whole cancer if at all possible, with a clear margin of unaffected tissue around it. Adjacent lymph nodes are also removed, especially if the tumour is large enough to indicate that it may well have spread.

Surgical interventions result in mutilation of the body; sometimes this is visible, as in the removal of a breast or the formation of a stoma but all alterations of the body will affect a person's self-image whether or not they are visible to others. Removal of the lymph nodes may not be visible but may result in the person developing a lymph-oedematous limb, which is clearly visible and extremely uncomfortable.

Sensitive nerve plexuses can be destroyed, resulting in altered functioning of the body; for example, a man may be left impotent or with incontinence following prostatectomy.

Surgical procedures are also used for:

- Bypassing an obstruction
- Reconstructing the body to improve body image, as in breast cancer
- Debaulking a tumour so that it does not press on other organs
- Relieving pain
- Palliative measures, as when a stent is inserted to keep the oesophagus open.

Nursing care for the person having surgery

Surgery may be the first step of a person's treatment for cancer; they may go on to have radiotherapy and/or systemic anti-cancer treatments, which are described below.

As when the person is undergoing diagnostic investigations, compassionate care is essential. Postoperatively, the person will experience pain and will require regular analgesia while the healing process is underway.

Nursing care requires preparing a person for surgery; educating them so they know what to expect from the surgery and the care they will have to take following surgery. If the person appears not to understand the consequences of surgery, it may be appropriate to arrange an appointment for that person with the surgeon.

Systemic Anti-cancer Treatments

Chemotherapy has for a long while been the main pharmacological treatment for cancer but increasingly, other types of drugs are used, so the term 'Systemic Anti-cancer Treatments' (SACTs) is now used, instead of referring to all of it as 'chemotherapy'. Included in the SACTs are biological therapies and immunotherapies designed to target the genes in the cells and alter their metabolism, so that cell death (apoptosis) occurs. Some of the immunotherapy drugs are used for non-cancer patients and are effective in treating rheumatoid arthritis, Crohn's disease, renal vasculitis and they have also been used to terminate ectopic pregnancies, thus saving the woman from invasive surgery that results in the loss of the fallopian tube, compromising future pregnancies. This chapter focusses on the use of these drugs in cancer, where the doses are different and the potential for severe side-effects occur.

Chemotherapy

Chemotherapy treatments developed as a consequence of war. Sulphur mustard gas was used in the trenches in the First World

War and had been refined by the Second World War to nitrogen mustard. A bombing raid on an Italian seaport resulted in blowing up a US ship carrying canisters of nitrogen mustard; the survivors had various symptoms from contamination with the gas, which included a rapid drop in blood lymphocytes. It was deduced that mustard gas may be useful in treating lymphomas, where there is an excess of white blood cells. The treatment was effective for a short time, extending life by several weeks and the results were sufficiently encouraging to warrant further research and refinement. Chemotherapy agents are referred to as being cytotoxic, that is they kill cells, attacking both normal and diseased cells. They also work by interfering in the process of cell regeneration, which is why the cell cycle is significant when considering cancer development. Some agents work in a particular phase of the cell cycle, so they are termed 'phase specific', while others act throughout the entire cell cycle of regeneration and are 'non-phase specific', however, cells that are not regenerating, including cancer cells, are unaffected.

Therefore, to target as many cells as possible, a combination of several chemotherapy agents are used together to obtain the greatest 'cell kill'. However, as the agents target normal and diseased cells together, a balance has to be achieved, so chemotherapy agents are given in cycles timed to allow normal cells to recover – which is about 3 weeks. Cancer cells have a longer recovery time. Chemotherapy is usually used in conjunction with surgery and radiotherapy; it is not universally effective against all cancers but can be significantly effective in curing leukaemia.

The cycles are also timed to coincide with the body's circadian rhythms (day to night-time patterns) as the drugs work better if allied to hormonal fluctuations and there are fewer side-effects experienced.

Several cycles are needed, as there is a percentage of cells that escape the effect of the chemotherapy because they were not at the responsive stage in their process of regeneration.

The cancers that respond best to chemotherapy are:

- Acute lymphoid leukaemia in children
- Acute myeloid leukaemia
- Hodgkin's disease
- Germ-cell testicular cancers
- Choriocarcinoma
- Ovarian cancer
- Wilms' tumour
- Embryonal rhabdomyosarcoma
- Ewing's sarcoma.

Chemotherapy agents

Chemotherapy agents (there are over 50 different ones) are grouped together in families representing either their similar chemistry or the way that they work. The main groups are:

- Alkylating agents, the first chemotherapy agents to be used, were developed from nitrogen mustard – they link directly to DNA molecules and cause mutations of the genetic information in the DNA and they are carcinogenic. While they can cause cancer, they are sufficiently effective against cancer, so the risk is outweighed by the benefit. These drugs stop the DNA helix unwinding so cell regeneration cannot take place. They can be either monofunctional, that is working on one phase of the cell cycle or bifunctional, working in two parts of the cycle. Some examples are:
  - Chlorambucil
  - Cyclophosphamide

  - Melphalan
  These drugs are used mainly for people with leukaemias, lymphomas or solid cancer tumours. Cyclophosphamide relies on an enzyme in the liver to activate it; if this is missing, it is not effective.

  Treatment can result in renal failure, haemorrhagic cystitis (inflammation in the bladder that causes bleeding) and infertility because it affects stem cells. Younger patients may need counselling if they have not yet started a family, as sperm and egg banking take time and may cause an unacceptable delay to treatment

- Platinating agents are very similar to alkylating agents in that they affect the cross-linking of DNA and these two groups of drugs are often linked together into one category. These drugs contain platinum and examples include:
  - Carboplatin
  - Cisplatin

- Antimetabolites are drugs that are similar to molecules that appear in the cells which attract enzymes to bind to them. When these enzymes bind to the drug rather than the 'metabolites' they should bind with, the synthesis phase of the cell cycle is interrupted, thus the cell is poisoned and dies. The drugs ensure that DNA cannot repair itself when damaged as through molecular influences of the cancer cells. Cancer cells also require folic acid to grow; antimetabolites block the action of folic acid. Examples of agents modifying DNA are:
  - Capecitabine
  - Gemcitabine
  - 5-flourouracil (5 FU)
  An example of an agent which affects folic acid levels is:
  - Methotrexate
  Antimetabolites are used to treat breast, colorectal and osteogenic and pancreatic cancers

  These drugs affect rapidly dividing cells as the endothelial cells that line the mouth and gastrointestinal tract resulting in mucositis, and the hair resulting in alopecia.

- Mitotic inhibitors are extracted from plant material, and bacteria such as the streptomyces. The mitotic inhibitors from streptomyces are called cytotoxic antibiotics. They target the DNA molecule and prevent an enzyme called topoisomerase from breaking down and rejoining the DNA helix. Examples are:
  - Anthracyclines, most active in the synthesis phase, such as Epirubicin and Doxorubicin
  - Non-anthracyclines such as Mitomycin and Bleomycin
  Other topoisomerase inhibitors that interrupt the uncoiling of DNA strands are:
  - Epipodophyllotoxins
  - Etoposide
  - Irinotecan

  Other mitotic inhibitors are those that affect the microtubules inside the cells that instigate changes when the cell is ready for regeneration; they affect the division of chromosomes, particularly the spindles that pull the chromosomes apart. Mitotic inhibitors infiltrate these tubules and examples are:
  - *Vinca* alkaloids, from the periwinkle plant, such as Vincristine and Vinblastine
  - Taxanes, from the bark of the yew, such as Paclitaxel and Docetaxel
  - Camptothecin analogs, from the Asian 'Happy Tree', such as Irinotecan.

299

These drugs are used in a variety of cancers such as non-small-cell lung cancer, breast, ovarian and prostate cancer. They affect the white blood cells and can cause neutropenia, a very serious side-effect, as the person has nothing left to fight off infection.

Resistance to chemotherapy

When the first dose of chemotherapy is administered, the person is monitored for any allergic reactions; these are rare but can occur. If a person does have an allergic reaction, treatment is stopped. The cancer tumour can also develop resistance to the treatment, as it produces cytokines, which block the action of the chemotherapy agent, and measurement of tumour markers indicate whether or not the cancer is responding to the treatment. The solution to the problem of resistance is to use a combination of drugs.

Combination therapies

Initially, chemotherapy treatment used single agents, however people can develop resistance to an agent just as in antibiotic therapy (Kelland 2005). The side-effects of a single agent may be sufficient to warrant discontinuation of the therapy. However, mixing several different agents that work differently together allows for more aggressive treatment, which results in a greater 'cell kill', because each can be used to the maximum level without the same toxic effect that occurs if used singly. Cancer cells are less likely to develop resistance from this combined assault. Research has worked to find which combinations are most effective; the mix includes phase-specific and non-phase-specific agents.

Within the combination, other drugs that are not specifically chemotherapy agents but improve their action can also be given. Combination therapies are usually known by their acronyms, which usually derive from the first letter of each drug used, e.g. BEP (a combination of bleomycin, etoposide and Platinol used to treat testicular cancer); CHOP which includes cyclophosphamide, doxorubicin (formerly called hydroxydaunomycin), vincristine (formerly called Oncovin) and prednisolone used to treat non-Hodgkin's lymphoma. Another combination is FEC – fluorouracil, epirubicin and cyclophosphamide used to treat breast cancer.

Side-effects of chemotherapy

Most people know of the side-effects of chemotherapy, making the treatment as dreaded as the disease itself and sufficient to make them question whether it is truly beneficial. Saltmarsh and De Vries (2008) write of the paradoxical image of chemotherapy that poses problems for patients and nurses – it provides a cure but at a cost, which is often called into question. Nurses administering chemotherapy which is usually given intravenously, have to remain positive for the person's sake, while knowing that they will experience side-effects which compromise their quality of life. Sometimes the side-effects are sufficiently severe to postpone or stop treatment, which is expensive for the patient and for the NHS. However, many of the side-effects are effectively controlled with the use of premedication, which is given routinely.

Nausea Chemotherapy-induced nausea (CIN) has been described as the worst side-effect; and affects approximately between 60% and 72% of people (Miller & Kearney 2004). Some drugs are more ematogenic (causing nausea and vomiting) than others; cisplatin being one of the worst and the vinca alkaloids being the least ematogenic. Nausea is sometimes accompanied by vomiting but this is not the most common experience.

Nausea is a subjective, individual experience, described as queasiness, unease in the stomach, a feeling of a need to vomit, retching or heaving. The feeling of nausea after chemotherapy may be classified as acute, occurring within 24 hours, or delayed, occurring 48 hours later. Untreated acute nausea may develop into anticipatory nausea, where the very thought of attending for chemotherapy may induce nausea so much that the person is reluctant to attend for treatment.

Nausea can be associated with other interrelated symptoms such as fatigue and constipation, anxiety, taste changes in the mouth and heightened perception of smells, thus making it difficult to manage. The person invariably has to cope with this at home on their own because it usually occurs after they have left the hospital; it is exhausting, disrupts sleep and prolongs the recovery period between treatments.

Thorough assessment is needed before treatment commences and should include questions, such as:

- Were you nauseous after your last treatment?
- How often do you feel nauseous?
- How long does it last?
- How severe is it?
- What other sensations and symptoms accompany it?
- What makes it better and what makes it worse?

The person may find keeping a record in a journal or diary is useful, as a pattern usually develops and it may be difficult to remember what has happened in between cycles of treatment.

As it is a usual side-effect, most people having chemotherapy will be given a premedication of an antiemetic, usually Ondansetron 8 mg and a steroid, Dexamethasone 8 mg up to an hour before the chemotherapy is given, as it easier to prevent the symptom than treat it once it has developed (Ng & Della Florentina 2008). Newer drugs, such as neurokinin type 1 receptors may be used as they remain in the body for a shorter time. Antiemetics cause drowsiness and constipation, which can be problematic.

There are non-pharmacological approaches that can be used to control nausea. Research evidence suggests that using music to distract people during the receipt of chemotherapy inhibits feelings of nausea. Progressive muscle relaxation; meditation and controlled breathing, may also be effective and acceptable coping strategies. Guided imagery, where the person focusses on a pleasant scene or an enjoyable calming experience can be effective because the person has a sense of control over their situation (Molassiotis *et al.* 2008). The research-based evidence for these interventions is limited but they do have the advantage of being relatively inexpensive, easy to learn and apply. These coping strategies can be used in other situations where a person experiences mounting tension and anxiety, such as waiting for test results.

Constipation Constipation is usually secondary to other side-effects, such as nausea, where the person has not eaten the right foods or has not felt like drinking enough fluids to remain hydrated. The use of premedication to minimise the experience of nausea, analgesics taken to control pain and treatment with the vinca alkaloids (vincristine and vinblastine) are also constipating because they slow down bowel transit time, resulting in more water being absorbed from the bowel.

Constipation can be a significant problem, requiring assessment to establish the cause. If it is related to the chemotherapy regime using vinca alkaloids, it is known that the problem disappears 10 days after treatment has stopped and management may include taking laxatives prophylactically but increasing fluids may be sufficient to resolve the problem. If the constipation is secondary to other treatment (iatrogenic), the person needs regular laxative therapy in combination with the analgesics and antiemetics. Bulk forming laxatives are not advised because they require the person to drink plenty of water, which may be difficult when feeling nauseous. Espresso coffee is a natural purgative and exercise also helps to maintain peristalsis and a healthy bowel.

Diarrhoea Diarrhoea occurs because chemotherapy agents affect rapidly dividing cells, which are those cells that line the gut.

Chemotherapy agents are most effective on cells that rapidly divide, which includes those lining the gut, resulting in diarrhoea. Some of the drugs most likely to cause diarrhoea are:

- Capecitabine
- Cisplatin
- Cyclophosphamide
- Daunorubicin
- 5-Fluorourcil
- Irinotecan.

Episodes of diarrhoea may start within hours of the first treatment and can prove acutely embarrassing. Its severity can result in dehydration, necessitating rapid treatment with drugs such as loperamide or codeine. If the diarrhoea does not subside, it may be necessary to reduce chemotherapy or stop treatment until the person recovers. The compromised immune status may mean the person is more susceptible to developing infections from *Clostridium difficile*.

Hair loss Hair loss (alopecia) is a symptom that most people associate with chemotherapy, some saying it is the worst side-effect; however, it does not occur with all agents (Randall & Ream 2004). In the recent Department of Health survey (DH 2012), 73% of respondents claimed they were not distressed by their hair loss, which suggests this side-effect is managed well. Hair loss occurs because the hair cells regenerate fairly quickly, so are very susceptible to the cytotoxic effect of the chemotherapy. The hair does regrow but it may well change in colour and texture. All body hair is affected, so eyebrows, eyelashes and pubic hair is lost as well as scalp hair. It is a visible sign that the person is unwell and draws unsolicited public attention, which may be embarrassing.

There are several ways to manage this side-effect. The person having chemotherapy is advised to have short hair; hair initially thins and the thinning is less noticeable than when the hair is worn long. Using very mild shampoos, not washing the hair frequently and letting the hair dry naturally also helps to preserve hair, a great deal depends on the aggressiveness of the treatment regime used and the agents involved.

The loss of eyebrows and eyelashes is problematic, as eyelashes and eyebrows protect the eyes from dust particles. The advice here is to wear sun glasses.

Scalp cooling There is some research-based evidence that scalp cooling can minimise hair loss. People used to wear gel filled caps that had been frozen, which were then periodically changed as they warmed up. Now most chemotherapy suites have machines that keep the cap at a constant temperature. The cap has to fit snugly to the head for the best results, so the right size cap needs to be selected for each person. A poor fit will result in hair loss – which may still occur with a correct fit. The cap has to be worn for at least

15 minutes before treatment starts and continues for at least 30 minutes after treatment has stopped. Cool caps lower the person's temperature and they need extra blankets to keep warm during the process. The caps are heavy as well as cold and some people opt not to continue with the treatment because of the discomfort. Scalp cooling is not a guarantee against hair loss; some people still experience hair loss or thinning, which can be very distressing having coped with all the discomfort. It is difficult for healthcare professionals to advocate for scalp cooling, knowing that it is not always successful. Cooling of the scalp reduces the uptake of the chemotherapy agents in the hair follicles, some people fear that the cancer will metastasise as a result but there is no research-based evidence to support this claim.

Men can be as traumatised by hair loss as much as women, so it is essential that everyone is offered the same advice. Some people opt to disguise the hair loss by wearing hats or scarves, while others opt to use wigs. Some acrylic wigs are available from the NHS; the Cancer Research website has a list of wig suppliers (Cancer Research UK 2011).

Neutropenia Neutropenia develops quickly and requires immediate action, because if untreated can prove fatal. As chemotherapy affects rapidly dividing cells, depresses the function of the bone marrow and the production of blood cells, in particular neutrophils. The person receiving chemotherapy is at risk of developing opportunistic infections and does not have the body's first-line of defence. The infections may come from the patient themselves, as when the oral mucosa is breached, the person can develop ulcers and sores, which are a source of infection. Cleaning teeth with a soft toothbrush reduces the risk of damaging the gums. The person receiving chemotherapy is also advised not to drink very hot beverages, which might also cause burns in the mouth.

A person is classed as being 'neutropenic' when their neutrophil count is lower than 1×10^9/L; febrile neutropenia is when the person's temperature is greater than 37.5°C. Approximately 40% of people receiving chemotherapy experience neutropenic events resulting in changes to the chemotherapy regime, which may be reduced in or stopped while until the person recovers. The first sign of neutropenia is a raised temperature, so the recipient of chemotherapy needs to record their temperature daily. In the event of a raised temperature, the person must contact their healthcare team immediately or report to hospital for a possible emergency admission. Everyone receiving chemotherapy is given a card detailing local arrangements and emergency telephone numbers. Neutropenia can escalate very quickly and the person can develop neutropenic sepsis and die within hours if untreated.

What To Do If...

A person arrives at the emergency department with a slightly raised temperature and tells you they had a chemotherapy treatment 48 hours previously. Some of the questions you may ask include:

- Have you got your 'chemotherapy alert card?' (this will have a record of the treatment and the consultant caring for the person and contact details)
- When did you last have treatment for chemotherapy?

It is imperative that the person receives treatment quickly and is not made to wait, as they will deteriorate very quickly and reach a point where they may die.

A course of granulocyte stimulating factor (GCSF) may be given to a person at particular risk over a period of 10 days, as this helps the neutrophil levels to recover quickly (Khan *et al.* 2008).

Some foods could possibly lead to a person developing infection, so it is advised that a 'neutropenic diet' is followed, in which uncooked foods such as salads, blue cheeses, unpasteurised milk products and undercooked meats are avoided.

People are also advised to avoid mingling in crowded areas when shopping or having visitors who have an infection while their immune system is lowered by chemotherapy, to prevent the risk of cross-infection.

Peripheral neuropathy Some 30–40% of people are affected by chemotherapy induced peripheral neuropathies, which occur following treatment with high doses of chemotherapy agents such as the platinum drugs, the taxanes and vinca alkaloids. Combination therapies, which include these agents can damage the nerves and this is felt in the feet and hands as tingling (paraesthesia) or altered sensations (dysaesthesia), numbness and shooting pain. This condition is painful and can be difficult to manage if the nerve endings are permanently damaged. Reporting this side-effect at once to the healthcare team will result in a reduction of the dose or stopping treatment for a short while, which reverses the problem, however, it is not always reversible and it can be a major factor in people opting out of further treatment. Taking supplements, such as vitamin E and B may help, but should only be taken following consultation with the medical team. Alcohol drinkers may be more susceptible to the condition.

Neuropathic pain responds better to treatment with analgesics, which are combined with antidepressants or anticonvulsant drugs, such as gabapentin which are more efficient in controlling nerve pain than analgesics alone.

'Chemobrain' and 'chemofog' Some people observe that during the treatment period, they experience memory problems, where they may forget words when they are talking or forget appointments. They usually find reliable solutions, such as making lists, keeping a diary, etc. Others report difficulty in concentrating on reading and absorbing information. There may be a variety of reasons for 'chemobrain' and 'chemofog'; people may be anxious, have sleep problems, feel fatigued, all of which can affect concentration levels. In general, people report this as a passing problem, either more significant side-effects detract from the focus on concentration, or they feel they will adapt to a world of treatment and recovery. Researchers into this topic found that it is a problem that is rarely shared with healthcare professionals but is openly discussed with others in a similar position in clinics in chemotherapy department waiting rooms.

Primary Care

Chemotherapy is usually administered while the person is an outpatient and most of the side-effects can occur once they have returned home, so they may feel vulnerable and alone.

Nursing care for the person receiving chemotherapy

The person with cancer, who is having chemotherapy treatment, requires support and understanding. Every person receiving chemotherapy is given a card, which details the drugs they are receiving and also lists key contact numbers so that they can get help as soon as they need it.

Red Flag

Only nurses who have been assessed annually as competent to do so can administer SACTs.

(Manual for Cancer Services, National Cancer Action Team 2011).

Before chemotherapy is administered

Receiving a diagnosis of cancer can be very devastating, so much so that the person fails to hear much more information. It is the usual practice to see the person at a later date (two to three days later), to discuss the treatment plan and gain consent for the treatment to proceed, as they are better able to focus on the information given. Pre-chemotherapy consultations are usually conducted by nurses who have had additional training in giving chemotherapy because they are better placed to deal with any queries.

Each person's treatment plan is customised to meet their specific needs and the person needs to understand what the treatment involves, the possible side-effects to consider and the strategies they can employ to keep well during this period. Preparation for treatment includes administration of drugs to prevent complications, such as the use of antiemetics to prevent nausea. Chemotherapy agents are expensive and it is traumatic for the patient if treatment has to be stopped or suspended while they recover from the side-effects of the treatment.

Administering chemotherapy

Chemotherapy is usually given as an intravenous infusion; however, there are a few oral preparations. Oral drugs have to be capable of withstanding the digestive process, which may alter their effectiveness and if a person is nauseous and vomits, it is difficult to establish what dosage has been absorbed. Patients prefer oral medication because this negates the need for frequent hospital visits; however, healthcare professionals are anxious that the regime may not be strictly adhered to. As both parties are anxious to maximise the effectiveness of the chemotherapy, intravenous infusions and frequent hospital visits remain the standard pattern. Chemotherapy drugs are usually given in cycles, which are repeated at intervals sufficiently long to enable normal cells to recover but short enough to hit cancer cells before they replicate. If the person requires several cycles, a permanent device, such as a Hickman catheter or a porta cath can be inserted and this prevents several cannulations.

The person is not hospitalised for the administration of chemotherapy unless they are suffering severe side-effects; most people attend specialist chemotherapy suites, which cancer centres have tried to make as comfortable as possible, furnishing them with recliner chairs. The feedback from users indicates that this environment is preferred as it normalises life, comparing it with a visit to the hairdressers, where they are hooked up to a giving set instead of a hair dryer.

Before each treatment is commenced, the person must attend a haematology clinic so that a full assessment can be taken of their blood. Box 15.1 outlines the blood values needed for chemotherapy to proceed.

A creatinine clearance test is also undertaken to establish whether the kidneys are functioning well, as most chemotherapy

---

Box 15.1 Blood values necessary for chemotherapy to proceed

Haemoglobin – greater than 10g/dL
Total white blood count – greater than 3.0×10^9/L
Total neutrophil count – greater than 1×10^9/L
Platelets – greater than 80×10^9/L
Creatinine.

---

agents are excreted through the kidneys. If these are not functioning properly, there will be a build up of toxic waste products in the body.

The time taken for tests to be completed and results noted may lengthen the day at hospital and some centres operate a 'two stop' system where patients attend day 1 for tests and return 24–48 hours later for treatment. This system is preferred because less time is perceived as 'wasted', although it necessitates two trips to hospital.

What the Experts Say

" It can be very dehumanising, I feel like being on a factory conveyor belt.

It's like KFC [Kentucky Fried Chicken] cancer ward.

(McIlfatrick et al. 2007)

Biological Therapies and Immunotherapies

Biological therapies including immunotherapies are the other branches to Systemic Anti-cancer Treatments (SACTs). Immunotherapy is not a new concept; William Coley, an American surgeon practising in the 1800s, found that one of his patients with a solid tumour went into remission from his cancer following erysipelas (a streptococcal bacterial infection). He experimented by injecting small amounts of streptococcal bacteria into bone tumours, to stimulate the body's immune system which targeted the cancer cells, causing them to die, which is called apoptosis (Copier et al. 2009). Other doctors used Bacille Calmette-Guérin (BCG) vaccine being used to treat bladder cancers once it was noted that people with active tuberculosis infections recovered from cancer. Grange et al. (2009) suggest that our current trend of living in hygienic environments means that we are not exposed to substances that help us develop a useful and protective immune system which enables our bodies to deal with disease and cancer, and offer it as an explanation of why more children are developing asthma and other allergic conditions, reaffirming the old wives tale that everyone needs to eat a speck of dirt to survive.

These treatments were used less and less at the turn of the 20th century, as radiotherapy and chemotherapy seemed to provide better options. However, they have re- emerged, sometimes being used as an adjuvant therapy, that is something that can be used alongside other treatments to effect a cure. When used in this way, it is possible to use higher doses of chemotherapy, as they reduce the side-effects of chemotherapy and are primarily used in the treatment of solid tumours, such as cancers of the breast, colon, lung, prostate and kidney (Copier et al. 2009).

Immunotherapies

Immunotherapy is a treatment that uses products made from either cloning cells of mice or using human cells, or a mixture of the two.

Immunotherapy works by targeting the cells during the cell cycle of regeneration and locking onto specific receptor sites on cell membranes and, for this reason, they are often called 'targeted therapies'. The receptor sites are protein molecules, either on the surface of the cell or within it that react with specific agents (e.g. immunoglobulins) to set up a chain of further chemical reactions within the cell, which enable the cell to grow and multiply or, check for deviations and mutations, which if present, will result in apoptosis.

Physiology of the immune response The body's immune system differentiates between what is the true self and what is foreign, i.e. non-self, includes cells that have mutated, foreign proteins as in transplanted organs and bacteria that has been ingested. It sets in motion a chain of reactions to rid the body of what is considered harmful and dangerous to the body's continued survival. The immune system comprises of lymph glands, nodes and lymphatic tissue, white blood cells, lymphocytes, antibodies, cytokines (protein molecules).

There are three types of lymphocytes:

- T cells, and by attacking foreign proteins, tumour cells and cells containing viruses provides cell mediated immunity. T cells change into four subtypes of cells:
- Helper cells
- Suppressor cells
- Cytotoxic cells
- Memory cells.

   T cells are activated by an antigen which locks onto a specific receptor on its surface. It promotes a chain of responses, helper cells produce interleukins, which mark the damaged cell for destruction which is undertaken by the cytotoxic cells. Suppressor cells deactivate B cells when no more T cells are needed.

- B cells produce antibodies and proteins called immunoglobulin's that target bacterial infections and provide humoral immunity; which are the building blocks to fight infection within the plasma and interstitial fluids. Once B cells connect with an antigen, they produce antibodies, which destroy the antigens and stimulate the production of T cells. B cells retain a memory of the antigen it has encountered, so that when it meets it again, it responds quickly.

- Natural killer cells provide immunosurveillance by checking the body tissue for foreign proteins which it proceeds to surround, engulf and destroy.

   Some lymphocytes live for a long time in the body, resulting in a life time of immunity, and the disease does not recur. Some diseases do recur, but the action of the antibodies means subsequent infections are not as severe as the first exposure, which is why it is better to get chickenpox as a child rather than in adulthood, where the condition is more serious.

Lymphocytes are produced in the bone marrow and the thymus gland, some, like the B cells, stay in lymph tissue until required. The immune system becomes less effective as we age, thus making us more susceptible to cancers developing.

Within the cells of the body (lymphocytes, in particular) and cancer cells, soluble proteins called cytokines are produced as a result of reaction within the cell and the cell membrane; these cell messengers sit on the cell surface attracting other protein

303

molecules and lymphocytes, which enter the cell, setting up a reaction, which leads to cells mutation or apoptosis. Over 80 different cytokines have been identified, and they work in different ways; some stimulate the immune response, while others dampen it down; others trigger the production of proteins that respond to a chemical stimulus depending on their concentrations, the more concentrated they are, the stronger the signal the emit. They are part of the body's normal response to inflammation controlling the function of the cells and tissues. The cell cycle of regeneration has five stages and the cell only proceeds through each stage if the splitting of the DNA strands and subsequent regrouping occurs without problems being detected by these enzymes and protein molecules, some referred to as kinases. When problems are detected, they initiate cell death (apoptosis). One such protein is called p53; this protein is missing in approximately 40% of cancers. The main groups of cytokines are:

- Interleukins, 20 different types have been identified, IL-1 and IL-2 are the main ones, which stimulate lymphocytes stored in lymph tissue to migrate into the blood stream
- Interferons, which consist of three types, alpha, beta and gamma, which are produced in response to a viral infection
- Tumour necrosis factors
- Colony-stimulating factors
- Growth factors
- Angiogenic factors.

When an infection occurs or in response to other changes such as mutations of cells, the body's proinflammatory process is triggered, stimulating cytokines to release interleukins and tumour necrosis factor, which act as cell messengers to stimulate the production of anti-inflammatory cytokines. In other words, there is a build-up of a chemical soup warning surrounding tissues of danger before other chemicals or enzymes and protein molecules build up to deal with the problem, this is called a biofeedback loop.

Cancer cells can also produce cytokines that work on adjacent cells, making the local cellular environment receptive to tumour growth. As the cancer grows, certain cytokines (tyrosine kinases) enable the development of blood vessels, which draws nutrients and oxygen into the centre of the tumour, thus allowing further growth. Many tumours contain a cytokine called granulocyte colony stimulating factor.

While a great deal is known about cytokines, no-one has identified a single cytokine that is present in all cancers. It is thought that cytokines have a role to play in the following complications of cancer:

- Cachexia, this syndrome develops in some cancers as discussed above
- Asthenia (muscle weakness) and chronic fatigue are produced by excess tumour necrosis which results in muscle soreness
- Pain is intensified especially in the bone as a result of cytokine action. The key principle of immunotherapy is to utilise cytokines to induce an inflammatory response to the cancer cells sufficient to weaken and destroy them.

Treatment using cytokines
Interferon alpha is used to treat:

- Hairy cell leukaemia
- Multiple myeloma
- Cutaneous T-cell lymphoma
- Malignant melanoma
- Carcinoid tumours
- Chronic myeloid leukaemia

- Non-Hodgkin's lymphoma
- Renal cell carcinoma
- Kaposi's sarcoma.

Interferon alpha stops tumour growth; it makes affected cells more responsive to an attack by the immune system and stops the cytokine's influence in the formation of a blood supply. It also makes tumour cells less aggressive and slows the rate of regeneration, specifically in the G_0 phase and so are 'tumouristatic' because the cells do not go on to divide; this is opposed to being 'tumouricidal', which means killing the cell. It is usually given as a subcutaneous injection, but can be given intramuscularly or intravenously (Ward 1995).

It can produce 'flu-like symptoms, a raised temperature, aches, shivering, fatigue and lethargy, all side-effects experienced when fighting infection. Usually, these symptoms are mild and disappear once treatment has stopped. Prophylactic treatment usually involves prescribing an antipyretic such as paracetamol.

Interleukin 2 is used to treat:

- Renal cell cancers
- Myeloid leukaemia
- Kaposi's sarcoma
- Metastatic malignant melanoma
- Non-Hodgkin's lymphomas.

Interleukin 2 is very toxic which limits its use. Like interferon alpha, it produces 'flu-like symptoms but can also produce angina (heart pain), severe hypotension (low blood pressure) and respiratory distress and multiorgan failure (Tadman & Roberts 2007).

Tumour necrosis factor (TNF) is used to treat:

- Melanoma
- Sarcoma.

Like interleukin 2, TNF is very toxic, producing severe side-effects, therefore is only used under experimental conditions (Tadman & Roberts 2007). Anderson *et al.* (2004) summarise the advantages and disadvantages of this treatment, pointing out that it is often used in combination with Doxorubicin, as it opens up the blood vessels so they are more receptive to the chemotherapy.

Haemopoietic growth factors, three different types are used:

- Erythropoietin
- Granulocyte colony stimulating factor (G-CSF)
- Granulocyte macrophage colony stimulating factor (GM-CSF).

Haemopoietic growth factors are used to influence the production of blood cells and counteract anaemia when the bone marrow is affected by chemotherapy. They are used to reduce the risk of the person developing neutropenia, which could result in the chemotherapy treatment being stopped for a short while. This means that higher doses of chemotherapy can be given, making them an adjuvant therapy rather than a treatment against cancer cells.

Biological therapies

The other biological therapies sometimes referred to as biotechnology therapies are:

- Monoclonal antibodies, which lock onto specific protein receptors excreted by the cancer cells, which leads to them being called 'targeted therapies', work by either:
  - Making the cancer cells responsive to attack from the body's own immune cells which then destroy them, *or*
  - Making the cancer cells resistant to enzymes that would help the cells to grow.

One example is rituximab used in the treatment of non-Hodgkin's lymphomas, another is trastuzumab (Herceptin) used in certain types of breast cancer. Monoclonal antibodies do not cause infection, so are unlike vaccines (Graham 2009).

These monoclonal antibodies are formed from a mixture of murine (mouse) and human immunoglobulins and are used to treat non-Hodgkin's lymphoma; a neoplasm of the B and T cells, in conjunction with chemotherapy. Rituximab, when used with cyclophosphamide, vincristine and prednisolone (CVP) as an adjuvant therapy, is at least twice as effective as using CVP alone. These antibodies target specific antigens (CD20) that are found on the surface of large B cell lymphomas. When the two combine, they attract natural killer (NK) cells (lymphocytes in the immune system), which release perforin (a small protein), which enters the targeted cell and causes apoptosis (Graham 2009).

Rituximab is usually given with other chemotherapy agents intravenously but can be given singly (monotherapy). The person receiving the treatment is given a premedication, which consists of an antipyretic (like paracetamol to keep the temperature down) and an antihistamine, usually chlorphenamine to pre-empt the development of side-effects. The rate of infusion administration is important – if given too quickly, it can cause a reaction referred to as 'cytokine release syndrome', which has been described as being similar to the onset of 'flu and a mild rash. Cytokine release syndrome is more prominent following the first dose, as this is when most cells are targeted and destroyed reducing the tumour burden. Subsequent treatments affect fewer cells, resulting in less cytokines being released.

The symptoms are graded on a scale of 1–4, with 1 and 2 being considered mild reactions that occur about two hours after treatment; and 3 and 4 being more severe. Grade 2 differs from grade 1, in that the rash is itchy and is accompanied by breathlessness. Once the symptoms abate, the treatment can be recommenced and infused over a longer period. The more severe reactions are similar to a severe allergic reaction, resulting in a low blood pressure, breathlessness, bronchospasm, which lead to a lack of insufficient oxygen intake and respiratory distress. This reaction usually occurs within minutes of the transfusion starting and affects about 10% of patients, constituting a medical emergency.

When a severe reaction occurs, the infusion is stopped immediately and the person is treated with bronchodilators' and oxygen therapy. A full investigation of urea, electrolyte and haemoglobin levels in the blood is undertaken. The reaction can cause thrombocytopenia (a decrease in the platelets, which affects the blood clotting system) and hypocalcaemia (low calcium levels, which result in a rash which is seen in the skin as small red pin pricks).

Half of the people who experience such an allergic reaction can have the treatment recommenced without any further reactions occurring.

Red Flag

The person's vital signs (temperature, pulse and blood pressure) need monitoring every 15 minutes for at least the first hour the infusion is in progress to spot an allergic reaction early. If the person does not show any signs of a reaction, the recordings can then be taken every half hour. If there is a change, stop the treatment and call for medical help.

Vaccines Vaccines, such as the human papilloma virus (HPV) vaccine, are given to prevent the development of cervical cancer. Vaccines are currently being developed from tumour cells for reinjecting into the body, they are not all made from viral material. The abnormal cells are harvested to make a vaccine, which is then injected into the body. This stimulates the immune system into producing antibodies to destroy the cancer.

The UK has recently introduced a vaccination programme for all girls aged over 13 years against the strains of human papilloma virus (HPV) type 16 and 18, as this is believed to result in 70% of cervical cancers (Davis 2008). Panlagua (2006) point out that unfortunately, the vaccine does not protect against all types of cervical cancers. Cervical cancer represents the second most common cancer affecting women worldwide and has received wide media coverage since the celebrity Jane Goody (a star of reality TV) died of the disease. While this vaccination programme does not directly target cancer cells, it has a role in the prevention of future cancers and therefore is classified as immunotherapy, as it promotes immune protection while it is biological in its nature.

Stanford *et al.* (2008) outline how other vaccinations, such as *Mycobacterium vaccae* are being used to treat adenocarcinomas of the lung. Although this treatment is still experimental, results suggest that for some people, life expectancy can be extended by 4 months.

Anti-angiogenesis agents

Anti-angiogenesis agents such as tyrosine kinase enzymes, combine with certain cytokines (soluble proteins) to prevent the formation and development of blood capillaries, thus starving the cancer of oxygen and nutrients which it needs to grow.

Knowing that tyrosine kinase enzymes are needed for the formation of small capillaries (angiogenesis) within the tumour, tyrosine kinase inhibitors, such as Sorafenib, an oral drug, have been developed to stop this process and are used to treat primary liver cancer (Hull & Chester 2008). Other anti-angiogenesis drugs are Sunitinib and bevacizumab, which are used in the treatment of renal cell cancers that are resistant to chemotherapy and radiotherapy.

When compared with interferon alpha treatment for renal cell cancers, Sunitinib extends survival by two years, thus leading to its recommendation by NICE (2009). Sunitinib 50 mg is taken as oral medication once a day for 4 weeks, followed by a 2-week gap and can be given with another drug, Pazopanib 800 mg or on its own (Thomson 2011).

These drugs produce the following side-effects:

- Fatigue
- Nausea, with or without vomiting
- Diarrhoea and
- Hypertension (raised blood pressure).

The side-effects disappear as soon as treatment is stopped; treatment could continue if preceded by giving an antiemetic prophylactically to manage the nausea, and anti-diarrhoeal drugs can be given to manage the diarrhoea.

Bevacizumab is a monoclonal antibody, and is another targeted therapy which stops the vascular endothelial growth factor (VEGF) from working and initiating a capillary network in the tumour. VEGF is produced when fetuses are growing and in adults, it is only present when there is a wound, so its effect on other parts of the body is minimal, unlike chemotherapy agents that affect normal and abnormal cells alike. It is used in combination with taxanes such as Paclitaxel and Docetaxel used to treat breast cancer. It is also used to treat colorectal (Lemmens *et al.* 2008) and renal cell cancers (Boxall & Nathan 2006).

Bevacizumab can cause hypertension, proteinuria (bleeding in the bladder and passed in the urine), epistaxis (nose bleeds) and thromboemboli (blood clots) and they can affect the heart leading to heart failure.

Radio immunotherapy

It is now possible to join a radioactive atom with the monoclonal antibody (rituximab); this preparation is called ibritumomab tiuxetan (Zevalin). The radioactive monoclonal antibody enters the B-cell lymphocyte by attaching itself to the CD20 protein sitting on the surface of the B cell. Once in the cell, it causes the cell to die; the energy emitted by the radioactive atom also spreads to adjacent cancer cells which are caught in the 'cross-fire' and is used in the treatment of indolent (slow to develop) no-Hodgkin's lymphomas, a disease of the immune system.

It is given intravenously in outpatients as two treatments over 4 hours, one week apart. The person is monitored closely while the infusion is in progress, as it can cause hypotension, shortness of breath, throat irritation including coughing, chills, fever, nausea, vomiting, dizziness and a rash, however, the side-effects are usually mild. Monitoring includes recording the person's blood pressure, pulse rate and temperature every 15 minutes. If these side-effects appear, the infusion is stopped immediately. A premedication of antihistamine and an antipyretic (e.g. paracetamol) is usually given.

The radioactive ingredient is so small that the person is not a threat to their family and friends, however, the patient needs to wear a condom for sexual activity and women should avoid becoming pregnant during the treatment period.

The dosage is determined by the person's weight and their platelet count. The treatment does affect the blood count and neutrophil levels drop, their lowest point can occur two months after treatment, leaving the person at severe risk from infection. Causer (2005) points out that the lowering of the red blood cells leave the person feeling fatigued.

Nursing care for the person receiving biological therapies

These therapies are also used for non-cancer conditions, such as rheumatoid arthritis, Crohn's disease and other autoimmune-related conditions, so it is vital that the person receiving these therapies is well informed and fully appreciates the reason for the treatment. Preparation is similar to that which is required for chemotherapy and as the therapies are often used in addition to chemotherapy, the care is as outlined above.

Reactions to biological therapies are less severe, yet they do occur and as they target the immune system, it is important that the person has a thermometer and takes and records their body temperature regularly, as an increase in body temperature is the first sign that something is not right. As with chemotherapy, all patients receiving SACTs, including biological therapies, need to carry a card detailing their treatment, which they can present if they need emergency care and this should ensure prompt treatment.

Radiotherapy

Radiotherapy has been used for over 100 years to treat cancer, either with intent to cure or to palliate and relieve symptoms that are causing distress. It can be used as the main, primary treatment or in conjunction with surgery and SACTs and may be used before surgery to contain the disease or after surgery, to mop-up any remaining cancer cells.

Radiotherapy is used to treat:

- Neuroblastomas
- Lymphomas
- Head and neck cancers.

Tumours that respond moderately well to radiotherapy are:

- lung cancers
- Oesophageal cancer
- Squamous cell carcinomas
- Prostate cancer
- Testicular cancer
- Cervical cancer.

Adenocarcinomas and fibrosarcomas do not respond well to this treatment.

Radiotherapy was developed following the pioneering work of Marie Curie, who discovered the radioactive elements in radium in the late 1800s, early 1900s. Cobalt and caesium are now used; these radioactive units are placed in huge machines, which are noisy, appear very frightening and feel claustrophobic. The person is required to lie very still during treatment.

Radiotherapy is delivered either by:

- Teletherapy or external beam radiation, *or*
- Brachytherapy, where the radioactive material is placed next to the tumour.

Dosages of radiotherapy are calculated as a Gray (Gy) and are divided up into units which are delivered at intervals; this is called fractionation. The aim with teletherapy is to ensure that the dose reaches the tumour. To do this, it has to pass through normal tissue and the machines deliver this at different angles into the body – a 3D effect. It is a very precise treatment and the person is measured up and the position where the beam needs to enter the body has to be marked with an indelible pen on the skin.

Red Flag

 It is crucial that the markings on the body are not washed off in-between treatments as the measurements will have to be recalculated and this takes approximately an hour to do.

Skin care

It is important that the skin through which the radiotherapy beam passes remains dry and so washing the area is not advised, nor is the application of creams or ointments as these will cause the skin to 'fry' when it is treated. The person is also advised not to shave or rub the area, nor to apply hot or cold packs. Wearing cotton clothing helps to keep the person cool.

Side-effects of radiotherapy

After a few doses of radiotherapy, the skin may blanch (look white) or become red (erythematosus). The surface layer may peel off, this may leave dry or wet skin exposed and this reaction is called desquamation.

The radiation to the head and neck cause ulceration of the mucosal lining of the mouth, causing severe pain. It also causes the oral secretions to decrease, resulting in a dry mouth, which is termed as xerostomia and the person may require artificial saliva to replace what has been lost. As with chemotherapy, it is advised that the person uses a soft toothbrush and avoids eating hot and spicy food.

> **Jot This Down**
> List as many other foods that might cause damage to the oral mucosa.

Nursing care for the person receiving radiotherapy

Most people receive radiotherapy as outpatients and nurses may only be involved if there are issues with the person's skin, which if it breaks down, that is if desquamation occurs, the area will need a dressing and the principles of aseptic wound care need to be followed.

The main problem posed by these wounds is the amount of exudate that is produced, which requires the attention of a tissue viability specialist nurse. The other key issue appertains to the person's sense of self, these wounds can be highly visible (as in head and neck cancers), which can lead to social withdrawal. These people require psychological support as well as physical care.

Other Problems Resulting from All Cancer Therapies

Weight Loss/Weight Gain

Weight loss has already been discussed earlier, as it is often the symptom that triggers a person to seek medical advice. In general, people expect a person with cancer to lose weight, so are not prepared for a person with cancer who gains weight.

Weight gain can cause the person almost as many problems as weight loss and it is interesting to note that in the recent research undertaken on the behalf of the Department of Health (DH 2012), 60% of people with breast cancer were disturbed by their weight gain.

Weight gain occurs in response to pharmacological treatment, steroids result in Cushingoid features with fat deposited on the shoulders.

Other symptoms such as fatigue impacts on a person's weight, as when they are feeling tired, they have less impetus to exercise.

Fatigue

Approximately two-thirds of people receiving cancer treatment experience fatigue, which is severe enough to compromise their quality of life. It is more than just tiredness resulting from insomnia. Cancer related fatigue (CRF) is a complex symptom that is not easily relieved by rest, and like other symptoms, such as pain, it is subjective – there is no way to measure the degree of fatigue felt and the symptom can persist for months after the treatment has been completed (Stone & Minton 2008). Very often, people experiencing this symptom fail to report it, believing nothing can be done to improve their quality of life and attribute the cause to their worry over their state of health and insomnia but fatigue can be as a result of being anaemic, having increased levels of cytokines

(enzymes produced by the tumour) and the body's reaction to excrete the toxins that build-up as a result of treatment, all of which are treatable.

A full assessment needs to be undertaken to establish the pattern the person's fatigue takes and this should include establishing whether or not they are anaemic (Wagner & Cella 2004).

The person receiving chemotherapy treatment is advised to drink plenty of fluids to flush these toxins out of the body but if they are feeling nauseated as a result of the treatment, this may be difficult to achieve.

While resting may seem like the most sensible advice, taking exercise is the better advice. Increased exercise offers a form of distraction and also improves mood and outlook, enhancing the general feeling of well-being. Some research undertaken with people with breast cancer found it beneficial.

The person may find cognitive behavioural therapy (CBT) beneficial as it helps them to re-frame they way they view their illness (Gielissen *et al.* 2007).

Survivorship

In the Introduction of this chapter, it states that over half the people diagnosed with cancer survive the disease for at least five years, yet the experience of cancer does affect people to the extent that they believe themselves to be changed forever. Nearly half of the people are afraid of dying from cancer and about the same proportion are fearful of the cancer returning. These fears do not entirely subside with time; 23% are still afraid even five years later, despite being asymptomatic (DH 2012). The government used patient reported outcome measures (PROMS) to assess the quality of life for people following their cancer treatment. This study had nearly 5000 participants with 3300 respondents, giving a 66% response rate from all over England; hence it provides fairly comprehensive data and is the largest study of this type to be conducted in Europe. The study targeted people who had experienced four types of cancer:

- Breast
- Colorectal
- Prostate
- Non-Hodgkin's lymphoma.

This choice perhaps reflects the cancers that are potentially detected early, thus treated early and have a better response rate to treatment than other cancers, such as lung and ovarian cancers, which are notoriously difficult to detect in the early stages of disease. The majority of people responding were aged between 50 and 75 years of age; 52% were men and 93% were white British; 40% reported having other long-term conditions besides cancer.

Quality of life after treatment for cancer is dependent on four things:

- Other concurrent long-term conditions
- Whether they are in full or partial remission
- Age, with those aged between 64-75 years mostly expressing that they are enjoying a good quality of life
- The extent to which they are physically active.

Most people questioned (82%) said their cancer had responded to treatment fully; 10% said their cancer was still present and 3% reported that the cancer had returned.

This survey demonstrates that most people enjoy a good quality of life, live independently and are relatively pain-free, they were not anxious or depressed and those who had a longer time from treatment to survey (i.e. 5 years post-treatment) reported more positively on these aspects. There is inadequate space to examine all the responses here but the report is worth reading in more detail.

Over half those surveyed knew their named nurse and had access to a healthcare provider should they have further health concerns and, on the whole, felt hospital staff had been supportive during their cancer experience but they would have preferred more advice on:

- Diet
- How to manage their finances
- Physical activity
- Free prescriptions
- Emotional aspects.

What is interesting from this survey, is that those people who undertook regular exercise, that is 30 minutes of walking daily, reported a much better quality of life on other aspects, such as sleeping, their mood, etc. and were overall more positive about life.

The other significant factor is that those who are 'socially deprived' have more negative responses to the questions asked.

From diagnosis and through treatment, people with cancer have an intensive interface with healthcare professionals. Once treatment is completed and the person is discharged from care, the period until the next check-up may seem like a yawning gap and in itself, may appear quite frightening. People with cancer may need to be prepared for this period to enable a smoother transition into survivorship.

Doyle (2008) writes:

We can no longer "save" people from drowning and then leave them on the dock to cough and splutter on their own in the belief that we have performed all we can.

Corner and Wagland (2013) analysed the free text comments found on the survey cited above and found that people commented on their feelings of isolation and being 'in limbo' once initial treatment had concluded. While the statistical analysis suggests most people recover well, the issues of survivorship emerge more from the qualitative comments made by the survey participants.

Younger people experienced more problems when they wished to return to work following treatment. It would appear that employers need to re-evaluate the perceptions of people who have been treated for cancer; many people felt that they were forced to return to work before they were ready and perhaps would have benefited from a longer convalescent stage.

Factors that enhance survivorship for people who have had cancer are:

- The person's cancer journey was well coordinated, in particular their experience of hospital care
- The preparation for their experiences included realistic appraisal of possible problems and side-effects
- Good support from professionals and family throughout the experience.

Negative experiences and social difficulties often resulted in poorer outcomes.

As a result of their analysis, Corner and Wagland (2013) make the following proposals:

Healthcare professionals should:

- Ensure that the person with cancer experiences well coordinated care with few delays to investigations and treatment, and that the person is kept informed of all their options at each stage

- Apprise the person of the physical impact of the investigations and treatment and provide the person with information that will help them to manage their own care
- Prepare the person for the period post-treatment, when they may feel vulnerable and experience psychological problems
- Give the person details of social benefits and financial services that are open to them and can support them after treatment.

The key point made is that for successful survivorship, individualised, personalised care is essential.

Link To/Go To

The Macmillan Cancer Support website can direct people to self-help groups and provide information on resources that are available to them. A recent innovation is their campaign, 'no one should face cancer alone'.

http://www.macmillan.org.uk

End of Life Care

Cancer is a chronic illness rather than a fatal illness, however, some people present late with an advanced cancer and can only be offered palliative care. It is difficult to have a conversation about end of life issues and advance care planning, if the intent of the medical and nursing team is to effect a cure, but it is often at this stage when the person first meets with healthcare professionals and receives the diagnosis of cancer that death is very much on their minds. If the prospect of their dying is dismissed, it is not an easy topic to handle; they may never broach the subject again until it is too late to make plans for future care.

Most specialist cancer nurses working with consultants have undergone an intensive course to develop their communication skills and are very adept at dealing with these difficult conversations.

The best strategy is to:

- Find out why the person is asking the question, what has been their past experience of people with cancer, do they know someone who has had cancer?
- Find out what they know about their cancer, have they looked it up on the internet, what have other healthcare professionals discussed about their cancer with them?
- Find out how they are currently feeling.

Having established their fears and concerns, you then know what the next step should be. If you do not have the answers, be honest and say so, however, refer them on to someone who does have the answers. Ideally, make an appointment for them to see someone who can give them the answers they need. Never dismiss their concerns or make a joke of the issue.

Professional and Legal Issues

 Nursing people with cancer requires skilled care; most nurses caring for people with cancer have undertaken additional studies at degree or Masters level to ensure that they are suitably equipped with knowledge and skills to provide care.

Cancer care is highly charged because people feel pressured to start treatment straight away; the earlier treatment starts, the better the chance of recovery. However, informed consent before treatment commences is vital and people can only give informed consent if they are fully apprised of what the treatment entails.

As we have seen earlier, the side-effects of treatment can lead to death. They can also be disfiguring and compromise life afterwards, so that life never returns to what it once was.

Conclusion

This chapter has considered cancer care without specifically referring to each individual cancer and has addressed the general approach taken to cancer care. Treatment of cancer is constantly changing and outcomes for people with cancer continue to improve, however, the outcome for some remains death, especially if the cancer is found in its late stages.

In the past, cancer research has attracted a great deal of funding, which has allowed for progress to be made; it still requires funding but the competition for money is still fierce.

Cancer still remains a very personal experience for the person with the diagnosis. It is the worst news they can be given and we should remember that even though the odds are stacked more favourably these days than in the past, the person still has to come to terms with the devastating impact that the news has for them. Nursing care demands that we are compassionate and caring and mindful of each individual's needs!

Key Points

- Cancer is a generic term for a host of different illnesses; some develop as a result of lifestyle choices we make and require different approaches to treatment.
- Cancer treatments can be debilitating and perceived as worse than the illness itself, leading to neutropenia and possible death, which requires rapid responses when they present for emergency care.
- Cancer is a chronic, rather than terminal, illness and many people survive cancer but are in need of support to adjust to life with disability and deformity.
- Cancer is a frightening experience and people need care and compassion but above all else, honesty from healthcare professionals and sensitive handling of their issues.
- Some people with cancer present too late for curative treatment and palliative care is their only option.
- Cancer is an illness that affects all of a person's social circle – families, friends and work colleagues, so we are not just caring for the person but people important to the person as well.
- Cancer research is at the cutting edge of medical science and to remain proficient in caring for people with cancer, we must ensure our knowledge is current and up-to-date.

Glossary

Apoptosis: this is when a cell dies. Cells regenerate as they age, through a process called mitosis; if the cells are deformed then a programmed death or apoptosis occurs

Bronchoscopy: the passing of a tube fitted with a camera into a person's lung which enables a view of the trachea and the bronchioles

Carcinogenic: a substance is said to be 'carcinogenic' if it causes alterations in a cell that lead to it becoming cancerous. For example, asbestos, if inhaled, irritates the lining in the lungs to produce mesothelioma

Cystoscopy: the passing of a tube fitted with a camera into the bladder to view the internal structure. It also has pincers to enable the collection of samples of the mucosa

Endoscopy: the passing of a tube fitted with a camera through the oesophagus to the stomach to view the organ internally. The procedure may be done with the person awake or anaesthetised

Mammography: the taking of an X-ray of the breast tissue to detect breast cancer

Nociceptors: the sensitive nerve endings that recognise chemical messengers released as part of an immune response to injury and tell us we are in pain

Proto-oncogenes: substances/chemicals in the cell that trigger the unwinding of the DNA helix in the nucleus, which signals that the cell is preparing to divide in two

Sigmoidoscopy: the passing of a tube through the anus and rectum to view the sigmoid section of the large bowel. It has a camera and pincers to enable the collection of specimens

References

Anderson, G.M., Nakada, M.T., DeWitte, M. (2004) Tumour necrosis factor alpha in the pathogenesis and treatment of cancer. *Current Opinion in Pharmacology*, 4, 314–320.

Boxall, J. & Nathan, P. (2006) Renal cell cancer: causes, prognosis, management and treatments. *Cancer Nursing Practice*, 5(3), 29–32.

Cancer Research UK (2011) http://cancerhelp.cancerresearchuk.org/about-cancer/cancer-questions/hair-loss-and-wigs (accessed 8 October 2011).

Cancer Research UK (2012) http://publications.cancerresearchuk.org/publicationformat/formatfactsheet/keyfactsall.html (accessed 3 October 2012).

Causer, L. (2005) Radioimmunotherapy in the treatment of non Hodgkin's lymphoma. *Cancer Nursing Practice*, 4(9), 27–33.

Copier, J., Dalgleish, A.G., Britten, C.M. *et al.* (2009) Improving efficacy of cancer immunotherapy. *European Journal of Cancer*, 45, 1424–1431.

Corner, J. & Wagland, R. (2013) National Cancer Survivorship Initiative: text analysis of patients' free text comments: Final Report. University of Southampton, Southampton.

Davis, C. (2008) Stopping cervical cancer in its tracks. *Cancer Nursing Practice*, 7(5), 19–21.

DH (2007) *Cancer Reform Strategy*. Department of Health, London. http://www.dh.gov.uk/publications

DH (2012) *Quality of Life of Cancer Survivors in England: report on a pilot survey using patient reported outcome measures (PROMS)*. Department of Health, London. https://www.gov.uk/government/uploads/system/uploads/attachment_data/file/127272/9284-TSO-2900701-PROMS.pdf.pdf (accessed 30 May 2013).

DH (2013) *The Handbook to the NHS Constitution for England*. Department of Health, London. http://www.nhs.uk/choiceintheNHS/Rightsandpledges/NHSConstitution/Documents/2013/handbook-to-the-nhs-constitution.pdf

Doyle, N. (2008) Cancer survivorship: evolutionary concept analysis. *Journal of Advanced Nursing*, 62(4), 499–509.

Fayed, L. (2009) *The History of Cancer*, updated 8 July. http://cancer.about.com/od/historyofcancer/a/cancerhistory.htm (accessed 3 October 2012).

Gielissen, M.F., Verhagen, C.A. & Bleijenberg, G. (2007) Cognitive behaviour therapy for fatigue cancer survivors: long term follow up. *British Journal of Cancer*, 97(5), 612–618.

Graham, A.H. (2009) Administering rituximab: infusion-related reactions and nursing implications. *Cancer Nursing Practice*, 8(2), 30–35.

Grange, J.M., Krone, B. & Stanford, J.L. (2009) Immunotherapy for malignant melanoma – tracing Ariadne's thread through a labyrinth. *European Journal of Cancer*, 45, 2266–2273.

Hamilton-West, K. (2011) *Psychobiological processes in Health and Illness*, Sage, London.

Hull, D. & Chester, M. (2008) Management of patient participation in a hepatocellular carcinoma clinical trial. *Cancer Nursing Practice*, 8(7), 35–39.

Khan, S., Dhadda, A., Fyfe, D. & Sundar, S. (2008) Impact of neutropenia on delivering planned chemotherapy for solid tumours. *European Journal of Cancer Care*, 17, 19–25.

Kelland, L.R. (2005) Cancer cell biology, drug action and resistance. In: D. Brighton & M. Wood (eds). *The Royal Marsden's Hospital Handbook of Cancer Chemotherapy*, Ch. 1. Elsevier, Churchill Livingstone, Edinburgh.

Lemmens, L., Claes, V. & Uzzell, M. (2008) Managing patients with metastatic colorectal cancer on bevacizumab. *British Journal of Nursing*, 17(15), 944–949.

McIlfatrick, S., Sullivan, K., McKenna, H. & Parahoo, K. (2007) Patients' experiences of having chemotherapy in a day hospital setting. *Journal of Advanced Nursing*, 59(3), 264–273.

Miller, M. & Kearney, N. (2004) Chemotherapy – related nausea and vomiting – past reflections, present practice and future management. *European Journal of Cancer Care*, 13, 71–81.

Molassiotis, A., Stricker, C.T., Eaby, B., Velders, L. & Coventry, P.A. (2008) Understanding the concept of chemotherapy – related nausea: the patient experience. *European Journal of Cancer Care*, 18, 444–453.

Ng, W.I. & Della Florentina, S.A. (2008) The efficacy of oral ondansetron and dexamethasone for the prevention of acute chemotherapy-induced nausea and vomiting associated with moderately ematogenic chemotherapy – a retrospective audit. *European Journal of Cancer Care*, 19, 403–407.

NHS Choices (2013) http://www.nhs.uk/choiceintheNHS/Rightsand pledges/Waitingtimes/Pages/Guide%20to%20waiting%20times.aspx (accessed 8 July 2013).

National Cancer Action Team (2011) *Manual for Cancer Services: chemotherapy measures*, Version 1.0, National Cancer Peer Review Programme, NHS. http://www.rcplondon.ac.uk/sites/default/files/final -chemotherapy-measures_0.pdf (accessed 5 July 2013).

NICE (2009) *Sunitinib for the First Line Treatment of Advanced and/or Metastatic Renal Cell Carcinoma*. Technology appraised 169. National Institute for Health and Clinical Excellence, London.

Panlagua, H. (2006) Knowledge of cervical cancer and the HPV vaccine. *British Journal of Nursing*, 15(3), 126–127.

Randall, R.J. & Ream, E. (2004) Hair loss with chemotherapy: at a loss over its management? *European Journal of Cancer Care*, 14, 223–231.

Saltmarsh, K. & De Vries, K. (2008) The paradoxical image of chemotherapy: a phenomenological description of nurses' experiences of administering chemotherapy. *European Journal of Cancer Care*, 17, 500–508.

Stanford, J.L., Stanford, C.A., O'Brien, M.E.R. & Grange, J.M. (2008) Successful immunotherapy with Mycobacterium vaccae in the treatment of adenocarcinoma of the lung. *European Journal of Cancer*, 44, 224–227.

Stone, P.C. & Minton, O. (2008) Cancer-related fatigue. *European Journal of Cancer*, 44, 1097–1104.

Tadman, M. & Roberts, D. (2007) *Oxford Handbook of Cancer Nursing*, Oxford University Press, Oxford.

Thomson, N. (2011) Multidisciplinary clinic for patients with metastatic renal cell carcinoma. *Cancer Nursing Practice*, 10(7), 22–27.

Ward, U. (1995) Biological therapy in the treatment of cancer. *British Journal of Nursing*, 4(15), 869–891.

Wagner, L.I. & Cella, D. (2004) Fatigue and cancer: causes, prevalence and treatment approaches. *British Journal of Cancer*, 91, 822–828.

Test Yourself

1. If someone who has smoked all his life fears he has cancer, what symptoms should he expect:
   (a) Coughing in the morning and breathlessness if he exercises
   (b) A persistent cough that he remembers having for more than 3 months
   (c) A cough that wakes him up at night and disturbs his sleep
   (d) A productive cough that produces green phlegm

2. Which substance is not a 'promoter' of cancer:
   (a) Rays of sunlight
   (b) Chemicals in cigarettes
   (c) Viruses
   (d) Red wine

3. Treatment of cancers depends on:
   (a) Patient's preferences, site of cancer and consultant preference
   (b) Consultant's preference, type of tumour and known response to treatment
   (c) Tumour type, and its staging and grading and MDT decision
   (d) Patient's preferences, MDT decision and tumour type

4. Chemotherapy refers to:
   (a) All treatments for cancer, including biological therapies
   (b) Immunotherapies and mitotic inhibitors
   (c) All treatments that have been man-made rather than originating from plants
   (d) Alkylating agents, mitotic inhibitors and platinating agents

5. People with cancer feel supported when:
   (a) They are called by name when attending clinic and see the same people each time
   (b) They have a named nurse who is their point of contact and who phones regularly to check on their progress
   (c) When they receive information about what to expect from treatment in terms of side-effects
   (d) When they receive advice about their diet, side-effects to expect and where to get financial support

6. Where in the cell cycle of regeneration does the DNA helix unwind into two strands:
   (a) G_0
   (b) G_1
   (c) S
   (d) G_2

7. The care for the area of skin that is irradiated with radiotherapy should be:
   (a) Washed daily with soap and water
   (b) Moisturised daily to keep it supple
   (c) Kept dry and clean whilst treatment is ongoing
   (d) Have talcum powder applied daily

8. Targeted therapy is:
   (a) A chemotherapy agent that are designed for use with a particular cancer
   (b) Radiotherapy that is directed to a particular point in the body
   (c) A radioisotope that is targeted to a particular organ of the body
   (d) Immunotherapy that targets a specific cell

9. One of the cancers below does not have a government-funded screening programme, which is it:
   (a) Breast cancer
   (b) Lung cancer
   (c) Colorectal cancer
   (d) Cervical cancer

10. Everyone being treated for cancer experiences:
    (a) Hair loss
    (b) Fatigue
    (c) Pain
    (d) Anxiety

Answers

1. b
2. c
3. c
4. d
5. b
6. d
7. c
8. d
9. b
10. d

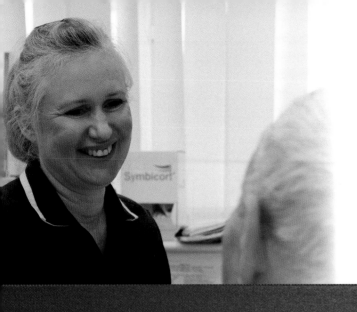

16

The Principles of Infection Control

Nigel Davies

Kingston University/St George's, University of London, UK

Learning Outcomes

On completion of this chapter you will be able to:

- Describe why infection control is essential in healthcare settings
- Detail the standard approaches to preventing the spread of infection
- Identify the most common healthcare associated infections
- Explain how the treatment of people with communicable diseases differs from that of other infections
- Understand common diagnostic tests and treatment approaches used by infection control practitioners
- Provide explanations to patients and their families about the prevention and control of infection

Competencies

All nurses must:

1. Practise in a holistic, non-judgemental, caring and sensitive manner
2. Manage risk, and promote health and well-being
3. Respect individual rights to confidentially. Also actively share personal information with others when the interests of safety and protection override the need for confidentiality
4. Recognise when the complexity of clinical decisions requires specialist knowledge and expertise, and consult or refer accordingly
5. Carry out comprehensive, systematic nursing assessments through interaction, observation and measurement
6. Practise safely by being aware of the correct use, limitations and hazards of common interventions

 Visit the companion website at **www.wileynursingpractice.com** where you can test yourself using flashcards, multiple-choice questions and more.

Nursing Practice: Knowledge and Care, First Edition. Edited by Ian Peate, Karen Wild and Muralitharan Nair.
© 2014 John Wiley & Sons, Ltd. Published 2014 by John Wiley & Sons, Ltd. Companion website: www.wileynursingpractice.com

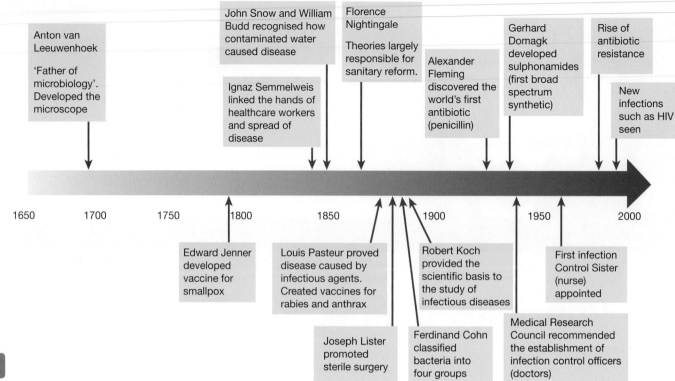

Figure 16.1 Infection control – a historical timeline.

Introduction

The control of infection is essential to the well-being of individuals and society. History teaches us that a lack of understanding of infection prevention and control measures can lead to disease and death, sometimes on a large scale, for example the epidemics of cholera and typhoid in the 19th century and more recently, the spread of blood-borne viruses, such as hepatitis C and human immunodeficiency virus (HIV).

In healthcare settings, such as hospitals and GP practices, policies and procedures are often used to guide practitioners treating patients with infections. These policies are written using the current evidence and research not only to ensure that the patient receives the best treatment for the infection but also to prevent the spread of the infection to others. Sometimes, in diseases that can be particularly serious or transmitted easily to others, the policies are laid down in law and patients are required to follow the treatment regimen, for example in cases of tuberculosis (TB). These diseases have to be reported to a national database and are known as 'communicable' or 'infectious diseases'.

Nurses working in all healthcare settings should have a good understanding of the principles of infection control, so they can apply guidelines to prevent further infection and also explain the reasons for tests and treatment to their patients. Concordance from patients is much greater when the reasons for treatment are understood; this often requires the nurse to interpret the patients' understanding and adapt often complex information in a meaningful way.

This chapter provides an introduction to infection prevention and control to enable you as a nurse to practise confidently and effectively, and to know when to refer to specialist infection control teams for further advice.

Development of Infection Control Practices

The science behind infection prevention and control measures has advanced a great deal in the last 150 years. Figure 16.1 outlines some of the milestones that have occurred, which have contributed to the development of infection control. The timeline refers to the revolutionary work of doctors and scientists, such as Pasteur, Lister and Koch but also to the work specifically related to hygiene by Semmelweis and Florence Nightingale. These discoveries still underpin many of the principles of infection control today, such as the importance of hand hygiene. Infection control teams are now common in all hospitals with their evolution traced back to the appointment of infection control officers in the 1920s. However, it was then not until the 1950s that the first infection control nurse was appointed, and they were not common in all hospitals until the 1980s.

In healthcare settings recently, there has been a renewed focus on the control of infections and especially those that are believed to be caused by the treatments people receive. These infections are often referred to as healthcare associated infections (HCAI).

Principles of Microbiology and Virology

In Chapter 22, the science behind infection is explained. This includes the body's response to infection. This chapter concentrates on the practical aspects of infection control; however, to appreciate your role as a nurse in controlling infection it is important to understand the principles of microbiology and virology. This is so you can discuss the care of patients confidently with colleagues and also explain to patients and relatives the implications of any infection they might have or the potential for cross-infection to and from others.

Jot This Down

Refer to Chapter 22 and read the section on bacteria and viruses.

- How would you describe what bacteria are to a patient?
- Can you explain to a student colleague what a virus is?
- Many bacteria have Latin names. What do you understand by the terms:
  - *Staphylococci*?
  - *Streptobacilli*?
- If bacteria are said to be Gram-positive, what does this mean?
- Name three common human diseases caused by viruses
- In relation to many common medicines and treatments can you explain the terms:
  - Antibiotic
  - Antimicrobial
  - Antiviral

Preventing the Spread of Infection

Broadly speaking, the spread of infections can be prevented at two levels: first, at the individual level using standard precautions and the isolation of patients; second, at a population level through public health measures, which include surveillance and preventative treatments, principally through vaccination programmes.

Standard Precautions

Standard precautions (previously referred to as universal precautions) should be applied across all healthcare settings to prevent the transmission of blood-borne and other infections in body substances where potentially infectious materials are present.

These precautions include:

- Routine use of barriers (such as gloves and/or goggles) when anticipating contact with blood or body fluids
- Washing hands and other skin surfaces immediately after contact with blood or body fluids
- Careful handling and disposing of sharp instruments during and after use
- Isolating infected patients.

Monitoring and surveillance are also undertaken to track infections and help prevent the spread of infection (Pratt *et al.* 2007).

Hand Hygiene

One of the most important aspects of infection prevention and control is good hand hygiene. Although seemingly a simple practice, ensuring health professionals clean their hands effectively is key to preventing cross-infection. The importance of hand hygiene was first noted by Semmelweiss in 1847, when he recognised that fever and subsequent death in large numbers of women following childbirth could be prevented by doctors and midwives washing their hands. Although the importance of good hand hygiene has been generally accepted by health professionals, over the past 10 years there have been campaigns across community and hospitals settings to increase the compliance and ensure heath professionals have greater awareness. This has partly been achieved through the introduction of alcohol hand gels, which are used to decontaminate the hands. The gels are often more convenient to use than standard hand washing and can be located at the bedside of all patients. Alcohol gel is not a substitute for hand washing.

Red Flag

Alcohol gels are only effective on visibly clean hands and are not effective against spores, present for example in *Clostridium difficile (C. diff)*. Therefore, if you are caring for a patient with *C. diff* you should ensure you wash your hands with soap and water. In some hospitals, if there is an outbreak of *C. diff* the alcohol gels may be removed. You may need to explain this to patients and relatives.

Cleaning hands in a clinically effective way requires a standard and methodical approach, to ensure all the surfaces on the hands are clean. Figure 16.2 describes the process.

It should be noted that the hands need to be wet before the soap is applied and that thorough drying is as important as the process of washing. In healthcare settings, hands should be dried with paper towels, as the warm air hand dryers can increase the spread of infection. (See "Evidence" box on page 318.)

It is also important that arms are 'bare below the elbows' to ensure effective hand washing. This was recognised by the Department of Health in 2008 within national guidelines for hand hygiene but caused some controversy as it meant some health professionals needed to amend dress codes, for example doctors no longer wearing long sleeved white coats. Complying with 'bare below the elbows' policies includes not wearing wrist watches, rings (other than plain wedding bands) or acrylic nails. Uniforms usually have short sleeves, however, often in community and some hospital and nursing home settings, uniform is not always worn and so thought needs to be given in these cases to ensure the 'bare below the elbows' principles can be applied if clinical care of any sort is performed. Some health professionals wish to keep their arms covered for cultural, religious or other reasons (e.g. extensive tattoos). In these cases, the local uniform policy should be consulted and advice sought from infection control nurse specialists.

When to Clean Your Hands

It is important to clean your hands at appropriate times to both protect the patient and protect yourself. The situations in which you should clean your hands either by washing with soap and water or by using hand gels have been summarised into 'five moments for hand hygiene', which are shown in Figure 16.3. These guidelines are based on evidence from the World Health Organization (WHO 2009). They define the key times for hand hygiene in a simple and standardised way.

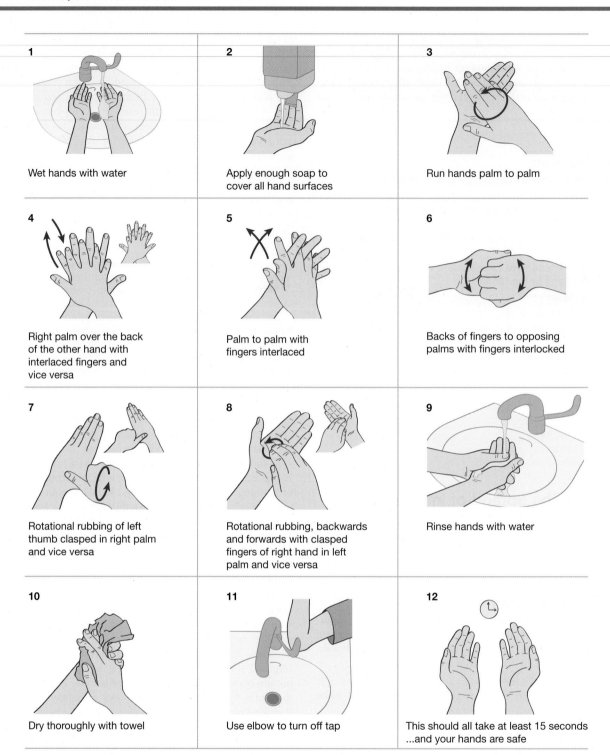

Figure 16.2 **Correct hand washing technique.** Reproduced with permission of WHO.

Your 5 moments for
HAND HYGIENE

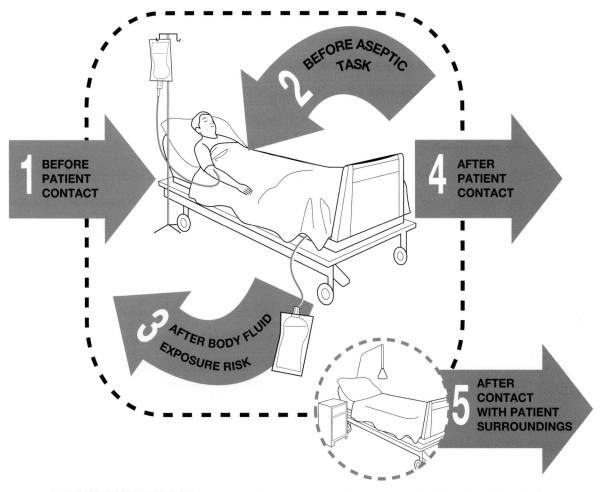

1 **BEFORE PATIENT CONTACT**	**WHEN?** Clean your hands before touching a patient when approaching him or her	
	WHY? To protect the patient against harmful germs carried on your hands	
2 **BEFORE AN ASEPTIC TASK**	**WHEN?** Clean your hands immediately before any aseptic task	
	WHY? To protect the patient against harmful germs, including the patient's own germs, entering his or her body	
3 **AFTER BODY FLUID EXPOSURE RISK**	**WHEN?** Clean your hands immediately after an exposure risk to body fluids (and after glove removal)	
	WHY? To protect yourself and the health-care environment from harmful patient germs	
4 **AFTER PATIENT CONTACT**	**WHEN?** Clean your hands after touching a patient and his or her immediate surroundings when leaving	
	WHY? To protect yourself and the health-care environment from harmful patient germs	
5 **AFTER CONTACT WITH PATIENT SURROUNDINGS**	**WHEN?** Clean your hands after touching any object or furniture in the patient's immediate surroundings, when leaving - even without touching the patient	
	WHY? To protect yourself and the health-care environment from harmful patient germs	

Figure 16.3 Five moments for hand hygiene (WHO 2009). Reproduced with permission of WHO.

317

The Evidence

A study completed at the University of Westminster (Redway & Fawdar 2008) compared the bacteria levels present after the use of paper towels, warm air hand dryers and modern jet air hand dryers. Of these three methods, only paper towels reduced the total number of bacteria on hands. The study also found that the jet air dryer was capable of blowing micro-organisms and potentially contaminating others up to 2 metres away.

Method Used	Mean Change in Bacteria Present (%)
Paper towels (2-ply 100% recycled)	−48.4
Paper towels (2-ply through-air dried, 50% recycled)	−76.8
Warm air dryer	+254.5
Jet air dryer	+14.9

What To Do If...

What would you do if a doctor refuses to clean their hands before examining a patient?

Personal Protective Equipment (PPE)

Gloves, masks, protective eyewear and chin-length plastic face shields are examples of personal protective equipment (PPE). PPE must be provided and worn by staff in all instances where they will or may come into contact with blood or body fluids. This includes, but is not limited to, dentistry, phlebotomy, processing of any bodily fluid specimen, and post-mortem procedures. (See Figure 16.4 for further information.)

Isolation or Barrier Nursing

Isolating a patient in a single room may take place either to protect others from infection (source isolation) or to protect the patient themselves from infection (protective isolation).

Source isolation is used for patients who are infected with, or are colonised by, infectious agents that require additional precautions over and above the standard precautions used with all patients. Common reasons for source isolation include infections that cause diarrhoea and vomiting and infections that are spread through the air. The patient's other nursing and medical needs must always be taken into account and infection control precautions may need to be modified accordingly, e.g. if a patient needs monitoring in high dependency or intensive care facilities. Patients requiring source isolation are normally cared for in a single room, although outbreaks of infection may require affected patients to be nursed in a cohort, that is, isolated as a group. The room should have all the equipment needed for the patient with equipment, such as blood pressure monitoring equipment remaining in the room. Where insufficient single rooms are available for source isolation, they should be allocated to those patients who pose the greatest risk with advice being given by infection control nurse specialists. As a general rule, patients with diarrhoea and vomiting, or serious air-borne infections, such as tuberculosis, will have the highest priority.

Protective isolation is used for patients who are particularly at risk of infection including people with compromised immune systems. These patients often have reduced numbers of white blood cells called neutrophils; this condition is known as neutropenia and those people suffering from it are described as neutropenic.

Jot This Down

Source a hard copy or online version of the *Royal Marsden Manual for Clinical Nursing Procedures* (many hospitals and universities have copies of the online version available).

Read the section on 'Source Isolation and Protective Isolation'

- If a patient is in source isolation how should meals be served? And how should crockery and cutlery be disposed of?
- How would you deal with spillages of urine or faeces if someone is in source isolation?
- If the patient requested a bath, do you think this would be possible?
- What colour of bag would you place infected linen in?
- What colour of bags should be kept in the room?

Care, Dignity and Compassion

Being nursed in a single room can literally be very isolating for patients. Consider ways in which isolation can be reduced, contact with the patient's wider network maintained and emotional support provided. Barratt et al. (2010) discuss the findings of their study, where they found that the overall experience of being in isolation for most patients was negative.

Surveillance of Common Healthcare Associated Infections

There are a number of healthcare associated infections that are monitored nationally. Every quarter, the data collected in the enhanced surveillance is used to produce epidemiological commentaries with the aim of contributing to a better evidence base regarding risk factors for infection. Public Health England, formerly the Health Protection Agency (PHE 2013) produces tables of counts of the common infections on a monthly and annual basis. The infections that are monitored include:

- **Staphylococcus aureus bacteraemia** – both meticillin-resistant *Staphylococcus aureus* (MRSA) and meticillin-sensitive *Staphylococcus aureus* (MSSA). The surveillance of MRSA bacteraemia has been mandatory for all NHS acute Trusts in England since April 2004. In January 2011, this scheme was extended to include surveillance of MSSA bacteraemia
- **Escherichia coli (E. coli) bacteraemia** – mandatory reporting has been in place since 1 June 2011, although many hospitals reported voluntarily before this. This was introduced following a year-on-year increase in Gram-negative bacteraemia, as reported by the voluntary surveillance system

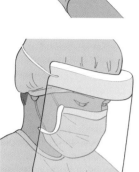

Latex gloves are recommended when dealing with blood or body fluids

- People with allergies to latex must be provided with other glove alternatives.
- Gloves must be changed after each client.
- Gloves should be worn:
  - When working with blood, blood products, semen, vaginal secretions, and any other potentially contaminated body fluids such as cerebrospinal fluid, amniotic fluid and saliva
  - When touching mucous membranes or breaks in the skin
  - When performing or assisting with any invasive procedures, such as venepuncture or surgery
  - When working in situations where hand contamination may occur, such as with an uncooperative patient
  - When the healthcare practitioner has cuts, scratches or other breaks in their own skin

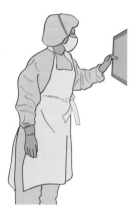

Masks, goggles or face shields should be worn

- During all invasive procedures and any procedure in which blood or body fluids may spatter or become airborne, e.g. during endoscopic procedures, during surgery
- During procedures in which heavy bleeding or other extensive fluid loss (such as peritoneal fluid) may occur

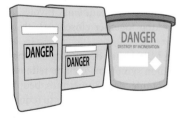

Gowns or aprons should be used when extensive fluid loss may occur

Reusable PPE must be cleaned and decontaminated or laundered by the employer. Lab coats and scrubs are generally considered to be worn as uniforms or personal clothing. When contamination is reasonably likely, protective gowns should be worn. If lab coats or scrubs are worn as PPE, they must be removed as soon as practical and laundered by the employer.

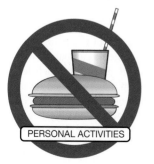

All equipment should be disposed of appropriately to prevent cross contamination

There is now a universal colour coded system in use across the UK health service.

Needles must not be re-sheathed or re-capped after they are used. Syringes, needles, and scalpel blades should be placed immediately in puncture-resistant containers ('sharps-bins'). Whenever possible small sharps boxes should be taken to the bed side or point of care.

Personal activities

- Eating (including sweets and chocolates), drinking, smoking, applying cosmetics or lip balm, and handling contact lenses should be prohibited in work areas that carry the potential for occupational exposure
- Food and drink must not be stored in refrigerators, freezers or cabinets where blood or body fluids are stored or in other areas of possible contamination

Figure 16.4 Protecting yourself and using personal protective equipment (PPE).

- *Clostridium difficile* (*C. diff*) **associated diarrhoea** – since April 2007 all acute NHS Trusts in England have been required to report all cases of *C. diff* infection in patients aged 2 years and over.
- **Glycopeptide-resistant *Enterococci* (GRE) bacteraemia** – this was previously known as 'vancomycin resistant *Enterococci* (VRE)' and is sometimes still referred to as such by clinicians. Mandatory monitoring was required in English NHS Trusts between 2003 and 2013 but is now collected on a voluntary basis.

Jot This Down

Access the Public Health England website (formally the Health Protection Agency) and review the data that has been collected on the infections listed above.

The following link accesses the mandatory surveillance data:

http://www.hpa.org.uk/web/HPAweb&HPA webStandard/HPAweb_C/1244763936373

- What strikes you about the data on MRSA? Why do you think the number of cases has fallen?
- Look at the quarterly data for *C. diff*. Find the data for the hospital or healthcare organisation you are associated with and compare their rates to other trusts.
- Look at the data for GRE bacteraemias. Can you think of any reasons why from April 2013, this data is no longer collected on a mandatory basis?

Similarly, data is collected in other countries:

- For Scotland, access the Health Protection Scotland website:

http://www.hps.scot.nhs.uk/haiic/newsdetail .aspx?id=563

- In Wales, the Public Health Wales website:

http://www.wales.nhs.uk/sites3/page .cfm?orgid=379&pid=13063

- In Northern Ireland, the HSC Public Health Agency website:

http://www.publichealthagency.org/publications/ summary-cdi-and-mrsa-incidence-tables-1st-april-2006 -present

Common Healthcare Associated Infections

There has been increased attention over the last two decades on the control of infections that may either be caused by, or associated with, the treatments people receive. These infections are often referred to as healthcare associated infections (HCAI) or iatrogenic infections, meaning that they are an adverse effect or complication arising from medical or healthcare treatment. Examples of these infections include meticillin resistant *Staphylococcus aureus* (MRSA) and *Clostridium difficile* (*C. diff*). Norovirus can spread quickly between people in close contact, including hospitals but is also evident in community settings.

Meticillin-Resistant *Staphylococcus aureus* (MRSA)

MRSA has been a major infection control challenge in the UK and internationally during the past decade. It has led to public concern about hospital safety and had a major effect on government health policy. Guidelines to reduce the risk of transmission (RCN 2005; Gould 2011) emphasise the importance of surveillance, decolonisation strategies, standard infection prevention and control precautions and antibiotic stewardship.

The Evidence Meticillin

Meticillin (or methicillin) is a narrow-spectrum type of penicillin. In 2005, the name of the drug was changed from methicillin to meticillin in accordance with the International Pharmacopoeia guidelines. It was developed in the late 1950s to treat infections caused by susceptible Gram-positive bacteria, in particular organisms such as *Staphylococcus aureus* that would otherwise be resistant to most other penicillins.

It is no longer used clinically and has been replaced by antibiotics such as flucloxacillin (Newsom 2004). Although no longer used to treat patients, it serves a purpose in the laboratory to determine the antibiotic sensitivity of *Staphylococcus aureus*. In this way, the drug name has become synonymous with the term meticillin-resistant *Staphylococcus aureus* (MRSA) as this continues to be used to describe *Staph. aureus* strains resistant to all penicillins.

MRSA – key facts

MRSA is a strain of *Staphylococcus aureus* which is resistant to meticillin and other antibiotics. It is an organism that colonises the skin, particularly the nose, skin folds, hairline, perineum and navel. It commonly survives in these areas without causing infection – a state known as colonisation. A patient becomes clinically infected if the organism invades the skin or deeper tissues and multiplies.

MRSA is prevalent in healthcare environments because individuals tend to be older, sicker and weaker than the general population, which heightens their vulnerability to infection through weakened immunity. In addition, these environments involve a great many people living and working together closely, which is perfect for transferring MRSA.

The symptoms of a person with MRSA vary depending on what part of the body is infected. Common symptoms include redness, swelling and tenderness at the site of infection. Sometimes, people may carry MRSA without having any symptoms. In order to reduce the spread of MRSA, healthcare staff should ensure that they wash their hands thoroughly between patients (RCN 2005).

Public concern about MRSA

During the early 2000s, public concern about the rising numbers of people with MRSA came to the fore. Media campaigns were led by patient groups and the press included stories which led the public to see MRSA as a new 'super-bug'.

The government responded by placing a target on the NHS to halve the number of cases over a 3-year period, an objective which many clinicians thought at the time was ambitious. Investment was made both by the government and by local hospitals to tackle MRSA which led to greater reductions than initially envisaged. Although the number of cases of MRSA has now reduced in most hospitals, the myths and stories that were abundant at its height, are still remembered by many patients and can cause concern and fear. This needs to be taken into account when patients are screened for MRSA and particularly if patients are colonised or infected.

> **Nursing Field** Mental Health
>
> Infection prevention and control is an important issue in all settings.
>
> Those people in mental health facilities will often have more underlying physical health problems than the general population, because of this, they are therefore predisposed to risk factors for HCAIs.
>
> Service-users should be offered support and training in order for them to feel able to contribute effectively. The nurse should ensure that service users are treated as equal partners in controlling and preventing HCAIs.

Patient information about MRSA

Because of the public concern about MRSA, most patients have some awareness of the term but often lack detailed knowledge. Hospitals and GP practices have developed patient information leaflets and DVDs to explain what MRSA is, importantly the difference between colonisation and infection and how it is treated.

> **Jot This Down**
>
> From your own experience personally or from clinical placements, reflect on how you would explain what MRSA is to a patient.
>
> Now read a patient information leaflet on MRSA or watch the NHS Choices (2012) video: 'How MRSA is caught, what happens when you have it, and how hospital staff and visitors can help prevent infection'. Presentation by Dr Brian Duerdan, DH Chief Microbiologist:
>
> **http://www.nhs.uk/Video/Pages/MRSA.aspx.**
>
> What are the three key messages you need to get across to patients?

MRSA screening and decolonisation

Screening people to detect whether they are carriers of MRSA was introduced in all NHS hospitals for elective admissions in 2009 and for emergency patients in 2011. There is some debate about the cost-effectiveness of screening all patients versus only screening high-risk patients. This therefore means that methods of screening and which patients are screened may vary slightly between hospitals and in the community and so reference should be made to local policies. However, typically, screening consists of taking swabs (see section on "Swabs" below) from the nose and groin. If the patient has a urinary catheter, intravenous lines or wounds, then these are also swabbed. In babies, the umbilicus is often swabbed.

If a patient is found to carry MRSA, then de-colonisation can take place to help prevent infection occurring. Complete eradication of MRSA is not always possible but a decrease in carriage can reduce the risk of transmission to others and the risk of surgical wound infection to the patient themselves (Coia *et al.* 2006). Decolonisation usually takes the form of two treatments; first, mupirocin or neomycin nasal cream and second, chlorhexidine shower and hair washes.

> **Medicines Management**
>
>
>
> The medications given to patients for MRSA de-colonisation typically include:
> - Either: **Mupirocin** (often referred to by its trade name of Bactroban), which is a cream applied to the anterior nares of both nostrils two–three times daily for 5 days, or: **Neomycin** (often referred to by its trade name of Naseptin), which is a cream or ointment applied to both nostrils four times a day for 10 days.
> - **Chlorhexidine 4%** skin wash/bath, daily for 5 days. Patient should be told to pay particular attention to washing the axillae, groin and skin folds and skin should be moistened with water before applying the chlorhexidine to reduce the likelihood of reactions. Hair should also be washed with the Chlorhexidine, at least three times during the 5 days, if possible. A normal shampoo can be used after the Chlorhexidine each time.
>
> Treatment should be prescribed or follow a patient group direction, and practitioners should note guidance in the British National Formulary (BNF 2013).

Clostridium difficile (C. diff)

Clostridium difficile, commonly referred to as '*C. diff*', 'CDI' (*C. diff* infection) or CDAD (*C. diff* associated diarrhoea) is the leading cause of hospital-acquired diarrhoea. Although it was first described in the mid-1930s, it has come to the fore more in the past three decades. In 1978, *C. difficile* was identified as the primary cause of pseudomembranous colitis and shown to be present in the faeces of patients undergoing antibiotic treatment with clindamycin. Further reports showed a strong correlation between pseudomembranous colitis, antibiotic therapy, *C. difficile* colonisation and toxin production. Collectively, these studies and observations revealed *C. difficile* as an emerging pathogen, capable of causing severe gastrointestinal disease in people having antibiotic therapy (Voth & Ballard 2005).

> **Care, Dignity and Compassion**
>
>
>
> Any diarrhoea-related care plan should address the following issues – safety and dignity and this includes the maintenance of privacy, appropriate and effective skin care, attention to nutritional needs, hydration and elimination.

There are several possible explanations for the increase in *C. difficile* disease during the past three decades, including:

- Better detection methods, which have led to an increase in reported cases of *C. difficile* including mandatory surveillance and reporting systems required by the Department of Health since the mid-2000s
- The high-frequency use of antibiotics and gastric suppressant medications (e.g. protein pump inhibitors, such as omeprazole) has increased the likelihood of people acquiring *C. difficile*-associated disease
- As the frequency of disease has increased, hospitals have become contaminated with spores of *C. difficile*, making infection of susceptible patients more probable.

321

(a) Hospital apportioned rates

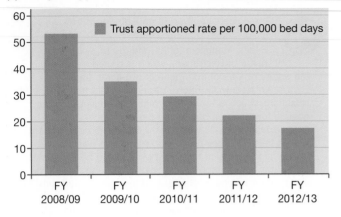

(b) All case rates

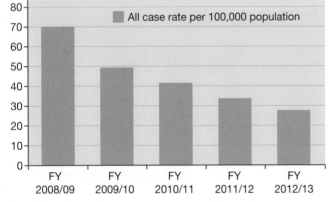

Source: *Public Health England (2013) used under the Open Government Licence v2.0. Summary Points on Clostridium difficile Infection (CDI) July 2013, available online at: http://www.hpa.org.uk/webc/HPAwebFile/HPAweb_C/1278944283388 (last accessed 20.9.13)*

Figure 16.5 Trends in rates of *Clostridium difficile*. Prevention and control measures appear to be working.

The government has sought to tackle *C. diff* by addressing these issues (DH 2012a), with emphasis on clean hospital campaigns and prudent antibiotic prescribing both in hospitals and by GPs.

Since 2000, more frequent and severe disease has emerged and large outbreaks in hospitals have necessitated ward closures and extensive infection control measures. However, a reduction in numbers has been seen in the past 4 years (see Figure 16.5) suggesting that prevention and control measures are beginning to work.

Clostridium difficile is present in the gut of up to 3% of healthy adults and 66% of infants. However, it rarely causes problems in children or healthy adults, as it is kept in check by the normal bacterial population of the intestine (the normal flora). When certain antibiotics disturb the balance of bacteria in the gut, *Clostridium difficile* can multiply rapidly and produce toxins, which cause illness.

Clostridium difficile infection ranges from mild to severe diarrhoea and in some cases, to severe inflammation of the bowel (pseudomembranous colitis). People at greatest risk are those who have been treated with broad spectrum antibiotics (those that affect a wide range of bacteria), people with serious underlying illnesses

and the elderly – over 80% of *Clostridium difficile* infections reported are in people aged over 65 years.

Preventing transmission

Clostridium difficile infection is usually spread on the hands of healthcare staff and other people who come into contact with infected patients or with environmental surfaces (e.g. floors, bedpans, toilets) contaminated with the bacteria or its spores. Spores are produced when *Clostridium difficile* bacteria encounter unfavourable conditions, such as being outside the body. They are very hardy and can survive on clothes and environmental surfaces for long periods. Good hand hygiene is needed (see earlier), with attention being given to washing hands with soap and water, as alcohol gel is not effective against spores.

Norovirus

Norovirus, sometimes referred to as acute non-bacterial gastroenteritis or winter vomiting disease, has increased in incidence in recent years. It is a severe but self-limiting infection causing nausea, forceful vomiting and watery diarrhoea, lasting for one to 3 days. Most people recover without treatment. However, dehydration can cause greater problems in the very young and those vulnerable because of other illnesses (e.g. patients with impaired immune system or the frail elderly). Norovirus can occur at any time of the year, however, it is much more prevalent during winter months, hence the use of the commonly used alternative name 'winter vomiting bug'.

Care, Dignity and Compassion

When a person is feeling nauseous or vomiting, the nurse should aim to offer that person emotional and physical support.

Norovirus is spread easily through air-borne droplet contamination, especially if someone has vomited. It is equally spread through contact as the virus can survive on hard surfaces for hours. Prevention through hand washing is vital. This is important for all clinical staff but also for the patients themselves and any visitors. In the past, lack of hand hygiene associated with food preparation has been shown to lead to infection.

In hospitals, a chlorine-based detergent should be used to clean hard surfaces. During outbreaks, this should occur more frequently than standard cleaning. Alcohol gels, while helping to clean hands, are not as effective as hand washing with soap and water (Gould 2008).

The incubation period is between 24 and 48 hours. During this time, people can be infectious to others, while not yet having symptoms themselves. Therefore, if people are exposed to others with norovirus, e.g. patients in the same hospital bay or passengers on the same cruise ship, care needs to be taken to isolate these patients, as well as those with symptoms to prevent the spread. In hospital outbreaks, this often means that wards will be 'closed' to admissions, transfers and discharges, to isolate both symptomatic patients and those potentially infected away from those not affected by norovirus. Hospitals also often impose restricted visiting to reduce the number of people having contact with patients. An escalation approach to closing wards is usually taken with affected bays being closed first and if necessary, restrictions being placed on the whole ward (Norovirus Working Party 2012). As well as patients becoming infected, there is also a risk to staff.

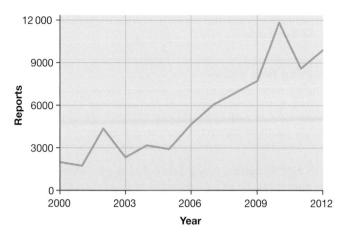

Figure 16.6 Laboratory reports of norovirus infections in England and Wales 2000–2012. *Source*: Norovirus Working Party 2012; Public Health England, used under the Open Government Licence v2.0.

Red Flag

If you suspect that you have norovirus (whether this is confirmed or because you have symptoms of diarrhoea and vomiting), you will need to stay away from the clinical placement while the symptoms are still active and for a further 48 hours after the symptoms subside, to ensure you do not pass on the infection to patients or other staff.

During the winter of 2012/2013, a large number of cases of norovirus was seen across the UK. Figure 16.6 shows how the number of cases in England and Wales has increased in recent years. This increase reports official laboratory testing for norovirus and so the increase may partly be explained by GPs and hospitals having easier access to testing as testing methods have improved recently.

Jot This Down
Using the internet to help you, find one example of a norovirus outbreak reported in the media associated with a:
· Hospital
· Nursing or residential care home
· Cruise ship
· School
Consider the similarities of these cases and how transmission is easier in closely confined environments.

Urinary Tract and Catheter Associated Infections

Urinary tract infections (UTIs) are very common. They can be painful and uncomfortable, but they usually pass within a few days or can be easily treated with a course of antibiotics. UTIs are more common in women than in men, with the main causal agent being *Escherichia coli* (commonly referred to as *E. coli*) bacteria.

It has been estimated that UTIs account for between 20% (DH 2007) and 40% (IHI 2013) of all hospital-acquired infections. The majority of hospital-acquired UTIs are attributable to indwelling urinary catheters. It is well established that the duration of catheterisation is directly related to risk for developing a UTI, therefore regular re-assessment is necessary. Good practice to prevent catheter associated UTIs falls into two domains: first, actions that

must be followed when the catheter is inserted; and second, on-going care (see Box 16.1 for guidelines). Greater awareness among healthcare practitioners in the UK has been promoted in recent years, to prevent catheter associated UTIs, with practice now

---

Box 16.1 Guidelines to Prevent Urinary Catheter-Associated Infections

Insertion actions

1. Procedure carried out using recognised aseptic non-touch technique
   · Gown, gloves and drapes (in-line with local policy), used for the insertion of invasive devices
2. Personal protective equipment
   · Disposable apron and gloves to be worn and disposed of following use and between patients
3. Catheter needed?
   · Catheterisation follows an assessment of clinical need, which includes considering alternative options
4. Clean the urethral meatus
   · Prior to insertion of catheter
   · With sterile normal saline or sterile water
   · Use correct wiping technique (front to back)
   · Use sterile single use lubricant.
5. Sterile, closed drainage system
   · Choice of urinary catheters, based on individual patient assessment and local policy
   · Correct size of catheter is selected; smallest size that will allow drainage
6. Hand hygiene
   · Hands are decontaminated immediately before and after each episode of patient contact using the correct hand hygiene technique. See Figure 16.3 – Five moments for hand hygiene
7. Documentation
   · Document, date, reason for insertion, catheter size, operator undertaking insertion and if insertion was high risk, with signature.

On-going care

1. Hand hygiene
   · Hands are decontaminated immediately before and after each episode of patient contact using the correct hand hygiene technique
2. Catheter hygiene
   · Catheter site should be cleaned regularly as stated in local policy
   · Catheter is emptied a minimum of twice daily into clean container
3. Sampling
   · All samples obtained using aseptic technique, via the catheter sampling port
4. Drainage bag position
   · Above floor but below bladder level to prevent reflux or contamination
   · Closed urinary drainage system intact or only disconnected as per manufacturer's instructions
5. Catheter manipulation
   · Examination gloves worn to manipulate a catheter, manipulation should be preceded and followed by hand decontamination
6. Catheter needed?
   · Review need for catheter daily
   · Document, date and time of removal of catheter, operator undertaking removal, with signature.

(*High Impact Intervention No. 6, Urinary Catheter Care Bundle*, DH 2007)

monitored in acute and community Trusts through a national tool known as the 'Patient Safety Thermometer' (DH 2012b).

> **Jot This Down**
>
> - Why do you think UTIs are more common in women than men?
> - Why do you think *E. coli* is the main causal bacteria?
> - Why does urinary catheterisation increase the risk of UTI?

Link To/Go To

http://www.nice.org.uk/guidance/QS61

In April 2014 the National Institute for Health and Care Excellence issued a new quality standard for infection prevention and control, with specific advice for quality improvement.

Care and Treatment for People with Infectious Diseases

Infectious diseases, also known as communicable diseases or transmissible diseases, are illnesses that result from the infection, presence and growth of bacteria or viruses, which are pathogenic (i.e. capable of causing disease). Infections may range in severity from asymptomatic to severe and fatal. This section will discuss the principles of prevention, diagnosis and treatment for measles, tuberculosis (or TB), HIV and Hepatitis C.

Measles

Measles is a viral infection spread by droplets passed on through direct contact with someone who is infected. It can be contracted easily in people who have not been vaccinated. People in close proximity are very much at risk, which is why outbreaks are often seen in schoolchildren. Measles is a notifiable infection.

The infectious period is from around four days before the appearance of the rash, to around four days after its appearance. It is most infectious before the rash is visible so the virus is often spread before people realise they are infected. Those most at risk of catching measles include babies under 1 year, people whose immune system is suppressed, for example by cancer or HIV, malnourished people, children with vitamin A deficiency and pregnant women – the infection may cause miscarriage or premature delivery. All children who have not been vaccinated are at risk from measles.

The symptoms take about 10–14 days to develop after exposure to the virus (the incubation period). At first, people develop symptoms like the common cold. This is followed by tiny white spots on the inside lining of the cheeks. A rash then develops a couple of days later, usually starting on the face and spreading across the body. Abdominal symptoms may occur, including nausea, vomiting and diarrhoea. Symptoms usually last about 2 weeks.

Measles is not usually serious but there are potential complications that can be fatal, even for otherwise healthy children. These include otitis media, pneumonia, hepatitis, conjunctivitis and encephalitis (inflammation of the brain, which occurs in about one in 5000 cases). Although complications involving the nervous

system occur in fewer than one in 1000 cases, the long-term effects can be devastating.

> **Nursing Field** Children
>
> The treatment for most children will be at home, with pain and fever-reducing syrups, such as paracetamol. They should be encouraged to drink fluids. Hospital treatment with antiviral drugs may be needed in the more serious cases.

In the UK, measles is now believed to be preventable through the implementation of a longstanding immunisation programme. Children are offered vaccination against measles as part of the MMR vaccine, which is given to children between 12 and 15 months of age, with a later booster dose before the child starts school. However, the uptake of the vaccination in the 1990s and into the 2000s was hampered by the now discredited concerns which linked the MMR to autism. The overwhelming body of evidence does not support those concerns, and experts are emphatic that the MMR vaccine is safe and effective, preventing illnesses whose real potential to cause damage is greater than many people remember. The lingering fears for some parents continue to mean the vaccination uptake is still low in some areas, with large numbers of children not being effectively vaccinated and thus there is potential for outbreaks to occur.

> **What the Experts Say**
>
> Dr Marion Lyons, director of health protection at Public Health Wales (PHW 2013) warned that a death was inevitable if parents did not take action to vaccinate children against the measles epidemic. She told the BBC: 'There were six deaths in France in 2011 and five of those were teenagers. If we don't vaccinate our children, it will happen'.
>
> ('BBC News', South West Wales, 14 April 2013)

> **The Evidence** A Case Study: South Wales Measles Outbreak, Spring 2013
>
> In the Spring of 2013, a measles outbreak was seen in South Wales, centring on Swansea, although cases were reported all across Wales. Over 1400 notifications of measles cases were made; approximately 10 times more than the usual number of cases. Nearly half of the notifications (664) came from Swansea alone. A total of 88 people had to be admitted to hospital for measles and one man, aged 25, died. Figure 16.7 shows the rise in cases over the Winter and Spring period.
>
> The outbreak attracted media attention across the UK. The Welsh health authorities set up special vaccination clinics in hospitals and schools to encourage parents to have their children immunised and prevent further spread.
>
> Much of the media attention focussed on the low vaccination uptake in the area. It was estimated that before the outbreak, 45% of children had not been vaccinated against measles. There was particular concern in this outbreak that the uptake of the MMR vaccination was low among children aged 10–17, who were babies during the vaccination scare.
>
> Another reason for the low effective vaccination rate, was that many children had not had the two necessary injections. It was estimated that 70 000 children in Wales had not had an effective dose of the vaccination.
>
> (PHW 2013)

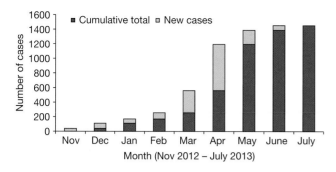

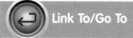

Figure 16.7 Measles outbreak – reported cases in South Wales (21012/13). *Source*: **Public Health Wales:** http://www.wales.nhs.uk/sitesplus/888/page/66389#b.

sal immunisation of all teenagers, which was the practice between the 1960s and 1990s no longer takes place, as rates are now low or non-existent in many areas.

> ### Link To/Go To
>
> http://guidance.nice.org.uk/CG117
>
> The National Institute for Health and Care Excellence (NICE 2011) has produced guidance on the management of TB, which includes vaccination advice based on current risk factors.

Tuberculosis

Tuberculosis (also called TB) is an infectious disease caused by various strains of mycobacteria, usually *Mycobacterium tuberculosis*, typically attacking the lungs, but can also affect other parts of the body. It is spread through the air when people who have an active infection, cough, sneeze or otherwise transmit respiratory fluids. Most infections are asymptomatic and latent; one in ten latent infections eventually progresses to active disease which, if left untreated, can be fatal in around 50% of those infected.

The typical symptoms of active TB infection are:

- A persistent cough with blood-stained sputum
- Fever
- Night sweats
- Weight loss
- Loss of appetite
- Tiredness and fatigue.

Diagnosis of active TB is made following a chest X-ray, as well as microscopic examination and microbiological culture of body fluids. In latent TB, diagnosis can be made using a tuberculin skin test (Mantoux test) and/or blood tests.

Globally, TB is a very common disease, particularly prevalent in sub-Saharan Africa and parts of Asia. In the UK, TB is seen more in socioeconomically deprived areas, with cities such as London having the highest rates (Pedrazzoli *et al.* 2012).

Risk factors for TB

A number of factors make people more susceptible to TB infections. The most important risk factor is HIV, with 13% of all TB cases associated with the virus. This is particularly the case in sub-Saharan Africa. Tuberculosis is closely linked to overcrowding and malnutrition, making it one of the principal diseases of poverty (Jarvis 2010).

An understanding of the risk factors helps to explain why different strategies are used to prevent and treat TB. For example, NHS commissioning organisations in some areas of England have targeted immunisation of babies based on the postcode of the parents, including those who live in poorer social economic areas, as rates of TB in these areas has been increasing. However, univer-

Prevention and treatment of TB

Tuberculosis prevention primarily relies on vaccination. The only vaccine currently available is the bacillus Calmette–Guérin (BCG) vaccine. The BCG is effective against disease in childhood but confers inconsistent protection against contracting pulmonary TB and the immunity it produces decreases after about 10 years. It is the most widely used vaccine worldwide; new vaccines are currently in development.

The treatment and management of TB is with antibiotics. Treatment usually lasts 6 months, with combinations of antibiotics. Sometimes, people find it difficult to take their medication every day. If this is the case, then some patients may be asked to join a programme of 'directly observed therapy'. This can include supervised treatment, involving regular contact between the patient and the treatment team (daily or three times a week) to support and prompt the antibiotics administration.

Preventing the spread of infection

While patients are contagious, which will usually be for up to three weeks into their course of treatment, precautions need to be taken to prevent the spread of TB to others. For most people, the best way to do this is in their normal home environment and not to be admitted to hospital. Patients do not normally need to be isolated during this time, but it is important that they take some basic precautions to stop TB spreading to their family and friends; these include:

- Staying away from work, school or university
- Always covering the mouth when coughing, sneezing or laughing
- Disposing of used tissues carefully in a sealed plastic bag
- Opening windows when possible, ensuring a good supply of fresh air
- Not sleeping in the same room as other people, as coughing or sneezing can occur without realising it.

Unless there is a clear clinical or socioeconomic need, such as homelessness, people with TB should not be admitted to hospital. However, if a patient needs to be admitted, then the NICE (2011) and RCN (Story & Cocksedge 2012) guidelines should be followed. The main component of care for people with TB in hospital, is that they should be isolated in a single, ideally negative-pressure room, where the air is continuously or automatically monitored and vented to the outside (*Nursing Times* 2012a).

325

Jot This Down

It is important to consider the healthcare advice relating to TB but also not to forget the impact the infection has on patients and carers.

Access both the NICE website to read the TB clinical guidelines produced by UK health professionals, and the 'Truth about TB', which is run by patients and carers of people who have contracted TB. Read their stories about their diagnosis and care.

· http://guidance.nice.org.uk/CG117
· http://www.thetruthabouttb.org/

From this information, what are your main priorities for care of a patient diagnosed with TB?

What advice would you give to someone who thinks they have been in contact with someone with TB?

What the Experts Say

I have treated many people with TB. Most patients have other needs in addition to their TB treatment, as they are vulnerable due to poverty and often don't speak English well. Being a TB nurse specialist allows me to combine the science and art of nursing as I need to understand the pathology of the disease and treatment but the role also requires care, compassion and creativity to tailor a plan of care that will be followed by the patient.

(Tracey a TB clinical nurse specialist)

The British HIV Association has published evidence-based standards of care for people with HIV (BHIVA 2012). The standards are grouped into 12 themes, prioritised as the most important issues for the care of people with HIV.

Jot This Down

There is a great deal of information available for patients about HIV and AIDS. Go to the NHS Choices website, read the information aimed at patients and follow some of the links to other sites, such as campaign groups and sexual health information pages.

NHS Choices:

http://www.nhs.uk/Conditions/HIV/Pages/Introduction.aspx

· List three new pieces of information that you have gleaned from reading this information.

Link To/Go To

If you are interested in learning more about the standards that people living with HIV should expect from health care, then read the British HIV associations standards:

www.bhiva.org/documents/Standards-of-care/BHIVAStandardsA4.pdf

Blood-Borne Pathogens

Blood-borne pathogens include any human pathogen present in human blood, but they may also be present in other body fluids. Blood-borne pathogens include human immunodeficiency virus (HIV), hepatitis B (HBV), hepatitis C (HCV), hepatitis D (HDV), malaria, syphilis, babesiosis, brucellosis, leptospirosis, arboviral infections, relapsing fever, Creutzfeldt-Jakob disease, adult T-cell leukemia/lymphoma (caused by HTLV-I), HTLV-I-associated myelopathy, diseases associated with HTLV-II and viral haemorrhagic fever.

Human immunodeficiency virus/acquired immunodeficiency disease

Many people including student nurses have some lay knowledge of HIV and AIDS. This may include knowledge or myths about the transmission of the virus as well as out-of-date information about prognosis and treatments. The aim of this section is to concentrate on the infection control principles associated with the transmission and prevention of HIV, especially precautions and procedures for controlling HIV infection among healthcare workers. In Chapter 22, the background to HIV and the effect it has on the immune system are explained. Other specialist texts or articles should be referred to in relation to the care of people living with HIV and treatment of AIDS (e.g. *Nursing Times* 2012b; Peate 2010, 2012a,b).

HIV transmission Three factors are needed for HIV to be transmitted (Evans 2011):

1. An HIV source
2. A sufficient dose of the virus (viral load)
3. Access to the bloodstream of another person.

Different levels and concentrations of HIV have been found in most bodily fluids of infected persons, however, **only** blood, semen, breast milk and vaginal and cervical secretions have been shown to transmit HIV infection.

Transmission occurs mainly through sexual contact with an infected person. The risk of transmission depends on sexual practices, with receptive anal contact without a condom carrying the greatest risk. This is due to the larger surface area of mucous membranes involved. Indeed receptive partners are at greater risk for transmission of any sexually transmitted infection (STI), including HIV.

As a nurse, you should remember that sexual identity and gender preference do not always predict behaviour, and that assumptions should not be made about risk of transmission. Safer sex practices should be advocated to all patients and clients.

Another common mechanism for transmission of HIV is injection drug use when needles, syringes and other drug use equipment are shared. More rarely, HIV may be transmitted through transfusions of blood or blood products. This is now very uncommon in developed countries, as blood is screened for HIV antibodies. HIV can also be transmitted during tattooing or during blood-sharing

Table 16.1 Preventing HIV transmission.

	MEASURES	COMMENTS
Safer sex	Safer sex practices include: · Abstinence · Mutual monogamy · Correct use of condoms	Both women and men may need instruction in the correct use of condoms
Injection drug-users	Injection drug-users need instructions about precautions: · Do not share needles or other paraphernalia · If sterile needles are not available, use bleach to clean needles · If you have sexual intercourse, use a condom to prevent infecting others	Needle exchange programmes are in place throughout the country to enable users to access sterile equipment
Uninfected partners	· Use of prevention strategies even if the partner is also HIV infected · Initial and periodic screening of partners	The partner may have a different strain of the virus
Complacency and risky behaviour	The following have been identified as challenges, particularly among younger gay men: · Unprotected sex · Use of alcohol and other drugs · Lack of awareness of HIV infection · Stigma and internalised homophobia · Social isolation · Racism, poverty and lack of access to health care · Complacency about HIV, based on ignorance	Complacency appears to stem from two key factors: · Lack of experience with the severity of the early HIV epidemic. · The mistaken belief that advances in treatment and decreased mortality mean that HIV is no longer a serious threat
Research	Pre-exposure prophylaxis (PrEP) is now being considered following recent drug trials	Controversial in some areas and high costs may prohibit wider use

activities such as 'blood brother' rituals, where blood is exchanged or contaminated equipment is shared.

An HIV-positive woman can transmit HIV to her baby either during pregnancy, at the time of birth or while breast-feeding. Women newly or recently infected with HIV or those in the later stages of AIDS tend to have higher viral loads and may be more infectious.

Other factors such as co-existing infections may increase the likelihood of infection and make its treatment more complex. People who are HIV-positive may have other sexually transmitted infections, such as syphilis, gonorrhoea, genital warts, human papilloma virus (HPV), trichomoniasis, scabies, herpes and chlamydia. Sores, lesions or inflammation from STIs make the skin or mucous membrane more vulnerable to other infections.

HIV prevention and risk reduction HIV/AIDS is preventable. Prevention should be part of a more general sexual health education programme, as the prevalence has risen of other preventable STIs. Screening for STIs is recommended, since many of those infected do not show symptoms.

The introduction of standard precautions in healthcare has unquestionably prevented thousands of cases of HIV/AIDS, but because the virus is transmitted through behaviours that many people find pleasurable (sexual activity and injection-drug use), prevention is more complex. Prevention needs to begin with education and counselling about sexual practices and injection-drug use. An unprejudiced approach needs to be adopted with recognition

that for many people 'just saying no' is not a realistic option and therefore, there is a need for basic, practical, 'how-to' information to reduce risk.

Table 16.1 sets out some of the recommendations and issues to be considered with regard to HIV prevention.

Preventing HIV exposure to healthcare practitioners The risk of transmission of occupational exposure is extremely low. There is a potential risk that healthcare workers could become infected with HIV through needle-sticks or direct contact with HIV-infected blood, for example through a break in the skin or through the eyes or the mucosal lining of the nose.

Needle-stick injuries and other occupational exposures to potentially life-threatening infections can be extremely stressful for the practitioner and therefore have implications for mental as well as physical health. This needs to be considered as a part of post-exposure prophylaxis (PEP). Specific guidelines for PEP for healthcare staff vary between different hospitals and community Trust settings but the principles are the same. Although specialist advice would always need to be sought, it is important that all nurses have a basic understanding of these guidelines (HIV post-exposure prophylaxis), so that they are self-aware and can provide initial information to patients or colleagues. In some cases, passing on this knowledge may prompt people to seek timely further advice, as it is believed there is a window of opportunity of up to 48–72 hours to prevent HIV infection with antiretroviral therapy (Benn *et al.* 2011).

The Evidence HIV Post-Exposure Prophylaxis (PEP)

The current UK guidance on HIV post-exposure prophylaxis (PEP) is in two forms:

1. The UK Chief Medical Officers' Expert Advisory Group on AIDS (EAGA), for recommendations following occupational exposure (DH 2008).
2. The British Association for Sexual Health and HIV, for recommendations following sexual exposure (Benn *et al.* 2011).

	Post-Exposure Prophylaxis (PEP) Following Occupational Exposure	Post-Exposure Prophylaxis Following Sexual Exposure (PEPSE)
Assessing the risk	The risk of occupational exposure to HIV-infected blood is **low**. Epidemiological studies have indicated that the average risk after percutaneous exposure to HIV-infected blood in healthcare settings is about 3/1000 injuries. After a mucocutaneous exposure, the average risk is estimated at less than 1 in 1000. It has been considered that there is no risk of HIV transmission where skin is intact Four factors are associated with increased risk of occupationally acquired HIV infection: · Deep injury · Visible blood on the device which caused the injury · Injury with a needle which had been placed in a source patient's artery or vein · Terminal HIV-related illness in the source patient where the source patient is not on therapy and has uncontrolled viral load	The risk of HIV transmission depends upon the exposure characteristics, the infectivity of the source and host susceptibility Prevalence of HIV in the UK is highest among men who have sex with men (MSM), living in London. The rate in the remainder of the UK is lower but equals that of heterosexual men from sub-Saharan Africa The following factors may increase the risk of HIV transmission: · A high viral load in the source · Breaches in the mucosal barrier, such as mouth or genital ulcer disease and trauma following sexual assault or first intercourse · STIs enhance HIV transmission · The risk of HIV transmission is likely to be greater if ejaculation occurs
Immediate action	· Immediately following any exposure the site, e.g. wound or non-intact skin, should be washed liberally with soap and water Antiseptics and skin washes should not be used · Free bleeding of puncture wounds should be encouraged gently · Exposed mucous membranes, including conjunctivae, should be irrigated copiously with water, before and after removing any contact lenses · Prompt reporting with risk assessment by an experienced clinician needs to occur · Assessment and testing of the source patient should be considered following guidelines	Those presenting for PEPSE must be seen in a GU medicine/sexual health/HIV department at the earliest opportunity so appropriate treatment and pre-test discussion (if HIV status is as yet unknown)
When PEP is recommended	· PEP should be recommended to healthcare workers if they have had a significant occupational exposure to blood or another high-risk body fluid, from a patient or other source either known to be HIV infected or considered to be at high risk of HIV · PEP should be commenced as soon as possible after occupational exposure, allowing for careful risk assessment · Ideally, this should be within 1 hour. PEP is generally not recommended beyond 72 hours post-exposure.	· Source individual is known to be HIV-positive. Consideration will include type of sexual exposure and viral load · Source individual is of unknown status and comes from a group or area of high HIV prevalence then PEP is recommended following receptive anal sex only. Where the source is not from a group or area of high HIV prevalence then PEP is not recommended · Sexual assault. It is believed that transmission of HIV is likely to be increased following aggravated sexual intercourse (anal or vaginal), such as that experienced during sexual assault. Clinicians may therefore consider recommending PEPSE more readily in such situations · Needle-stick injuries in the community following an injury from a discarded needle. In general, PEP is not recommended following these exposures
Recommended therapy	· A triple agent combination regimen is advised based on the evidence from treatments given to people with established HIV infection · This consists of oral medication which is given for 4 weeks. Every effort should be made to facilitate adherence to a full 4-week regimen · Since nausea is a common problem, the prescription of prophylactic anti-emetics should be considered · Anti-motility drugs may be helpful if diarrhoea develops – a common side-effect	

	Post-Exposure Prophylaxis (PEP) Following Occupational Exposure	Post-Exposure Prophylaxis Following Sexual Exposure (PEPSE)
Advice and support	• The exposed healthcare worker should have the opportunity to consider whether or not to continue PEP. Their decision should be informed by all that is known about the source patient in terms of past exposure to risk of HIV infection and also the nature and severity of the exposure • These aspects should be considered together with the potential for unpleasant short-term adverse effects and unknown long-term effects of taking PEP drugs. • Follow-up should be for at least 12 weeks after the HIV exposure event or, if PEP was taken, for at least 12 weeks from when PEP was stopped.	Following initial discussion, follow-up should take place in a GU medicine/sexual health/HIV department, so the following issues can be addressed: • The need to continue with a further 4-week course of PEPSE if the baseline result is negative • The need to have a follow-up HIV test 12 weeks post-completion of PEP • The side-effects of the drugs and the support available in the clinic and in the community to help adherence • The need to utilise generic social support over the following 4 months • The need for safer sex for the following 4 months • Issues around disclosure • Coping strategies • For patients concerned about sexual risk-taking, health advisers can offer on-going risk reduction work or referral to psychology if appropriate

Diagnostic Tests and Treatment

There are many diagnostic tests and treatment approaches used by infection control practitioners to identify the cause of infection and determine the best treatment. Diagnostic tests frequently involve a specimen being obtained and then the laboratory performing a series of tests to isolate the organism responsible for the infection and which antibiotics the organism is sensitive to. This enables treatment to be well informed and based on evidence about what will be effective.

Medicines Management

 When helping people with their medicines, it is essential that you provide advice that the person understands in order for the therapeutic effects of the medicines to have greatest effect. People should be reminded that they must complete the full course of antibiotic therapy prescribed, even if after a few days their symptoms may appear to be relieved.

In this section, some common diagnostic tests are explained and the way in which specimens are obtained is discussed, as this is frequently either a nursing task or if the patient is self-caring, requires a nurse to explain how the specimen is obtained.

Common Laboratory Tests

Microbiology and virology laboratories in hospitals carry out different tests. Increasingly, some tests can now be performed outside the laboratory using equipment that enables 'near-patient testing'. This is very helpful in clinical settings, such as walk-in centres, emergency departments and sexual health clinics, where diagnoses can be made more rapidly and decisions about treatment or whether a patient needs to be isolated, can be made. Examples of near patient testing for infection control can range from simple urine 'dipstick' test for the presence of protein, suggesting a urinary tract infection, to HIV and CD4 count tests.

Obtaining Specimens

Specimens are obtained most frequently in five ways:

- Blood tests
- Swabs including wound, ear, eye, nose and throat swabs.
- Urine samples
- Stool samples
- Sputum samples.

Other less common specimens which may be collected, include cerebrospinal fluid (CSF) during a lumbar puncture, tissue from biopsies or bronchial 'washings' in cases of suspected TB.

As with any type of laboratory specimen, there are certain criteria that need to be met for proper collection and transportation of specimens (*Nursing Times* 2008). This will ensure proper stability of the specimen and more accurate test results. Containers need to be clean or in some cases, sterile to prevent substances interfering with the analyses. The container needs to have a secure lid and be leak resistant, this is particularly important, as other healthcare professions and ancillary staff should not be exposed to body fluids when handling or transporting the specimens. The local laboratory will issue guidelines and ensure staff know which containers should be used, e.g. specific blood bottles or 24-hour urine collection containers. If in doubt, ring the laboratory or speak to the infection control nurse for advice. In some cases, a preservative is added to the container. If this is the case, the guidelines need to be read and followed, for example it may be necessary to refrigerate the sample or to ensure it is sent to the lab within a specific period of time. Equally, the volume of the specimen needs to be correct, otherwise the concentration of the preservative may be too low or too high.

Red Flag

All specimens should be labelled correctly: this includes the patient's name and identification/hospital number. Care should be taken to ensure that the information on the label and on the requisition form match. Labels should be placed on the container, not the lid of the container as this can be removed and mixed-up.

All specimens should be labelled correctly. Care should be taken when a sample is being placed in a fridge, that the label is compatible with this storage choice, i.e. the ink does not leach. This may be relevant when printed labels are used with some printers.

The collection date and time needs to be included on the specimen label. This will confirm that the collection was done correctly. For some timed specimens, e.g. 24-hour urine collection, the start and stop times should be documented.

Blood Tests for Infection

Blood sampling should be performed by a healthcare worker trained and competent in the procedure. In nursing, this is usually a registered nurse, although un-registered practitioners, such as phlebotomists can be trained to successfully take blood. As there are many different blood tests, information needs to be obtained about the appropriate laboratory containers (blood bottles) required for specific tests and the amount of blood required. Protective clothing, such as gloves and aprons (and facial protection when appropriate) must be used along with an aseptic non-touch technique.

Blood Cultures

Detection of micro-organisms by culture of blood is essential in the diagnosis of bloodstream infections. Accurate positive results provide valuable information to guide antibiotic prescribing, which can improve the outcome from blood-borne infections. However, contaminated blood cultures can cause considerable diagnostic confusion and lead to unnecessary antimicrobial therapy, so careful collection of the blood using an aseptic non-touch-technique is needed.

Swabs

Swabs are used to determine whether there is local infection or colonisation across a variety of different parts of the body. Swabs are commonly used to obtain specimens from wounds, ears, eyes, nose and throat.

- **Wound swabs** – results from wound swabs should be interpreted alongside clinical signs of infection. In the absence of any clinical signs of infection, positive wound swabs generally just indicate colonisation.
  - Obtain the specimen prior to any dressing or cleaning procedure of the wound. This will maximise the material obtained and prevent killing of the organism by the use of antiseptics
  - Use a sterile swab and gently rotate on the area to collect exudate from the wound and place into transport medium. Where there is pus, collect as much as possible in a sterile syringe or sterile container (do not use a swab) and send to the laboratory.
- **Ear swabs**
  - No antibiotics or other therapeutic agents should have been in the aural region for about 3 hours prior to sampling the area as this may inhibit the growth of organisms

- If there is discharge from the ear this should be sampled
- Place a sterile swab into the outer ear and gently rotate to collect the secretions
- Place swab in transport medium
- For deeper ear swabbing a speculum may be used. Experienced medical staff only should undertake this procedure as damage to the eardrum may occur.
- **Eye swabs**
  - The patient should be asked to look upwards and gently pull the lower lid down or gently part the eyelids
  - Use a sterile cotton-wool swab and gently role the swab over the inside of the lower lid. Hold the swab parallel to the cornea to avoid injury if the patient moves
  - Place the swab in the transport medium.
- **Nose swabs**
  - Specify on the lab form if this is a routine admission screen for MRSA or for the investigation of a suspected infection
  - If the nose is dry, moisten the swab in sterile 0.9% saline solution beforehand
  - Insert the swab into the anterior nares and direct it up into the tip of the nose and gently rotate. Both nares should be swabbed using the same swab to obtain adequate material
  - Place in transport medium.
- **Throat swabs**
  - Place the patient in a position with a good light source. This will ensure maximum visibility of the tonsillar bed
  - Either depress the tongue with a spatula or ask the patient to say 'aahh'. The procedure is likely to cause gagging and the tongue will move to the roof of the mouth. This can prevent accurate sampling, therefore it is important to quickly but gently rub the swab over the tonsillar fossa (tonsillar bed) or area where there is exudate or a lesion
  - Care should be taken not to contaminate the swab by contact with the tongue or the oral mucosa on removal
  - Return swab to the container with transport medium.

Urine Samples

Urine is an important tool for clinical diagnosis (Skobe 2004). The clinical information obtained from a urine specimen is influenced by the collection method, timing and handling. A vast assortment of collection and transport containers for urine specimens are available. Determining which urine collection method and container should be used depends on the type of laboratory test ordered. Types of collection include routine urinalysis completed at ward or department level to complex laboratory tests. The tests tend to be classified, according to the type of collection required:

- **Random specimen** – This is the specimen most commonly sent to the laboratory for analysis, primarily because it is the easiest to obtain and is readily available. Random specimens can sometimes give an inaccurate view of a patient's health if the specimen is too diluted. As the name implies, the random specimen can be collected at any time.
- **Early morning urine (EMU)** – this is the specimen of choice for urinalysis and microscopic analysis, since the urine is generally more concentrated (due to the length of time the urine is allowed to remain in the bladder) and, therefore, contains relatively higher levels of cellular elements, such as protein, if present. The specimen is collected when the patient first wakes up in the morning, having emptied the bladder before going to sleep.

Proper collection practices and accurate recording of the collection time are important.

- **Midstream specimen of urine (MSU)** – this is the preferred type of specimen for culture and sensitivity testing because of the reduced incidence of contamination. Patients are required to first cleanse the urethral area. The patient should then void the first portion of the urine stream into the toilet. These first steps significantly reduce the opportunities for contaminants to enter into the urine stream. The urine midstream is then collected into a clean container (any excess urine should be voided into the toilet). This method of collection can be conducted at any time of day or night.
- **24-hour urine collection** – a timed specimen is collected to measure the concentration of substances affected by diurnal variations, over a specified length of time, usually 24 hours. In this collection method, the bladder is emptied prior to beginning the timed collection. Then, for the duration of the designated time period, all urine is collected and pooled into a collection container, with the final collection taking place at the very end of that period. The specimen should be refrigerated during the collection period, unless otherwise requested. Accurate timing is critical to the calculations that are conducted later in the labs.
- **Catheter specimen urine (CSU)** – this method may either be used for a patient with an existing urinary catheter or in some cases, a catheter may be inserted to obtain the specimen. Specimens are collected directly from a special port in the catheter tubing using an aseptic sterile technique using a syringe.

Nursing Field Children's Specimens

For infants and small children, a special urine collection bag is adhered to the skin surrounding the urethral area. Once the collection is completed, the urine is poured into a collection cup or transferred directly into an evacuated tube with a transfer straw. Urine collected from a nappy is not recommended for laboratory testing, since contamination from the nappy material may affect test results.

Stool Samples

- The specimen form should state whether the sample is a routine (admission) screening sample or an investigation for suspected intestinal infection
- If viral gastroenteritis (e.g. norovirus, rotavirus) is suspected, the stool specimen should be sent to the virology laboratory. To exclude a bacterial cause, a second stool specimen can be sent to the microbiology laboratory
- A faecal specimen is more suitable than a rectal swab
- A specimen can be obtained from a nappy or clean potty
- Use the scoop attached to the inside of the lid of the specimen container to place faecal material into the container
- In babies and young children where diarrhoea is present, a small piece of non-absorbent material lining the nappy can be used to prevent material soaking into the nappy
- Examine the sample for consistency, odour or blood and record observations to monitor changes
- If segments of tapeworm are seen, send to the laboratory. Tapeworm segments can vary from the size of rice grains to a ribbon shape, one-inch long.

Sputum

Good quality sputum samples are essential for accurate microbiological diagnosis of chest infections, pneumonia and bronchitis. Samples contaminated with secretions and saliva are difficult to interpret and can be misleading. The patient should be encouraged to cough, especially after sleep, and expectorate into a container. Physiotherapy may be needed to help facilitate expectoration. You should ensure that the material obtained is sputum and not saliva, before sending the sample to the laboratory.

Conclusion

This chapter has introduced the reader to the principles of infection prevention and control. It is intended that this will enable you to have the knowledge and evidence that underpins this fundamental aspect of nursing care. However, it should be recognised that infection control is a complex and specialised subject and in some cases, the information here will not be sufficient and you should refer to a specialist infection control nurse or consultant medical microbiologist for more information and advice.

The chapter has considered why infection control is essential in healthcare settings to prevent disease and promote recovery. The standard approaches to preventing the spread of infection have been described, with emphasis given to hand hygiene. The chapter also includes information about the treatment of people with communicable diseases (e.g. tuberculosis) and how their treatment differs from that of people with other infections. The most common healthcare-associated infections that you may come across in practice are discussed, including, MRSA, *Clostridium difficile* and norovirus, and the common diagnostic tests and treatment approaches used by infection control practitioners are presented. The chapter has included approaches to providing explanations to patients and their families about the prevention and control of infection.

Key Points

- The importance of infection prevention and control has been described providing the reader with an historical perspective.
- A discussion concerning the most common healthcare-associated infections has been provided.
- The requirement to use a person-centred, evidence approach to the treatment of people with communicable diseases has been discussed.
- The unique role and function of the nurse as central in the prevention, monitoring and control of infection has been reiterated.
- The chapter has provided insight and understanding concerning a number of ways of collecting specimens.
- Information giving is a key factor in the fight against infection prevention and control.

Glossary

Aseptic technique: this refers to any procedure that is performed under sterile conditions. The most common example of where an aseptic technique is used is in hospital operating theatres but it is also needed in ward areas when invasive procedures are undertaken, e.g. urinary catheterisation, cannula insertion, wound dressing changes

(Continued)

Bacteraemia: the presence of bacteria in the blood

Bacteria: bacteria are micro-organisms typically a few micrometres in length and have a wide range of shapes, ranging from spheres to rods and spirals. Large numbers of bacteria can be found on the skin and as gut flora. Most are rendered harmless by the protective effects of the immune system; however, a few species are pathogenic and cause infectious diseases

Barrier nursing: this occurs when a patient with an infectious disease is isolated usually in a side-room. The most effective form of isolation is in a single room with a self-contained toilet and its own hand basin

Cohort nursing: patients suspected of having the same organism are looked after in bays together. This is an alternative form of isolating infected patients that should be considered if there are not enough single rooms

Communicable disease: communicable diseases, also known as infectious diseases or transmissible diseases, are illnesses that result from the infection, presence and growth of pathogenic (capable of causing disease) biologic agents in an individual. Infections may range in severity from asymptomatic to severe and fatal

Contagious: infectious diseases are sometimes called 'contagious' when they are easily transmitted

Disinfection: the application of substances to non-living objects to destroy micro-organisms that are living on the objects. Disinfection does not necessarily kill all micro-organisms, especially resistant bacterial spores and is less effective than sterilisation. Disinfectants work by destroying the cell wall of microbes or interfering with the metabolism

Iatrogenic: an inadvertent adverse effect or complication resulting from medical treatment or advice, including that of nurses, therapists, pharmacists, doctors and dentists. Healthcare-associated infections are a subset of iatrogenic conditions other examples include surgical complications and drug interactions

Infectivity: refers to the ability of a pathogen to establish an infection. More specifically, how frequently it spreads from host to host. The measure of infectivity in a population is called the 'incidence'

MC&S: microscopy, culture and sensitivity (MC&S) is the term often used when sending samples or swabs to the laboratory. It refers to the sample being viewed under a microscope, then grown or cultured to enable further identification of an organism. The sensitivity or resistance of the organism to antibiotics is also tested

Nosocomial: a hospital-acquired infection is frequently referred to in the medical literature as a nosocomial infection. It is an infection whose development is favoured by a hospital environment, such as one acquired by a patient during a hospital visit or one developing among hospital staff

Outbreak: outbreak is a term used in epidemiology to describe an occurrence of disease greater than would otherwise be expected at a particular time and place. It may affect a small and localised group or impact upon thousands of people across an entire continent. Two linked cases of a rare infectious disease may be sufficient to constitute an outbreak

Pathogenic: capable of producing disease

Period of increased incidence: this term is used to differentiate between an outbreak and when two or more cases of a disease occur, which may be related. Typically, used in *C. diff* cases it would refer to two or more new cases occurring in a 28-day period on a ward

Quarantine: used to separate and restrict the movement of well people who may have been exposed to a communicable disease, to see if they become ill. The term is often erroneously used synonymously with isolation, which refers to separating ill people who have the disease from those who are healthy

Standard precautions: guidelines recommended and agreed nationally for reducing the risk of transmission of blood-borne and other pathogens in hospitals. They apply to all patients receiving care in healthcare environments, regardless of their diagnosis or presumed infection status. Standard precautions apply to: (1) blood; (2) all body fluids, secretions, and excretions *except sweat*; (3) non-intact skin; and (4) mucous membranes

Virus: a small infectious agent that replicates only inside the living cells of other organisms

References

Barratt, R., Shaban, R. & Moyle, W. (2010) Behind barriers: patients' perceptions of source isolation for methicillin-resistant Staphylococcus aureus (MRSA). *Australian Journal of Advanced Nursing*, 28(2), 53–59.

BBC (2013) *BBC News, South West Wales*, 14 April. http://www.bbc.co.uk/news/uk-wales-south-west-wales-22146173 (accessed 15 April 2013).

BHIVA (2012) *Standards of Care for People Living with HIV 2013*, British HIV Association, London. www.bhiva.org/documents/Standards-of-care/BHIVAStandardsA4.pdf (accessed 31 August 2013).

Benn, P., Fisher, M. & Kulasegaram, R. (2011) *UK Guideline for the Use of Post-Exposure Prophylaxis for HIV Following Sexual Exposure*. http://www.bashh.org/BASHH/Guidelines/Guidelines/BASHH/Guidelines/Guidelines.aspx?hkey=072c83ed-0e9b-44b2-a989-7c84e4fbd9de (accessed 31 August 2013).

BNF (2013) *BNF 65* (March 2013). BMJ Publishing Group Ltd and Royal Pharmaceutical Society, British National Formulary, London.

Coia, J.E., Duckworth, G.E., Edwards, D.I. *et al.* (2006) Guidelines for the control and prevention of meticillin resistant Staphylococcus aureus (MRSA) in healthcare facilities. Joint Working Party of the British Society of Antimicrobial Chemotherapy, Hospital Infection Society and Infection Control Nurses Association. *Journal of Hospital Infection*, 63(Suppl 1), S1–44.

DH (2007) *High Impact Intervention No 6. Urinary Catheter Care Bundle*. Department of Health for England, London. http://webarchive.nationalarchives.gov.uk/20120118164404/hcai.dh.gov.uk/files/2011/03/Document_-Urinary_Catheter_Care_High_Impact_Intervention_FINAL_100907.pdf (accessed 30 September 2013).

DH (2008) *HIV Post-exposure Prophylaxis: guidance from the UK Chief Medical Officers' Expert Advisory Group on AIDS*. Department of Health, London. https://www.gov.uk/government/news/hiv-post-exposure-prophylaxis-guidance-from-the-uk-chief-medical-officers-expert-advisory-group-on-aids (accessed 31 August 2013).

DH (2012a) *Updated Guidance on the Diagnosis and Reporting of Clostridium Difficile*. Department of Health, London. https://www.gov.uk/government/uploads/system/uploads/attachment_data/file/146808/dh_133016.pdf (accessed 15 April 2013)

DH (2012b) *Guidance to Support the NHS in Implementing the NHS Safety Thermometer*. Department of Health, London. https://www.gov.uk/government/news/guidance-to-support-the-nhs-in-implementing-the-nhs-safety-thermometer-published (accessed 30 September 2013).

Evans, N. (2011) *HIV/AIDS Transmission and Infection Control*. Wild Iris Medical Education Nursing, CEU. http://www.nursingceu.com/courses/353/index_nceu.html (accessed 31 August 2013).

Gould, D. (2008) Management and prevention of norovirus outbreaks in hospitals. *Nursing Standard*, 23(13), 51–56.

Gould, D. (2011) MRSA: implications for hospitals and nursing homes. *Nursing Standard*, 25(18), 47–56.

IHI (2013) *Catheter-associated Urinary Tract Infections*. Institute for Healthcare Improvement. http://www.ihi.org/explore/cauti/Pages/default.aspx (accessed 30 September 2013).

Jarvis, M. (2010) Tuberculosis 1: exploring the challenges facing its control and how to reduce its spread. *Nursing Times*, 106(1), 23–25.

Newsom, S.W.B. (2004) MRSA – past, present, future. *Journal of the Royal Society of Medicine*, 97(11), 509–510.

NHS Choices (2012) *How MRSA is Caught, What Happens When You Have it, and How Hospital Staff and Visitors can Help Prevent Infection*. Video presentation by Dr Brian Duerdan, DH Chief Microbiologist. http://www.nhs.uk/Video/Pages/MRSA.aspx (accessed 24 February 2014).

NICE (2011) *Tuberculosis: clinical diagnosis and management of tuberculosis, and measures for its prevention and control. Clinical Guideline 117*. National Institute for Health and Clinical Excellence, London. http://guidance.nice.org.uk/CG117

Norovirus Working Party (2012) *Guidelines for the Management of Norovirus Outbreaks in Acute and Community Health and Social Care Settings*. Joint working party of the Hospital Infection Society, Infection Prevention Society, NHS Confederation, British Infection Association, National Concern for Healthcare Infections, Health Protection Agency.

Nursing Times (2008) *Nursing Times* specimen collection series 1–6. *Nursing Times*, March–May, Issue 1. http://www.nursingtimes.net/nursing-practice/clinical-zones/infection-control/specimen-collection-1-obtaining-a-midstream-specimen-of-urine/1295662.article

Nursing Times (2012a) Case management for tuberculosis. Nursing practice guidance in brief. *Nursing Times*, 108(28), 15.

Nursing Times (2012b) HIV infection – identifying and testing patients. *Nursing Times Learning*. http://www.nursingtimes.net/online-nurse-training-courses/HIV-Infection-Identifying-and-Testing-Patients# (accessed 31 August 2013).

Peate, I. (2010) Living with HIV: mental health and well-being. *British Journal of Well-being*, 1(6), 34–37.

Peate, I. (2012a) Guidelines for the management of HIV infection in pregnant women. *British Journal of Midwifery*, 20(3), 215.

Peate, I. (2012b) World AIDS Day 2012: are you missing the signs of an HIV infection? *British Journal of Community Nursing*, 17(12), 604.

Pedrazzoli, D., Fulton, N., Anderson, L., Lalor, M., Abubakar, I. & Zenner, D. (2012) *Tuberculosis in the UK: annual report on tuberculosis surveillance in the UK*. Health Protection Agency, London.

Pratt, R.J., Pellowe, C.M., Wilson, J.A. *et al.* (2007) Epic 2: national evidence-based guideline for preventing healthcare-associated infection in NHS hospitals in England. *Journal of Hospital Infection*, 65 (Suppl 1), S1–64.

PHE (2013) *Summary Points on Clostridium difficile Infection (CDI)*. Public Health, England. http://www.hpa.org.uk/webc/HPAwebFile/HPAweb_C/1278944283388 (accessed 30 September 2013).

PHW (2013) *Measles Outbreak: Data, NHS Wales/Public Health*. Public Health, Wales. http://www.wales.nhs.uk/sitesplus/888/page/66389#b (accessed 30 September 2013).

RCN (2005) *Methicillin-resistant Staphylococcus aureus (MRSA): guidance for nursing staff*. Royal College of Nursing, London.

Redway, K. & Fawdar, S. (2008) A comparative study of three different hand drying methods: paper towel, warm air dryer, jet air dryer. *European Tissue Symposium* (November). http://www.europeantissue.com/pdfs/090402–2008%20WUS%20Westminster%20University%20hygiene%20study,%20nov2008.pdf (accessed 28 December 2012).

Skobe, M.T. (2004) The basics of specimen collection and handling of urine testing. *Lab Notes*, 14(2). http://www.bd.com/vacutainer/labnotes/Volume14Number2/ (accessed 12 June 2013).

Story, A. & Cocksedge, M. (2012) *Tuberculosis Case Management and Cohort Review – Guidance for Health Professionals*. Royal College of Nursing, London.

Voth, D.E. & Ballard, J.D. (2005) Clostridium difficile toxins: mechanism of action and role in disease. *Clinical Microbiology Reviews*, 18(2), 247–263.

WHO (2009) *WHO Guidelines on Hand Hygiene in Health Care: a summary*. World Health Organization, Geneva.

Test Yourself

1. Semmelweiss was responsible for noting the importance of hand hygiene, when he recognised fever and subsequent death in large numbers of women following childbirth could have been prevented by doctors and midwives by washing their hands. In which year did he note this?
   (a) 1827
   (b) 1847
   (c) 1947
   (d) 1927

2. One of the most important aspects of infection prevention and control is:
   (a) Good hand hygiene
   (b) Washing hands with antibacterial soaps
   (c) Washing hands with antiviral soaps
   (d) Not allowing the hair to fall below the collar line

3. Which of the following is not considered an item of personal protective equipment?
   (a) Gloves and masks
   (b) Protective eyewear
   (c) A hair net
   (d) Chin-length plastic face shields

4. When caring for a patient with *C. Difficile*, you should:
   (a) Always wear PPE
   (b) Ensure hands are washed with soap and water
   (c) Ensure hands are cleaned with alcohol gel
   (d) Never wash with soap and water

5. Infections caused by, or associated with the treatments people receive are known as:
   (a) Patient-induced infections
   (b) Unavoidable infections
   (c) Iatrogenic infections
   (d) Healthcare-associated infections

6. The only vaccine currently available for tuberculosis is:
   (a) BCG vaccine
   (b) CTG vaccine
   (c) MMR vaccine
   (d) HCV vaccine

7. The risk of transmission of occupational exposure is:
   (a) Extremely high
   (b) Extremely low
   (c) None existent
   (d) No longer an issue

8. If you are in doubt about a specimen you have been asked to collect you should:
   (a) Take the specimen anyway
   (b) Take the specimen anyway and inform the laboratory
   (c) Seek advice
   (d) Ask the patient

9. When taking a swab from the aural region:
   (a) Do this first thing in the morning
   (b) Only ever do this last thing at night
   (c) Ensure that no topical antibiotics or other therapeutic agents have been administered for approximately three hours prior to sampling the area
   (d) Ensure that no topical antibiotics or other therapeutic agents have been administered for approximately one hour prior to sampling the area

10. Aseptic technique refers to:
    (a) Any procedure that is performed under sterile conditions
    (b) Any procedure that is performed under clean conditions
    (c) Any procedure involving blood
    (d) Any procedure that is only performed in the operating theatre

Answers

1. b
2. a
3. c
4. b
5. d
6. a
7. b
8. c
9. c
10. a

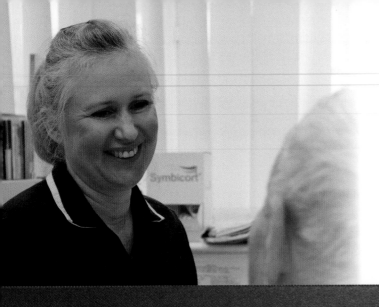

17

The Principles of Nutrition

Laureen Hemming

University of Hertfordshire, UK

Learning Outcomes

On completion of this chapter you will be able to:

- Outline why nutrition is a vital component of health care and essential for recovery from illness
- Describe the digestive system and the associated organs that aid digestion and the absorption of nutrients
- List the social and psychological factors that affect a person's ability to maintain an optimum nutritional status
- Explain the role of nutritional screening, particularly with the older population
- Discuss dietary options that will optimise a person's nutritional status whatever the underpinning pathology
- Explain why nutrition and hydration need to be considered when a person is at the end of their life

Competences

All nurses must:

1. Identify people who are at greater risk of being malnourished, either through undernourishment or obesity, using a nationally recognised screening tools when they are admitted to health care services
2. Advise carers how to supplement inadequate diets for those who need additional nutrients
3. Explain the impact illness has on a person's nutritional status, and the requirements needed to expedite recovery
4. Assist people who are ill to maintain their nutritional needs
5. Debate the values of continued nutritional support for vulnerable adults, including those who are at the end of life
6. Explain the roles of the multiprofessional team (dieticians, pharmacists and speech and language therapists) in supporting a person's nutritional status

 Visit the companion website at **www.wileynursingpractice.com** where you can test yourself using flashcards, multiple-choice questions and more.

Nursing Practice: Knowledge and Care, First Edition. Edited by Ian Peate, Karen Wild and Muralitharan Nair.
© 2014 John Wiley & Sons, Ltd. Published 2014 by John Wiley & Sons, Ltd. Companion website: www.wileynursingpractice.com

Introduction

Nutrition is vital for health – without food and water, we die; it is the process of ingesting, absorbing and utilising nutrients from the food and drink, and includes the elimination of the waste products resulting from these processes. The phrase 'to nurse' in America means to breast-feed your child; however, 'to nurse' in health care signifies much more and looking after a person's nutritional needs is an essential part of the nursing role – or it should be. Denny (2006) writes that too little emphasis has been placed on the importance of diet in medical and nurse education, which has resulted in significant problems for those who are ill. It was a point Florence Nightingale also made in 1859 but still rings true today!

What the Experts Say

" *Thousands of patients are starved annually in the midst of plenty from the want of attention to the ways which alone make it possible to take food.*
(Florence Nightingale's *Notes on Nursing*, cited in Brogden 2004)

Evidence from the National Confidential Enquiry into Patient Outcomes and Death (NCEPOD 2011) found a third old people (over 80 years of age) admitted to hospital were malnourished.

(Stewart 2011)

In the Rajasthan province of India, long ago, the Raj had doctors working with the chefs to determine the menus for the family to ensure that meals contained elements of ayurvedic medicine, which is found in food to maintain a healthy family. Rick Stein's India (televised 15 July 2013, on the BBC), reinforced the link that has always existed between nutrition and health. Spices contain many trace elements that are essential for a healthy body and the diet ideally should be balanced – that is, it should include proteins for tissue building and repair, carbohydrates for energy, fats for insulation and the production of cartilage, and fibre from fruit and vegetables to maintain a healthy gut and get rid of toxins and waste material that accumulates in the body. When we do not have a healthy balanced diet, we are at risk of developing diseases. Obesity is the cause of many diseases:

- Diabetes mellitus
- Hypertension
- Heart disease
- Cerebral vascular accidents
- Cancer.

There are also diseases that affect our ability to digest food and obtain nourishment from food, such as:

- Crohn's disease
- Folic acid deficiency
- Diverticular disease
- Cancer of the gastrointestinal organs.

What we eat and drink is largely determined by personal preferences, but is also significantly influenced by our culture, the society in which we find ourselves and for some, by religious doctrine. Nutrition is more than just 'refuelling the body', it has psychological, social, spiritual and cultural significance that remains, whether we are healthy or unwell. For some, meal times are a social event, a time when people gather to share part of their day and special occasions are marked with specific foods, for example there is feasting after Ramadan and Christians have special meals for Easter where eggs signify rebirth and re-emergence and a new beginning. We use food to demonstrate affection – special meals are organised to celebrate birthdays, weddings and funerals. Some cultures have stricter rules than others on what should be eaten when we are unwell, and beliefs about the foods that should be eaten to optimise health. There are also culturally determined rituals that need to be observed for food preparation and the eating of food. If a person is unable to wash their hands before eating, they may well decline food offered, thus compromising their nutritional status.

There are two significant healthcare problems related to malnutrition:

- Undernourishment: 1:3 older people admitted to hospital or care homes are malnourished (Todorovic 2011)
- Obesity.

These will be discussed in more depth later.

The Nutrients

Nutrients are classified as either:

- *Organic*, that is they have a chemical compound that contains carbon, such as carbohydrates, proteins, fats and vitamins
- *Inorganic*, that is they do not contain carbon, such as water, minerals and oxygen.

Some nutrients are needed in large quantities, such as carbohydrates and proteins and these are referred to as macronutrients; while others are needed in much smaller quantities, such as minerals and these are referred to as micronutrients. The body requires a balance of nutrients for optimal health and when it is under stress from illness or infection, it will require a different proportion of nutrients for repair and regrowth. The cells in the body produce cytokines, which are chemical messengers that instigate changes in cellular metabolism, so that the cells can access the nutrients they require for growth and repair. Initially, there is a **catabolic phase** where chemical reactions occur to break down complex compounds in the body, to produce energy and fuel for repair of the tissues, resulting in a surge of blood glucose levels. The body's insulin levels are not sufficiently high enough to cope with this surge and the raised blood sugar levels are noted by cells in the brain. By a process of feedback loops, the hypothalamus recognises this and depresses the appetite urge, resulting in the person experiencing anorexia. This reaction also stops the use of carbohydrates, which are stored in the liver as glycogen as the main source of energy and the body then utilises proteins from skeletal muscle as its main source of energy and fuel. In cancer, the cancer cells produce cytokines that enhance this action, which is why many people with cancer lose weight while still eating normally, which is referred to as cachexia (see Chapter 15). It is estimated that a person can lose up to 2.3 kg of weight in the first four postoperative days and this will affect their ability to recover, as it affects wound healing and the body's immune response, making them more susceptible to postoperative infections and hospital-acquired infections. This is why after a period of bed rest, people are very weak and lack muscle tone.

As the body recovers, it enters the **anabolic phase** where complex compounds are rebuilt and stored in the body. The rebuilding of proteins into skeletal muscle takes time and exercise helps the regeneration.

Nutrients are grouped as follows:

- Carbohydrates
- Fats
- Proteins
- Vitamins
- Minerals.

Carbohydrates

Carbohydrates are found in milk, honey, fruits, sugar cane and sugar beet in the form of monosaccharide's and disaccharides. They are also found in starchy foods, such as grains, pulses and root vegetables, in the form of polysaccharides. Once food is ingested, digested and metabolised, the carbohydrates are converted into glucose, the basic molecule, which is used in the body to form adenosine triphosphate (ATP) and that, in turn, produces the energy the cells require. Excess glucose is converted into glycogen and stored primarily in the liver. If the body does not have sufficient glucose circulating in the blood, it converts this glycogen in a process termed gluconeogenesis. Reserves of glycogen are also stored in the muscle and in fat as adipose tissue. Approximately 50% of our daily diet should consist of carbohydrates.

Proteins

Proteins are found in eggs, meat, fish, milk and products made from these, and are referred to as complete proteins because it is a form of protein the body can easily assimilate. These proteins are altered through the digestive process to become amino acids, which the body uses for growth and repair, the building of cells and development of enzymes. Other sources of proteins are found in legumes, nuts, grains, cereals and vegetables and are referred to as incomplete proteins. The process of altering these proteins into amino acids in the body is a little more complex; however, while not considered the optimum source of protein, they are perfectly adequate. People choosing a meat-free diet do not suffer any adverse consequences, providing they have sufficient protein from alternative sources such as these.

Fats (Lipids)

Fats are described as either *saturated* – and these are the fats that are found in animal products; or *unsaturated* fats – which are found in plants, as in seeds, nuts and vegetable oils. Fats are required in the diet because:

- They are the building blocks for the cell membranes
- They are in the form of triglycerides the a major source of energy in the muscle
- They are needed for the absorption and metabolism of fat soluble vitamins
- They are needed for the production of bile salts
- In the form of adipose tissue, they protect organs in the body and provide a layer of insulation under the skin, which keeps us from feeling the cold.

However, we can have too much and an excess fat (lipids) in the blood stream is termed *hyperlipidaemia*. There are two types of lipoproteins:

- *Low density lipoproteins (LDPs)*, which can be thought of as 'less desirable lipoproteins'. LDPs carry cholesterol (derived from metabolised animal fats) and any excess is deposited in artery walls as atheromatous plaques. These plaques can grow sufficiently large to occlude the blood vessels and lead to myocardial infarction or cerebral vascular accidents

- *High density lipoproteins (HDLs)* or 'highly desirable lipoproteins', which have a protective effect as they remove cholesterol from the arteries and transport it to the liver for excretion. HDLs are found in cold water fish, such as tuna, salmon, mackerel and we should consume at least three portions of fish a week to maintain a healthy balance in the body. HDL levels above 35 mg/dL have a protective effect, reducing the risk of coronary heart disease, while HDL levels lower than 35 mg/dL are associated with an increased risk.

A Mediterranean diet is often advocated, as it is based on the inclusion of olive oil in food preparation and this monounsaturated fat lowers LDLs and cholesterol, which is a healthy option. It also contains tomatoes rich in the antioxidant lycopene, a protective ingredient against prostate cancer, among others.

Vitamins

Vitamins are either *fat soluble* or *water soluble*. Fat soluble vitamins (A, D, E and K) are bound to ingested fats, so a fat-free diet would eliminate these vitamins and result in illnesses, such as rickets disease, where the bones soften and bow. Vitamin D is essential for the construction of bone, as it is required in the metabolism of calcium that is part of its formation. Vitamin D is also made in the body when cholesterol in the skin is radiated by ultraviolet rays from the sun. The use of suncreams with a high factor can prevent this happening and incidences of rickets in children are increasing (Patience 2013b). These fats are stored in adipose tissue in the body and an excess may lead to toxicity and ill health.

Vitamins C and B complex are water soluble, and these vitamins, usually found in green leafy vegetables, tomatoes and fruit, can leech out during a long cooking process and deteriorate during a long period of storage. These vitamins are absorbed in the gastrointestinal tract; excess amounts are excreted in the urine. Vitamin B_{12} requires special mention as it requires the presence of the intrinsic factor (a substance secreted by the gastric mucous membrane) before it can be absorbed. Absence of this leads to the person developing anaemia.

Vitamins are not required in large quantities but are vital to the maintenance of homeostasis.

Minerals

Essential minerals are:

- Calcium
- Iron
- Magnesium
- Phosphorus
- Potassium
- Sodium
- Sulphur.

All are required by the body and are found in food. Some manufacturers add extra minerals, such as sodium (salt), in their products, so we may unwittingly consume more than is necessary, which can have implications for health.

Minerals are essential for:

- Maintaining fluid balance in the cells and interstitial spaces
- Building and maintaining bones and health teeth
- Metabolising food and converting it to energy.

Minerals are found in all types of food, meat, fish, dairy, vegetables, fruit and nuts.

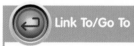

Figure 17.1 Proportions of nutrients for a healthy lifestyle.

Pie chart sections:
- Fruit and vegetables 5 different portions which include green, red and yellow coloured items
- Carbohydrates Bread, pasta, cereal, starchy foods
- A third of this section should be protein from either meat, fish, beans Another third should consist of dairy products and another third is reserved for food and drink high in fats and sugar.

A Healthy Diet

A healthy diet requires a balance of the nutrients listed above. To help everyone assess their dietary needs, the NHS advocates the 'eatwell plate', which gives an idea of the proportions of nutrients we need for a healthy lifestyle (Figure 17.1). Meals are generally divided into three a day, but when people are ill, they may not be able to face three meals but prefer smaller, more frequent meals or three meals with additional snacks in-between.

Link To/Go To

'Eatwell plate', NHS Choices

http://www.nhs.uk/Livewell/Goodfood/Pages/eatwell-plate
.aspx

A Protective Diet

There are three biochemical processes that occur in the body as part of metabolism or in response to environmental stressors and they are:

- Glycation, where glucose molecules bind with amino acid tissue, such as collagen and cause a breakdown at a cellular level, resulting in the loss of elasticity in the skin – in other words, it leads to the development of wrinkles
- Oxidation, a by-product of metabolism, where free radicals, that is chemicals, are released which have a free electron. The free electron clings to an electron of a fatty acid and results in lipid oxidation which causes ageing
- Inflammation is part of the body's response to toxic substances that it wishes to clear; however, it can be overwhelmed when there is too much glucose in the body.

A protective diet is one that is rich in protective nutrients and certain foods are known to be antioxidating, such as red fruits and vegetables, green leafy vegetables and broccoli. Lycopene and caro-

tenoids found in tomatoes are particularly protective of skin tissue against ultraviolet radiation damage.

An anti-inflammatory diet would be low in fats, dairy products, processed meats, alcohol and sugar. Shitake mushrooms, green tea, avocado, turmeric and ginger are rich in antioxidants and have anti-inflammatory properties (Pearson 2013).

People who suffer recurrent episodes of infection find a change in diet can halt the repetitive cycle.

Physiology of the Alimentary System

The alimentary or digestive system starts at the mouth and ends at the anus; it is called the gastrointestinal (GI) tract (Figure 17.2). It includes the oesophagus, stomach duodenum, jejunum, small intestine, the ascending, transverse and descending and sigmoid colon, the rectum and anal canal. In addition there are accessory organs that assist the digestive process: the liver, gall bladder, bile duct and pancreas.

The digestive system has six processes:

- The ingestion of food or, simply, eating and drinking
- The secretion of chemicals and enzymes that help break down the food into nutrients. The GI tract produces 7 litres of fluid a day
- The mixing and propulsion of food through the GI tract to prevent stasis at any point
- Digestion of food and this involves two processes:
  - Mechanical digestion, which is the teeth grinding the food prior to it being swallowed, and the churning of the food in the stomach and small intestine, to break it down further into a liquid
  - Chemical digestion, which is the action of various enzymes and chemicals to reduce the food to its nutrients in a form that can be absorbed by the cells
- Absorption of nutrient through the villi that line the colon into the lymph system
- The removal of waste products that are not absorbed through the process of defecation.

The Mouth

The mouth or buccal cavity is enclosed by the teeth, cheeks and palate and houses the tongue. It is lined with mucous membrane. Salivary glands in the floor of the mouth secrete saliva containing amylase in response to the chewing action, which starts the process of mixing food and breaking down the starches, so both mechanical and chemical digestion is taking place. There are three sets of glands:

- Parotid
- Submaxillary
- Sublingual.

The teeth (adults have 32 permanent teeth) masticate (chew and grind) the food, mixing it with saliva and altering the pH levels to being slightly alkali. If chewing bread for a little while, it takes on a sweeter flavour as a result of this. The chewed food passes into the oesophagus passing the pharynx.

The Oesophagus

The oesophagus is a conduit for food into the stomach, approximately 25 cm long and passes through the thorax and the diaphragm. It is a muscular tube lined with squamous and at the lower

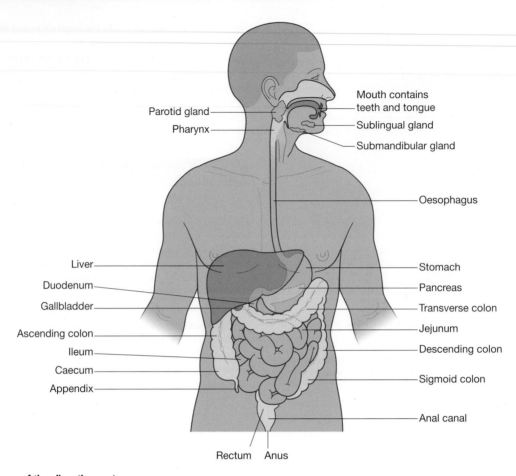

Figure 17.2 Organs of the digestive system.

end, simple stratified columnar epithelium. At the end, there is the gastro-oesophageal sphincter, which remains closed when food is not being swallowed to keep the contents of the stomach from flowing back into the oesophagus. The stomach contents are acid and when this flows back into the oesophagus (as it does after a large meal or after exercising too soon after a meal), it is felt as a burning sensation often referred to as 'heartburn'.

Red Flag

The heart lies above the stomach, and coronary pain can be misinterpreted and believed to be 'heartburn', which is usually treated by taking antacids. A myocardial infarction requires emergency treatment.

What other signs and symptoms would you look for if the patient was having a 'heart attack'?

The Stomach

The stomach is a large muscular sack with sphincters at either end, which can expand to accommodate 4 litres of food and fluid. It is divided into three regions:

- Cardiac
- Fundus
- Pyloric.

At the pyloric end, there is the pyloric sphincter, which is closed. This enclosed sack churns the food, mixing it with gastric juices produced from the secreting cells and gastric glands that line the inner wall, which is made up of columnar epithelial cells. The secretory cells are:

- *Mucus secreting cells*, which produce an alkaline mucus that protects the inner lining of the stomach from the acidic gastric secretions
- *Zymogenic cells*, which produce pepsinogen, a precursor to pepsin which is needed for the digestion of proteins
- *Parietal cells*, which secrete hydrochloric acid that is bactericidal and also helps with protein breakdown. These cells also produce the 'intrinsic factor', which is needed for the absorption of vitamin B_{12}
- *Enteroendocrine cells*, which produce hormones and hormone-like substances, such as gastrin, histamine, endorphins, serotonin and somatostatin. Gastrin affects the motility (movement) of the stomach, which churns and mixes food up.

There are three phases of gastric activity, or mechanical and chemical digestion:

1. *The cephalic phase*, when the stomach prepares to receive food triggered by the sight, smell and taste of food. The vagus nerve transmits motor impulses to the stomach
2. *The gastric phase* starts as food enters the cavity. Distension of the stomach, which activates stretch receptors in the stomach wall and chemical stimuli from the gastric glands, results in an influx of gastric juices from the cells listed above.

3. *The intestinal phase* occurs when the food is partially digested and ready to move into the small intestine. The food at this point is referred to as 'chyme'.

The whole process takes approximately 4–6 hours depending on the content of the meal eaten. If the meal is particularly fatty or high in fibre, it takes longer.

Thus, the stomach responds to endocrine and parasympathetic controls and the length and strength of motility depends on the secretion of gastrin and the amount of food ingested.

The Small Intestine

The small intestine is about 6 meters long and 2.5 cm wide and starts at the pyloric sphincter, coils around the abdominal cavity suspended by the mesentery and enters the ileocaecal junction, where it becomes the large intestine (see Figure 17.3). It is divided into three sections:

- The duodenum, which is 25 cm long and ends around the head of the pancreas. Pancreatic enzymes and bile from the liver via the bile duct enter the duodenum to mix with the chyme to continue with the digestion of lipids and sugars
- The jejunum is 2.4 m in length where further digestion and absorption of nutrients takes place
- The ileum is approximately 3.6 m long and meets the large intestine at the ileocaecal valve and continues with absorption of nutrients.

The inner lining of the small intestine is comprised of hundreds of folds, which increase the surface area of the intestine facilitating the absorption of nutrients through the intestinal wall into the blood stream. Throughout the lining, there are a variety of cells with special functions:

- *Absorptive cells*, which are fringed with microvilli (small hair-like projections), which filter out nutrients
- *Goblet cells*, which secrete mucus
- *Enteroendocrine cells*, such as those in the stomach which secrete hormones to aid digestion
- *Paneth cells*, which produce bacteriocidal lysozyme that has a phagocytic action and engulfs waste and unwanted products; it continues the cleansing action that started in the stomach with the production of hydrochloric acid.

The chyme entering into the small intestine still requires a great deal of work to break it down into nutrients that are capable of being absorbed and used by the cells of the body. The pancreatic juices, bile and enzymes produced in the small intestine, break down carbohydrates into monosaccharides; proteins into peptides and amino acids and fats into lipids and fatty acids. Of the nutrients, 90% are absorbed in the small intestine.

The Large Intestine or Colon

The final section of the digestive system is the large intestine or colon and is often described anatomically as the ascending colon, from the ileocaecal valve up to under the ribcage, where it turns across the abdomen and is called the transverse colon and at the left side, turns down to become the descending colon. As it nears the base, it turns inwards and is referred to as the sigmoid colon, which then becomes the rectum and ends at the anus. The colon has several functions:

341

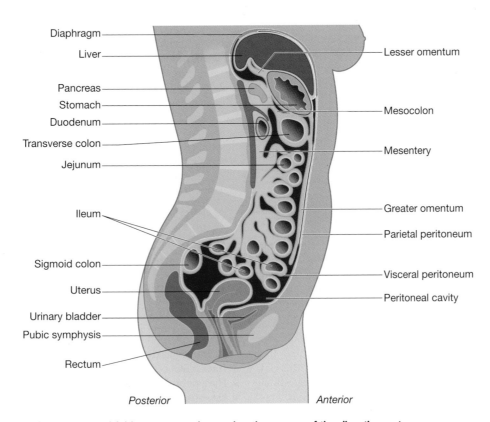

Diaphragm
Liver
Pancreas
Stomach
Duodenum
Transverse colon
Jejunum
Ileum
Sigmoid colon
Uterus
Urinary bladder
Pubic symphysis
Rectum

Lesser omentum
Mesocolon
Mesentery
Greater omentum
Parietal peritoneum
Visceral peritoneum
Peritoneal cavity

Posterior   *Anterior*

Figure 17.3 Relationship of the peritoneal folds to one another and to the organs of the digestive system.

- It continues to absorb nutrients but absorbs a great deal of water, turning the contents into a semi solid mass
- It produces vitamin K, vitamin B_1 and B_2 using folic acid
- It secretes mucus to lubricate faeces
- It stores indigestible foodstuffs until the time for defecation.

The difference in the large intestine compared with the small intestine, is the muscular layer in the walls. The large intestine has circular muscle and longitudinal muscles and they work together in a peristaltic movement, churning and pushing the contents towards the rectum and anus. Peristalsis is a wave of muscular movement, like ripples over the sea. The way the muscle is configured gives the colon a puckered appearance with pouches called haustra. When these pouches fill, the distension triggers muscle contractions. In babies, this is experienced as colic for the first three months of their lives, with some babies suffering more than others. The lining of the colon is similar to the small intestine and within it are intestinal glands that secrete mucus to lubricate the contents as they pass through; however, the colon has fewer folds or villi in its lining.

Chyme entering the colon is very fluid; however, the colon absorbs 90% of the water from this liquid, resulting in a semi-solid mass of matter, which becomes faeces. The process is aided by bacteria which break down proteins and decompose bile salts and the fermentation of the chyme results in the production of gas or flatulence. An excessive build up of flatulence can be painful; drinking warm water can help reduce the pain, as anything entering the stomach initiates the gastrocolic reflex, which triggers the peristaltic movement.

Peristalsis pushes the faecal matter into the sigmoid colon and then the rectum. As the rectum distends, sensory messages are received by the sacral spinal cord and in return, motor impulses influence the longitudinal muscles, which shorten and build up pressure in the rectum resulting in signals to the brain of a need to defecate.

The anal sphincter is under voluntary control, if it is voluntarily constricted, the sphincter does not open and defecation does not occur; however, when it is relaxed, defecation occurs and the rectum is emptied. Contraction of the diaphragm and abdominal muscles assist in propelling the faeces through the anus. If control is exerted, water continues to be absorbed from the faecal mass resulting in hard and dry faeces, which are harder to expel. This results in constipation. Constipation also occurs due to:

- Insufficient fluids being taken
- Insufficient fibre in the diet
- Lack of exercise
- Emotional stress being experienced
- A reaction by certain drugs – all analgesics are constipating as they bind with μ receptors that line the intestines. This has a direct affect on the muscular contractions, affecting the longitudinal muscles, slowing down the rate of peristaltic movement and allowing more water to be absorbed from the chyme.

Diarrhoea occurs when the chyme passes through the intestine too quickly. There is also increased peristaltic action and the volume reaching the rectum triggers the urge to defecate. This can be caused by food poisoning, where microbes irritate the intestinal lining, and it is the body's response to achieve homeostasis. Frequent bowel movements (or diarrhoea) results in electrolyte imbalance and dehydration.

Undernourishment and Malnutrition

Undernourishment is often referred to as malnutrition yet obesity is also malnutrition, because people are not eating the right foods for health or they are not eating the right quantities of the appropriate nutrients for health. There are identifiable groups of people who are at risk of being undernourished, the largest being the elderly and by this, we refer to those over the age of 75 years of age, however, many writers classify anyone over the age of 65 years as being old/elderly. Ageing is often associated with the development of the following chronic conditions and malnutrition can be both a cause and consequence of these:

- Diabetes
- Cancer
- Cardiovascular disease
- Osteoporosis
- Cognitive decline
- Anorexia of ageing
- Sarcopenia, which is the loss of muscle protein, which in turn leads to fatigue from loss of muscle function.

Undernourishment also affects:

- Recovery from illnesses
- Wound healing
- Immune response
- Respiratory efficiency
- Muscle strength

It can lead to feeling:

- Fatigued
- Depressed.

It can also lead to anaemia as a result of inadequate iron intake, which leaves the person feeling weak and at risk of falling, thus incurring other problems, such as fractures to wrists and hips (Shepherd 2009).

Malnutrition from undernourishment is defined as an inadequate intake of nutrients to provide sufficient energy to sustain body tissue and function and is associated with prolonged hospitalisation, however, it is estimated that 27% of elderly people admitted to hospital are already undernourished.

People who are undernourished spend an extra three days in hospital to recover and costs the NHS over £13 billion pounds per annum, twice as much as caring for people with obesity (Blaikley 2012). Most of these people are already undernourished when they are admitted to acute care (van der Kramer 2011; Timms 2011).

Jot This Down

Why do you think older people might have a poorer diet?
Besides physical illness and chronic conditions, such as those listed above, what else might impact on their attitude to food and their ability to provide food for themselves?

Elderly people can be at risk of undernourishment because they:

- Have a reduced appetite and therefore reduce their intake of food
- Have a reduced sense of taste, so food is no longer pleasurable
- Have poor dentition and cannot eat food that is hard to chew
- Have reduced manual dexterity and cannot manage cutlery
- Have poor posture, so cannot reach their food
- Have poor sight, so cannot see what they have to eat

- Have dysphagia and have difficulty in swallowing food
- May be taking medication that affects their flow of saliva and results in a dry mouth
- Have been recently bereaved and do not feel like eating
- May be suffering from depression
- May be lonely
- May not want to care for themselves
- May be unable to purchase and prepare food.

Elderly people residing in care homes have been found to be at greater risk of undernourishment than those living in the community on their own (Smith 2008).

Primary Care

Nurses working in primary care are in the best position to identify those elderly people that are undernourished and advise them to promote healthier living.

Shepherd (2009) points out that 38% of people aged over 65 years have low plasma levels of vitamin D; this is significant because vitamin D is needed for the absorption of dietary calcium from the intestines and metabolism of calcium and bone health. Insufficient vitamin D leads to osteomalacia and osteoporosis; it also plays a significant role in our ability to fight off infections. As people age, the immune system becomes less efficient, which results in the development of autoimmune diseases, chronic inflammatory disorders and cancer.

Normally, vitamin D is derived from milk and dairy products and sesame seeds; however, it is also produced in the body following exposure to sunlight. If the older person does not venture outside much, they are compromised. This is an example of how lifestyle can impact on a person's nutritional status.

If the older person reduces their activity and exercise levels, they also alter their metabolic needs, which may result on a reduced intake of food. Reducing the protein intake as well as the reduction of exercise leads to sarcopenia; reduced muscle strength has a cyclical effect on their ability to perform simple tasks, such as housework, going for walks, etc. The more sedentary the person becomes, the more at risk they are of developing malnutrition.

Van der Kramer (2011) highlights other significant factors that affect appetite and the desire to eat. The ambiance in which food is presented and the very presentation of food itself can affect the desire to eat. It may seem illogical, but food presented on china tastes better than when it is presented on disposable paper plates. The taste of drinks is altered by the use of plastic and paper utensils and for a person whose taste buds have been affected by their illness, the altered taste is sufficient to make them refuse drinks. Disposable plastic and wooden cutlery can also change the taste of food, which is unappetising. The size of food portions can also overwhelm a person who is ill.

Appetite is stimulated by the smell of food cooking; however, some smells can have the opposite effect if it is a food that the person does not like. Hospital wards can have various aromas, the one that is missing is of food being cooked as the food arrives precooked in trolleys or sealed packets.

Weight loss and cancer

Approximately 80% of people developing cancer notice weight loss as the first symptom that all is not well; this and pain is what prompts them to seek medical advice (Holder 2003). The weight loss is termed 'cancer cachexia' because the triggers and responses are different to weight loss from starvation. In cancer, the tumour produces cytokines (chemical messengers) that alter cellular metabolism, so that the tumour has the requisite nutrients to grow and develop. The changes affect the liver's ability to convert stored glucose and promote resistance to insulin. As a consequence, the person has a raised basal metabolic rate (BMR) and has a higher blood sugar level, which depresses the appetite. The cytokines can also alter the motility of the digestive tract, so food takes longer to process and this also affects a person's appetite; they still feel full from the previous meal.

Cancer treatments can also affect a person's nutritional status. Chemotherapy regimens lead to:

- Feeling nauseous
- Dysgeusia (altered taste)
- Xerostomia (dry mouth – as seen above, saliva is needed to commence digestion of food in the mouth)
- Mucositis (inflammation, possibly with infection, of the mucosa from the mouth to the bottom of the oesophagus, which is very painful)
- Dysphagia (difficulty in swallowing)
- Hyperosmia (altered sense of smell, which can affect the desire to eat).

Loss of more than one-fifth of the person's body weight means they have a poor prognosis and they are much less likely to respond to treatment. Approximately one in five people with cancer die because of malnutrition, rather than the cancer itself.

343

Screening for malnutrition

Undernourishment and malnutrition have been identified as a serious problem in the UK, particularly in the older population, which is often undetected and untreated. It is estimated that 3 million people in the UK are malnourished (Wilson & Blackett 2012). Two bodies: the National Institute for Health and Clinical Excellence (NICE) and the British Association of Parenteral and Enteral Nutrition (BAPEN) recommend the use of the Malnutrition Universal Screening Tool (MUST), as it has proved to be valid, reliable and suitable for use in all healthcare settings, and it can be used as a self-assessment tool (Parsons 2011).

Link To/Go To

For a free download of the screening tool, go to:
www.bapen.org.uk/pdfs/must/must-full.pdf

The screening tool is based on working out the person's body mass index (BMI), which is a simple calculation of dividing the person's weight by their height squared: kg/m^2. The MUST tool has this calculated and tabulated for ease of use (Fletcher 2009). However, screening requires a holistic perspective and should include assessment of the following:

- Physical assessment
  - History of recent weight loss
  - Whether the person has dentures and if these fit
- The person's ability to prepare food or feed themselves

- Social assessment
  - Do they live at home or are they in residential care
  - Do they live alone
  - Can they shop for food
- Psychological assessment
  - Has the person recently experienced a bereavement
  - Are they depressed
  - Is there any cognitive impairment
- Clinical assessment
  - What is their medical status
  - Does this affect the person's ability to feed themselves
  - Does it affect their ability to eat
  - Does it affect their ability to digest food?

While nurses can undertake screening, a full nutritional assessment needs to be undertaken by a qualified dietician, who uses biochemical and anthropometric measurements in addition to the data collected above.

Some people will require additional assessment from a Speech and Language Therapist (SALT assessment) as they determine whether the swallowing reflex is capable of coping with eating and drinking. This is particularly important for people who have had a cerebral vascular accident (CVA) or for people with advanced dementia.

Red Flag

When weighing patients:
- It is important that the scales are calibrated and well maintained
- People who are being weighed should be in similar clothes each time, as this makes a difference
- Check whether the person has developed oedema or if they are dehydrated, as this can change their weight.

What the Experts Say

Mitchell (2011) citing work undertaken by Age UK, offers the following 7-step guide to reducing incidences of hospital-acquired malnutrition:

1. Hospital staff must actively listen and record dietary advice given by relatives of those in their care
2. Everyone working in the health service should be 'food aware'
3. Everyone admitted to hospital should be assessed for signs of malnutrition
4. Where possible, meal times should mean that no treatments, investigations, tests are conducted during this time
5. A 'red tray' system should be introduced to highlight who needs help with feeding
6. Trained volunteers should be recruited to help with meal times
7. Healthcare professionals should abide by their professional codes of conduct and ensure no harm befalls those in their care.

Red tray system

The 'red tray system' has been introduced to highlight those people in acute care settings who have difficulty in feeding themselves. The aim is bring to the attention of staff in acute care that a person

cannot feed themselves and needs assistance and that uneaten food needs to be brought to the attention of the healthcare professionals (Fletcher & Carey 2011).

Appetite stimulants

As seen above, the smell of food cooking is an appetite stimulant, and unpleasant smells has the opposite effect. There are other ways in which the appetite can be stimulated; chefs in restaurants offer an 'amuse-bouche', which is a small, tasty bite-sized piece of food that stimulates the taste buds in the tongue and stimulates the salivary flow. Alcohol in small measures as an aperitif has been used for years and also works in a similar manner. There are drugs that can be prescribed:

- Megestrol acetate
- Dexamethasone
- Progestagens
- Cannabinoids.

However, these do produce side-effects and may not improve quality of life significantly.

Nutritional Support

There are three levels of nutritional support:

1. Giving oral supplements to enhance the dietary intake
2. Enteral feeding
3. Parenteral feeding.

Food Fortification

It is better to keep a person eating if at all possible before resorting to invasive measures, such as enteral or parenteral feeding. There are many reasons why someone is not taking in an adequate diet, ranging from feeling despondent and not wanting to eat to having poorly-fitting dentures, which make eating difficult.

Food can be fortified by adding extra proteins, such as adding cheese to mashed potatoes, or eggs to sauces; extra carbohydrates can be added with the addition of cream; extra fats can be added by using butter.

Nutritional supplements often come as pre-packed branded formulas; some people tolerate them very well but others find the taste, smell and texture difficult. Some taste better at room temperature, while others prefer them to be very cold or even frozen and served as ice-cream. They should always been given after food rather than before food, as they can depress the appetite (Shepherd 2009).

Fish oils

A great deal of interest has been shown in the use of fish oils as a supplementary product. Fish oils are rich in omega 3 fatty acids (eicosapentaenoic acid, EPA) and are thought to interfere with the metabolic changes that occur, especially the use of skeletal muscle protein as an energy source. Although research into this has mixed results, adding omega 3 fatty acids to the diet in the early stages of cancer, do seem to slow down the weight loss.

Enteral Feeding

Enteral feeding is introduced when a person has swallowing difficulties and requires a tube to be passed through the nose or mouth and down into the stomach. People requiring this type of feeding may have head and neck cancer or they may have had a cerebral vascular accident or some type of brain injury or illness that affects their neurological control of the swallowing reflex, putting them at risk of choking on food and fluids. There are a variety of enteral feeding tubes currently available on the market, the two main types are:

- *Nasogastric tubes*, which are used as a short-term method of feeding; these can have a fine bore but are more susceptible to blocking, while wider bore tubes are more uncomfortable for the person
- *Percutaneous endoscopic gastrostomy (PEG or gastrostomy 'button') tubes*, which are inserted under general anaesthetic into the stomach and are more permanent, as they are sutured in place. The majority of people requiring enteral feeding have a PEG tube fitted. The tube may be inserted into the jejunum (percutaneous endoscopic jejunostomy, PEJ). The gastrostomy 'buttons' protrude less, they rest flush with the abdominal wall and are less noticeable under clothing than the PEG tube.

Feeds can be given intermittently or over a longer period of time controlled by a pump. It is usual not to feed during the night, as this represents circadian rhythms.

Enteral feeding is undertaken in all care settings: hospital, home, residential care and there are home enteral nutrition (HEN) teams, comprising nutrition nurses specialists, district nurses, dieticians and speech and language therapists, who monitor and advise on care given in the community (Omorogieva 2010).

What the Experts Say

People receiving oral or enteral feeding in the community need to be assessed every 3 months by healthcare professionals trained in his field, to determine whether their needs have changed.

There are complications to this type of feeding. While a dietician can ensure the person has their full daily requirement of nutrients, this type of feeding does not depress the appetite and the person can still experience hunger pangs, even after being recently fed. Complications can be divided into those that are feed-related, stoma-related or tube-related.

Feed-related complications Long-term feeding can result in:

- Diarrhoea
- Constipation
- Bloating
- Nausea.

The dietician may need to adjust the content of the feed to prevent diarrhoea and constipation and antiemetics may be administered to control the nausea.

Stoma-related complications While the tube is inserted under aseptic conditions, it is difficult to maintain sterility of the area. The skin around the tube entrance to the stomach (stoma) requires being kept clean and dry to prevent infection developing at the site.

Tube-related complications The tube can dislodge, become blocked or the end can become buried in the wall of the stomach.

Nasogastric tubes are easier to become dislodge, especially if the person vomits or has a fit of coughing, as they may be only secured by tape across the bridge of the nose, which means that before giving any feed, the nurse must check that the tube is indeed in the stomach and not in the lungs or coiled at the back of the throat. If the person has dysphagia, they may not be able to feel the tube, and certainly will have difficulty in coughing up fluid that is going down into the trachea. A simple way to determine whether the tube is in the stomach is to withdraw some fluid using a syringe and test its pH level using pH strips as the stomach contents are usually acidic. If the PH recording is less than 5.5 it is advisable to check that the tube is correctly placed by X-ray.

To prevent blockages of the tube, warm water should always follow a feed (called 'flushing') to keep the tube patent. Moving the person may help to dislodge the tube if it is resting on the wall of the stomach but if the tube is suspected of being buried in the stomach lining, an X-ray needs to be taken to establish this and a gastroenterologist will remove the tube.

Psychosocial affects of enteral feeding

The person being fed in this manner may experience feelings of frustration, loss of control and anger at the perceived alterations to their body image. They may interpret being fed as a return to their childhood and these feelings may impinge on the way they react socially, resulting in isolating themselves from others (Holmes 2010).

Nursing care and management

The nurse is responsible for managing enteral feeding, as they have to ensure that the feeding tube is correctly sited before the feed commences; other staff may be involved if they have the requisite knowledge and skills. The procedure for administering a feed is as follows:

- Wash hands thoroughly. Hygiene is important, as nutritionally compromised people are more at risk of acquiring an infection. The person receiving the feed may also require their hands to be washed, even though they may not be feeding themselves, as it is part of the routine preparation people engage in before eating. For some, this may have cultural significance and not washing their hands is perceived as being disrespectful and dirty
- Clean the patient's mouth using a soft toothbrush, as this stimulates the gastric juices in preparation for digesting the feed
- Ensure the person having the feed has been adequately prepared and they are in a sitting position if their medical condition permits this, or they are lying on their left side. The person should remain at an upright angle following the feed for at least an hour, to prevent reflux (the feed flowing back into the oesophagus from the stomach)
- Ensure that the correct feed for the individual being fed is used, as feeds are calculated to meet individual nutrient requirements by the dietician
- The nasogastric (NG) tube requires flushing with either cooled boiled water (in the home setting) or sterile water in the hospital setting to ensure that it is patent
- A 50/60 mL syringe without a barrel is attached to the NG tube and the feed is poured in gradually, this is referred to as gravity feeding, as the feed flows down the tube by gravitational pull. The feed should never be forced in with a syringe barrel.

345

Red Flag

Syringes and giving sets used for enteral feeding are specifically designed for non-intravenous use.

They are coloured purple to distinguish them.

This is to minimise the risk of giving the wrong type of feed to a person by the wrong method, which could lead to death (Fletcher 2011).

The alternative to gravity feeding is to use a pump, which administers the feed at a slower, controlled rate.

Once the feed has been administered, the nurse needs to:

- Flush the tube with water as undertaken at the beginning of the procedure, to ensure the tube is clear and clean following the feed
- Remove the syringe or pump and spigot of the end of the tube
- Ensure the person is comfortable and remaining with head and shoulders raised higher than the stomach
- Clear away equipment used and leave clean equipment available for the next feed
- Wash hands thoroughly at the end
- Record the amount of feed given and the time of the feed in the person's nursing documentation.

Care, Dignity and Compassion

While giving a person a feed via the tube, remember it is their feeding time. Eating and drinking is usually a pleasurable, and often a social event, so it is important to replicate this as far as possible and communicate directly with the person, even if they cannot respond verbally.

It is essential not to appear rushed, even if you are under pressure of work.

Parenteral Feeding

Parenteral feeding is introduced when a person's gastrointestinal tract is not functioning or accessible for feeding by other methods. Parenteral feeding is inserting nutrients directly into the bloodstream. The solutions infused contain amino acids, glucose, fats, electrolytes, vitamins and minerals. Some commercial preparations do not contain all the minerals and vitamins but these can be supplemented, according to individual need.

Parenteral nutrition can be administered through a peripheral cannula or a peripheral inserted central catheter (PICC line) in the short term, but if the person requires longer-term therapy, a Hickman line or Broviac device is inserted into the subclavian or internal jugular vein, proving central venous access. These lines/ devices are usually inserted in theatre or X-ray environments, as they are checked for accurate placing by X-ray and it is a surgical procedure. The line is held in place by a Dacron cuff, which provides a barrier to infection as it binds with the subcutaneous tissue.

Inserting lines centrally carries the risk of causing pneumothorax, as well as the possibility of introducing infection. The person requires close monitoring, as electrolyte imbalances can occur.

Professional and Legal Issues

As it is technically possible to keep someone alive through parenteral nutrition; the question arises about when to stop treatment

The dilemmas occur when a person is in the terminal stages of cancer or if they are in the advanced stages of dementia, while families may wish to influence decisions, they are not legally entitled to do so, unless they have a 'Lasting Power of Attorney' negotiated and in place (see Chapter 20)

Parenteral feeding does not necessarily extend life expectancy, so the issue concerns 'quality of life' (Holmes 2011).

However, it is difficult to measure quality of life; it is a subjective determinant:

- How would you determine 'quality of life'?
- When do the risks of parenteral nutrition outweigh the benefits to the person?

Obesity

Obesity is a growing problem in both developing and developed countries with over a billion people affected. Ashwell (2010) predicts that by 2025, over half of all men and one-third of all women will be obese. Obesity is associated with the development of non-communicable chronic conditions such as:

- Type 2 diabetes
- Hypertension
- Cardiovascular disease
- Cancer
- Raised blood cholesterol level, which leads to arteriosclerosis, resulting in occlusion of vessels.

Meetoo (2010) offers one explanation for the growth of this problem, as being the extent to which globalisation has occurred. That is, the international economic expansion with its associated political and social interdependence has resulted in a flow of people from rural areas and lifestyles into urban living. Urban living requires less energy expenditure than rural living, it also necessitates a different lifestyle, where food is bought, and convenience food or 'fast' food is easier to obtain and prepare for consumption. Meetoo claims that traditional diets are replaced by 'obesogenic' diets; India now has the highest number of people with type 2 diabetes and a record number of people with cardiovascular disease. He believes that marketing campaigns promote cheap food with high fat and calorie content, fast-food chains that contribute to a 'toxic' environment and altered patterns of living.

Wright (2011) points out that obesity, while being a significant problem now, has been a health problem in the past as well. Hippocrates, in 400BC associated certain deaths with obesity; William Harvey, who dissected obese cadavers from 1679, realised that obesity had a significant shortening of life-expectancy. Savarin, writing in 1854, noted that the difference between animals and humans was that humans ate for pleasure, rather than just hunger and thirst.

Obesity is defined as having a BMI over $30 \, kg/m^2$, however, there is debate over this classification and waist measurements are a more significant indicator of obesity. A preferred indication is either waist to hip ratio or waist to height ratio, where the waist measurement should be half of the height (Ashwell 2010).

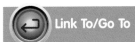

Link To/Go To

Work out your waist to height ratio using the chart at:

http://www.ashwell.uk.com/shapechart.pdf

Causes of Obesity

A simplistic explanation is to say that a person consumes more food than their energy expenditure requires but raising their energy expenditure to match the calories consumed does not totally rectify the problem. Lazarou and Kouta (2010) point out that the propensity to developing obesity can start in the womb; obesity in pregnancy results in alternations to neuroendocrinological function and energy metabolism in the fetus. Babies fed on formula milk rather than being breast-fed are more likely to develop obesity, as are children who are offered larger than needed meals. Children and adolescents who eat regularly are less likely to become obese.

Breakfast Consumption and Its Relationship with Obesity

A review of research trials held by the Cochrane Central Register of Controlled Trials, reveals that people (adults and children) who regularly eat cereal for breakfast have, on the whole, a lower BMI and are more likely to eat regular meals and less likely to snack or graze in between mealtimes. However, 'breakfast skippers' are more likely to be obese. The statistical differences are not as significant for those who have a fruit and vegetable breakfast or a meat or egg breakfast, however, these people are also less likely to be obese (Ashwell 2010).

Obesity and Poverty

Families on low incomes are more likely to have a poorer diet and are more susceptible to illnesses connected to this. This was first highlighted by Joseph Rowntree in 1901 (Glasper 2010). Low-income families tend to eat more processed foods, with a lower nutrient content than the rest of society. According to the Child Poverty Act (2010), there are 2.8 million children living in poverty in the UK (Patience 2013a). This may mean they are undernourished but they may also be obese because they are eating more carbohydrates than fruit and vegetables. These families rely more on local corner shops, because they do not own a car or drive, where prices are higher and choices are fewer than in the large 'out of town' supermarkets, and where stock of fresh produce is limited because that not sold is wasted. The government has set up a financial incentive under the title 'Change4life' in order to improve the situation for corner shops. Change4life also includes advice for families on diet, shopping tips, menu swaps and exercises to promote healthier lifestyles but the website relies on families having access to home computers.

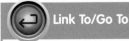

Link To/Go To

To find out more and access free posters, games and activities that can be used with all age groups to promote healthier living, see the Change4life website:

http://www.nhs.uk/Change4Life/Pages/why-change-for-life.aspx

It is possible to maintain healthy nutrition on a low income if:

- Meals are planned in advance and impulse buys are avoided
- Cheaper cuts of fresh meat are bought and cooked longer
- Fresh fruit and vegetables are bought in smaller quantities and kept refrigerated
- Meat sauces are bulked up with pulses, beans and high fibre vegetables
- Water is drunk instead of commercial sugary drinks
- Cereal breakfast is eaten every morning.

Diabetes and Nutrition

It is estimated that 2.9 million people in the UK have diabetes, 90% of these have what is referred to as type 2 diabetes and it is predicted that these numbers will rise with the obesity 'epidemic'. This occurs when the body does not produce enough insulin in the pancreas to meet the demand and is strongly associated with obesity. It is treated with a drug that stimulates the pancreas to produce more insulin and block the factors that produce insulin resistance within the body. Type 1 diabetes occurs when the body does not produce any insulin and this is treated with insulin injections or continuous infusion via a pump.

Nutrition is the corner stone for managing diabetes and weight reduction may mean that pharmacological interventions are not required for type 2 diabetes. People with diabetes are at greater risk of developing eating disorders, depression and can be at risk of malnutrition. Hyperglycaemia (raised blood sugar levels) is linked to poor wound healing, dehydration and depressed immune function (Hughes 2012). Medication to reduce glucose levels may result in hypoglycaemia (low blood sugar levels), so nutritional intake needs to be finely balanced to maintain an optimum level of blood glucose in the body. If the person with diabetes develops depression and does not eat as a result, it has consequences for their diabetes. Jennings (2011) points out that 85% of people with diabetes do not get much needed psychological support to help them to adapt to their condition. Nutritional advice for the person with diabetes is:

- Eat three meals a day
- Eat high protein diet and avoid low fat versions
- Eat at least two portions of fish a week
- Drink plenty but avoid sugary drinks
- Increase fruit and vegetable consumption
- Include beans and pulses in the diet
- Include starchy carbohydrates but reduce sugar and sugary foods
- Reduce saturated fats
- Reduce salt
- Limit alcohol
- Avoid using manufactured diabetic drinks and foods.

The focus should be on what the person can eat rather than on what they should avoid, as this approach is more motivational (Mellor 2012). Chocolate and cake is permissible in moderation, as long as a balance is achieved (Hughes 2012).

Nutrition and Mental Illness

Research studies demonstrate the interrelationship between food and our emotional state and people with mental health issues adopt dietary practices that are not conducive to health (Dunne 2012). There is evidence that demonstrates that those with severe mental health illnesses, such as schizophrenia and bipolar disorders have a poor nutritional status: people with schizophrenia tend to be less active, have irregular meals, have inadequate amounts of fruit and vegetables in their diet. The antipsychotic medication they receive can also result in these people gaining weight and there is an increased risk of acquiring type 2 diabetes (Jennings 2011). Weight gain is most noticeable in younger, newly diagnosed people and this altered body image further impacts on them when they already have a lowered self-esteem, making supporting them difficult. A great deal depends on their readiness to change their lifestyle and eating patterns. To work effectively, the brain requires:

- *Carbohydrates*, especially the complex starchy variety as this maintains a constant blood level longer
- *Amino acids*, serotonin levels are lower in people with depression and this affects mood and sleep patterns. Serotonin is a chemical messenger that transmits nerve impulses
- *Essential fatty acids*, particularly omega 3 and omega 6, which are found in oily fish also help with the transmission of nerve impulses
- *Vitamins*, particularly the B vitamins
- *Minerals*, iron and selenium, which is found in nuts, broccoli and chicken
- *Water*.

Caffeine, while it stimulates the brain and neuronal activity, may also affect sleeping and the brain does need to rest as part of the circadian body rhythm.

Harbottle (2011) points out that there is now evidence that a sugar-rich diet is positively correlated to the incidence of clinical depression. Sugar has addictive properties and is used in convenience foods, such as biscuits, to make food more palatable. Caffeine is used as an energy boost when the person is feeling lethargic but it increases levels of agitation and anxiety, thus increasing symptoms of depression. Alcohol consumption tends to increase when a person is feeling depressed, but its diuretic effect leads to dehydration, which increases irritability and low mood.

Antidepressant and antipsychotic treatments also have an impact on people that results in weight gain: antidepressants decrease the basal metabolic rate, antipsychotics make people feel hungry, so they eat more. Weight gain has a negative impact on body image and self-esteem, prompting the person to try and diet to lose the excess weight but it usually ends in a repetitive cycle, with associated mood swings.

Nutrients that Improve Depression

Studies have shown the people who are depressed have lower levels of certain nutrients and there is a beneficial effect when these are provided in the diet. Nutrients that are required are:

- Vitamin B_{12}
- Zinc
- Selenium
- Vitamin D.

These nutrients are found in nuts and cereals, fruit and vegetables and pulses, in short, in a balanced diet. Advice to a person suffering with depression is to:

- Eat regular meals
- Always start with breakfast, which includes cereals and milk; cereals three times a day is better than snack feeding on food with high sugar content
- Include protein at each meal to provide tryptophan, which enhances mood
- Have fish three of four times a week as the fatty acids (omega 3 and 6)

- Drink at least 2 litres of fluid a day
- Restrict caffeine and alcohol intake.

The nerves are made up of fats and there is now some suggestion that insufficient fat intake may be linked to the onset of dementia but this has yet to be proven. The neurotransmitters, the chemical messengers transmitting signals from one nerve to another require amino acids.

People with Dementia

Dementia is an umbrella term covering over 100 different types of progressive, incurable conditions that affect memory, recall and language, which result in altered behaviour patterns. It is the fourth leading cause of death in those over the age of 65 years. The most common types are Alzheimer's disease and vascular dementia. People with dementia exhibit:

- Amnesia, where they fail to remember names, where they are, what they were about to do
- Agnosia, where they fail to recognise familiar people and objects
- Aphasia, where they fail to recognise words or find words to express themselves
- Apraxia, where they can no longer coordinate movement
- Associated psychological and social behavioural symptoms of distress.

All of the above can affect their nutritional status, as they may forget to eat, forget what to use in the way of cutlery, fail to perceive what is presented as food and fail to feed themselves because of lack of coordination. The dementia may cause changes to the sense of smell and taste, so the person does not recognise the food they are being given, adding sugar or honey to sweeten food may make it more appetising and the extra calories do not make a significant impact.

People with dementia may also have a greater need for more calories than an older person might require, as they may expend more energy through constant walking and agitated behaviours; have a raised basal metabolic rate; they may exhibit aggressive behaviour when they are hungry and in pain but cannot express their needs to others. They frequently suffer from night hunger and should have fortified warm drinks (with skimmed milk powder added) at bedtime to sustain them through the night. Meal times should be regular, and adhere to a similar ritual or pattern. Finger food is easier to manage than cutlery.

As the disease progresses, they may develop dysphagia, difficulty in swallowing and will require a SALT assessment. They may also refuse to eat, which is extremely distressing for their families. This is usually a sign that they are now in an advanced stage of dementia, however, it is difficult to predict if they have reached the dying phase, which makes decisions about nutritional support difficult and contentious. However, tube feeding has been shown to:

- Not improve functional status
- Not to prolong survival
- Not to improve pressure sore outcomes
- Not to reduce infection
- Add a risk of aspiration pneumonia
- Increase agitation
- Result in distress and discomfort to the person.

Care does not stop when feeding does; the families need support when coming to terms with the fact that this signals the dying phase and that the person no longer needs nourishment, as their body is now effectively shutting down (Barber & Murphy 2011).

Hydration

A chapter on the principles of nutrition is incomplete without mention of fluid intake. In addition to nutrients, a person requires 1.5–2 litres of fluid a day. Some fluid is obtained through the diet, as food is not dry, but drinks are essential to life. Unfortunately, children are offered sugary drinks and become customised to taking fluid in that form. As adults, we may take fluid in the form of tea and coffee, which contain caffeine and that has a deleterious effect if consumed in large quantities. Fluids are needed to enable the body to flush out harmful toxins that accumulate as part of the metabolic pathways. When fluids are not given, acute kidney damage may occur and in the elderly and this may be irreversible.

A recent newspaper headline:

Thousands dying of thirst on NHS.

Borland, *Daily Mail* Wednesday, 28 August 2013

While headlines are designed to capture sales, the report that ensues causes concern. It reports that 210 000 people are estimated to have died in the last year from dehydration. Guidelines are to be issued by the government that details routine testing of everyone admitted to health care, and in particular all those over the age of 65, of their hydration levels and to instigate methods of rehydration, whether orally or intravenously. It is important that nurses keep accurate records, on fluid balance charts, of the person's intake and urinary output and alert medical teams if there is significant imbalance, especially if the person is critically ill.

If a person is unable to drink until the cause of their problems have been established, then intravenous fluids need to be administered.

Nutrition and Wound Healing

Wounds heal by either primary or secondary intention (Nazarko 2013). Wounds healing by primary intention are clean, usually surgical, where the two skin edges are joined, either by sutures, staples or tape and it is a simple matter of connective tissue building up to seal the wound. Healing by secondary intention is far more complex, as these wounds are open as in ulcers and burns, where the healing edges are not closed and granulation has to occur from the wound bed. These wounds are significantly difficult to heal if the person is malnourished.

A severe grade 4 pressure ulcer will cost the NHS up to £10 551 before healing takes place. It also affects a person's quality of life, as they will experience pain and loss of physical ability, which has repercussions on their social life (Medlin 2012).

Wound healing has three distinct stages:

1. The inflammatory stage where fluid and cells flood into the areas part of the immune response and this lasts 3–6 days. During this time, adjacent healthy cells may become damaged. Vitamin K and calcium are required to build a fibrin mesh that is the basis for cell regeneration. Vitamin C protects vitamin E, a lipid soluble antioxidant, which is needed to protect cellular membranes. Zinc and copper are also needed for the formation of granulation tissue, which seals the wound. Zinc is bacteriocidal and enhances the immune response. These micronutrients are important because without them, wound healing takes longer.

2. The proliferative or building stage starts approximately 3 days after the injury and lasts up to 3 weeks. During this phase, the body requires all nine essential amino acids, arginine and glutamine (which are cytokines), glucose, vitamin C and iron to produce collagen, which makes new connective tissue. Vitamin C helps white blood cells to flood into the area, enhancing a resistance to developing infection. If there is not enough glucose, the body utilises fat and sugars in muscle to meet its needs, resulting in muscle wastage and fatigue developing.

3. The remodelling stage follows this and is where tissue returns to normal homeostasis. This can take up to two years, depending on the wound (Sherman & Barkley 2011).

Nutritional needs for wound healing are dependent on:

- *The type and severity of the wound*: surgical wounds heal relatively quickly, whereas, pressure ulcers, burns and chronic wounds take much longer
- *Comorbidities*: diseases of the liver, kidney, heart and gastrointestinal tract can alter metabolic nutrient requirements and the available nutrients for wound healing
- *The nutritional state of the person at the time the wound occurred*: if the person is well nourished, they will heal quicker but if they are already malnourished or undernourished, it will take longer.

It is estimated that a person's protein needs are 1–1.4 g/kg ideal body weight, and for wound healing, this rises to 2 g/kg ideal body weight, in cases of severe wounds. Wounds that have a high exudates loss will require 3 g/kg ideal body weight of protein. The person also requires 100–200 mg/day of vitamin C, which is available if they can eat at least 5 portions of fruit and vegetables (excluding potatoes) a day. This diet would also give the person sufficient zinc, iron and copper to facilitate wound healing.

In addition to proteins, a person requires an adequate carbohydrate intake, as the body's cells will use protein for energy if there is insufficient carbohydrate, thus depleting the reserves of protein for wound healing to take place.

If a person cannot manage this diet, then the nutrients need to be gained from food supplements, of which there are many preparations and it is largely a matter of personal choice. There are many commercially prepared nutritious drinks that are either milk or fruit based, which contain all the essential amino acids.

In addition to diet, the person needs to be kept well hydrated as dehydrated skin does not heal well and is liable to tear; it also helps to clear the body of waste products.

Nutrition for the Person Who Is Dying

As people reach the end of their life and their condition is deemed terminal, whatever their disease, their nutritional status alters in the following ways:

- Bodily functions slow down, this includes gastric emptying and absorption of nutrients, so there is less need for food and drink
- Medication used, such as analgesics and sedatives, alter their sense of taste and desire for food
- Fatigue and lack of energy also depresses the appetite
- Psychologically, the person just does not feel like eating; it ceases to be important to them.

This can cause great distress, particularly to those (family and friends) who care deeply and would like to see the person make every effort to stay alive (Holmes 2011). Some cultures do not hold with 'giving up' as death approaches and this can cause increased tension between all involved.

The Liverpool Care Pathway has not made decisions about nutrition easy either, as there is some debate as to whether tube-feeding is a medical treatment or not. It raises several ethical questions, such as:

- Should people die because of lack of nourishment?
- Should nutritional support be withdrawn knowing it will lead to death?
- Will the withdrawal of nutritional support cause suffering rather than offer relief of suffering?

The aim of end of life care is to:

- Provide relief of physical symptoms, such as pain, breathlessness, terminal agitation
- Provide social, psychological and spiritual support to the person and those closest to them
- Allow the person to live until they die and maintain their 'quality of life'
- Not artificially hasten death but allow death with dignity.

Exemplary palliative care shifts the focus from the disease to the person, enabling them to live until they die, and participate in making choices as to how their symptoms are managed and supporting them in their choices where it is possible to do so. This includes respecting their wishes with regard to their diet and fluid intake.

While nutrition does not prolong life, it does allow the person:

- Strength and time to meet their goals and objectives they have set
- Death with dignity and not from starvation
- Control over their disease process; dehydration can cause pain as the inactive metabolites of morphine are not flushed out of the body, thus blocking active metabolites from linking to the pain receptors and suppressing the painful stimuli (Acreman 2009).

Nutritional Nursing Care for the Person at the End of Life

Nursing care commences with assessment, the MUST tool has been outlined above. In addition, the nurse needs to establish:

- How the person views their nutritional status – what are their priorities?
- How those closest to the person view nutrition; how realistic are their expectations for the person at the end of their life? Aggressive persuasion to eat results in conflict and distress for all involved. One carer shared that she had thrown food at her dying husband; shocking as this may sound, it is not uncommon. Caring for someone who is dying is stressful, mentally and physically exhausting and feeding is associated with showing love and compassion. When the person being cared for rejects food, it may feel like you are also being rejected
- What the person would like – taste changes.

The goal of care should be to make meal times an enjoyable experience and at the end of life, it is important that memories are created that are pleasant and worthy of keeping. Nurses can help create a caring atmosphere by ensuring:

- Bedpans and vomit bowls are cleared away and the environment smells clean
- The person is positioned so that they can eat with ease
- The food tray or table is set attractively; disposable tray clothes, china crockery all help to create a special atmosphere

- Food portions are small and set attractively on the plate; using smaller plates helps with this
- Use of proper cutlery and china as opposed to disposable paper and plastic utensils.

The dying person has little time left, while we have all the time in the world, therefore we should make every effort to deliver compassionate care.

Dehydration at the End of Life

While people can accept that a dying person may not require nutrition at the end of life, it is more difficult to accept the reduced need for fluids, especially if the dying person has a dry mouth and cracked lips. The research-based evidence for providing medical hydration, either by intravenous or subcutaneous infusion at this stage is very mixed and studies are flawed for various reasons, such as sample sizes being too small and parameters for measurement too vague or subjective (Van der Riet *et al.* 2008).

Providing some hydration (1 litre a day) via subcutaneous infusion does lessen terminal agitation and twitching (myoclonus), improves the analgesic effect of morphine and affects levels of sedation. Some people want and need to be more aware, so they can say 'goodbye' and respond to people they love and care for. This level of hydration may not assuage their feelings of thirst because the sensation of thirst is associated with a dry mouth. The best way to deal with this symptom is to provide meticulous mouth care.

What the Experts Say

Very often, the thirst is a sensation around the mouth, lips and tongue that can be palliated with good oral care, salivary stimulations, like ice cubes made of crushed pineapple.

However, maintaining hydration artificially does mean the person has invasive tubes, which they may find distressing. It is perceived by some as the 'medicalisation' of the natural process of dying. Excess fluids retained in the body can add to the symptom burden, it may increase breathlessness and bubbly, noisy breathing, which is very distressing for the person and their family. It may increase oedema, which can also be uncomfortable.

Families and those close to the person who is dying may perceive the withdrawal of nutrition and fluids as abandonment of the person; the giving up of hope by the healthcare professionals and interpret it as a lack of care. Families require support at this difficult time and reassurance that withdrawal of nutrition and fluids does not increase suffering. Replacing feeding the person with regular mouth care reassures everyone that the healthcare professionals are maintaining vigilant care at the end of life.

Nursing Care When the Person Is Not Drinking

Mouth care is essential when the person is not drinking, as the mucosa lining the mouth becomes dry and cracked. The best way to clean the mouth is to use a soft toothbrush and a little toothpaste, brush the teeth gently and use a moistened sponge swab to clear away the debris.

If the person is wearing dentures, then these need to be removed and cleaned, the mouth is swabbed with a sponge swab soaked in clean water before dentures are replaced.

If the person is dying and unconscious, they may well respond to the insertion of the swab and suck on it, demonstrating their need for some moisture, even if they cannot swallow.

Once the mouth care has been completed, remove the toothbrush and swabs, ensure the mouth is dry and apply a little Vaseline to the lips to keep them clean and supple.

What the Experts Say

> It is easy to administer small drops of water to keep the oral mucosa moist by using a straw.
> You will need a glass with a small amount of water, a clean straw and a towel to protect the person and the sheets.
> Place the towel under the person's chin.
> Place the straw in the water and the index finger over the open end of the straw. As you remove the straw from the water, you will see a small amount of water retained in the straw. You will only need a quarter of a centimetre of water in the straw. As you remove your finger slightly, a small drop of water will escape from the end of the straw.
> Using this method, you can insert a drop of water into the front of the mouth.
> This is sufficient to offer respite and quench the sensation of thirst.

Hospital Nutrition Services

It is estimated that the NHS spends £300 million on food and £500 million on catering, yet reports in national newspapers (e.g. *The Independent*, 5 January 2013) reveal that at least a quarter of food prepared is binned, which amounts to throwing away £27 million. The average spend is between £2.19 and £18.14 a day per patient. Most staff, when asked, said they would not eat the food they serve. Yet, we see from the above that food is essential for good health and recovery from illness. Various chefs have attempted to influence and improve the situation. James Martin has recently worked with hospitals in Scarborough and Birmingham (this hospital had 40% food wastage) with some success at introducing locally sourced foods and introducing nutritious menus because the teams he was working with provided on-site catering. Some hospitals use a cook/chill facility, with food being prepared off-site, which means there is little choice.

One hospital has introduced the concept of a 'nutrition champion' on each area. The nutrition champion in this instance, is a healthcare assistant who liaises with the nurses when a person is admitted, to ascertain what the medical diagnosis is and whether a nutritional assessment (MUST) has been completed. The nutritional champion meets with the patient and their family to find out what their food preferences are, what they have been eating and helps to devise a food plan; they will help with menu choices and identify those people who will need assistance with feeding. People who require assistance with feeding have their meals served on a 'red tray', thus indicating to all members of staff that the person needs help and that food left on the plate may be because they have yet to receive help. The nutrition champion endeavours to ensure that meal times are 'protected' and that the person does not have any procedures or investigations carried out at this time. They also ensure that the environment is clean, bedpans removed, hand washing facilities are offered and the person is comfortably positioned to enjoy a meal and they can assist with feeding (Potterton 2012).

Conclusion

Nursing has advanced in complexity and technicality over the years and nurses have developed skills that once were the remit of medical practitioners; yet 'to nurse' is inherently to nourish and sustain a person, especially when they are ill. Many of the articles that have been used to inform this chapter have pointed to the low priority nurses attribute to nutrition – as stated at the beginning, insufficient emphasis is placed on nutrition in nurse education. Florence Nightingale would be appalled to read the headlines in many of the newspapers, especially after making her edict in *Notes on Nursing*.

Nutrition is pivotal to the well-being of a person. It is needed to sustain life, it is needed to recover from illness and it is needed when a person is dying. Inadequate and poor nutrition makes us ill and contributes to the ageing process. There is mounting evidence to suggest that poor nutrition is one of the reasons for the development of dementia but this is as yet, unproven.

This is a field of care where nurses can make a significant impact and reap rich rewards from the satisfaction of seeing people recover more quickly from illness and disease.

Key Points

- What we eat and drink is vital to maintaining a healthy body and a poor diet results in ill health.
- The nutrients need to be balanced for homeostasis and when an element is missing, ill health including mental health occurs.
- The nutrients we eat are as important as the medical treatment received; wounds only heal if the nutrients are available to sustain this.
- Nurses have a crucial role to ensure that the people they are caring for are adequately nourished; ignoring this aspect of care is detrimental to their patient's well-being.
- There are professional, legal and ethical dilemmas to consider when feeding artificially continues and adversely affects quality of life.
- A dying person still requires nutrition to ensure a comfortable and dignified death but the type and amounts are different.

Glossary

Anabolic phase: the rebuilding of complex compounds within the cells

Ayurvedic medicine: a traditional medical approach practised in Asia

Catabolic phase: the breaking down of complex compounds within the cells

Enteral feeding: feeding by tube into the digestive system either in stomach or the small intestine

Malnutrition: results from either too little food of not enough of the right kind of food and also applies to over eating, which results in obesity

Nutrients: the compounds found in food, e.g. carbohydrates, proteins, etc.

(Continued)

Obesity: a condition where the person exceeds their nutrient requirements and excess fats and carbohydrates are deposited as fat in the subcutaneous tissues, muscle and liver

Parenteral feeding: is feeding intravenously with nutrients, such as amino acids

Sarcopenia: the loss of muscle protein mass

Undernourishment: not having sufficient food to maintain body weight and results in lost weight

References

Acreman, S. (2009) Nutrition in palliative care. *British Journal of Community Nursing*, 14(10), 427–431.

Ashwell, M. (2010) An examination of the relationship between breakfast, weight and shape. *British Journal of Nursing*, 19(18), 1155–1159.

Barber, J. & Murphy, K. (2011) Challenges that specialist palliative care nurses encounter when caring for patients with advanced dementia. *International Journal of Palliative Nursing*, 17(12), 587–591.

Blaikley, C. (2012) Mind the hunger gap: a review of malnutrition in the community. *British Journal Community Nursing*, 17(Suppl), S10–S14.

Borland, S. (2013) Thousands dying of thirst on NHS. *Daily Mail*, Wednesday 28 August 2013, front page.

Brogden, B.J. (2004) Clinical skills: importance of nutrition for acutely ill hospital patients. *British Journal of Nursing*, 13(15), 914–920.

Denny, A. (2006) New NICE guideline on nutrition support. *Nursing and Residential Care*, 8(9), 396–400.

Dunne, A. (2012) Food and mood: evidence for diet-related changes in mental health. *British Journal of Community Nursing*, 17(Suppl 7), S20–S24.

Fletcher, A. & Carey, E. (2011) Knowledge, attitudes and practices in the provision of nutritional care. *British Journal of Nursing*, 20(10), 615–620.

Fletcher, J. (2009) Identifying patients at risk of malnutrition: nutrition screening and assessment. *Gastrointestinal Nursing*, 7(5), 12–17.

Fletcher, J. (2011) Nutrition: safe practice in adult enteral tube feeding. *British Journal of Nursing*, 20(19), 1234–1239.

Glasper, A. (2010) Let them eat kale: tackling dietary inequalities in deprived areas. *British Journal of Nursing*, 19(21), 1370–1371.

Harbottle, L. (2011) Nutrition and mental health: the importance of diet in depression. *British Journal of Well-being*, 2(7), 19–22.

Holder, H. (2003) Nursing management of nutrition in cancer and palliative care. *British Journal of Nursing*, 12(11), 667–673.

Holmes, S. (2010) Nutrition in the palliative care of chronic and life threatening conditions. *British Journal of Nursing*, 15(Suppl 7), S24–S30.

Holmes, S. (2011) Principles of nutrition in the palliation of long-term conditions. *International Journal of Palliative Nursing*, 17(5), 217–222.

Hughes, S. (2012) Diabetes: support for those at risk of malnutrition in the community. *British Journal of Community Nursing*, 17(110), 529–534.

Jennings, E. (2011) Diabetes and severe mental illness. *British Journal of Well-being*, 2(3), 21–26.

Lazarou, C. & Kouta, C. (2010) The role of nurses in the prevention and management of obesity. *British Journal of Nursing*, 19(10), 641–647.

Medlin, S. (2012) Nutrition for wound healing. *British Journal of Nursing, Tissue Viability Supplement*, 21(12), S11–S15.

Meetoo, D. (2010) The imperative of human obesity: an ethical reflection. *British Journal of Nursing*, 19(9), 563–568.

Mellor, D. (2012) A review of the current nutritional guidelines for diabetes. *Practice Nursing*, 23(5), 234–239.

Mitchell, M. (2011) Elderly still hungry to be heard: a nutrition update from Age UK. *British Journal of Community Nursing*, 16(7), 347.

Nazarko, L. (2013) Helping wounds to heal by improving nutrition. *NRC*, 15(6), 416–420.

Omorogieva, O. (2010) Managing patients on enteral feeding in the community. *British Journal of Community Nursing*, 15(Suppl 7), S4–S10.

Parsons, E. (2011) Nutritional care and the Malnutrition Universal Screening Tool (MUST). *British Journal of Community Nursing*, 16(Suppl 3), S16–S21.

Patience, S. (2013a) Supporting low-income families with nutrition. *Journal of Health Visiting*, 1(6), 336–341.

Patience, S. (2013b) The importance of maintaining appropriate vitamin D levels. *Journal of Health Visiting*, 1(5), 260–264.

Pearson, K. (2013) Nutrition and skin ageing: the impact of oxidation, glycation and inflammation. *Journal of Aesthetic Nursing*, 2(4), 178–183.

Potterton, J. (2012) Role of healthcare assistant as nutritional champion. *British Journal of Healthcare Assistants*, 6(4), 164–168.

Shepherd, A. (2009) Nutrition through the lifespan. Part 3: adults aged 65 years and over. *British Journal of Nursing*, 18(5), 301–307.

Sherman, A.R. & Barkley, M. (2011) Nutrition and wound healing. *Journal of Wound Care*, 20(8), 357–367.

Smith, A. (2008) Nutrition in care homes: going back to basics. *Nursing and Residential Care*, 10(2), 68–72.

Stewart, J. (2011) Nutritional status of older patients admitted to hospital for surgery. *British Journal of Community Nursing*, 16(Suppl 7), S18–S20.

The Independent (2013) Nine million hospital meals thrown out. *The Independent*, 5 January 2013.

Timms, L. (2011) Effect of nutrition on wound healing in older people: a case study. *British Journal of Nursing, Tissue Viability Supplement*, 20(11), S4–S10.

Todorovic, T. (2011) The growing problem of malnutrition in the community. Editorial Comment. *British Journal of Community Nursing*, 16(Suppl 3), S5.

Van der Kramer, V. (2011) Nutrition for older people: building immunity over the winter season. *British Journal of Community Nursing*, 16(11), S22–S24.

Van der Riet, P., Good, P., Higgins, I. & Sneesby, L. (2008) Palliative care professionals' perceptions of nutrition and hydration at the end of life. *International Journal of Palliative Nursing*, 14(3), 145–151.

Wilson, N. & Blackett, B. (2012) Parenteral nutrition: considerations for practice. *British Journal of Community Nursing*, 17(Suppl 5), S16–S19.

Wright, J. (2011) Looking at Nutrition, part 2: obesity and body image. *British Journal of School Nursing*, 6(2), 96–97.

Test Yourself

1. Which foods produce essential amino acids in the best form for absorption?
   (a) Beans and lentils
   (b) Green vegetables
   (c) Meat and eggs
   (d) Butter and cream

2. Organic nutrients are found in:
   (a) Biscuits
   (b) Broccoli
   (c) Cakes
   (d) Salt

3. Food needed for an anti-inflammatory diet should include:
   (a) Avocado
   (b) Cream
   (c) Butter
   (d) Potatoes

4. The GI tract produces:
   (a) 4 litres of fluid a day
   (b) 5 litres of fluid a day
   (c) 6 litres of fluid a day
   (d) 7 litres of fluid a day

5. A person who requires help with feeding when in hospital will have their food served on a:
   (a) Blue tray
   (b) Green tray
   (c) Brown tray
   (d) Red tray

6. A person with a BMI of $28\,kg/m^2$ is considered to be:
   (a) Obese
   (b) Undernourished
   (c) Normal
   (d) Mildly obese

7. A person with depression puts on weight because they are:
   (a) On medication
   (b) Have lost interest in food
   (c) Have mood swings
   (d) Are lazy

8. A person with type 2 diabetes asks your advice about eating diabetic jam; you respond with:
   (a) All carbohydrate food should be avoided
   (b) Diabetic jams contain substances that can be harmful
   (c) Homemade jam is better than shop bought jam
   (d) Diabetic jam contains sugar

9. A protective diet would include:
   (a) Butter, cream and eggs
   (b) Tomatoes, broccoli and carrots
   (c) Cheese, beef and chicken
   (d) Mushrooms, rice and peas

10. Which statement reflects the situation of a person who is dying:
    (a) Someone who is dying does not need food and drink
    (b) Someone who is dying needs parenteral nutrition
    (c) Someone who is dying may eat and drink if they want to
    (d) Someone who is dying is not interested in food and drink

Answers

1. c
2. d
3. a
4. d
5. d
6. d
7. a
8. b
9. b
10. c

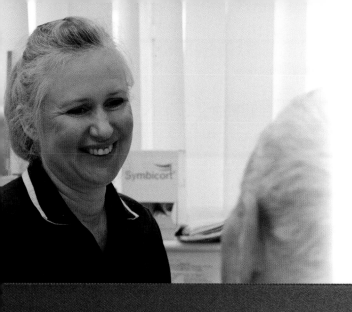

18

The Principles of Skin Integrity

Melanie Stephens

University of Salford, UK

Learning Outcomes

On completion of this chapter you will be able to:

- Identify and describe the structures of the skin, hair and nails, explaining the processes involved in wound healing
- Explain the functions of the skin
- Review the psycho-socioeconomic aspects of wound care
- Categorise the factors that affect skin integrity and breakdown and how these impact on wound healing processes
- Recognise and review common wounds, including the assessment of the wounds, their clinical management and the involvement of the interdisciplinary team

Competencies

All nurses must:

1. Take a person-centred, personalised approach to care
2. Possess a broad knowledge of the structure and functions of the human body, and other relevant knowledge from the life, behavioural and social sciences, as applied to health, ill health, disability, ageing and death
3. Assist in providing accurate information to people and their carers on the management of a device, site or wound to prevent and control infection and to promote healing wherever that person might be, for example, in hospital, in the home care setting, in an unplanned situation
4. Use up-to-date knowledge and evidence to assess, plan, deliver and evaluate care, communicate findings, influence change and promote health and best practice
5. Make person-centred, evidence-based judgements and decisions, in partnership with others involved in the care process, to ensure high quality care
6. Manage resources effectively to ensure the quality of care is maintained or enhanced

 Visit the companion website at **www.wileynursingpractice.com** where you can test yourself using flashcards, multiple-choice questions and more.

Nursing Practice: Knowledge and Care, First Edition. Edited by Ian Peate, Karen Wild and Muralitharan Nair.
© 2014 John Wiley & Sons, Ltd. Published 2014 by John Wiley & Sons, Ltd. Companion website: www.wileynursingpractice.com

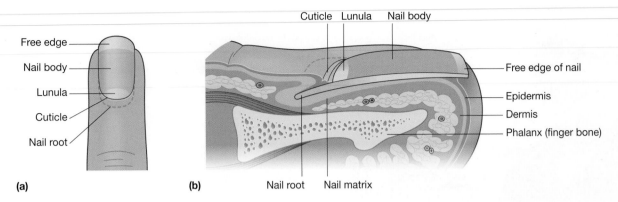

Figure 18.1 Structure of the fingernail.

Introduction

Nurses who are aware of the changes in skin integrity through the lifespan and the phases of healing are more likely to take an active role in the prevention and management of wounds of the patients for whom they care. Although the largest organ of the body, the skin is the first organ that can often be ignored when patients are acutely ill or experiencing an exacerbation of their chronic illness. Care of the skin is part of the fundamental aspects of nursing care, however it is often overlooked. The multifaceted factors that can lead to skin breakdown make the challenge of prevention and management of the skin a testing but rewarding specialism of nursing.

Anatomy and Physiology of the Skin

The skin, often referred to as the 'integumentary system', is made up of the hair, nails and skin, which provides the body with an external cover, acting as a divider between the organs of the body and the external environment. The skin is the largest organ of the body and weighs 2.7–3.6 kg, with an average surface area of 1.9 m². It has many functions related to the structures that make up the layers of the skin.

The Hair

A hair bulb, with a root enclosed in a hair follicle produces hair. It is situated in the dermis of the skin, however in the scalp this is below the dermis. Visible hair named the 'shaft' is mainly made up of dead cells. Only the palms of the hands, soles of the feet, nails, parts of the external genitals, lips and nipples do not have hair. The function of hair is protection and many factors influence its growth, including nutrition, genetics and hormonal influences. Protection of the skin by hair is constrained, but its role is to protect the scalp in particular from the ultraviolet rays, heat loss and injury. Eyebrows and lashes protect foreign bodies from entering the eye, as do hair in the nostrils and ears. Hairs through touch receptors in the hair root, sense light touch.

The Nails

Dead cells arising from the stratum germinativum of the epidermis, make up the keratinised plates called 'nails'. The cells form clear, solid coverings to the dorsal and distal section of fingers and toes. The role of nails is to aid the development of fine motor skills such as grasping, scratching and manipulation. A nail also provides protection against trauma to the fingers and toes.

A nail has three segments: body, free edge and root (Figure 18.1). The body often looks pink in colour due to the flow of blood in the underlying capillary network and is the visible portion of the nail. The free edge is the part of the nail that may extend past the end of a finger or toe. The nail root is that aspect of the nail that is buried in the fold of the skin.

There is also the 'cuticle', a thin strip of epidermis that stretches over the nail margin, the 'matrix', the proximal portion of epithelium deep to the nail root and the 'lunula', the whitish crescent-shaped end of the nail.

> **Jot This Down**
>
> Why is the care of hair and nails important to nurses as practitioners and also in the care of patients?

The Skin (Figure 18.2)
The epidermis

The epidermis is the outermost layer of the skin and is made up of epithelial cells; it is slightly acidic, with a pH of 4.5–6. These cells, depending on their location on the body, are normally 4–5 layers thick, the most layers being present on the palms of the hands and the soles of the feet. The epithelium has 4–5 layers depending on the anatomical part of the body; the stratum corneum, the stratum granulosum, the stratum lucidum, the stratum spinosum and the stratum basale (Figure 18.3).

The stratum corneum consists of 20–30 sheets of keratin fragment filled dead cells arranged in what is termed as 'shingles', which flake off as dry skin. This layer is the thickest of the epidermis, making up 75% of the epidermis total thickness.

The stratum granulosum helps reduce loss of water from the epidermis as it contains a glycolipid. Keratinisation, a process by which the cells' plasma membranes thicken, also begins in this layer. In areas of thick skin, flattened, dead keratinocytes are present and this is known as the *stratum lucidum*.

The innermost layer of the epidermis is where keratin and melanin is produced by melanocytes. The role of melanin is to shield the skin from the harmful effects of ultraviolet light, by protecting the underlying keratinocytes and nerve endings. This melanocyte activity possibly explains the variation in skin colours in humans. The tough, protective quality of the epidermis is due to the fibrous and water repellent nature of the protein keratin. Keratinocytes move up through the layers of the epidermis as they

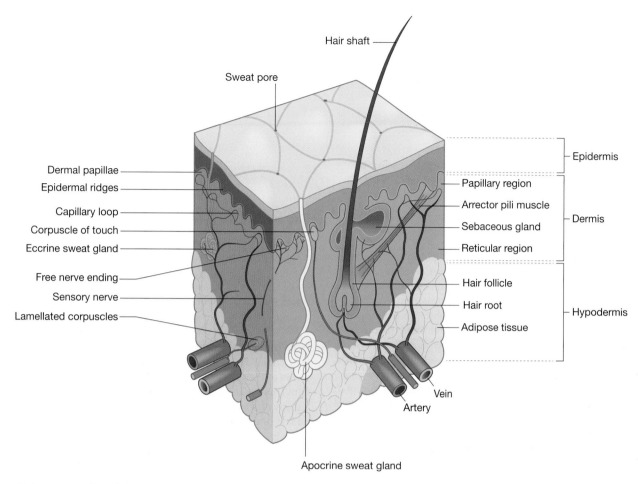

Figure 18.2 Cross-section of the skin.

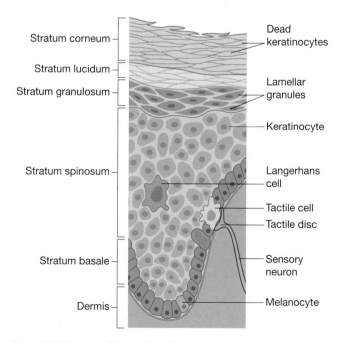

Figure 18.3 Layers of the epidermis.

mature, eventually becoming the dead cells that flake off as dry skin. Flaking of these millions of cells occurs daily when rubbing of the skin takes place, for example when drying with a towel or removing a piece of clothing. As flaking occurs, so does the production of their replacement cells in the *stratum spinosum*, which is 8–10 cells thick. In this layer mitosis occurs, although not as abundantly as the stratum basale, and cells that began in the bone marrow migrate to the epidermis.

Other cells found in the epidermis include Langerhans cells (found in the stratum spinosum) and tactile cells. Langerhans cells help other immune system cells to detect an infecting microorganism and destroy it. Tactile cells contain a disc that detects touch and are located in the deepest part of the epidermis. They are numerous in number around parts such as the fingertips, armpits, genital region and soles of the feet and are found in the *stratum basale*.

The dermis

The subsequent deeper layer of the skin that contains hair follicles, sebaceous glands (glands that secrete sebum, an oil) and sweat glands is the 'dermis'. It is made up of flexible irregular connective tissue, from woven collagen and elastin fibres, opulently abounding with blood vessels, nerve fibres and lymphatic vessels. The dermis

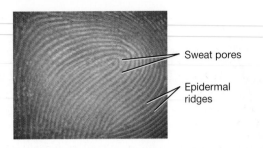

Figure 18.4 Epidermal ridges and sweat pores. Source: Jenkins & Tortora (2013). Reproduced with permission of John Wiley & Sons Singapore Pte. Ltd.

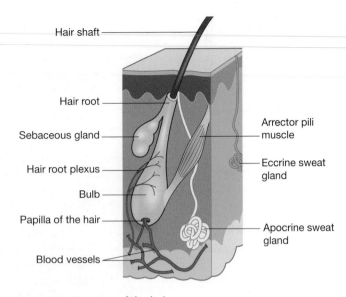

Figure 18.5 Structure of the hair.

has two layers: papillary and reticular. The *papillary* layer contains thin collagen and fine elastin fibres. This layer consists of projections that serrate the overlying epidermis, and contains capillaries and receptors for touch and pain. The *reticular* layer, which is deeper, contains dense bundles of collagen fibres (that provide the skin with tensile strength of elasticity and extensibility), deep pressure receptors, sweat and sebaceous glands and blood vessels. Ridges formed from these bundles of collagen run downwards, forwards and horizontally around the body and are named 'cleavage lines', are genetically determined and are unique for each person. When surgeons operate, they ensure any incision runs parallel to the cleavage lines as they heal more easily and with less scarring than incisions or traumatic wounds across cleavage lines. Macrophages, known as 'wandering cells', are contained within the reticular region (Figure 18.4).

Hair Follicles

A hair follicle, made up of stem cells, produces hair in three cycles: growth, cessation and rest. Each hair follicle goes through this cycle. *Growth* is when cells of the hair matrix divide, adding new cells to the hair root and this is when hair grows fast, around 1 cm every 28 days and scalp hair in particular stays in this phase for 2–7 years. *Cessation* occurs at the end of the growth stage and as yet, the stimulus for this is unknown. This is a short phase 2–3 weeks and the blood supply to the hair is cut-off and the hair becomes fully keratinised; the hair becomes a 'club hair' and enters the final stage. The *rest* phase is when the hair begins to fall out and can prematurely enter this phase in periods of extreme stress. This stage can last up to 3 months; 50–100 club hairs are shed daily from the scalp.

The structure of a hair follicle includes: a papilla, a matrix, a root sheath, a hair fibre and a bulge (Figure 18.5). The *papilla* is a large structure at the base of the follicle made up of connective tissue. The *matrix* is a collection of epithelial cells scattered with melanocytes and is where the hair *sheath* and *fibre*, made of keratin is formed through cell division, which is the fastest cell growing population in the human body (this can be affected however, by radiotherapy and chemotherapy). The *bulge* accommodates stem cells, providing the hair follicle with new cells for growth and if needed also takes part in the wound healing process.

Attached to the hair follicle is the arrector pili muscle, which when stimulated allows the hair to stand perpendicular to the skin and protrude slightly to create goose bumps. Sebum and sweat are secreted by the sebaceous glands and apocrine glands on to the hair follicle for protection, lubrication and pliability.

Hair-follicle pigmentation

Hair colour is due to the amount of melanin in the cells. Various forms of melanin produce a range of hair colours: dark hair contains true melanin; blonde and red hair contain variants of melanin; and grey hair contains less melanin due to a decline in its production. White hair is due to air bubbles in the hair shaft and a lack of melanin.

Blood Vessels

Blood vessels contained within the skin include arterioles, capillary networks and venules. Flow of blood through the capillaries is controlled by hormones and the nervous system. Blood vessels in the skin transport and distribute oxygen, nutrients and hormones and remove waste products.

Nerve Fibres

The dermis contains both sensory and motor nerves. Sensory nerve endings are sensitive to touch, or initiate signals that produce sensations of warmth, coolness, pain, pressure, vibration, tickling and itching. The sensory receptors are found throughout the skin and include tactile discs in the epidermis, corpuscles of touch in the dermis and hair root plexus around hair follicles. Motor nerves aid the vasodilation and vasoconstriction of blood vessels and glands and the contraction and relaxation of muscle tissues, i.e. the arrector pili.

Lymphatic Vessels

The lymphatic system parallels the blood vessels supply and function, but as their permeability is greater than capillaries, they frequently absorb proteins, lipids and interstitial fluid, which is often when pressure is greater in the interstitial fluid, the fluid that surrounds cells of the body tissues, than in the lymph. The role of the lymphatic system is to transport lymphatic fluid, aid in circulating body fluids and help guard against disease triggering agents.

Subcutaneous Tissue

Primarily adipose tissue (fat) lies under the dermis and helps the skin adhere to underlying structures.

Glands of the Skin

There are many glands of the skin and each has its own particular function: ceruminous (earwax), sebaceous (oil) and sudoriferous (sweat).

Cerumen is the yellow-brown waxy secretion of ceruminous glands, which are located in the external auditory canals. Their role with hair follicles is to prevent the entry of foreign substances. Cerumen also waterproofs the canal and aids prevention of bacteria and fungi from entering the cells.

Sebaceous glands are located all over the body, however, they are not found on the palms and soles and are mostly connected to hair follicles. The glands are stimulated by androgens (sex hormones). Their role is to secrete an oily substance called sebum, a mixture of triglycerides, cholesterol, proteins and salts, which lubricate and soften the skin and hair and lessens water evaporation in low humidity. Sebum also destroys bacteria, protecting the skin from infection. Related medical conditions include sebaceous cysts and acne vulgaris.

Sudoriferous glands are small tubular structures that produce perspiration. There are two types: eccrine and apocrine. The forehead, soles and palms contain a higher number of *eccrine* glands, which is situated in the dermis and has a duct that opens in a pore at the surface of the epidermis. The sweat produced by the eccrine glands is mainly compiled of water, however, it does contain antibodies, sodium, chloride, urea, uric acid, ammonia, amino acids, glucose and minute amounts of vitamin C and lactic acid. A person may sweat in response to their emotional state, for example when anxious or to maintain homeostasis, or to maintain homeostasis through the regulation of body temperature through perspiration. This is all regulated by the sympathetic nervous system. *Apocrine* sweat glands are located in the armpits (axillary) anal and genital area and are considered remnants of mammalian sexual scent glands. The sweat produced in these areas varies slightly, as fatty acids and proteins are also secreted, but is odourless, however when bacteria on the skin metabolise, the sweat produced from these glands has a musky, unpleasant odour.

Skin Pigmentation

Pigmentation levels affect the colour of the skin a human is born with; skin colour can vary from black and brown skin to pinkish white. The pigments that affect skin colour are haemoglobin, carotene and melanin. Those born with a golden skin tone such as persons of Asian ancestry have large amounts of carotene (a yellow to orange pigment) and melanin (a yellow to brown pigment). However, in all persons, carotene is found where the stratum corneum is thickest. Those born with brown or black skin have greater levels of melanin; however lengthened exposure to the sun can cause an accumulation of melanin, resulting in darkening or tanning of the skin. A pink skin tone, conversely, is due to the lack of melanin, which allows red blood cells carrying haemoglobin in the blood vessels of the skin to show through the almost translucent epidermis of Caucasians. Regardless of a person's racial origin, all scar tissue heals pink.

Jot This Down
Take some time out and think of the different illnesses and emotions that can affect skin colour.
• What could make the skin change to the following colours: red, bluish, paleness, yellow to orange, black hard leather appearance?

In the 'Jot This Down', exercise above, you might have thought about the skin being influenced by emotions and illness. A reddening of the skin may be due to embarrassment, fever, hypertension or inflammation. Other causes are a drug reaction, sunburn or rosacea. Poor oxygenation and a lack of haemoglobin may give a blue colour to lips, ears and the nose (cyanosis). Pallor may appear with shock, fear or anger. Jaundice may give a yellow to orange colour of the skin. Pink may appear in the healing of skin in Afro-Caribbean patients.

Function of the Skin

The skin, hair and nails each have many functions and these are categorised in Box 18.1.

Wound Healing (Figure 18.6)

When there is loss of the integrity of the skin, a chain of events are signalled in order to return the skin to as near normal structure and function. The process of wound healing includes four main phases: haemostasis, inflammation, proliferation and maturation.

Haemostasis

The initial reaction of the skin to injury is bleeding and the body saturating the wound bed with blood. The purpose of this is to release platelets to the injured area so that they will adhere to the exposed collagen of the damaged vessel(s). The platelets then become sticky and fibrin connects with the platelets and any circulating red blood cells form a plug and haemostasis occurs. Fibrinolysis (the breaking down of the clot) then occurs and other cells, such as macrophages and new platelets, arrive at the wound bed and jolt the wound into the next phase of healing.

Inflammation

The inflammatory stage of wound healing requires the release of many cells, substances, hormones and growth factors to aid wound healing processes. Granulation tissue, ground substance and collagen are formed. Typically during this stage of wound healing, the wound is cleansed, bacteria, debris and devitalised tissue are removed preparing the wound for the next phase of wound healing. Often this stage of wound healing is linked to the patient complaining of pain, heat, swelling and redness at the wound bed.

 Link To/Go To

http://ewma.org/fileadmin/user_upload/EWMA/pdf/Position _Documents/2006/English_pos_doc_2006.pdf
This report provides a best practice position statement on diagnosing a wound infection.

Proliferation

Growth factors that are released by macrophages stimulate angiogenesis and cell migration to aid the formulation of granulation tissue during this phase of wound healing. Tissue made from collagen, fibrin, fibronectin, proteoglycans, glycosaminoglycans and glycoproteins develops. The function of the tissue produced at this stage is to provide shape and offer metabolic and structural support to the surrounding cells. The wound bed is often seen as red and

Box 18.1

Protection	Nails protect the extremities of the fingers and toes Hair insulates the skin and scalp in cold weather Keratin protects the underlying skin from chemical, biological and physical damage Lipids inhibit water loss and thus provide protection against dehydration and hinder access of water across the skin surface when bathing, showering or swimming Sebum keeps skin and hair from drying out and destroys bacteria on the surface Acidic pH of the skin from sweat slows the growth of some bacteria Melanin offers some defence against ultraviolet light Langerhans cells (LC) and macrophages (M) aid immunity by alerting the immune system (LC) to invading microbes and phagocytosing those that get through (M) Eyelashes and cilia protect against foreign materials entering the eyes, nose and ears
Sensation	Transmitting of messages via nerve endings to the central nervous system; tactile, thermal, pressure, injury and pain
Synthesis of vitamin D	When exposed to sunlight, a precursor molecule in the skin is activated and converts cholesterol to vitamin D (only 10–15 minutes, twice a week is required)
Excretion	Elimination of water, salts, carbon dioxide, ammonia and urea from the body. On average, the skin loses 400 mL of perspiration through evaporation per day
Absorption	Certain lipid soluble substances can be absorbed through the skin, including fat soluble vitamins, medicines, oxygen and carbon dioxide, toxic materials
A storage reservoir	8–10% of total circulating blood flow is accommodated in the skin The skin also stores fats as adipose tissue and water
Regulation of body temperature	Eccrine glands aid the regulation of body temperature through secretion of sweat, which is then evaporated from the skin In response to the temperature of the environment, blood vessels in the skin dilate or constrict to radiate or conserve heat Erector pili muscles adjust the angle of hair follicles to trap air around the hairs to provide insulation

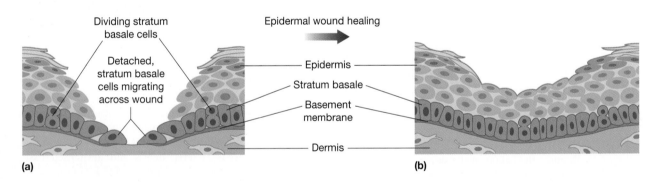

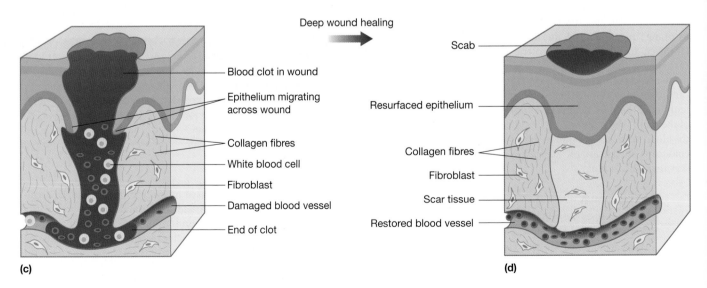

Figure 18.6 **Healing of epidermal and deep wounds.**

granular and wound edges start to close together, as muscle fibres are contracting. On occasion, pink epithelial sites are noted, as basal cells have travelled from the stem cells of the hair bulge across the moist wound bed, stopping only when they meet another basal cell (contact inhibition).

Maturation

Cell migration, cell growth and collagen deposition occurs at this phase of wound healing, increasing the tensile strength of the wound. Blood supply and cellular activity is reduced and the final outcome for some wounds is scar formation. Some patients however, have abnormal scarring such as keloid and hypertrophic.

Jot This Down

Which race or group of persons are more prone to keloid and hypertrophic scars?
    As all scar tissue heals pink, what implications might this have for a patient's body image and what support and advice is available?

 Link To/Go To

https://www.changingfaces.org.uk/Skin-Camouflage

This charity provides advice and support for people and families who are living with conditions, marks or scars that affect their appearance.

Psycho-Socioeconomic Aspects of Wound Care

According to the European Wound Management Association (EWMA 2008) a large proportion of wounds are considered 'hard to heal', this is where wound healing is often prolonged or never occurs, despite advances in clinician's knowledge, skills and the treatments offered. This can lead to frustration and anxiety for all involved and the healthcare burden on resources is increased.

Many factors can impact on the healing or non-healing of any wound and have been explored and the evidence appraised by members of EWMA and although they are only presented as supporting practice in the care of hard to heal wounds, the information presented is useful for all wounds when considering the patient receives timely and prompt treatment. The factors are classified as: wound complexity and healing (Vowden *et al.* 2008), psychosocial factors and wound healing (Moffatt *et al.* 2008) and the economic burden of hard to heal wounds (Romanelli *et al.* 2008).

Wound Complexity and Healing

Predicting the likely healing time of any wound is often very difficult to determine. Usual methods include regular wound measurement and assessment. This informs the practitioner of the progression of the wound as the radius and wound edges decrease.

In venous leg ulcers, Margolis *et al.* (2004) found that duration and size of the ulcer was a good indicator and from this, developed a simple scoring system to indicate the likely outcome of wound

healing for the majority (over 70%) of leg ulcers to be 24 weeks. However, decreasing of wound size or epithelial advancement is only one indicator of wound healing and other indicators are required as healing rates among patients varies greatly (Hill *et al.* 2004). Four main factors have been highlighted as affecting wound healing and include: patient-related factors, wound-related factors, skill and knowledge of the professional and resources and treatment-related, and are categorised in the EWMA table, which is linked below.

 Link To/Go To

The link to the EWMA table:

http://ewma.org/fileadmin/user_upload/EWMA/pdf/Position _Documents/2008/English_EWMA_Hard2Heal_2008.pdf

---

Patient-related factors

A vital component of wound healing is to assess the patient holistically and therefore, prior to even assessing the wound and the dressing currently being used, it is imperative that the clinician assesses the physical, social and psychological factors that may impinge on wound healing.

Physical factors include any comorbidities that affect body systems that in turn influence the rate of healing at the wound bed. These can be issues such as oxygenation, blood supply, nutrition, sleep, the release of hormones, neurological impairment, the impact of any medication, to name but a few. Psychosocial factors that can impair the wound healing process include pain, gender, stress, economic status, body image, concordance, health beliefs and social isolation.

Many patients with large wounds will develop coping strategies, but these may not be effective enough to prevent any real impact on the wound healing process.

The effect of both the psychological and physical impact of the hard to heal wound can be detrimental to the quality of life for a patient and their significant others. The whole outcome can cause a spiralling effect of pain, sleep deprivation and reversed sleep, wake cycle, anxiety, depression and social isolation. These problems can lead to reduced socioeconomic status, low income, loss of relationships and friendships, and meaning and purpose in life. As a result of their wound, these individuals suffer from leading restricted lives, experiencing further social isolation, being discredited and burdening others (Charmaz 1983).

What the Experts Say

 Whenever I carry out a full assessment of a patient with a wound, in particular ones that are on visible parts of the body, I ask the patient to complete the Edinburgh Depression Scale. I do this, as often those with the smallest of wounds suffer the most emotional stress and those with larger wounds have better coping mechanisms. The score helps provide objective data to the subjective data I have been assessing and collecting and then I can speak with the patient and their GP to consider other therapies such as counselling, occupational therapy, psychotherapy and medication for depression.

(Rachel Smith, District Nurse)

361

Wound-related factors

Many wound characteristics affect the rate of healing, including wound duration and wound senescence.

Jot This Down

Think about the wounds that you have seen that do not seem to heal readily.

· What is contributing to this delay in healing?

A number of reasons account for the slow healing of chronic wounds, and you might have thought of factors such as the size of the wound, its position and how much healthy blood supply the wound has.

The more chronic the wound is, the longer it takes to heal and this has correlations with the amount of senescent cells that develop, that is, the amount of cells in a wound bed that are unable to replicate. According to Harding et al. (2005), if the wound contains over 15% of senescent fibroblasts, wound healing will be dramatically affected and therefore 'hard to heal'.

The size and depth of wound can impact on the healing process and due to the biological nature of wound healing, large, deep cavity wounds will take longer to heal than smaller, superficial wounds. However, the type of wound can be a variable, such as a fistulae or sinus; these are often small but deep wounds and only have one of the two compounding factors.

The condition of the wound bed in particular in the presence of necrotic and sloughy tissue can not only affect the correct assessment of a wound but also delay the wound healing process, as this type of tissue requires thorough assessment and consideration of the implications of debridement. As many hard to heal wounds have high bacterial counts, more than one bacteria infiltrating the wound bed and the presence of a biofilm, it is easy to understand why wound infection can fuel a chronic inflammatory response, delaying the healing process. This amplified inflammatory response causes inhibition of cell growth and angiogenesis and an increase in tissue degradation.

Another wound-related factor is poor perfusion of the skin from diseases and surgical complications such as atherosclerosis, atheroma, thrombus, calcification, dehydration and hypothermia. These can deprive the wound bed of oxygen and nutrients required for metabolic and cellular activity, delaying the healing process.

The location of the wound is often critical to the success of healing, if the anatomical location is in an area where there is a point of direct pressure or around a joint, then it is imperative to choose the right dressing, secured with the right material and which may require even off-loading or having the pressure to the area redistributed.

The final wound-related factor is the ability of the wound to respond to initial treatment. A report by Vowden et al. (2007) suggests that when using topical negative pressure, if there is a reduction of wound size by 15% in the first 2 weeks, then predictable outcomes for the chronic wound are favourable. However, it is essential to reassess the patient holistically if the wound does not heal in the accepted time frame, and amend management accordingly.

Skill and knowledge of the nurse

It would make common sense that if a practitioner has high level skills and knowledge, then the outcome of the wound management received by the patient would be optimal. However, in hard to heal wounds, professionals often become frustrated and often dislike facing patients with their concerns and expectations, or are overwhelmed at the patients who are experiencing suffering and discomfort for wounds which they cannot manage. In these instances, it is imperative to know one's limitations and seek further support, as advocated by the Nursing and Midwifery Council (NMC 2010), rather than risk withdrawing visits, avoiding difficult conversations and providing poor care. With the recent introduction of 'Patient Reported Outcome Measures' (DH 2009b), measures of a patient's health status or health-related quality of life are a means of assessing effectiveness of care from the patient's perspective. Patients are asked to provide health status information before and after an intervention and provide indications of the quality and outcome of care received. This may offer problems when caring for patients with chronic long-term wounds, as practitioners need to be clear about the goals set in relation to wound healing being a reality and justification of their treatment choices, as PROMs are now being closely linked to payment by results, as up to 10% of a Trust's income can be dependent on patient experience (DH 2009b).

Resource Treatment-Related Factors

Over the last two decades, wound management products and services have developed rapidly, both in number and design. Practitioner's knowledge of these advances varies and patients can receive either appropriate timely evidence-based interventions or ritualistic, traditional practice, based on habit. Wound care resources in relation to guidelines, formularies, access to equipment and staff have created an 'atlas of variation' across the UK and therefore, where a patient lives will depend on the wound management they receive. Consistency in practice will only occur according to Bux and Mahli (1996) and Preece (2004), when there is appropriate education of staff. In the future, however, potential treatment and the allocation of resources may be targeted in relation to the assessment of biochemical characteristics such as gene expression and protease levels, allowing the provision of a quality-based, objective-measured service.

The Quality Agenda and Wound Management

Quality care is clearly embedded into the healthcare arena and has already impacted the field of wound management (Ousey & White 2010).

Documents such as QIPP, *Quality, Innovation, Productivity and Prevention* (DH 2010c); *NHS 2010–2015: from good to great. Preventative, People-centred, Productive* (DH 2009a); and *Revision to the Operating Framework for the NHS in England* (DH 2010b), are placing an emphasis on promoting productivity without affecting quality both in the primary and secondary sector. Not only is quality at the centre of everything clinicians do within these documents, but also the provision of cost-efficient practice.

The Evidence

The cost of wound care is rising, and according to Posnett and Franks (2007) around 200 000 people in the UK have a chronic wound, which costs approximately £2.3–3.1 billion/year.

Prescription costs for wound dressings alone in primary care was estimated at £116 million in September 2009, therefore there is an ambitious drive by the government to reduce this expenditure by £600 000 to £3 million per year, which has led to the publication of documents such as *High Impact Actions for Nursing and Midwifery* (NHS Institute for Innovation and Improvement, NHS-III 2009), a manuscript that sets actions for nurses in improving the delivery of care; *State-of-the-Art Metrics for Nursing*, indicators that measure performance on a range of aspects of care to improve patient outcomes (NNRU 2008), and the *NHS Safety Thermometer*, a tool to measure, monitor and analyse patient safety issues (NHS 2012). These three documents in particular focus on the prevention of avoidable pressure ulcers, through the correct risk assessment and implementation of pressure relieving measures. As the UK population has now reached 62 million and the number of people over 60 has exceeded those who are 16 and with five times as many people over the age of 85 than there were in 1951 (ONS 2010), the risk of developing pressure ulcers is increasing and according to the Health and Social Care Bill (2012), the aim of the NHS is to achieve results that are among the best in the world. Quality in the NHS is part of everyday practice and therefore, it is imperative that practitioners involved in wound management regularly evaluate and audit practice to demonstrate the delivery of high quality care to all.

Link To/Go To

QIPP

http://webarchive.nationalarchives.gov.uk/20130221101407/
http://improvement.nhs.uk/default.aspx?alias=www
.improvement.nhs.uk/qipp

This is link to the online resource for the QIPP agenda and information.

Interdisciplinary Care

From the French doctor, Charcot, and perhaps even today in policy such as Harm-free Care, the development of pressure ulcers is considered the result of poor nursing care. However, other documents, such as those produced by the National Institute for Health and Care Excellence (NICE), European Wound Management Association (EWMA), European Pressure Ulcer Advisory Panel (EPUAP) and National Pressure Ulcer Advisory Panel (NPUAP), all share themes that wound management is complex and that an interdisciplinary approach is vital to aid prevention and management.

It is essential that professions work together to optimise the patients well-being, but also work across sectors and boundaries to ensure the delivery of seamless service (Bellingham & Stephens 1999). Not only does interprofessional working put the patient at the centre of their care, it also enables best practice that is cost-effective and efficient (Barr *et al.* 2002). All staff are accountable for ensuring that a patient's condition does not unavoidably worsen within their care, so all have a duty for the safe provision of the prevention and management of tissue breakdown when caring for patients from the equipment they use and the care delivered.

Jot This Down

Review the role of the members of the interprofessional team, referring back to the development of wounds and the stages of wound healing, where would each profession's role impact these processes?
Which other members of the team can you add to this list?

You may have considered any of the following members of the interprofessional team:

Patients

The DH (2010a) in the White paper 'Equity and Excellence: liberating the NHS' considered patient choice and patient involvement paramount to the delivery of care, 'no decision about me, without me'. Patient involvement is essential to the delivery of good care, as the goal is for the patient to be responsible for their own health gains and avoid damaging their health.

The Tissue Viability Nurse

The tissue viability nurse's role is a key lead position in wound prevention and management, undertaking the four key roles of a nurse specialist duties working alongside other members of staff and acting as consultant, researcher, educator and manager. Developing policy and guidance; educating staff; reviewing chronic and hard to heal wounds; appraising and carrying out research and managing budgets; writing bids and monitoring expenditure for the benefit of patient care.

Directors, Leads and General Managers

Final accountability for the implementation and management of patient care lies with professional leads, managers and directors, the provision of which is directed through the allocation of resources and education of staff.

Medical Staff

Doctors have overall responsibility for patients care and therefore must work with others to address the potential and actual complications of acute and chronic illness that may impede skin breakdown or wound healing. Addressing factors that affect the prevention and management of wounds allows the provision of appropriate care and enhanced reported patient outcomes.

Nurses

Nurses are in the ideal position to offer holistic care that addresses the needs of the patient, be that in hospital, the home, hospice or nursing and residential home. Utilising the nursing process, the nurse can assess, plan, implement and evaluate the care delivered to patients and their significant others, working collaboratively with other members of the interprofessional team.

Support Workers, Trainee Assistant Practitioners, Healthcare Assistants

Support workers, trainee assistant practitioners and healthcare assistants assist and support registered nurses in the delivery of care. It is essential that they do not accept duties that are beyond their roles and responsibilities or have them delegated to them within the field of wound management.

Podiatry

The role of the podiatrist is essential in the prevention and management of wounds in the foot. They provide advice, support and treatment for many patients and should be the first point of call for any diabetic patients for full examination of the foot. Callus, lesions and ulcers in patients with the diabetic foot, should be cared for alongside a podiatrist and not cared for by the nurse alone and a rapid referral is paramount.

Dieticians

The role of the dietician is to provide detailed advice and support to the patient, their family and other members of the interprofessional team on nutrition and hydration. This is in order to plan suitable nutritious meals and if necessary supplements, to prevent skin breakdown and aid wound healing.

Occupational Therapists

The role of the occupational therapist is to assess and maximise function and independence, promoting meaning and purpose of the activities of daily living a patient may undertake in his or her normal day-to-day routine. Their role can include recommendations for equipment with regular follow-up.

Physiotherapists

The role of the physiotherapist is vital, as not only do they promote independence and movement, they can also offer advice on repositioning, correct body alignment and posture. Physiotherapists work closely with the occupational therapist in the provision of equipment to aid independence.

Prosthetist and Orthotist

A prosthetist will ensure the patient is fitted and made with the most appropriate artificial limb. An orthotist, however, will provide equipment such as splints, braces and casts to aid movement, resolve alignment and relieve pressure.

Radiographers

Radiographers provide a service in which underlying pathology of wounds can be explored through X-rays, scans and imaging.

Healthcare Scientists

Of all healthcare decisions, 80% are influenced by healthcare scientists' findings, according to NHS Careers (2013). There are three broad areas.

- *Life sciences*: investigating the causes of illness and how it progresses in blood diagnostics, infection services, tissue and cellular science and genetics
- *Physiological sciences*: investigating the functioning of organ/body systems to diagnose abnormalities, and find ways to restore function and/or reduce disabling consequences to the patient
- *Clinical engineering and medical physics*: develop methods of measuring what is happening in the body, devise new ways of diagnosing and treating disease and ensure that equipment is functioning safely and effectively.

Bioengineers and Estates

The maintenance and management of equipment is managed by bioengineers and estates teams. Their role is to ensure the equip-

Table 18.1 The four main categories of wound.

CLASSIFICATION	TYPE OF WOUND
Malignant	Fungating wound
Mechanical	Surgical or traumatic wounds
Burns	Chemical or thermal
Chronic	Leg ulcers, diabetic foot ulcers, pressure ulcers

ment used for patients is cleaned, serviced and maintained, in compliance with the Medical Devices Agency. Some Trusts however, have outsourced this service to suppliers. All staff have a duty to report faulty equipment, replace it and remove it from the workplace until reviewed by these members of staff.

Wound Care and Management

There are many reasons why the skin integrity of a person may be torn, pierced, cut or broken and often, clinicians classify wounds in order to provide uniformity in the future assessment and management of the wound. There are many ways in which to classify a wound, including in categories: aetiology, morphology and tissue colour, to name but a few. The four main categories of wounds, as suggested by Collier (2003), include: mechanical, chronic, burns and malignant, and are presented in Table 18.1, although the list for chronic wounds is not exhaustive.

However, Collier's classification system does not account for iatrogenic/factitious wound types or what is called self-inflicted wounds, even though arguably one could consider them traumatic.

Wounds can also be classified by the process, in which they are healing, for example: primary, secondary and tertiary intention. *Primary intention* occurs in surgical or traumatic wounds where there is no tissue loss and the edges of the wound are brought together for suturing, gluing or taping. *Secondary intention* is when the edges of the wound are too far apart and, because of the degree of tissue loss, the wound needs to fill with granulation tissue before epithelialisation occurs. *Tertiary intention* is when the wound is primarily left open for up to 5 days before closing with sutures or staples, allowing the drainage of exudate or infected pus.

Other classification tools are based upon the severity and depth of tissue damage and are known as superficial, partial thickness and full-thickness wounds, and can involve the epidermis, or tissue destruction occurs right through the epidermis and dermis to underlying structures, exposing bone and body tissues.

Wounds can also be classified on the length of time they have been present upon a person. These are often referred to as acute or chronic. Wounds that result in timely restoration of anatomical and functional integrity without complication are considered *acute* wounds. *Chronic* wounds however, are those that last longer than 6 weeks, take longer to heal than normally expected and may provide full restoration in anatomical and functional integrity. One type of wound that cannot be classified as acute or chronic is a *palliative* wound, which is when wound healing is unattainable and care is based upon symptom management not common management such as moist wound healing and wound bed preparation. Table 18.2 highlights a list of wounds that can be attributed to the terms *acute, chronic* or *palliative*.

Table 18.2 Classification of wound types.

CLASSIFICATION OF WOUND	TYPE OF WOUNDS
Acute	Surgical incisions, traumatic injuries: lacerations, bites, abrasions, burns and avulsions
Chronic	Pressure ulcers, leg ulcers, burns, dehisced surgical wounds, diabetic foot ulcers
Palliative	Malignant lesions of the skin, epidermolysis bullosa and progressive arterial disease

Jot This Down

Reflect back on the care of a recent patient with a wound. How would you classify the depth and type of the wound based on the two systems above? Which structures of the skin were involved? What psycho-socioeconomic factors impacted on the wound management for this patient? Was the wound acute, chronic or palliative?

Wound Assessment

According to Posnett *et al.* (2009) a wound assessment that addresses the holistic assessment of the patient is imperative to good wound management. The assessment process should discover any contributing or causative factors that could impinge on the wound healing process, consider the state of the wound bed and peri-wound area and then plan appropriate interventions. These interventions should be regularly evaluated and continually reassessed, as this underpins clinical decision-making, helps set appropriate goals and reduces waste and potentially morbidity.

The World Union of Wound Healing Societies (WUWHS 2008) supports the work of Posnett *et al.* and recommends that a comprehensive wound assessment: determines the cause of the wound; identifies any underlying conditions that may contribute to wound healing; assesses the status of the wound; and develops a management plan.

Clinical information needed in order to make the assessment comprehensive includes:

- A full medical and surgical history
- Information that assesses the patient holistically, taking into consideration the bio-psychosocial model (Engel 1977)
- The patient is not seen in isolation and the impact of the family, work life, social life, etc. is taken into consideration
- Any contributing factors such as comorbidities that may impinge on skin breakdown or wound healing.

Many healthcare services now have comprehensive wound assessment charts, however there are national and international charts that have been created to aid practice in clinical areas where there is not yet any coordinated documentation such as those devised by Healthcare Improvement Scotland (HIS 2009; Gray *et al.* 2009; Fletcher 2010). These charts contain the necessary information to undertake a full assessment and include:

Cause of the wound

It is important to identify the cause of the wound, for example: was it due to urine and faeces falling on to the skin causing nappy rash? A sharp instrument pushed into a person's skin, creating a traumatic injury? An avulsion injury caused from catching a digit on a piece of machinery? Alongside the cause, the clinician should ask how long the wound has been present (acute, chronic or palliative) and what previous interventions have been used. Inappropriate assessment of the cause will lead to poor management in the future.

Wound size

No method of wound measurement is 100% accurate, however all wounds should be measured for length, width and depth at each dressing change as an initial baseline for assessment and for further wound progression. The three commonest guides are: the linear measurement or the 'clock face'; the greatest width × greatest length; or wound tracing.

- The *clock face* measures the wound by carrying out the following actions: when measuring length, the head is at 12 o'clock and the feet at 6 o'clock. When measuring width, measure perpendicular to the length, i.e. measure the widest part from 3 o'clock to 9 o'clock. The depth can be measured in a variety of ways, however a simple tool is to use a swab to measure the deepest depth from epidermis to end of the cavity, which may be through dermis and down to bone. To measure undermining, you would assess the depth for each hour of the clock beginning at 12 and moving round to 11 in a clockwise direction. Tunnelling would be measured by using the clock face for direction, i.e. the tunnelling occurs at 4 o'clock and is 3 cm in depth from the epidermis to the end of the tunnel.
- *Greatest width × greatest length* is measured by making sure the wound is measured that length-ways is from head to toe and width-ways is perpendicular to this. The measurements are then multiplied to give the surface area of the wound.
- The third method is to complete an acetate grid *wound tracing* and count up the squares in the outline of the wound.

Many health services use photography as a method to support the documentation of a wound assessment, the advantages are a visual guide and image of the progression and state of the wound, however disadvantages are the skill and competence of the photographer (Are the same rules applied for each repeat photograph?) and also the issue of consent.

Red Flag Consent and Medical Photography

Is the photograph to be used just for the patient's notes, or for teaching or even publication? Clinical governance issues must be followed in-line with your local policy.

Wound site

The wound site can assist in the identification of any comorbidities or processes that could be connected with the occurrence of the wound, for example a diabetic foot ulcer, occurs on the foot, usually were there has been uneven pressure distribution and a venous ulcer is common in the gaiter region. Naming and documenting the site of the wound is vital, specifically if there is more than one area of loss of skin integrity.

Colour and type of tissue at the wound bed

The colour and type of tissue at the wound bed can often indicate the stage of wound healing or the presence of a complication. Those wounds healing by secondary intention can be classified as: necrotic, infected, sloughy, granulating and epithelialising.

Wounds can contain more than one tissue type and colour and present as a mixed wound, but prior to assessment of colour and tissue type, the old dressing should be removed and the wound should be cleansed.

Necrotic tissue is where ischaemia has occurred and the tissue has died, forming an eschar or scab, presenting as hardened black or brown coloured tissue. Other necrotic tissue can present as thick layers of slough and can be grey, brown, off white or dark purple. It is necessary to remember that the wound underneath the eschar may be more extensive than can be visibly seen as the scab masks the actual size of the wound, often after debridement (if advocated), the true extent of damage is seen and can be shocking to both staff and patient.

Infected wounds normally produce a purulent discharge and in most cases, a host reaction. The type of bacteria causing the infection can affect the colour of the exudate, which can be yellow, green or fluorescent in colour and may even contain old or new blood. In many instances, a wound swab may be taken, but this is not to prove an infection is present as assessment has demonstrated this, the swab is to aid identification of the bacteria present. The discharge from an infected wound may also be large in amount and have an offensive odour. Granulation tissue in an infected wound may be a darker red in colour and the peri-wound area may show signs of infection, however in neuropathic diabetics or immune compromised patients, the natural immune response may not be visible.

Sloughy tissue is characteristically yellow/white in colour, however a note of caution here as tendons and ligaments are a shiny, creamy white and should not be classified as slough. Slough is the collection of dead cells collected in the exudate and is related to the end-stage of the inflammatory phase of healing. It can easily be removed by macrophages and disappears as the wound heals.

Granulation tissue was first described by John Hunter in 1786 and is seen as red and granular in appearance, consequently the name. This is actually the tops of the capillary loops that develop during proliferation phase of wound healing. This tissue is often friable and can bleed easily if touched. If granulation tissue is dark red, this could signify an infection or poor tissue perfusion.

Epithelialising tissue is pinky white in colour and is seen as the wound margins start to contract and island sites are visible on the surface of the wound bed. As noted earlier all scars heal pink and careful consideration of the care of the scar is needed and involvement of other services depending on the patient's natural skin tone and the site of the scar itself.

Suitable dressings for different wound types are shown in Figure 18.7.

Level of exudate

Exudate is normally clear and amber coloured and has no odour. The WUWHS (2007) report four categories when assessing and documenting wound exudate; these comprise of colour, consistency, odour and amount. It can be difficult to measure the amount of exudate a wound has; the symbols +, ++ and +++ have been used to signify mild, moderate and heavy exudate. Instead of using subjective methods, a more reliable way is to weigh dressings before and after use to measure the amount of exudate. This may not be feasible, so it is suggested that data must be made of the type and amount of dressings used over a certain time frame including any staining, the presence of strike through, maceration or leakage around the dressing, which may be signifying an increase, decrease of exudate levels or that it is remaining the same.

The level of exudate can impede the wound healing process as too little leads to the wound drying out and too much causes maceration or excoriation of the peri-wound area.

Signs and symptoms of infection

During assessment, the clinician should explore the potential of a wound infection; identification should make clear if the wound bed is contaminated, colonised or infected, and this should also be differentiated from the inflammatory response of wound healing. Prompt diagnosis aids optimal treatment and requires both clinical assessment and if necessary, diagnostic testing. There are classic signs such as pyrexia, oedema, pain, inflammation and an increase in exudate production, but there are also additional signs such as delayed healing, increased watery exudate rather than pus, pocketing at the wound base, bridging, increased pain, malodour, friability of tissues, a change in the colour of granulation tissue and wound breakdown, although some patients with diabetes may fail to present with any symptoms apart from closer observation of a delay in wound healing (Patel 2010). A routine and simple method of diagnosing the offending bacteria, is via a wound swab, however, the reliability of this method depends on the method used. Deep tissue biopsy is considered the most reliable method of diagnosing the causative agent of wound infection, but its use in day-to-day wound care is restricted due to the trauma to the patient and the professional, who is allowed to take the biopsy, as this is often limited only to doctors and podiatrists.

Jot This Down
What is your local policy for taking a wound swab? How does this compare with best practice?
Discuss your findings with the infection control team.

Pain at the wound bed

Often, patients with a wound will experience some pain during the care received. Pain at the wound bed can be due to a variety of causes, such as neuropathic in the patient with diabetes, anticipatory as the patient waits for the dressing to be removed, and iatrogenic due to self-harm. Carrying out a full assessment that includes a full pain history, body map and location/site of the pain can aid appropriate dressing selection and pain management approach (WUWHS 2008). Regular reassessment is imperative to reassess strategies and progress, as are the use of visual analogue scales commonly added to wound assessment charts in clinical practice. Pain does not always correlate with the size and depth of wound and the cause of the pain can often be psychological than physical, however its management is imperative to the wound healing process and both pharmacological and non-pharmacological approaches should be explored.

Surrounding skin

The margins of the wound will be liable to change as the wound progresses through the phases of wound healing. Changes in colour

Woud type		Characteristics	Examples of suitable dressings
Epithelialising	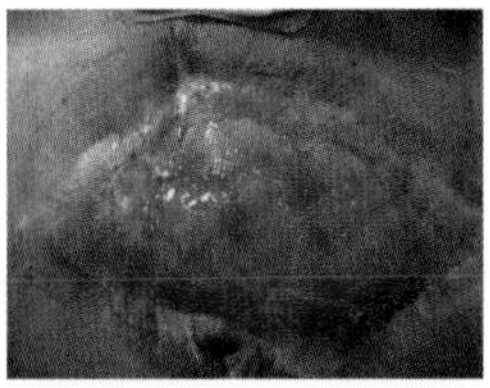	Clean, superficial, low to medium exudate, pink in colour	Low and non-adherent dressings, knitted viscose, paraffin gauze, film dressings
Granulating	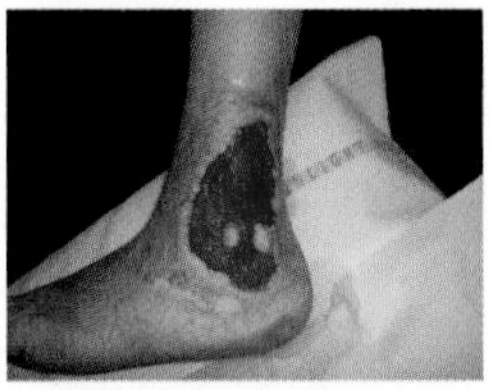	Clean, low to medium exudate, red in colour with granular appearance	Alginates , hydrocolloids, foams
Sloughy	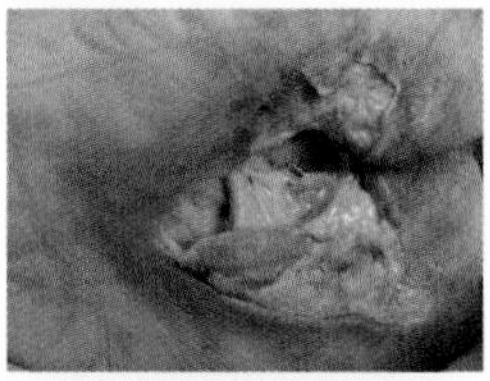	Medium to high exudate, yellowish-grey in colour, partially or completely covered in slough	Hydrogels, alginates, spun hydrocolloids
Necrotic wounds	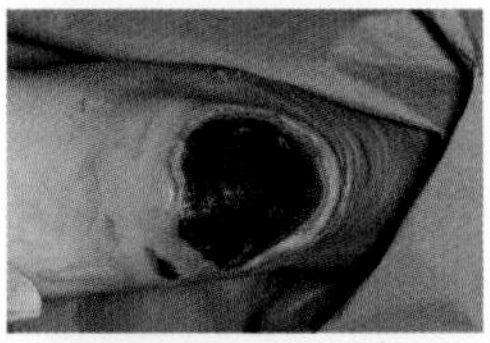	Black, dry, eschar devitalized tissue	Hydrogels, hydrocolloids
Infected wounds	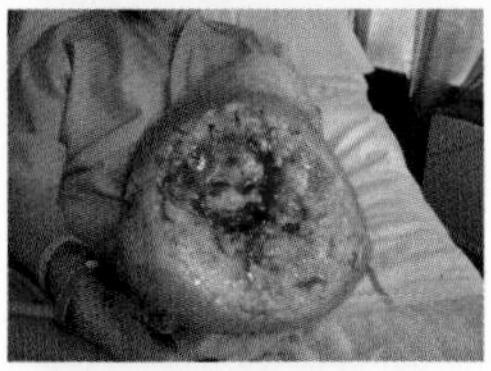	Painful, moderate to high exudate, malodorous, crusting	Silver-impregnated dressings, hydrogels, spun hydrocolloids
Blistering	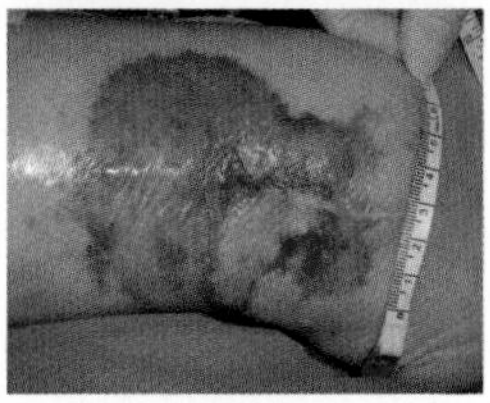	Clean, superficial, low to medium exudate	Non-adherent dressings

Figure 18.7 **Suitable dressings for different wound types.** Source: Buxton & Morris-Jones (2009). Reproduced with permission of John Wiley & Sons Ltd.

and appearance can indicate healing or wound breakdown, for example redness may indicate infection. The peri-wound area can become macerated or excoriated if the wound produces too much exudate for the dressing to handle and the clinician then needs to explore the use of either more absorbent dressings, more frequent dressing changes and protective barrier skin products for the peri-wound area (Figure 18.8).

Other clinical data

Not only will the practitioner record in the assessment the clinical information mentioned earlier, but also the type of wound, the phase of wound healing, any grading, staging or classification for that particular type of wound, factors affecting wound healing, diagnostic tests and any current management.

Types of Wound
Minor injuries

Many wounds are trivial in nature and include common wounds seen in minor injury units, walk-in centres, practice nurse clinics and accident and emergency. These can include, and are classified as:

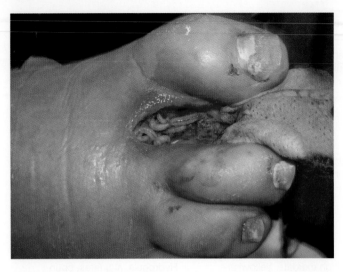

Figure 18.8 Using larvae to clean a peri-wound area. Source: Buxton & Morris-Jones (2009). Reproduced with permission of John Wiley & Sons Ltd.

368

Avulsions: these occur when the skin has been pulled off with or without the involvement of bone by doors and machinery. This can include digits, however they can occur in the legs and arms of patients who have previously had steroidal treatment, as their skin is friable and easily avulsed.

Contusions: are bruises, and these occur from trauma to the skin and bleeding arises in the tissue spaces. Bruising can be graded from 0–5, 5 being a critical bruise from bleeding into the brain or compartment of a muscle and 0 being a light bruise with very little damage. Underlying medical conditions can cause bruising, such as leukaemia, coagulation problems and infection, so the clinician needs to carry out a full assessment to exclude these and explore other factors such as physical abuse.

Cuts: these are wounds with well-defined edges, little bruising and usually straight in alignment. They usually occur due to sharp implements and are easily repaired with sutures, staples, glue or Steri-Strips.

Abrasions: scrapes to the knee when falling on gravel, for example are brought about by the action of friction and shear between a blunt item and the skin. These types of wounds often dry out, scab over and heal without scarring, however if gravel is embedded into the skin, it should be removed to prevent tattooing of the skin permanently.

Bites: human or animal bites can cause heavily contaminated wounds, which require thorough assessment for the type of toxins and bacteria present, so correct antibiotics can be prescribed. These types of wounds are healed through tertiary wound healing.

Skin tears: shear and friction forces that separate the epidermis from the dermis or dermis from the subcutaneous layers lead to skin tears. They mainly occur in the elderly, because of the fragility of the skin from medication, age and altered skin function. Healing May be lengthened due to comorbidities, however treatment can vary from dressings, Steri-Strips, compression bandaging and surgery. Skin tears can be classified (see later).

Lacerations: falls, blows to the skin and crushing injuries from blunt instruments cause a break in the skin with an irregular wound edge, which heals by secondary intention.

Table 18.3 Description of types of surgical wound.

TYPE OF SURGICAL WOUND	DESCRIPTION
Clean	An incision in which no inflammation is encountered in a surgical procedure, without a break in sterile technique and during which the respiratory tract, alimentary or genitourinary tracts are not entered
Clean contaminated	An incision through which the respiratory, alimentary or genitourinary tract is entered under controlled conditions but with no contamination encountered
Contaminated	An incision in which there is a major break in sterile technique, or gross spillage from the gastrointestinal tract, or an incision in which acute, non-purulent inflammation is encountered as well as open traumatic wounds that are more than 12–24 hours old
Dirty or infected	An incision in which the viscera (internal organs) are perforated or when acute inflammation with pus is encountered, e.g. emergency surgery for faecal peritonitis) and for traumatic wounds where treatment is delayed, there is faecal contamination or devitalised tissue

Surgical wounds

Post-surgery wounds can be classified as: clean, clean contaminated, contaminated and dirty or infected (NICE 2008, p. 9). The descriptions are given in Table 18.3.

Classification of surgical wound complications Fistulas

can occur when patients have a malignancy and inflammatory bowel disease, however, others have no one cause. A passage is formed between two organs for example bowel and the vagina (recto-vaginal) and faeces from the bowel will pass out of the vagina. Common fistulas occur between the bowel and skin (enterocutaneous).

A cavity or bursae that leads from the outside of the body inside is known as a sinus. It is lined with epithelial cells and is caused by infection, a foreign body or breakdown of dead tissue. Patients with sinuses often have surgical intervention, as recurrence rate is high. Epidemiology shows that factors that increase the vulnerability of a sinus include recent blunt trauma and haematoma formation, immobility, sedentary job and lifestyle, previous abscess formation and surgery at the site.

Dehiscence or the unplanned opening of a wound post-surgery is often triggered by poor surgical technique, haematoma formation, insufficient number of sutures, infection, age, diabetes and trauma to the wound. Wound healing is often by secondary or tertiary intention and grafts made of Teflon are used to add strength to the peritoneal lining.

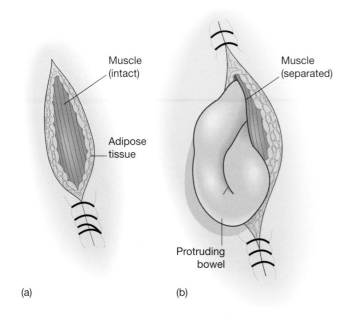

Muscle
(intact)

Adipose
tissue

Muscle
(separated)

Protruding
bowel

(a)   (b)

Figure 18.9 Evisceration of a wound can be frightening for the patient.

Evisceration is a very frightening experience for both patient and clinician. It occurs in 30% of all surgical wounds and is when the gastrointestinal tract protrudes the wound opening (Figure 18.9). The patient should be observed for signs of shock, the open wound and bowel covered with moist sterile dressings, the person let down with the foot of the bed elevated 20 degrees and medical attention sought immediately. Again, as in a dehisced wound, a return to theatre and the use of Teflon grafts is often advocated.

Factitious wounds

Wounds caused by self-harm are routinely peculiar, with sharp geometric margins surrounded by normal looking skin (Gupta *et al.* 1987). How these wounds present on assessment depends on the cause, for example burn, tourniquet, excoriation or chemical injury and can present as blisters, purpura, ulcers, erythema, oedema, sinuses or nodules. At times, skin loss can be so significant that the person requires plastic surgery. Timely identification is vital to avert unnecessary surgery and morbidity (Tantam & Huband 2009). The wounds tend to occur in areas that are easily accessible, i.e. the opposite arm to the dominant writing hand, the abdomen or legs. They are often asymmetrical and appear quickly, with no previous history of injury or disease. Patients are often those with dermatological conditions (Harth *et al.* 2010) and have no intent to any suicidal intent. NICE (2004) guidance is provided for clinicians who care for patients who have wounds due to self-harm. Self-harm wounds are categorised into two types: pathological and non-pathological.

Culturally sanctioned, *non-pathological* self-harm consists of body modification practices such as tattoos or piercing.

Pathological self-harm, typically, is a method of emotional regulation and is further categorised into four types: major, stereotypic, compulsive and impulsive (Favazza 2012).

- *Major* comprises of the infrequent destroying of major body tissue, for example amputation

- *Stereotypic* consists of tissue injury, e.g. from head banging, eye gouging, lip biting and face slapping
- *Compulsive* includes recurring behaviors such as skin scratching and nail biting
- *Impulsive* involves cutting, burning and carving.

Leg Ulcers

Leg ulcers affect 1% of the population at a particular point in time and can be defined as 'the loss of skin below the knee on the leg or foot, which takes more than 6 weeks to heal' (NHS Centre for Reviews and Dissemination, NHS-CRD 1997).

Classification of leg ulcers

Factors that make a patient prone to the development of leg ulcers include venous hypertension, peripheral vascular disease, diabetes, rheumatoid arthritis and systemic vasculitis.

Venous leg ulcers

For most patients, the major cause of leg ulceration, between 60% and 80%, is due to venous hypertension and is treatable. Valves in the superficial, deep and perforator veins become damaged and impair the flow of blood returning to the heart, initiating a back-flow. This backflow leads to varicosities, venous stasis, lower leg oedema and a change in the colour and integrity of the skin. The tissue becomes fibrous and woody in nature and brown staining appears (lipodermatosclerosis). Many patients complain of itchiness, pain and tenderness, especially when walking. This creates immobility and then adds further complexities to the situation, with ineffective use of the calf muscle pump to aid venous return. Ankle flare (dilation of the superficial veins of the leg near the ankle) and atrophie blanche (white plaque spots near the ankle) can often be visible on examination. Past medical and surgical history that increase the susceptibility to venous leg ulceration includes: family history, a sedentary job and lifestyle, gender (women more than men), pregnancy, diet, obesity, reduced mobility, malnutrition and intravenous drug use.

Clinical indicators of a venous leg ulcer Leg ulcers that are venous have classic indicators: they are found on the medial malleolus and gaiter region of the leg; pain is often dull, aching and relieved by elevation (Figure 18.10). The skin has staining, atrophie blanche and ankle flare. Oedema reduces with management and elevation, veins of the leg are distended and varicosities are seen. The ulcer is usually shallow, flat and has high levels of exudates; there is often wet or dry eczema in the peri-wound area. Ankle brachial indices reading would be between 0.9 and 1.2.

Arterial leg ulcers

Arterial disease affects 22% of the persons who have a leg ulcer and is attributed to smoking, a history or family history of cardiovascular problems, high cholesterol, high alcohol intake, diabetes, aged over 50, sedentary lifestyle and male. Arterial disease is caused by hardening and narrowing of the arteries due the deposition of fat (atheroma and atherosclerosis), which leads to tissue death of the extremities of the limbs. A cascade effect occurs, where a lack of oxygen and nutrients to the leg occurs, causing ischaemia and cell death, or total occlusion of a blood vessel and thrombosis, which leads to gangrene and mummification of the toes.

When assessing patients with leg and foot ulcers, classic signs and symptoms aid the clinician in detecting arterial disease. These

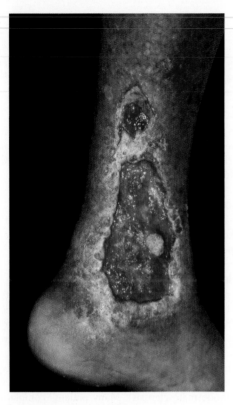

Figure 18.10 **Venous leg ulcer.** Source: Buxton & Morris-Jones (2009). Reproduced with permission of John Wiley & Sons Ltd.

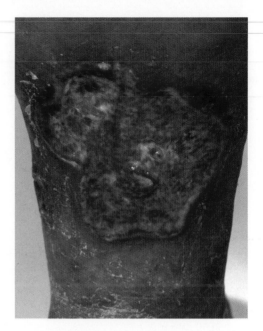

Figure 18.11 **Arterial leg ulcer.** Source: Buxton & Morris-Jones (2009). Reproduced with permission of John Wiley & Sons Ltd.

include a history of rest pain, which is pain experienced at night when lying in bed with elevated legs. It is relieved when the legs are dangled out of bed or the person goes to sit in the chair. Intermittent claudication, triggered on exercise, is caused by cramping pain in the hips, thighs, buttocks and calf muscles, due to inadequate supply of oxygenated blood. Absence of foot pulses, coldness, hairless, mottled appearance of the skin (bluish/red in Caucasians, purple/bluish/black in black people and ashen grey/yellow in Asians), brittle toenails, breaks that do not heal and sunset rubra (skin turns red on dependence). The person may also complain of numbness and tingling in the toe, foot or leg.

Clinical indicators of an arterial leg ulcer

The ulcer can appear anywhere on the foot. Pain is increased at night or on exercise, with rest or when elevated. The skin is pale and hairless; oedema is seen in the dependent leg. There is poor capillary refill with a punched out deep ulcer with extensive tissue loss (Figure 18.11). Ankle brachial indices reading would be below 0.8. Often referral to a vascular surgeon is necessary or indeed, urgent.

Rheumatoid arthritis and systemic vasculitis

Of all leg ulcers, 9% occur in patients with rheumatoid arthritis and the ulcer has other underlying components, such as an arterial, venous or a vasculitic component.

Diabetic ulcers

Five per cent of all people with leg ulcers have diabetic ulcers. These are usually ulcers that have multiple aetiology and result from a combination of diabetes and venous disease or diabetes and arterial disease.

Iatrogenic leg ulcers

Some elderly patients with a history of leg ulceration may become classified as having a 'hard to heal' wound. On a full reassessment, it may be noticed that there is no significant reason for the person's ulcer not to heal; however the only contact the patient receives is the weekly visit from the district nurse due to social isolation and lack of family and friends. It can be discovered that the patient is removing the dressing, picking at the wound or causing other wounds (self-harming), due to a lack of company in their life. In these instances, referral to social and local services is necessary to increase contact with others in their local community. A 'Leg Club' may be part of the local service provision and referral to this service will assist with improving the quality of life for the patient with this type of wound and promoting healing and addressing meaning and purpose in the lives of elderly and vulnerable.

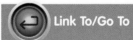 Link To/Go To

http://www.legclub.org/about.shtml

The Lyndsey Leg Club website: a charity that was set up by a district nurse from Suffolk in response to the social factors and isolation caused by leg ulceration.

Pressure Ulcers

According to the European and National Pressure Ulcer Advisory Panels (2009, p. 7): 'A pressure ulcer is localised injury to the skin and/or underlying tissue usually over a bony prominence, as a result of pressure, or pressure in combination with shear. A number of contributing or confounding factors are also associated with pressure ulcers; the significance of these factors is yet to be elucidated'.

As pressure ulcers affect 10.2–10.3% of the population in hospital (Phillips & Buttery 2009), they correspond to considerable costs to the NHS, or £1.4–2.1 billion per year (Bennett *et al.* 2004) and to the patient, in relation to quality of life, sickness, morbidity and mortality. The introduction of cost-effective, evidence-based practice is therefore imperative. Three key methods for delivering good quality care to reduce the number of avoidable pressure ulcers are to: use pressure – relieving surfaces, have access to a tissue viability nurse and introduce prevention protocols and guidance.

Causes of pressure ulcers
The causes of pressure ulcers are either extrinsic or intrinsic.

Intrinsic Intrinsic factors include those that affect the physical, social and mental well-being of a patient and can include factors such as nutrition, body temperature, dehydration, age, medication, immobility, sleeping, elimination, anxiety and depression (this list is not exhaustive).

Extrinsic The three main extrinsic causes of pressure ulcers are pressure, friction and shear.

Pressure: When the skin is compressed between a hard surface and a bony prominence, either from a high pressure for a short period of time and a low pressure for a long period of time, pressure damage can occur. This often leaves a wound that is circular in shape and can often affect the epidermis, dermis and underlying structures and bone. A cascade effect takes place when the pressure impedes the flow of blood in the underlying layers of the skin. Initial tissue hypoxia occurs, which if unrelieved, becomes ischaemia and then cell death occurs. Initial damage may often not be visible, as the damage occurs at the bony prominence. Days later, a large necrotic wound is present and the extent of the damage is now visible. In instances where patients have been admitted to hospital after being found collapsed at home, it is imperative to ask which position where they found in and for how long they had been in that position. This should be documented clearly, as within days of admission, pressure ulcers may develop in those areas and harm-free care may have been unavoidable, but therapeutic interventions should have already commenced.

In health, a person will reposition themselves in response to pressure exerted on the skin, however it is the vulnerable, immobile, frail, elderly and acutely sick or chronically ill patient whose risk of skin damage from pressure is intensified.

Tissue tolerance, i.e. the ability of the skin to tolerate pressure without adverse problems, depends upon capillary closing pressures. Healthy individuals can normally tolerate 32 mmHg exerted on the capillaries without detrimental effect, i.e. blood flow being disturbed and harm taking place. However, this does not take into account other mechanical and intrinsic forces or the closing pressure of the lymphatic system, whose role is to drain away excess fluid in the interstitial spaces.

Friction: Abrasions or blisters occur when the skin's surface rubs across another surface, such as a heel along a hospital sheet. The damage created is worsened if the skin is moist and exacerbates the risk of further damage, when other mechanical forces are involved.

Shear: The repositioning of patients can greatly increase the risk of wounds from shearing forces. During moving and handling,

the surface of the skin can become fixed while the rest of the body tries to move, causing underlying structures to be stretched, distorted and torn. This can often be seen as puckering of the skin and occurs when sliding patients up the bed incorrectly or from patients sliding down the bed. The shape of the wound is often tear-shaped and has a deep cavity.

Risk assessment
According to NICE (2005) guidance, all patients should have an initial and ongoing assessment of their risk of developing pressure ulcers. There are many risk assessment tools to choose from, however the local policy will dictate which tool is used and how. Most importantly for clinicians, is that they use their clinical judgement alongside the assessment, as many tools have limitations in relation to over or under prediction.

Classification of pressure ulcers
In order to provide consensus across Europe in the care and management of pressure ulcers, NPUAP developed a common classification system (NPUAP 2007; NPUAP & EPUAP 2009):

Category/stage I: non-blanchable erythema Intact skin with non-blanchable redness of a localised area usually over a bony prominence. Darkly pigmented skin may not have visible blanching; its colour may differ from the surrounding area. The area may be painful, firm, soft, warmer or cooler, when compared with adjacent tissue. Category/stage I may be difficult to detect in individuals with dark skin tones. May indicate 'at risk' persons.

Category/stage II: partial thickness Partial thickness is loss of dermis presenting as a shallow open ulcer with a red pink wound bed, without slough. May also present as an intact or open/ruptured serum-filled or serosanguineous filled blister. Presents as a shiny or dry shallow ulcer without slough or bruising (bruising indicates deep tissue injury) (Figure 18.12). This category should not be used to describe skin tears, tape burns, incontinence associated dermatitis, maceration or excoriation.

Category/stage III: full thickness skin loss Full thickness tissue loss. Subcutaneous fat may be visible but bone, tendon or muscles are *not* exposed. Slough may be present but does not obscure the depth of tissue loss. *May* include undermining and tunnelling. The depth of a category/stage III pressure ulcer varies by anatomical location. The bridge of the nose, ear, occiput and malleolus do not have (adipose) subcutaneous tissue and category/stage III ulcers can be shallow. In contrast, areas of significant adiposity can develop extremely deep category/stage III pressure ulcers. Bone/tendon is not visible or directly palpable.

Category/stage IV: full thickness tissue loss Full thickness tissue loss with exposed bone, tendon or muscle. Slough or eschar may be present. Often includes undermining and tunnelling. The depth of a category/stage IV pressure ulcer varies by anatomical location. The bridge of the nose, ear, occiput and malleolus do not have (adipose) subcutaneous tissue and these ulcers can be shallow. Category/stage IV ulcers can extend into muscle and/or supporting structures (e.g. fascia, tendon or joint capsule), making osteomyelitis or osteitis likely to occur. Exposed bone/muscle is visible or directly palpable.

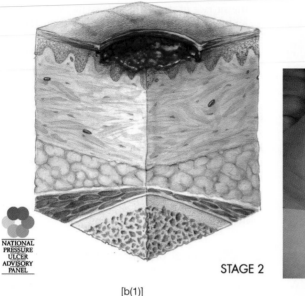

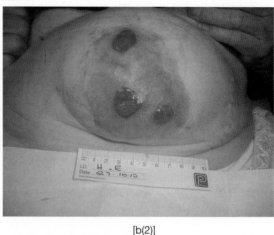

STAGE 2

[b(1)]

[b(2)]

Figure 18.12 **Stage II pressure ulcer.** Source: Flanagan (2013). Reproduced with permission of John Wiley & Sons Ltd.

Additional categories/stages for the USA

Unstageable/unclassified: full thickness skin or tissue loss – depth unknown Full thickness tissue loss in which actual depth of the ulcer is completely obscured by slough (yellow, tan, gray, green or brown) and/or eschar (tan, brown or black) in the wound bed. Until enough slough and/or eschar are removed to expose the base of the wound, the true depth cannot be determined; but it will be either a category/stage III or IV. Stable (dry, adherent, intact without erythema or fluctuance) eschar on the heels serves as 'the body's natural (biological) cover' and should not be removed.

Suspected deep tissue injury – depth unknown Purple or maroon localised area of discolored intact skin or blood-filled blister due to damage of underlying soft tissue from pressure and/ or *shear*. The area may be preceded by tissue that is painful, firm, mushy, boggy, warmer or cooler, when compared with adjacent tissue. Deep tissue injury may be difficult to detect in individuals with dark skin tones. Evolution may include a thin blister over a dark wound bed. The wound may further evolve and become covered by thin eschar. Evolution may be rapid, exposing additional layers of tissue, even with optimal treatment.

Pressure ulcer or moisture lesion?

As many hospital-acquired pressure ulcers develop in the sacral area, there has been much debate surrounding the classification of pressure ulcers, which previously have been categorised as stage I or II, when in fact the skin breakdown is actually a moisture lesion. In order to identify whether a wound to the sacral/anal area is a pressure ulcer or moisture lesion, the EPUAP (2005) published a position statement and asks the clinician to consider the following questions, if the answer is yes to all of them, the wound is to be considered a moisture lesion:

- Is there moisture present and is the skin shiny and wet?
- Is the wet skin caused by incontinence?
- Is the moisture lesion over a bony prominence?

- Has shear and pressure been excluded as a causative factor?
- Is the lesion linear, in a cleft of skin or around the perianal area?
- Is the shape of the lesion diffuse, e.g. lots of spots in the area, irregular edging?
- Is the lesion a copy or kissing lesion and a replica of the other cleft?
- Is the depth superficial, the lesion red, not uniformly distributed and is there no necrosis?
- Is there maceration around the edges?
- Does the lesion improve with skin barrier products designed to manage incontinence issues?

Reactive Hyperaemia

The characteristic bright red flush of skin in a patient with white/pink skin, which occurs when pressure is released from the skin is reactive hyperaemia. It can be assessed by applying light fingertip pressure to the area affected for 10 seconds and then observing the reaction. The skin initially should be white, which should then turn to its original colour, demonstrating to the practitioner that the skin is healthy and has a good blood supply. If the skin does not react and remains the same bright red flush, this is indicative of a stage I pressure ulcer and a revised approach to care should be taken. Reactive hyperaemia is difficult to distinguish in patients with black or brown skin; pressure ulcer development will be indicated by areas where there is localised heat that does not dissipate, or where there is damage, coolness, purple/black discolouration, localised swelling (oedema) or tissue hardness (induration) (NHS Quality Improvement, NHS-QI 2003).

Burns

A burn is an injury to the skin caused by heat, electricity, chemicals, radiation or friction (see Table 18.4). Over 250 000 people each year suffer a burn injury and 330 of these people die (Edwards 2012). Most are accidental in nature and many involve children, the elderly and adults who are obese, have cardiovascular and neurological conditions.

Table 18.4 Burn injuries.

TYPE OF BURN	INJURIES SUSTAINED	SYMPTOMS
Radiation from sunburn, radiotherapy and radiation	Affect the epidermis and dermis, mainly superficial in nature	Headache, chills, local discomfort, nausea and vomiting. Reddened blistered skin
Electrical from high voltage of electricity	Entry and exit wounds which are small and mask the true extent of damage	Tissue necrosis, gangrene, cardiac monitoring for ventricular fibrillation and cardiac arrest
Thermal from fire, combustible products, fireworks, excessive heat, steam, cold, liquid and surfaces	Can be superficial epidermis to deep wounds down to bone and underlying structures	Charring of the skin, blood vessels, muscle tissue, nervous tissue and bone
Chemical from corrosive substances (acid and alkali)	Can be superficial to deep wounds	Depends on the agent and the mechanism of action, duration of contact and body surface exposed

Table 18.5 Classification of burns.

CLASSIFICATION OF BURN	APPEARANCE	PAIN	HEALING TECHNIQUES AND TIMES
Full thickness	Pale, waxy, yellow, brown, mottled, charred or non-blanching red. Surface is dry, leathery and firm to touch, thrombosed blood vessels are visible	No sensation of pain or light touch	Require excision and skin grafting and are hard to heal. Often require initial fasciotomy and escharotomy. Often have contractures and hypertrophic scarring
Deep partial thickness	Pale and waxy, moist or dry, ruptured blister may occur that appear as tissue paper	Less pain than superficial thickness as areas of decreased sensation	Excision and grafting. More than 21 days healing time often with contractures and hypertrophic scarring
Superficial partial thickness	Bright red, moist glistening appearance with blisters. Blanches on pressure	Pain is severe in response to air and temperature. Pain and touch response intact	Dressing products and skin substitutes. Healing within 21 days with minimal or no scar formation
Superficial	Pink to bright red in colour	Stinging sensation	Water-soluble lotions and dressings. Healing in 3–6 days; no scar

373

Classification

The classification of burns is in accordance with the depth of tissue damage (see Table 18.5 for appearance and estimated healing times).

- Full thickness burns involve all layers of the skin and extend into the adipose, muscle, connective tissue and bone layers
- Deep partial thickness burns involve the epidermis and dermis but hair follicles, sebaceous glands and sweat glands are left intact
- Partial thickness burns affect the epidermis, dermis and the papillae of the dermis
- Superficial burns affect only the epidermis.

Burns assessment

There are two major methods of assessing a burn injury, one is used for adults (the Rule of Nines) and the other for children (the Lund and Browder tool), due to changes in body size with age. Alongside a comprehensive wound assessment, other pertinent information particular to burns nursing includes history of the burn, time of injury, causative agent, early treatment, age and body weight. Most questions are asked quickly, as initially on arrival, burns patients are awake, but conscious states can alter quickly in a major burn injury.

Assessing the extent of damage of a burn in a child is through the use of the Lund and Browder tool. Damage to the surface area

is measured by body parts affected (see Figure 18.13). In adults, the Rule of Nines, by division of the body into five surface areas (see Figure 18.13), only partial or full thickness burns are included in the estimation.

Any patient with a burn who meets any of the following criteria should be transferred to a specialist burns unit for further management (National Network for Burn Care 2012):

- Burns to the face, hands or feet
- Burns to a person aged 5 years and under and 60 years and over
- Burns circumferential to a joint
- Chemical and electrical burns
- Inhalation injuries
- More than 5% total body surface in children
- More than 10% body surface in an adult
- Any burn not healed in 14 days.

The Diabetic Foot

Nearly three million people in the UK have diabetes, and the number of patients requiring diabetic foot amputations has been increasing by 26% (Diabetes UK 2012). On average, 125 amputations are carried out each week, 80% of which are preventable and the cost in treating diabetic foot injuries and amputations is £600–700 million/year (Kerr 2012).

A diabetic foot ulcer is defined as 'a full thickness lesion of the skin, i.e. a wound penetrating through the dermis; lesions, such as

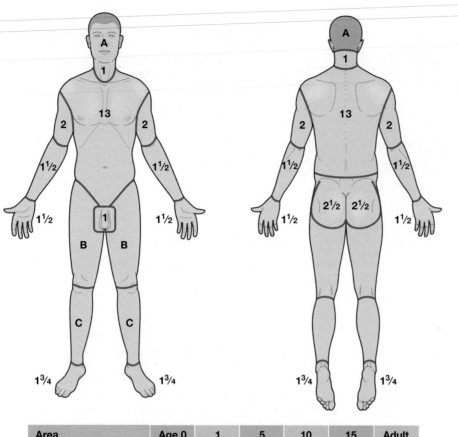

Region	% PTL	FTL
Head		
Neck		
Ant. trunk		
Post. trunk		
Right arm		
Left arm		
Buttocks		
Genitalia		
Right leg		
Left leg		
Total burn		

Area	Age 0	1	5	10	15	Adult
A = ½ of head	9½	8½	6½	5½	4½	3½
B = ½ of one thigh	2¾	3¼	4	4½	4¼	4¾
C = ½ of one lower leg	2½	2½	2¾	3	3¼	3½

Figure 18.13 Lund and Browder tool.

Box 18.2 Signs and Symptoms

- *Loss of sensation*: might not feel heat, cold, pressure, friction or shear
- *Dry skin*: from autonomic neuropathy, which leads to cracks, fissures and callus formation
- *Infection and osteomyelitis*: may not be visible but can be seen as mummification of toes and gangrene in the foot
- *Foot deformities*: Charcot's foot, claw toes, prominent metatarsal heads, altered gait and muscle atrophy.

blisters or skin mycosis (infection) are not included' (International Working Group on the Diabetic Foot, IWGDF 2003). This type of foot does not just contain an ulcer but an assortment of pathological changes such as loss of sensation (neuropathy), reduced blood flow (ischaemia and calcification), deformities of the foot (Charcot) and uneven distribution of pressure. Signs and symptoms are shown in Box 18.2.

Diabetic foot assessment

Interprofessional working is the key to affective diabetic foot ulcer assessment and management. Any patient who is admitted to healthcare services and presents with diabetes should have a thor-

ough assessment of the foot. If this assessment is not within the role of the clinician, podiatrists are at hand to help. The assessment is based upon a thorough holistic assessment but pertinent aspects include the examination of the foot based upon the IWGDF (2003) Pedis system, which takes into consideration, perfusion of the foot, extent and size of ulcer/damage, depth of tissue loss, infection and sensation. Podiatrists who usually carry out this assessment investigate the patients gait, mobility, posture, balance, reflexes, sensory function (vibration perception, protective pain sensation and neuropathy), foot pulses, Doppler and toe pressures (Figure 18.14).

Malignant and Fungating Wounds

Malignant wounds are frequently found in head and neck and breast cancers; however, they can also occur in the skin. They develop at the primary site of the cancer or at lymph nodes for example the groin or axillae. A fungating wound occurs when the tumour has invaded the epithelial layer of the skin and breaks through the surface, forming an ulcerative area (crater) or proliferative area (cauliflower-like nodules) (Dealey 2005). It is imperative to assess if the ulcer is malignant, especially as management would be focussed on symptoms rather than healing. In leg ulcers, it is recommended that if an ulcer fails to improve within a 12-week period, then a biopsy for malignancy should be taken,

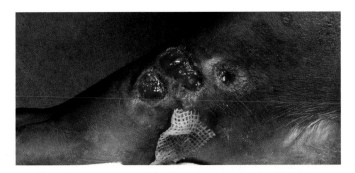

Figure 18.14 The diabetic foot. Source: Buxton & Morris-Jones (2009). Reproduced with permission of John Wiley & Sons Ltd.

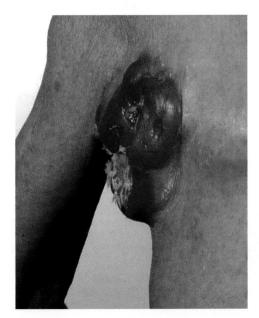

Figure 18.15 Malignant and fungating wound. Source: Buxton & Morris-Jones (2009). Reproduced with permission of John Wiley & Sons Ltd.

as often the ulcer is cancerous and not a typical venous one (Scottish Intercollegiate Guidelines for Nurses, SIGN 2010). Some patients are offered radiotherapy, chemotherapy or surgery for short-term symptom relief, however because cancer cells continue to grow, the wound will not disappear and will regress at a later stage (Figure 18.15).

Nursing Management

After a thorough holistic patient and wound assessment, it is imperative for the clinician to plan, implement and evaluate the care provided. If after the initial assessment the patient requires more advanced care than the clinician can provide, referrals for advice, support and guidance must be sought immediately and if necessary a transfer of care.

Moist Wound Healing

From 1962 onwards, the principles of moist wound healing challenged pervious presumptions of leaving a wound to dry out and scab over. George Winter (1962) and his study on pigs highlighted that if wounds were kept moist and the scab removed, cell migration is encouraged. His work has been repeated and is the basis of treatment for most wounds, as the advantages of moist wound healing include reduction in infection, less injury to the wound bed, less pain, assist debridement and cost-effective treatment.

Wound Bed Preparation

In order to optimise wound healing and ensure the dressings and equipment function at their best, it is imperative that the practitioner manages and prepares the wound bed. Wound bed preparation, according to Falanga (2000, p. 1) is 'the management of a wound in order to accelerate endogenous healing or to facilitate the effectiveness of other therapeutic measures'. Falanga suggests that effective wound bed preparation is achieved through the following actions: restoration of bacterial balance; management of necrosis; management of exudate; correction of cellular dysfunction; restoration of biochemical balance.

TIME

The TIME principle (Schultz *et al.* 2003) is a systematic approach to aid clinicians in the management of the wound bed. The method allows the nurse to focus on the stages of wound healing and eliminate any obstacles to facilitate healing processes. The abbreviation stands for:

T – Tissue non-viable or deficient
I – Infection or inflammation
M – Moisture imbalance
E – Epidermal margin – nonadvancing or undermined.

The nurse would consider, by answering questions at each stage, whether the wound requires debridement, infection treating, exudate managing and, is the wound improving?

Wound Cleansing

Wound cleansing should only be considered if the wound contains a previous dressing, foreign material or to loosen surface debris (Dealey 2005), as the procedure, if not necessary, can reduce the wound bed temperature and remove vital cytokines, growth factors and cause a delay in wound healing. The choice of method of cleaning a wound should be based upon a full assessment and a no-touch technique. Some wounds are suitable for cleaning with warm tap water, in the shower, bath or a bowl, others require 0.9% saline solution.

Dressing Selection

The sheer number of dressings available in order to create prompt and cosmetically acceptable healing can often be baffling and lead to the wrong type of dressing being chosen and a delay in the healing process. However, understanding the category in which the dressing is classified can help aid appropriate dressing choice. The selection will be based upon a full patient and wound assessment, the goals of the wound intervention, knowledge of the dressing to be used, its uses, side-effects and contraindications, the evidence base, the clinician's personal choice, the patient's concordance with treatment, known allergies and cost. Most organisations have developed wound care formularies and guides to aid prescribing and selection; manufacturer's guidelines should be followed regarding application, wear time and removal. However, a guide to actions and dressings for consideration are included in Table 18.6.

Not only must the clinician choose the correct dressing for the type of wound and appropriate wound bed management, a nurse must also consider addressing other factors that are affecting

Table 18.6 Dressings.

CLINICAL OBSERVATION	ACTION TO ACHIEVE WOUND BED PREPARATION	TYPE OF DRESSINGS TO BE CONSIDERED	OTHER ACTIONS FOR CONSIDERATION
Tissue non-viable or deficient	Debridement of necrosis or slough	Consider debridement via autolytic, sharp surgical, enzymatic, mechanical or biological methods	Seek further advice before intervening on foot ulcers for patients who present with impaired vascular flow, diabetes and neuropathy. Consider surgical and vascular opinion. Utilise podiatry
Infection or inflammation	Remove infection or biofilm	Topical antimicrobials, antibacterial, anti-inflammatories, protease inhibitors. Charcoal dressings to manage malodour	As above and ensure diagnosis of infection is correct. Try a 2-week antimicrobial challenge
Moisture imbalance	Moisten dry wounds or remove excess exudate	Moisture rebalancing: Dry wounds; use films, hydrocolloids, hydrogels and foams. Heavily exuding wounds; compression therapy, foams, alginates, hydrofibres, wound managers, topical negative pressure	Consider skin protection to the peri-wound area in heavily exuding wounds
Edge of wound – non-advancing or undermined	Reassess cause and consider debridement, advanced therapies or surgical intervention	Debridement skin grafts Biological agents	Consider biopsy if non-healing. Utilise adjuvant therapies such as hyperbaric oxygen, referral to other members of the MDT. Consider palliative wound and symptom management. Consider peri-wound area is it viable, does it require management/protection, is it suitable for adhesive dressings or tapeless/non-adhesive ones?

376

wound healing, for example nutrition, pressure relief, repositioning, lack of sleep and pain. There should be consideration of other members of the interprofessional team aiding diagnosis and management, use of specialist equipment and adjuvant therapies such as hyperbaric oxygen, medication, pressure relieving and reducing devices and cosmetic camouflage.

 Link To/Go To

Wounds UK offer position statements and consensus statements from International, European and National Wound Care Expert Groups to aid decision-making in wound care.
http://www.wounds-uk.com/best-practice-statements

Multiple Pathology and Wound Care

Care of the Older Person's Skin

Age is a contributing factor in the potential for skin breakdown and the delay in wound healing. As a person ages they also develop other intrinsic and extrinsic factors that further interfere with this process. Although ageing cannot be prevented, it is important for the nurse to reduce harm by ensuring good skin care strategies are put in place. Common skin conditions that affect the elderly include: eczema, psoriasis, infections, infestations and pruritus (Davies 2008), however skin tears, pressure ulcers and incontinence-related damage can occur. Skin conditions, like general health

issues, often go under-reported in the elderly as they almost seem defeatist to health and well-being issues or prefer to be stoical. It is therefore important on admission and at regular intervals to assess the skin of the older person and also regularly enquire for further problems that may be considered trivial, as often the skin problem is a sign or symptom of an underlying condition for example diabetes, renal failure, thyroid dysfunction or iron deficiency anaemia. In 2008, a best practice statement was developed by a team of specialists on behalf of *Wounds UK*, this was updated in 2012 and advocates some of the following summarised key principles in care of the older person:

1. Holistic assessment of the older person is key to further management and treatment.
2. Exploration of underlying conditions is often necessary due to the skin problem being a result of a systemic disease.
3. Emollients applied twice per day to rehydrate the skin, are a practical solution for protection.
4. Ensure an older person's nails are kept short to minimise trauma when scratching.
5. NICE (2004) best practice should be followed for the prevention and management of pressure ulcers.
6. Early detection of moisture and subsequent management in relation to maceration in the chronic wound is essential; the use of suitable barrier creams and films may be necessary.
7. As incontinence can increase skin breakdown, appropriate measures for the management of urine and faeces is required.
8. Skin tears (Figure 18.16) can occur from handling, equipment and the environment. It is important to classify a skin tear (see Table 18.7): realign the skin tear immediately after injury if possible and utilise appropriate non-adhesive dressings to optimise healing.

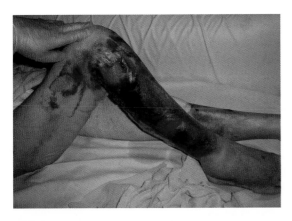

Figure 18.16 Skin tear. Source: Flanagan (2013). Reproduced with permission of John Wiley & Sons Ltd.

Table 18.7 Classification of skin tears. (Carville *et al.* 2007)

SKIN TEAR CLASSIFICATION (STAR)	SKIN DAMAGE
Category 1a	A skin tear where the edges can be realigned to the normal anatomical position (without undue stretching) and the skin or flap colour is not pale, dusky or darkened
Category 1b	A skin tear where the edges can be realigned to the normal anatomical position (without undue stretching) and the skin or flap colour is pale, dusky or darkened
Category 2a	A skin tear where the edges cannot be realigned to the normal anatomical position and the skin or flap colour is not pale, dusky or darkened
Category 2b	A skin tear where the edges cannot be realigned to the normal anatomical position and the skin or flap colour is pale, dusky or darkened
Category 3	A skin tear where the skin flap is completely absent

9. At life's end, despite all the best care possible, the skin may be at risk to unavoidable pressure ulcers, previously known as the Kennedy terminal ulcer (Kennedy 1989). They are butterfly-shaped and situated predominately, but not exclusively, on the buttocks. However, since 2010 (Sibbald *et al.* 2010), the term for the changes in the skin of an older person at the end of life is 'skin changes at life's end' (SCALE) and if a pressure ulcer does develop, then the tissue viability nurse should be contacted as to ascertain if the pressure ulcer was unavoidable or not.

Neuroischaemic Diabetic Foot Ulcer

Of all diabetic foot ulcers, 60% are neuroischaemic in nature (Gershater *et al.* 2009). Patients with these types of ulcers present late and often have involvement of gangrene, due to poor vascular supply to the foot. The focus of their care should be on revasculari-

sation, but because of the gangrene, patients are often considered unsuitable and tend not to be listed for surgery but for amputation instead. The IWGDF (2007) highlight the issue that clinicians need to be assessing the vascular flow of diabetic patients with neuropathy earlier on in their care, prior to the development of ulcers and gangrene. They suggest the assessment of toe pressures and ankle pressures to indicate earlier vascular intervention and call for a new classification system that takes into consideration these patients with microangiopathy, so as to ascertain treatment options such as reconstruction, vascular surgery or pharmacology (Apelqvist 2010). Debridement of these types of wounds may be initially delayed due to the risk of trauma. If the gangrene is dry and mummified, the practitioner may leave the wound alone and seek an urgent vascular opinion (Wounds International 2013).

Conclusion

The prevention and management of wounds has progressed over the last 30 years from a simple wound assessment to the biological, psychological and economical impact of the wound on the patient, the carers, the clinicians and healthcare providers. Practitioners more than ever need to acquire the necessary knowledge, skills and attitudes in order to assess, plan, implement and evaluate the care delivered for this group of patients. As technology moves forward, so does the need to critically appraise the evidence provided within the realms of cost- effectiveness and efficiency. The quality agenda will promote the collection of outcomes measures and metrics, in order for clinicians to quantify their decisions to ensure the right treatment for the right patient at the right time.

Key Points

- The cost of wound care is rising and according to Posnett and Franks (2007), around 200 000 people in the UK have a chronic wound, which costs approximately £2.3–3.1 billion per year.
- The tissue viability nurse's role is a key lead position in wound prevention and management, undertaking the four key roles of a nurse specialist duties working alongside other members of staff and acting as consultant, researcher, educator and manager.
- A vital component of wound healing is to assess the patient holistically and therefore prior to even assessing the wound and the dressing currently being used, it is imperative that the clinician assesses the physical, social and psychological factors that may impinge on wound healing.
- The wound site can assist in the identification of any comorbidities or processes that could be connected with the occurrence of the wound, for example a diabetic foot ulcer occurs on the foot, usually were there has been uneven pressure distribution and a venous ulcer is common in the gaiter region. Naming and documenting the site of the wound is vital, specifically if there is more than one area of loss of skin integrity.
- A wound assessment that addresses the holistic assessment of the patient is imperative to good wound management. The assessment process should discover any contributing or causative factors that could impinge on the wound healing process, consider the state of the wound bed and peri-wound area and then plan appropriate interventions.

(Continued)

- The causes of pressure ulcers are either extrinsic or intrinsic. According to NICE (2005) guidance, all patients should have an initial and ongoing assessment of their risk of developing pressure ulcers.
- Age is a contributing factor in the potential for skin breakdown and the delay in wound healing. As a person ages, they also develop other intrinsic and extrinsic factors that further interfere with this process.

Glossary

Abrasion: an injury caused by rubbing or scraping that results in the loss of the superficial layer of skin or epidermis and or dermis and may involve the mucous membrane

Acid mantle: the body's natural protection of the outer layer of skin having a pH between 4.0 and 5.5

Angiogenesis: the process of forming new blood vessels

Autolysis: the process where devitalised or dead tissue is self-digested through the action of enzyme

Bacterial burden or load: the number and virulence of bacteria in a wound

Blanching: when pressure is applied to a reddened area the area under the pressure becomes white

Charcot: (Char Coe) foot, a progressive condition affecting the musculoskeletal system of the foot in persons with diabetes. Fractures of the bones in the foot joint dislocation and deformities can occur. The bottom of the foot has the appearance of the base of a rocking chair due to the arch of the foot collapsing

Contraction: shrinking in size. In wound healing, contraction occurs around the edges of the wound causing the wound size to become smaller

Debridement: the removal of devitalised or dead tissue and foreign material from the wound bed

Dependent: opposite of elevated

Dependent rubor: a redness or purple colour of a leg when it is in the dependent or lowered position

Dermis: the second layer of the skin, under the epidermis

Epidermis: outermost layer of the skin

Epithelialisation: the process of epithelial cell formation and migration from the wound edges

Erythema: redness of the skin

Eschar: necrotic tissue that forms a black thickened covering over wounds

Exudate: fluid that comes from wounds

Fibrin: a protein involved in the blood clotting process and the granulation phase of healing

Fascia: a band or sheet of connective tissue found throughout the body

Fibroblast: an important cell in wound healing

Friable tissue: tissue that bleeds easily

Granulation tissue: tissue that forms in the wound base, which fills in wounds with scar tissue as healing with secondary intention

Induration: a process where the skin becomes firm, often surrounds a wound as a healing ridge or can be a sign of building biofilm

Inflammatory phase of healing: the body's initial response to injury and lasts between 2–4 days

Intermittent claudication: often identified as a pain in the lower limbs related to poor or compromised blood supply

Ischemia: a deficiency of blood supply to an area

Lipodermatosclerosis: a thickening in the tissues of the lower legs

Maceration: a softening and whitish look to the intact skin around wounds caused by excessive moisture

Macrophage: a white blood cell that ingests dead cells, micro-organisms, foreign material and other debris

Malleolus: the ankle bone

Necrotic tissue: dead tissue that usually presents as black or brown

Neuropathy: any abnormal degenerative or inflammatory state of the peripheral nervous system.

Occlusive: when referring to a dressing, it closes the wound from the external environment

Offload: to reduce or eliminate pressure from an area

Peri-wound: the tissue that surrounds the wound

Slough: dead tissue, usually yellow in colour and can be stringy in appearance

STAR: Skin Tear Audit Research

Tensile strength: the strength of a closed or healed wound in terms of the greatest stress the tissues can bear without tearing

Total contact cast: a fibreglass device/cast often used to support the healing of diabetic foot ulcers (neuropathic ulcers) by redistributing the weight along the entire surface of the foot

Ulcer: a break in the skin or mucous membrane with the loss of the surface tissue

References

Apelqvist, J. (2010) A paradigm shift is needed in diabetic foot care. *Wounds UK.* http://www.woundsinternational.com/practice-development/a-paradigm-shift-is-needed-in-diabetic-foot-care/page-1 (accessed 29 June 2013).

Barr, H., Freeth, D., Hammick, M., Koppel, I. & Reeves, S. (2002) *A Critical Review of Evaluations of Interprofessional Education.* HEA, London.

Bellingham, J. & Stephens, M.(1999) Bridging the hospital/community gap. *Community Nurse,* 5(8), 51–52.

Bennett, G., Dealey, C. & Posnett, J. (2004) The cost of pressure ulcers in the UK. *Age and Ageing,* 33(3), 230–235.

Bux, M. & Mahli, J.S. (1996) Assessing the use of dressings in practice. *Journal of Wound Care,* 5(7), 305–308.

Carville, K., Lewin, G., Newall, N. *et al.* (2007) STAR: a consensus for skin tear classification. *Primary Intention,* 15(1), 18–28.

Charmaz, K. (1983) Loss of self: a fundamental form of suffering in the chronically ill. *Sociology of Health & Illness,* 5(2), 168–195.

Collier, M. (2003) The elements of wound assessment. *Nursing Times,* 99(13), 48.

Davies, A. (2008) Management of dry skin conditions in older people. *British Journal of Community Nursing,* 13(6), 250–257.

Dealey, C. (2005) *The Care of Wounds.* Wiley Blackwell, Oxford.

DH (2009a) *NHS 2010–2015: from good to great. Preventative, People-centred, Productive.* Department of Health, London.

DH (2009b) *Patient Reported Outcome Measures.* Department of Health, London.

DH (2010a) *Equity and Excellence: liberating the NHS.* Department of Health, London.

DH (2010b) *Revision to the Operating Framework for the NHS in England.* Department of Health, London.

DH (2010c) *Quality, Innovation, Productivity and Prevention.* Department of Health, London.

Diabetes UK (2012) *The State of the Nation 2012 England.* http://www.diabetes.org.uk/Documents/Reports/State-of-the-Nation-2012.pdf.

Edwards, J. (2012) Burn wound and scar management. *Nursing in Practice.* http://www.nursinginpractice.com/article/burn-wound-and-scar-management

Engel, G.L. (1977) The need for a new medical model: a challenge for biomedicine. *Science,* 196(4286), 129–136.

EPUAP (2005) *Pressure Ulcer Classification: differentiation between pressure ulcers and moisture lesions.* European Pressure Ulcer Advisory Panel. http://www.epuap.org/archived_reviews/EPUAP_Rev6.3.pdf.

EPUAP (2009) *Pressure Ulcer Treatment: a quick reference guide.* European Pressure Ulcer Advisory Panel. http://www.epuap.org/guidelines/Final_Quick_Treatment.pdf.

EWMA (2008) *Hard to Heal Wounds: a holistic approach.* European Wound Management Association. http://ewma.org/fileadmin/user_upload/EWMA/pdf/Position_Documents/2008/English_EWMA_Hard2Heal_2008.pdf.

Falanga, V. (2000) Classifications for wound bed preparation and stimulation of chronic wounds. *Wound Repair Regeneration,* 8, 347–352.

Favazza, A.R. (2012) Non suicidal self-injury: how categorization guides treatment. *Current Psychiatry,* 11(3), 21–26.

Fletcher, J. (2010) Development of a new wound assessment form. *Wounds UK,* 6(1), 92–99.

Gershater, M.A., Löndahl, M., Nyberg, P. *et al.* (2009) Complexity of factors related to outcome of neuropathic and neuroischaemic / ischaemic diabetic foot ulcers: a cohort study. *Diabetologia,* 52(3), 398–407.

Gray, D., White, R. & Kingsley, A. (2009) *Applied Wound Management Assessment Chart.* http://www.wounds-uk.com/applied-wound-management/applied-wound-management-assessment-and-continuation-chart (accessed 29 June 2013).

Gupta, M., Gupta, A. & Haberman, H. (1987) The self-inflicted dermatoses: a critical review. *General Hospital Psychiatry,* 9(1), 45–52.

Harding, K.G., Moore, K. & Phillips, T.J. (2005) Wound chronicity and fibroblast senescence – implications for treatment. *International Wound Journal,* 2(4), 364–368.

Harth, W., Taube, K.M., & Gieler, U. (2010) Factitious disorders in dermatology. *Journal der Deutschen Dermatologischen Gesellschaft,* 8(5), 361–373.

Hill, D.P., Poore, S. & Wilson, J. (2004) Initial healing rates of venous ulcers: are they useful as predictors of healing? *American Journal of Surgery,* 188, 22–25.

HIS (2009) *General Wound Assessment Chart.* Healthcare Improvement Scotland. http://www.healthcareimprovementscotland.org/our_work/patient_safety/tissue_viability_resources/general_wound_assessment_chart.aspx (accessed 29 June 2013).

IWGDF (2003) *Definitions and Criteria.* International Working Group on the Diabetic Foot. http://iwgdf.org/consensus/definitions-and-criteria/ (accessed 30 June 2013).

IWGDF (2007) *Peripheral arterial disease and diabetes: International Consensus.* International Working Group on the Diabetic Foot (accessed 6 March 2014). http://iwgdf.org/consensus/peripheral-arterial-disease-and-diabetes/

Kennedy, K.L. (1989) The prevalence of pressure ulcers in an intermediate care facility. *Decubitus,* 2(2), 44–45.

Kerr, M. (2012). *Foot Care for People with Diabetes: the economic case for change.* NHS Diabetes and Kidney Care.

Margolis, D.J., Allen-Taylor, L., Offstad, O. & Berlin, J.A. (2004) The accuracy of venous leg ulcer prognostic models in a wound care system. *Wound Repair Regeneration,* 12(2), 163–168.

Moffatt, C., Price, P., Vowden, K. & Vowden, P. (2008) Psychosocial factors and Wound healing. In: European Wound Management Association. *Hard to Heal Wounds: a holistic approach.* http://ewma.org/fileadmin/user_upload/EWMA/pdf/Position_Documents/2008/English_EWMA_Hard2Heal_2008.pdf.

National Network for Burn Care (2012) *National Burn Care Referral Guidance.* http://www.specialisedservices.nhs.uk/library/35/National_Burn_Care_Referral_Guidance.pdf

NHS Careers. (2013) *Careers in Healthcare Science.* National Health Service Careers. http://www.nhscareers.nhs.uk/explore-by-career/healthcare-science/careers-in-healthcare-science/ (accessed 29 June 2013).

NHS (2012) *NHS Safety Thermometer.* National Health Service. http://harmfreecare.org/measurement/nhs-safety-thermometer/ (accessed 29 June 2013).

NHS-CRD (1997) *Compression Therapy for Venous Leg Ulcers.* NHS Centre for Reviews and Dissemination, University of York, York.

NHS-III (2009) *High Impact Actions for Nursing and Midwifery.* NHS Institute for Innovation and Improvement. http://www.institute.nhs.uk/building_capability/general/aims/ (accessed 29 June 2013).

NHS-QI (2003) *Best Practice Statement for the Prevention of Pressure Ulcers.* NHS Quality Improvement, Scotland.

NICE (2004) *Self Harm: short term treatment and management: CG16.* National Institute for Health and Clinical Excellence, London.

NICE (2005) *Pressure Ulcers: the management of pressure ulcers in primary and secondary care: CG29.* National Institute for Health and Clinical Excellence, London.

NICE (2008) *Prevention and Treatment of Surgical Site Infections: CG74.* National Institute for Health and Clinical Excellence, London.

NMC (2010) *The Code.* Nursing and Midwifery Council, London.

NNRU (2008) *State-of-the-Art Metrics for Nursing: a rapid appraisal.* National Nursing Research Unit. http://academia.edu/461331/State_of_the_art_metrics_for_nursing_a_rapid_appraisal.

NPUAP (2007) *Pressure Ulcer Category/Staging Illustrations.* National Pressure Ulcer Advisory Panel. Washington, DC, USA. http://www.npuap.org/resources/educational-and-clinical-resources/pressure-ulcer-categorystaging-illustrations/

NPUAP & EPUAP (2009) *Pressure Ulcer Prevention Quick Reference Guide.* http://www.epuap.org/guidelines/Final_Quick_Prevention.pdf (accessed 6 March 2014).

ONS (2010) *Population Estimates for England and Wales 2010.* Office of National Statistics, Newport.

Ousey, K. & White, R. (2010) Embedding the quality agenda into tissue viability and wound care. *British Journal of Nursing,* 19(11), 18–22.

Patel, S. (2010) Investigating wound infection. *Wounds Essentials.* http://www.wounds-uk.com/pdf/content_9489.pdf.

Phillips, L. & Buttery, J. (2009) Exploring pressure ulcer prevalence and preventative care. *Nursing Times,* 105(16), 34–36.

Posnett, J. & Franks, P.J. (2007) The costs of skin breakdown and ulceration in the UK. In: *Skin Breakdown: the silent epidemic.* Smith and Nephew Foundation, London.

Posnett, J., Gottrup, F., Lundgren, H. & Saal, G. (2009) The resource impact of wounds on health care providers in Europe. *Journal of Wound Care,* 18(4), 154–161.

Preece, J. (2004) Development of a wound management formulary for use in clinical practice. *Professional Nurse,* 20(3), 27–29.

Romanelli, M., Vuerstaek, J.D., Rogers, L.C., Armstrong, D.G. & Apelqvist, J. (2008) Economic burden of hard to heal wounds. In: European Wound Management Association. *Hard to Heal Wounds: a holistic approach.* http://ewma.org/fileadmin/user_upload/EWMA/pdf/Position_Documents/2008/English_EWMA_Hard2Heal_2008.pdf

Schultz, G., Sibbald, G., Falanga, V. *et al.* (2003) Wound bed preparation: a systematic approach to wound management. *Wound Repair Regeneration,* 11, 1–28.

Sibbald, R.G., Krasner, D.L. & Lutz, J.B. (2010) *SCALE: Skin Changes at Life's End.* Final Consensus Document. *Advances in Skin Wound Care,* 23(5), 225–236.

SIGN (2010) *SIGN Guideline 120: management of chronic venous leg ulcers.* Scottish Intercollegiate Guidelines for Nurses. http://www.sign.ac.uk/guidelines/fulltext/120/recommendations.html (accessed 29 June 2013).

Tantam, D., & Huband, N. (2009) *Understanding Repeated Self-injury: a multidisciplinary approach.* Palgrave Macmillan, Basingstoke.

Vowden, K., Teot, L. & Vowden, P. (2007) Selecting topical negative pressure therapy in practice. In: European Wound Management Association

379

Position Statement, *Topical Negative Pressure in Wound Management.* EWMA, London.

Vowden, P., Apelqvist, J. & Moffatt, C. (2008) Wound complexity and healing. In: European Wound Management Association. *Hard to Heal Wounds: a holistic approach.* http://ewma.org/fileadmin/user_upload/EWMA/pdf/Position_Documents/2008/English_EWMA_Hard2Heal_2008.pdf.

Winter, G.D. (1962) Formation of the scab and the rate of epithelization of superficial wounds in the skin of the young domestic pig. *Nature* 193, 293–294.

Wounds International (2013). *Guidelines: Wound Management in Diabetic Foot Ulcers.* http://www.woundsinternational.com/pdf/content_10803.pdf.

Wounds UK (2012) *Best Practice Statement: care of the older person's skin,* 2nd edn. *Wounds UK,* London.

WUWHS (2007) *Wound Exudate and the Role of Dressings. A Consensus Document.* World Union of Wound Healing Societies, MEP, London.

WUWHS (2008) *Wound Infection in Clinical Practice. A Consensus Document.* World Union of Wound Healing Societies, MEP, London.

Test Yourself

1. What is the other name the skin, hair and nails are known as?
   (a) Integumentary system
   (b) Integrity system
   (c) Epidermis and dermis
   (d) Genitourinary system

2. What is the pH of the skin?
   (a) Acid
   (b) Alkaline
   (c) Neutral
   (d) None of the above

3. Which vitamin is synthesised by the skin?
   (a) A
   (b) B
   (c) C
   (d) D

4. How many phases of wound healing are there?
   (a) 1
   (b) 3
   (c) 4
   (d) 6

5. What % of senescent fibroblasts would dramatically affect wound healing?
   (a) 5%
   (b) 10%
   (c) 25%
   (d) 15%

6. Which member of the interprofessional team will provide equipment such as splints, braces and casts to aid movement, resolve alignment and relieve pressure?
   (a) Physiotherapist
   (b) Occupational therapist
   (c) Prosthetist
   (d) Orthotist

7. If a wound does not have correct moisture balance what 2 complications can occur at the peri-wound area?
   (a) Inflammation and granulation
   (b) Proliferation and maturation
   (c) Maceration and excoriation
   (d) Excoriation and incontinence

8. How long should a wound have been present on the body before it can be deemed as chronic?
   (a) 2 weeks
   (b) 4 weeks
   (c) 6 weeks
   (d) 12 weeks

9. Which is not classed as a tissue type in wound assessment and classification?
   (a) Granulation
   (b) Slough
   (c) Exudate
   (d) Necrosis

10. What is the classification system used to assess skin tears?
    (a) SCALE
    (b) TIME
    (c) Rule of Nines
    (d) STAR

Answers

1. a
2. a
3. d
4. c

5. d
6. d
7. c
8. c
9. c
10. d

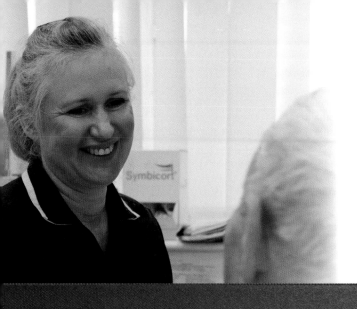

19

The Principles of Medicine Administration and Pharmacology

Muralitharan Nair

University of Hertfordshire, UK

Learning Outcomes

On completion of this chapter you will be able to:

- Define the term pharmacology
- Differentiate between the terms 'pharmacokinetics' and 'pharmacodynamics'
- Evaluate up-to-date information on medicine management and work within national and local policies
- Administer medicines safely in a timely manner, including controlled drugs
- Discuss the advantages and disadvantages of various routes of drug administration
- Keep and maintain records within a multidisciplinary framework and as part of a team

Competencies

All nurses must:

1. Demonstrate an understanding of legal and ethical frameworks relating to safe administration of medicines in practice
2. Use knowledge of commonly administered medicines in order to act promptly in cases where side-effects and adverse reactions occur
3. Demonstrate an ability to safely store medicines under supervision
4. Ensure safe administration of medications
5. Work within the ethical and legal framework that underpins safe and effective medicine management
6. Work in partnership with other healthcare teams

 Visit the companion website at **www.wileynursingpractice.com** where you can test yourself using flashcards, multiple-choice questions and more.

Nursing Practice: Knowledge and Care, First Edition. Edited by Ian Peate, Karen Wild and Muralitharan Nair.
© 2014 John Wiley & Sons, Ltd. Published 2014 by John Wiley & Sons, Ltd. Companion website: www.wileynursingpractice.com

Introduction

Drug administration does not mean just giving out medication to patients; it involves working with the person, their relatives and other healthcare professionals in the safe administration of medicine. Nurses also have to follow the local, national and professional guidelines to ensure that they carry out their duties confidently and professionally. Nurses have an important role and responsibility in drug administration. They are in the forefront in the delivery of care, which includes drug administration. Knowing about pharmacology is one important aspect of nurses' knowledge base. Knowing how to incorporate that knowledge into clinical judgements is equally paramount. Nurses are also responsible for the safe preparation of patients to return to the community after treatment or investigation in the hospital. Nurses are delivering care to a better informed person group. The nurse's roles in pharmacology include ensuring medications are concordant with patients, educating patients about the drugs they are sent home with and providing information about them. Many pharmacology textbooks for student nurses include comprehensive information about medications, which students may find too daunting. The content in this chapter, therefore, will reflect on situations that nurses will most likely come across in practice and are required to know about.

Pharmacology

What Is Pharmacology?

Pharmacology is the science that studies the origin, nature, chemistry, effects, and uses of drugs; it includes pharmacokinetics, pharmacodynamics, therapeutics and toxicology. It also includes the body's reaction to drugs and how drugs cause desired and undesired effects. Drugs have been in existence for a very long time. They have been used for medical reasons in treating diseases, for example diabetes and heart failure, and for recreational purposes, such as the use of cannabis and anabolic steroids.

There are many pharmacology textbooks written for nurses. However, no textbook will cover all the medications that are being prescribed in the UK. The *British National Formulary* (BNF 2012) is a good resource. The BNF is also available online.

Link To/Go To

www.bnf.org

This book will provide information such as the group the drug comes under, the action of the drug, dosage, side-effects and contraindications.

Pharmacokinetics

Pharmacokinetics is the study of how drugs enter the body, reach their site of action and are removed from the body, which includes absorption, distribution, metabolism and excretion.

Absorption

When the drug is administered, absorption needs to take place before it reaches the cells. Drugs are administered via different routes of absorption. Some of the routes of absorption include:

- Sublingual
- Oral
- Rectal
- Inhalation
- Injections = intramuscular (i.m.)/intravenous (i.v.)/subcutaneous (s.c.)
- Vaginal
- Buccal
- Aural (ear).

Red Flag

Students are not allowed to administer drugs via the i.v. route. Only qualified nurses who have had special instructions on i.v. drug administration are allowed to give drugs through this route.

The chemical nature of the drug determines how and where the absorption takes place. Absorption takes place through the intestinal wall and into the plasma before it reaches the site of action. Any drug given through the oral route is absorbed from the gastrointestinal (GI) tract and then it is transported to the liver via the portal circulation (hepatic portal vein) (Figure 19.1).

In the liver, the drug is metabolised by the hepatic enzymes before it is returned to the general circulation. One of the liver's functions is to detoxify some of the drugs, which may reduce the effect of the drug; this process is called 'first pass metabolism' or 'first pass system' (Figure 19.2). The amount of drug that returns into general circulation after it has gone through the liver is now available for therapeutic use. Not all the drugs are available for action, particularly if they have gone through protein binding (see later). Some drugs go through the liver without any biotransformation (Crouch & Chapelhow 2008).

Drugs administered by other routes, such as by injection and rectally, will bypass the first pass metabolism. Drugs given using these routes go directly into the bloodstream and therefore the bioavailability of drugs using these routes is much higher compared with medications taken orally.

The presence of food in the GI tract at the time of taking medications can affect the absorption of the drug. This is due to the fact that the digested food particles compete with the drug molecules at the same absorption site. This can result in low plasma concentration causing delayed action of the drug. Therefore, unless it is indicated that the medication should be taken with food, drugs should be administered an hour before eating.

Jot This Down

Can you think about conditions or surgery that the person may have had that can affect absorption of drugs from the GI tract?

Absorption is facilitated by certain transport systems in the body:

- The active transport system (Figure 19.3) – requires cellular energy to move drugs from an area of low concentration to high concentration
- The passive transport system (Figure 19.4) – does not require cellular energy. Drugs move from an area of high concentration to an area of low concentration

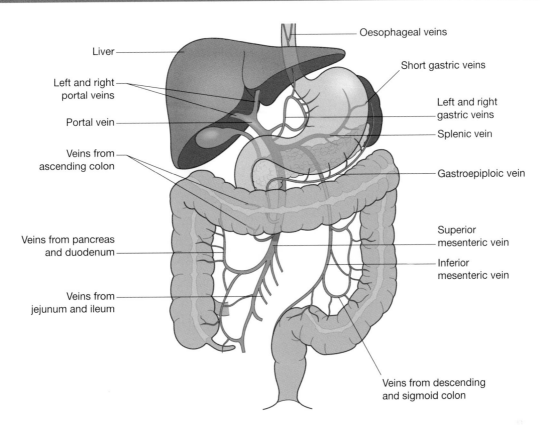

Figure 19.1 Portal circulation.

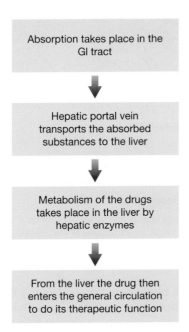

Figure 19.2 First pass metabolism.

- Facilitated diffusion (Figure 19.5) – drugs are transported into the cells by carrier proteins found on the surface of the cells.

Distribution

Drug distribution refers to the movement of a drug to and from the blood and various tissues of the body (e.g. fat, muscle and brain tissue) and the relative proportions of drug in the tissues. After a drug is absorbed into the bloodstream it rapidly circulates throughout the body. The average circulation time of blood is 1 minute. As the blood circulates, the drug moves from the bloodstream into the body's tissues. Drugs pass more readily between the intravascular and interstitial compartments than between other compartments in the body, for example the central nervous system. There are many factors that affect drug distribution in the body. Examples of these are:

- Lipid solubility – the greater the lipid solubility, the greater the distribution
- Drug molecule size – smaller molecules are distributed more extensively throughout the body than larger molecules
- Cellular binding – drugs may exist in free or bound form. Bound forms of drugs exist as reservoirs. The free and bound forms co-exist in equilibrium. Cellular binding depends on the plasma binding proteins
- Plasma protein binding – the level of plasma proteins affects the distribution. The most important and abundant plasma protein is albumin. Others include globulins, glycoproteins and lipoproteins.

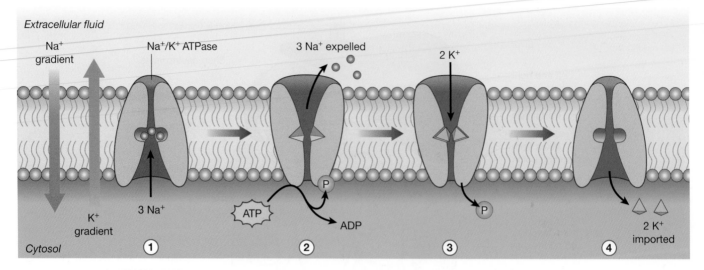

Figure 19.3 **Active transport system.**

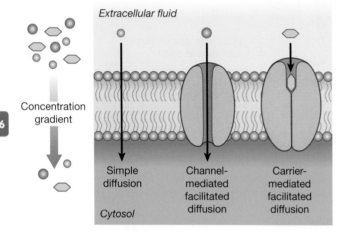

Figure 19.4 **Passive transport system.**

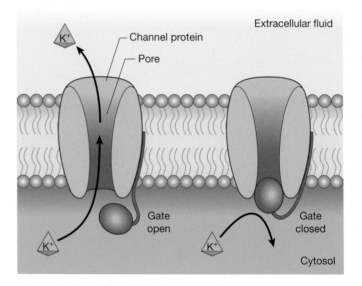

Figure 19.5 **Facilitated diffusion.**

Once the drug reaches the general circulation after going through the liver, the drug molecules are distributed mainly by four methods:

- Blood flow
- Plasma protein binding
- Solubility of the drug
- Storage sites.

Blood flow Drugs are distributed to many or all parts of the body by the circulation. Therefore the distribution of drugs is dependent on vascular permeability, blood flow, tissue uptake of the drug and plasma protein binding. Organs that are highly vascular, such as the heart, liver and kidneys, will rapidly acquire a drug because of the rich blood supply. However, the levels of a drug in bone, fat, muscle and skin may take some time to rise due to reduced vascularity and perfusion. The person's level of activity and local tissue temperature may also affect drug distribution to the skin and muscle. Other factors that can affect drug distribution include heart diseases, blood pressure and blood volume.

> **Jot This Down**
>
> Can you think about any other conditions that may affect drug distribution by increased or decreased blood flow?

Plasma protein binding In the circulation, a drug is bound to circulating plasma proteins or is 'free' in an unbound state. The plasma protein usually involved in binding a drug is albumin. If a drug is bound, then it is said to be inactive and cannot have a pharmacological effect. Only the free drug molecules can cause an effect. As free molecules leave the circulation, drug molecules are released from plasma protein to re-establish the ratio between the bound and the free molecules. Certain drugs do compete with other drugs for drug-binding sites on albumin.

Binding tends to be non-specific and competitive. This means that plasma proteins will bind with many different drugs and these drugs will compete for binding sites on the plasma proteins. Displacement of one drug by another drug may have serious consequences. For example, warfarin (anticoagulant) can be displaced by tolbutamide (an antidiabetic drug), producing a risk of haemorrhage as the level of warfarin in plasma increases, while tolbutamide can be displaced by salicylates (used as an analgesic agent for the treatment of mild to moderate pain), producing a risk of hypoglycaemia.

Red Flag

Certain diseases such as nephrotic syndrome, severe burns and malnutrition can affect the availability of plasma protein binding sites. In these conditions, the level of plasma protein is reduced, thus increasing the plasma concentration of drug and leading to a greater effect of the drug on the systems of the person.

Solubility of the drug Capillaries supplying the central nervous system differ from those in most other parts of the body. They lack channels between endothelial cells through which substances in the blood normally gain access to the extracellular fluid. This barrier constrains the passage of substances from the blood to the brain and cerebrospinal fluid. Lipid-soluble drugs, e.g. diazepam, will pass fairly readily into the central nervous system, whereas lipid-insoluble drugs will not. This is due to the fact that the cell membrane is made up of lipid (Figure 19.6) and lipid-soluble drugs cross the cell membrane much more readily than water-soluble drugs.

Storage sites Fatty tissue will act as a storage site for lipid-soluble drugs, e.g. anticoagulants. Drugs that have accumulated in the fatty tissue may not be released until after administration of the drugs has ceased. Calcium-containing structures such as bone and teeth can accumulate drugs that are bound to calcium, e.g. tetracycline (antibiotic). Drugs such as those that accumulate in fatty tissues leave the tissues so slowly that they circulate in the bloodstream for days after a person has stopped taking the drug. Distribution of a given drug may also vary from person to person. For instance, obese people may store large amounts of fat-soluble drugs, whereas very thin people may store relatively little. Older people, even when thin, may store large amounts of fat-soluble drugs, because the proportion of body fat increases with ageing.

Metabolism

Metabolism is the transformation of drugs in preparation for excretion from the body. This mainly occurs in the liver by the hepatic enzymes and, to some extent, in other areas such as the intestines, lungs and plasma (Crouch & Chapelhow 2008). The enzymes responsible for the biotransformation of drugs belong to the group of cytochrome P459. These enzymes are found in the smooth endoplasmic reticulum of a cell. The products of drug metabolism are called 'metabolites'. The inactive metabolites are excreted from the body. If these metabolites are not excreted, they can be toxic. Metabolism occurs in two phases: Phases I and II.

Phase I metabolism can involve reduction or hydrolysis of the drug, but the most common biochemical process that occurs is oxidation (oxidation is the chemical reaction that occurs when cut apples turn brown when exposed to the oxygen in air).

Phase II metabolism involves conjugation – that is, the attachment of an ionised group to the drug. These include glutathione, methyl or acetyl groups. These metabolic processes principally

387

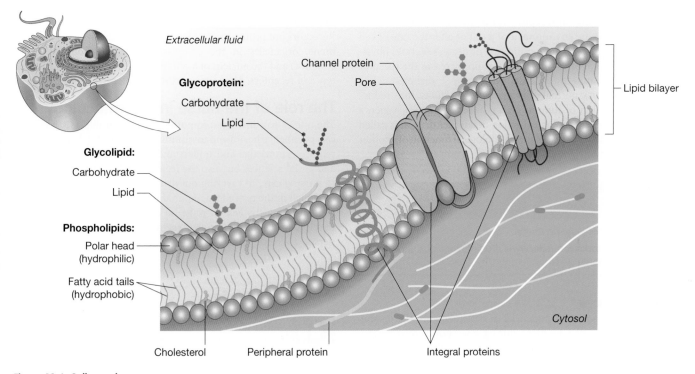

Figure 19.6 Cell membrane.

occur in the hepatocyte cytoplasm. Other sites of drug metabolism include epithelial cells of the gastrointestinal tract, lungs, kidneys and the skin.

Excretion

Excretion is the removal of a drug from the body. Some of the organs of excretion include the kidneys, GI tract, skin through sweat (for example vitamin B), the breast and the lungs. The rate of excretion is dependent on the physical status of the person. If the person suffers from renal or heart failure the drug may stay in the system longer, resulting in drug toxicity. The lungs are the main route of excretion for anaesthetic gases and, to some extent, alcohol. The kidneys are the principal organs of excretion for drugs. Most water-soluble drugs are excreted by the kidneys and fat-soluble drugs in the faeces.

Jot This Down

Can you name any conditions that may affect drug excretion?

Half-life

Half-life is the period of time required for the concentration or amount of drug in the body to be reduced by one-half. This is important information when calculating the dosage and frequency of the drug for a person. The half-life of a drug is affected by absorption, metabolism and excretion. Half-life varies between drugs. For example, penicillin has a half-life of 1 hour, while that of digitoxin is about 1 week. This information is also important when administering drugs that may interact to enhance or decrease physiological response.

Pharmacodynamics

This is the study of drug action at the biochemical and pharmacological level and the effect of the drugs on the body. This activity is carried out by acting on receptors (proteins) on a cell. The drug can either change the environment of a cell or alter the rate of cell function. Thus, drugs can either increase or decrease certain physiological functions. For example, metformin increases the receptor sensitivity to insulin in patients with type 2 diabetes, while tamoxifen can block normal cell function and activity, thus reducing the proliferation of tumour cells (Cummings 2008). When a drug enhances the physiological action of another drug, it is called an agonist. One that decreases the physiological function of another drug is called an antagonist.

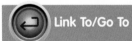 **Link To/Go To**

You may find this website useful:

http://www.xmarks.com/site/www.druginfozone.nhs.uk/home/ (accessed 8 March 2014).

Drug interactions

Drug interactions may be beneficial or detrimental to the person. The interaction may take place during absorption, distribution, metabolism and excretion. The interaction can take place between drugs or between drugs and chemicals in food (Galbraith *et al.* 2007). See Table 19.1 for some drug–food interactions.

Table 19.1 Drug–food interactions.

FOOD STUFF	INTERACTIONS
Grapefruit juice	
• Calcium channel blockers (felodipine)	Grapefruit juice increases the effectiveness of calcium channel blockers, meaning blood pressure could drop to dangerously low levels. In extreme cases, the heart could stop beating
• Simvastatin	Grapefruit juice increases the level of simvastatin in the blood and makes side-effects more likely
• Entocort	Entocort is a medicine that contains budesonide and is used to treat Crohn's disease, a condition that affects the digestive system. Grapefruit or grapefruit juice can increase the level of budesonide in the blood
Grilled meat and theophylline	Intake of grilled meat accelerates the elimination of theophylline
Liquorice and antihypertensives	Liquorice reduces the effectiveness of antihypertensive drugs. Liquorice enhances sodium retention and potassium excretion in the distal tubule of the kidneys, thereby elevating blood pressure
Warfarin and leafy vegetables (vitamin K)	Leafy vegetables such as cabbage and spinach can reduce the effect of warfarin. These vegetables contain vitamin K, which is an antidote for warfarin. Warfarin is also affected when taken with grapefruit or grapefruit juice
Tetracycline and calcium	Calcium ions are found in many food sources. Taking tetracycline with cheese or milk will affect the absorption of the drug

Receptors

Receptors are protein molecules found embedded in a cell membrane, organelles in the cytoplasm (e.g. mitochondria, Golgi complex) and the nucleus of a cell (Figure 19.7). There are different types of receptors. They transport drug molecules into the cell.

The role of the nurse in pharmacology

The nurse's role involves promoting the responsible use of chemicals to enhance health and to minimise side-effects (Box 19.1). This requires knowledge and understanding, not only of the physical and social sciences but also the legal and ethical issues pertaining to nursing care. In carrying out drug administration, nurses must be skilled in the procedure required to handle, control and administer drugs safely. Nurses must be able to work cooperatively in developing care plans and drug regimens that are acceptable to the person and their family.

What the Experts Say

 People don't always get their medicine and it wasn't always given at an appropriate time, coordinated with meal times, which was interfering with their glycaemic control.

(Caroline, a Diabetes Specialist Nurse)

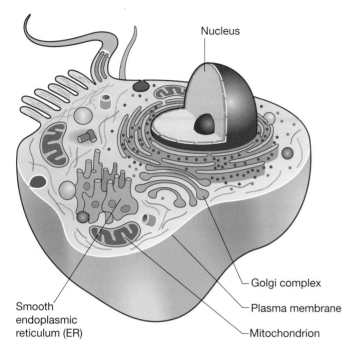

Figure 19.7 Anatomy of a cell.

The nurse is responsible for knowing about anything that affects nursing care in relation to drug use such as timing of doses, special techniques for administration, precautions to take before administering a drug, assessment of the toxicity, drug interactions and the side-effects (NMC 2008a, Standard 8).

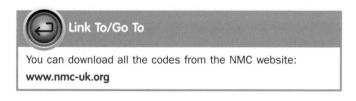

Link To/Go To

You can download all the codes from the NMC website:

www.nmc-uk.org

Side-effects are undesirable physiological effects exerted by the drug other than the intended therapeutic effect. Some drugs have a multitude of side-effects. The nurse needs to know about the serious side-effects, for example suppression of respiration, retention of urine, as in the case of opioid drugs, and also the common side-effects such as nausea and vomiting.

The number of drugs in current use is far too great for anyone to memorise. However, the nurse must be able to find reliable information pertaining to the drugs that a particular person is prescribed. This information is available in the *British National Formulary* (BNF).

Nurses should be aware of the contraindications and precautions of the drugs they are administering to the person. Contraindications are symptoms that alert the healthcare professionals to potential dangers of the drug. For example, glaucoma is a contraindication for anticholinergic drugs. The danger is that these drugs may increase intraocular pressure and precipitate or aggravate glaucoma. Precautions are measures taken to prevent or reduce adverse effects of the drug.

Box 19.1 Outline of the Nurse's Role in Medicine Management

- *Knowledge of therapeutic uses of medicines*. Nurses should refer to the BNF if they are sure of the therapeutic use, side-effects and contraindications of the drug they are giving the person
- *Awareness of the person's care plan*. Nurses need to check the care plan regularly to make sure that the person's care has not changed as a result of the drug or that the person has developed any adverse reactions
- *Consent from the person that it is acceptable to administer the medication*. The person may refuse to take the medication they are prescribed if they are not sure why they have to take it
- *Check the identity of the person*. A hospital number is unique to every person. No two patients have the same hospital number but you may have two patients with the same surname on your ward. Check against their identity bracelet and their treatment chart
- *Check the orientation level of the person* (by asking them for their name and date of birth). This is to ensure that the correct person is receiving the medication
- *Check the prescription chart*. To ensure that you have the correct treatment chart corresponding to the correct person
- *The prescription must be clearly written and legible*. It is a requirement for the prescriber to prescribe all medications legibly using capital letters, otherwise the nurse can query and refuse to give the medication until it is legibly written
- *Double-check that the medication has not been administered at an earlier time*. Check the signature box for the corresponding time and date
- *Check allergies*. Nurses must check with the person and their medical notes to ensure that the person is not allergic to the medication. Any allergies should be notified immediately to the doctor and it should be documented in the person's notes
- *Clear prescription label* on the medicine to be administered
- *Check expiry date* of the medicine being administered
- *Consider dosage* is in line with weight, method of administration, route and timing
- *Administer/withhold* in light of the person's condition
- *If medication has been administered orally*, ensure that all medication has been taken by the person
- *Observe for effects/side-effects* and report accordingly
- *Clear, accurate and immediate record* of:
  - Medicines administered
  - Medicines withheld (giving rationale)
  - Medicines refused
  - Delegation of the task

Nurses need to check that dose range and route are specified for all the medications prescribed. Many factors are taken into account before a dosage is prescribed for the person. Factors such as weight, nutritional status, the nature of the person's illness and the physical state of the person should be considered before prescribing the drug.

Drugs are considered as poison by the body. Many drugs are deactivated by the liver enzymes and excreted by the kidneys. Most water-soluble drugs are excreted by the kidneys and some in the faeces. Fat-soluble drugs are mainly excreted in the faeces. Other organs of excretion for drugs include the lungs and the skin. Thus, nurses need to be aware that people with liver and or kidney disorders are at risk of developing complications related to their drug treatment.

Standards for Medicines Management (NMC 2008a) sets certain criteria that must be fulfilled by every practising nurse practitioner. Some of the criteria in Standard 8 include:

- You must be certain of the identity of the person to whom the medicine is to be administered
- You must know the therapeutic uses of the medicine to be administered, its normal dosage, side-effects, precautions and contraindications
- You must check the expiry date of medicines to be administered
- You must have considered the dosage, weight where appropriate, method of administration, route and timing
- You must contact the prescriber or another authorised prescriber without delay when contraindications to the prescribed medicine are discovered, where the person develops a reaction to the medicine, or where assessment of the person indicates that the medicine is no longer suitable

For the full list of the criteria see The Code.

Red Flag

Instructions by telephone to administer a medicine should not be accepted by any nurse practitioner. However, in exceptional circumstances, where medications have been previously prescribed, the use of fax, text message or e-mail may be used to confirm any change to the original prescription.

What the Experts Say

It is easy to neglect communication about medicines when you have only a few minutes with each patient, so attitudes need to change to recognise that taking the time to discuss medicines now will help to prevent errors and worsening health – saving more time in the long run.

There needs to be a cultural change across the healthcare professions to raise awareness.

(A Nurse Consultant in thrombosis and anticoagulation)

Primary Care

Advise the patient on the following:

- Learn the name of medications they are taking and why they have to take them. Know the unwanted effects of the drugs they are prescribed
- Advise the patient to keep all medication in a cupboard and out of reach of children
- Always check the medication label to ensure they are taking the correct medication at the correct time
- If unsure of any medication, check with the local pharmacist
- Check for the expiry date of the drug and dispose of any unwanted in a safe manner, for example returning unwanted drugs to the chemist or the pharmacy department. Drugs should not be disposed down the drain because of concerns about trace levels of drug residues found in surface water, such as rivers and lakes, and in some community drinking water supplies
- If they miss a dose, do not double the dose for the next intake. Always seek advice from the doctor, pharmacist or the practice nurse

- Never stop prescribed medications unless advised to do so
- Do not crush or open capsules without checking with the pharmacist or doctor
- Take the medications as directed by the doctor
- Order repeat medication in good time before the medication runs out. Most doctors' surgeries will repeat medications 1 week before they run out
- Always check with the pharmacist when taking non-prescription medications with prescribed medications, for drug interactions.

(Adapted from Kozier *et al.* 2008)

Person Group Directions

Person Group Directions (PGDs), in existence since August 2000, constitute a legal framework that allows registered healthcare professionals to supply and administer medicines to groups of patients who fit the criteria laid out in the PGD. A healthcare professional can supply (e.g. provide an inhaler or tablets) and/or administer a medicine (e.g. give an injection or a suppository) directly to a person without the need for a prescription or an instruction from a prescriber. The legislation applies to the NHS, including private and voluntary sector activity funded by the NHS. The legislation specifies that each PGD must contain the following information:

- *The name of the business to which the Direction applies*
- *The date the Direction comes into force and the date it expires*
- *A description of the medicine(s) to which the Direction applies*
- *Class of health professional who may supply or administer the medicine*
- *Signature of a doctor or dentist, as appropriate, and a pharmacist*
- *Signature by an appropriate organisation*
- *The clinical condition or situation to which the Direction applies*
- *A description of those patients excluded from treatment under the Direction*
- *A description of the circumstances in which further advice should be sought from a doctor (or dentist, as appropriate) and arrangements for referral*
- *Details of appropriate dosage and maximum total dosage, quantity, pharmaceutical form and strength, route and frequency of administration, and minimum or maximum period over which the medicine should be administered*
- *Relevant warnings, including potential adverse reactions*
- *Details of any necessary follow-up action and the circumstances*
- *A statement of the records to be kept for audit purposes.*
  (**http://www.mhra.gov.uk/Howweregulate/Medicines/ Availabilityprescribingsellingandsupplyingofmedicines/ ExemptionsfromMedicinesActrestrictions/ PersonGroupDirectionsintheNHS/index.htm**) (accessed 15 August 2013)

Examples of where PGDs may be appropriate are services where assessment and treatment follow a clearly predictable pattern (e.g. immunisation, family planning). In general practice, they can be used to enable registered nurses to administer a prescription-only medicine to a group of patients who fit the criteria specified in the PGD, for example to administer vaccinations. The following healthcare professions can supply and administer medications:

- *Registered nurses*
- *Midwives*
- *Health visitors*
- *Optometrists*
- *Pharmacists*
- *Chiropodists*
- *Radiographers*
- *Orthoptists*
- *Physiotherapists*
- *Ambulance paramedics*
- *Dieticians*
- *Occupational therapists*
- *Speech and language therapists*
- *Prosthetists*
- *Orthotists.*

**(http://www.elmmb.nhs.uk/patient-group
-direction-primary-care/** (accessed 8 March 2014)

Changing Demography of the UK

The demography of the UK is changing. People are now living longer and consequently many of them are living with comorbidities (Crouch & Chapelhow 2008). In addition to this, a large number of migrant workers are now working in the UK temporarily or on a permanent basis and some of the migrants bring health problems, such as tuberculosis, while others adopt a Western lifestyle that increases their risk of developing heart disease and stroke. In addition to this, the birth rate has increased while the death rate has decreased. The death rate is low because of new medicine and better healthcare facilities in the UK. The elderly who get ill and cannot look after themselves at home may be admitted to care homes, where they are cared for by others. All the changes will continue to reshape the health system in the UK and nurses need to ensure that they too are developing the skills and knowledge in delivering high quality care.

Generic and Brand Names

All drugs produced have a generic and one or more brand names. A generic name is a drug's common scientific name. A brand name drug is a medicine that is discovered, developed and marketed by a pharmaceutical company. Once a new drug is discovered, the company files for a patent to protect against other companies making copies and selling the drug. An example of a generic drug, one used for diabetes, is metformin hydrochloride. A brand name for metformin hydrochloride is Glucophage. A generic drug, one used for hypertension, is metoprolol, whereas a brand name for the same drug is Lopressor. Another example is a drug called sildenafil. Sildenafil is the generic name of a medicine used to treat erectile dysfunction (the inability to get an erection). Pfizer, the company that makes sildenafil, sells it under the brand name Viagra. Medicines sold under their generic name are usually cheaper because the research and development costs are lower. However, they contain the same active ingredient as the equivalent branded medicines.

The brand name is usually clearly given on any packaging and the generic name is written somewhere on the packet in small print. Prescribers are encouraged to prescribe using the generic name of the drug. This is because:

- The generic name is the one doctors are encouraged to use. There are sometimes many brand names for one medicine. Possible

confusion or mistakes are reduced if all prescribers use the same names when talking about and prescribing medicines
- Generic medicines are often cheaper for the NHS. Even for medicines over the counter, such as paracetamol, there is often a big price difference between brands.

Legislation and Policies Governing Drug Administration

The NMC Standards for Medicine Management clearly state:

The administration of medicines is an important aspect of the professional practice of practitioners whose names are on the Council's register. It is not solely a mechanistic task to be performed in strict compliance with the written prescription of a medical practitioner. It requires thought and the exercise of professional judgement…

(NMC 2008a)

> **Jot This Down**
>
> During your clinical placement, have you witnessed any situation where professionals do not exercise their professional judgement when giving out medicines to patients?

If this is the case, what must the professionals do if they come across a treatment chart that is not properly completed by the doctors? Do they carry out their duties and guess what is written? When administering medications to patients, it is important that nurses have an understanding of the relevant legislation and policies they have to comply with. The legislation relates to the prescribing, supply, storage and administration of medicines. The Medicine Act 1968 provides a legal framework that takes into account the manufacture, licensing, prescription, supply and administration of medicines. The Act classifies medicines into:

- *General sales list* (GSL) – these do not need a prescription, are sold in a general store and direct pharmaceutical supervision is not required, e.g. paracetamol
- *Pharmacy only medicines* (P) – these are sold only under control of a pharmacist
- *Prescription only medicines* (POMs) – these are supplied or administered to a person under the direction of a UK registered doctor, dentist or nurse prescriber, e.g. morphine. A person may not administer a POM unless he or she is a practitioner or acting in accordance with the direction of a practitioner. The restriction on sale and control of some POMs do not apply to a registered midwife in the course of their professional duty. Some midwives may also administer parenterally in the course of their duty certain POMs such as oxytocin and pethidine.

 Link To/Go To

For more up-to-date classifications, see:

**http://www.rpharms.com/mep/legal-classification-of
-medicines.asp**

Misuse of Drugs Act 1971

This Act controls the import, export, production, supply, possession and manufacture of controlled drugs to prevent abuse. It is also designed to promote research and education relating to drug dependence (Dougherty & Lister 2011). The level of control depends on the potential for abuse or misuse. The drugs subject to control are termed 'controlled drugs'. These drugs are classified into three groups:

- *Class A (Part I)*, examples are Ecstasy, LSD, heroin, cocaine, crack, magic mushrooms, amphetamines (if prepared for injection)
- *Class B (Part II)*, examples are amphetamines, cannabis (in January 2009), methylphenidate (Ritalin), pholcodine
- *Class C (Part III)*, examples are tranquillisers, some painkillers, gamma hydroxybutyrate (GHB), ketamine.

The Evidence

Fergusson *et al.* (2003) reported that cannabis may interfere with a person's capacity to concentrate, organise and use information. This effect can last several weeks after taking cannabis. Students form a large proportion of cannabis users.

The level of control is dependent on the potential for abuse or misuse. Under the current legislation, the control drugs are classified into five schedules (see Legislation.gov.uk 2001). see Legislation 2001; **https://www.gov.uk/government/policies/reducing-drugs-misuse-and-dependence/supporting-pages/classifying-and-controlling-drugs**). See Table 19.2 for the schedules and some of the drugs in the schedules.

 Link To/Go To

For more information on the misuse of drug regulation, visit: **http://www.legislation.gov.uk/uksi/2001/3998/contents/made**

Safe Custody of Drugs

With the exceptions of drugs in Schedules 4 and 5, controlled drugs must be kept in a locked cupboard and the keys kept by the person in charge of the ward or their deputy. All drugs administered are recorded in a controlled drugs register. Every drug must have its own page with the drug's name as the heading, the date and time

of administration, name of the person, signatures of the nurse administering the drug and the witness. The number of ampoules or tablets or the amount of elixir before and after is recorded. No cancellation or deletion must be made and all entries must be in ink.

Preparation of Drugs

Drugs come in many forms: tablets, liquids, suppositories, ointments, patches and creams. Tablets are sugar-coated, starch-based or film-coated. They are formulated in this format because they are either broken down in the stomach or the intestine. Sugar-coatings are used to improve appearance and palatability. In all starch-based tablets, the breakdown of the starch coating takes place in the mouth by the salivary enzyme amylase. Tablets have to disintegrate in the GI tract before they can be broken down and absorbed. Tablets may be formulated to achieve controlled release as they pass through the GI tract.

Enteric-coated tablets

Some tablets are coated with a hard shell so that the breakdown of these tablets takes place in the intestine where the pH is alkaline, and not in the stomach where it is acidic. These tablets are known as enteric-coated tablets. Some of the drugs in enteric-coated tablets are gastric irritants and therefore should be taken with food or after a meal. Thus nurses should never crush enteric-coated medications as it may render the drug ineffective (*British Pharmacopoeia* 2008). The NMC (2008a) also recommends caution, as crushing or opening capsules can potentially change the therapeutic properties of the medication, including rendering the medication ineffective. Crushing should only occur in the best interest of the person.

Red Flag

 Do not crush enteric-coated tables; to do this will render the drug ineffective.

Capsules

Some drugs are prepared in a capsule so that they are easy to swallow. The capsule is made of gelatine and the contents may be a powder, solid, liquid or even paste. If the capsule is difficult for the person to swallow, the capsule should not be removed and the contents sprinkled on food to give to patients (Dougherty & Lister

Table 19.2 A schedule table with examples of drugs within the schedules.

SCHEDULE 1	SCHEDULE 2	SCHEDULE 3	SCHEDULE 4	SCHEDULE 5
Cannabis, raw opium	Most opiates commonly used, such as diamorphine, morphine, fentanyl, pethidine	Minor stimulant drugs and barbiturates, pentazocine, temazepam	Benzodiazepines, such as diazepam, anabolic and androgenic steroids	Minimal risk of abuse. Drugs such as low strength morphine, cocaine, morphine
Must be kept in a locked cupboard where access is restricted	Must be kept in a locked cupboard where access is restricted	Varies – some drugs are required to be kept in a locked cupboard, such as buprenorphine	No requirement	No requirement
Controlled drug register must be used	Controlled drug register must be used	No requirement	No requirement	No requirement

2011). Breaking the capsule could render the drug ineffective. Masking the drug with food before feeding elderly or confused patients is then causing harm to the patient. Patients have the right to know what they are taking and the effects it may have on them. It is the nurse's duty to inform the person what the medication is for and the *Standards of Conduct, Performance and Ethics for Nurses and Midwives* clearly states that:

> You must always act lawfully, whether those laws relate to your professional practice or personal life.
>
> Failure to comply with this code may bring your fitness to practise into question and endanger your registration.

(NMC 2008b)

Medicines Management

If you are not allowed to crush or break a capsule or a tablet, are there any other ways you could administer the medication? Refer to the *Standards for Medicine Management* (NMC 2008a).

However, nurses do come across situations where patients are confused and/or refuse to take their medications. So what can nurses do to act in the best interest of the person? The *Standards of Conduct, Performance and Ethics for Nurses and Midwives* offers the following position statement:

> As a general principal, by disguising medications in food or drink, the person or client is being led to believe that they are not receiving medication when in fact they are. The registered nurse, midwife or health visitor will need to be sure that what they are doing is in the best interests of the person or client and be accountable for this action.

(NMC 2008b)

Thus, when undertaking such a task, nurses need to seek advice from the doctor or pharmacist and support from the person's relatives or advocates. All action taken must be clearly documented in accordance with *Record Keeping: guidance for nurses and midwives* (NMC 2009).

Slow-release preparations

If a drug is eliminated rapidly, the plasma concentration will also fall rapidly and therefore the person may have to take the drug more frequently. This is avoided by giving the person medications in a slow-release preparation. Such drugs are formulated using a complex matrix coating that dissolves slowly in the GI tract. Tablets such as aspirin and omeprazole are manufactured using this format (Galbraith *et al.* 2007). Crushing these tablets will render the drug ineffective.

Red Flag

Never handle any tablets with your fingers when administering medications to patients.

Liquid preparations

Some people, especially children, find it difficult to swallow tablets because of their unpleasant taste. Many drugs, especially antibiotics, are prepared in liquid format. These preparations are prepared using certain flavourings such as strawberry; even sugar may be

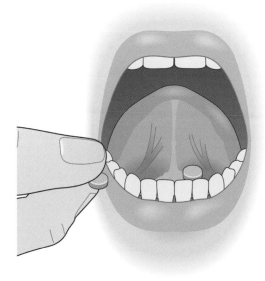

Figure 19.8 Sublingual route.

added to make it more palatable. However, you must remember that some medications, such as penicillin, are unstable in solution and therefore they are prepared in a powder format and water is added to the powder to make a suspension. These drugs should be left in the drug fridge and used within two weeks of preparation.

Creams and ointments

The preparation of creams and ointments is different, in that creams are water-based while ointments are oil-based. Water evaporates quickly once it is applied. Some of the water with the drug molecule gets absorbed via the aqueous pores. On the other hand, ointments are lipid-based and absorption can be significant, depending on the application. If a dressing is applied over the ointment, the absorption is better as the skin under the dressing becomes soft and the drug penetrates into the skin much more quickly.

Sublingual and buccal drugs

Although the mucous membrane of the mouth is not highly vascular, certain drugs, such as glyceryl trinitrate (vasodilator given to treat angina and heart failure), are administered using the sublingual route (Figure 19.8). The drug gets absorbed quickly and is available for action within a short time. The other important factor is that drugs given via this route bypass the first pass metabolism. Moreover, in mixing the drug with food, gastric enzymes and juices are avoided as they may interfere with the drug metabolism and absorption. Oxytocin is a drug that can also be administered via the buccal route (cheek of the mouth) (Figure 19.9). This drug is used in labour as it assists uterine contraction in childbirth.

Rectal route

Many drugs in the UK are now available to be administered rectally. They include non-steroidal anti-inflammatory drugs, such as diclofenac, mild tranquillisers, such as diazepam, glycerol suppositories (for treating constipation) and many others. There are many advantages and disadvantages to using this route, some of which are listed in Table 19.3.

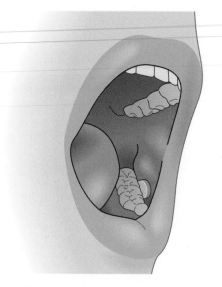

Figure 19.9 Buccal route.

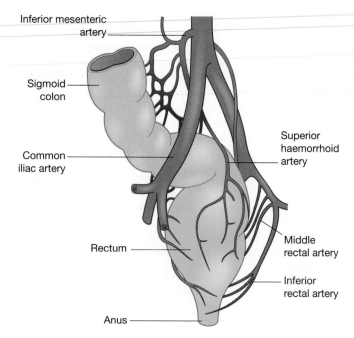

Inferior mesenteric artery

Sigmoid colon

Common iliac artery

Superior haemorrhoid artery

Rectum

Middle rectal artery

Inferior rectal artery

Anus

Figure 19.10 Rectal anatomy.

Jot This Down

A medication given rectally may work better than one given orally. Why is this so? Think about the anatomy of the rectum (see Figure 19.10).

Retention enemas as bowel evacuants and in some cases medications such as diazepam are administered via this route (Dougherty & Lister 2011). The advantages of this route include bypassing first pass metabolism, avoiding gastric irritation as seen with some medications and the abundant supply of blood vessels (Figure 19.10). Enemas for bowel movement are hypertonic. When admin-istered into the rectum, an enema causes water to move from the body into the rectum, which aids defecation.

When inserting suppositories or an enema, the nurse must instruct the patient to:

- Lie on the left side with their knees brought right up to the chest. This facilitates insertion of the suppositories or an enema
- Retain the suppository or the enema for approximately 15 minutes before opening their bowels.

Some patients may find the rectal route unacceptable and expel the suppository or the enema before it has had a chance to work.

What To Do If...

 What if the person refuses to have an enema or a suppository? How might you deal with this situation? Some nursing actions you may consider include:

- Discussing with the patient their anxieties and worries
- Discussing the benefits of taking the prescribed bowel laxatives.

Table 19.3 Advantages and disadvantages of using the rectal route.

ADVANTAGES	DISADVANTAGES
Bypasses the first pass metabolism	Constant use of the rectal route may cause anal trauma and even perforation
If a person is unconscious, this route can be used to administer drugs when other routes such as i.v., i.m. are not easily accessible as the person may be very thin	Person may find it uncomfortable
If the person is vomiting, then the oral route will be a problem, so the rectal route could be used in preference to i.m. or i.v.	Patient cooperation is needed to retain the suppository
Some patients may have difficulty in swallowing, in which case the rectal route is available	The procedure can be painful for the person if they suffer from anal stricture or have haemorrhoids, in which case some bleeding may take place

Jot This Down

A person has had an abdominoperineal (AP) resection and formation of a colostomy for rectal cancer. The person is prescribed metronidazole (antibiotic) suppositories as a prophylactic treatment for infection. What will you do?

Vaginal administration

The vaginal route may be used for the treatment of vaginal infection with antibiotics such as metronidazole. The suppository or pessaries need to be inserted high up the vagina and therefore manufacturers often supply an applicator in the package. Women

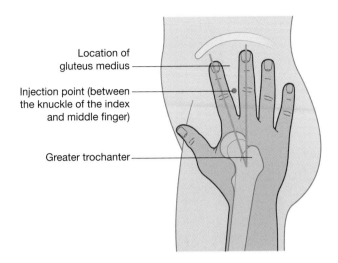

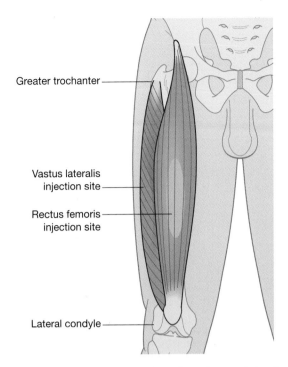

Figure 19.11 Location of the gluteus medius muscle.

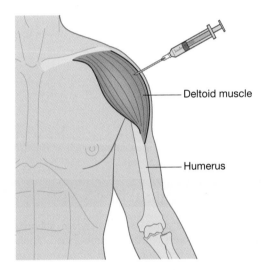

Figure 19.12 Location of the deltoid muscle.

Figure 19.13 Location of the rectus femoris and vastus lateralis muscles of the thigh.

should be advised to wear a small pad or panty liners so that their clothing will not be soiled as the medication may leak out as it dissolves. Remember that the vagina does not have sphincters like the anus.

Intramuscular/intravenous routes

Many medications are administered using these routes. When a person is unable to take oral medication as a result of nausea and vomiting or they are nil by mouth, they may need drugs to be administered using one of these routes. Intramuscular (i.m.) injections are given using the dense muscles. The muscles used are the gluteus medius in the buttocks (Figure 19.11), the deltoid muscle of the upper arm (Figure 19.12) and the rectus femoris and vastus lateralis (Figure 19.13) of the thigh. Nurses need to adhere to local policies when giving intramuscular injections. The advantage of using this route is that it bypasses the first pass metabolism. The disadvantage is that i.m. injections can be painful, depending on the drug. If the correct procedure is not adhered to the injection can cause more harm than good and may cause bleeding if the blood vessel is damaged in the process.

Intravenous (i.v.) injections are administered by doctors and qualified nurses who have had instructions in the administration of intravenous drugs. When giving medication through this route, the drug is given straight into the bloodstream and therefore the bioavailability of the drug is 100%. The first pass metabolism is avoided, resulting in very fast action of the drug. The i.v. route is also used to administer chemotherapy drugs, antibiotics and others when a quick action is needed. If the drug is given too quickly, it can result in circulatory shock or even death of the person (Galbraith *et al.* 2007).

Nurses need to remember that they have to adhere to the Nursing and Midwifery Council's (NMC) guidelines in the safe preparation and administration of injections. The NMC clearly states that:

It is unacceptable to prepare substances for injection in advance of their immediate use or to administer medications drawn into a syringe or container by another registrant when not in their presence.

(NMC 2008a)

However, in an emergency, for example during cardiopulmonary resuscitation (CPR), nurses may be required to mix medications or prepare them for others to administer; this is recognised by the NMC.

Red Flag

Nurses must always wear gloves when preparing or administering i.m. or i.v. injections.

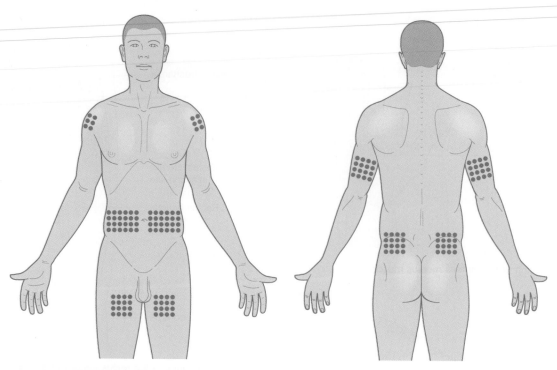

Figure 19.14 Subcutaneous injection sites.

Subcutaneous injections

The subcutaneous (s.c.) route is used to administer a small amount of drug into the subcutaneous tissue for slow absorption. This method is used to give drugs that otherwise cannot be given orally, such as insulin, which is rendered ineffective by the gastric juices. Another drug commonly given subcutaneously and postoperatively to prevent complications such as deep vein thrombosis, is enoxaparin (Clexane), which is an anticoagulant. The sites recommended are the abdomen, the lateral and posterior part of the upper arm, the thighs and the buttocks (Figure 19.14).

Inhalers

Certain drugs, such as salbutamol inhaler and oxygen, are administered via the respiratory tract by inhaling the medications via the oral or nasal route. This method is preferred when a quick and local action is required. Salbutamol works by acting on receptors in the lungs called beta 2 receptors. When salbutamol stimulates these receptors it causes the muscles in the airways to relax. This allows the airways to open, making breathing easier for the person. In conditions where there is narrowing of the airways, such as asthma or chronic obstructive pulmonary disease (COPD, e.g. emphysema and chronic bronchitis), it is difficult for the person to exhale because of the narrow airways. By opening the airways, salbutamol makes it easier for the person to breathe.

Link To/Go To

You may find this guideline from NICE, on 'Involving patients in decisions about prescribed medicines and supporting adherence', useful.

http://www.nice.org.uk/nicemedia/live/11766/43042/43042.pdf

Aural route

This route is used to administer medications such as ear drops to treat ear infection, or to soften ear wax.

Medical Abbreviations

In practice, you will come across some standard abbreviations that are being used by doctors when prescribing medications. See Table 19.4 for some of the common medical abbreviations used in hospitals.

Some Common Drugs Used in Practice and Their Action

Antibiotics
What are antibiotics?

The word 'antibiotic' comes from the Greek *anti* meaning 'against' and *bios* meaning 'life' – life of the bacteria. Antibiotics are also known as antibacterials, and they are drugs used to treat infections caused by bacteria. The early antibiotics were the natural products of other microorganisms – fungi or other bacteria. Many antibiotics are chemicals secreted by one organism that are toxic to another. It is these chemicals that are used to produce antibiotics.

Today most of the antibiotics are synthesised in medical laboratories. Antibiotics may be classed as 'broad-spectrum', which means they can affect a wide range of different bacteria. Examples of these include amoxicillin and cefotaxime. Other antibiotics only work against specific types of bacteria and are known as 'narrow-spectrum' antibiotics. Examples of these include vancomycin and teicoplanin.

Although there are a number of different types of antibiotic they all work in one of two ways:

Table 19.4 Common medical abbreviations.

ABBREVIATIONS	WHAT IT MEANS
p.o.	orally/by mouth
s.c.	subcutaneous
i.m.	intramuscular
i.v.	intravenous
p.r.	per rectum
b.d.	twice a day
o.d.	once a day
t.d.s.	three times a day
p.r.n.	given as necessary
q.d.s.	four times a day
stat	give immediately
p.v.	per vagina
nocte	at night
t.t.a./t.t.o.	tablets to take away/tablets to take out
s/l	sublingual
mg	milligram
mL	millilitre
mcg or μg	microgram
kg	kilogram
e.c.	enteric-coated
caps	capsule
neb	nebuliser

Antibiotics in this group include penicillin, cephalosporins and vancomycin.

Blocks protein synthesis Drugs can work on the ribosome of a cell or on the nucleus. The drugs interfere with the replication of deoxyribonucleic acid (DNA) or ribonucleic acid (RNA), preventing bacteria from being able to multiply and grow in number. Protein synthesis is important for bacteria to increase in number to cause the infection. There are many antibiotics that are part of this group and they include erythromycin, chloramphenicol and aminoglycosides.

Disrupts cell membrane These types of antibiotics affect the cell membrane system of the bacteria. Electrolytes and water leak out of the cytoplasm, thus rendering the cell unstable, and cellular death takes place. Antibiotics that disrupt the cell membrane include polymyxin B and nystatin.

Interferes with nucleic acid synthesis Nucleic acid production is important for microbial cells. Any antibiotics that interfere with nucleic acid production will disrupt microbial cell reproduction. Some of the antibiotics in this group include ciprofloxacin and nalidixic acid.

Prevents synthesis of folic acid Bacteria cannot use preformed folic acid as human cells do. They manufacture folic acid by using a compound called para-aminobenzoic acid (PABA). PABA is a B complex vitamin that is synthesised by intestinal bacteria. PABA assists friendly bacteria to produce folic acid. Bacteria need to use this folic acid to grow and reproduce. Antibiotics that interfere with folic acid synthesis include trimethoprim and sulphonamides.

397

- A 'bactericidal' antibiotic kills the bacteria. Penicillin is a bactericidal. A bactericidal usually either interferes with the formation of the bacterium's cell wall or its cell contents.
- A 'bacteriostatic' stops bacteria from multiplying. This group of antibiotics works with the host's immune system to get rid of the organisms that are in the body.

How do antibiotics work?

Antibiotics work by interfering with the growth of the bacteria. This can take place in five different ways:

- Inhibiting cell wall formation
- Blocking protein synthesis
- Disrupting cell membranes
- Interfering with nucleic acid synthesis
- Preventing synthesis of folic acid

Inhibits cell wall formation Bacteria have much thicker walls than human cells. This rigidity is a result of a substance called 'mucopeptide'. Mucopeptide is a polymer made of polysaccharide and peptide chains found in the cell walls of bacteria. Some antibiotics work by interfering with the formation of mucopeptide, resulting in weakness of the bacterial cell. This makes the bacterial cell wall more porous. As the fluid inside the cell is hypertonic, water from outside the cell moves into the cell. This causes the bacterial cell to swell and burst, thus destroying the bacteria.

Jot This Down

What do you understand by the terms broad- and narrow-spectrum antibiotics?

Side-effects

All antibiotics have adverse effects. These vary from drug to drug. Some of them can be very severe and can cause severe toxic effects to the person. The drugs may damage body tissue or organs and interfere with body function. In some cases, they destroy the normal flora of the body, resulting in an increase of bacteria that cause illness. Apart from the common side-effects, such as nausea and vomiting, diarrhoea and upset stomach, the person may develop symptoms such as allergy, drug toxicity, meticillin (methicillin) resistant *Staphylococcus aureus* (MRSA) and antibiotic-related colitis.

Allergy

One of the commonest side-effects of any antibiotic is an allergic reaction. These reactions may be minor or severe. In some patients, a small allergic reaction such as diarrhoea is not uncommon. Patients who have never had any drug therapy may develop allergic reactions when they are treated with antibiotics. This may be due to a variety of factors, for example the body's reaction to foreign chemicals or contamination of the drug by environmental factors.

If the reactions to the drugs are severe, such as cardiac problems, then the treatment should be discontinued immediately and documented in the person's notes. The person should also be informed of their allergic reaction so that they are aware of their allergy.

Jot This Down

Can you think about any other allergic reactions that the person may have as a result of antibiotics?

What To Do If...

What should you do if the person develops an anaphylactic reaction during antibiotic therapy? Some of the nursing actions include:

- Stop the antibiotic therapy immediately
- Report the patient's condition to the person in charge
- Stay with your patient and monitor their vital signs
- Document all outcomes in the patient's care plan

Link To/Go To

For information on anaphylaxis visit:
www.anaphylaxis.org.uk

Drug toxicity

Apart from fighting infection, antibiotics can also damage the body as a result of toxic effects. Some toxic symptoms include kidney failure, liver failure, bone marrow defects and nerve damage. Other less severe symptoms include diarrhoea, nausea and vomiting. The kidney and the liver are the two main organs that are affected by drug toxicity. This is because of their roles in drug metabolism and excretion. Drugs such as the sulphonamides can cause renal problems when they crystallise in the kidneys and form kidney stones. Some drugs given together with diuretics, such as gentamicin (an antibiotic) and furosemide (a diuretic), can be nephrotoxic if they are not regulated properly. Liver problems can develop as a result of drug toxicity. The liver is the principal organ of drug metabolism and excretion. Diseases such as liver cirrhosis may occur, thus affecting liver function, which can be fatal to the person.

Some drug toxicity may affect the central nervous system, resulting in the person developing convulsions, ataxia, nervousness, insomnia and temporary blindness. The most common symptom is acoustic nerve damage, resulting in tinnitus and deafness.

Antibiotic resistance

Bacteria are termed drug-resistant when they are no longer inhibited by an antibiotic to which they were previously sensitive. The emergence and spread of antibacterial-resistant bacteria has continued to grow, due to both the over-use and misuse of antibiotics. Treating a patient with antibiotics causes the microbes to adapt or die; this is known as 'selective pressure'. If a strain of a bacterial species acquires resistance to an antibiotic, it will survive the treatment. As the bacterial cell with acquired resistance multiplies, this resistance is passed on to its offspring. In ideal conditions, some

bacterial cells can divide every 20 minutes; therefore, after only 8 hours, in excess of 16 million bacterial cells carrying resistance to that antibiotic could exist. Also, antibiotics can destroy many of the harmless strains of bacteria that live in and on the body. This allows resistant bacteria to multiply quickly and replace them.

MRSA

MRSA stands for meticillin-resistant *Staphylococcus aureus*. It is sometimes known as a super bug. There are various subtypes (strains) of *S. aureus* and some strains are classed as MRSA. MRSA strains are very similar to any other strain of *S. aureus*. That is, some healthy people are carriers and some people develop MRSA infections. *Staphylococcus aureus* is a bacterium (germ). It is often abbreviated to '*S. aureus*' or '*Staph*'. *S. aureus* bacteria are often found on the skin and in the nose of healthy people. These people are called *S. aureus* carriers. In healthy people who are carriers, *S. aureus* is usually harmless.

However, *S. aureus* bacteria sometimes invade the skin to cause infection. This is more likely if you have a cut or graze, which can allow bacteria to get under the surface of the skin. *S. aureus* is the cause of skin infections such as boils, pimples, impetigo and skin abscesses, and is a common cause of wound infections. Sometimes, these germs get into the bloodstream and can cause septicaemia (blood infection), pneumonia (lung infection) and endocarditis (heart valve infection).

MRSA bacteria are difficult to treat with any antibiotic as they have developed resistance to these drugs. This may have resulted from uncontrolled use of antibiotics, both in the hospital and community, or excessive use of antibiotics on animals bred for meat. The constant use of antibiotics can also kill the normal flora of the GI tract, thus leaving the bacteria to grow and cause problems.

Antibiotic-related colitis

The normal flora of the gut protects the lining of the GI tract. As mentioned above, uncontrolled use of antibiotics may destroy the normal flora. This is more evident in persons treated with oral antibiotics. Some of these antibiotics include penicillin, cotrimoxazole and tetracyclines. One of the most widely spoken about infections in hospital is caused by a bacterium called *Clostridium difficile* (*C. difficile*, or *C. diff*). This is a normal bacterium in the gut, which protects the lining of the GI tract. As a result of misuse of some antibiotics, these bacteria multiply in great numbers and produce toxins, resulting in the person developing severe diarrhoea and fever.

Red Flag

When caring for patients with MRSA or *C. diff*, always wear protective clothing such as mask, apron and gloves and wash your hands before and after attending to the person.

New strains

There are already signs of new strains. New Delhi metallo-β-lactamase (NDM-1) is a gene carried by some bacteria that is capable of destroying antibiotics. NDM-1 is encoded for by sections of bacterial DNA known as 'plasmids', which can be transferred between types of bacteria, hence more than one type of bacteria can acquire this type of resistance. It is most often seen in

Klebsiella pneumoniae and *E. coli*. Another super bug that is giving great concern is the bacterium that causes multi-drug-resistant tuberculosis (MDR-TB). Multi-drug-resistant tuberculosis strains are generally considered to be those resistant to at least two drugs, such as isoniazid (INH) and rifampin (RIF).

Anticoagulants

Blood clotting is a mechanism by which the blood sticks together to form small solid clots. It is a natural and vital function of the body, without which a person would bleed to death after an injury. The blood has a complex system that regulates when or how clots form. More than 30 factors in the blood are known to affect clotting and it is essential that the balance of these clotting factors is at the right level. Blood clotting is triggered by small blood cells called 'platelets'. The clotting blood goes through a series of chemical reactions before clots are formed.

Anticoagulants are prescribed for patients who suffer from clotting disorders, postoperatively and after a myocardial infarct (MI). In the UK, aspirin, warfarin and heparin are currently the drugs of choice of oral anticoagulant therapy for most blood coagulation problems (**http://www.person.co.uk/doctor/Oral -Anticoagulants.htm**). Anticoagulant medicines reduce the ability of the blood to clot. This is necessary if the blood clots too quickly, as these blood clots can block blood vessels and lead to conditions such as a stroke or an MI. Some of the conditions where anticoagulants are used include:

- Deep vein thrombosis (DVT) – blood clot in the veins resulting from poor circulation, for example in patients who are on prolonged bed rest after a major surgery
- Pulmonary embolism (PE) – blood clot in the lungs
- Atrial fibrillation (AF) – irregular heart beat. AF increases the risk of stroke. Patients with AF are prescribed anticoagulants such as warfarin to protect them from developing a stroke
- High or moderate risk of cerebrovascular accident (CVA) – stroke.

Aspirin

As well as its anti-inflammatory, analgesic and antipyretic properties, aspirin is used as an anticoagulant. It works by its action on the platelets – aspirin prevents platelets from clumping together and starting the formation of a clot, and is known as an 'antiplatelet agent'. Aspirin is one of the earliest analgesics and it is synthesised from willow bark in the form of salicylic acid (Galbraith *et al.* 2007). These days, aspirin is produced in various forms as fast-release, slow-release and enteric-coated. As aspirin is acid based, this medication is better absorbed from the GI tract with food. Taken on an empty stomach, it can cause gastric problems.

Side-effects Some of the side-effects associated with aspirin include:

- Gastric bleeding
- Allergy (rare)
- In large doses, papillary necrosis of the kidney
- The risk of children developing Reye's syndrome as a result of aspirin treatment to control pyrexia
- Aspirin induced asthma.

Elimination Aspirin is freely excreted in urine, however the excretion rate is better in an alkaline than in an acidic urine.

Table 19.5 Warfarin – Drug–drug interactions.

DRUGS THAT INCREASE WARFARIN ACTION	DRUGS THAT DECREASE WARFARIN ACTION
Aspirin	Phenytoin
Non-steroidal anti-inflammatory drugs	Oestrogen
Liquid paraffin	Antacid
Propranolol	Phenobarbitone
Co-trimoxazole	Carbamazepine

Warfarin

Warfarin is the main oral anticoagulant used in the UK for long-term anticoagulant therapy. Warfarin structurally resembles vitamin K, which is essential for blood clotting and is mainly found in leafy vegetables such as spinach, broccoli, vegetable oil and cereals. Warfarin inhibits the action of vitamin K and thus lengthens the clotting time. Vitamin K has an essential role to play in the production of prothrombin, which is a protein found in the blood. Prothrombin plays an important part in the process of the formation of clots. If the production of vitamin K is slowed down, the production of prothrombin is also reduced. This means that it will take longer for blood clots to form. Warfarin is used to treat patients with MI, DVT and AF. The dosage of warfarin is regulated by blood test using the international normalisation ratio (INR).

Other drugs can interfere with the action of warfarin. Some of the drugs can increase, while others can reduce, the effects of warfarin. See Table 19.5 for some of the drug–drug interactions of warfarin.

Side-effects

- Passing blood in the urine or faeces
- Passing black faeces (melaena)
- Severe bruising
- Prolonged nose-bleeds (lasting longer than 10 minutes)
- Bleeding gums
- Blood in the vomit or coughing up blood
- Unusual headaches
- In women, heavy or increased bleeding during menstruation, or any other bleeding from the vagina.

Elimination The elimination of warfarin is almost entirely by metabolism. Warfarin is eventually metabolised to reduced metabolites (warfarin alcohols) and excreted in the urine, and some through the GI tract.

Red Flag

 All patients discharged on warfarin **must** be referred to an anticoagulation clinic for continued INR monitoring and dosage.

Heparin

Heparin is a mucopolysaccharide naturally found in the body in the mast cells, plasma and the endothelial cells of blood vessels. Heparin is given systemically, that is in i.v. or s.c. form, as it is easily digested by the GI tract. Heparin is a medicine which is used in a number of conditions – an example is treatment and prevention of thromboembolic diseases.

As mentioned before, the clotting process is complicated and begins when blood cells called 'platelets' clump together and produce chemicals that activate the clotting process. The final part of this process involves a substance called 'thrombin' being activated to produce a protein called 'fibrin'. Fibrin binds the platelets together, forming a blood clot. This is the body's natural way of repairing itself.

Heparin works by inactivating thrombin in the clotting process. This stops the formation of fibrin and so stops blood clots forming. Heparin is used to treat blood clots that have formed abnormally inside the blood vessels. It can also be used to prevent these dangerous blood clots, known as 'thrombus'. If the person is overdosed with heparin, then they are administered protamine sulphate, which has a rapid action in neutralising the action of heparin.

A thrombus can be dangerous because the clot may detach and travel in the bloodstream (where it becomes known as an 'embolus') and may eventually get lodged in a blood vessel, thereby blocking the blood supply to a vital organ, such as the heart, brain or lungs. This is known as a 'thromboembolism'.

Side-effects There are numerous side-effects of heparin. Some of these are:

- Anaphylactic shock
- Angioedema
- Asthma
- Bleeding
- Chills
- Cyanosis
- Hypersensitivity reactions
- Local irritation or skin problems at the injection site
- Metabolic problems
- Osteoporosis
- Rhinitis
- Soft tissue necrosis
- Thrombocytopenia
- Thromboembolism
- Urticaria.

Elimination Heparin is mainly excreted by the kidneys.

What To Do If…

What will you do if the person refuses to take their medication? Consider some of the reasons why the person may refuse to take their medication. Some issues may include:

- Not knowing what the medication is for
- Feeling that he/she may be seriously ill
- May not like the taste of medications

Fibrinolytic drugs

Fibrinolytic or thrombolytic drugs are used to treat blood clots formed as a result of tissue injury. Once the drug is administered, it starts the process of dissolving clots. These drugs are administered by intravenous infusion. Fibrinolytic drugs catalyse the conversion of the proenzyme plasminogen to plasmin, which, when in proximity to a thrombus or embolus, degrades fibrin into soluble peptides, which then dissolve the clot. Streptokinase, the first thrombolytic drug, has now been replaced by the second generation agent, tissue type plasminogen activator (t-PA).

Third-generation thrombolytic drugs, which are recombinant mutant variants of t-PA and have been shown to have comparable efficacy with that of t-PA, have also now reached clinical practice. These include reteplase and tenecteplase. They differ from native t-PA by having increased plasma half-lives that allow more convenient dosing. Before starting the person on fibrinolytic anticoagulation, heparin must be discontinued and the activated partial thromboplastin time (aPTT) ratio calculated.

Thrombolysis is mainly used in patients with:

- Acute MI
- Ischaemic stroke
- (Sub)acute peripheral arterial thrombosis
- Acute massive PE
- Occluded haemodialysis shunts.

Side-effects The most common side-effect of fibrinolytic drugs is bleeding. The bleeding can take place from most of the body systems, including the GI tract, urinary system, in the central nervous system and respiratory tract. Other side-effects associated with the fibrinolytic drugs are cholesterol embolism and reperfusion arrhythmias.

Excretion The main organs of excretion are the kidneys.

Analgesia

Strategies for coping with pain vary greatly from person to person. Coping methods that were perceived as helpful in the past are often used by the person and may become habitual. Nurses caring for patients should remember that pain is a personal experience and is unique to the individual. There are different pain assessment tools used in clinical practice to assess the level of pain in patients, such as the visual analogue scale and numerical intensity scale. If pain is not assessed properly and appropriate analgesia administered as prescribed, the patient will remain in pain and their progress will be affected (Peate *et al.* 2012). There are different types of analgesics:

- Non-opioid analgesics such as paracetamol used to treat mild to moderate pain
- Non-steroidal anti-inflammatory drugs (NSAIDs) such as aspirin, which acts on the peripheral nerve endings, inhibiting prostaglandin synthesis
- Opioids such as morphine used to treat severe pain
- Synthetic opioids such as codeine, tramadol and fentanyl.

The World Health Organization developed a three-step 'ladder' (Figure 19.15) for cancer pain relief. If pain occurs, there should be prompt oral administration of drugs in the following order: non-opioids (aspirin and paracetamol); then, as necessary, mild opioids (codeine); then strong opioids, such as morphine, until the person is free of pain. To calm fears and anxiety, additional drugs – 'adjuvants' – should be used. To maintain freedom from pain, drugs should be given 'by the clock', that is every 3–6 hours, rather than 'on demand'. This three-step approach of administering the right drug in the right dose at the right time is inexpensive and 80–90% effective (WHO 1986).

Opioids

Opioid drugs exert their action on the central nervous system (CNS). These drugs stimulate receptors in the CNS. These receptors are opioid agonists, which means these receptors will allow opioids to attach to them and produce a response. The three main CNS

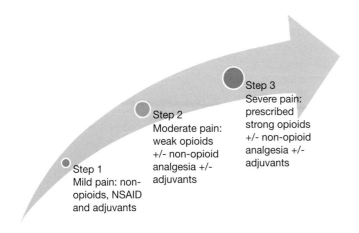

Figure 19.15 Analgesic steps.

In the figure:

Step 1
Mild pain: non-opioids, NSAID and adjuvants

Step 2
Moderate pain: weak opioids +/- non-opioid analgesia +/- adjuvants

Step 3
Severe pain: prescribed strong opioids +/- non-opioid analgesia +/- adjuvants

Table 19.6 CNS opioid receptors.

RECEPTOR TYPE	WHERE IN THE CNS	FUNCTIONS
μ (mu)	Dorsal horn of the spinal cord in the substantia gelatinosa and the thalamus	They can exist either in the pre-synaptic or post-synaptic neurones, depending upon cell types. They can cause respiratory depression, hypothermia and a state of euphoria. These receptors are also found in the GI tract. Constipation is a major side-effect of μ-agonists, due to inhibition of peristaltic action
κ (kappa)	Hypothalamus, spinal cord in the substantia gelatinosa	Cause drowsiness, respiratory depression. They alter the perception of pain, consciousness, motor control, and mood
δ (delta)	Limbic system	Respiratory depression and mood changes

receptors for opioid analgesia are the mu, kappa and delta receptors (see Table 19.6 for their location and functions).

Opioid drugs interact with these receptors in the CNS to control pain response and modify a person's mood and psychological state. Opioids may also alter the chemical levels, for example these drugs may decrease the calcium ion concentration and inhibit its uptake into the brain cells. Other opioids may inhibit the release of nor-epinephrine and modify dopamine release.

Opioid drugs are readily absorbed from the GI tract, nasal mucosa and the peripheral tissues after an injection. These drugs are administered orally, rectally, s.c., i.m., i.v., by epidural and by transdermal routes. Once absorbed, they are widely distributed in the body. Increasingly, analgesics are administered by PCA (person-controlled analgesia) pumps, which allow the person to control the amount of drug administered.

Side-effects Some common side-effects of opioid analgesia include:

- Constipation
- Retention of urine
- Suppression of respiration
- Drowsiness
- Pupil constriction
- Dry mouth
- Nausea and vomiting
- Cough suppression

> **Jot This Down**
>
> In hospital, can patients receiving opioid analgesia be addicted to the drug? Is there a difference between dependency and addiction?

Elimination Most of the water-soluble metabolites are excreted in the urine.

NSAIDs

These drugs are given for mild to moderate pain and they have an analgesic and anti-inflammatory effect. Some of these drugs are aspirin, paracetamol, ibuprofen, diclofenac and indometacin. These drugs inhibit prostaglandin synthesis. Prostaglandins are mediators of inflammatory response, production of pain, and fever. When tissues are damaged, white blood cells flood to the site to try to minimise tissue destruction. Prostaglandins are produced as a result, which then cause pain at the site of injury.

Other roles of prostaglandins include the augmentation of histamine and other chemicals in causing vasodilatation and increasing vascular permeability to fluids. Prostaglandins also play a role in channelling the pain sensation to the CNS.

Other roles of NSAIDs include:

- The release of lysosomal enzymes – lysosomes are cellular organelles that contain acid hydrolase enzymes that break down waste materials and cellular debris
- Neutrophil aggregation and adhesion at the site of injury
- Leukotriene production – compounds derived from arachidonic acid that function as regulators of allergic and inflammatory reactions
- Cartilage metabolism.

Side-effects Some of the side-effects of NSAIDs include:

- Abdominal pain
- GI bleeding
- Melaena
- Kidney damage
- Hypotension
- Fluid retention.

Non-pharmacological Therapies

There are many complementary therapies available instead of using drugs (Ellson 2008). Some of the non-pharmacological interventions for pain management include:

- *Transcutaneous electrical nerve stimulation (TNS)*: whereby a pair of electrodes are applied to the skin and the area is stimulated by a small electric current. TNS machines are available for use in the hospital or in the community, and then can be used as needed. It is mainly used for chronic pain.
- *Acupuncture*: needle insertion into acupuncture points of the body. It is an ancient Chinese treatment. Acupuncture is based

on the belief that an energy, or 'life force', flows through the body in channels called 'meridians'. This life force is known as *Qi* (pronounced 'chee').

 Link To/Go To

You will find the following website useful in finding out more about acupuncture:

http://www.nhs.uk/conditions/Acupuncture/Pages/Introduction.aspx

- *Massage*: manual stimulation of muscles is used as pain relief
- *Yoga*: a meditative technique; breathing and posture is used as a healing process. Originated from ancient India
- *Aromatherapy*: the use of essential oils on the body through gentle massage technique.

  Other techniques include:

- Herbal medicine
- Music therapy
- Reflexology
- Homeopathy.

Bronchodilators

In the UK, diseases that cause airflow obstruction are common. About 5.1 million people receive treatment for asthma and about 600 000 people are diagnosed as having chronic obstructive pulmonary disease (COPD), although this is likely to be an underestimate (British Thoracic Society, BTS 2006). In COPD, the constriction of airway smooth muscle gives rise to symptoms such as chest tightness, wheezing and breathlessness. Patients are administered bronchodilators to relieve these symptoms.

Drugs administered as gases penetrate the cell linings of the respiratory tract easily and rapidly. These include sprays and aerosols. They are absorbed almost as fast as they are inhaled, because the blood and the lung membrane are in close proximity. Drugs given in this form are bronchodilators, such as salbutamol. Patients who suffer from chronic obstructive pulmonary disease (COPD) include those with:

- Asthma (extrinsic and intrinsic)
- Chronic bronchitis
- Emphysema
- Cystic fibrosis.

Bronchodilator medicines are available in short-acting and long-acting varieties. The three most widely used bronchodilators are:

- Beta-2 agonists
- Anticholinergics
- Theophyllines.

Beta-2 agonist

Beta-2 agonists can be short-acting or long-acting. They are usually taken through an inhaler. Beta-2 agonists work by relaxing muscles in the lungs, which allows the airways to dilate (widen). Long-acting beta-2 agonists also reduce the amount of mucus in the lungs by increasing the motion of cilia. Cilia are tiny hairs that line the airway walls and 'sweep' mucus out of the airways. Kaufman (2010) reports that the beta-2 agonists reduce the dead space in the trachea by reducing resistance. The most familiar short-acting beta-2 agonists are:

- Salbutamol
- Terbutaline.

The action of short-acting drugs is rapid and the effect can last 4–6 hours. They are given in high doses in cases of acute, severe asthma. Long-acting beta-2 agonists are often used in combination with inhaled corticosteroids. Examples of long-acting beta-2 agonists are formoterol and budesonide (Symbicort) and salmeterol and fluticasone (Advair). The effect of long-acting beta-2 agonists could last for at least 12 hours and therefore they are useful in treating nocturnal (night) symptoms.

Side-effects The most common are nervousness, restlessness and trembling. Some people also find they get a dry, irritated throat after using the medication. Less common side-effects include palpitations, muscle cramp and headaches.

Anticholinergics

Anticholinergic or muscarinic agents are often prescribed in conjunction with beta-2 agonists. When the parasympathetic nervous system is activated, it releases norepinephrine and acetylcholine, causing constriction of the airways. Anticholinergic inhalers complement the beta-2 agonists by preventing acetylcholine from binding with anticholinergic receptors in the smooth muscle and submucosal glands. This prevents the development of cholinergic effects such as increased mucus secretion, and it also relaxes smooth muscle cells causing a widening of the airways.

Anticholinergics are mainly used to treat COPD and are usually taken through an inhaler. However, patients with severe COPD may need to use a nebuliser. This is a device that uses air pressure to turn the medicine into a fine mist, which the person breathes in through a mask. Like beta-2 agonists, anticholinergics also relax the muscles in the lungs. Short- and long-acting varieties are available and they are ipratropium bromide and oxitropium bromide. Short-acting anticholinergic medications work in about 15 minutes and last for 6–8 hours. Tiotropium, a long-acting anticholinergic, takes about 20 minutes to work and can last for 24 hours; therefore it is taken only once a day for maintenance.

Side-effects Compared with beta-2 agonists, anticholinergics are better tolerated by most people and serious side-effects are rare. A dry mouth is the most commonly reported side-effect. Less common ones are nausea, constipation, palpitations and headaches.

Theophyllines

Theophyllines are long-acting bronchodilators that are usually used to treat COPD. It is not clear exactly how theophyllines work, but they seem to relax the muscles in the lungs while reducing possible inflammation (swelling) in the airways. Hanania and Donohue (2007) state that theophylline is considered to be a respiratory stimulant. It works by improving contractility of the diaphragm and assists corticosteroids through its anti-inflammatory properties. Theophyllines are usually taken in tablet or syrup form. Due to a risk of associated side-effects, such as nausea and dizziness, theophyllines are often only used if other bronchodilators have proven ineffective.

Side-effects Theophyllines can cause serious side-effects if too much of the medication builds up in the body. Regular blood tests are needed to ensure levels of theophylline in the body are safe. The elderly are more at risk of developing side-effects from theophyllines, because their liver may not be able to remove the medication from their body. Other side-effects include increased heart rate, palpitations, tremor, seizures and headaches.

The Evidence Fish Oil and COPD

Omega-3 (fatty acid) has anti-inflammatory properties. New research has identified that it may be beneficial for COPD patients. The American Heart Association recommends omega-3 in the diet of COPD patients. Other benefits of omega-3 include:

- Treatment of dermatitis
- Reduces risk of cardiovascular disease: increased vasodilation, reduction of triglycerides, cholesterol, blood pressure and risk of thrombosis
- Anti-inflammatory action
- Improves glucose metabolism in diabetes
- Strengthens the immune system
- Increases fertility
- Increases vigor
- Strengthens certain neuronal functions
- Reduces the risk of cardiovascular disorders
- Combats eye health problems
- Controls body weight.

   Interactions of omega-3 include:
- Can slow clotting when used with herbs, e.g. cloves, garlic, ginger, turmeric

   For more information visit:

   http://www.inkanat.com/en/arti.asp?ref=salmon-oil

Cardiac Glycosides

Cardiac glycosides (CG) are termed inotropic agents. Inotropic drugs can either have positive or negative properties. Positive inotropic drugs improve contraction force of the heart muscle thus increasing cardiac output. They are used in the treatment of heart failure with atrial fibrillation. One of the common drugs used in practice to treat heart failure is digoxin. Digoxin is extracted from the leaves of purple foxgloves and, in practice, it is often called 'digitalis'. Digitalis is a generic term for all 'cardiac glycosides'. Digoxin acts on the autonomic nervous system to slow down the heart rate and also on the atrioventricular node of the heart to slow down the conduction of the ventricles.

However, negative inotropic drugs decrease myocardial contractility and are used to decrease cardiac workload in conditions such as angina. Examples of drugs that have a negative inotropic effect include beta blockers, such as metoprolol, and calcium channel blockers (CCB), for example nifedipine. Metoprolol is a beta-adrenergic receptor blocker. It blocks the beta version of epinephrine (adrenaline) from attaching and sending signals to the cardiac tissue, thus lowering pulse rate, stroke volume and cardiac output. The action of negative inotropic drugs also results in a decrease in the electrical activity in the heart. CCB inhibit inward movement of calcium ions through the slow channels of active membranes, thus reducing the afterload of the heart.

How do cardiac glycoside drugs work?

CG work by regulating the movement of calcium ions in and out of the myocardium and the activity of the autonomic nervous system. Calcium is an essential ion for muscle contraction. These drugs inhibit the activity of the enzyme ATPase at the sodium-potassium pump. This results in an increase in intracellular sodium ions. This then affects the sodium-calcium pump, whereby less calcium ions are removed from the myocardial cells, thus increasing the levels of calcium ions in the intracellular space. Stores of calcium ions from the mitochondria are also released into the intracellular space, thus further increasing the level of calcium in the cell. Calcium is an important ion for muscle contraction. The increased level of calcium improves myocardial contraction, thus increasing cardiac output.

Side-effects As the margin between the therapeutic and toxic levels of CG is so narrow, nurses need to be cautious when administering CG. Side-effects include:

- Nausea and vomiting
- Visual disturbance
- Headache
- Confusion
- Diarrhoea
- Bradycardia (slow heart rate – below 60 beats/minute)
- ECG changes, for example prolonged P-R interval and shortened Q-T complex.

Red Flag

Nurses must always take the person's pulse rate before administering digoxin. If the pulse rate is below 60 beats/minute, the drug must not be given. It should be documented in the person's care plan and in the treatment chart that the drug has been omitted and the doctor informed. The person should be assessed, their pulse rate checked hourly, and advised to stay in bed until it is safe for them to mobilise.

Care, Dignity and Compassion

Old people, especially the very old, require special care and consideration from prescribers (BNF 2012). Department of Health (DH 2001) guidance on 'Medicines for Older People' describes how to maximise the benefits and how to avoid excessive, inappropriate consumption of medicines by older people.

- *Before administering the medication, consider whether the person needs the drug*
- *Limit the range of drugs*
- *Prescribe lower dosage of drugs than for a younger adult*
- *Review medications regularly. Discontinue if not needed*
- *Write down precise instructions on how and when to take the medications*
- *Advise the person on the proper disposal of unwanted drugs*

Drug Calculations

Nurses have to use mathematical calculations in practice to administer medications to patients, and some of these calculations occur during an emergency. The calculations are made for tablets and fluids. Many of these calculations involve converting larger units to smaller units and smaller to larger units. To convert larger units to smaller the larger is multiplied, for example:

- kilograms (kg) to grams (g) = kg × 1000
- litres (L) to millilitres (mL) = L × 1000
- milligrams to micrograms (mcg or μg) = mg × 1000.

To convert smaller units to larger, the smaller is divided, for example:

- grams to kilograms = g/1000
- millilitres to litres = mL/1000
- micrograms (mcg or μg) to milligrams = mcg/1000.

By definition, 1 gram = 1000 milligrams and 1 milligram = 1000 micrograms.

SI Units

Some examples of conversions:

- 200 mg = 0.2 g; 0.6 g = 600 mg; 600 mcg (or μg) = 0.6 mg
- 2000 mL = 2 L; 0.030 m = 30 mm; 0.03 mg = 30 mcg (or μg).

In practice, most of the drugs supplied from pharmacy have already been adjusted by the pharmacist, and nurses ensure that they administer the medication correctly, adhering to local and national policies. However, there are times when nurses may need to calculate the dosage of a drug before dispensing, especially when administering i.v. fluids to patients. This is when nurses need to use their calculating skills to obtain the correct dosage for the person.

Jot This Down Exercise 1
1. Convert 550 mg to g
2. Convert 0.1 g to mg
3. Convert 50 mcg (or μg) to mg
4. Convert 100 mL to litres
5. Convert 0.125 g to mg
Answers to Exercise 1: **1.** 0.55 g; **2.** 100 mg; **3.** 0.5 mg; **4.** 0.1 litres; **5.** 125 mg

Jot This Down Exercise 2
A person is prescribed 120 mg of verapamil but the tablets are available as 40 mg each. How many tablets are required? The solution involves finding how many 40s are in 120 or in other words, 120 divided by 40.
Always remember this formula for calculating tablets:
Number of tablets = what you want/what you have
So in the above example, 120/40 = 3

Jot This Down Exercise 3
1. 600 mg is prescribed, tablets are 300 mg each: how many tablets will you give?
2. 50 mg is prescribed, tablets are 12.5 mg each: how many tablets will you give?
3. 1 mg prescribed, tablets are 500 micrograms: how many tablets will you give?
4. 625 mg prescribed, tablets are 1.25 g each: how many tablets will you give?
5. 3 tablets each contain 250 mg. What is the total dose in milligrams?
Answers to Exercise 3: **1.** 2 tablets; **2.** 4 tablets; **3.** 2 tablets; **4.** ½ tablet; **5.** 750 mg.

Liquid Medications

When a medication is in a liquid form, you should consider the concentration of the drug in that liquid. For example, pethidine hydrochloride is available as 50 mg/mL. This means that 50 milligrams of pethidine hydrochloride are dissolved in every millilitre of liquid. In this case, it is the volume you need to consider.

For example: A drug is available as 25 mg/mL and 75 mg is required. What volume will be given in mL?

Formula: volume of the drug = amount prescribed/

amount per measure

So in the above example: 75/25 = 3 mL

Another example: A child is prescribed amoxicillin 250 mg every 6 hours. The liquid medicine dispensed is 125 mg in 5 mL. What volume of medicine should be dispensed?

Using the above formula: 250/125 × 5 mL = 2/1 × 5 = 10 mL.

Red Flag

 Any liquid medicine needs to be shaken thoroughly to make sure that the suspension is mixed evenly, otherwise the person will get too much or too little of the drug.

Jot This Down Exercise 4
1. Drug available as 10 mg/mL: prescription is for 20 mg, how many mL will be given?
2. Drug available as 10 mg/2 mL: prescription is for 5 mg, how many mL will be given?
3. Drug available as 20 mg/5 mL: prescription is for 40 mg, how many mL will be given?
4. Drug available as 10 mg/mL: how many mg will there be in 3 mL?
5. Drug available as 20 mg/5 mL: how many mg will be in 7.5 mL?
Answers to Exercise 4: **1.** 2 mL; **2.** 1 mL; **3.** 10 mL; **4.** 30 mg; **5.** 30 mg.

Intravenous infusions

Sometimes patients are administered medication via the parenteral route because either the person cannot swallow any tablets or the drug may be destroyed by chemicals in the stomach (Shihab 2009). Intravenous (i.v.) infusions are administered to patients, and nurses are required to ensure that the infusion runs on time. One needs to bear in mind that the drops per minute will vary between an adult and a child. It is estimated that there are 20 drops per mL for the adult i.v. administration tubes. However, this is slightly less for blood. In the case of blood, it is calculated that there are 15 drops in 1 mL of blood. One reason for this is that blood is thicker than clear fluid and therefore there are slightly fewer drops in 1 mL. In order to calculate the flow rate, you can use the following formula to calculate drops per minute.

Formula for calculating drop rate:

Drops per minute = (volume × 20 drops)/(time × 60 minutes)

Example: The person is prescribed 1 litre of normal saline over 4 hours. How many drops per minute should the drip rate be? The drip factor is 20 drops per mL.

Using the formula above:

Drops per minute $= (1000 \times 20)/(4 \times 60) = 2000/24$

$\qquad\qquad = 83$ drops/minute

You are allowed to round the figure to a whole number.

Jot This Down Exercise 5

Using the formula above, calculate, the drip rate for the following:

1. The person is prescribed 500 mL of normal saline over 6 hours, what is the drop rate?
2. If a person requires 1000 mL in 6 hours, what is the rate?
3. If a person is to be given 500 mL by i.v. infusion using a controller with a drip factor of 20 drops/mL over 6 hours, what would you set the drip rate to?
4. If a person is to be given 750 mL by i.v. infusion using a controller with a drip factor of 20 drops/mL over 12 hours, what would you set the drip rate to?
5. The person is written up for 1 unit (475 mL) of blood over 3 hours through an adult blood administration set. What is the drip rate?

Answers to Exercise 5: **1.** 28 drops; **2.** 56 drops; **3.** 28 drops; **4.** 21 drops; **5.** 40 drops.

Conclusion

This chapter has explored some aspects of drug administration and policies and legislation governing the drug administration. Nurses should always adhere to the local, professional and national policies in the safe administration of medicine. The nurse's role involves more direct care compared with other healthcare professionals and therefore nurses need to ensure a high standard of nursing care with respect to drug administration.

Key Points

- All drugs produced have a generic and one or more brand names. A generic name is a drug's common scientific name. A brand name drug is a medicine that is discovered, developed and marketed by a pharmaceutical company.
- Drug administration does not just involve giving out medication to patients; it involves working with the person, their relatives and other healthcare professionals in the safe administration of medicine. Nurses also have to follow the local, national and their professional guidelines to ensure that they carry out their duties confidently and professionally.
- The chemical nature of the drug determines how and where the absorption takes place. Absorption takes place through the intestinal wall and into the plasma before it reaches the site of action.
- Drugs administered orally have a major hurdle to go through before they reach the general circulation. This is called 'first pass metabolism'.
- Some of the enteric-coated tablets are gastric irritants and therefore should be taken with food or after a meal. Thus, nurses should never crush enteric-coated medications as it may render the drug ineffective.

- Anticoagulant medicines reduce the ability of the blood to clot. If the patient is overdosed with an anticoagulant, prompt action is needed to reverse the action of the drug. Some of the serious side-effects include bleeding from the GI tract, haematuria, bleeding from the gums and epistaxis.

Glossary

Adjuvants: drugs that have few or no pharmacological effects by themselves, but may increase the efficacy or potency of other drugs when given at the same time
Administration: giving out
Aggregation: clumping together
Agonist: drug that stimulates a receptor
Aminoglycosides: a group of antibiotics
Anabolic: refers to a substance that aids in the repair of body tissue, particularly protein
Antagonist: drug that does not activate a receptor
Anticoagulants: drugs that delay or prevent clotting
Aqueous pores: water channels
Ataxia: a condition that causes a loss of physical coordination
Atrial fibrillation: a heart condition that causes an irregular and often abnormally fast heart rate
Biotransformation: chemical alteration of a substance, especially of a drug, within the body, as by the action of enzymes
Buccal: the space between the cheek and the gum
Enzymes: substance which hastens or brings about a chemical change without itself undergoing any alterations
Epistaxis: nose bleed
Exhale: breathe out
Glaucoma: raised intraocular pressure
Hypertension: high blood pressure
Intracellular: the space inside the cell
Lipid-based: substances that are insoluble in water but soluble in non-polar organic solvents and are oily to touch
Metabolism: the chemical processes occurring within a living cell or organism that are necessary for the maintenance of life
Metabolites: substances produced by metabolism
Microorganisms: bacteria
Nephrotic syndrome: a clinical syndrome in which there is low plasma albumin and albuminuria
Parenterally: direct infusion into a vein
Polymer: a large molecule (macromolecule) composed of repeating structural units
Prostaglandin: chemical that enhances pain
Reye's syndrome: a rare form of encephalopathy with liver damage
Subcutaneous tissue: the third layer of the human skin
Sublingual: under the tongue
Synthesis: the combining of separate elements or substances to form a coherent whole
Therapeutics: the science and art of healing and the treatment of disease
Tinnitus: ringing in the ears
Toxicology: the science dealing with poisons
Vascularity: pertaining to blood vessels

References

BNF (2012) *British National Formulary*. BMJ Publishing, London.
British Pharmacopoeia (2008) *British Pharmacopoeia*. The Stationery Office, London.

BTS (2006) *The Burden on Lung Disease.* British Thoracic Society, London.

Crouch, S. & Chapelhow, C. (2008) *Medicine Management.* Pearson Education, Harlow.

Cummings, J. (2008) The administration of medicines. In: R. Richardson (ed.) *Clinical Skills for Student Nurses – Theory, Practice and Reflection.* Reflect Press Ltd, Devon.

DH (2001) *National Service Framework for Older People.* Department of Health, London.

Dougherty, L. & Lister, S. (eds) (2011) *The Royal Marsden Hospital Manual of Clinical Nursing Procedures,* 8th edn. Wiley-Blackwell, Chichester.

Ellson, R. (2008) Pain management. In: R. Richardson (eds) *Clinical Skills for Student Nurses – Theory, Practice and Reflection.* Reflect Press Ltd, Devon.

Fergusson, D.M., Horwood, L.J. & Beautrais, A.L. (2003) Cannabis and educational achievement. *Addiction,* 98(12), 1681–1692.

Galbraith, A., Bullock, S., Manias, E., Hunt, B. & Richards, A. (2007) *Fundamentals of Pharmacology – an Applied Approach for Nursing and Health,* 2nd ed. Pearson Education, Harlow.

Hanania, N.A. & Donohue, J.F. (2007). Pharmacologic interventions in chronic obstructive pulmonary disease: bronchodilators. *Proceedings of the American Thoracic Society,* 4, 526–534.

Legislation.gov.uk (2001) http://www.legislation.gov.uk/uksi/2001/3998/contents/made (accessed 8 March 2014).

Kaufman, G. 2010. Inhaled bronchodilators for chronic bronchitis and emphysema. *Nursing Standard,* 25(5), 61–68.

Kozier, B., Erb, G., Berman, A., Snyder, S., Lake, R. & Harvey, S. (2008) *Fundamentals of Nursing: concepts, process and practice.* Prentice Hall, Harlow.

NMC (2008a) *Standards for Medicines Management.* Nursing and Midwifery Council, London.

NMC (2008b) *Standards of Conduct, Performance and Ethics for Nurses and Midwives.* Nursing and Midwifery Council, London.

NMC (2009) *Record Keeping: guidance for nurses and midwives.* Nursing and Midwifery Council, London

Peate, I., Nair, M., Hemming, L. & Wilde, K. (2012) *Adult Nursing – Acute and Ongoing Care.* Pearson Education, Harlow.

Shihab, P. (2009) *Numeracy in Nursing and Healthcare – Calculations and Practice.* Pearson Education, Harlow.

WHO (1986) *Cancer Pain Relief.* World Health Organization, WHO, Geneva.

Test Yourself

1. Hepatic portal vein transports the absorbed substances to the:
   (a) Spleen
   (b) Liver
   (c) Pancreas
   (d) Small intestine

2. Heparin is an:
   (a) Anticoagulant
   (b) Antipyretic
   (c) Analgesic
   (d) Antiemetic

3. Patients receiving a suppository or an enema should lie:
   (a) On their right side with their knee right to the chest
   (b) On their left side with their knee right up to the chest
   (c) On their back
   (d) It does not matter in which position the person lies

4. Enemas for bowel movement are:
   (a) Hypotonic
   (b) Isotonic
   (c) Megatonic
   (d) Hypertonic

5. Methadone is a:
   (a) Class B drug
   (b) Class A drug
   (c) Class C drug
   (d) None of the above

6. Buccal is:
   (a) The space between the cheek and the gum
   (b) The space in the inner ear
   (c) Another name for the mouth
   (d) Under the tongue

7. Protamine sulphate is an antidote for:
   (a) Warfarin
   (b) Aspirin
   (c) Opioid drugs
   (d) Heparin

8. Enoxaparin is:
   (a) An antibiotic
   (b) An antiemetic
   (c) A narcotic
   (d) An anticoagulant

9. If a person is prescribed digoxin, you must always:
   (a) Take their pulse before giving the drug
   (b) Measure their blood pressure
   (c) Measure their hourly urine output
   (d) Check for any bleeding

10. A person is admitted to your ward with nephrotic syndrome. It is:
    (a) A clinical syndrome in which there is high levels of plasma albumin
    (b) A clinical syndrome in which there are low plasma albumin and albuminuria
    (c) A clinical syndrome in which the person develops high blood pressure
    (d) A clinical syndrome in which the patient develops high blood urea

Answers

1. b
2. a
3. b
4. d

5. b
6. a
7. d
8. d
9. a
10. b

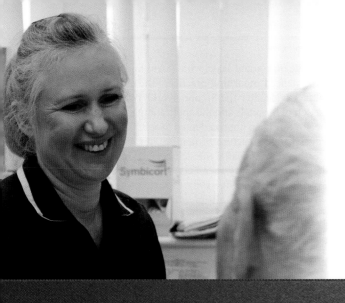

20

The Principles of Death, Dying and Bereavement

David Garbutt

University of Salford, UK

Learning Outcomes

On completion of this chapter you will be able to:

- Identify the factors influencing the modern way of dying in the UK today
- Identify the role of the nurse in supporting dying patients and their families
- Demonstrate the core skills of:
  - Communication
  - Assessment skills
  - Symptom control
  - Advance care planning
- Apply the principles of ethics to End of Life Care (EoLC) nursing practice
- Demonstrate an insight into the application of modes of care delivery in promoting effective EoLC nursing care
- Describe the main principles of loss, grief and bereavement

Competencies

All nurses must:

1. Promote the autonomy and choices of individuals as they approach death
2. Work in partnership to facilitate patient and carers needs in all healthcare settings
3. Communicate in an effective, person-centered way
4. Assess physical, psychological, social and spiritual needs of dying patients and their families
5. Plan care that is 'concerns led' and promotes quality of life for patients and families
6. Practice in a holistic manner

 Visit the companion website at **www.wileynursingpractice.com** where you can test yourself using flashcards, multiple-choice questions and more.

Nursing Practice: Knowledge and Care, First Edition. Edited by Ian Peate, Karen Wild and Muralitharan Nair.
© 2014 John Wiley & Sons, Ltd. Published 2014 by John Wiley & Sons, Ltd. Companion website: www.wileynursingpractice.com

Introduction

This chapter will explore the principles of care at the end of life for those personally facing death and their families and loved ones. It will examine the historical context of death and dying and look at the sociological development of its current place in contemporary society. It will investigate the wider philosophical and psychosocial context surrounding death, dying and bereavement as well as the principles and practice of its effective delivery. The complex area of grief, loss and bereavement and the conceptual models that underpin modern grief theory will be explored and their implications for health care today presented alongside the implications of loss and grief for professional caregivers.

Where Do Our Ideas about Death and Dying Come From?

It is suggested that our current experiences of death and dying have been shaped by the historical ideas and views of previous generations and so to understand our own modern perspective, we must first look to the past (Kellehear 2007). Our society's relationship with death has changed a lot over the past 500 years. Death in the middle ages for example, was seen as a normal part of daily life and often came swiftly and without the warning that chronic illness and medical diagnostic skills and treatment affords today. The industrial revolution saw more workers leaving rural areas, moving to the cities and living closer together, overcrowding and poor living conditions and sanitation meant deaths from diseases such as cholera, typhoid and typhus were all too common. In Victorian and Edwardian Britain, death was a familiar event to most families, usually due to infectious diseases, accidents or during childbirth. During this time, society's reactions to these types of events were closely aligned to a clear set of rules and rituals that helped people more clearly understand how to act, think and behave when faced with death (Box 20.1). The First World War and the subsequent

loss of life on a grand scale, with absent bodies and foreign graves, also influenced mourning practices. The creation of the National Health Service after the Second World War encouraged the construction of hospitals and the application a technological approach to health care at an unprecedented pace. Over time, these and other changes in the structure of families, the role of women and the increasing move towards the sick being cared for by professionals rather than by family members, saw a shift in where and how people died (Seale 1990, 1998).

Today, in part due to advances in living conditions and improved standards and access to health care, the main causes of death are long-term conditions, such as organ failure, dementia and cancer, usually occurring in later life. Dying has therefore become a longer, slower process, with death occurring predominantly in hospitals and nursing or residential homes. Today, over half of all deaths occur in hospital and it is suggested that if trends continue, fewer than 1 in 10 of us will die at home by 2030, despite many of us wishing to do so (Gomes & Higginson 2008). Dying in a hospital or nursing home has therefore become the modern way for death in the UK today (Box 20.2).

Jot This Down

- How do Thomas's and Mary's deaths differ?
- What are the main differences in:
  - The reasons they died?
  - How and where they were cared for?
  - The role of medicine and healthcare professionals?
  - The role of the family?

Death as Taboo?

The shift from death being a more natural and familiar experience to one that occurs in institutions and is facilitated by professionals such as doctors, nurses and undertakers has been said by some to have removed death from the midst of everyday life and hidden it away – to have 'professionalised' it. Consequently, as a society, it is argued that we have become unfamiliar with death and dying and

---

Box 20.1

Thomas was a 44-year-old mine worker, in 1900, who lived with his family and his mother-in-law in a small terraced house in a mining town in the Northwest of England. Over the previous year, he had experienced increasing difficulty in breathing and for the past two weeks had been bedridden. Thomas was cared for by his wife and mother-in-law and eldest daughter, who was 13 years old. Thomas's breathing steadily got worse and after a short period of being very unwell (he could not afford a doctor to visit), his parish priest visited him and gave him the Sacrament of the Sick. Thomas died with his family around him. His body was prepared by 'the woman at the end of the street' (who was also usually attendant at the birth of the children of the local area) and he was duly dressed and placed in a simple coffin. His body remained at home, with the local community, including children, visiting to pay their respects and receive hospitality from Thomas's family in the form of a piece of 'death cake'. All the curtains in the houses of the street were drawn to show respect. The following day, he was buried at the local cemetery and his funeral was paid for by a 'penny policy' – a form of insurance often paid by people to cover the expenses of a funeral and to avoid a pauper's burial.

Box 20.2

Mary was an 88-year-old woman who was admitted to hospital in 2013, following a fall in the care home where she had lived for the past 2 years. Mary had suffered from ill health for many years; however she had been living alone independently since her husband died 8 years ago. Mary moved into the care home, as she was becoming increasingly forgetful and needed more help. She has one daughter, Alison, who lives a 3-hour car journey away. Mary has two grandchildren who she sees at Christmas and on birthdays. Mary was recently been diagnosed with dementia and has had a series of strokes, the last one of which made it difficult for her to speak. When Mary's carers went to wake her this morning, she was unresponsive. After discussion with her GP over the phone, the carer rang an ambulance and Mary was admitted to the local hospital. Mary was put on intravenous fluids, had a CT brain scan and a nasogastric tube inserted. Mary died that evening, without waking up, before her family could get to the hospital.

struggle to talk about it or discuss our views, feelings and preferences for how and where we might choose to die. Increasing secularism in society, it could be suggested, has also impacted on our traditional ways of understanding death and dying. Some people suggests that death has become a 'taboo' subject that we feel uncomfortable discussing openly (Gorer 1955; Ariès 1974). Others, however, have challenged the notion that death is a taboo subject in modern Western culture and propose that its discussion is experiencing a revival as individuals seek to take more control over the circumstances of their life and subsequently their death (Kellehear 2009; Walters 1994).

Jot This Down

- Do you think death and dying is still a taboo subject in our society, as people like Ariès and Gorer state?
- Is death and dying something you readily talk about with your family and friends?
- Why do you think people find it so hard to discuss things like this?
- How might your personal thoughts and feelings about death influence how you care for dying patients and their families?

What Is Death?

When are we dead? On the face of it, this appears to be a simple question with a straightforward answer. Most people would probably agree that a person is dead when the brain no longer functions or when the heart stops beating; however in many traditional societies death is not viewed as a single event but rather as a process. This might suggest that that although we may have a clear clinical definition of death, the process of dying may involve a series of social and psychological stages that a dying person may move through before being viewed as socially dead (Barley 1995; Helman 1994).

What the Experts Say

Simon was only 24 when he had his accident. I never liked him riding that thing but couldn't stop him, he loved it so much. When I got the call I was at work and rushed to the hospital. Simon was in intensive care and wired up to all kinds of machines and had a tube down his throat that the doctor said was breathing for him. I sat there day and night for the best part of a week, talking and reading to him. He just looked asleep, he looked so healthy with pink cheeks and everything. When they said that his brain had been so badly damaged that he was never going to wake up, I couldn't believe it. They said that they had done 'tests' that showed his brain was never going to recover and that really it was just the machine that was breathing for him that was keeping his body going. They said they thought it best for him to turn his machine off, I was stunned he looked so well – he still had a tan from his holidays.

Later, a woman came to talk to us about donating his organs to help other people.

(Joyce, Simon's mother)

What the Experts Say

When Frank was first diagnosed with dementia, it was the simple everyday things that he couldn't remember but he always could recall things that happened years ago. As he got more unwell he started to forget the names of people he had known for years. Eventually, he couldn't remember who people were at all. When he forgot who I was, it was devastating. I'd sit at his bedside in the care home and it was as though he didn't know me, as though we had never met, we were strangers. It made me not want to go to see him; at times I had to force myself as it was so hard. Most of his friends had already stopped going by this time too. It was almost as though he wasn't my Frank, as though he had gone and someone else was there in his place. When he died I was sad of course but I'd got used to the idea of 'my Frank' not being here a long time ago.

(Mary, Frank's wife)

Jot This Down

- How do Joyce and Mary's accounts make you feel about how we view death?
- How might the different definitions of death help us (or not) to think about how carers and patients themselves may view death and dying?
- What implications might this have for how you think about dying, death, loss grief in the future?

Biological Death

The ability to prolong biological life with modern technology has raised questions about where the boundaries between life and death are drawn, thus changing the technical definition of death (Veatch 1976). As advances in resuscitation and artificial ventilation have developed over the past few decades, so the shift in the nature of clinical death from cardiac death (i.e. the heart stops beating) to brainstem death (when the brain becomes unable to autonomously control the physical processes required for life, i.e. respiration). Modern medical understanding of what constitutes death usually focusses on when the brainstem has been irreversibly damaged. Consciousness and the ability to breathe autonomously are permanently lost but the heart is still beating and the body is kept alive by a ventilator (AOMRC 2008).

The Death of Personhood

However, dying is not just a biological act. As we have seen, it is also a personal and a social one. When does a person cease to be a person? In a philosophical sense, a person is someone who has a physical body, is conscious, has relationships with others, has a sense of themselves as an individual, can think about their place in the world and can make plans and act on those plans (Taylor 1985). Given these criteria, it is interesting to perhaps think about how the process of dying can impact on the ability to be a person in the fullest sense.

Social Death

The term 'social death' has come to represent the manner in which those facing death can be seen by others as having a diminished social existence (Glaser & Strauss 1965; Sudnow 1967) It is suggested by these commentators that social death precedes biological death, as the individual is gradually removed both metaphorically and literally from everyday life, taking less and less of an active social role and increasingly likely to be cared for by professionals in an institutional setting. Yet Mulkay (1993) argues that often, biological death can come before social death, with the deceased maintaining a prominent role in the life of others, influencing how the living act and behave, thus maintaining a social presence.

It is important to understand that the reality of death cannot be understood purely as a physical event – it has deep social and psychological meaning for both the individual and society. Death and dying are both socially negotiated phenomena and a personal, individual journey. As professional caregivers, we must appreciate and understand this if we are to move away from a biomedically defined notion of death as a biological event to a person-centered, individualised one, which encompasses a more humanistic, holistic view.

A Good Death?

Death is one of the attributes you were created with; death is part of you. Your life's continual task is to build your death.

(Montaigne 1993)

> ### Jot This Down
> - What would be your idea of a good death?
> - What could you do to ensure you achieved your 'good death'?
> - What have been your experiences of a good death?
> - Have you witnessed what you felt to be a 'bad death'?

The concept of a 'good death' may seem strange to many but how and where people die is often very important to individuals and their families. Within today's modern society, the idea of what constitutes a good death might vary according to the particular cultural group one is aligned to and the view of death that comes from either a religious or more non-religious view (O'Gorman 1998) Traditionally, religion gave a structure to the preparation for death but within an increasingly secular society a new more individual response to the understanding of the meaning of death appears to be emerging.

In individualistic societies such as ours in the 'modern West', a 'bad death' is perhaps seen as that of the person with no autonomy, for instance the patient with dementia who cannot communicate his or her wishes. Our society's concept of a 'good death' is perhaps therefore one characterised by choice and control – a death that occurs where one would choose it, in one's own home with loved ones around and one that was free of pain, anguish and fear – a death that was anticipated but not one that came after a protracted time of disability and increasing weakness, confusion or dependence.

> ### The Evidence
> A **good death** is . . .
> - To know when death is coming, and to understand what can be expected
> - To be able to retain control of what happens
> - To be afforded dignity and privacy
> - To have control over pain relief and other symptoms
> - To have choice and control over where death occurs (at home or elsewhere)
> - To have access to information and expertise of whatever kind is necessary
> - To have access to any spiritual or emotional support required
> - To have access to specialist palliative care in any location
> - To have control over who is present and who shares the end
> - To be able to issue advance directives, which ensure wishes are respected
> - To have time to say goodbye, and control over other aspects of timing
> - To be able to leave when it is time to go, and not to have life prolonged pointlessly.
>
> (Age Concern 1999)

There is much discussion about the nature of death and dying and its social regulation. Some commentators advocate that each individual should be free to define the nature of their own death and call for the introduction of assisted suicide for those unable to take their own life. This view is often presented as a natural extension of choice and control that is increasingly valued in our society, while others advocate that to sanction intentional ending of life would threaten the inherent value of life itself and could lead to vulnerable members of society to be pressurised into ending their lives prematurely, perhaps seeing themselves as a burden on their family and society as a whole. Further arguments abound that the nature and development of palliative and end of life care would be severely affected by the legalisation of physician assisted suicide and that the legal and ethical challenges for health carers would present an unacceptable burden on the professional and philosophical values of medicine and health care itself.

Care at the End of Life

Approaches to Delivery of End of Life and Palliative Care
What is end of life care?

'End of Life Care' is care that helps all those with advanced, progressive incurable illness to live as well as possible until they die. It enables the supportive and palliative care needs of both patient and family to be identified and met throughout the last phase of life and into bereavement. It includes management of pain and other symptoms and provision of psychological, social, spiritual and practical support.

(NCPC 2006; *End of Life Care Strategy*, DH 2008)

End of life care is commonly referred to as care that is required during the last 6–12 months of life, regardless of the individuals diagnosis (GMC 2010). Traditionally, care of the dying has been more clearly aligned to those with a cancer diagnosis, however it is becoming increasingly recognised that other diseases, such as organ failure, cardiovascular disease and dementia, dominate the

Link To/Go To

Department of Health, *End of Life Care Strategy*:

https://www.gov.uk/government/uploads/system/uploads/attachment_data/file/136431/End_of_life_strategy.pdf

Department of Health, *End of Life Care Strategy*: fourth annual report:

https://www.gov.uk/government/publications/end-of-life-care-strategy-fourth-annual-report

'Dying Matters', Raising awareness of dying, death and bereavement:

http://dyingmatters.org/

NICE, Quality Standards, QS13: End of life care for adults:

http://guidance.nice.org.uk/QS13

Advance Care Planning

Advance care planning is a voluntary process of discussion about future care between an individual and their care providers, irrespective of discipline. It is the process of identifying how an individual wishes to be cared for, before they lose capacity and can inform such things as where a person may wish to die, what their view regarding certain treatments or interventions may be, who they want to be present and perhaps what may be important to them to maintain their dignity.

Jot This Down

· How would you feel about exploring advance care planning with a patient you were caring for?

· What skills or approaches would you use to help the discussion take place?

· When would be the best time to have these discussions?

Red Flag

 It is important to remember that not all patients may wish to enter into such discussions and many may well prefer not to talk about such things and should not be pressed to do so; however for some it will be very important and a way of maintaining autonomy and control over their care.

What the Experts Say

 Simon was 18 when he told me that he had had enough and didn't want to go back into hospital. He'd had cystic fibrosis all his life and there was little hope of a transplant now. He had been getting weaker and losing weight for while now and he kept getting these chest infections, which meant another stay in hospital, where he was completely miserable. He struggled with not being able to be with his family and friends, his dog and he missed not being able to use his phone. Each time he came out, he seemed that bit worse, he was breathless most of the time now. We sat down and wrote out what he wanted if he became too ill to say it for himself and discussed it with his nurses and our GP. Simon wrote down what he wanted in his care plan and when the time came, everything was in place and he died in his own bed, with his family and his dog, with his phone in his hand. Just the way he wanted.

(Frances, Simon's mum)

An advance care plan (ACP) can take many forms – it could be a verbal discussion or documenting wishes in a person's healthcare records; however the more clearly and explicitly documented and the more members of the care-giving team across the different organisations involved are aware of the ACP, the more likely it is that an individual's wishes will be realised. If the individual wishes, family and friends can be involved but it may be important to point out that if the person's wishes for end of life care involve or are in some way dependent on other members of the family, opening up discussion around this is very important. For example if a person wished to die at home but this made other members of the family anxious about their abilities to cope with caring for them, it is important to identify this early and discuss this difficulty and any possible solutions to it. The value of ACP is that it opens up a dialogue between the patient, their family and the professionals involved in their care, without this, preferences are unknown and families and professionals are left to try to guess what a person may have wanted. As a person's illness progresses, so may their views on the type of care they may want or need, this is why it is important to regularly review advance care plans to ensure that they remain in line with what the person is thinking and feeling at the time.

Advance care planning promotes patient-centred care, as it tailors their wishes and preferences to their care. It also opens up the possibility of discussion around prognosis – 'how long have I got' and also possibly, what the immediate and longer-term future may hold 'What is going to happen to me?' and also help them plan and predict what they feel they may need; 'What support will I need, who will be able to look after me and my family?' It can help the professional to anticipate what resources may be needed and promotes a dialogue between patients, family and carers, addressing any fears or concerns early in the process. By asking people what they want, we can continue to put their wishes at the heart of the plan of care and ensure that they remain in control, even when they become too ill to tell us what they want. By dealing with these issues, an ACP can provide people with hope that at least their views and wishes are recognised as important and will be respected.

Best Interest Decision-Making

When a person loses capacity and their wishes are not clearly known, there is an expectation that health professionals, guided by the views of the family, should make a decision that is in the individual's best interests. The Mental Capacity Act clearly states that any previously stated views and preferences must be taken into account when making such a decision but ultimately, following a discussion with all the key people involved, including a relative (or appointed representative if there is no family), it would fall to an individual who is in the best position to understand the implication of various courses of action and can see the overall picture.

417

What the Experts Say

> John had lived at Ford house for about 5 years. He was 50 and had lifelong severe learning disabilities. He loved being in the house with the other tenants. But I had seen John getting worse, as his breathing worsened due to his heart condition. He was struggling to manage diet and fluids as he kept coughing and the nurses were worried that they were going into his lungs and that this was why he kept getting chest infections. When he was admitted to hospital. I went with him and after a couple of days the doctors called a meeting. Myself and John's mum and dad were there and the doctors wanted to know how we felt about John's worsening condition and what John would most likely want to happen if he could tell us. The doctors felt that if John's heart were to stop beating then it would not be appropriate to try to resuscitate him. Both John's parents and myself felt that given how poorly John was he would want to kept comfortable and not be kept alive by tubes and machines if he wasn't going to get back to how he was. So we all agreed this was for the best and John died peacefully a few days later.

(Barbara, Learning Disability Domiciliary Care Manager)

In the example above a capacity assessment had been made and found that John lacked capacity due to his learning disability and physical condition. He was unable to understand, retain and weigh information material to the decisions and any alternatives. John was also unable to communicate a decision, therefore a 'Best Interests' decision meeting was held with the key people involved: the healthcare team looking after him, his parents and his care manager. The meeting looked at John's condition, his prognosis and options for care. The outcome was that given John's deteriorating condition and poor prognosis and the views of his family regarding what he would wish if he were able to choose himself, he should be kept comfortable and to attempt cardiopulmonary resuscitation would be futile and not in his best interests.

Lasting Power of Attorney

If an individual wants to ensure that their wishes are unequivocally stated and that someone they identify is able to make decisions on their behalf, then they can choose to appoint another person as their 'Lasting Power of Attorney' (LPA). Previously, this role has been concerned with financial affairs and arrangements, however since 2007 an individual can be appointed as an LPA (through officially being recorded as such with the Office of the Public Guardian) and has the power to make proxy decisions concerning a person's care and medical treatment. It is important to identify if an LPA has been appointed and if so, that this decision was made in accordance with the LPA process superseding any other previously recorded wishes or views, for example in an ACP or an advance decision to refuse treatment (ADRT).

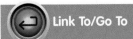

Link To/Go To

Lasting Power of Attorney for Health and Welfare:
https://www.gov.uk/power-of-attorney

Advance Care Planning Guidance: **http://www.gmc-uk.org/ guidance/ethical_guidance/end_of_life_advance_care _planning.asp**

http://www.nhs.uk/Planners/end-of-life-care/Documents/ Planning-for-your-future-care.pdf

The Preferred Priorities for Care

The Preferred Priorities for Care (PPC) document is one way of identifying and recording a patient's wishes. It comprises a patient-held record, which records the patient's wishes, the socioeconomic circumstances of the family, the services being accessed, reasons for changes in their care and a needs assessment that documents care on an ongoing basis. It has been used in the home and is now being trialled in care homes with older people.

Advance Decisions to Refuse Treatment

An Advance Decision to Refuse Treatment (ADRT) replaces previously used terms such as 'Living Wills' and 'Advance Directives'. It is a clearly documented statement of wishes and preferences regarding the withholding and withdrawing of treatment. It comes into effect in the event of an individual's losing his or her capacity to make such decisions; until this time, the normal process of consent applies. An ADRT forms part of an Advanced Care Plan in that it identifies individual wishes and preferences regarding treatment and can be used to open discussions with health and social care professionals about how best to plan for the future.

What the Experts Say

> When Tony was brought in, the first thing his wife told us was that he had an ADRT. He had been admitted a couple of times previously with his worsening symptoms due to his heart failure and been treated with diuretics and other medication. Tony was too ill to discuss this himself but we sat down with his wife and she told us about his wishes and what he had written in his ADRT. She showed us the document and it clearly stated that if Tony suffered a cardiac arrest due to his heart failure, he did not want anyone to attempt cardiopulmonary resuscitation. The form had been printed from the ADRT website, it was signed by Tony, dated last week and witnessed by his friend. It also clearly stated that he wanted to refuse resuscitation even if it meant that he would die if we didn't attempt it. We discussed it as a team and we were happy to respect it. Tony died peacefully a couple of days later.

(John, Cardiac Consultant)

What Tony's story tells us is that as healthcare professionals, we must be sure that what is written in an ADRT meets a number of essential criteria that reinforces its validity.

- **Has the person lost capacity?**
  - All efforts must be made to maximise a person's ability to make an informed decision but in the event that capacity has clearly been lost, then the ADRT comes into force
- **Is the decision valid?**
  - Is the situation in-keeping with what the person was anticipating; have they changed their mind or done or said anything that might be inconsistent with the ADRT? Have they appointed a Lasting Power of Attorney since the ADRT was written?
- **Is the advanced decision applicable?**
  - Does the ADRT specify which treatment the person wishes to refuse and is the treatment in question specified in the ADRT?
- **Does the decision refer to life-sustaining treatment?**
  - Does the ADRT clearly refer to a decision by the patient to refuse life-sustaining treatment? Is it signed by the person and also by a witness?

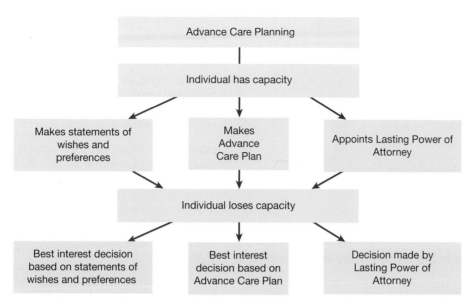

Figure 20.3 The relationship between Advance Care Planning, Best Interest decision-making, ADRT and Lasting Power of Attorney.

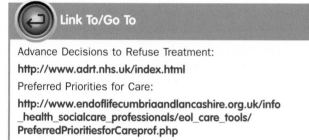

Link To/Go To

Advance Decisions to Refuse Treatment:

http://www.adrt.nhs.uk/index.html

Preferred Priorities for Care:

http://www.endoflifecumbriaandlancashire.org.uk/info
_health_socialcare_professionals/eol_care_tools/
PreferredPrioritiesforCareprof.php

Mental Capacity

The Mental Capacity Act came into force in 2005 and became fully effective in 2007. It aims to empower and protect people who lack capacity and to ensure that the decision-making process remains focussed on their best interests and that their wishes and preferences remain at the centre of the decision-making process. It allows people to plan ahead in the eventuality that they may lose capacity in the future and clarifies who should be involved in decision-making and what the process should entail.

The MCA is underpinned by five key principles:

1. A person must be assumed to have capacity unless it is established that he lacks capacity
2. A person is not to be treated as unable to make a decision unless all practicable steps to help him to do so have been taken without success
3. A person is not to be treated as unable to make a decision merely because he makes an unwise decision
4. An act done, or decision made, under this Act for or on behalf of a person who lacks capacity must be done, or made, in his best interests
5. Before the act is done, or the decision is made, regard must be had to whether the purpose for which it is needed can be as effectively achieved in a way that is less restrictive of the person's rights and freedom of action.

The application of the Mental Capacity Act to end of life care is clearly apparent, as the progressive nature of terminal process will undoubtedly lead to a person losing capacity to make decisions at some point.

Figure 20.3 highlights the relationship between advance care planning, best interest decision-making, ADRT and lasting power of attorney.

Care in the Last Few Days of Life

Diagnosing Dying: Signs and Symptoms of Approaching Death

Understanding the clinical indications of the dying process is an important skill if nurses are to support patients' family members effectively. Communicating honestly and appropriately at this time is important if families are to have important conversations or act on a patient's preference about how and where they die. Predicting when a patient might die is difficult (Christakis 2001). Some patients survive for a long period, despite a poor initial prognosis, while others may deteriorate rapidly and unexpectedly. Families often seek some indication from professionals about 'how long?' It is prudent to avoid guessing or to be pressured to be too exact. Often if pushed, it is best to support the family with the uncertainty of the situation and talk in terms of 'days', 'weeks' or 'months', accordingly, perhaps focussing on the immediate present and what might be done to improve the patient's comforts and dignity. However, there are common signs and symptoms that often present that signify that a patient is approaching the terminal stages of their illness and that death is imminent.

Signs and symptoms of approaching death

- *Profound tiredness and weakness*
  - *Reduced interest in getting out of bed*
  - *Needing assistance with all care*
  - *Less interest in things happening around them*
- *Diminished intake of food and fluids*
- *Drowsy or reduced cognition*
  - *May be disorientated in time or place*
  - *Difficulty concentrating*
  - *Scarcely able to cooperate and converse with carers*
- *Gaunt appearance*
- *Difficulty swallowing medicine.*

(*Changing Gear*, NCPC 2010)

419

Other signs of impending death may include
- Decreasing blood perfusion
- Neurologic dysfunction
- Decreasing level of consciousness
- Decreased ability to move
- Joint position fatigue
- Increased need for care
- Tachycardia, hypotension
- Peripheral cooling, cyanosis of extremities
- Mottling of skin
- Loss of ability to swallow, sphincter control
- Diminished urine output
- Terminal delirium
- Changes in respiration
- Weak/no radial pulse.

Common symptoms in the last 48 hours of life
- Pain
- Restlessness/agitation
- Upper airway secretions
- Dyspnoea
- Nausea and vomiting.

Pain It is important to ensure that these common symptoms are anticipated and addressed proactively. As the patient may well be unable to swallow, any analgesia they may have been taking previously will need to be converted to a non-oral preparation and route and administered parenterally; this is usually done through a syringe driver via an indwelling subcutaneous 'butterfly' needle in order to maintain a steady dose of analgesia over a 24-hour period. When a person is unable to verbally communicate their pain due to their condition, it is important that staff look for non-verbal signs, such as facial expressions (grimacing), groaning or moans. The patient's relatives may communicate that they feel the patient is in pain, they know the person better than ourselves and we must address their concerns and administer analgesia appropriately, however we must also be aware that terminal agitation and restlessness may also be present and not to confuse the two symptoms, as they require different approaches to their management.

Restlessness/agitation Restlessness and agitation are recognised symptoms of the terminal phase and will require management through the use of sedative and anxiolytic medication. However, all possible reversible reasons for this must be excluded or addressed before such a diagnosis can be made.

Common reversible causes of terminal agitation

- *Pain*
- *Urinary retention*
- *Full rectum*
- *Nausea*
- *Cerebral irritation*
- *Anxiety and fear*
- *Side effects of medication*
- *Poor positioning.*
  (*Oxford Handbook of Palliative Medicine*, Watson et al. 2009)

Upper airway secretions Profound weakness at the end of life can lead to the accumulation of upper airway secretions that the patient is too weak to expectorate and results in moist, noisy breathing. This is often referred to as the 'death rattle' and occurs in 50% of patients. The noise made can be distressing for those

witnessing it from the bedside and often family members will feel the patient is choking or can't breathe, though if deeply unconscious, the patient may be unaware. It is best to try to avoid this symptom occurring in the first place if possible, as once established, secretions are more difficult to remove than to prevent. Repositioning can help but if treatment is required antimuscarinic drugs, such as Hyoscine hydrobromide or Glycopyrronium can be given subcutaneously to prevent further secretions.

Dyspnoea Breathlessness in the terminal stages can be addressed through the use of oxygen if the person is hypoxic but largely, its effectiveness in reducing symptoms of breathlessness at this stage is considered to be little better than room air (Abernethy *et al.* 2010). Also the use of oxygen can make mouth care more difficult, as it can further dry out the oral mucosa and can act as barrier between the patient and their loved ones.

Often, simple measures, such as the use of a fan to move air across the patient's face and reducing anxiety by promoting a calm and comforting atmosphere, can work to reduce the patient's perception of breathlessness. Pharmacological measures include the use of opioid and anxiolytic drugs to help reduce the sensation of breathlessness and minimise anxiety.

Nausea and vomiting There are many causes of nausea and vomiting in advanced disease, such as gastric stasis/obstruction, drug induced and metabolic, i.e. hypercalcaemia/renal failure; however in the final stages of life it is sometimes not possible or appropriate to identify a specific cause and broad spectrum antiemetics to cover the main possible causes may be the most prudent approach. Drugs such as cyclizine and levomepromazine are commonly administered continually via syringe driver and as required via subcutaneous injection.

Promoting comfort is the main aim of any management at the end of life and a holistic approach must be taken that acknowledges the interrelationship between the emotional, psychological, spiritual and the physical. A person may be frightened, which will cause their pain to be worse; they may feel spiritually distressed, which presents as anxiety and agitation. We may have a greater degree of knowledge and expertise in the clinical management of symptoms at the end of life but they must be used alongside a compassionate and empathic approach – we should never underestimate the power of a reassuring touch or calming voice.

Psychosocial Care
Psychosocial care is a core component of good palliative care. It promotes the importance of viewing each individual holistically and acknowledges the impact of a person's illness on their psychological, emotional, social and spiritual well-being. It includes the giving of bad news, respecting and developing coping strategies and acknowledging fears and maintaining hope. It plays an important role in determining how patients and families respond to the impact of the illness and aids in coping with the experiences of loss and change, as well as in expanding the sense of what is possible.

Holistic Assessment
Effective psychosocial care is dependent on an approach to assessment that identifies these issues and acknowledges them equally alongside the medical, symptom and treatment related aspects of care. According to The National End of Life Care Programme (NEoLCP) (now part of NHS Improving Quality, NHSIQ), holistic assessment is vital in order to identify where a person's needs are currently not being addressed and indicates where other health and

social care professionals could be involved to address this. Individual preferences and wishes can also be highlighted, enabling them to be more in control of what's happening and promote dignity and choice. The Holistic Common Assessment tool provides guidance for holistic assessment of the supportive and palliative care needs of adults. All people who have been recognised as approaching the end of their life should be offered this type of assessment.

Thinking back to the end of life care pathway in Figure 20.1, there are particular milestones within a persons end of life care journey that may indicate when an assessment may be appropriate. A structured approach to holistic assessment is valuable at key points in a person's care pathway, such as at diagnosis when the person is identified as approaching the end of life or when the individual is thought to be entering into the dying phase (actively dying) or at any other time that a patient, family member or a professional carer may deem necessary. A holistic assessment can be carried out by any professional who knows the person, their condition and its management and has the appropriate skills.

Domain 1: Background information and assessment preferences

Demographic and contact details, history of illness, treatment plan, professional involved, next of kin. Consent to assessment, previous assessments undertaken, preferences for setting of assessment and family involvement

Domain 2: Physical well-being

Impact of illness on physical well-being, symptoms such as pain, nausea and breathlessness, affect on sleep, energy levels, nutrition, weight loss

Domain 3: Social and occupational well-being

Type of accommodation, who they live with, level of dependency and sources of help with shopping meal preparation, etc. Work and financial issues, family and close relationships, needs related to children (talking to them about death)

Domain 4: Psychological well-being

Mood, anxiety, adjustment to worsening illness or treatment, knowledge, understanding of disease/treatment sources of emotional support, unresolved concerns, coping strategies and strengths, perception of the future

Domain 5: Spiritual well-being and life goals

Identification of views on faith or belief, impact of illness on faith/belief, practical support or other needs related to religion or spiritual matters (contact with faith leader, opportunity/space to pray); discussion of important life goals, or exploring what endows life with meaning and purpose.

(NEoLCP 2010)

Psychosocial Assessment at the End of Life Points to Remember

- Assessment should be patient concerns-led
- It should be carried out **with** patients and families not **on** them
- It should be done in a conversational style, rather than viewed as a series of boxes that must be ticked
- Helping patients to assess their own needs should be central to the process
- Patient consent is necessary to the assessment process
- Professionals undertaking assessment should have reached an agreed level of competency in key aspects of assessment
- Patient preference for communicating with particular professional, their family and friends should be taken into account.

Link To/Go To

Holistic common assessment of palliative care needs for adults requiring end of life care:

http://www.endoflifecumbriaandlancashire.org.uk/CubeCore/.uploads/New%20Website%20Info/2.%20Info%20for%20H&SCPS/End%20of%20life%20care%20tools/HCA_guide.pdf

Communication

Communication underpins virtually all nurse–patient interactions and is the bedrock of any therapeutic relationship. It perhaps comes into even sharper focus when dealing with the challenges of such an emotionally charged situation as caring for a dying patient and their family. Effective care at the end of life depends heavily on the ability of the individual practitioner to develop a trusting relationship with both patients and those close to them. Patient and family-centered communication that is honest and sensitive is therefore essential.

What the Experts Say

I had a handover and found out that in the bay where I was working was Vinnie, a 45-year-old man who was diagnosed with a malignant brain tumour 18 months ago. He had been admitted to our medical ward, as he had deteriorated rapidly overnight and is now thought to be dying. His wife Michaela is with him and I really didn't know to say, so I just asked her if she was comfortable or needed anything. She said she was fine but just as I was about to leave, she asked me if I thought Vinnie was looking better?

(Anna, 2nd year student nurse)

Jot This Down

- Have you ever not known what to say? How did this feel?
- How might you have answered Michaela's question?
- What do you think are the skills required to communicate effectively with Michaela?

Core Conditions

Effective communication is based on what are known as the core conditions. These are the foundations of a therapeutic encounter and it is suggested that without these, it is difficult to have a full and open relationship and may lead to a closing off and a creation of barriers between people.

Congruence Genuineness, honesty with the patient or family member

Empathy The ability to understand and appreciate what the other person is feeling and to convey this understanding in a relationship

Respect Acceptance, unconditional positive regard towards the other person.

Communication Microskills

While it is essential to have the core conditions in place, there are a number of practical skills and approaches to both verbal and non-communication that can positively enhance communication with patients and family members.

Picking up on cues

A cue is often a verbal or non-verbal hint that there is something more to be explored. It could take the form of a direct question, a comment or body language or facial expression. Picking up on cues is important, the patient or family member will be reluctant to offer further cues if their initial ones are not picked up. Linking an open question to a cue is much more likely to promote further disclosure than when not linked to a cue, as it is not focussing on the main concern of the patient or relative.

> **Michaela:** *Do you think he's looking better?*
> **Anna:**　　 *What do you mean by better?*

Here the cue is the word 'better'. It suggests to Anna that Michaela is unsure about the situation and that to explore more about what she understands would be the best way to go.

As Anna and Michaela's conversation continues, Anna uses more microskills to respond to Michaela and facilitate the discussion, to show Michaela that she is interested and listening and that her concerns are important to her.

Reflective responding

Reflecting back the words used by a patient or relative can suggest that you have been listening carefully. It can be presented in the form of a question seeking more clarity or merely as an acknowledgement and indication of your attention and engagement. It allows the other person to hear their own words and that you are focussed on what they are saying.

> **Michaela:** *His colour seems better, so I'm kind of hoping he's coming round*
> **Anna:**　　 *Coming round?*

Here, Anna may begin to understand what Michaela's perception of the situation is. Is she unaware and lacking information or is she struggling to accept the emerging reality that Vinnie is now thought to be entering into the last few hours or days of life.

Educated guesses

An educated guess is an attempt to clarify that your view of the situation is correct by picking up on cues and other information. If, given her responses, Anna thinks Michaela is unclear about what is happening about Vinnie and his condition, she may present this as a question.

> **Anna:**　　 *I'm getting the feeling Michaela that you're a bit unsure as to what's going on regarding Vinnie's condition, is that right?*
> **Michaela:** *Well when we arrived last night he seemed really poorly, fitting and everything and it all happened really fast and now he seems much better than when we arrived.*

An educated guess is different from making an assumption, as it is based on indicators from the person themselves, such as verbal and non-verbal cues, and demonstrates a wish to understand and be clear about the person's concerns. Our educated guesses may not always be correct but the important thing is to communicate our willingness to try to understand and can open up further discussion. If we do 'guess' wrongly, then the individual will hopefully correct us and thus lead to further discussion.

Paraphrasing/summarising

Paraphrasing is similar to reflective responding but instead of using the other person's words you reflect back what they have said using your own. This demonstrates that you have heard what has been said and that you have thought about it and communicated that understanding.

> **Anna:**　　 *So you've had a long night, things seem to be happening really fast, but you think that Vinnie is looking better, have I got that right?*
> **Michaela:** *Yeah I'm really tired and I didn't take in a lot of what the Doctor said last night, I can remember he said something about 'symptom control' and 'comfort measures' but I don't know what that meant.*

Summarising is an important skill to help both the health and social care professional to take stock of where a conversation is going, what has been discussed and how to proceed. It also demonstrates that you have been listening carefully and by summarising the points discussed so far and checking that you have understood them correctly, you are both clear about what is the issue or difficulty.

> **Anna:**　　 *I can see your tired, and it must be hard to take in everything that's happening, but it seems to me that you're not sure what is happening regarding Vinnie's care at the moment.*

Giving information

Open, honest discussion with family and, whenever possible, patients about the aims of care is vitally important and should occur as soon as is practically possible. However, at this point it has been established that Michaela is not clear about what the aims of care for Vinnie are. Previous conversations have unfortunately not clarified her understanding of the situation and have left her unsure and with further questions. It is therefore left to the team currently caring for Vinnie and Michaela to explore this further.

When we have established a person's concerns and identified their information needs, we must provide that information in a way that is tailored to the individual: not too much and not too little, not too fast and not too slow. It is easy to view communication as purely a one-way process when we give information to another; however checking that other people truly understand what has been said, and that they are comfortable with receiving more before going on is vital – this is known as the 'Chunk and Check' approach.

In the scenario, this may be the opportunity to discuss the fact that Vinnie is in fact dying and that the aims of care are now to focus on his comfort and supporting Michaela and the rest of the family.

Empathic response

An empathic response is one which demonstrates that you have some insight into the feelings being experienced by another. Having broken the news to Michaela that Vinnie is dying, it is important that we acknowledge and attend to her feelings and emotions.

> **Michaela:** *I just don't know what to think. It's all too much to take in.*
> **Anna:**　　 *This must be a very confusing time for you, it must seem overwhelming. (Anna lightly touches Michaela's shoulder)*

By acknowledging how someone is feeling and communicating this to them, you are demonstrating empathy, one of the core conditions. Touch, be it holding a hand or a hand on a shoulder, if done within the construct of the core conditions, can be a powerful conveyor of empathy, concern and compassion.

Identifying main concerns

Patients and families often appreciate someone who can help them make sense of difficult situations and help them identify some kind of order to what are often confusing and unclear thoughts and feelings.

> **Anna:** *What's the most difficult part of all of this Michaela?*
>
> **Michaela:** *I'm not ready for this (Michaela becomes upset). I wasn't expecting this when we came in! How am I going to tell the children? Do I need to make some calls?*
>
> **Anna:** *I'm sorry this has been such a difficult conversation and it wasn't the news you were hoping for (pause). I can see you're very upset (pause). If you like we could talk about where we can go from here.*

By asking her to identify her main concerns Anna has helped Michaela to prioritise the most important thing for her to address. She has demonstrated empathy by identifying that she can see Michaela is upset. The use of pauses and silences give both parties time and space to think about what has been said, communicates that we are listening rather than wanting to speak and allows room for further disclosure.

From the beginning of the conversation, Anna has used many skills and approaches that have allowed Michaela to explore the unfolding situation at her own pace whilst also being supported. By asking an open question linked to the cue that Michaela is finding the situation difficult to deal with and by using verbal and non-verbal skills such as open questions, picking up on cues, empathic responses, pauses and silences Anna has remained a supportive presence while ensuring that the control within the conversation always rested with Michaela and focussed on her priorities and concerns. Anna may go on to help Michaela to plan a way forward or liaise with a more experienced senior member of staff about a strategy to help Michaela discuss the situation with her children and other family members.

Handling difficult emotions

Often when dealing with such emotionally challenging situations, we can be concerned about whether we have the right skills or abilities to support people. We may be anxious that we could be asked difficult questions that we are unable to answer. We might be fearful of making things worse or unleashing an emotional reaction that we are unable to deal with. We may worry that a patient or relative may in some way blame us for the things that have gone wrong for them. We may have concerns about whether we are able to manage our own emotional reaction and that we may become upset as the situation reminds us of our own mortality or experiences of loss.

Communication Barriers
Blocking behaviours

Often, because of the difficulties described above, we can find it hard to engage with patients and families who are dealing with difficult emotions. This often results in unintentional (or intentional) blocking of communication. This is where certain strategies are employed that disrupt the communication and can send messages to the patient or family that we are unwilling or reluctant to enter into a discussion about certain topics.

Attempts to lessen or reduce the seriousness of concerns

We can at times send messages to people that their concerns are something that we may not consider as all that serious or difficult, for instance by using such phrases as *'Don't worry everyone feels*

that way at first'. This may be done in order to attempt to reassure or make someone feel better when actually it can have the opposite effect, making the other person feel as though their concerns don't matter or that they should not be feeing what they are feeling. This obviously can discourage people from wanting to discuss this further with us or disclose any more concerns they may have.

Providing reassurance and advice too early We can often feel the need to solve problems and deal with patient's difficulties before we have fully elicited what those concerns may be. By offering advice and reassurance too early in a conversation, we are in danger of not fully exploring the issues or helping the other person identify their own views and possible solutions. This can block communication before any real discussions of what may be troubling someone before they even start.

Handing challenging encounters over to more senior staff

As discussed earlier, our anxieties about our perceived lack of skills and knowledge can lead us to avoid opening up difficult conversations and instead seek to avoid or remove ourselves from the situation; this is an understandable reaction, particularly for a student who is unsure of their level of responsibility and abilities in such a situation. One way that this can often be done, is to refer the person to someone else.

Changing the subject It can often be difficult to truly hear what another is saying. Actively listening and helping the other person stay focussed on their concerns can be difficult and it is all too easy to move the focus of the conversation to one which we assume is more relevant or that makes us feel more comfortable.

Jot This Down
· Think of a time when you have needed support.
· Think about the person you chose to go and speak to about your problem.
· Why did you choose them?
· What qualities did they have?

Spirituality

The National Institute for Health and Clinical Excellence (NICE 2004, p. 10) states that 'patients and carers should have access to staff who are sensitive to their spiritual needs', however spiritual needs are often seen as some of the more challenging aspects of a person's life to ask about. Spiritual support for patients and their families at the end of life are often not assessed or addressed. Often the main the focus of care at the end of life is on physical symptoms, as this is considered to be the main cause of suffering for dying patients (Jeffery 2003) and the psychological, social and spiritual aspects of care are seen as of secondary importance (Dunlop & Hockley 1997). Although we are becoming increasingly competent at managing difficult physical symptoms, such as pain, neglecting the role that the psychological, emotional and spiritual domains play in the patients 'total pain' would mean we are only partially addressing the problem.

Jot This Down
· How would you define spirituality?
· What gives your life meaning and purpose?
· How important are religious or spiritual beliefs to you and how you live your life?

Many health and social care professionals lack confidence in addressing this important aspect of care (NCPC 2010). They often struggle to see what their role is and may feel they are intruding into a private area of someone's life and only offer the most basic of spiritual care that essentially relates to identification of a person's religion and observation of religious practices. A person's religious needs are often seen as the same as their spiritual needs; however they are not necessarily the same thing.

Spirituality is a personal search for meaning and purpose in life, which may or may not be related to religion. It entails connection to self-chosen and/or religious beliefs, values and practices that give meaning to life, thereby inspiring and motivating individuals to achieve their optimal being. This connection brings faith, hope and empowerment. The results are joy, forgiveness of oneself and others, awareness and acceptance of hardship and mortality, a heightened sense of physical and emotional well-being, and the ability to transcend beyond the infirmities of existence.

(Tanyi 2002)

Spirituality is…

- Searching for meaning
- Relationships – God/s, others, ourselves
- Being human – part of the human condition
- Unique to the individual – paramount
- Comes into focus when were ill/distressed
- Can be a force that affects the way we live and how we act
- Can be experienced within or without a religious framework.

The Evidence

Spirituality is the dynamic dimension of human life that relates to the way persons (individual or community) experience, express and/or seek meaning, purpose and transcendence, and the way they connect to the moment, self, to others, to nature, to the significant and/or sacred.

(Task Force on Spiritual Care in Palliative Care, EAPC 2011)

The notion of spiritual care is a difficult one to quantify or explain and largely because of this, has perhaps become sidelined within the healthcare encounter or seen, at least by health professionals, as a less vital part of the illness experience. Problems of the spirit, however, transcend all distinctions between separate experiences; it is both body and mind, self and others. It remains a largely intangible issue that many struggle to understand or know how to assist someone in spiritual distress. The term is widely used yet is notoriously vague and obscure.

Cobb (2001) also comments on the lack of attention that spiritual care receives in relation to care of the dying. He feels that, although spirituality is difficult to describe, it is fundamental to the understanding of well-being, suffering, life and death. It is unavoidable, as it shapes our own lives and our relationship with others. It is the means of making sense of human existence. When faced with death, our understanding of the spiritual nature of our lives can often come into sharper focus. Lunn (1993) perhaps most eloquently describes spirituality as concerning the essence of what it means to be human, ultimate concerns, questions about meaning and values, and our deepest relationships, whether with others, with God or Gods or with ourselves.

What is often difficult is to identify whose role within the healthcare team it is to deliver spiritual care. It is difficult to argue

that it is not part of everyone's job; however it is often overlooked in favour of more tangible practical types of support.

The HOPE Questions for a Formal Spiritual Assessment

H. Sources of hope, meaning, comfort, strength, peace, love and connection

O. Organised religion

P. Personal spirituality and practices

E. Effects on medical care and end-of-life issues.

(Anandarajah & Hight 2001)

As we have seen, the philosophy of palliative and end of life care is focussed on the holistic care of patients that takes into account their psychological emotional and spiritual as well as physical needs. This approach is often referred to as 'psychosocial care'. The National Council for Palliative Care (NCPC) has defined psychosocial care as being 'concerned with the psychological and emotional well being of the patient, their family/carers, including issues of self esteem insight into an adaptation to the illness and its consequences, communication, social functioning and relationships' (NCPC 2000).

What the Experts Say

 I know I'm going to die, my Mum's really upset and she and her friends say they'll pray for me and I think that's nice but it's just not what I'm into. I don't believe in God or heaven or anything. I've been writing a blog and had some amazing discussions with other people, some in my situation, some not. I've also been writing letters to my daughter. I know she can't read yet but I want her to know me when she's older, open them on birthdays or when she gets married. I want to share with her what I've learned from all of this. If I didn't, then I would just think what's the point – me dying wouldn't mean anything. I'm spending as much time as I can with my family, every minute with them seems so important and valuable. It's really important for me to do all of these things, let people know how much I love them. Some people ask do I ever feel angry or wonder why it's happened to me and I say no not really, I just think well why not me?

(Kylie, 32, cancer patient)

Jot This Down

- Without any religious belief, where do Kylies spiritual beliefs and values lie?
- What gives her life meaning and purpose?
- What are her sources of strength?
- Might her beliefs and values play a role in her decisions about how and where she is cared for?

What the Experts Say

 I can't believe Kylie is so calm about all of this. I'm in bits, it's just not right that your children should die before you. I'm just so angry. Why should it happen to this family? What have we done to deserve this?

There are murderers walking the streets with their whole lives ahead of them, it doesn't seem fair. I keep thinking maybe it's my fault, I smoked while I was pregnant, could that be it? I go to church but it doesn't help, I just keep think if you could have stopped this, then why didn't you? Since her dad died she has been my life, I don't know if I can cope when she's gone, and then there's Lucy?

(Carol, Kylies mum)

It is often difficult for people to see a reason why things have happened. This search for meaning can be hard for people facing the loss of a loved one. Often a religious belief can be a comfort but sometimes people can begin to question their beliefs when a sense of fairness or justice in the world is challenged. Our relationships with others, family, friends or God, as we have identified, is often at the core of our spirituality and when this is threatened, it can lead to a sense of spiritual distress. Spiritual care is the responsibility of all professional carers and can be delivered through sensitive, thoughtful communication, helping others explore and attempt to understand their feelings and emotions.

 Link To/Go To

The National Council for Palliative Care (NCPC): **http://www.ncpc.org.uk/**

Breaking Bad News

Jot This Down

- Have you ever had to tell someone something that perhaps they didn't want to hear?
- How did it make you feel?
- Did you think about the way you might tell them? The place? The words you used?
- How might these considerations be applied to difficult discussions with patients?

The notion of breaking bad news often seems to conjure up the idea of a professional (usually a doctor) imparting information about a patient's diagnosis and subsequent (poor) prognosis. Although this is the archetypal image, the progressive nature of life-shortening illness means that patient's and family's encounter many situations where the patient's disease and treatment will not be progressing as hoped for and occasions when various health and social care professionals will be involved in such discussions. It is important that as professionals, although we may recognise these changes and may consider them as a common occurrence, we must always appreciate the profound effect they can have on people.

 What the Experts Say

When they said I needed a bed downstairs I knew what that meant. I was never going to sleep in my own bedroom again. The room I had shared with my husband all our married life. I was never going to lie next to him anymore. It was the room where I had nursed my children, we had each one's cot next to us when they were tiny. I knew it meant I was getting worse, that I needed more help, that I wouldn't be able to use my own toilet anymore. It felt like I was losing everything, all the things that just about made me feel normal. I was going to need a commode, a hoist, a hospital bed, my lovely home was going to be turned into a hospital ward. When they told me I burst into tears and couldn't stop crying, I don't think they realised why I was so upset.

(Barbara, living with end-stage heart failure)

When communicating anything that may make a person view their future in a negative way, it is important that we communicate this thoughtfully and sensitively. One of the most well known and widely used models of breaking bad news is the six-step approach, developed by Dr Rob Buckman:

S.P.I.K.E.S a Six Step Guide to Breaking Bad News

S. *Setting, listening Skills*
P. *Patient's Perception*
I. *Invite patient to share Information*
K. *Knowledge transmission*
E. *Explore Emotions and Empathise*
S. *Summarise & Strategise.*

(Buckman 1992)

Step One: Setting

It is important initially to remember general courtesies and to clarify who everyone involved is. You should be sure you know all the facts about the situation to avoid any ambiguities or uncertainties. It also is important to get the physical context right, i.e. is there a private room that can be used? Is the seating set out correctly, have other staff been informed so as to minimise unnecessary disturbances, are bleeps turned off? Have staff allocated time? Privacy is vital; however, this can be difficult in a hospital setting or even at home if other family members and friends are present, and this raises questions about who should be there and whether their presence is appropriate. Staff may have concerns about alerting the individual to the fact that bad news is coming by asking if they want someone to be present. However, by knowing the family and understanding the relationships, it is possible to identify sources of support early and clarify if and when it would be important to inform them; they may wish to be present at all important discussions about treatment and care.

Step Two: Perceptions

It is vitally important to find out how much the individual knows, what they have been told and what they understand, as these may be entirely different things. A patient may be told that their treatment is 'palliative' but what is their understanding of this term? How serious does he/she think it is? We must gather information that allows us to identify where a patient's gaps in their knowledge lie or if indeed they already have some suspicion of the seriousness of the situation. We should assess the person's emotional and psychological state from their verbal and non-verbal behaviour. It is important not to rush this stage and it may take time; however, by using the skills already mentioned, such as clarifying and summarising and picking up on cues, we will gain a better sense of the individual (and perhaps family's) understanding, which will aid greatly in the subsequent stages.

Step Three: Invitation for Information

This step is essential if we are to truly understand the patient's preferred role in the process and allow them to control rate and level of detail of information they wish to receive. By asking questions such as 'are you the type of person who prefers to have all the details or a rough outline', you are putting the individual in charge and providing them with the opportunity to stem the flow or request more detail. If you do not include this stage, you may end up having an interaction with the patient which is delicate and insecure. Some people just do not want to know at the time – but they might do later.

Step Four: Knowledge Transmission

Starting from the patient's starting point (aligning) and providing a warning shot, such as 'I'm sorry I have some bad news to tell you' allows the person to ready themselves for the actual news. By pausing and gauging the reaction, we can see if it is appropriate to continue. Some people express a clear desire for full information and if you are sure about this, then it may well be appropriate to move quickly to this to avoid further anxiety. It is important to keep the words you use simple and avoid 'medspeak' or jargon and communicate sensitively, avoiding harsh words or statements. Putting the individual in control of the flow of information is crucial and we must respect to right of the person **not** to know. This is known as 'negotiated disclosure' and means that we should never tell someone something they do not want to know or are not ready to hear.

Step Five: Explore Feelings and Empathise

It is important to be aware that some people can react in very emotional ways – an outburst of tears, even anger. In this step, we are concerned with acknowledging the patient's reactions and empathically communicating that this must be difficult news to hear. It is important that we do not judge or sanction someone's emotional reaction, for instance by saying things like 'there's no need to get angry' or 'please don't cry'. The way we communicate empathically may involve some of the microskills we have already discussed, such as empathic responding, educated guesses, pauses and silences and touch.

Step Six: Summarise and strategise

This stage is about moving on and planning for the future. The patient may feel bewildered and dispirited and will look to you to make sense of the confusion and to offer options and a way forward. This is an opportunity to jointly make a plan or strategy, identify short and medium team goals and answer any outstanding questions. It may be important to provide practical support in terms of signposting patients to other services or sources of help, providing further, perhaps written, information and identifying individual coping strategies and how to reinforce them.

Culture and Ethnicity

Helman (1994) defines culture as a collection of guidelines that are socially inherited and influence the way in which members of social groups act, perceive and emotionally experience the world. It encompasses, but is not necessarily the same as, religion although many of our cultural understanding of death and dying have their origins in a religious framework. For many people, the cultural context of death and dying is closely linked to ethnicity and faith and influences how they understand and find comfort and hope in the face of death. There is as much diversity within given cultures as there is between them. Ritualistic beliefs and behaviours are deeply engrained in our cultural approaches to death and dying.

Ethics and Decision-Making at the End of Life

The very nature of end of life care and the profound ethical questions it raises for health and social care practitioner demands an understanding of the underpinning ethical theories and the part they play in clinical decision-making. A common framework often applied in the healthcare arena is the 'four principles' approach (Box 20.3; Beauchamp & Childress 2009). These principles reflect four core moral principles and should each be acknowledged and evaluated in relation to each other and their importance to the ethical challenge in question.

Ethical Challenges at the End of Life
Artificial hydration and nutrition

> ### What the Experts Say
>
> We were sat in the relatives' room, Mrs Rogers was very upset, I had just explained to her that her husband was dying and that the main aim now was to keep him comfortable. She said 'but he isn't drinking, that's why he's dying, if you gave him a drip, surely he would get better'. I tried to explain to her that fluids wouldn't be helpful at this point and might even make her husband more uncomfortable but she was so upset, she thought we were letting him die of thirst.
>
> (Raj, Medical Registrar)

Box 20.3 Four Principles of Biomedical Ethics.

Autonomy – Is concerned with the ability of the individual to act freely and not to be constrained or restricted. It relates to the right of the individual to self-determination. Respect for autonomy is fundamental for informed consent and advance directives

Beneficence – To do good, to act in such a way that promotes the best interests and well-being of others. This is a fundamental aspect of our care-giving role

Non-maleficence – To do no harm, to ensure that no action or omission of action to a patient is detrimental to the health and well-being of patient

Justice – Fairness, to ensure that people are treated without prejudice and are seen as equal. It also relates to the allocation and distribution of resources.

Jot This Down

Autonomy – How could we act in a way that we were confident we were in accordance with Mr Rogers' views?

Beneficence – What is in Mr Rogers' 'best interests' – would artificial fluids make him more comfortable?

Non-maleficence – Would withholding or commencing artificial fluids at this point do harm to Mr Rogers?

Justice – Should we treat Mr Rogers and all other patients in this situation exactly the same? Should we pay equal weight to Mrs Rogers concerns?

What the Experts Say Truth Telling/Collusion

Mr Patel stopped me in the corridor just before I was about to go into his mother's room. He said that the Doctor had told him that Mrs Patel's cancer had spread and that he would appreciate it if I didn't tell her this. He said that they had discussed it as family and decided that it would be best if she didn't know, they knew her best and she couldn't cope with this news. Everyone in the family was worried that she would give up and die sooner if she knew.

(Wendy, Macmillan Nurse)

Mr Rogers cannot tell us what he would wish, as he is too unwell, therefore Raj and the rest of the team must make a decision that they believe is in his best interests, in that it will minimise any harm and maximise any good that Mr Rogers may experience. This is best identified from any previously expressed views that are recorded or by discussing it with his family. However, Mrs Rogers feels that artificial fluids will make her husband better (or at least more comfortable), when actually evidence suggests that giving artificial hydration at the very end of life when someone is unable to tolerate oral fluids affects neither the length of remaining life or the patient's comfort (NCPC 2007), and current literature suggests that the benefits of providing artificial hydration are limited and do not clearly outweigh the burdens (Raijmakers *et al.* 2011) Therefore, not commencing them would be doing good and minimising harm. Administering artificial fluids may lessen Mrs Rogers' immediate distress, however the reality remains that her husband is dying. It is possible to give mixed messages to relatives about the goals of care at this point and this can lead to inconsistencies in approaches to Mr Rogers' care by different members of the team, and perhaps facilitating false hope, thus doing more harm. It may be best to make an evidence-based decision as to the benefits of hydration for Mr Rogers, as this will be in his best interests. It would not be ethically justifiable to treat Mr Rogers in order to minimise distress to Mrs Rogers but it would be important to sensitively discuss this with Mrs Rogers and explore her understanding and feelings around this and allay any fears she may have.

Red Flag

A blanket policy approach of either always initiating or always withholding or withdrawing artificial fluids for people in this situation is ethically indefensible. Each situation must be looked at individually and the benefits and burdens of such treatment must be weighed up against the particular needs of the individual.

Nursing Fields of Practice

How would these issues relate to other people who had impaired capacity, such as:

· People with dementia or mental health problems?
· Individuals with learning disabilities?
· Young children and babies?

Jot This Down

Autonomy – To promote autonomy, should we give Mrs Patel the information? Would being given this information allow her to make her own decisions about future care and treatment? Does Mrs Patel also have the right not to know and would respecting this be promoting autonomy?

Beneficence – What is in Mrs Patel's 'best interests'? Would having this information do good in that she could make the decisions that were best for her?

Non-maleficence – Would telling Mrs Patel the truth cause her distress? Would it rob her of hope and upset her family?

Justice – Should we treat Mrs Patel and all other patients in the situation the same way? Should we always tell the truth, as this is the fairest way to deal with this type of dilemma? Should we consider the wishes and needs of the family equally with Mrs Patel's?

Wendy does not know what Mrs Patel understands about her condition at this point. She does, however, know that her son is devoted to his mother and does not want to see her upset. Wendy has a duty of care to Mrs Patel (NMC 2008), however she understands that family-centered care at the end of life is very important and that Mrs Patel's needs will undoubtedly overlap with those of her family. Wendy could discuss with Mr Patel his thoughts and feelings about discussing the diagnosis with his mother, perhaps somewhere private. By using good communication skills, she could elicit his concerns and address why he feels his mother should not be told; families are often concerned that the news will harm patients. Wendy could explain to Mr Patel that she would respect Mrs Patel's autonomy and that to make informed decisions about the future, she would need to understand the nature of her illness; giving her the information she required would therefore be doing good, however Mrs Patel also had a right not to discuss this if she did not wish to and found it too difficult, not telling Mrs Patel anything she did not wish to know would also be respecting her autonomy. She could negotiate with Mrs Patel how much information and in what detail she wanted to know about her current condition and would not disclose anything that she did not want to explore, thus minimising harm. This can then be documented and communicated to the rest of the care-giving team.

Red Flag

Often an individual's preferences and wishes can change over time and in relation to how their illness is progressing. It is therefore vital that any assessment of need or decision is reviewed regularly to ensure it remains aligned with the person's current views.

Mental Capacity

What the Experts Say

> We had been looking after Shirley for about 12 months, since her motor neurone disease had progressed to the stage where she needed more nursing care. Only last month we had sat together while she told me what she wanted to put in her advanced care plan. She had just had a couple of spells in the hospice with chest infections but there wasn't always a bed and she was worried that if it happened again, she would have to go to hospital. She had been getting weaker recently and her breathing was more compromised after each episode, she told me she was frightened that she might not come out and that she didn't want to die there. We wrote down in her PPC that she didn't want to go to hospital or have antibiotics if she got another infection, she just wanted to be cared for at home, even if it meant it might shorten her life. I heard this morning that she had been seen by the doctor over the weekend, as she had become confused and been admitted to hospital due to a urinary tract infection.

(Pauline, District Nurse)

Jot This Down

Autonomy – Has Shirley's autonomy been compromised? When she became confused how did her advance care plan influence the decision-making of the professionals?

Beneficence – What is in Shirley's 'best interests'? Did the GP do what he thought was in her best interests and did this differ from her views?

Non-Maleficence – Would more harm have come to Shirley if the GP had not organised hospital admission or is not respecting her views harmful in itself?

Justice – Should we always respect an advance care plan in every instance? Should such a document be legally binding, so that clinicians must respect everyone's advance care plan as it is written?

Shirley had expressly stated that she didn't not want to go to hospital in the event of another infection. However, the GP was presented with the dilemma of trying to balance Shirley's best interests with what she had written in her advance care plan. Sometimes circumstances arise that patients and families may not foresee. Did Shirley anticipate that she may get a different kind of infection than the chest infection she had experienced previously? Would a urinary infection have as much an effect on her prognosis

as a respiratory infection? Was this the situation that she had predicted when she wrote her ACP? These are the questions that the doctor should have been asking himself as he was considering what to do. In the end, the doctor after weighing up the facts and discussing with the family, decided that this was not quite the situation that the ACP was intended for and that Shirley's best interest would be best served by going to hospital. This was felt to promote the most good, as with treatment she would probably return to her pre-infection state and minimise harm by lessening the chances of her dying prematurely.

Grief, Loss and Bereavement

How could you go about choosing something that would hold the half of your heart that you had to bury?

(Mercy, Jodi Picolt 1996)

The process of dying often involves a series of losses and emotional reactions to those losses. This often affects all those involved from the individual themselves to family and friends and often the professional caregiver. This section discusses the nature of such loss and possible grief reactions and the theoretical and practical issues that often arise.

There has been a clear and dramatic change in the ways that society reacts to death and bereavement in the UK over the past 100 years (Klass *et al.* 1996). Living in a more secular society has reduced the importance of communal rituals and beliefs in favour of more individualistic ones.

Definitions

Loss is the state of being deprived of, or being without, something one has had and the death of a loved one is perhaps the most traumatic loss of all (Parkes 2006).

Grief is the multifaceted psychological response of pain and suffering experienced after loss (Walter 2009).

Bereavement is the process of losing a close relationship and mourning is the period of time during which signs of grief are made visible (Small 2001).

Models

Numerous models have been developed that seek to help us understand the complexity of thoughts and emotions that are often experienced when we are bereaved. Elizabeth Kübler-Ross has been credited with developing one of the most influential conceptual models of loss and grief; the five stages of grief model (Kübler-Ross 1969) (see Figure 20.4). This model proposes that there are a number of stages that bereaved people and those facing loss through the diagnosis of a terminal illness experience and has influenced contemporary thinking and education around the subject for many years. Her five stages of grief model proposed that people experience progressive stages of denial, anger, bargaining, depression and acceptance.

Other proponents of the stage or phase theory of grief include John Bowlby and his four stages of grief model (Bowlby 1961) and Colin Murray Parkes phases of grief theory (Murray Parkes 1975).

Worden (1991) suggested that the bereaved need to complete certain tasks, namely to accept the reality of the loss, experience the pain of grief, adjust to an environment with the deceased missing and to withdraw emotional energy and reinvest it into

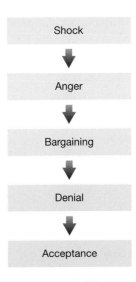

Figure 20.4 **Kübler-Ross 5-stage model.**

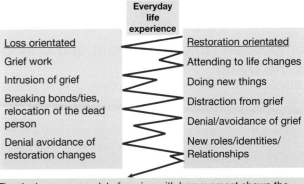

The dual process model of coping with bereavement shows the relationship between dealing with the stresses of the loss itself (Loss orientated) and moving on with ones life (Restoration orientated)

Figure 20.5 **Grief and restorative-oriented states.** *Source:* Stroebe and Schut 1999.

other relationships. This 'task' model describes the importance of individuals 'working through' their grief to find a place of resolution and acceptance and the expression of grief was seen to be central to this.

However, other perspectives attribute less significance to the idea of leaving the deceased behind and suggest that it is important to relocate them and find a place for them in a new reconstructed life. The theory of 'continuing bonds' (Klass *et al.* 1996) describes this concept as a natural response to losing a loved one. In Victorian England it was common for the memorialisation of the deceased through elaborate monuments in municipal ceremonies. Post-mortem photographs of the deceased, often children, were frequently displayed and even shared as postcards, as a means of maintaining bonds with the dead (Burns & Burns 2002). This idea of continuing bonds focusses on the importance of individuals and community maintaining a relationship with the deceased. Rather than living in the past, mourners find a new place for the dying within their new life.

Despite its longevity, some have sought to question the validity of the stage model view and explicate a different view of the process of grief and resilience (Thomson *et al.* 2002; Bonanno 2004). These newer perspectives on the understanding of grief and loss have challenged some of the accepted views of traditional grief theory. Stage models have often been interpreted as a linear progression and give a clear if somewhat tacit suggestion that grief must be worked through on a pathway, from distress to acceptance and that to not display signs of distress or to maintain an emotional relationship to the dead was not just abnormal but almost pathological. George Bonanno (2004) proposes that traditional theorists have sought to pathologise grief and that individuals are actually naturally resilient, that the absence of a grief reaction is not abnormal and that the notion of working through grief by revisiting traumatic events can actually be harmful (Bonanno 2004).

Stroebe and Schut's Dual Process model builds on the stage theory of grief but adds a degree of dynamism to explain how a grieving individual may move back and forth between grief-orientated and restorative-oriented states (as shown in Figure 20.5) (Stroebe & Schut 1999).

Some commentators contend that grief-like depression has become a medical 'problem' to be diagnosed and treated, rather than a natural human response to challenging life events (Illich 1975; Parker 2007). However, it is clear that sometimes the traumatic experience of losing a loved one or the realisation that one's own life may be coming to an end can cause serious clinical problems, such as anxiety and depression, and that a distinction should be made between normal and complicated grief reactions. This 'complex grief' can cause severe psychological reactions in those individuals, can be associated with adverse health outcomes and should be treated medically (Hawton 2007).

429

Jot This Down

Think of a time when you lost something (this does not have to be about bereavement, something as simple and as everyday as losing your keys or purse will suffice).

- **What did it make you feel?** – What emotions did it create? What physical feelings did it create?
- **What did it make you think?** – What were the thoughts going around in your head?
- **What did it make you do?** – How did the loss make you act, what behaviours did it encourage?

Think about these for a while and then imagine how someone faced with the loss of a loved one may feel about such a loss or the reality of such a loss in the near future.

 Link To/Go To

VOICES survey of bereaved relatives: **http://www.ons.gov
.uk/ons/rel/subnational-health1/national-bereavement
-survey–voices-/2011/stb-statistical-bulletin.html**

Who Cares for the Carers?

Compassion Fatigue, Burnout and Caring for the Dying

Healthcare workers are repeatedly faced with loss and grief and caring for dying patients for a sustained period of time can develop intense feelings of grief (Genevro 2004). Staff grieve for patients lost and these feelings can contribute to the failure in achieving quality care and complicating unresolved personal grief and recent personal bereavement. Over time, multiple losses can impact negatively on individuals and develop into accumulative loss (Adams *et al.* 1991).

Figley (1995) discusses the effects of compassion fatigue, describing them as promoting a sense of hopelessness and a decrease in experiences of pleasure, constant stress and anxiety, pervasive negative attitude, decrease in productivity, inability to focus and development of feelings of incompetency and self-doubt.

Jot This Down

· How does caring for dying patients make you feel?

· How do you deal with these feelings?

· What are your strategies for coping with difficult feelings?

Twycross (1995) identified a number of areas that were challenging for professionals involved in caring for dying patients.

- *Facing your own limitations personally and professionally*
- *Sharing control*
- *Learning to be with patients rather than doing things for them*
- *Dealing honestly with your emotions*
- *Facing your own mortality.*

(Twycross 1995)

As nurses, when patients are dying, our natural sense of accomplishment of helping someone to return to independence or to heal from an episode of injury or illness, is missing. It can be hard to see through the pain and the distress and appreciate the positive and helpful work that we do. It is often tempting to set very high standards for ourselves and the care we give that are difficult to achieve both as a person and as a professional and consequently leads to sense of dissatisfaction, when we fail to do so.

As professionals, we may feel the need to assume the position of expert and feel the need to control or be influential in caring situations; this sense of control is often an illusion and it is better to be led by patients and their needs. Doing our job as best we can and setting ourselves realistic expectations of ourselves is important to avoid this. Often in end of life situations, it is the 'being' rather than the 'doing' that is important. Presenting a supportive presence, rather than focussing on tasks, is important to promote independence, choice and control until the end. It is vital to recognise the challenge of facing multiple losses and the emotional cost of this, in order to manage our own emotions and recognise and attend to our needs. Understanding our views and emotions surrounding death can be helpful in empathising with others facing loss and to appropriately manage our personal feelings in such interactions.

Coping Strategies

- Seeking help is not a weakness
- Find out if supervision is available
- Education
- Recognise your development needs
- Manage your workload
- Reporting systems
- Remember, you are not alone!
- Make time to play and engage in life-affirming activities.

What the Experts Say

"I had been looking after Simon for a few weeks on the ward and we got on really well, he reminded me so much of my dad. He was funny and we used to have a laugh when I was on duty. He always seemed really positive and full of life and although his leukaemia wasn't curable, I never expected him to die. I was on duty that day, I was part of the team in that bay and when I came on duty and heard that he had deteriorated overnight and they had phoned his wife, I was stunned. I actually couldn't go into the side ward where he was, as I was too frightened. When his wife arrived, I saw her coming onto the ward and I just felt overwhelmed and though we had spoken many times, I just couldn't face her, I started to cry and had to run into the store room.

(Vicky, 1st year student nurse)

It is important that as professional caregivers that we are able to engage and disengage in therapeutic relationships (NMC 2008). This means that we must be able to support others and to be aware of the possibility that our own emotions may emerge when we are caring for dying patients and their families. This type of nursing can remind us of our own losses and grief and may well raise difficult feelings for us. It is important to remember that the safety and care of others is our prime concern and, although to be empathic may mean to understand the feelings and emotions of others, we must be aware of when we are predominantly dealing with our emotions rather than those of our patients and their families.

Twycross (1995) discusses the need to develop strategies to address professional compassion fatigue, such as facing your own limitations personally and professionally and dealing honestly with your emotions. Without an understanding of our own views about mortality, it may be difficult for us to engage therapeutically with those who are facing death themselves.

It is both the privilege and the penalty of being part of a healthcare team that we will meet people who are suffering in the face of loss. If we back off or fail to recognise their needs we may miss the opportunity to help them through a turning point in their lives. We may also miss the opportunity to learn from them that losses are often integrating factors in family life and, in the end, a source of new meaning and hope.

(Parkes 1998)

Conclusion

This chapter has highlighted how the pattern and trajectory of death and dying has changed significantly over the past few generations. Death has been said by some to have become medicalised, professionalised and institutionalised and therefore hidden from society; others, however, have suggested that are we are becoming re-acquainted with death and dying, which is becoming less of a taboo subject.

The hospice and palliative care movement has done much to improve the care of people who are dying, providing a clear evidence base for many of its approaches and the *End of Life Care Strategy* has highlighted how all individuals with progressive diseases can have access to the right kind of care at the end of life, irrespective of what condition they have.

Nurses and other health and social care workers require a good knowledge, not just of the physical and symptom control needs of the patients who are dying, but also psychosocial and spiritual healthcare needs as well as the underpinning issues related to loss, grief and bereavement. A clear understanding of the legal, ethical and professional issues that can arise when caring for dying patients and their families is also prerequisite to effective care.

Through advance care planning and a systematic approach to coordinating care for patients at the end of life, more people can have a peaceful dignified death in the place of their choosing. Sensitive, honest communication at the end of life will ensure that more people will have not just their physical care needs addressed but also their emotional, psychological and spiritual needs.

Working in this particular field of care can demand a degree of emotional commitment on the part of professional carers and it is essential for such individuals to understand the importance of ensuring their own psychological health through the development of appropriate support strategies.

Key Points

- The concept of a 'good death' may seem strange to many but how and where people die is often very important to individuals and their families.
- Promoting comfort is the main aim of any management at the end of life and a holistic approach must be taken that acknowledges the interrelationship between the emotional psychological, spiritual and the physical.
- It can often be difficult to truly hear what another is saying. Actively listening and helping the other person stay focussed on their concerns can be difficult and it is all too easy to move the focus of the conversation to one which we assume is more relevant or that makes us feel more comfortable.
- The very nature of end of life care and the profound ethical questions it raises for health and social care practitioners demands an understanding of the underpinning ethical theories and the place they play in clinical decision-making.
- As nurses, when patients are dying, our natural sense of accomplishment from helping someone to return to independence or to heal from an episode of injury or illness is missing.
- Numerous models have been developed that seek to help us understand the complexity of thoughts and emotions that are often experienced when we are bereaved.
- Healthcare workers are repeatedly faced with loss and grief and caring for dying patients for a sustained period of time can develop intense feelings of grief.

Glossary

End of life care: End of life care enables the supportive and palliative care needs of both patient and family to be identified and met throughout the last phase of life and into bereavement. It includes the management of pain and other symptoms and the provision of psychological, social, spiritual and practical support

Palliative care: Palliative care is an approach that improves the quality of life of patients and their families facing the problem associated with life-threatening illness, through the prevention and relief of suffering by means of early identification and impeccable assessment and treatment of pain and other problems, physical, psychosocial and spiritual

Best interests: When a person lacks the capacity to state what they wish to happen or not happen to them, often it is necessary to make a decision based on what is believed to be in their 'best interests'. It is important that these decisions are based on any available information (such as Advance Care Plans or Advance Decisions to Refuse Treatment documentation) and take into account the perspective of those who may know the person best. If no-one is available to take on the role of advocate, then an independent person (known as an IMCA, Independent Mental Capacity Advocate) from a nominated body can be included in the discussions and represent the person's views to those who are working out their best interests (MCIP 2007)

Mental capacity: Mental capacity means to have the ability to make decisions autonomously and without impairment, understanding the implications of those decisions. It involves the individual being able to understand information being given to them, retain that information long enough to be able to make a decision, weigh up the information available and communicate that decision

Psychosocial care: Care that considers the emotional psychological, spiritual, social, cultural and physical domains of a person health, the interconnectedness of these domains and how their particular illness or condition may be affecting these

431

References

Abernethy AP, McDonald CF, Frith PA, *et al.* (2010) Effect of palliative oxygen versus room air in relief of breathlessness in patients with refractory dyspnoea: a double-blind, randomised controlled trial. *Lancet*, 376, 784–93.

Adams, J.P., Hershatter, M.J. & Moritz, D.A. (1991). Accumulated loss phenomenon among hospice caregivers. *American Journal of Hospice and Palliative Care*, 8, 29–37.

Age Concern (1999) Debate of the Age Health and Care Study Group. The future of health and care of older people: the best is yet to come. Age Concern, London.

Anandarajah, G. & Hight, E. (2001) Spirituality and Medical Practice: using the HOPE questions as a practical tool for spiritual assessment. *American Family Physician*, 63, 81–89.

AOMRC (2008) *A Code of Practice for the Diagnosis and Confirmation of Death.* Academy of Medical Royal Colleges, London.

Ariès, P. (1974). *Western Attitudes Toward Death: from the middle ages to the present.* Johns Hopkins University Press, Baltimore.

Barley, N. (1995) *Dancing on the Grave.* John Murray, London.

Beauchamp, T.L. & Childress, J.F. (2009) *Principles of Biomedical Ethics.* Oxford University Press Inc., Oxford.

Bonanno, G. (2004) Loss trauma and human resilience. *American Psychologist*, 1, 20–28.

Bowlby, J. (1961). Processes of mourning. *International Journal of Psychoanalysis*, 42, 317–339.

Buckman R. (1992) *Breaking Bad News: a guide for health care professionals*, p. 15. Johns Hopkins University Press, Baltimore.

Burns, S. & Burns, E.A. (2002). *Sleeping Beauty II: grief, bereavement in memorial photography American and European traditions.* Burns Archive Press.

Christakis, N.A. (2001) *Death Foretold: prophecy and prognosis in medical care.* University of Chicago Press, Chicago.

Cobb, M. (2001) *The Dying Soul: spiritual care at the end of life.* Open University Press, Buckingham.

Corner, H. & Thomas, K. (2010) The Gold Standards Framework in acute hospitals. *End of Life Care*, 4(4).

DH (2008) *End of Life Care Strategy: promoting high quality care for adults at the end of their life.* Department of Health, London.

DH (2012) *End of Life Care Strategy. Fourth annual report.* Department of Health, London.

Dunlop, R.J. & Hockley, J.M. (1997) *New Approaches to Palliative Care*, p. 289. Open University Press, Maidenhead.

EAPC (2011) Task force on spiritual care in palliative care. European Association of Palliative Care, Milan.

Figley, C.R. (1995). Compassion fatigue as secondary stress disorder: An overview. *Compassion Fatigue: coping with secondary traumatic stress disorder in those who treat the traumatized*, pp. 1–20. Brunner/Mazel, New York.

Genevro, J.L. (2004) Report on bereavement and grief research. *Death Studies*, 28(6), 491–575.

Glaser, B. & Strauss, A. (1965) *Awareness of Dying.* Aldine, Chicago.

GMC (2010) Treatment and care towards the end of life: good practice in decision making. General Medical Council, London.

Gold Standards Framework Programme (2006) Prognostic Indicator Guidance to aid identification of adult patients with advanced disease in the last months/year of life, who are in need of supportive and palliative care. Version 1.24. Prognostic Indicator Paper vs 1.21, Birmingham. http://www.goldstandardsframework.org.uk/.

Gomes, B. & Higginson, I. (2008) Where People Die (1974—2030): past trends, future projections and implications for care. *Palliative Medicine*, 22(1), 33–41.

Gorer, G. (1955) The pornography of death. *Encounter*, October, 49–52.

Hawton, K. (2007) Complicated grief after bereavement. *British Medical Journal*, 334(7601), 962–963.

Healthcare Commission (2008) Spotlight on complaints. A report on second-stage complaints about the NHS in England. Healthcare Commission, London.

Helman, C.G. (1994) *Culture, Health and Illness, An Introduction for Health Professionals*, 3rd edn. Butterworth Heinemann, London.

Illich, I. (1975) The medicalization of life. *Journal of Medical Ethics*, I, 73–77.

Jeffery, D. (2003) *Psychosocial Issues in Palliative Care*, Oxford University Press, Oxford.

Kellehear, A. (2007) *A Social History of Dying.* Cambridge University Press, Cambridge.

Kellehear, A. (2009) *The Study of Dying: from autonomy to transformation.* Cambridge University Press, Cambridge.

Klass, D, Silvermann, P.R. & Nickman, S. (eds) (1996) *Continuing Bonds. New understandings in grief.* Taylor & Francis, London.

Kübler-Ross, E. (1969) *On Death and Dying.* Routledge, London.

Lunn, L. (1993) From: Sheldon, F. (1997) *Psychosocial Palliative Care: Good Practice in the Care of the Dying and Bereaved*, p. 23. Cengage Learning, Andover.

MCIP (2007) OPG606: Making decisions. The Independent Mental Capacity Advocate (IMCA) service (10.07), 2nd edn. Mental Capacity Implementation Programme. https://www.justice.gov.uk/downloads/protecting-the-vulnerable/mca/making-decisions-opg606-1207.pdf

Mental Capacity Act (2005) *Code of Practice* (2007). The Stationery Office, London.

Montaigne, D.M. (1993) *The Complete Essays.* M.A. Screech (Translator) Penguin, Harmondsworth.

Mulkay, M. (1993) Social death in Britain. In: D. Cark (ed.) *The Sociology of Death: theory, culture, practice,* pp. 31–49. Blackwell, Cambridge.

NAO (2008) End of Life Care Report. National Audit Office, The Stationery Office, London.

NCPC (2000) What do we mean by 'psychosocial'? A discussion paper on use of the concept within palliative care. National Council for Palliative Care, London.

NCPC (2006) *End of Life Care Strategy: the National Council for Palliative Care submission.* National Council for Palliative Care, London.

NCPC (2007) *Artificial Nutrition and Hydration: summary guidance.* National Council for Palliative Care, London.

NCPC (2010) *Changing Gear: guidelines for managing the last days of life in adults.* National Council for Palliative Care, London.

NEoLCP (2010) National End of Life Care Programme. Holistic common assessment of supportive and palliative care needs for adults requiring end of life care. National Cancer Action Team.

NICE (2004) *Improving Supportive and Palliative Care for Adults with Cancer: spiritual support services*, pp. 95–104. National Institute for Health and Care Excellence, London.

NMC (2008) *The Code: Standards of Conduct, Performance and Ethics for Nurses and Midwives.* Nursing and Midwifery Council, London.

O'Gorman, S.M. (1998) Death and dying in contemporary society: an evaluation of current attitudes and the rituals associated with death and dying and their relevance to recent understandings of health and healing. *Journal of Advanced Nursing*, 27, 1127–1135.

ONS (2011) *Leading Causes of Death in England and Wales, 2009.* Office of National Statistics, London.

Parker, G. (2007) Is depression overdiagnosed? Yes. *British Medical Journal*, 335(7615), 328–329.

Parkes, C.M. (1975) *Bereavement: studies of grief in adult life.* Penguin, Harmondsworth.

Parkes, C.M. (1998) *Coping with Loss.* Wiley-Blackwell, Oxford.

Parkes, C.M. (2006) *Love and Loss. The roots of grief and its complications.* Routledge, London.

Picolt, J. (1996) *Mercy.* Washington Square Press; Later Printing edition.

Raijmakers, N., van Zuylen, L., Costantini, M. *et al.* (2011) Artificial nutrition and hydration in the last week of life in cancer patients. A systematic literature review of practices and effects. *Annals of Oncology*, 22, 1478–1486.

Seale, C. (1990) Demographic change and the care of the dying, 1969–1987. In: D. Dickenson & M. Johnson (eds) *Death Dying and Bereavement*, pp. 45–54. Sage, London.

Seale, C. (1998) *Constructing Death: the sociology of dying and bereavement.* Cambridge University Press, Cambridge.

Small, N. (2001) Theories of grief: a critical review. In: J. Hockey, J. Katsz & N. Small (eds) *Grief, Mourning and Death Ritual.* Open University Press, Buckingham.

Smith, C.F., Hough, L., Cheung, C., *et al.* (2012) Coordinate My Care: a clinical service that coordinates care, giving patients choice and improving quality of life. *BMJ Support in Palliative Care*, 2, 301–307.

Stroebe, M. & Schut, H. (1999) The dual process model of coping with bereavement: rationale and description. *Death Studies*, 23, 197–224.

Sudnow, D. (1967) *Passing On: the social organisation of dying.* Prentice Hall, Engelwood Cliffs.

Tanyi, R.A. (2002) Towards clarification of the meaning of spirituality. *Journal of Advanced Nursing*, 39(5), 500–9.

Taylor, C. (1985) *The Concept of a Person, Philosophical Papers*, pp. 97–114. Vol. 1. Cambridge University Press, Cambridge.

Thomson, R., Bell, R., Holland, J., Henderson, S., McGrellis, S. & Sharpe, S. (2002) Critical moments: choice, chance and opportunity in young people's narratives of transition to adulthood. *Sociology*, 36, 335–54.

432

Twycross, R. (1995) *Introducing Palliative Care*. Radcliffe Publishing Ltd, Abingdon.

Veatch, R. (1976) *Death, Dying and the Biological Revolution: our last quest for responsibility*. Yale University Press, New Haven.

Walter, C.A. & McCoyd, L.M. (2009) *Grief and Loss Across the Lifespan: a biopsychosocial perspective*. Springer, New York.

Walters, T. (1994) *The Revival of Death*. Routledge, London.

Watson, M., Lucas, C., Hoy, A, & Wells, J. (2009) *Oxford Handbook of Palliative Care,* 2nd edn. Oxford University Press, Oxford.

WHO (2009) *WHO Definition of Palliative Care*. World Health Organization, Geneva.

Worden, J.W. (1991) *Grief Counselling and Grief Therapy*, 2nd edn. Routledge, London.

Test Yourself

1. When is it suggested that end of life care should be first considered?
   (a) 6–12 hours before death
   (b) 6–12 days before death
   (c) 6–12 weeks before death
   (d) 6–12 months before death

2. Approximately what percentage of people die in a hospital setting?
   (a) 20%
   (b) 50%
   (c) 70%
   (d) 80%

3. Thinking ahead regarding patient's wishes and preferences for end of life care is known as?
   (a) Improved Care Planning
   (b) Advance Care Planning
   (c) Advanced Care Planning
   (d) Enhanced Care Planning

4. The Elizabeth Kübler-Ross stages of loss include:
   (a) Weariness
   (b) Denial
   (c) Frustration
   (d) Sadness

5. The core conditions that underpin therapeutic communication are:
   (a) Sympathy
   (b) Honesty
   (c) Congruence
   (d) Pity

6. The principles of biomedical ethics include:
   (a) Truth telling
   (b) Advocacy
   (c) Autonomy
   (d) Confidentiality

7. Stroebe and Schut's model of grief and loss is known as the:
   (a) Double system model
   (b) Dual process model
   (c) Duo structure model
   (d) Twin process model

8. One tool to assist in identifying future wishes for care is the:
   (a) Preferred Principles of Care tool
   (b) Preferred Priorities for Care tool
   (c) Preferential Precedence for Care tool
   (d) Positive Place of Care tool

9. The Mental Capacity Act came into full effect in which year?
   (a) 2005
   (b) 2006
   (c) 2007
   (d) 2009

10. What are common symptoms in the last 48 hours of life
    (a) Restlessness/agitation
    (b) Deafness
    (c) Upper airway secretions
    (d) Pins and Needles

Answers

1. d
2. b
3. b
4. b
5. c
6. c
7. b
8. b
9. c
10. a & c

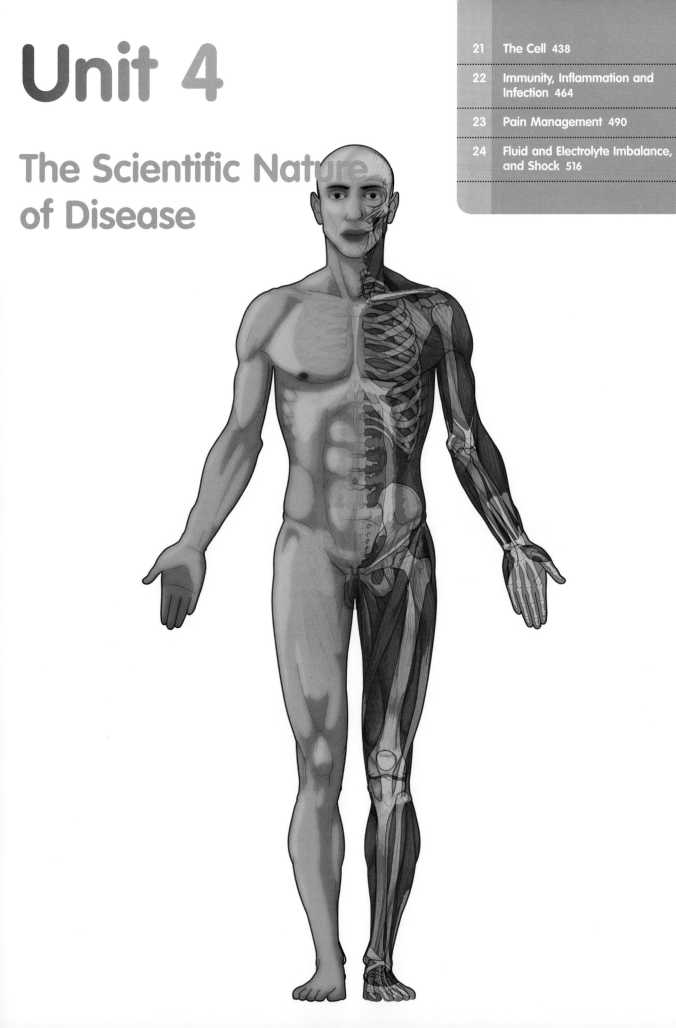

Unit 4

The Scientific Nature of Disease

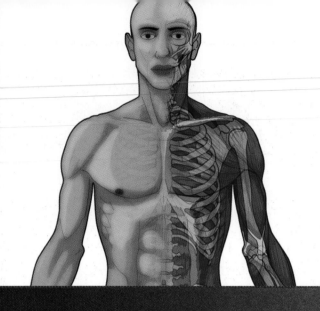

21

The Cell

Frances Gascoigne

University of Salford, UK

Learning Outcomes

On completion of this chapter you will be able to:

- List the organelles in the cell and explain their structures and functions
- Describe the terms, 'internal' and 'external environments' and explain the significance of these compartments for the health of the cells
- Relate cell development, maturation and death to genetics and health
- List and describe the body tissues
- Explain how a knowledge of the chemical, genetic and cellular levels of organisation in the body relate to the assessment of the human body and the implementation of nursing practice
- Gain an insight into the significance of cell and health promotion

Competencies

All nurses must:

1. Use knowledge of the cell, so that the appropriate interventions are implemented to provide an appropriate environment for cell growth and repair
2. Assess functional health status and provide information to the patient based on the assessment to avoid cell and tissue damage and promote health
3. Use evidence-based practice to plan and structure individualised care to protect cell and tissue damage
4. Recognise signs in ill health and the manifestation of cell malfunctioning
5. Evaluate nursing care of patients with genetic disorders and implement effective interventions to promote ongoing management
6. Revise the plan of care for patients with altered cell functioning

 Visit the companion website at **www.wileynursingpractice.com** where you can test yourself using flashcards, multiple-choice questions and more.

Unit 4 image source: Red_frog/iStock
Nursing Practice: Knowledge and Care, First Edition. Edited by Ian Peate, Karen Wild and Muralitharan Nair.
© 2014 John Wiley & Sons, Ltd. Published 2014 by John Wiley & Sons, Ltd. Companion website: www.wileynursingpractice.com

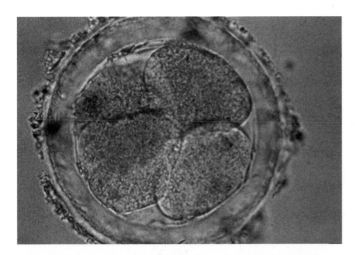

Figure 21.1 Four-cell stage of the first-cell divisions of a fertilised egg. These first-cell divisions set the stage for all subsequent development, structure and function.

Introduction

Life begins with cells (Figure 21.1). The cell is the basic unit of life and the workhorse of all living systems. Although life starts as a single cell, the developed human body is made up of trillions of cells of which there are about 200 different types. These cells function differently, depending on their location. For example, pancreatic cells have a very different function in comparison to that of cardiac muscle cells.

All of these contribute to the overall structure and functioning of you and the people you care for, in a coordinated manner. These cells share common features such as a nucleus that contains 46 chromosomes, and organelles such as mitochondria, lysosomes and Golgi bodies.

Knowledge of the structure and life of the cell is fundamental for the delivery of effective therapeutic nursing care in terms of providing basic human needs, both practical and psychological needs and medication. Cells are organised into tissues, and tissues are organised into complex structures and organs. Cells also form part of the communication network in the body and are able to exist as either single cells or groups of cells. Cells can be hard like bone tissue, soft like some muscle tissue or spongy like nose and ear tissues.

Jot This Down

What do you think the basic needs are for an appropriate standard of living and being?

In the 'Jot This Down' exercise above, you might have thought about the following:

1. Food and drink
2. Elimination
3. Personal hygiene
4. Breathing normally
5. Having choices
6. Thinking and thoughts
7. Being able to express yourself and your perceptions

8. Mobility, which may involve:
   - Comparatively simple movements such as pressing a buzzer or call button
   - More detailed movements such as walking and sitting
   - Negotiating the pouring of water into a beaker.
     These all use the same sources of energy and coordination for the control of movements.
9. Not to be in pain or have any discomfort when carrying out daily tasks or at best, be in control of pain and or discomfort
10. Entertainment
11. Companionship
12. Feeling safe
13. Having spiritual needs met
14. Being respected and having dignity
15. Sleep and rest.

The Evidence

Virginia Henderson (1991) emphasised the importance of increasing the patient's independence and described the nurse's role as:

- Substitutive (doing for the person)
- Supplementary (helping the person)
- Complementary (working with the person)

Feeling 'down in the dumps' is miscommunication between the cells in the brain (http://www.health.harvard.edu/special_health_reports/Understanding_Depression)

Each cell functions both as an individual and part of a community of structures and can grow, reproduce, process information, respond to stimuli and perform a vast number of chemical reactions and interactivities. The cell resides in a fluid, which is called the **tissue fluid**, the **intracellular fluid** or the **interstitial fluid**.

This serves as the channel of communication for the cells and is called the body's **internal environment** and the cell's **external environment**. (Your external environment is the world around you.)

The human body is composed of seven levels of structural organisation and in this chapter, we will be looking at the first four levels in some detail and relating them to the higher levels in relation to nursing care through the sections.

1. **The chemical level:** begins by introducing the individual chemical elements and compounds that are the building materials used to create the cells and maintain them.
2. **The genetic level:** explores the genetic materials and their patterns of instructions. Each cell and all of its structure and functioning is genetically coded and the relative genetic influence on growth and development is woven into this text.
3. **The cellular level:** explains the structure of the cell along with its chemical composition, its organelles and the ways it communicates with its neighbours, both those cells that are in close proximity and those that are some distance away. The structure and physiology of the cell in relation to maintaining homeostasis in the internal environment of the body will be related to nursing practice.

4. **The tissue level:** there are four basic types of tissues in your body, which are groups of cells that collect together to make up tissues:
   - Epithelial tissue
   - Connective tissue
   - Muscle tissue
   - Nerve tissue

   Within these four types of basic tissues there are subtypes such as cardiac muscle tissue and smooth muscle tissue.

5. **The organ level:** different types of tissue unite to form a body structure such as your bones, stomach, pancreas and heart.

6. **The system level:** related organs that have a common function, such as the digestive system that is made up of your mouth, salivary glands, pharynx, oesophagus, stomach, small intestine, large intestine, liver, gall bladder and pancreas. Sometimes an organ contributes to more than one system. For example the pancreas has two roles: it is part of the digestive system and the hormone producing endocrine system.

7. **The organisational level** is all of the levels working together with the cell in charge.

In essence, **the cell** is simply like a village and all its buildings on a showery day that is separated from the external environment by a perimeter of hedges and fences. In reality, the cell is a complex unit, which consists of the principal structures known as the **cytoplasm** and the **nucleus** encased in the **plasma membrane**. The cytoplasm can be likened to a moist gel, in which the **organelles** and the nucleus survive. The nucleus contains all the **genetic codes** and directs the creation of all of the cells which then make the tissues and organs. The cell must be able carry out the basic life processes of metabolism, responsiveness, movement, growth, differentiation and reproduction.

The Chemical Level

The chemical level is the lowest level of structural organisation and consists of '**matter**', chemical elements, atoms and molecules. Atoms and molecules are the building blocks of the cells. The survival and 'way of life' of the cell depends on thousands of interactions and reactions between all the chemical and structural elements. Molecules include carbohydrates, lipids, proteins, amino acids and the universal cellular unit of currency, adenosine triphosphate (ATP).

Matter

When we talk about the chemical structure of cells we start with the word 'matter', which is described as a particle and also as a substance that makes up all objects; those that are visible to the naked eye and those that are only visible with a magnifier. Matter has weight and occupies space and can exist in three states: as a solid, a liquid or a gas.

Jot This Down

Can you think of an example of 'matter' for each state?

In the 'Jot This Down' exercise above, you may have thought of the following:

1. Solids have a fixed volume and shape and include:
   - Bones and teeth which are compact and have a definite shape
   - Ice

2. Liquids have a fixed volume but no definite shape and include:
   - Blood plasma
   - Water

3. Gases have neither a definite shape nor volume and the particles are always in a random haphazard motion and include:
   - Oxygen and carbon dioxide
   - Steam.

Atoms

All forms of matter are made up of chemical elements, which are composed of small units called atoms. Each atom consists of different subatomic particles, three of which, protons, neutrons and electrons, are relevant to the human cell and physiology. The protons, which carry a positive charge and the neutrons, which are neutral, are found in the dense core nucleus of the atom. The nucleus is surrounded by orbits containing the electron particles that are held within a certain distance from the nucleus by their negative charge. This is because the opposite charges, positive protons and negative electrons, attract. Each atom has to be balanced, for example there must be an equal number of positive (protons) and negative (electrons) charges. The neutrons provide weight only.

Each atom is identified by either a single or two letters and is unique in terms of its contents, as each type is made up of different numbers of protons and neutrons, for example oxygen has eight protons, eight electrons and eight neutrons, whereas chlorine has 17 protons, 17 electrons and 18 neutrons. The atoms that are important in the human body are hydrogen (H^+); oxygen (O); carbon (C); nitrogen (N); iodine (I); calcium (Ca^{2+}), potassium (K^+); chlorine (Cl^-); sodium (Na^+); magnesium (Mg^{2+}), iron (Fe) sulphur (S) and phosphorus (P^-).

Knowledge of chemical elements and atoms comes in handy when you look at the electrolytes in the body. When atoms combine or dissolve, such as in sodium chloride, they share their electrons that are on the outer orbit. The orbit is also called a shell. There are some specific properties in relation to the nature of these outer shells and there is a maximum number of electrons that each shell can contain, for example the inner shell can contain two, the next shell can contain up to eight and each shell after that can contain up to 18. The outer shell is the significant one in reactions that take place in the body, as it on this shell where electrons are shared between atoms.

When you look at the chemical structure (Figure 21.2; formula of salt, it is NaCl), which tells you that it is sodium chloride. When you look at the diagram you can see that there is a single electron on the outer shell of sodium and chlorine has seven. We know that an atom can carry eight electrons, so sodium and chlorine share and then each has eight on the outer orbit or shell and it is now sodium chloride.

Jot This Down

Can you think of an example of when sodium chloride is used in the body?

In the 'Jot This Down' exercise above, you might have thought about the chloride shift. When the cell breathes, it produces carbon dioxide as waste, which has to be transported to the lungs to be exhaled. One of the ways carbon dioxide is transported involves a series of chemical reactions that occur in the red blood cell and the

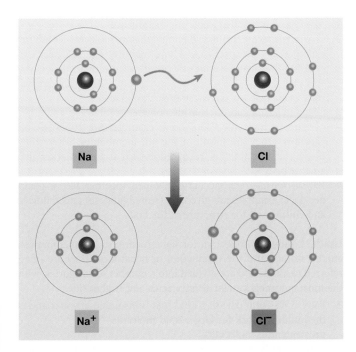

Figure 21.2 Individual sodium and chlorine atoms combine to make an NaCl molecule.

serum and they are all dependent on the chloride, which is attached to the sodium in the serum. If you have a low level of chloride in the serum, there is less for carbon dioxide to swap with in the cells and tissues and so be transported to the lungs for exhalation. This means that the carbon dioxide level in the cells and tissues may build up, which is called hypoxia.

Jot This Down

Can you think of a situation in health when your sodium chloride level may be low?

In the 'Jot This Down' exercise above, you may have thought about when somebody is dehydrated.

The action of combining sodium with chlorine is an example of ionic bonding and is a chemical reaction that generates or conducts electricity and is an 'electrolyte'.

Electrolytes are found in the body fluid, which is water-based and present in intracellular and extracellular compartments. Plasma and interstitial fluid make up the extracellular compartments. Some 60–70% of body weight is made up of water. When the electrolytes are dissolved in water, ions are formed, positively charged ions (Na^+) are called 'cations', whereas those that are negatively charged (Cl^-) are called 'anions'.

Atoms combine in different ways and amounts, to form different **molecules**, for example when two hydrogen (H_2) atoms combine with one oxygen (O) atom, they form one molecule of water (H_2O). Glucose is a larger molecule and is made up of 24 atoms: 6 carbon, 12 hydrogen and 6 oxygen atoms, to make one molecule of sugar ($C_6H_{12}O_6$). The Vitamin C molecule has 20 atoms: 6 carbon, 8 hydrogen and 6 oxygen atoms to make one molecule of vitamin C ($C_6H_8O_6$).

Diabetes

Jot This Down

Think about a patient you are caring for who has diabetes and how they presented clinically (the clinical signs). What do you think nurses need to know about diabetes?

In the 'Jot This Down' exercise above, you might have thought about the patient suffering from:

- Acute
  - feeling tired and lethargic
  - being thirsty
  - passing urine frequently
  - feeling dizzy
  - fainting
  - being unconscious
  - sweating
  - thrush
  - ketonuria – ketones in the urine
  - ketoacidosis – smelling ketones on their breath
  - hyperglycaemia – high blood sugar
  - hypoglycaemia – low blood sugar
- Chronic
  - peripheral neuropathy – foot ulcers
  - retinopathy and blurred vision
  - nephropathy
  - obesity or weight loss and loss of muscle
  - atherosclerosis
  - hypertension.

Sugar (glucose) and water are important components in the body and are essential for life. When you are thirsty your cells are asking for a drink. Water is the vital component of the internal environment, the environment in which the cells live, and accounts for almost two-thirds of body weight. If the cell becomes dehydrated, it is not able to carry out essential chemical reactions and functions and will die (Tortora & Jenkins 2013).

When your blood sugar is low you feel dizzy or giddy and if you do not fix the level of your blood sugar, you will faint and go into a coma. This is the cells telling you that they do not have enough energy to function properly. If your blood sugar is high, it means that the sugar is staying in the blood and the cells still do not have enough to function and you will feel dizzy. If there is too much sugar in the circulating blood, the blood vessels become clogged. There are two types of diabetes mellitus:

Type one This is the result of a deficiency in the production of insulin. It is an autoimmune condition, which occurs when the natural (innate) defence cells (the T cells) that protect the body against infection mistake the cells in the pancreas as foreign and attack them, either damaging them, so that they are unable to produce insulin, or destroying them completely. It is usually hereditary and runs in families, so the autoimmune reaction may also be genetic. It is not known what triggers the T cells to respond in this way but it has been suggested that it may be due to a viral infection.

Type two This occurs when the cells in the pancreas do not produce enough insulin or there is an inability of the cells and tissues to respond to insulin, and is often referred to as 'insulin resistance' diabetes.

The **pancreas** is an organ that has two distinct functions: it makes and produces enzymes, which are necessary for digestion; and it produces insulin.

Insulin is a specific protein called a hormone that has the role of facilitating the transport of glucose across the cell membranes of the liver and the skeletal muscles into these cells. Once in the cells of the liver, the mitochondria use it for the production of energy (adenosine triphosphate – ATP), which the cells need to function and survive. Any excess glucose is converted into glycogen and stored in the skeletal muscle cells and in the cells of the liver. The cells that make up the liver are called 'hepatocytes'.

Thus, insulin controls the amount of glucose in the bloodstream and maintains the normal levels (homeostasis of glucose in the internal environment). When you eat sugar the specific pancreatic cells, called 'beta cells', produce the insulin. Without insulin, the glucose you eat will remain in the bloodstream and will also pass across those cell membranes that allow it to move across easily, such as cells in the kidneys and the eyes, causing retinopathy and nephropathy.

If you do not eat enough sugar, the insulin will convert the stored glycogen in the skeletal muscle cells and hepatocytes into glucose for the cells of the body to use in order to produce energy and stay alive.

Homeostasis and hormones, which have been introduced in the pathophysiology above, will be discussed later in this chapter.

Molecules

Molecules (sugar and water were the examples used above) combine to form larger **organic** and **inorganic** molecules (Table 21.1).

Organic molecules contain **carbon** and are essential for the maintenance of the growth, structure and function of the cells and thus tissues and organs. Categories of organic molecules are **carbohydrates, lipids, amino acids, proteins, nucleic acids** and **adenosine triphosphate (ATP)**. Inorganic molecules contain **little or no carbon atoms**, and include water, salts, acids and bases and contribute towards the optimal conditions to maintain homeostasis in the internal environment.

Organic molecules

Carbohydrates Carbohydrates (saccharides) function as building blocks in the cells and tissues and are sources of energy. They are divided into four groups: monosaccharides, disaccharides, oligosaccharides and polysaccharides.

1. *Monosaccharides* are simple sugars (glucose)
2. *Disaccharides* are formed when two glucose molecules combine; examples are sucrose, lactose and maltose. The cell needs to separate the two molecules before it can use them for energy (convert sucrose into glucose, for example using an enzyme such as sucrase to convert sucrose into glucose).
3. *Oligosaccharides* are saccharide polymers containing a number of glucose molecules combined; examples are fructose and galactose. They are found in the cell membranes, where they play a role in cell to cell recognition such as a cell marker, like a name badge.
4. *Polysaccharides* are saccharides joined together like a chain necklace; examples are glycogen (stored glucose) and cellulose and chitin used for structure in the body.

Lipids Lipids are important for the structure of cell membranes, energy storage and the production of hormones. They are often referred to as fats and are divided into a number of categories, with the most common known as fatty acids and triglycerides.

1. Fatty acids form part of a lipid that is insoluble in water and is the building block for larger lipid molecules, examples are the prostaglandin molecules.
2. Glycerolipids are formed from one, two or three glycerol molecules of lipids to make mono-, di- or triglycerides.
3. Glycerophospholipids are phospholipids, which are the key components of the cell membrane – phospholipid bilayer. They are also involved in communication between cells and cell metabolism.
4. Sterol lipids are:
   - Cholesterol
   - Steroids, which function as hormones, examples are oestrogens, androgens (testosterone)
   - Signalling molecules
   - Forms of vitamin D
   - Bile acids derived from cholesterol.

Proteins Proteins are the building blocks for all the structures and the functioning mechanisms in the body. They are large, complex molecules comprised of amino acids and the chemical elements, carbon, hydrogen, oxygen and nitrogen. Many of these protein molecules will be stabilised with sulphur bridges. They have a wide diverse range of functions in the body depending on their structure, such as hormones, enzymes and transport molecules. For example the **iron** atom is transported in the blood stream by the protein transferrin and bilirubin is bound and transported by albumin.

Table 21.1

ORGANIC	INORGANIC
Make up one-third of the body	Make up two-thirds of the body
Carbohydrates (made up of smaller simple sugars)	Water
Lipids	Acids and bases
Proteins	Oxygen
Amino acids	Carbon dioxide
Nucleic acids	Nitrogen
Adenosine triphosphate (ATP)	

Jot This Down

Can you think of another function of serum albumin?

In the 'Jot This Down' exercise above, you might have thought about its role in maintaining the osmotic pressure of the blood. It acts like a sponge and holds onto the water in the blood. If your serum albumin level is reduced, the water content of the blood passes out of the blood stream into the interstitial fluid and the blood is unable to pull it back in from the tissue spaces, resulting in tissue oedema.

In the 'Jot This Down' exercise above, you might have thought about

- Glucose
- Ketones
- Blood
- Protein
- Specific gravity.

In the 'Jot This Down' exercise above, you might have thought about nephrotic syndrome (NS). Albumin is normally restricted from passing into the urine by cells called podocytes in the Bowman's capsule of the kidney. Nephrotic syndrome is a nonspecific kidney disorder, in which the podocytes have little holes in them and the albumin leaks through into the urine. This syndrome can be genetic in origin; other causes include inflammation in the kidney and nephropathy, caused by high blood sugar associated with diabetes.

Amino acids **Amino acids** play strategic roles as the building blocks of **proteins**. An individual amino acid is called a 'monomer' and when two or more combine, they form a more complex structure, which is often called a 'polymer'. There are 20 amino acids, which combine in a variety of ways to form all the different proteins. The body makes some amino acids – the others must be provided in the daily diet, as the body is unable to store them.

Amino acids made by the body are called **non-essential amino acids**:

- Alanine
- Arginine
- Aspartic acid
- Asparagine
- Cysteine
- Glutamic acid
- Glycine
- Proline
- Serine
- Tyrosine
- Selenocysteine.

Amino acids that need to be provided in the diet are called **essential amino acids**:

- Histidine
- Isoleucine
- Leucine
- Lysine
- Methionine
- Phenylalanine
- Threonine
- Tryptophan
- Valine.

In the 'Jot This Down' exercise above, you might have thought about:

- Animal proteins such as milk, cheese, eggs and meat
- Nuts and grains.

Adenosine triphosphate (ATP) ATP is the molecular unit of energy and is required for numerous cellular activities, such as muscle contraction, transport of substances across cell membranes, movement of chromosomes during cell division and making larger molecules from smaller units. Three phosphate atoms are bound to an adenosine molecule in aerobic cellular respiration. Glucose and oxygen are the fuels that the mitochondria use to drive the process which occurs in three key stages:

1. Glycolysis
2. Krebs cycle and the
3. Electron transport chain.

Moving on in the wave of molecules the way the amino acids are used to build proteins is planned and controlled by your genes.

The Genetic Level

Genes consist of another group of large molecules, called **DeoxyriboNucleic Acid** and **RiboNucleic Acid** (abbreviated as **DNA** and **RNA**, respectively). **Nucleic acids**, which are stored as these polymers, are the genetic machinery used by all cells, except mature red blood cells.

Red blood cells, which are devoid of any DNA, are produced in the red bone marrow from stem cells (see Figure 22.4). The development process of red blood cells (erythrocytes) is called erythropoieses and is stimulated by the hormone, erythropoietin, which is produced by epithelial cells in the kidney.

443

Erythrocytes are cells which have a specialised structure for transporting oxygen from the lungs to the cells. They also carry a percentage of carbon dioxide away from the cells to the lungs for exhaling. As they do not contain a nucleus or any organelles:

- They have more space for carrying haemoglobin and oxygen. Each erythrocyte contains about 280 million haemoglobin molecules. A haemoglobin molecule is made up of globin, composed of four polypeptide (long protein) chains, each of which is attached to a ring-like molecule called 'heme'
- They are not able to reproduce or carry out metabolic activities and so are not able to repair any damaged parts. They live for 120 days and then are destroyed and their parts recycled by the liver, spleen and red bone marrow
- They cannot be targeted by a virus (see Chapter 16).

Jot This Down

Can you think of a genetic condition which is linked to haemoglobin?

In the 'Jot This Down' exercise above, you might have thought of sickle cell disease, which is discussed below, by relating the structure of the red blood cell to its function. This is to introduce you to genetics and highlights the impact that the genetic level has on the behaviour of the cell and the general health of the individual. You may encounter words such as 'allele' that are unfamiliar to you and these will be explained after this section.

Sickle cell disease

The Evidence

Sickle cell disease affects 1 in every 2400 live births in England and in November 2010, was the most common genetic condition at birth.

Link To/Go To

Sickle Cell Disease in Childhood Standards and Guidelines for Clinical Care NHS 1332-SC-Clinical-Standards-WEB Public Health England.

http://www.sct.screening.nhs.uk/getdata.php?id=11187

Link To/Go To

Consultant haematologists stress it is important to have a knowledge of this condition in order to improve the patient experience by offering effective treatment outcomes for individuals with sickle cell disease and thalassaemia.

South Thames Sickle Cell & Thalassaemia network: http://www.ststn.co.uk/

British Society for Haematology: http://www.b-s-h.org.uk

King's College Hospital NHS, 1 January 2013: http://www .kch.nhs.uk/Doc/pl%20-%20591.1%20-%20the%20sickle%20 cell%20and%20thalassaemia%20service.pdf.

Sickle cell disease is an inherited blood disorder characterised by defective haemoglobin that occurs as the result of a mutation of the gene responsible for the structure of the protein, haemoglobin. The mutation varies and the number of haemoglobin cells that are involved varies according to the number of alleles with a mutation. Erythrocytes, which are carrying normal haemoglobin (Hb) are smooth, disc-shaped and flexible, which enables them to move through the blood vessels easily. After they are squeezed, as they pass along narrow capillaries, they stretch and relax back into shape. They are also able to alternate their shape from a normal–tight to a normal–relaxed conformation, as they pick up and unload oxygen.

Erythrocytes carrying abnormal haemoglobin are sticky and are formed into abnormal shapes like a sickle (crescent) or a C-shape after they have unloaded the oxygen they are carrying to the cells. This means that:

- The oxygen is unable to move into the erythrocyte and bind with the haemoglobin
- The erythrocytes stick together in clusters and block the smaller blood vessels (arteries and capillaries), which restricts the movement of normal oxygen carrying haemoglobin
- Clusters of the misshapen cells block larger blood vessels and thus impair blood supply to the cells
- Sickle cells have a shorter life span and are destroyed by the spleen because of their abnormal shape. The spleen is also damaged by the abnormal cells which in turn compromise the spleens ability to function normally and fight infections.

The most common variations of the sickle cell gene include:

1. *Sickle cell trait*: 1 'sickle allele' + 1 normal haemoglobin allele, whereby an individual has both normal haemoglobin (Hb) and sickle cell haemoglobin (HbS)
2. *Sickle cell anaemia*: 2 'sickle alleles', whereby an individual has all sickle haemoglobin (HbSS)
3. *Sickle cell-haemoglobin C and E* are variations either in the structure of the erythrocyte or the haemoglobin and are relatively rare
4. *Haemoglobin S-beta-thalassaemia*: 1 'sickle allele + 1 thalassaemia allele, whereby an individual has both sickle and thalassaemia haemoglobin.

Jot This Down

Can you think of the complications that an individual with sickle cell disease may experience?

In the 'Jot This Down' exercise above, you might have thought about:

- Fatigue
- Breathlessness
- Dizziness
- Delayed wound healing
- Delayed growth and development due to anaemia (reduced life span of abnormal erythrocytes and haemoglobin) and the lack of oxygen as the abnormality inhibits the ability of haemoglobin to carry oxygen
- Pain, which occurs when the cells do not receive enough oxygen

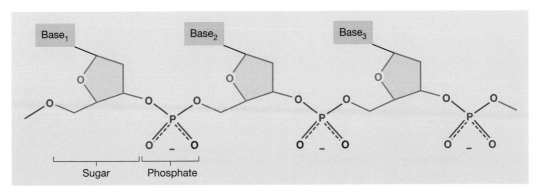

Figure 21.3 Showing the alternating deoxyribose (sugar) molecule and phosphate group with the nucleotides (bases) attached in a small portion of the DNA molecule.

What the Experts Say

Patients describe the pain as sharp, throbbing, shooting or burning.

Nursing Fields Paediatrics

In children younger than 3 years of age, dactylitis (painful swelling of the fingers and toes) can occur. Pain can affect any area, although as the child grows, pain is most often in the sternum and ribs (chest), arms and legs, pelvis and abdomen.

- Violent coughing and fever, called 'acute chest syndrome', when the small blood vessels in the lungs are blocked with clusters of sickle cells causing damage to the cells and tissues in the lungs
- Stroke, due to impaired blood supply as the misshaped erythrocytes can block larger blood vessels
- Jaundice, as sickle cells have short life spans and are destroyed by the spleen more readily. The liver is unable to recycle them quickly enough and the bilirubin (by-product of erythrocytes) builds up in the filtering system and blood stream
- Increased incidence of infections
- Leg ulcers
- Bone damage
- Gall stones
- Impaired eye sight due to eye damage.

All these physiological impairments come from **one** misplaced amino acid in a single protein in **one** type of cell! This abnormality is caused by a mutation, which is a permanent change in the DNA sequence of the gene responsible for the structure of haemoglobin.

We have discussed the exception to the rule and apart from the erythrocytes, all human cells contain a complete set of the DNA and RNA molecules, which consist of sugars, phosphates and nucleosides. There are five different nucleo**sides**; adenosine, guanosine, cytidine, thymidine and uridine. When a nucleoside is combined with a sugar, deoxyribose or ribose, and a phosphate group, they are called nucleo**tides** and are commonly referred to as nitrogenous bases. These bases, now labelled adenine (A), guanine (G), cytosine (C), thymine (T) and uracil (U), are either purines or pyrimidines and are the building blocks of the DNA and RNA nucleic acids.

RNA is present in the cytoplasm of the cell and in particularly high concentrations in the nucleolus of the nucleus. DNA, on the other hand, is found mainly in the chromosomes, which are in the nucleus. DNA is formed from the bases A, G, C and T, whereas RNA is formed from A, G, C and U.

DNA

The four bases are arranged in long sequences attached to a backbone, which consists of the monosaccharide molecule, deoxyribose and a phosphate group of molecules attached alternatively in a chain and gives the molecule its name – deoxyribonucleic acid (Figure 21.3).

The arrangement of the bases in the DNA molecule is not random. The purines are structured with two aromatic rings and the pyrimidines have a single aromatic ring. The number of rings in the structures determines the size of the bases (Figure 21.4a) and it is the size of the bases that dictates the pairing in the DNA structure. The DNA molecule consists of two complimentary strands, with the bases significantly paired, one large base (purine) with one small (pyrimidine) base to create the two strands. The purine bases are 'G' and 'A', and the pyrimidine bases are 'T' ('U' in RNA) and 'C'. The hydrogen bonding between the two bases further determines the specific purine and pyrimidine bonding, which forms the complimentary base-pairs:

- 'A' always pairs with 'T' ('U' in RNA) because they join with two hydrogen bonds and
- 'G' always pairs with 'C', with three hydrogen bonds.

As in linking fingers – A and T (U) link with two fingers and G and C have three fingers (Figure 21.4b).

Picture a staircase with the deoxyribose as the banisters and the nucleotides (bases) as the steps (Figure 21.5). The banisters run in opposite directions and if you split the two strands apart, you will know how to create a new strand as opposite A you will always pair a T and vice versa and opposite a G you will always pair a C and vice versa, so each strand acts as a template for the other. This is the way the patterns for genes are stored.

As the DNA is too large to be stored as an open staircase, it is coiled into a helical structure, which resembles a spiral staircase and like a spiral staircase the banisters must be symmetrical.

If you pair two of the smaller single ring bases the step will be narrower and create a bend or kink inwards, similarly if you pair

445

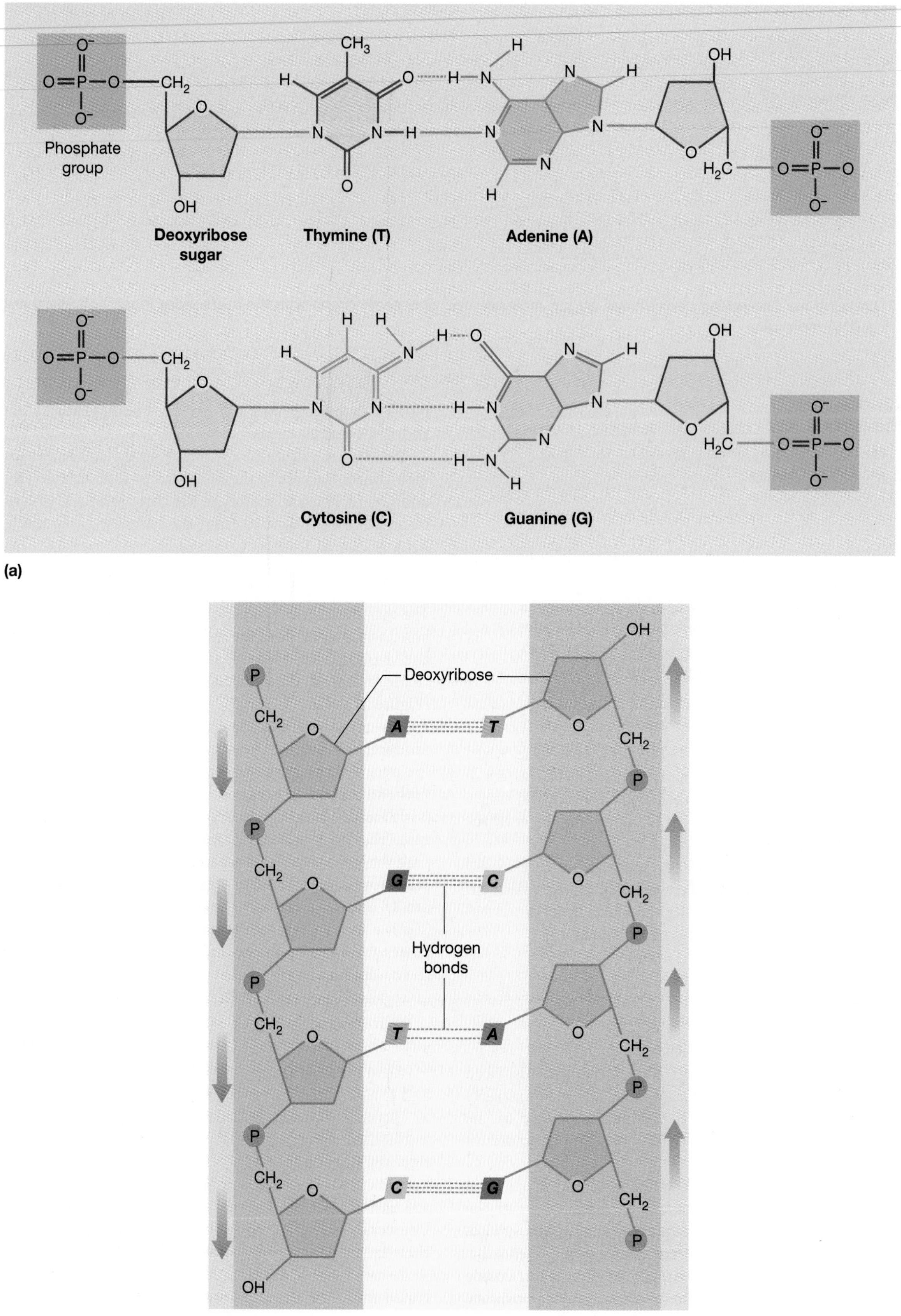

(a)

(b)

Figure 21.4 (a) A nucleotide consists of a base, 5-C sugar and a phosphate group. (b) A and T pair with 2 hydrogen bonds, while C and G pair with 3 bonds.

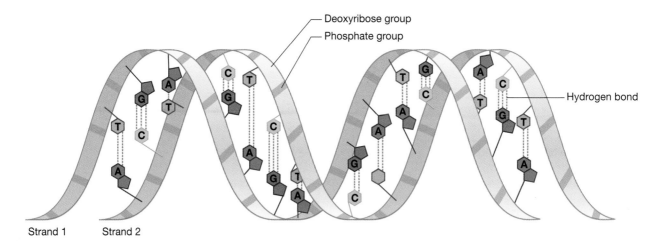

Figure 21.5 **DNA base-pairing: paired bases face towards the centre of the double helix. The structure is stabilised by the hydrogen bonds between base-pairs.**

two of the larger molecules together it will be wider and create a bulge outwards. Both of these mismatches are called lesions and are visible when the molecule folds. When the protein, DNA, is put away for storage, it is termed **folding** into the helical structure, which is a uniform double stranded helix.

Jot This Down

Can you think of an environmental factor that induces lesions in the DNA pairing?

In the 'Jot This Down' exercise above, you might have thought about toxic chemicals or radiation (UV light and X-rays).

When a lesion occurs, two pathways can occur (Pagès & Fuchs 2002).

1. Enzymes allow the lesions to be bypassed so that they are not copied

2. They are copied and cause mutations, which can cause cancer.

When the DNA is folded into the helical structure, the helix is wound round proteins called histones, which together form nucleosomes. 'Scaffolding proteins' organise the nucleosome-bound DNA into the structures that we see under a microscope as a chromosome. Each (double) strand of DNA along with its associated scaffolding proteins and its folds gives the chromosome its shape.

These proteins help to keep the DNA 'condensed' in much the same way that a spool keeps a long length of thread condensed. The spool termed the 'nucleosome' is the functioning part of DNA, the lengths of DNA in between the nucleosomes is termed the 'linker DNA'. When the DNA is stored it is termed a 'genome'.

It is estimated that there are approximately 30 000 genes in the nuclear genome. The distribution of these genes varies greatly between chromosomal regions, for example chromosomes 19 and 22 are gene-rich, whereas 4 and 18 are relatively gene-poor. The size of genes also shows great variability from small genes, with single exons to genes with up to 79 exons. An **exon** is that part of the DNA that is used both for the coding and support of a gene, the rest of the DNA that is not being used at the time of coding is called an intron. In an undividing cell, the genetic material is known as chromatin.

There are two types of nuclear division in a dividing cell: **mitosis** and **meiosis**.

Mitosis is the process of cell duplication or reproduction with nuclear division when one cell divides and reproduces two genetically identical daughter cells in one step.

Meiosis is a very specialised type of nuclear division and reproduction in which the number of chromosomes are reduced (halved), resulting in four gametes (sperm or ova). Meiosis occurs in two steps. The genetic material is diverse and occurs only in cells that will become **gametes**.

Mitosis

There are two distinct events named 'interphase' and 'mitosis', often discussed under the heading of **mitosis**.

The DNA is replicated each time the cell divides. The DNA is the control centre and issues all the instructions when building proteins. The process of cell division or cell reproduction in somatic cells (a somatic cell is any cell that is not a gamete or stem cell) involves the division of the nucleus termed **mitosis** and division of the cytoplasm called **cytokinesis**. This creates two new 'daughter' cells, which are identical to the original cell, each with the same number of chromosomes: 46 in total, made of 23 pairs. As they have two sets (23 pairs) of chromosomes, they are called 'diploid cells' with the two chromosomes that make up each pair called **homologous** chromosomes and, apart from the sex chromosomes, are viewed microscopically as very similar. In the female, the homologous pair of sex chromosomes consists of two X chromosomes, whereas in the male, the pair consists of an X and a Y chromosome.

447

The Evidence

Homologous chromosomes are pairs of chromosomes that are in the same position on the DNA and have genes of the same characteristic in the same loci (location); one chromosome inherited from the mother and one chromosome from the father. They are not necessarily identical but carry the same type of information. For example the gene that codes for hair colour from the maternal chromosome will pair with the gene for hair colour from the paternal chromosome and the dominant gene with respect to hair colour will dictate the hair colour of the gamete (child). All genes have a continuum, ranging from dominant to recessive with dark blue-black hair as dominant and white as recessive.

Before the cell can divide, all the chromosomes must be copied, which is termed **DNA replication**.

This process of producing two identical copies occurs during the interphase, which consists of three stages, G_1, G_2 and S, each lasting for 8 hours. During this interphase, the cell is producing additional organelles and cytosolic components along with DNA replication over this period. This is in readiness for when the cell divides into two daughter cells during the mitotic phase (mitosis). These two phases (the interphase and mitotic phase) make up the cell cycle, which is an orderly sequence of events, guided and controlled by enzymes.

During division of the nucleus, two enzymes, helicase and polymerase, work in unison with the helicases, preparing the DNA for the polymerase to guide the copying of the DNA.

Link To/Go To

Click on *Exercise 23: DNA Replication* at:

http://www.wiley.com/college/pratt/0471393878/instructor/exercises/index.html

- The DNA helicases unwind and separate the two strands of the DNA double helix at multiple positions along the strands called 'origins', forming a series of bifurcated Y-shaped structures known as **replication forks**.
- The DNA polymerases then initiate and guide the copying of the DNA strand at these points known as 'origins of replication'. Polymerase is thus responsible for the making of a complementary DNA strand through specific base-pairing, resulting in two daughter DNA helices that are identical to the original parent molecule.

DNA replication in these individual replication units takes place at different times in the S stage of the interphase of the cell cycle (Figure 21.6).

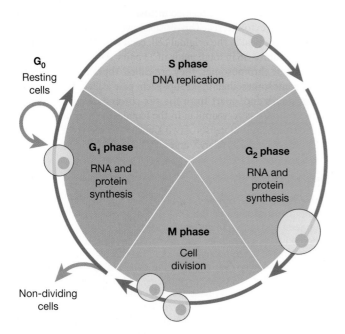

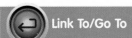

Figure 21.6 Stages of the cell cycle.

There are 15 different DNA polymerases and, while they are specialised for replication, it is evident that many point (origins of replication) mutations that occur in malignancies arise when the polymerases either misread the signposts or misguide the copying (Lange *et al.* 2011). Enzymes are subjected to wear and tear, just like the rest of the body cells and tissues, with use and ageing and sometimes they become worn out.

On the opposite side of the coin, some of the polymerases are beneficial and can suppress the potential cancer sites.

What the Experts Say

" Polymerases are potential targets for therapeutic strategies.

Link To/Go To

http://www.nature.com/nrc/journal/v11/n2/abs/nrc2998.html

During the G_1, which is the interval between the mitotic and the S phase, the cell is actively replicating its organelles and cytosolic components. After cell division, the G_2 phase, which is the interval between the S phase and the beginning of the mitotic phase, cell growth continues. Enzymes and other proteins are made, all in preparation for cell division. Centrosomes, which organise and regulate the cell cycle progression, have completed their replication, which started during the G_1 phase.

When cells divide, the genetic information is conserved and transmitted unchanged to each daughter cell during the mitotic phase of the cell cycle.

The chromatin condenses into discrete chromosomes, which can then be seen clearly through a microscope during cell division. During most stages, we see the chromosomes as X-shaped objects composed of two chromatids, which are like arms and legs. One arm and one leg makes one chromatin and the other arm and leg, then forms the chromatid. Because they are identical, the two chromatids are called sister chromatids. The ends of the chromatids are called **telomeres** (*telos* is Greek for 'end') and the point where they are joined is called a **centromere**, although it is not always at the centre.

Along with the nuclear division (mitosis), cytoplasmic division (cytokinesis) is also completed.

During mitosis (Figure 21.7), which is a continuous process over four stages: **prophase, metaphase, anaphase and telophase**, the duplicate copies of the contents of the nucleus are moved into discrete separate poles within the cell, supported by microtubules called 'mitotic spindles'. In the final stage of telophase, the identical sets of chromosomes revert to the chromatin from within a newly formed nuclear envelope. The spindles break up and the cytoplasm is divided into two by the indentation of the plasma membrane, with a nucleus in each. At the end of telophase, we have two complete identical 'daughter cells'.

When you damage a cell due to injury or it wears out naturally, the process of interphase and mitosis produces new replacement cells. Mitosis is a crucial part of the cell cycle, dependent on a series of crucially timed movements and activities, which are controlled

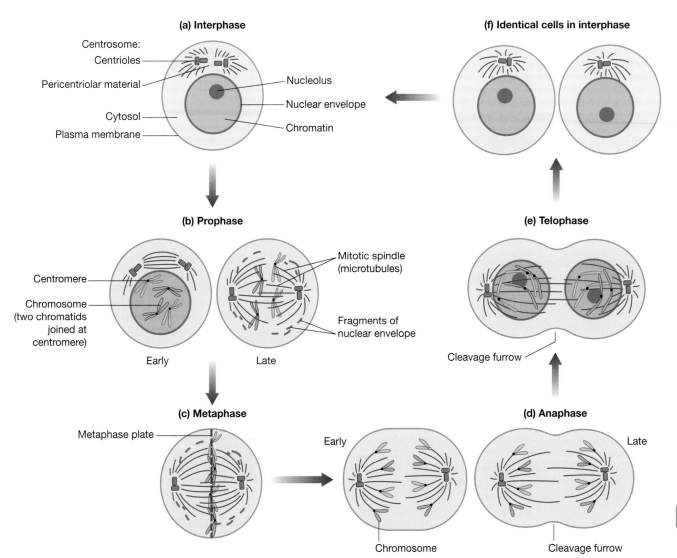

Figure 21.7 Stages of mitosis.

by the genes within the cells that are replicating and dividing. If this control goes wrong, it can replicate itself to make new cells that are incorrectly made, which then become out of control. It is these out of control cells that can become cancerous with unstable chromosomes. Remember we looked earlier at the effects of UV radiation and DNA polymerase. Sometimes, the polymerases do bypass these mistakes or even negate them.

Jot This Down

Can you think of the sources of UV radiation (light) that can damage the DNA and what you would tell someone who is sunburnt to watch out for?

In the 'Jot This Down' exercise above, you might have thought about sunlight and tanning beds. One of the first signs of significant damage, is an alteration in any of your moles. These may change colour, size or texture.

Red Flag

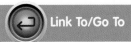

If a mole changes in any way or a new mole appears, go to your GP.

Moles are small patches on your skin and are collections of cells called 'melanocytes'. Moles are potentially cancerous and can cause melanoma if the sunlight damages those genes that control how and when the cells grow and divide in the mole.

Link To/Go To

Be sun smart NHS videos.

http://www.nhs.uk/Conditions/cancer-of-the-skin/pages/Introduction.aspx

Meiosis

The production of gametes, gametogenesis, is termed 'spermatogenesis' in the male and is the process by which male primordial germ cells undergo meiosis, and produce sperm cells. In the female, a similar process termed oogenesis occurs with the production of an ovum.

In sexual reproduction, the union between a sperm cell and an ovum cell (called **gametes**) produces a 'zygote'. We know that each cell has a total of 46 chromosomes (23 pairs) and if you had that number of chromosomes in the gametes you would have a zygote with 92 chromosomes (46 pairs), which is not viable. A process of meiosis, also known as 'reduction division', occurs in specialised organs known as the 'gonads'. Meiosis halves the number of chromosomes in the egg and sperm cells with the production of four haploid gametes. 'Haploid' means they contain 22 pairs of chromosomes with the set of sex chromosomes making a total of 23 pairs. They are called 'sex chromosomes' as they determine the sex of the baby. While the female always produces an X, the male can produce either an X or a Y and thus it is the male who determines the sex of the baby; XX is female and XY is male (Figure 21.8). The male

gonads are called 'testes' and in the female, the gonads are called 'ovaries'.

Meiosis (Figure 21.9) is divided into the four phases: **prophase I, metaphase I, anaphase I, telophase I**.

During the first phase or step of meiosis, the paired chromatids are split. Prior to the start of meiosis I, there is an interphase period when DNA replication occurs with each chromosome having two genetically identical chromatids attached at their centromere (a total of 46 chromosomes written as '2n'). During prophase 1, the two sister chromatids of each pair of homologous chromosomes come together and then pair off and segregate into separate cells, so that gametes finish up with only one set of each type of chromosome, instead of the normal two. Parts of the chromatids of two-paired homologous chromosomes may be exchanged with one another, which is termed 'crossing over'.

This mixing and matching (Figure 21.10) produces genetically different chromatids, different both from those in the starting cell and from each other. The net effect of meiosis I is that each cell has one of the replicated chromosomes from each homologous pairs of chromosomes (23 chromosomes written as 'n').

During meiosis when chromosomes become intertwined, there is plenty of opportunity for various kinds of structural aberration to take place.

For example:

- A chromosome may break in two places and the section in between may drop out, taking all its genes with it. The two ends then join up giving a shorter chromosome with a chunk missing in the middle which is called **deletion**
- A chromosome may break in two places and the middle bit then turns round and joins up again, so the normal sequence of genes is reversed, which is called **inversion**
- A section of one chromosome breaks off and becomes attached to another chromosome, which is called **translocation**
- A section of the chromosome replicates so that a set of genes is repeated and this is called **duplication**
- The addition or loss of one or more whole chromosome – the two homologous chromosomes, instead of separating go off into the same gamete. This results in half of the gametes having two of the chromosomes and the other half of the gametes having none.

The fusion of the first kind of gamete that has two of the chromosomes with a normal gamete of the other sex, will give an extra one and is known as **trisomy**.

The fusion of the second kind of gamete without the chromosome with a normal gamete, will give an individual with only one of this particular type of chromosome.

- **Down's syndrome** is caused by the presence of an extra chromosome number 21.

Also caused by non-disjunction are various sex-chromosome abnormalities such as:

- **Klinefelter's syndrome** – caused by the genetic constitution XXY when the X chromosome has failed to separate during oogenesis
- **Turner's syndrome** – where an X or Y chromosome is missing.

Meiosis I proceeds directly, without going through interphase, to meiosis II, which has four stages analogous with meiosis I: prophase II, metaphase II, anaphase II and telophase II.

This second part of meiosis, meiosis II, begins with two haploid cells and through a process similar to mitosis, produces four haploid cells. These four haploid cells are genetically different from

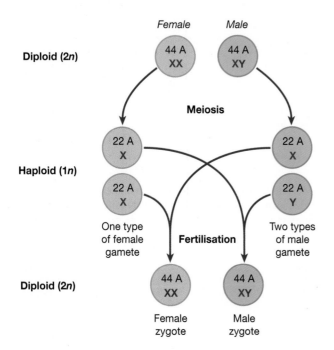

Figure 21.8 Stages of meiosis.

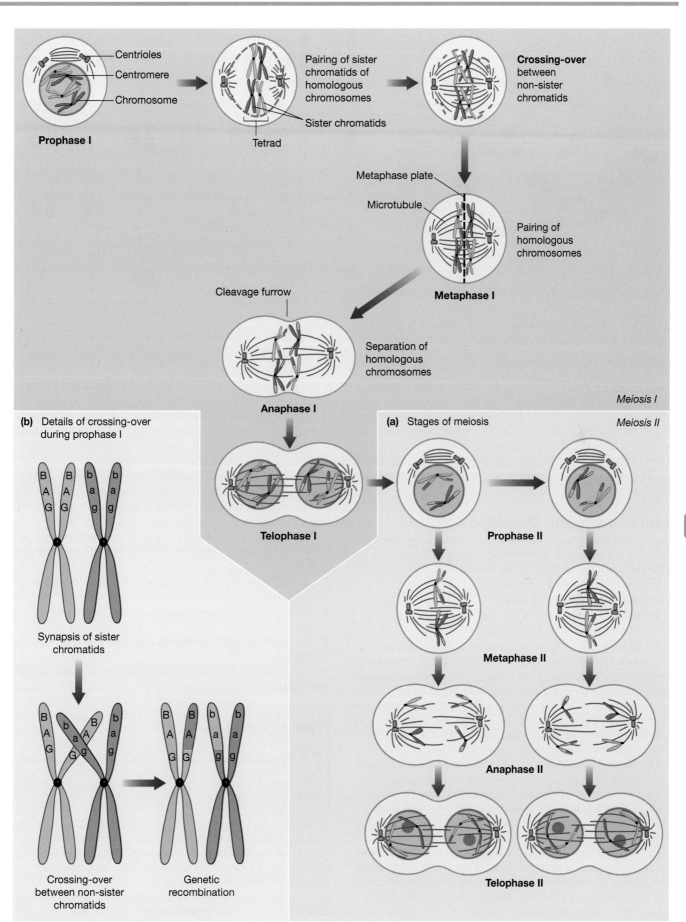

Figure 21.9 **Meiosis, reproductive cell division.**

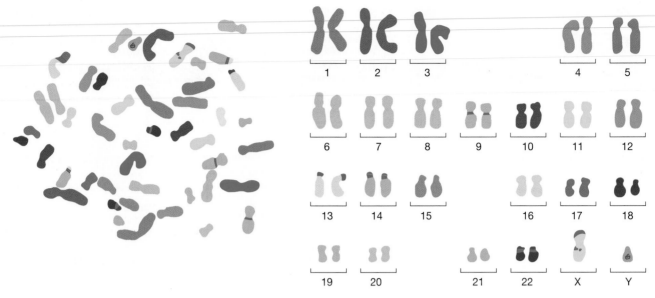

Figure 21.10 Mixing and matching: note chromosome 13 and 22.

one another, with the number of chromosomes remaining unchanged from the beginning until the end of meiosis II ($n = 23$) with single chromatics. These haploid cells become unfertilised eggs in females and sperm in males. The genetic differences, due to random arrangements during crossing-over in meiosis, lead to the genetically different composition in each cell and ensure that siblings of the same parents are never entirely genetically identical.

Fetal Growth and Development

A zygote will grow into a fully functioning human being and is the beginning of growth and development. It contains information for making all the different types of cells characteristic of you and me.

Life *in utero* consists of three phases:

1. Pre-embryonic (the first 3 weeks)
2. Embryonic (until the end of the eighth week)
3. Fetal (from eight weeks until term).

Soon after fertilisation, the zygote enters a phase of mitotic division, called cleavage, which is an essential part of the formation of the blastomere and leads to the creation of a population of cells that are all the same. By the end of the third day, there are 16 blastomeres and with successive cleavage, a solid sphere of blastomeres called the 'morula' is produced. The cells in the blastomere still carry all the genetic details to make all the different cells, both in terms of structure and function, in the human being.

The number of cells in the morula continues to multiply until at the 32-cell stage, the fluid that has been nourishing the cells is accumulated internally into a fluid filled sac and forms the 'blastula'. The blastula is a hollow ball of cells, the cavity is called a 'blastocoele' and the ball of cells and the cavity is now called a 'blastocyst'. About six days after the zygote is formed, the blastocyst attaches to the endometrium (the wall of the uterus) and implantation begins. The developing embryo eventually receives its nourishment from the area of implantation. During the formation of the blastocyst, the cells begin to take on different characteristics and two distinct cell populations arise:

- The embryoblast cells on the inside of the blastocyst
- The trophoblast cells form the outer superficial layer that completes the sphere like wall of the blastocyst. These cells will form the 'chorion', which is the basis of the fetal part of the placenta. The developing cells will receive nutrients from the placental cells.

During the third week of development, there is a clear difference in the way different classes of cells grow and mature, which is the start of cell differentiation. During this stage, cells begin to lose the ability to produce all the different cell types in the body.

The blastocyst – the cells begin to differentiate into three primary germ layers, each of which develops into a particular mass of cells:

1. The outermost layer, **the ectoderm** – forms the skin and nervous system
2. The middle layer, **the mesoderm** – forms the muscles and skeletal structures
3. The innermost layer, **the endoderm** – forms the internal organs and gut.

This process of movement into the three layers is called 'gastrulation'.

What the Experts Say

" Gastrulation is the period in embryonic development when the cells form the embryo, when the body plan of you is established; the most important time of your life – more important than birth, marriage and death. (Lewis Wolpert 1969)

A **homeobox** is a DNA sequence found within genes that are involved in the regulation of development (morphogenesis) of you and I. Genes that have a homeobox are called **homeobox genes** and are from the **homeobox gene family**.

A homeobox is about 180 base-pairs long and it encodes a protein domain (the **homeodomain**), which can bind DNA.

452

Homeobox genes encode transcription factors, which typically switch on cascades of other genes, for instance all the ones needed to make a leg. Hence, if one of the genes in a homeobox is faulty, it is likely to affect the cascade of genes, resulting in a pattern of abnormalities in development when compared with a single gene.

A particular subgroup of homeobox genes are the **Hox genes**, which are found in a special gene cluster, the **Hox cluster** (also called the 'Hox complex'). Hox genes function in patterning the body axis and tell the home cell where in the body it is. Thus, by providing the identity of particular body regions, Hox genes determine where limbs and other body segments will grow in a developing fetus. Mutations in any one of these genes can lead to:

- The growth of extra typically non-functional body parts, such as the duplication of a digit (polydactyl) resulting in six or more fingers or toes on one hand or foot, respectively
- Disruption in the development of the brainstem, inner ear or cardiovascular system
- Autism
- Malformed genitals
- Limb malformations
- Premature actions, such as early fusion of cranial sutures, which impairs brain growth and development
- Failure of cells to fuse together resulting in growth defects.

Nursing Fields Paediatrics

Anencephaly is the absence of a major portion of the brain, skull and scalp that occurs during development. Most fetuses do not survive.

Anencephaly is a neural tube defect caused by the interaction of multiple genetic and environmental factors. One of these genes is one that provides instructions for making a protein that is involved in processing the B vitamin folate called folic acid (Safra *et al.* 2013).

Jot This Down

Can you think of another neural tube defect which is a central nervous system malformation secondary to a failure of closure or development of the neural tube?

In the 'Jot This Down' exercise above, you might have thought of spina bifida.

The neural tube starts to develop when some of the mesodermal and endodermal cells signal some of the ectodermal cells to change shape (elongate) to form the neural plate cells. These cells grow into a tube-like structure, which later represents the spinal cord with the top end growing into your brain and the bottom end, the tail of your spine. If the top end is malformed or does not close, the brain is malformed as in anencephaly, and failure of the bottom end results in spina bifida.

Cell Differentiation

If the two cells from the first cell division are separated using a fine hair, each will go to form a complete embryo. This separation sometimes happens naturally and results in the formation of identical or monozygotic twin fetuses. Although each cell would normally go on to produce only half an embryo, separated they produce a whole one. Any cell isolated from an embryo up to the eight-cell stage has the remarkable ability to reconstitute a complete embryo. A single cell separated and isolated from the embryo after the eight-cell stage will not generate a whole embryo.

What this means is that up until the eight-cell stage (that is the third-cell division in mitosis) the individual cells are still sufficiently similar so that any one of them can develop into a complete embryo.

However, if this were the only mechanism of differentiation, then a cell that had been removed from the eight-cell stage embryo would not replace the seven missing cells before continuing to divide and develop – it would simply divide and differentiate from the stage it had reached but would not develop into a whole embryo.

This shows that the early embryo is not made up of a defined set of cells, each of which follows its own predetermined course of differentiation. The environment of each cell is significant and this is relevant in all areas of cell growth. Throughout development, the interactions of cells play an important role in controlling differentiation. The inability of cells isolated from the embryo after the eight-cell stage indicates that, as development proceeds, the capacity of cells to change their course of development decreases.

This cell regulation (the ability of the pre eight-cell isolated cell to develop normally) is not confined to the pre eight-cell stage. For example, if part of the forebrain of a rabbit is removed from the developing embryo at day 13, then the adult rabbit will have a normal brain – the remaining cells adjust their development to replace the missing cells. However, if the whole forebrain rudiment is removed or it is removed at too late a stage, the animal will be missing its forebrain.

This suggests that particular populations of cells act together to form specific regions of the brain and that damage to part of such a cooperative system will result in regulation and regeneration of the damaged region.

This illustrates that the developing cell is influenced by its immediate environment and that cells must be able to detect and respond to the presence of adjacent cells. There is some sort of communication between cells. This interaction involves messages, which are chemical in nature, passing between cells.

Experimentation reveals that tissue from regions other than the blastopore (the blastocyst becomes a 'blastopore' when the three layers of cells appear) does not produce a second complete embryo. Also, that tissue taken at a later stage of development from the mesodermal and endodermal blastopore regions does not produce a complete embryo.

This result suggests that the chemical messages produced by the mesodermal and endodermal blastopore region are different from those produced by the ectodermal blastopore region and other regions in the developing embryo.

This suggests that not only do we have a tissue sending a message but also a tissue able to receive that message. Cellular differentiation is complex and involves the timing of transcription and translation at particular times during development coordinated by communication between developing cells. The environment, mentioned earlier, of the cell also determines its development and differentiation.

Now consider shapes – your hand and arm are different for example. The process of formation of shapes and the generation of new patterns is called 'morphogenesis' and involves cells having different structures and shapes, for example a neuron has an axon whereas a hepatocyte (liver cell) is oblong in shape.

453

Although the genetic make-up of the fetus principally determines its growth and development, other influences – both stimulatory and inhibitory – are superimposed on the genetic program. During the first half of pregnancy, the fetus's own genetic program is the primary determinant of growth, constraining patterns of growth. During the second half, the patterns of growth and development are more variable. The four primary epigenetic factors at work during the second half of pregnancy are placental, hormonal, environmental (such as maternal nutrition, disease, drugs, altitude) and metabolic (such as diabetes). Epigenetic means the control of changes in gene function that do not involve changes in DNA sequences so the DNA produces a normal gene that has its way of working altered. If the DNA was altered, the gene would be a mutation.

Genetic Disorders

Gene tests (also called 'DNA-based tests'), the newest and most sophisticated of the techniques used to test for genetic disorders, involve direct examination of the DNA molecule itself. Other genetic tests include biochemical tests for such gene products as enzymes and other proteins and for microscopic examination of stained or fluorescent chromosomes.

Some DNA-based gene tests

- **Adult polycystic kidney disease** (APKD; kidney failure and liver disease)
- **Alpha-1-antitrypsin deficiency** (AAT; emphysema and liver disease)
- **Amyotrophic lateral sclerosis** (ALS; Lou Gehrig's disease; progressive motor function loss leading to paralysis and death)
- **Alzheimer's disease** (APOE; late-onset variety of senile dementia)
- **Ataxia telangiectasia** (AT; progressive brain disorder resulting in loss of muscle control and cancers)
- **Gaucher disease** (GD; enlarged liver and spleen, bone degeneration)
- **Inherited breast and ovarian cancer** (BRCA 1 and 2; early-onset tumors of breasts and ovaries)
- **Hereditary non-polyposis colon cancer** (CA; early-onset tumors of colon and sometimes other organs)
- **Charcot–Marie–Tooth** (CMT; loss of feeling in ends of limbs)
- **Congenital adrenal hyperplasia** (CAH; hormone deficiency; ambiguous genitalia and male pseudohermaphroditism)
- **Cystic fibrosis** (CF; disease of lung and pancreas resulting in thick mucous accumulations and chronic infections)
- **Duchenne muscular dystrophy/Becker muscular dystrophy** (DMD; severe to mild muscle wasting, deterioration, weakness)
- **Dystonia** (DYT; muscle rigidity, repetitive twisting movements)
- **Fanconi anaemia, group C** (FA; anaemia, leukaemia, skeletal deformities)
- **Factor V-Leiden** (FVL; blood-clotting disorder)
- **Fragile X syndrome** (FRAX; leading cause of inherited mental retardation)
- **Haemophilia A and B** (HEMA and HEMB; bleeding disorders)
- **Hereditary haemochromatosis** (HFE; excess iron storage disorder)
- **Huntington's disease** (HD; usually midlife onset; progressive, lethal, degenerative neurological disease)
- **Myotonic dystrophy** (MD; progressive muscle weakness; most common form of adult muscular dystrophy)
- **Neurofibromatosis type 1** (NF1; multiple benign nervous system tumors that can be disfiguring; cancers)
- **Phenylketonuria** (PKU; progressive mental retardation due to missing enzyme; correctable by diet)
- **Prader Willi/Angelman syndromes** (PW/A; decreased motor skills, cognitive impairment, early death)
- **Sickle cell disease** (SS; blood cell disorder; chronic pain and infections)
- **Spinocerebellar ataxia, type 1** (SCA1; involuntary muscle movements, reflex disorders, explosive speech)
- **Spinal muscular atrophy** (SMA; severe, usually lethal progressive muscle-wasting disorder in children)
- **Thalassaemias** (THAL; anaemias – reduced red blood cell levels)
- **Tay–Sachs disease** (TS; fatal neurological disease of early childhood; seizures, paralysis).

As the mitochondrium has its own set of DNA, referred to as mitochondrial DNA, it has its own set of inherited diseases, known as primary mitochondrial diseases.

Mitochondrial Inheritance

Each cell contains thousands of copies of mitochondrial DNA, with more being found in cells that have high energy requirements, such as brain and muscle. 'Mitochondria', and therefore their DNA, are inherited almost exclusively from the mother through the oocyte. Mitochondrial DNA has a higher rate of spontaneous mutation than nuclear DNA and the accumulation of mutations in mitochondrial DNA has been proposed as being responsible for some of the somatic effects seen with ageing.

In humans, *cytoplasmic* or *mitochondrial inheritance* has been proposed as a possible explanation for the pattern of inheritance observed in some rare disorders that affect both males and females but are transmitted only through females, so-called maternal or matrilineal inheritance A number of rare disorders with unusual combinations of neurological and myopathic features, sometimes occurring in association with other conditions, such as cardiomyopathy and conduction defects, diabetes or deafness, have been characterised as being due to mutations in mitochondrial genes. An example is muscular dystrophy.

Jot This Down
What do you think muscular dystrophy is?
Can you think of three interventions that you would implement in a patient with this disease?

In the 'Jot This Down' exercise above, you might have thought about:

Muscular dystrophy – It is a genetic (inherited) progressive condition that gradually causes the muscles to weaken. It often affects a particular group of muscles, before moving on to other muscles. This leads to an increasing level of disability. There are a number of types of muscular dystrophy, such as Duchenne and Becker. Patients with muscular dystrophy need regular exercises and assistance with mobility to maintain independence. They also require emotional support, which must be tailored for each individual.

Mitochondria have an important role in cellular metabolism through oxidative phosphorylation – it is not surprising that the organs most susceptible to mitochondrial mutations are the central nervous system, skeletal muscle and heart. In most persons, the mitochondrial DNA from different mitochondria is identical, or shows what is termed **homoplasmy**. If a mutation occurs in the mitochondrial DNA of an individual, initially there will be two populations of mitochondrial DNA, so-called **heteroplasmy**. The proportion of mitochondria with a mutation in their DNA varies between cells and tissues and this, together with mutational heterogeneity, is a possible explanation for the range of phenotypic severity seen in persons affected with mitochondrially inherited disorders. While matrilineal inheritance applies to disorders that are directly due to mutations in mitochondrial DNA, it is also very important to be aware that mitochondrial *proteins* are mainly encoded by nuclear genes. Mutations in the nuclear genes can have a devastating impact on respiratory chain functions within mitochondria. Examples include genes encoding proteins within the cytochrome-c (COX) system, which follow autosomal recessive inheritance, and the *G4.5* (*TAZ*) gene that is X-linked and causes Barth syndrome (endocardial fibroelastosis) in males.

1. Mendelian, or single-gene, disorders can be inherited in five ways: autosomal dominant, autosomal recessive, X-linked dominant, X-linked recessive and Y-linked inheritance.

2. Autosomal dominant alleles are manifest in the heterozygous state and are usually transmitted from one generation to the next but can occasionally arise as a new mutation. They usually affect both males and females equally. Each offspring of a parent with an autosomal dominant gene has a one in two chance of inheriting it from the affected parent. Autosomal dominant alleles can exhibit reduced penetrance, variable expressivity and sex limitation.

3. Autosomal recessive disorders are only manifest in the homozygous state and normally only affect individuals in one generation, usually in one sibship in a family. They affect both males and females equally. Offspring of parents who are heterozygous for the same autosomal recessive allele have a one in four chance of being homozygous for that allele. The less common an autosomal recessive allele, the greater the likelihood that the parents of a homozygote are consanguineous.

4. X-linked recessive alleles are normally only manifest in males. Offspring of females heterozygous for an X-linked recessive allele have a one in two chance of inheriting the allele from their mother. Daughters of males with an X-linked recessive allele are obligate heterozygotes but sons cannot inherit the allele. Rarely, females manifest an X-linked recessive trait because they are homozygous for the allele, have a single X chromosome, have a structural rearrangement of one of their X chromosomes, or are heterozygous but show skewed or non-random X-inactivation.

5. There are only a few disorders known to be inherited in an X-linked dominant manner. In X-linked dominant disorders, hemizygous males are more severely affected than heterozygous females.

Unusual features in single-gene patterns of inheritance can be explained by phenomena, such as genetic heterogeneity, mosaicism, anticipation, imprinting, uniparental disomy and mitochondrial inheritance.

Genetic diseases – caused by an error in a single gene in the DNA. These are 'pure' genetic diseases. They are strongly inherited from parents, and usually have very clear patterns of inheritance – cystic fibrosis, muscular dystrophy and dwarfism (achondroplasia).

Chromosome diseases – caused by a major error in the DNA, with an entire chromosome having a problem. Chromosomes have hundreds and thousands of genes, so these diseases have major errors in the DNA code. The most common example is Down syndrome.

Polygenic diseases – 'multiple genes' influence of multiple genes as opposed to a single gene. Usually this means that a disease does not have a high level of genetic causes, and is not strongly inherited down families, but there may be a slight familial inheritance pattern. In fact, saying a disease is polygenic is almost like saying it is 'mostly non-genetic'. Many of the big name diseases are in this class of diseases including cancers, heart disease, autoimmune diseases, and many others. With most of these conditions, they are not regarded as being caused by genetics, nor are they directly inherited from parents. However, a family history of disease is a risk factor for the disease, indicating that there is some inherited risk in the genes.

Inheritance is the passage of hereditary traits from one generation to another. It is the process by which you acquired your characteristics from your parents and will transmit your characteristics to your children.

We have looked at growth and development and now we will look at the repair and maintenance of our cells and tissues with protein replacement, which involves copying portions of our DNA.

Protein Replacement

If individual proteins are to be made, only the portion of the DNA that contains that specific information will be unwound. Enzymes direct the specific location and activity of unwinding. There are four overall sequential stages involved in the production of a protein as shown in Figure 21.11. However there are a series of steps within some of these stages, for example transcription is guided by promoter genes.

There are three types of RNA: messenger, transfer and ribosomal RNA, abbreviated to, mRNA, tRNA and rRNA, respectively involved:

- DNA holds the genetic information in the double helix
- RNA polymerase enzymes direct the unwinding of the specific part of the DNA
- mRNA reads and copies the genetic information guided by a transcription factor
- tRNA takes this copy out of the nucleus to the ribosomes and
- rRNA then directs and translates the detail and directs the making of the protein in the cytosol of the cell
- A newly made protein is then sent out of the cell to its location.

In copying a particular gene or set of genes, T C still lines up with G and vice versa **but** A lines up with U (instead of T) and vice versa.

Most descriptions of the code are given in terms of mRNA because experiments for deciphering the code have involved mRNA and not the more inaccessible DNA. For example:

UUU UUC codes for phe – has two codons
GCU GCC GCA GCG codes for alanine – has four codons

There are three bases in a gene and each trio is called a **codon**. Some proteins consist of several genes, others may only have one.

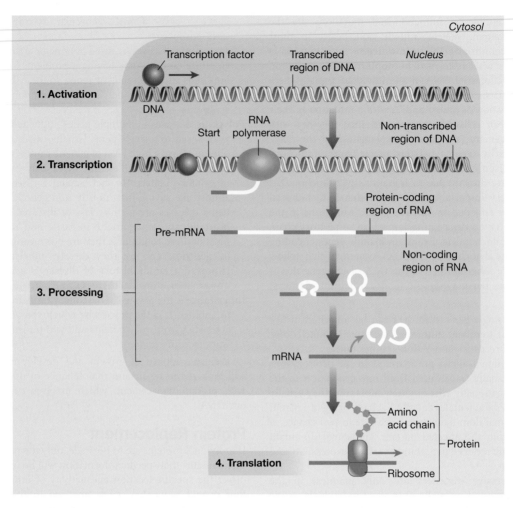

Figure 21.11 The process of making a new strand involves the pairing of the bases, although these are slightly different in RNA.

Three Stages in Transcription
Promoter

A **promoter** is a DNA sequence that enables a gene to be transcribed. The promoter is recognised by RNA polymerase, which then initiates transcription. In RNA synthesis, promoters are a means to demarcate which genes should be used for messenger RNA creation – and, by extension, control which proteins the cell manufactures.

Core promoter The Core promoter directs the:
- Transcription Start Site (TSS)
- Points out the binding site for RNA polymerase
  - RNA polymerase I: transcribes genes encoding ribosomal RNA
  - RNA polymerase II: transcribes genes encoding messenger RNA and certain small nuclear RNAs
  - RNA polymerase III: transcribes genes encoding tRNAs and other small RNAs
- General transcription factor binding sites.

Distal promoter
- Anything further upstream (but not an enhancer or other regulatory region whose influence is positional/orientation independ-

ent which means that it will not work effectively if it is closer to the gene)
- Specific transcription factor binding sites.

Promoters represent critical elements that can work in concert with other regulatory regions (enhancers, silencer (DNA), boundary elements/insulators) to direct the level of transcription of a given gene (Figure 21.12). If a promotor 'gets it wrong' and initiates copying before the gene starts or does not recognise the stop end, the protein is very likely to be incorrectly structured.

Most diseases are heterogeneous in aetiology, meaning that one 'disease' is often many different diseases at the molecular and cellular level, though the symptoms exhibited and the response to treatment might be identical. Diseases respond differently to treatment as a result of differences in the underlying molecular level features.

The Cellular Level

Most of the cells in the body contain many of the structures, components and organelles although the numbers of organelles may vary, depending on the function of the cell (Figure 21.13). For example, active cells such as those found in muscles will use ATP at a high rate and so will contain a large number of mitochondria.

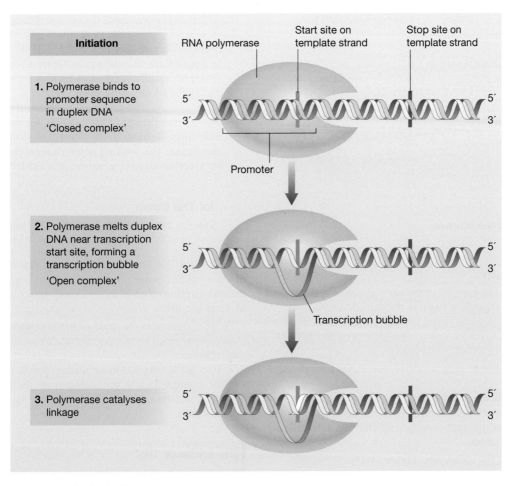

Figure 21.12 **The three stages of transcription.**

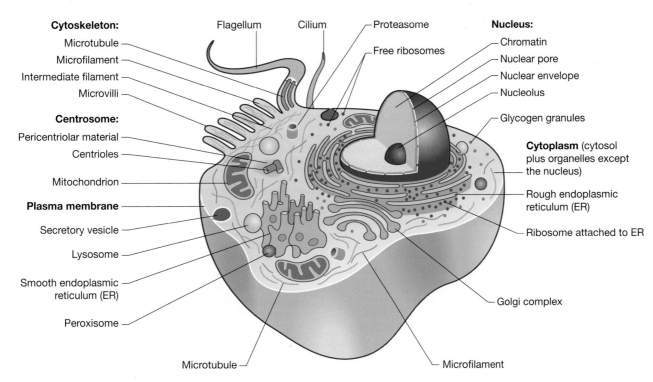

Figure 21.13 **Structure of the cell and its organelles.**

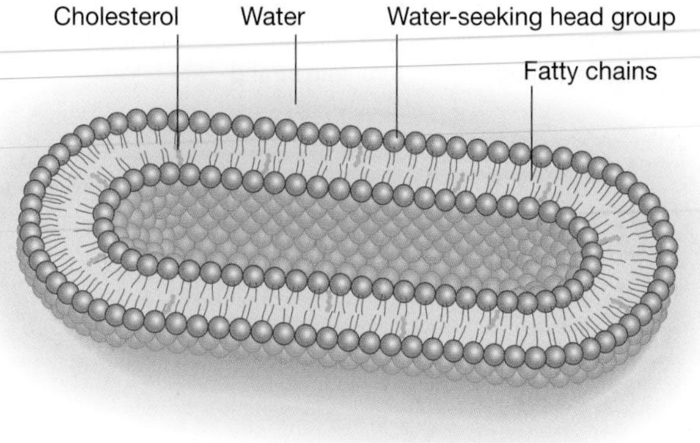

Cholesterol   Water   Water-seeking head group

Fatty chains

Figure 21.14 Membrane structure.

Jot This Down

List some of the features of the cell's structure and some of the organelles found in the cell and their functions.

In the 'Jot This Down' exercise above, you might have thought about:

The plasma or cell membrane, which is an essential perimeter barrier for maintaining the integrity of the cell, separates the cells intracellular, internal environment from its extracellular, external environment.

The structure of the membrane (Figure 21.14)

- The membrane is a sturdy, flexible 'mosaic fluid arrangement' of molecules and is referred to as a 'phospholipid bilayer', within which there are cholesterol and numerous protein molecules
- The phospholipids are positioned with their 'water liking' polar heads that contain phosphorus, facing towards the watery extracellular and intracellular watery compartments. Their fatty acid fat 'liking' and water 'hating' tails, fill the inside of the membrane. This is because they fold away from the water
- Together, the phosphates and lipid molecules form a head to tail feature.

The plasma membrane acts as a barrier and controls the substances that enter and leave the cell.

- The lipid tails allow several types of lipid soluble molecules through but block the entry or exit of any water like substances
- The amount of cholesterol, which helps to strengthen the cell membrane, make it more flexible but less fluid in its movement, varies in different cell types. Cholesterol molecules also reduce the permeability of the membrane to water-soluble elements such as ions (charged chemical elements) and monosaccharides.

Proteins within the cell membrane vary in size and structure. Some of them are fixed and others move freely within the lipid portion of the membrane.

They carry out a number of essential functions with respect to keeping the cell alive, such as acting as communicators, markers and transporters, and are classified as integral or peripheral.

- Integral proteins generally span across the membrane. They are referred to as transmembrane proteins, positioned with their 'water liking' regions on either side of the membrane and their

water hating regions inside the cell membrane. They have several functions:
- Provide selective specific ion channels, for example a sodium or a potassium channel across the membrane, like a tunnel
- Transport specific substances such as amino acids across the membrane by changing shape
- Act as a receptor and relay a function as directed by the ligand that fits into the site of the receptor, for example the antidiuretic hormone binds to the receptor of protein in the renal cell membrane. This binding action changes the water permeability of certain plasma membranes in the kidneys.

Jot This Down

Can you think of a situation when this would occur?

In the 'Jot This Down' exercise above, you might have thought of when a patient is dehydrated. The antidiuretic hormone increases the reabsorption of water in the kidney, thus reducing the amount of water lost in the urine.

- Peripheral proteins are attached to the surface polar heads of the membrane lipids or to integral proteins on either side of the cell membrane
- They act as enzymes by catalysing specific chemical reactions, for example lactase protruding from the membranes of the small intestine splits lactose into simple sugars which are then absorbed.

The Evidence Diet

If a person has lactase insufficiency, they must be advised not to drink or eat foods containing lactose. The unabsorbed lactose passes into the colon where it is fermented by bacteria with the production of fatty acids and gases such as carbon dioxide, hydrogen and methane. This results in abdominal discomfort with diarrhoea, flatulence and nausea.

This is primarily an inherited genetic, although it can be caused by gastroenteritis, coeliac disease, ulcerative disease and chemotherapy.

What the Experts Say

A teenager with primary lactose intolerance and who is a vegetarian has followed her nutritionist's advice and has an interesting balanced diet consisting of beans, pulses, tofu, vegetables, fruit, chips and soya milk. Marmite also provides added taste.

Chinese and Indian food is tolerated well, as it is usually lactose free.

- They act as linkers by anchoring membrane proteins of neighbouring cells to each other or to protein filaments both intra and extracellularly (both integral and peripheral proteins act as linkers to provide stability to the cell). They also provide temporary binding sites that help with the movement of materials and organelles within the cell and the cell itself. In dividing and contracting cells they support the changes to cell shape
- Glycoproteins act as cell markers, which enable cells to recognise cells of the same type during tissue formation and any foreign cells such as foreign tissue or cells.

The **cytoplasm** consists of the 'cytosol' and the 'organelles'. The cytosol is a gel-like substance enclosed within the cell membrane. It forms the fluid portion of the cytoplasm and is the intracellular environment, in which the organelles live. The cytosol contains water, dissolved solutes and suspended particles, such as atoms, glucose, proteins, lipids, ATP and cell waste products and makes up between 55% and 70% of the cell volume. Cytoskeleton filaments within the cytosol provide the cellular scaffolding, which maintains the shape of the cell just as your skeleton provides your shape. The cytosol is the site for several chemical reactions, such as glycolysis and those that provide the building blocks for cell growth and maintenance. The cytoplasm provides the medium for signal transduction from the cell membrane to the intracellular organelles such as the nucleus

The nucleus contains all of the genetic information, which is stored in DNA. It also has a high concentration of RNA in the nucleolus

Nuclear membrane – often called the 'nuclear envelope', as it opens to permit molecules to enter and leave the nucleus

Golgi apparatus – packages and sends molecules, such as steroids, out to other cells in the body

Lysosome – destroys/degrades unwanted molecules such as bacteria and damaged proteins

Phagosomes take bacteria into the cell and transport them safely to the lysosome. The phagosome encloses the bacterium so that it does not infect the cell intracellularly

Mitochondrium – provides energy ATP, uses oxygen and glucose, breaks up fatty acids into water and carbon dioxide called 'metabolic water' and carbon dioxide

Peroxisome – helps the lysosome clean up unwanted particles, breaks up large molecules so that they can be broken down into smaller molecules, fatty acids into smaller fatty acids by the mitochondrium

Endoplasmic reticulum – a series of canals that run through the cytoplasm connecting the cell membrane to the organelles such as the nucleus and Golgi apparatus

Smooth endoplasmic reticulum – synthesises fatty acids and steroids

Rough endoplasmic reticulum is continuous with the nuclear envelope. Ribosomes are attached to the outer surface and are the sites for protein synthesis

Ribosomes are made in the nucleolus – some are attached to the endoplasmic reticulum and these proteins are exported out of the cell; other ribosomes are free in the cytosol and make proteins for local use. Ribosomes are also in the mitochondrium where they make proteins for use by the mitochondrium

Endosomes take up molecules from outside the cell, the cell's external environment and the body's internal environment and deliver them to the lysosome

Secretory vesicles form part of the intracellular transport system – they act as a storage depot for proteins that may have been synthesised in the endoplasmic reticulum and then processed in the Golgi apparatus, before they are released out into the tissue fluid.

The Tissue Level

Tissues are collections of similar cells with their structure relating to their function. They work in unison towards a goal, for example all the cells that are in muscle tissue will contract or relax together or in a defined sequence to either lengthen or shorten the muscle. There are four basic, main types of tissues: **epithelial, connective, muscle and nerve**.

Epithelial Tissue

Epithelial tissue is avascular and covers most of the external and many internal parts of the body. The cells are packed tightly together, forming a sheet. There are four classifications of epithelial tissue depending on their shape and the way they are arranged:

- Squamous epithelial cells are flat or scale like
- Cuboidal as the name implies are cube-shaped
- Columnar are column like
- Transitional are stretchy and variably shaped.

When any one of these cell shapes is arranged in a single layer, they are classified as simple cuboidal or simple squamous epithelial tissue for example. When they are arranged in layers, they are stratified and they are named by the type of cell that is on the outer layer, such as stratified cuboidal or stratified columnar epithelial tissue. The function required of the cell dictates which type of cell is used.

Jot This Down

Can you think of two functions that the lungs carry out?

In the 'Jot This Down' exercise above, you might have thought about breathing. More specifically, the cells in the lungs need to make it easy for oxygen and carbon dioxide to cross their cell membranes. They are also exposed to foreign particles, such as pollutants in the air that we may breathe in (inhale). So they must provide protection. In other locations, they will be required to secrete mucous or enzymes, absorb substances and filter body fluids.

Epithelial tissue also serves as epithelial membranes and has a layer of epithelial tissue on top of a specialised connective tissue. This base provides strength and stability for the epithelial cells. Epithelial membranes are classified as:

- Cutaneous tissue – commonly known as your skin
- Serous epithelial tissue, which provides a two layered membrane with a potential space in between. Examples are the parietal and visceral layers around internal organs that need space to move such as the heart and lungs
  - **Parietal** epithelial tissue lines the wall of the cavity
  - Produces serous fluid, which reduces friction between different tissues and organs
  - **Visceral** layer wraps round the individual organs
  - Produces serous fluid
- Mucous lines the tracts that are open to the external environment, such as the upper respiratory, digestive, urinary and reproductive tracts
  - Contain specialised cells that produce and secrete mucus.

Jot This Down

Can you think of a complication that may occur between the visceral and parietal tissue layers?

In the 'Jot This Down' exercise above, you might have thought about pericarditis, which is an infection of the fluid-filled sac between the two epithelial tissue layers around the heart. When the fluid and tissues lining the sac become inflamed, the tissues become tight, which causes chest pain. This is because the heart is pumping and moving against other tissues – like rubbing your hands together continuously.

Pleurisy is inflammation in the pleural space around the lungs, which similarly causes pain on breathing.

Connective Tissue

Connective tissue is the most abundant tissue found throughout the body in organs, bones, nerves, muscles, membranes, blood and lymph and skin. As the name implies, it connects things together and provides structural support, holding them in place.

Types of connective tissue include:

- Loose connective tissue, such as:
  - Areolar tissue in the lungs, which provides support for and contains the alveolus in a delicate webbed sac, like oranges in weaved bags
  - Collagen and elastic fibres
- Dense connective tissue found in tendons and ligaments to provide strength
- Adipose tissue, which gives shape in the form of subcutaneous tissue and storage for fat cells
- Bone, which gives structure and provides a support to attach your skin and other tissues to
- Cartilage gives support and protection
- Synovial tissues, which give structure and movement.

> ### Jot This Down
> Can you think of a disease involving the synovial joint?

In the 'Jot This Down' exercise above, you might have thought about arthritis.

Muscle Tissue

Muscle tissue provides the means for movement by and within the body. There are three types of muscle tissue:

- Skeletal muscle, which is frequently described as striated due to its striped appearance. It is attached to bones and gives movement as it has fibres, actin and myosin, that are able to contract and relax by lengthening and shortening the muscle tissue
- Cardiac muscle
- Smooth muscle.

Nerve Tissue

Nerve tissue is the messenger within the body. These tissues provide the link between the peripheries and the central brain tissue, as they are structured to relay messages. They also provide the communication between different parts of the central brain tissue.

> ### Jot This Down
> Can you think of a disease involving nerve tissue?

In the 'Jot This Down' exercise above, you might have thought about Parkinson's disease, which is a type of movement disorder when nerve cells in a specific part of the brain do not produce

enough dopamine. Dopamine is a chemical that relays messages from one nerve cell to another nerve cell. You are able to pick up a cup of tea and drink it – imagine not being able to get the cup up to your mouth because your nerve cells are unable to coordinate the movement.

Other disorders of nervous tissue that you might have thought about are Huntington's disease and spinal muscular dystrophy.

> ### Jot This Down
> Are mutations friend or foe?

With thalassaemia, the person who has the mutation, has a certain amount of protection against malaria and the inherited gene is prevalent where the mosquito is most abundant.

What the Experts Say

This subject provides the most compelling example of natural selection and, hence, 'survival of the fittest' in humans. It has been suggested that there is a link between thalassaemia and malaria protection, e.g. 'Darwinism', on 'survival of the fittest', is where mutations emerge triumphant as the individuals without the mutation become unfit due to an outside factor. In the case of thalassaemia, individuals without the mutation die from malaria because the mosquito selectively targets to bite those individuals with the correct form of haemoglobin.

Currently, with inherited disorders such as breast cancer, the options are either to remove the faulty gene completely prior to it causing the disease or to eradicate it once it has emerged. This is a dilemma faced by numerous individuals.

What the Experts Say

One young female said, 'I have chosen to remove the threat completely and have a bilateral mastectomy because I don't want to be constantly on the look out'.

Another female in her 20s said, 'I have decided to see what happens because it may never occur and then I have mutilated my body for nothing'.

When proteins are being made, they are controlled and protected by chaperone molecules that protect proteins against excessive heat, cold and any toxic molecules. At times of stress, proteins can misfold, which then causes disease (Figure 21.15).

If a chaperone is not working properly, the misfolded protein causes illness and also if the protein that it ought to have either corrected or destroyed is from a mutated gene, illness can occur. For example in Alzheimer's, a beta protein is misfolded, which disrupts the activities of surrounding proteins. This misfolding results in a tangle of beta sheets, which increase as the disease progresses. Normally, misfolded newly synthesised (MADE) proteins, proteins that have done their job, and old proteins that lose their native conformation, are dispatched to shredders for hydrolysis to small peptides (building blocks) and amino acids. In the case of Alzheimer's, the beta proteins are not destroyed and build up, causing the progressive confusion.

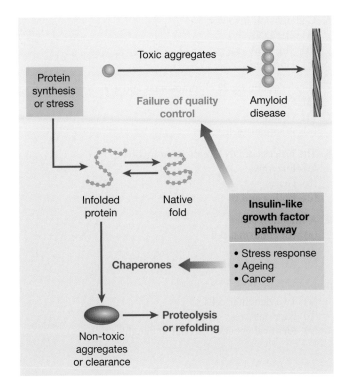

Figure 21.15 Stress response can lead to protein misfolding and on to disease.

What the Experts Say

> Several healthcare professionals in the community say it is essential to research possible cures or prevention of Alzheimer's and other forms of dementia, as these diseases provoke a great deal of stress for both the sufferers and their loved ones.

Conclusion

This chapter has looked at the cell and tissues by considering the chemical and genetic influence on cell growth and survival. The tissues are collections of individual cells that have the same characteristics to form a tissue structure. All the cells communicate to create a functioning human being and nursing involves communicating with the cells.

Key Points

- The different types of cells.
- The cell as a communicator, both locally and throughout the body.
- The impact of genetics on the cell.
- The constituents of the cell and their individual roles.
- The cell as the target for the maintenance of health.
- How the cells grow and develop into a fully functioning human being.

References

Henderson, V. (1991) *The nature of nursing – Reflections after 25 years.* Macmillan, New York.

Lange, S., Takata, K. & Wood, R. (2011) DNA polymerases and cancer. *Nature Reviews Cancer*, 11(2), 96–110.

Pagès, V. & Fuchs, R. (2002) How DNA lesions are turned into mutations within cells? *Oncogene* 21(58), 8957–8966.

Safra, N., Bassuk, A., Ferguson, P. *et al.* (2013) Genome-wide association mapping in dogs enables identification of the Homebox gene, NKX2–8, as agenetic component of neural tube defects in humans. *PLoS Genetics* 9(7), e1003646.

Tortora, G. & Jenkins, G. (2013) *Anatomy and Physiology.* John Wiley & Sons, Singapore.

Wolpert, L. (1969) Positional information and the spatial pattern of cellular differentiation. *Journal of Theoretical Biology*, 25(1), 1–47.

461

Test Yourself

1. The cell membrane consists of:
   (a) A polymer of sugars
   (b) A structural protein
   (c) Lipids

2. Ribosomes are found in the:
   (a) Nucleus
   (b) cytoplasm
   (c) a and b

3. The Golgi body is involved in:
   (a) Transporting proteins that are to be released from the cell
   (b) Altering or modifying proteins
   (c) Producing genes

4. Lysosomes are responsible for:
   (a) Producing steroids
   (b) Destroying unwanted molecules
   (c) Providing energy

5. Genes are found in:
   (a) the cytoplasm
   (b) the nucleus
   (c) both a and b

6. Cell division involves:
   (a) The DNA
   (b) The RNA
   (c) Hormones

7. A cell containing 22 chromosomes and a Y chromosome is a:
   (a) Sperm
   (b) Ovum
   (c) A somatic cell

8. The process of DNA replication involves:
   (a) Enzymes
   (b) Genes
   (c) Both a and b

9. A mutation is:
   (a) An abnormal cell
   (b) A normal cell
   (c) An altered gene

10. Meiosis produces:
    (a) Two daughter cells
    (b) Four gametes
    (c) Identical genetic material in daughter cells

Answers

1. c
2. c
3. b
4. b

5. b
6. a
7. a
8. c
9. c
10. b

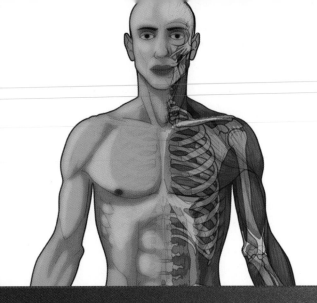

22

Immunity, Inflammation and Infection

Frances Gascoigne

University of Salford, UK

Learning Outcomes

On completion of this chapter you will be able to:

- Describe the major organs and tissues of the lymphatic system and their functions
- List and describe the functions of the cells and chemical proteins that are the tools for protecting the body against foreign invaders
- Understand the classification of microorganisms: eukaryotes, bacteria, archaea and viruses, so that the appropriate interventions can be implemented to provide a safe environment in a healthcare setting
- Discuss the physiology of innate immunity and explain how inflammation links to infection and fever and wound healing
- Compare and contrast the processes of cell-mediated and antibody-mediated immunity
- Understand the aetiology and pathophysiologies of autoimmune disorders and allergies to assess physical and psychological needs and support

Competencies

All nurses must:

1. Use knowledge of how microbes behave so that the appropriate interventions are implemented to provide a safe environment and prevent infection
2. Assess the functional health status of patients and provide information to the patient based on the assessment to avoid infection and promote health
3. Use evidence-based practice to plan and structure individualised care to protect patients whose natural defences against infection are compromised
4. Recognise signs of inflammation and the manifestation of infection
5. Evaluate nursing care of patients with infection and implement effective interventions to promote recovery
6. Revise plan of care for patients with altered immunity

 Visit the companion website at **www.wileynursingpractice.com** where you can test yourself using flashcards, multiple-choice questions and more.

Nursing Practice: Knowledge and Care, First Edition. Edited by Ian Peate, Karen Wild and Muralitharan Nair.
© 2014 John Wiley & Sons, Ltd. Published 2014 by John Wiley & Sons, Ltd. Companion website: www.wileynursingpractice.com

Introduction

Microbes are everywhere and, while we are not able to see them with the naked eye, they are an important part of the environment when they are in their rightful habitats. If they are ingested, inhaled or enter into your tissues through cuts or any other form of skin damage, they can become pathogens, causing either local tissue infection or entering into the bloodstream and causing a systemic infection. Despite our constant exposure to microbes, most of us remain relatively healthy, 'warding them off' or 'fighting against them', and recover within an acceptable period of time. The chief function of the lymphatic system with its tool kit of specialised cells and chemical proteins is to protect the body against attack, fight against invasions and build up a targeted immunity.

Consequently all health professionals must have a good knowledge and understanding of the cells, tissues and organs that make up this system of protection and fight so that they can anticipate and recognise any signs of infection. This will then enable the implementation of the necessary interventions to support the lymphatic system in its activity to 'fight' and 'expel' the invader, promote healing and the repair of damaged body tissues.

This chapter begins with a question followed by a brief overview of the classification of microbes and then leads into the structures and functions of the lymphatic system and the 'tools of its trade'. The mechanisms of innate and acquired immunity are explored and explained. The diseases associated with a malfunctioning immune system are highlighted and discussed throughout the chapter.

Jot This Down

Think back to when you have had a cold or a sore throat.

You may have had a runny or stuffy nose, felt congested, been sneezing or coughing and had a dry mouth. Your throat may have felt raw and irritable, your nasal secretions or sputum may have been discoloured. You may have gone to the GP who, during the consultation, will have looked at your throat, checked your temperature and felt your neck. He or she may have listened to your chest with a stethoscope, taken your pulse, asked you about the colour and consistency of any secretions such as sputum and asked if you had any pain or discomfort anywhere.

- What do you think the GP was looking for?
- What medication did you expect and what medication might you have received?

These clinical signs will be answered and explained once you have explored and understood the anatomy and physiology of innate immunity.

In the 'Jot This Down' exercise above, you might have had the following thoughts. A common cold is caused by a viral infection of the upper respiratory tract (nose, sinuses and throat) and the symptoms are related to the inflammatory response of innate immunity, and it is this that the GP would have been looking for. The tissues become inflamed and the mucous membranes secrete excess mucus in order to trap the virus and sneezing then expels it from the body. Coughing is a result of the increased mucus dripping down the back of the throat. Low-grade fevers associated with the symptoms of a cold in young adults are not an indication of infection (**http://www.nhs.uk/conditions/cold-common/pages/symptoms.aspx**).

There is no cure for the common cold, antibiotics will not help.

Treatment is to help relieve the symptoms and support the innate immunity by:

- Replacing any fluids you may have lost due to sweating and a runny nose, with plenty of fluids
- Rest
- Eat healthily: a low-fat, high-fibre diet with fresh fruit and vegetables (Kau *et al.* 2011)
- Steam inhalation
- Gargling with salt water.

A Cochrane review (Singh & Das 2011) suggests that zinc supplements within a day of the symptoms starting will speed up recovery and lessen the severity of the symptoms.

If the virus manages to survive and suppress and overcome these initial defence mechanisms, a secondary infection with a new virus or bacteria can occur, although the risk is low (Johnson *et al.* 2007). Examples include: sinusitis, otitis media, bronchitis and pneumonias, which cause:

- The secretions to become discoloured, typically yellow-green and thick
- Persistent fever with a 'red' inflamed sore throat; white patches on your throat or tonsils
- Painful swelling of neck glands
- Pain in your chest, face, head or ears
- Breathlessness, wheezing.

 Link To/Go To

It is noted in the prescribing guidelines in the UK (2006) that these symptoms do not indicate the need for antibiotic therapy. However, there is one exception where studies have shown that in elderly patients presenting with bronchitis, the risk of developing pneumonia is high and this risk can be substantially reduced by the use of antibiotics.

http://www.npc.nhs.uk/merec/infect/commonintro/resources/merec_bulletin_vol17_no3_acute_otitis_media.pdf

Inflammation

The symptoms of inflammation are brought about by the organised activity of the cells and chemicals of the immune system. Inflammation has different levels of intensity, varying from mild discomfort and irritability to life-threatening assaults on health. As it is a response to tissue damage, it can be localised or systemic, depending on the extent and the cause of the damage. Inflammation is characterised by warning signs of redness, swelling, heat and pain, which are indicators that the body is mustering the body's innate response to disarm any foreign invaders that take advantage of the breakdown in the body's defences. It also indicates the start of the healing process and tissue repair (Figure 22.1).

Innate senses and defences (i.e. those that we are born with), such as skin and mucous membranes, are on constant guard and taking stock of what they can see, hear, smell, feel and taste.

Langerhans cells, which are a type of dendritic cell (DC), in the epidermis and mucosal tissues, serve as the sentinels of immunity

465

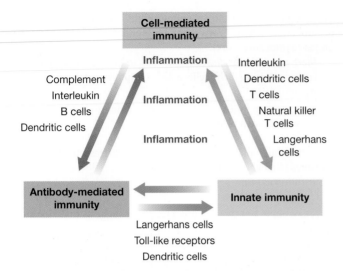

Figure 22.1 **Inflammation, highlighting the key cells and chemical mediators involved in the process of inflammation. The immune response has three distinct interlinked phases: innate (green box), cell-mediated (red box) and antibody-mediated (purple box).**

and are at the forefront of our defences. They are referred to as Toll-like receptors as they are able to recognise potential pathogens and when they are alerted to the presence of microbes, they activate the signalling pathways to start the immune response (Miller 2008).

When the Langerhans cells are alerted by a breakdown in the our defences or detect a possible intruder, they stimulate signalling dendritic cells and natural killer T cells (CD8), which are resident in the dermal layer of the skin. Communication is via signalling chemicals that are released locally by the dendritic cells.

The signalling dendritic cells then stimulate the inflammatory dendritic cells, which then orchestrate the inflammatory response by activating the inflammatory cytokines (inflammatory chemicals).

This inflammatory response can go one of three ways:

1. If the Langerhans cells on look-out recognise the possible intruder, they take a digital picture, label it antigen and send it to the dendritic cells, who relay it to the memory B cells archive. These B cells extract the specific antigen-antibody and send it to the surface. If the antigen is not too near, the antigen will shoo it away. If the antigen is in your nose or gut the antibody will activate interleukin and interleukin will start the relevant mild inflammatory process such as coughing, sneezing or diarrhoea.

2. If tissue damage occurs and the sentinel cells do not detect an intruder, the inflammatory dendritic cells will orchestrate the inflammatory response and will only use the cells and proteins needed for healing and repair.

3. If the cells on look-out do detect an intruder but do not recognise this intruder, they send a message to dendritic cells, which start the inflammatory process locally and a number of reactions occur:
   - Neutrophils are the first cells to be called and, by attracting chemical proteins such as histamine and complement, inflammation can isolate the microbe in the tissues. The chemicals in the bloodstream bring about:
     - vasodilation, which increases the blood flow to the area of damage

- Increase in the permeability of the blood vessel wall, which permits the neutrophils and other inflammatory chemicals to pass out of the bloodstream into the tissues.
- The neutrophils then kill the microbe by phagocytosis and expose its DNA on its surface (the neutrophil which carries out the phagocytosis is referred to as a phagocyte)
- The neutrophils will expel the remnants of the microbe and waste from the tissue damage, which includes the tired and worn out neutrophils, in the form of droplets, sputum or wound exudates
- The T cells in the tissues and chemical messengers will take the DNA that has been exposed from the tissues into the bloodstream and the process of cell-mediated immunity will then proceed onto antibody mediated immunity without the microbe entering the bloodstream.

However, if the microbe has managed to survive this initial onslaught and bypass the neutrophils and enter into the bloodstream, it has now become a pathogen and the dendritic cells will increase the intensity of the inflammatory response by activating further cells such as monocytes and chemical proteins to fight it. The monocytes enlarge and are termed macrophages.

The inflammatory response becomes more aggressive and the innate immune response links to the cell-mediated immune response when the microbe, which is now called an antigen, DNA is presented to the T lymphocyte by the macrophage:

- The monocytes enlarge into macrophages and take over from the neutrophils
- The T lymphocytes become more active and differentiate into different types of T lymphocytes by inserting different receptors (labels) into their membranes. These labels indicate what they are capable of and what they will do. For example:
  - *Cytotoxic T cells* are the destroyers and
  - *Helper T cells* assist with the overall continuation of the fight
- The release of tumour necrosis factor and additional interleukins.

The sequel progresses to antibody-mediated immunity when the T lymphocytes release chemical proteins that activate the B lymphocytes. The process of antibody-mediated immunity is similar to that of cell-mediated immunity but the T lymphocyte is the antigen presenting cell and the B lymphocyte the receptor cell. This B cell will differentiate into an antibody and a B memory cell.

If the microbe is a virus, dendritic cells will have called in a special antiviral chemical protein, called interferon and you will not be able to build up immunity naturally. The process of cell-mediated and antibody-mediated immunity is conducted in a laboratory and the antibody is given in the form of a vaccination.

Red Flag

 The most effective barrier against microbes is preventing them from becoming pathogens and all health professionals must have sufficient awareness and comprehension of the effective measures needed to prevent cross-infection (Figure 22.2).

Jot This Down

What do you think nurses need to know about microbes?

Use tissues when you sneeze A single sneeze propels germs over a distance of 32 feet	**Harmless bacteria and fungi live naturally on your skin** If they multiply your skin can become infected – keep skin clean and dry (www.nhs.uk/Conditions/Athletesfoot/Pages/Introduction.aspxwww.nhs.uk/Conditions)
Wash your hands between patients (www.wales.nhs.uk/sites3/.../739/rcn%20infection%20control.doc.pdf)	**Wash your hands before any procedures** e.g. mouth care, eye care, bathing (Collins 2008)
Put your hand over your mouth when you cough (www.wales.nhs.uk/sites3/.../739/rcn%20infection%20control.doc.pdf)	**Drink plenty of fluids** (Eccles 2004)
Cover any cuts or grazes when looking after patients (Collins 2008)	**Clean surfaces and any spillages** (Collins 2008)

Safety with microbes – washing your hands with soap and warm water – the physical action of scrubbing loosens up the microbes, the soap picks them up and binds them together and the water washes them away (Collins 2008)

Figure 22.2 **Simple preventative measures.**

In the 'Jot This Down' exercise above, you may have considered the following:

1. They are safe when in their normal environment
2. Many species colonise the human body and are called normal flora
3. Normal flora are found on the skin, mucous membranes and the gastrointestinal tract
4. Some benefit the human host, for example:
   - *Staphylococcus epidermis* protects against colonisation by pathogenic bacteria on the skin through microbial competition. It dominates the location
   - *Lactobacillus species*, which grow in the vagina and the gastrointestinal tract are 'probiotic' or 'good germs' as they produce lactic acid as a by-product of their metabolism. This creates an acidic environment which prevents other microbes such as the fungus *Candida* (commonly known as thrush), from sticking and growing on the mucous membranes.

The Evidence

Natural yoghurt is a good source of lactobacilli and has been used successfully to treat vaginal and oral thrush infections. Amber Williams (2002) recommends using natural, soy-base or organic yoghurt, as flavoured yogurts contain sugars which feed the fungus.

- *Escherichia coli* in the bowel secretes essential vitamins such as K and B12 and prevents pathogenic bacteria from establishing themselves in the bowel. This organism is a frequent cause of urinary tract infections.

Jot This Down

Provide an example of a situation when you will have to implement care to prevent possible infection by *E. coli*. Explain your answer and detail the required interventions.

In the 'Jot This Down' exercise above, you are likely to have thought about the impact that *E. coli* has on the individual. An example might be bowel incontinence, which can result in contamination of the urethra. In this situation, the nurse can:

- Regularly observe for soiling with cleaning and washing the perineal and external urethral areas with soap and water when required
- Encourage the patient to drink adequate fluids, providing help if needed, to flush any microbes in the urethra away
- Observe for signs of infection.

An Introduction to the Classification of Microbes/Microorganisms

The most precise method of classification of microbes is their genetic analysis, as each species of bacteria and virus has a unique genetic make-up. Another way of placing microorganisms in categories is according to their cell structure and organelles.

 Link To/Go To

The Three-Domain system (page 4) at:
http://lpc1.clpccd.cc.ca.us/lpc/zingg/Micro/lecture%20notes/M_T_Ch10_Classification_SS10.pdf is the most frequently used in microbiology.

Eukarya

Eukarya (eukaryotic cells) include all animal cells and fungi.

Jot This Down

Can you think of a common fungal infection?

In the 'Jot This Down' exercise above, you might have thought about: Athlete's foot (*tinea pedis*).

This fungus, a dermatophyte, feeds off other organisms, such as dead skin cells, and lives in a moist, warm, dark, humid environment. It causes infection when it multiplies. If it is not treated effectively, it can spread to other areas such as toenails causing fungal nail infections. It is also possible to spread it on your hands and if you have any cracked skin it can enter your body and spread to exposed tissue.

Jot This Down

As a health professional you need to be aware of how and where this infection may be 'picked up' and the interventions you would implement to avoid and treat contamination.

In the 'Jot This Down' exercise above, you might have considered:
- May have been picked-up from contaminated towels, clothing and surfaces, such as communal bathrooms and showers

  Interventions could be:
- Washing the feet regularly with soap and water and drying them thoroughly, particularly between the toes
- Advise against placing bare feet on the ground
- Advise changing socks regularly and wearing cotton socks
- Washing your hands.

Topical antifungal creams, powders and sprays and oral medication are used to kill the fungus.

Bacteria

Bacteria have cells that are equipped with all the structures and ingredients necessary for reproduction, growth and survival which they do in a highly organised manner. The way to destroy them is to damage the cell wall and disrupt their intracellular machinery. However, with the frequent use of antibiotics, the bacterial cell has learned and develops ways of combating elimination. By modifying its cell membrane and metabolism, it mutates into a strain such as MRSA (methicillin resistant *Staphylococcus aureus*), which is resistant to penicillin.

All healthcare professionals will be aware of the phrase:

'bacteria develop resistance to antibiotics'

The Evidence

Over 50% of the bacteria that cause infections in hospitals are resistant to at least one of the drugs most commonly used for treatment.

http://www.nhs.uk/news/2010/08August/Pages/drug-resistant-superbug
-in-UK.aspx

Archaea

Archaea are within the classification of microorganisms but no pathogenic Archaea have as yet been clearly identified. They tend to be found in extreme environments such as freezing tundra or hypersaline.

Viruses

Viruses are considered separately, as they differ from the other microorganisms, in that they require a living host to multiply and are not alive. They are a strand of DNA without a cell or metabolism of their own. Once they are inside a host cell, they treat it like a 'bed and breakfast', using host DNA for reproducing themselves and host enzymes or nutrients for food and energy. The way to eliminate a virus is to block its entry into the host cell and remove any enzymes and nutrients that it may be 'pinching' in order to reproduce, grow and survive.

The Lymphatic System and Immunity

The lymphatic system (see Figure 22.3) is part of the circulatory system and has three basic functions:
- Transporting intercellular fluid, initially formed as a blood filtrate, back into the bloodstream
- Transporting absorbed fat from the small intestine to the blood
- Playing a vital role in providing immunity against pathogens.

The lymphatic and circulatory systems function in unison to maintain the internal environment. They are comparable in structure, in that they both have vessels which serve to transport liquid and the cells and chemicals of immunity.

The organs and tissues of the lymphatic system serve as storage depots for the principal specialised cells and chemical proteins that work collectively, to protect the body against the invasion by microbes, fight pathogens and build-up permanent immunity.

The skin and the red bone marrow are seen as associated organs of immunity:

The skin, which is part of the integumentary system, is considered an active associated organ of immunity. It is composed of two layers, a superficial epidermis and a deeper dermis. The outer epidermis acts as the principal structural barrier to any microbes in the environment and is the first-line of defence. The hormone, epidermal growth factor, stimulates the replacement of damaged epidermal cells as a result of abrasions and minor burns.

As it is avascular, you do not bleed when you damage the epidermal layer, and microbes on the skin do not have direct access to the blood or lymphatic circulation. The specialised epidermal Langerhans dendritic cells work in unison with other cells in the dermis, such as T helper cells (CD4), as part of the surveillance network (Salmon *et al.* 1994; Cua & Tato 2010). The dermis is a deeper, thicker layer of connective tissue criss-crossed with a network of lymphatic and blood vessels. It is equipped with a kit of resident lymphocytes and migrant mast cells, leukocytes, macrophages and chemical proteins such as cytokines.

Repair of the dermis is referred to as 'deep wound healing' and involves a more structured process directed by the inflammatory response.

The red bone marrow, a connective tissue located chiefly in spongy bone tissue, contains pluripotent stem cells, which have the ability to develop into several different types of cells. All of the formed elements for immunity in the blood originate, develop and are structured in the red bone marrow (Figure 22.4).

Before exploring the organs and tissues of the lymphatic system, we will look at the channels that connect them, which are the lymphatic capillaries and lymphatic vessels.

Capillaries

The **capillaries** are tubes lined with endothelium that run between the cells of connective tissue. Unlike blood capillaries that are closed tubes with an arterial 'in'-flow and a venous 'exit', lymphatic capillaries are open ended. The reason they are structured with an open end is because they are the drains of the intercellular spaces. Most of the components of the blood plasma, apart from red blood cells and proteins, filter from the blood capillary network into the

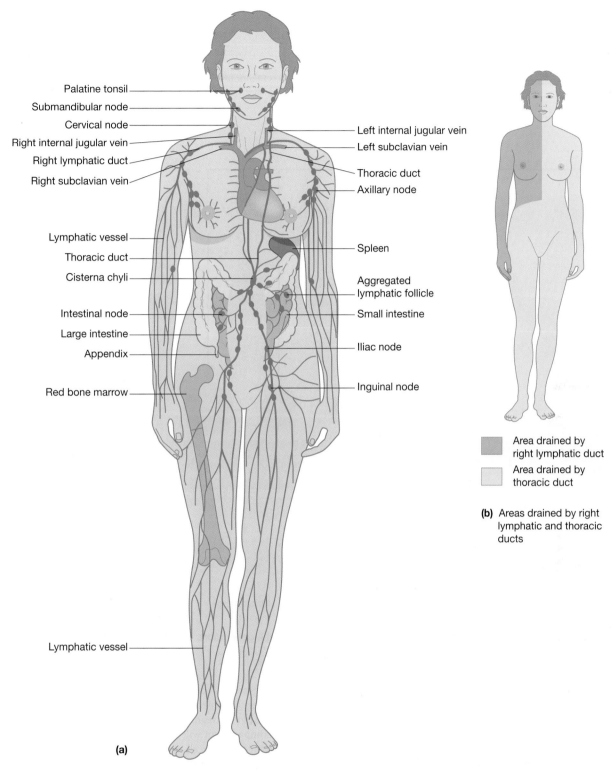

Palatine tonsil
Submandibular node
Cervical node
Right internal jugular vein
Right lymphatic duct
Right subclavian vein

Left internal jugular vein
Left subclavian vein
Thoracic duct
Axillary node

Lymphatic vessel
Thoracic duct
Cisterna chyli

Spleen

Aggregated
lymphatic follicle
Small intestine

Intestinal node
Large intestine
Appendix

Iliac node

Red bone marrow

Inguinal node

Lymphatic vessel

(a)

Area drained by
right lymphatic duct

Area drained by
thoracic duct

(b) Areas drained by right
lymphatic and thoracic
ducts

469

Figure 22.3 Components of the lymphatic system.

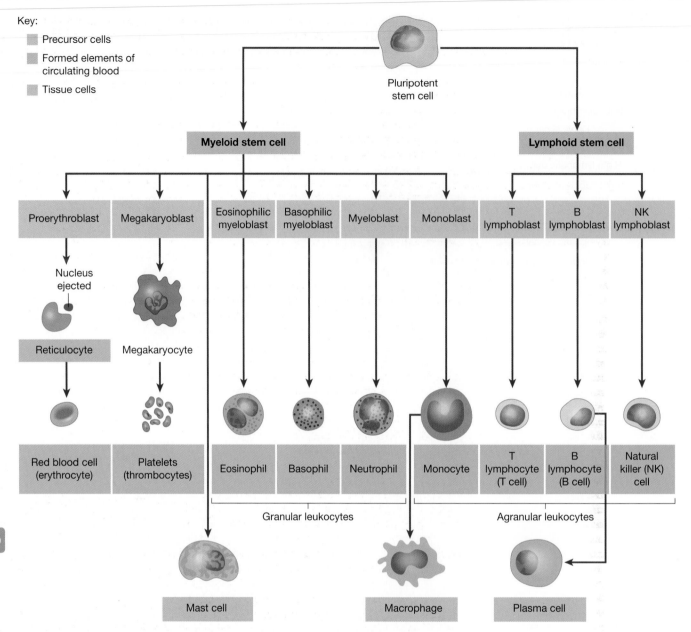

Key:

■ Precursor cells

■ Formed elements of circulating blood

■ Tissue cells

Figure 22.4 Origin, development and structure of formed elements. Some of the generations of some cell lines have been omitted.

intercellular spaces at the arterial end of the capillary and then are returned back into the bloodstream at the venous end of the capillary. Any excess fluid (about three litres a day), drains into the lymphatic vessels and is called **lymph**.

Dietary fats and fat soluble vitamins, absorbed by specialised lymphatic capillaries in the small intestine, called 'lacteals', give lymph a milky white colour.

(Some tissues which include cartilage, the epidermis, central nervous system and red bone marrow are not drained by lymphatic capillaries).

As well as containing the filtered constituents of plasma, it also provides an exit for any proteins that may have escaped from the bloodstream into the intercellular spaces. If proteins have leaked out of the bloodstream into the intercellular spaces, they cannot be reabsorbed back into the venous capillary because of the concen-

tration gradient across the capillary wall. The proteins become trapped in the intercellular space. The proteins then absorb fluid from the bloodstream by osmosis (see Chapter 24) and the intercellular compartment will swell.

Each epithelial cell is capable of responding to this increased intercellular pressure and they move further apart to allow an increased amount of fluid and proteins to drain into the lymphatic system when necessary. Pressure sensitive elastic fibres which anchor the drain to the vessel keep the cells apart until the pressure in the intercellular space has returned to normal. The proteins and fluid is returned to the circulatory system via lymphatic ducts.

To prevent overflow, when the pressure in the lymphatic system becomes higher than in the intercellular spaces, each epithelial cell acts like a swing door. Pushed open from the intercellular side and then held shut by pressure in the lymphatic vessel.

The flow of lymph is maintained by the:

- 'milking pump' action of skeletal muscles as they contract they compresses the vessels and the fluid is pushed forwards and the
- 'respiratory pump'.

When we inhale, the negative pressure in the thoracic cavity pulls the fluid forward; when we exhale, the pressure in the thoracic cavity increases and the valves in the lymphatic vessels prevent back flow.

Valves in the lymphatic capillaries and lymphatic vessel maintain the one way flow of lymph, which originates in the intercellular spaces and circulates into lymphatic capillaries, lymphatic vessels, lymph nodes, lymphatic vessels and then via lymphatic ducts back into the venous bloodstream and the cardiovascular circulation.

Jot This Down

Think back to when you may have seen a build up of proteins in the intercellular compartments and how it may present in a patient.

- What is it called and what care would you implement to help the patient feel more comfortable?

In the 'Jot This Down' exercise above, you may have recognised a condition that is called **oedema** – swelling in the tissues, as the proteins are like sponges and draw the liquid out of the bloodstream into the intercellular spaces and absorb it. The fluid has then become trapped in the intercellular spaces until it can all be drained by the lymphatic vessels. The flow of lymphatic fluid and thus drainage of intercellular fluid is facilitated by increasing venous return, which is achieved with exercise.

Lymphatic Vessels

Several lymphatic capillary networks empty into lymphatic vessels, which are lined by endothelial cells, have a thin layer of smooth muscle and an outer adventitia that binds them to the surrounding tissues . In the skin, they lie in the subcutaneous tissue and generally follow the same route as veins. In the deeper tissues, they form plexuses around the arteries.

- At intervals along their route, these vessels flow through fibrous encapsulated bean shaped organs, which are the lymph nodes and masses of lymphoid tissue called lymphatic follicles.

Lymph Nodes

Capsular trabeculae (Figure 22.5) divide the node into compartments with each compartment containing a superficial cortex and a deeper medulla surrounded by lymphatic sinuses.

471

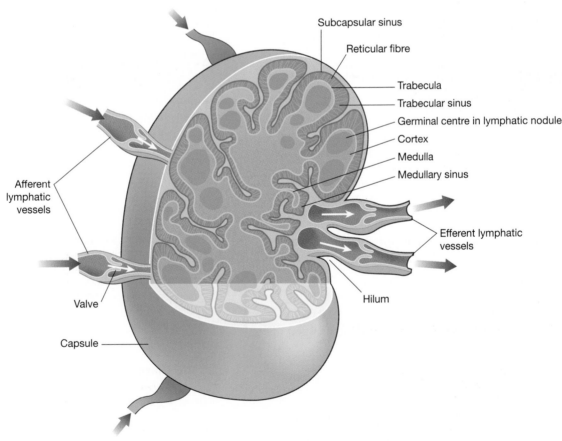

Route of lymph flow through a lymph node:

Afferent lymphatic vessel ⟶ Subcapsular sinus ⟶ Trabecular sinus ⟶ Medullary sinus ⟶ Efferent lymphatic vessel

Figure 22.5 Structure of a lymph node. Arrows indicate direction of lymph flow through a lymph node.

Within the cortex, there are aggregates of dividing B lymphocytes called lymphatic nodules.

Within the nodules, there is a germinal centre where B lymphocytes proliferate and develop into antibody-producing plasma cells or develop into memory B cells.

Strategically, lymph flows through the node in one direction, entering via a number of afferent lymphatic vessels, which penetrate the surface of the node at various points. Within the node, the lymph flows into a series of channels containing branching reticular fibres called sinuses, which surround the cortex, like an orange in a mesh bag. Lymphocytes and resident macrophages are embedded in the reticular fibres, which in essence, ensures that all lymph fluid will pass through a lymph node and be filtered:

- The reticular fibres trap the pathogens
- Macrophages destroy some of them
- Lymphocytes destroy the others with immune responses.

As there are only two efferent vessels for the flow of lymph out of the nodes, the flow is slow enough to allow the lymph to circulate through several sinuses, which means that it is filtered several times before it can leave the node.

Jot This Down

Think about patients that have had painful and/or swollen lymph glands
   Why did they have swollen glands?
   What is it called?
   Are all swollen glands painful?

In the 'Jot This Down' exercise above, you might have thought about:

1. **Infection**: bacterial, viral, fungal
   - Localised infection – with either one or two swollen glands; typical examples are common cold, tonsillitis, cellulitis
   - Systemic infection – with several swollen glands; a typical example is glandular fever
      Swollen glands are called 'lymphadenopathy' and are an indication that they are having to work excessively to filter and destroy pathogens and produce antibodies
2. **Immune disorder**
   - Rheumatoid arthritis with continuous inflammation (autoimmune disease)
3. **Malignancy**
   - Lymphoma
   - Leukaemia.

Not necessarily painful but 'discomforting'.

Lymph nodes are concentrated in a number of locations and are identified by this locality, such as axillary in the axilla.

Jot This Down

Thinking back to clinical practice and infection, where do you think the locations of lymph glands are in the body?

In the 'Jot This Down' exercise above, you may have thought of any of the following:

- Cervical
- Inguinal
- Axillary
- Pelvic
- Abdominal
- Thoracic
- Supratrochlear.

All these locations are in locations where they are needed more readily, which is where pathogens are most likely to enter the body – through the mouth, nose, lungs, gastrointestinal and reproductive tracts.

Jot This Down

The lymphatic system, just as any type of drainage system, can become blocked. Think about any clinical practice situation, where you might have seen a build up of lymphatic fluid called 'lymphoedema'.

In the 'Jot This Down' exercise above, you may have cared for someone with a swollen arm following surgery, which involved the lymph glands in the axilla, such as a 'modified radical' mastectomy.

A 'modified radical mastectomy' involves the surgical removal of the breast tissue, the lining of the chest muscle (pectoralis major) and the lymph nodes of the axilla. When the lymph nodes are removed, it is essentially damage to the lymphatic system, which then impairs the drainage of any excess fluid from the interstitial compartments.

Link To/Go To

Cancer Research UK estimate that about 20% will have lymphoedema of the arm after breast cancer treatment.

http://www.cancerresearchuk.org/cancer-help/type/breast-cancer/treatment/lymphoedema-after-breast-cancer-treatment

What the Experts Say

The patient is finding it difficult to mobilise and, although the patient said he/she understood what might happen, that his/her arm may become swollen after the surgery, he/she had not envisaged it becoming so uncomfortable and heavy.

- The patient said that he/she had been shown the arm compression but it is uncomfortable and hot to wear
- The patient is doing exercises but they are not working.

Jot This Down

Think about the nursing interventions you might implement to help alleviate the patient's discomfort?

The interventions aim to push the excess fluid out of the arm back into the lymphatic and circulatory system. This often takes a few weeks.

- The elastic sleeve covers the arm from the wrist to the top of the arm; care must be taken to make sure it is not too tight under the arm and restrict the flow in the axilla. The arm must be measured and assessed at regular intervals as a badly fitting sleeve can make the lymphoedema worse

- A 'stretchy' bandage may be more comfortable
- Manual lymphatic drainage facilitates the movement of the fluid manually
- Facilitate and encourage exercises to assist the drainage of the fluid from the arm
- Support the arm on a pillow when resting, ensuring that the arm is not too tight against the chest, as this will impede the drainage
- Keep the skin clean and dry, apply oil or cream to prevent the skin from becoming dry and cracked.

Lymphatic Follicles

Unlike the lymph nodes, which are encapsulated in a dense connective tissue layer, lymphatic follicles are not surrounded by a capsule and are scattered throughout the mucous membranes. They are referred to as mucosa-associated lymphatic tissue (MALT), lining the respiratory airways, the gastrointestinal, urinary and reproductive tracts, where they intercept microbes that enter the body through externally opened passageways. Larger collections of follicles are the tonsils (adenoid and palatine) and the lingual tonsils at the base of the tongue, which are positioned to participate in immunity responses against inhaled or ingested microbes. There are also lymphatic follicles called Peyer's patches in the ileum for protecting the intestinal wall and the appendix which is involved in the production of immunoglobulin A (IgA) antibodies, helping with the maturation of B lymphocytes and the direction of lymphocytes around the body.

Lymphatic Trunks

Lymphatic vessels pass lymph, node to node, through a sequential chain of lymph nodes. When they exit from this chain, they unite with other vessels from a particular region to form a 'lymphatic trunk':

- Lumbar trunk drains lymph from the legs, pelvis, kidneys, adrenal glands and the abdominal wall
- Intestinal trunk drains the stomach, intestines, pancreas, spleen and liver
- Bronchomediastinal trunk drains the thoracic wall, lungs and heart
- Intercostal trunk drains the chest
- Subclavian trunk drains the arms and
- The jugular trunk drains the head and neck.

The way the trunks are structured means that if one trunk becomes blocked, it will affect all the respective linked chain of nodes that drain into it. Lymph trunks empty into one of two collecting ducts (see Figure 22.3).

There are two **lymphatic ducts**. The lumbar, intestinal, left bronchomediastinal and intercostal trunks empty into the thoracic duct, which runs from the abdomen up through the diaphragm into the left subclavian vein. This is the main duct for the return of lymph to the blood with more than two-thirds of the lymphatic system draining into it. The right bronchomediastinal, subclavian and jugular trunks empty the other third of the lymph into the much smaller right lymphatic duct, situated within the right thoracic cavity. This duct returns the lymph into the junction of the right internal jugular and right subclavian vein

The spleen is the largest single mass of lymphatic tissue located in the upper left quadrant of the abdominal cavity between the stomach and the diaphragm. It is similar to lymph nodes in structure, with the splenic artery and splenic vein entering and exiting through a hilum but it has blood sinuses instead of lymphatic sinuses. It consists of two distinct types of tissues called white pulp and red pulp:

- The white pulp consists of lymphocytes, monocytes and macrophages and is structured as islands of white tissue surrounded by the blood sinuses. Blood flowing into the spleen through the splenic artery enters the central arteries of the white pulp and pathogens are filtered from the blood. Within the white pulp, the B and T lymphocytes carry out immune responses and the resident macrophages destroy the filtered pathogens by phagocytosis
- The red pulp is made up of blood-filled venous sinuses and splenic tissue cells arranged into cords (splenic cords), which consist of red blood cells, macrophages, lymphocytes, plasma cells and granulocytes (see Figure 22.4).

Within the red pulp, the spleen:

- Stores platelets
- Carries out a 'clearing up' role by removing aged and defective, fragile or deformed, blood cells and platelets
- During fetal life it produces red blood cells.

Nursing Fields Child and Family

The spleen is not a vital organ and sometimes has to be removed following damage from trauma. While a splenectomy in adults has much less effect on immunity, why is it more of a problem in children?

In the Nursing Fields box above, you might have thought about the building up of immunity.

As we age, the body becomes more adept at fighting against invaders and infections that it has seen in the past. The immunity is still being built up in children as they encounter more microbes and it is more of a challenge for the young immune system to fight off invaders and invasion. A splenectomy compromises this process

---

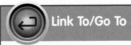

Link To/Go To

http://www.gosh.nhs.uk/medical-conditions/procedures-and-treatments/splenectomy/

The **thymus gland** is an encapsulated organ located in the mediastinum, between the aortic arch and the sternum, and extends from below the thyroid in the neck into the thoracic cavity superior to the heart.

It is packed with a large number of immature T lymphocytes and provides the environment for these to:

1. Mature into immunocompetent T lymphocytes
2. Differentiate into their functioning roles such as cytotoxic and helper T lymphocytes.

Only about 2% of the lymphocytes mature, the rest of them die by apoptosis (programmed cell death) and are 'cleared up' by thymic macrophages.

Apart from the immature and maturing T lymphocytes, the thymus gland consists of:

Dendritic cells, which assist in the differentiation process of the T lymphocyte, are derived from monocytes (agranular leukocytes) (see Figure 22.4).

Because they have a projection similar to that of an axon in the nervous system, they share the name, however dendritic cells in the lymphatic system have a different function

Epithelial cells, which have several long processes that extend outwards in a circle. They

- produce hormones called thymosins that stimulate the development of antibodies (immunoglobulins)
- have several long processes, which extend outwards in a circle.

The dendritic cells use these extending processes like 'pictures' to teach the T cell how to distinguish between self and foreign tissue.

This learning process involves the T lymphocytes.

- Making the markers derived from the 'pictures'
- Inserting these markers into their membranes, which are now called antigen receptors
- Being able to recognise these markers as their own label. This recognition includes detecting if:
  - the markers are made correctly
  - the T cell is recognising them as correct
  - the T cell is recognising them as self.

If they are incorrectly made or the T cell doe not recognise them as self, the T cell is recognised as a malfunctioning T cell and destroyed by the thymic macrophages.

Each epithelial cell has enough 'pictures' for as many as 50 T cells in each session of producing and teaching at any one time.

The thymus gland is large in children and continues to grow until it reaches maturity at puberty. This is because during childhood, it meets and fends off a great number of new infections for the first time. By puberty, it has fought off a large population of infections and a large archive of antibodies, thereafter as it expands with experience, so the thymus gland gets smaller. In adulthood, our immunity has matured and become more able to fight off infections and the thymus gland continues to shrink. Before it atrophies and disappears, it has populated the lymphatic tissues with functioning T cells that have the ability to differentiate and function. Throughout its working life, it is like a T cell factory, nurturing the developing T cells and then moving them on.

> ### Jot This Down
> Write down those autoimmune diseases that you know of and the type of tissue(s) involved.

In the 'Jot This Down' exercise above, you might have thought about 'systemic lupus erythematosus' often referred to as 'lupus', which is an inflammatory connective tissue disorder characterised by the presence of antinuclear antibodies.

Normally, we do not react against our own tissues, which is a concept known as 'self-tolerance'.

If the T cell is unable to distinguish self body tissues, it will instigate self-destruction, which is the basis of autoimmune diseases.

While the T cell is growing and maturing, it undergoes several tests and in the majority of cases, when it fails to pass a test, it is destroyed by thymic macrophages. However:

1. If the thymic macrophages make a mistake and destroy the T cells that are self-tolerant, instead of those that are not, the defective T cells will be sent out into the lymphoid tissue. This is classified as 'central tolerance'.

2. If the tests fail to be vigorous enough and some T cells that are not self-tolerant are sent out into the periphery, they are either muzzled by local 'back-up' mechanisms or are allowed to cause local disease classified as 'peripheral tolerance'
   - Peripheral intolerance can occur another way: not all genes are available in the thymus gland, so developing T cells cannot be exposed and tested for all self-antigen reactions (developed from the MHC genes, which are discussed later). This means that some of the T cells, even if they passed all the tests in the thymus gland, once they have been activated by an infection, turn out to be intolerant of specific self-tissue in some of the tissues. If the local macrophages fail to recognise and destroy these intolerant T cells, a more focussed disease occurs following an infection.

Those defective self-destructive T cells that slip past are sent out into the lymphatic tissues and will:

- be incapable of developing an immune response to a specific antigen and so will not be able fight an invader, which means that the individual will have a compromised immunity
- be intolerant of self, which means that an individual will develop an autoimmune disorder.

Autoimmune disorders or diseases can be:

- More organ or more tissue specific, for example:
  - Hashimoto's thyroiditis – a chronic progressive inflammatory disease of the thyroid with lymphocyte infiltration and gradual destruction of the gland
  - Primary myxoedema – thyroid deficiency resulting from destruction of the thyroid gland
  - Thyrotoxicosis – hyperthyroidism resulting from thyroid-stimulating immunoglobulins that stimulate activity of the gland
  - Pernicious anaemia – resulting from absence of intrinsic factor associated with loss of parietal cells; most individuals have antibodies to parietal cells
  - Addison's disease characterised by atrophy and hypofunction of the adrenal cortex
  - Myasthenia gravis resulting from the build up of antibodies to the acetylcholine receptor of the neuromuscular junction
  - Insulin-dependent diabetes mellitus causes impaired insulin secretion, often the result of islet cell destruction by antibodies directed at the cell surface or cytoplasm
  - Goodpasture's syndrome, which is a type II hypersensitivity disorder with pulmonary haemorrhage and progressive glomerulonephritis characterised by circulating antiglomerular basement membrane antibodies
  - Multiple sclerosis is a probable autoimmune process resulting in disseminated patches of demyelination in the brain and spinal cord and varied neurologic manifestations
  - Idiopathic thrombocytopenic purpura is a chronic disorder characterised by petechiae, purpura, mucosal bleeding, and antibodies against platelets
  - Primary biliary cirrhosis – inflammation and fibrosis of the bile ducts, which may be of autoimmune origin

- Active chronic hepatitis, which results in hepatic failure and/ or cirrhosis; may be autoimmune with infiltration by T cells and plasma cells.
- Not organ specific, for example systemic lupus erythematosus
- Less organ specific, for example:
  - Scleroderma, where there is diffuse fibrosis, degenerative changes and vascular abnormalities of skin, joint structures and internal organs; probably of autoimmune origin
  - Rheumatoid arthritis is a chronic syndrome with inflammation of peripheral joints and generalised manifestations, characterised by infiltration of synovium by lymphocytes and plasma cells
  - Sjögren's syndrome is a systemic inflammatory disorder characterised by dryness of the mouth, eye and other mucous membranes with lymphocyte infiltration of affected tissues
  - Ulcerative colitis is a chronic inflammatory disease of colon mucosa and is thought to be of autoimmune origin.

The Cells of Immunity

T lymphocytes and **B lymphocytes** develop from stem cells in the red bone marrow (Figure 22.4).

T cells are called T cells because they mature in the **Thymus**.

Immature **T lymphocytes** migrate from the red bone marrow to the thymus gland, where they mature into immunocompetent cells. As with the B lymphocytes, maturity is signalled when the T cells make and insert proteins into their cell membranes. These cell surface proteins function as receptors and distinguishing protein markers (CD) define its function and enable the T cell to carry out specific roles in immunity, thus identifying the cell class.

Examples of some of the more common specific types of T cells that you will encounter:

1. Helper T cell CD4
2. Cytotoxic T cell CD8
3. Suppressor T cell CD 8
4. Surveillance T cells CD3 and CD28
5. Memory T cell has both CD4 and CD 8 proteins on its cell membrane.

CD4 cells are the most numerous of the T lymphocytes, making up 70% of the circulating population. **CD** stands for 'cluster of differentiation', which indicates a definite subset of protein surface receptors that identify cell type, like a name badge.

B cells take their name from the *Bursa equivalent* originating from an avian feature. Once the **B lymphocytes** have developed and reached the pre-B (precursor B cell) or immunoglobulin (IgM) stage, they migrate to the thymus gland and lymphoid tissues (spleen, lymph nodes and lymphatic follicles), where they develop into functional maturity and carry out immune responses. Maturity is achieved when they have produced and inserted proteins, called antigen receptors, into their cell surface and they have the ability to further differentiate into:

- Plasma B cells, which produce antibodies (**Immunoglobulin**'s, abbrev. **Ig**)
- Memory B cells.

Immunoglobulins

Immunoglobulins are like a pincer, which folds around an antigen (a foreign invader, pathogen) and **squashes** it, which destroys it.

We have five classes of immunoglobulins, which have the ability to differentiate and produce specific antigen antibodies. Each class is found in slightly different regions of the body and has different functions:

- IgE
- IgM
- IgG
- IgD
- IgA.

IgE

IgE is secreted by plasma cells in skin, mucous membranes of gastrointestinal and respiratory tracts and the tonsils. It is the least common immunoglobulin in serum as it binds very tightly to receptors on basophils and mast cells even before interacting with antigens. The binding activity triggers the release of various chemical proteins such as histamine that mediate inflammation.

IgM

IgM is the first immunoglobulin to be made in the fetus and the first to be made by a 'novice' B cell, when it is stimulated by an antigen. This means it is the first Ig class to be released into the plasma by the plasma B cells during the primary response. It is found in two places:

- Free in the plasma, the third most common in serum
- Attached to the B cell membrane. When it is attached to the B cell it serves as an antigen receptor. It forms natural antibodies, such as those for ABO blood group antigens when it presents as a wheel shape with five prongs (Figure 22.6).

It fixes complement and is a potent agglutinating agent and thus efficient in clumping microorganisms for elimination.

> **Jot This Down**
>
> In which situation would this property of **agglutination** be disadvantageous?

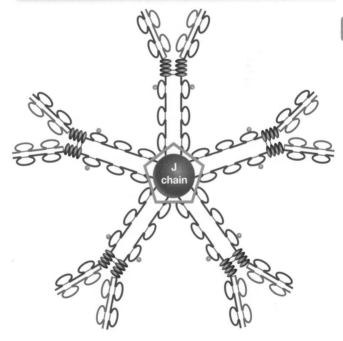

Figure 22.6 The middle J chain of IgM immunoglobulin regulates its five-pronged wheel structure. All immunoglobulins have heavy and light chains (coloured green and blue, respectively) with a hinge or central region.

475

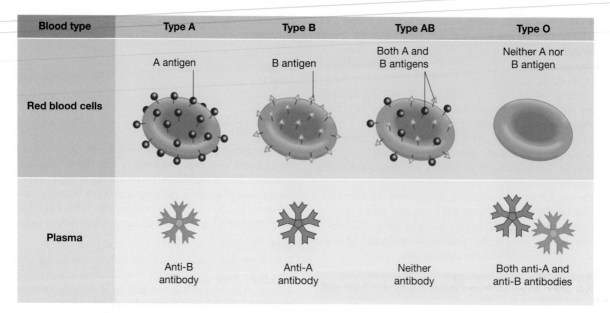

Blood type	Type A	Type B	Type AB	Type O
Red blood cells	A antigen	B antigen	Both A and B antigens	Neither A nor B antigen
Plasma	Anti-B antibody	Anti-A antibody	Neither antibody	Both anti-A and anti-B antibodies

Figure 22.7 Antigens and antibodies involved in the ABO blood groups.

In the 'Jot This Down' exercise above, you might have thought about blood groups and blood transfusion mismatch.

When you have a blood transfusion mismatch, an inflammatory reaction termed haemolytic reaction occurs when the donor erythrocytes are destroyed by preformed recipient antibodies. The red blood cells stick together (agglutinate) and block the blood flow.

A massive inflammatory reaction can be fatal!

Blood groups   Red blood cells (erythrocytes) are produced in the bone marrow (see Figure 22.4).

The surfaces of erythrocytes have genetically determined groups of antigens on their membranes. Based on the characteristic combinations of these antigens, we have three main blood groups, A, B and O. Two of the major antigens are designated A and B; those with the A antigen are designated as blood type A; those with blood type B have the B antigen. When neither antigen is found on the RBCs, the person is identified as type O. If you are type A you will have antibodies that react with type B, if you are type B you will have antibody A in the plasma. If you are type AB you will have neither antibody, if you are type O you will have type A and B antibodies (Figure 22.7).

Sometimes you may get a reaction if a foreign blood group A is introduced to a group A. This is because the antigens are not always put together in exactly the same way and although two people may be group A that does not mean that they are exactly the same type of A.

A third major RBC antigen is the Rh antigen. Persons with this antigen are called Rh-positive; those without are Rh-negative.

IgD

- Low levels in serum as it is primarily found on B cell surfaces functioning as a receptor for an antigen, and it is capable of anchoring to the membrane. Significantly, it does not bind complement.

IgG

- Most versatile, as it is capable of carrying out all the functions of the immunoglobulins, which makes it the main antibody of both primary and secondary responses

- Most abundant antibody in serum and in extra vascular spaces – represents 75–85% of circulating antibodies in serum
- Crosses the placenta mediated by a receptor on the placental cells and provides passive (the transfer of active antibody-mediated immunity in the form of readymade antibodies from the mother to the baby) immunity to the fetus
- Fixes complement
- Binds to macrophages, monocytes and some lymphocytes.

IgA

- Second most common
- Major class of Ig in secretions – tears, saliva, colostrums, intestinal juices and mucus – and thus important in local mucosal immunity
- Bathes and protects mucosal surfaces as it prevents pathogens from adhering.

The immunoglobulins vary in structure but all structures have antigen recognition sites formed by the interaction of light chain and heavy chain variable regions which provide a conical structure.

It is like a pair of forceps – open them up and pick up a pea! The pea represents the antigen. The open end of the forceps is capable of changing its shape to recognise different types and shapes of peas. IgA is the versatile 'forceps' (Figure 22.8) capable of picking up any shape or size pea, the B cell will then make a more specialised type of forceps, which are now pea-shaped.

Natural Killer Cells

Natural killer (NK) cells are lymphocytes that target cells. They reside in the spleen, lymph nodes and red bone marrow and will attack and destroy any body cells that they sense as being imperfect. These imperfect cells are those that display unusual or abnormal plasma membrane proteins. Cells that have become infected or are abnormal (as in tumour cells) become target cells. Sometimes the behaviour of the natural killer cells is a little erratic and they target normal uninfected cells – often experienced as a transient irritable throat or runny nose.

The natural killer (NK) cell: **A good cell or a bad cell or a nuisance cell?**

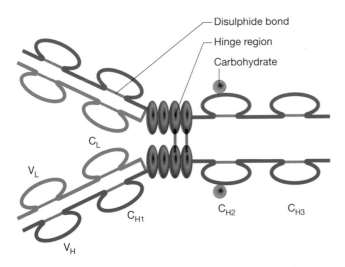

Figure 22.8 **Immunoglobulin(s) blue light chain represented by open forceps; green heavy chain represents the forceps fixed end and the hinge region enables the forceps to open and close.**

- When a natural killer cell binds to a target cell, it releases toxic granules such as **perforin** that puncture the membrane of the target cell, which allows excess fluid to flow into the cell and the target cell bursts and dies. This process is called cytolysis. If it was an infected cell, as it bursts, it releases the microbe, which is then destroyed by phagocytosis.
- It releases **granzymes** that digest proteins and induce the target cell to self-destruct by apoptosis. This destroys the cell that is infected but not the microbe inside the cell; however this can be destroyed by phagocytosis.

Natural killer T cells

Natural killer T (NKT) cells are cells that originate from the T lymphocyte and appear to have properties that resemble both those of the T lymphocyte and the natural killer cell.

They are found in the skin and mucous membranes and induce the release and action of interleukin 17.

Macrophages

These are modified monocytes, a type of agranular lymphocyte, which migrates to the tissues, such as the skin, liver, lungs, brain, spleen, red bone marrow and lymphatic nodes, where they reside as monocytes or fixed macrophages. They stand guard and emerge when they are alerted by chemicals telling them of the presence of a pathogen. As they emerge, they enlarge and become aggressive wandering macrophages, taking over from the neutrophils. They release chemicals that stimulate further inflammatory activity and play a part in the process of wound healing.

Granular white blood cells (see Figure 22.4) are produced in the red bone marrow and are different to the lymphocytes and monocytes which are agranular.

All granular leukocytes release **chemical proteins**. Chemical proteins act as chemical messengers, which can stimulate body tissues to react either by:

- modifying their structure, such as increasing the spaces between the cells and increase vascular permeability
- modifying their behaviour, such as increasing their metabolism, or by

- releasing further chemical proteins such as histamine and cytokines.

Neutrophils

Circulate in the circulation, waiting for an intruder, as their primary function is phagocytosis. They respond swiftly in response to the alert by the inflammatory dendritic cell when the outer defences are compromised and are the first cells to be attracted to the site of tissue damage.

> **Jot This Down**
>
> When we have an infection or an inflammatory reaction, blood samples are taken.
> What do you think we are looking for?

A full blood count will tell us what cells have increased in numbers, if the neutrophils are high, it indicates the infection is 'early'. If mast cells are raised it may indicate an allergy.

An exception when the neutrophil level may not be raised and when a person has an obvious infection is if the red bone marrow is not producing the neutrophils or they were not being developed, as in types of leukaemia or from medication such as chemotherapy.

As soon as the neutrophils arrive, they:

1. Release granules that enhance the inflammatory response by increasing vasodilation and vascular permeability
2. Activate the endothelial cells to express surface proteins that are 'leg like' projections that enable the neutrophil to move by diapedesis along the inner lining of the capillary and move into the tissues via gaps in the vascular capillary wall
3. Release extracellular traps (NETs) for the containment of infection and inflammation (Kumar & Sharma 2010)
4. Express complement receptors that aid phagocytosis
5. Begin to destroy any microbes in the tissues by phagocytosis and are now called 'phagocytes'.

Basophils and Mast Cells

Basophils circulate in the bloodstream and their numbers are generally very low unless an active infection is present, when they migrate towards the infected area and release chemical proteins.

Mast cells are not mobile and are found stationed in connective and mucosal tissue. They contain granules rich in histamine; those in the connective tissue are activated in response to activated complement and those in the mucosal tissue by T cells.

Oeosinophils

Eosinophils counteract the inflammatory response of basophils and mast cells by breaking down the chemicals these leukocytes release. Their numbers are generally low in the blood, unless there is an inflammatory response to a microbe or an allergic antigen.

Their main function is to stop the inflammatory process from going too far. They also have a role in fighting invasion by parasitic worms.

Dendritic Cells

These are modified monocytes and function as weak phagocytes. We have discussed their role in the thymus, where it is recognises that their most important role is as an antigen displaying cell (ADC). They are able to ingest a foreign cell and display the foreign antigen onto their own cell membrane. The dendritic cells then passes through the lymph nodes displaying the antigen 'like carrying a placard' and searching for the lymphocytes that match that antigen. This ADC triggers adaptive immunity as it is like a 'fog horn' shouting for it to 'get active' and is a significant bridge link between innate and acquired immunity.

There are several different types of dendritic cells with different roles, such as Langerhans, inflammatory and signalling, which reside in the dermal layer of the skin.

Chemical Proteins That Are Involved in Immunity

C-reactive protein (CRP) is a protein which is made and released by the liver in response to chemical released by macrophages and adipocytes in the acute phase of inflammation. It binds to a protein on the surface of dead or dying cells and bacterial cells, which activates the compliment system. The serum level is raised in the presence of a bacterial infection.

Prostaglandins are released by the damaged tissue and bring about vasodilatation. They also intensify the activity of **histamine** and **kinins**, which further increases vasodilatation. There are numerous different types of prostaglandins, for example PGE2, PGD2 and prostacyclin, all with vascular activities (not discussed in this chapter). They cause pain indirectly by sensitising the C fibres, which makes these pain receptors more sensitive to the effects of the **kinins**, for example **bradykinin** and **kallikrein**, which are released by the damaged tissues. They induce vasodilation and the contraction of smooth muscle.

The stinging sensation when you prick your finger is caused by the 'kinins' and the 'prostaglandins'.

Leukotrienes produced by white blood cells cause vasodilatation and increased vascular permeability.

Lipoxins are formed by platelets and neutrophils working together and released into the bloodstream. They direct macrophages to clean up dead cells and inhibit chemotaxis so stop the inflammatory process.

Complement is a group or complex of 20 proteins that are normally inactive. They are produced by the liver and found in the bloodstream and tissues throughout the body and are labelled according to their places in the complex as C, numbered C1–C9, factors B, D and P and some other regulatory proteins. They act in a cascade manner, i.e. C1 activates C2 and so on, when stimulated.

They are activated by tissue damage and the subsequent invasion of a pathogen and react in one of two ways:

1. The classical pathway, which depends on antibodies binding to invading microbes to form antigen-antibody complexes and then one of the C proteins, usually C1 binds to the antigen-antibody complex, which is called complement fixation OR
2. The alternative pathway, when there is interaction between the factors B, D and F with a surface protein on the microbe.

Both these pathways cause an orderly cascade of events. The complement proteins:

- Puncture the microbe, which disrupts the membrane and the cell bursts as it fills with fluid entering through the puncture 'wounds'
- Coat the microbe with a sticky protein that aids adhesion for phagocytosis – this is called **opsonisation** 'ready to eat'
- Encourage further phagocytes and macrophages, which increases inflammation

- Bind to mast cells, which in turn causes them to release histamine.

Cytokines are produced by damaged tissues and leukocytes and help to neutralise the invaders by intensifying the process of inflammation. They do this by attracting phagocytes into the area by chemotaxis (chemical attraction).

Examples of specific cytokines are as follows:

1. **Interleukins (IL1- IL30)**, of which there are several (at least 30), released by leukocytes and act on leukocytes and participate in the regulation of inflammation. They act as messengers and are involved in almost every aspect of immunity
2. **Interferons**, which are specifically antiviral chemicals and are produced by cells infected by a virus. It is protective as it travels to and binds to both nearby neighbour and distant cells that are not infected and stimulates these non infected cells 'telling them' to produce chemical proteins. These proteins then either block any potential receptors or cover their cell membrane. They may release chemicals that prevent the virus from approaching them as they become invisible to it. These actions prevent the virus from entering their cell membrane and so protect themselves. Interferon is currently being explored as a form of chemotherapy
3. **Histamine** is released by damaged tissues and increases local vasodilatation and vascular permeability, attracts leukocytes by chemotaxis to the site of injury. Plays a core role in the inflammatory response
4. **Tumour necrosis factor (TNF)** is a key regulator in the inflammatory process by attracting neutrophils, monocytes, T and B lymphocytes and macrophages in response to various stimuli. It also stimulates monocytes to secrete interleukins and more TNF, thus playing a role in the continuation of the inflammatory activity.

Fever

TNF released from stimulated macrophages and T-lymphocytes enters the bloodstream and as an **endocrine hormone**, it acts as a **pyrogen** and stimulates further cytokine liberation from mononuclear cells.

These circulating cytokines enter the brain, where they interact with a receptor on the hypothalamus and the hypothalamus then raises the body's temperature set point – the body's thermostat.

At first, your body will feel cold and will take measures to make you feel warmer. These measures are shutting down the peripheries and shivering until the new temperature is achieved. This experience is what is called a 'fever' – feeling cold with an elevated temperature!

It is a deliberate attempt by the chemicals that are mediating the fight activity as the increase in temperature increases the intensity of the inflammatory fight against the pathogen.

> ### Jot This Down
>
> The hypothalamus controls body temperature by resetting the thermostat, which brings about a number of body responses to raise the temperature.
>
> List these activities and explain what you would do to help the body reach the new set temperature and make the patient comfortable.

In the 'Jot This Down' exercise above, you might have listed these suggestions:

1. Provide extra clothing if the patient shivers
2. Give extra drinks or sugar if necessary as the body will need extra fuel. You may need to check 'blood sugar' levels if the patients is beginning to feel tired, the blood pressure is 'dropping too low' and or the heart rate is too fast. The heart rate will increase with body temperature as it will need to get the fuel round the body so that it can fight
3. Check vital signs
4. Once the body has reached the new set level, the patient will begin to feel more comfortable.

In severe infection, the subsequent systemic overproduction of TNF and cytokines leads to vascular instability and will eventually lead to septicaemia and shock.

Inflammation is like a circle of events, and will continue to go round and round until it is stopped. Lipoxins stop the inflammatory process and clean up the mess.

Phagocytosis

Phagocytosis occurs in five steps (Figure 22.9).

Phagocytes are specialised cells that perform phagocytosis:

1. **Chemotaxis** of phagocyte to the site of damage
2. **Adhesion**, the attachment of the microbe to the phagocyte
3. **Ingestion**, the cell membrane of the phagocyte extends projections that engulf the microbe and encase it in a phagosome (vesicle) in the cytoplasm. Imagine eating a sweet.
4. The phagosome then fuses with a lysosome to form a phagolysosome. The microbe is then **digested** by lysozyme and other lysosomal digestive enzymes.

5. **Destroyed or stored.** If the phagocyte did not manage to digest all of the microbe it stores the remnants in residual bodies.

If there are a large number of microbes the red bone marrow is stimulated and it will increase the number of neutrophils – 'production increases to meet the demand'.

Immunity in Action

We have looked at the structure of the lymphatic system and all the cells and chemicals it has at its disposal. We will now discuss these structures and cells in action.

All the activities are fighting ones aimed at preventing microbes from becoming a nuisance. The bacteria, which become pathogens and viruses, either feed on our bodies or liberate toxic substances. This destructive and toxic activity changes the internal environment and upsets the smooth everyday working life of the cells and thus the coordinated running of the body.

Innate Immunity

Recalling the triangle of immunity, we will look at **innate immunity** first.

Innate immunity consists of two sets of barriers – an outer perimeter and a back up secondary chemical 'fence'. We are born with all the structures and features of the 'innate' immune system (see Figure 22.10), which are our barriers to prevent invasion. They are situated in those places that the microbes are likely to target and are divided into three categories of barriers depending on their:

479

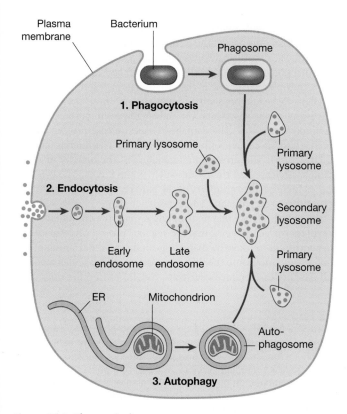

Figure 22.9 Phagocytosis.

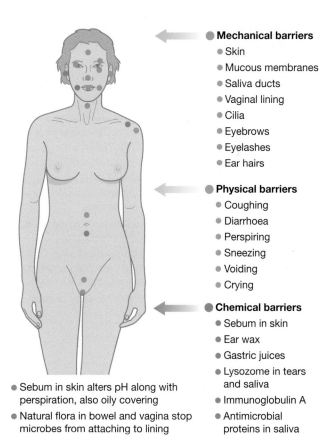

Figure 22.10 The structures and features of the innate immune system.

- **Structure**, classified as mechanical
- **Activity** classified as physical and
- **Make-up** under the category of chemical.

Jot This Down

List the components and their functions of the first-line defences, which are part of the innate immune system?

In the 'Jot This Down' exercise above, you might have thought about:

EXTERNAL PHYSICAL AND MECHANICAL BARRIERS	CHEMICAL BARRIERS AND INTERNAL DEFENCES
Skin, which comprises the outer epidermal tissues and the keratinised cells, which strengthen the outer layer of the skin	Sebum provides an oily protective coating that prevents microbes from settling and multiplying
Mucous membranes of: upper respiratory tract – nasal passages, pharynx and larynx lower respiratory tract – trachea, bronchi and lungs	Secrete mucus that moistens surfaces and traps microbes which are then dispelled by coughing and sneezing
Cilia – hair like projections that line the upper respiratory tract	Traps and expels inhaled microbes with wave like movements
Eyebrows and eye lashes protect the eyes from perspiration and foreign particles	Tears dilute and wash away irritants, keep the eye tissues moist and contain lysozyme, an antibacterial enzyme
Salivary glands and saliva	Saliva keeps mouth moist and contains lysozyme and immunoglobulin A, antimicrobial proteins
Vaginal secretions	Discourage microbial growth as they are acidic, move microbes out of the vagina
Defecation and vomiting	Expel ingested microbes
Perspiration	Washes microbes off the skin and contains the antimicrobial protein, lysozyme
Urinating	Washes the urinary tract and retards microbial growth
Ear lobes, hairs and wax	Obstruct microbes and prevents them from entering the ear, wax traps microbes
Stomach	Acidic gastric juices destroy microbes

Jot This Down

List the nursing interventions that may be necessary to support innate immunity and prevent infection.

In the 'Jot This Down' exercise above, you may have thought about:

1. **Oral hygiene:** keeping the mouth and nasal passages clear and moist. Provide and encourage fluids and assist with drinking if help is required. Give mouth care if the person you are caring for is unable to eat and drink or if the mouth becomes dry for any other reason. For example you may be caring for someone who is breathless and breathing through their mouth. When oxygen is delivered it makes the mucous membranes dry. Keep the mouth clean and moist to prevent the salivary ducts becoming clogged and to prevent cracked lips and gums.

2. **Eye care:** prevent the eyes from becoming dry with eye care if required and prevent the tear ducts from becoming clogged.

3. **Maintaining fluid balance** to ensure adequate hydration which assists in preventing the skin becoming dry with the possible formation of sores. It also aids urination

4. **Adequate nutrition** to maintain the mucous membranes lining the respiratory and gastrointestinal tracts and outer surface skin tissues

5. **Personal hygiene** which promotes general well-being of the skin and prevents microbes from germinating in areas where the skin is creased or hidden (groin, axilla).

As innate immunity is nonspecific it is able to respond rapidly to tissue damage caused by disturbance of skin cells, abrasions, cuts, exposure to extreme temperatures and chemical irritants before the onset of infection.

You will recall that the prime role of the innate immune response is to prevent infection by stopping any opportunistic microbes from entering into the bloodstream. All its actions are aimed at trapping any microbes that may have entered into the damaged tissues via the compromised outer defences. Innate immunity involves alerting interleukin 17 and getting the neutrophils into the area. Vasodilatation and increased permeability provide a wider route of access for the neutrophils into the tissues by diapedesis. Once they are there the area is sealed off by complement, the neutrophils destroy the microbes by phagocytosis and the damaged tissue is repaired. When the damaged area is sealed off, any microbes and neutrophils, dead or alive, are trapped within the tissues and become part of the serous exudate. The response is initiated by the sentinel Langerhans cells and the dendritic cells.

Neutrophils are the first cells to respond and arrive. Once they arrive, they play a lead role in the inflammatory response by releasing chemical mediators such as complement. These chemical proteins bring about vasodilatation and increase the permeability of the blood vessel wall. The damaged tissues release prostaglandins which attract more neutrophils into the area by chemotaxis (chemical attraction). The prostaglandins augment the activity of other chemicals released by the tissues such as the kinins. The prostaglandins increase the sensitivity of the pain receptors and the kinins irritate these receptors and you experience pain.

You will also recall that neutrophils activate the endothelial cells to express surface proteins that are 'leg like' projections that enable the neutrophil to move by diapedesis along the inner lining of the capillary and move into the tissues via gaps in the vascular capillary wall AND release extracellular traps (NETs) to trap the microbe.

Red Flag

The vasodilation and increased vascular permeability increases the blood flow to the area of damage, which causes **swelling**, **redness**, **warmth** and **pain**. The accumulation of the prostaglandins and the bradykinins increase the sensation of pain. The clinical presentation is 'classically' one of **inflammation**.

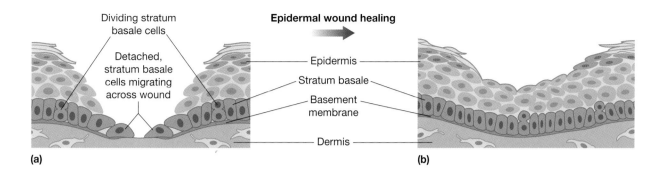

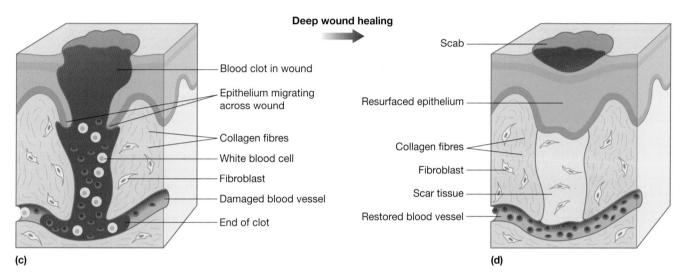

Figure 22.11 Skin wound healing.

Wound Healing
Deep wound healing

There are four phases of wound healing.

The exudate from the inflammatory process contains neutrophils, some of which will still be active and they will continue to kill any microbes by phagocytosis. This means that any exudates is sterile and will promote healing. As part of the innate immunity, the damaged tissues release platelet activating and tissue growth factors, thus wound healing is instigated immediately following the tissue damage with the **inflammatory phase (1)**.

Following injury (Figure 22.11), there is an immediate platelet aggregation (they stick together) and they release thromboplastin, which facilitates haemostasis. After the first phase, when bleeding has been controlled and the tissues are cleaned optimum wound healing requires a well structured and orderly progression of tissue repair by:

- cell migration and proliferation, and
- extracellular matrix deposition and remodelling.

This granulation is achieved by the tissues themselves with the use of chemical mediators and growth factors.

Granulation starts from 2 days after injury and lasts up to 3 weeks with fibroblasts laying beds of collagen and fills the defect with the production of new capillaries. Once granulation has occurred, there is contraction of the skin and the edges of the wound are pulled together. Finally **epithelilisation** (growing of

epithelial cell) crosses moist surfaces and cells travel about 3 cm from the point of origin in all directions, which completes the **proliferative phase (2)**.

At about 3 weeks the **remodelling phase (3),** with new collagen forming which increases tensile strength to wounds, will complete the process.

Red Flag

Scar tissue is only 80% as strong as original tissue.

Cell-Mediated Immunity

You will recall that as the need for defence intensifies (Figure 22.12) the neutrophils recruit the help of the **monocytes**, stored in the spleen and circulated towards other lymphatic tissues. As the monocytes migrate to the area of invasion, they enlarge and develop into phagocytic cells, termed wandering **macrophages**. Other stored monocytes are termed 'fixed macrophages', as they stand guard in several specific tissues such as the skin, liver, lungs, brain, spleen, lymph nodes and red bone marrow. The macrophages are larger and more aggressive towards the microbes in comparison to the size and behaviour of the neutrophils.

481

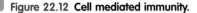

Figure 22.12 **Cell mediated immunity.**

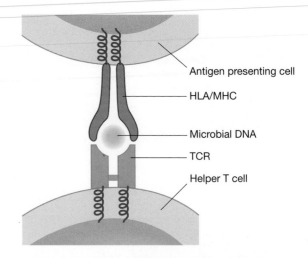

Figure 22.13 Showing the binding of the helper T-cell receptor with major histocompatability complex (MHC)/human leukocyte antigen receptor and the microbial DNA.

Recall T-cell maturity is signalled when the T cells make and insert antigen receptors on their cell surface as they develop in the thymus gland. T-cell antigen receptors (TCR) on the surface of T cells recognise the microbe fragments as foreign only when they are bound to the HLA and form HLA-microbial DNA complexes:

- When the T cell recognises the foreign DNA, it binds to the self-receptor and the microbial DNA on the macrophage and releases interleukin 1, which in turn mobilises the CD4 helper T cells
- The CD4 cell is activated and releases interleukin 2, a co-stimulator, which enables:
  - the helper T to recognise the microbial DNA as foreign
  - this 'educated' helper T cell to clone, thus there will be more helper T cells that recognise this foreign DNA
  - the helper T cell to differentiate into regulatory T cells and cytotoxic T cells
  - the regulatory T(R) cell to differentiate into memory T (M) and suppressor T (S) cells
  - alerting of the B cells to the presence of foreign DNA.
- The memory T cells will now recognise that foreign DNA if it turns up again
- The cytotoxic T cells CD8 go on the rampage and circulate looking for infected cells and eliminating them. They do this by releasing granules, granzymes, which puncture the infected cell membrane and the cell destructs
- In addition, cytotoxic cells will secrete chemical proteins that attract neutrophils and encourage phagocytosis and prevent them from leaving the area.

The suppressor T cells stop the process when all the infected cells have been destroyed. After **tissue transplantation** the donor tissue is sometimes recognised as foreign and macrophages present donor DNA to the interleukin activated lymphocytes (B and T cells), which brings about both antibody- and cell-mediated effects. Killer T cells bind with cells of the transplanted tissue, resulting in cell cytolysis and death. Helper T cells stimulate the multiplication and differentiation of B cells, and antibodies are produced to graft endothelium. To reduce the chances of this happening, donors and patients must be matched so that their proteins are as similar as possible. The greatest genetic diversity between different individuals occurs in the MHC region and particular care must be taken to

Linking Innate Immunity to Cell-Mediated Immunity

Following digestion of the microbe, the macrophage retains the microbe's DNA and displays it on its outer membrane surface next to its 'self' marker protein, known as the **human leukocyte antigen (HLA)** or **self-antigen**. When the macrophage presents the DNA to the T lymphocyte the macrophage is referred to as an **antigen presenting cell (APC)**. The activity links innate immunity to cell-mediated immunity.

These self-antigens are commonly referred to as **the major histocompatibility complex (MHC)** as they are coded within a large cluster of genes from a region in the genome (DNA), known as the 'major histocompatibility' complex. As chromosomes are paired, each person inherits one member of the pair from each parent and with each chromosome pair containing multiple genes, each carrying instructions for the production of one part of the self-antigen the possibility of two people having the same HLA type is extremely remote (Figure 22.13).

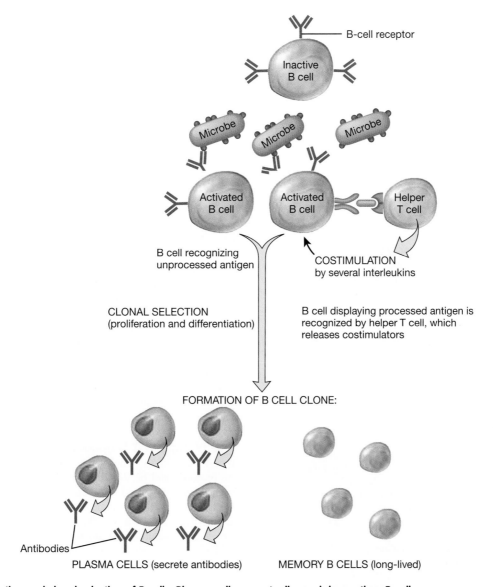

B-cell receptor

Inactive B cell

Microbe Microbe Microbe

Activated B cell Activated B cell Helper T cell

B cell recognizing unprocessed antigen

COSTIMULATION by several interleukins

CLONAL SELECTION (proliferation and differentiation)

B cell displaying processed antigen is recognized by helper T cell, which releases costimulators

FORMATION OF B CELL CLONE:

Antibodies

PLASMA CELLS (secrete antibodies) MEMORY B CELLS (long-lived)

Figure 22.14 Activation and clonal selection of B cells. Plasma cells are actually much larger than B cells.

match the MHC molecules of patients and donors as accurately as possible.

Antibody Adapted Immunity

The B lymphocytes are the key cells for mediating the antibody-mediated immune response (Figure 22.14). The interleukin, secreted by the helper T cells functioning as antigen presenting cells in the cell-mediated immune response stimulate the growth and differentiation of B cells into memory cells and plasma cells B cells. They are further activated by contact with an antigen. The plasma B cells produce specific antibodies, also known as antigen specific immunoglobulins, which serve to inactivate an invading antigen. The memory B cells 'remember' a specific antigen, and, when exposed to it a second time, immediately initiate the immune response.

Antibodies may bind to viruses or bacteria and inhibit their pathogenic activity. Different B cells generally produce different immunoglobulin sequences and this enables our B-cell repertoire to deal with almost any pathogenic molecule.

Disorders of the Immune System

We have learned how **inflammation** warns, fight, destroys and evicts unwanted residents in our bodies. Recall the classic presentation of inflammation; as redness, swelling, warmth and pain, all of which, in the case of **hypersensitivity** will be exacerbated both in terms of speed of onset, intensity and duration. Classification of reaction is:

- Primarily by the type of immune response that occurs on contact with the allergen; severe or mild
- Immediate or delayed
- By cell interaction: antigen–antigen or antigen–lymphocyte. Antigen–antigen are immediate, characterised as types I, II and III, also known as immediate hypersensitivity responses. Type IV hypersensitivity is an antigen–lymphocyte reaction, resulting in a delayed hypersensitivity reaction.

Immunological response is the preferred means of studying allergies, even though there may be two types of reaction occurring simultaneously

In the 'Jot This Down' exercise above, you might have thought about:

- Arthritis – rheumatoid or joint injury
- Psoriasis
- Crohn's disease
- Asthma – allergy.

There are four types of hypersensitivity responses, classified as below.

Type I IgE-mediated hypersensitivity

Common hypersensitivity reactions, such as allergic asthma, allergic rhinitis (hay fever), allergic conjunctivitis and anaphylactic shock, are typical of type I or IgE-mediated hypersensitivity. This type of hypersensitivity response is triggered when an allergen, which is 'perceived as a threat but in reality is relatively harmless' such as animal hair or a dust mite, is inhaled and it interacts with IgE bound to mast cells and basophils. The potency of the perceived threat by the IgE dictates the intensity of the response. This antibody–allergen complex prompts the mast cells to release histamine and complement.

Red Flag

With **anaphylaxis** the response is a rapid and intense one and is life-threatening.

Anaphylaxis is an acute systemic type I response that occurs in highly sensitive persons. The reaction begins within minutes of exposure to the allergen and may be almost instantaneous. The release of histamine and other mediators causes vasodilation and increased capillary permeability, smooth muscle contraction, and bronchial constriction. These chemical mediators cause the client to experience the typical manifestations of anaphylaxis. Initially, a sense of foreboding or uneasiness, light-headedness, and itching palms and scalp may be noted. Hives may develop, along with localised tissue swelling of the eyelids, lips, tongue, hands, feet and genitals. Swelling can also affect the uvula and larynx, impairing breathing. This is further complicated by bronchial constriction. The patient will be struggling to breathe, using the accessory muscles and gasping for air, stridor and wheezing, and a barking cough. These respiratory effects can be lethal if the reaction is severe and intervention is not immediately available. Vasodilation and fluid loss from the vascular system can lead to impaired tissue perfusion and hypotension, a condition known as anaphylactic shock.

Type II cytotoxic hypersensitivity

Antibody A haemolytic transfusion reaction to blood of an incompatible type is characteristic of a type II or cytotoxic hypersensitivity reaction. IgG or IgM antibodies are formed to a cell-bound antigen, such as the ABO antigen. When these antibodies bind with the antigen, the complement cascade is activated, resulting in destruction of the target cell. Haemolytic disease of the newborn is caused by this type of reaction.

Type II reactions may be stimulated by an exogenous antigen, such as foreign tissue or cells, or a drug reaction, in which the drug forms an antigenic complex on the surface of a blood cell, stimulating the production of antibodies. The affected cell is then destroyed in the resulting antigen–antibody reaction; for example haemolytic anaemia is sometimes associated with the administration of drugs such as penicillins.

Endogenous antigens can also stimulate a type II reaction, resulting in an autoimmune disorder such as Goodpasture's syndrome, in which antigens are formed to specific tissues in the lungs and kidneys. Hashimoto's thyroiditis and autoimmune haemolytic anaemia are additional examples of autoimmune type II reactions.

Type III immune complex-mediated hypersensitivity

Type III immune complex-mediated hypersensitivity results from the formation of IgG or IgM antibody–antigen immune complexes in the circulation. When these complexes are deposited in vessel walls and extravascular tissues, complement is activated and chemical mediators of inflammation, such as histamine, are released. Neutrophils are attracted to the area and increase the intensity. When neutrophils phagocytise the immune complexes, lysosomal enzymes are released, increasing tissue damage.

Localised responses may occur at a number of different sites. As immune complexes accumulate in the glomerular basement membrane of the kidneys, for example following a streptococcal infection or with systemic lupus erythematosus, glomerulonephritis develops.

Type IV antigen–T lymphocyte

Type IV antigen–T lymphocyte is a cell-mediated process and so the response will be slow in comparison to an antibody-antigen interaction and so it is documented as a 'delayed response'. It occurs due to an exaggerated interaction between an antigen and normal cell-mediated mechanisms. This exaggerated interaction results in the release of soluble inflammatory and immune mediators (from the lysozymes within the macrophages) and recruitment of killer T cells, causing local tissue destruction.

In the 'Jot This Down' exercise above, you may have thought about:

- Establishing the allergen
- The response to the allergen(s)
- Minimising the exposure to the allergen.

What are the aims of your interventions?

- To prevent a hypersensitivity response
- Provide prompt, effective interventions if an allergic response occurs
- Observe for evidence of an allergic response.

With a hypersensitivity response, supportive care is important to relieve discomfort. This may involve the administration of selected antihistamine or anti-inflammatory medications.

NOTE: Reassure the patient that all measures have been implemented to try and stop an allergy reaction. The patient may not trust that all staff will take care to remove the allergen for example and may keep asking if all the members of staff know about the allergy and are taking the correct care. To allay the individual's fear, suggest placing the information in a prominent place so that the patient and everyone else can read it.

Red Flag

Identifying allergens for the individual to reduce the likelihood of exposure is a key aspect of management. A complete history of the client's allergies is obtained, including medications, foods, animals, plants and other materials. The type of hypersensitivity response is documented, as are its onset, manifestations and usual treatment.

The nurse in the allergy clinic tells the patient what is going to happen.

Allergy clinics do tests to identify allergens and you may have seen patients with red dots in a line on the anterior aspect of the forearm. The potential allergens have been applied on the skin to test for an inflammatory response.

Initially, the blood will be tested before the allergen is put on the skin because if the patient is hypersensitive it may cause an extreme response even if it is only on the skin.

To identify possible allergens or hypersensitivity reactions, the following laboratory tests may be ordered:

- White blood cell (WBC) count with differential can detect high levels of circulating eosinophils. Normally, eosinophils constitute a very small percentage (1–4%) of the total WBCs. Oeosinophilia, however, is often present in clients with type I hypersensitivities
- *Radioallergosorbent test (RAST)* measures the amount of IgE directed toward specific allergens. Test results are compared with control values and used to identify hypersensitivities. RAST poses no risk for an anaphylactic reaction. It is particularly useful in detecting allergies to some occupational chemicals and toxic allergens (Goldsby *et al.* 2003)
- *Blood type and cross-match* are ordered prior to any anticipated transfusions. Because a blood transfusion is actually a transplant of living tissue, antigen matching is vital to prevent significant hypersensitivity reactions. Once blood type is determined, a sample of the client's blood is mixed with a sample of matching donor blood and observed for antigen–antibody reactions in the cross-match portion of this test. Although this procedure greatly reduces the risk of a haemolytic transfusion reaction (type II hypersensitivity), it does not totally eliminate it
- *Indirect Coombs' test* detects the presence of circulating antibodies (other than ABO antibodies) against RBCs. The client's serum is mixed with the donor's RBCs. If the client's serum contains antibodies to an RBC antigen, agglutination (clumping together) will occur. This is called a 'positive response'. The normal value is negative, or no agglutination. This test is also part of the cross-match of a blood 'type and crossmatch'.
- *Direct Coombs' test* detects antibodies on the client's RBCs that damage and destroy the cells. This is used following a suspected transfusion reaction to detect antibodies coating the transfused RBCs. It can also identify haemolytic anaemia when the cause is unknown. In the direct Coombs' test, the client's RBCs are mixed with Coombs' serum, which contains antibodies to IgG and several complement components. Agglutination will occur if the client's RBCs are coated with antibodies, resulting in a positive test. As with the indirect Coombs' test, the normal test result is negative

- Immune complex assays may be performed to detect the presence of circulating immune complexes in suspected type III hypersensitivity responses. The assays are particularly useful in diagnosing suspected autoimmune disorders. Nonspecific assays of IgG-, IgM-, and IgA-containing immune complexes, which do not detect specific antibodies, as well as specific antibody assays may be done. The normal result is a test negative for circulating immune complexes. A negative test does not, however, rule out an immune complex hypersensitivity response. In some cases, a negative result may indicate that the disease process has reached a later stage, in which complexes are no longer circulating but have initiated extensive tissue damage, such as glomerulonephritis (Kasper *et al.* 2005).

Complement assay is also useful in detecting immune complex disorders.

The opposite to hypersensitive reactions is a very slow or impaired response.

Immunodeficiency

Immunodeficiency is when the inflammatory response is impaired or absent. This may happen if one of the components is missing or damaged.

Genetic and inherited

Common variable immune deficiency (CVID) is characterised by humoral immunity deficiency. A genetic mutation that impairs the development of the B cells, resulting in deficient and insufficient numbers of IgG, IgA and IgM

Jot This Down

A patient has an impaired immunity due to a genetic mutation.

What do you think their needs are?

In the 'Jot This Down' exercise above, you might have thought about:

- Prevention of infection
- Prenatal diagnosis
- Genetic counselling.

Management involves careful and caring consideration and investigation so that the correct information can be provided as it has serious implications for future pregnancies and other relatives. Genetics consultation can help.

What the Experts Say   Help the Patient and Families

- Understand the cause of the condition
- Understand the expected prognosis
- Understand the implications
- Explain the need for genetic testing
- Explain the process of genetic testing
- Explain the coordination of the multidisciplinary team

Link To/Go To

Genetics – genetic testing and counselling – NHS Choices.
http://www.nhs.uk/Conditions/Genetics/Pages/genetic-testing -and-counselling.aspx

Immunodeficiency acquired through infection

AIDS is an immunodeficiency disorder caused by a virus that destroys the helper T cells (CD4).

Recall CD4 helper T cells are involved in cell-mediated immunity and without them the immune response is 'truncated'. As you know, a virus enters a cell and uses it as a 'bed and breakfast', multiplies incessantly and invades the helper T cells and attacks the macrophages. The virus plants its DNA into these cells and they then produce more of the virus; they are like squatters.

Produced by drug therapy as an unwanted side-effect

Methotrexate (chemotherapy) is an example of a drug which has the potential to impair the immunity as it interferes with the production of white blood cells.

Diseases that reduce the source of immunity, such as lymphomas and leukaemias

These impair the production of white blood cells or their development.

Conclusion

This chapter has provided the reader with an insight into the major organs and tissues of the lymphatic system and their functions. It has explored the basic processes of immunity and the chapter provides all the structures and tools (cells and chemicals) that the body uses to protect itself. There are several examples of when the immune system starts off with a fault, develops a fault or is damaged, and the reader is invited to explore the functions of the cells and chemical proteins that are the tools for protecting the body against foreign invaders.

Eukaryotes, bacteria, archaea and viruses are examined, so that the appropriate interventions can be implemented to provide a safe environment in a healthcare setting, and the reader is provided with examples of application to nursing interventions. As such, the chapter explores the physiology of innate immunity and explains how inflammation links to infection and fever and wound healing. The reader is also invited to compare and contrast the processes of cell-mediated and antibody-mediated immunity, and to understand the aetiology and pathophysiologies of autoimmune disorders and allergies to assess physical and psychological needs and support of patients in their care.

Key Points

- The difference between the innate immune response and those of the cell-mediated and antibody-mediated responses.
- The lymphatic system – the structure and its components – how they function and communicate to fight infection.
- The impact of genetics on immunity.
- The chemical proteins involved in immunity.
- Immunoglobulins and antibodies.
- Autoimmune diseases.
- Cancer.

Glossary

Adaptive immunity: the immunity we build up against infections, made up of cell-mediated immunity and antibody-mediated immunity

Antibodies: specialised specific immunoglobulins adapted to a specific microbe

Human leukocyte antigen: a cluster of proteins on the cell membrane that are produced by the major histocompatibility complex; the terms human leukocyte antigen and major histocompatibility antigen are often used interchangeably

Antibody-mediated immunity: adaptive immunity involving the B cells with the manufacture of specific antibodies

Antigen: a microbe that has been recognised by the body T cells as foreign

B cells: lymphocytes that are produced by stem cells in the bone marrow and mature in the thymus gland and lymphoid tissue

Cell-mediated immunity: the link between innate and antibody-mediated immunity and involves the T cells

Immunoglobulins: molecules produced by lymphocytes. There are five distinct classes

IgM: the first immunoglobulin to be made in the fetus and the first to be made by a 'novice' B cell when it is stimulated by an antigen. This means it is the first Ig class to be released into the plasma by the plasma B cells during the primary response

IgG: most versatile immunoglobulin, as it is capable of carrying out all the functions of the immunoglobulins, which makes it the main antibody of both primary and secondary responses

IgA: second most common immunoglobulin. Major class of Ig in secretions – tears, saliva, colostrum

IgE: the most common immunoglobulin, involved in allergy

IgD: least known immunoglobulin. Its functions are still being discovered

Innate immunity: the immunity that we are born with

Microbe: any microorganism that is not part of the human body

Major histocompatibility complex (MHC): a group of genes that code for specific cluster of proteins that are the markers on the surface of the cell membrane. They are unique to each individual

Pathogen: a microbe that has entered the body and caused inflammation

T cells: lymphocytes that are produced by stem cells in the bone marrow and mature in the thymus gland

References

Cua, D. & Tato, C. (2010) Innate IL-17-producing cells: the sentinels of the immune system. *Nature Reviews Immunology*, 10, 479–489.

Goldsby, R., Kindt, T., Osborne, B. & Kuby, J. (2003) *Immunology*, 5th edn. W.H. Freeman, New York.

Johnson, A., Islam, A., Duckworth, G., Livermore, D. & Hayward, A. (2007) Protective effect of antibiotics against serious complications of common respiratory tract infections: retrospective cohort study with the UK General Practice Research Database. *British Medical Journal*, 335(7627), 982.

Kasper, D., Longo, D., Fauci, A., Hauser, S., Jameson, J. & Loscalzo, J. (2005) *Harrison's Principles of Internal Medicine*, Vol. 1. McGraw Hill, Maidenhead.

Kau, L., Ahern, P., Griffin, N, Goodman, A. & Gordon, J. (2011) Human nutrition, the gut microbiome and immune system: envisioning the future. *Nature*, 474(7351), 327–338.

Kumar, V. and Sharma, A. (2010) Neutrophils: Cinderella of innate immune system. *International Immunopharmacology* 10, 1325–1334.

Miller, L. (2008) Toll-like receptors in skin. *Advances in Dermatology*, 24, 71–87.

Salmon, J., Armstrong, C. & Ansel, J. (1994) The skin as an immune organ. *Western Journal of Medicine*, 160(2), 146–152.

Singh, M. & Das, R. (2011) Zinc for the common cold. *Cochrane Database Systematic Reviews*, (2):CD001364.

Williams, A. (2002) Yogurt: still a favorite for vaginal candidiasis? *Journal of the National Medical Association*, 94(4), A10.

Further Reading

Katsnelson, A. (2006) Kicking off adaptive immunity: the discovery of dendritic cells. *Journal of Experimental Medicine*, 203, 1622.

Steinman, R. (2007) Dendritic cell: versatile controllers of the immune system. *Nature Medicine*, 13, 7–11.

Stockinger, B., Veldhoen, M. & Martin, B. (2007) Th17 T cells: linking innate and adaptive immunity. *Seminars in Immunology* 19(6), 353–361.

Test Yourself

1. We are born with some immunity, which is called:
   (a) Cell-mediated immunity
   (b) Innate immunity
   (c) Antibody-mediated immunity

2. Innate immunity involves:
   (a) The B cells
   (b) The T cells
   (c) Both a and b

3. The lymphatic system circulates:
   (a) Plasma
   (b) Lymph
   (c) Neither a nor b

4. Lymph nodes are found:
   (a) In the axilla
   (b) In the groin
   (c) In both a and b

5. Interferon is found in the body, it is:
   (a) An antimicrobial chemical
   (b) An antiviral chemical

6. Neutrophils are:
   (a) Red blood cells
   (b) White blood cells
   (c) Neither a nor b

7. There are several immunoglobulin classes in the body:
   (a) True
   (b) False

8. Antibodies are:
   (a) Specific
   (b) Non-specific
   (c) T cells

9. B cells are part of:
   (a) Antibody-mediated immunity
   (b) Innate immunity
   (c) Cell-mediated immunity

10. An autoimmune disease is:
    (a) An infection
    (b) Acute disease
    (c) Chronic disease

Answers

1. b
2. b
3. b
4. c
5. b
6. b
7. a
8. a
9. a
10. c

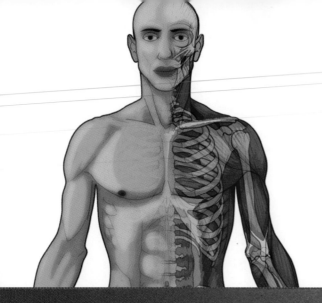

23

Pain Management

Anthony Wheeldon

University of Hertfordshire, UK

Learning Outcomes

On completion of this chapter you will be able to:

- Describe the physiology of pain
- Demonstrate an understanding of the Gate Control Theory of Pain
- Explain the difference between acute and chronic pain
- Identify the physiological consequences of unresolved pain
- Discuss the impact of psychosocial issues on the individual with pain
- Identify the major causes of pain

Competencies

All nurses must:

1. Recognise the importance of pain recognition as part of a comprehensive patient assessment
2. Demonstrate the ability to perform a comprehensive assessment of an individual's pain
3. Recognise the cardinal signs and symptoms of acute pain
4. Plan effective pain management, which incorporates both pharmacological and non-pharmacological methods of pain control
5. Work collaboratively with other members of the multidisciplinary team to ensure that patients receive care interventions that are based on the best available evidence
6. Promote self-management strategies in individuals living with chronic pain

 Visit the companion website at **www.wileynursingpractice.com** where you can test yourself using flashcards, multiple-choice questions and more.

Nursing Practice: Knowledge and Care, First Edition. Edited by Ian Peate, Karen Wild and Muralitharan Nair.
© 2014 John Wiley & Sons, Ltd. Published 2014 by John Wiley & Sons, Ltd. Companion website: www.wileynursingpractice.com

Introduction

Everyone throughout their lifetime will experience pain at various times to varying degrees; indeed, pain is the most common reason for people to seek medical assistance (McCaffery & Beebe 1994). Pain is a complex phenomenon that can be difficult to conceptualise. Pain is often defined as an unpleasant or uncomfortable sensation that acts as a warning of tissue damage, as occurs as a result of injury, strain or disease for example. However, there are times when pain lacks such a useful purpose and continues long after healing is completed. Pain is a common factor shared by all human beings but it should be treated as a personal and individual experience. This is because it is widely recognised that the way individuals express and cope with their pain is influenced by a multitude of determining factors, which may include culture, life experiences and personality but could equally be difficult to determine or characterise. Pain can also be an emotional experience unrelated to tissue damage. Pain is often used to describe feelings of loss, grief and even unrequited love for example. Whatever the cause or nature of pain, it is vital that nurses recognise that, if inadequately controlled, pain can be detrimental to the individual's physiological and psychological well-being. Although pain management is often associated with the use of analgesia, there are a number of non-pharmacological methods of pain management that can help patients live with and cope with their pain. Successful assessment and control of pain is, therefore, reliant upon an individualised holistic plan of care that utilises a range of treatments.

The Physiology of Pain

Pain physiology involves both physiological and psychological concepts and, as a result, is a complex phenomenon that has some aspects that are not fully understood. The transmission and sensation of pain follows very distinct processes. Firstly tissue damage is detected by the peripheral nervous system by specialised nerve cells called nociceptors. Peripheral sensory neurones are then innervated and nerve signals are sent towards the central nervous system. On receiving pain signals the brain then interprets the meaning and location of the pain (Figure 23.1).

Nociceptors

Nociceptors are free nerve endings that are found throughout the body. They are present in every tissue, except for the brain. Nociceptors are stimulated by noxious stimuli, of which there are three broad types – thermal, mechanical and chemical. Thermal stimuli are sensations of severe heat or cold and mechanical stimuli are produced by tissue damage caused by the following:

- Trauma or minor injury
- Ischaemia and hypoxia
- Ulceration
- Infection
- Nerve damage
- Inflammation.

While mechanical stimuli detect tissue damage, chemical stimuli detect the chemical products of tissue damage. Damaged tissue results in the release of pro-inflammatory cytokines, such as histamine, kinins and prostaglandins – all of which stimulate nociceptors as well as promoting an inflammatory response. The precise actions of nociceptors are not fully understood, however two dis-

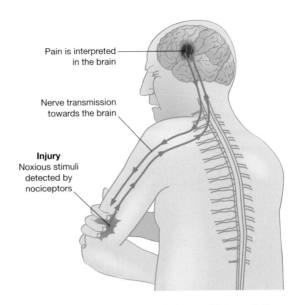

Figure 23.1 Pain pathway of transmission and interpretation.

Pain is interpreted in the brain

Nerve transmission towards the brain

Injury Noxious stimuli detected by nociceptors

tinct types have been identified. Polymodal nociceptors detect mechanical, thermal and chemical stimuli, whereas mechanoreceptors sense intense mechanical stimuli only (Julius & Basbaum 2001).

The Ascending Pain Pathway

The ascending pain pathway describes the transmission of pain messages from the site of injury to the areas of the brain that interpret their meaning. The stimulation of nociceptors sets in motion a chain reaction, which leads directly to the transmission of a pain impulse along sensory fibres from the site of injury towards the spinal cord, through the central nervous system and eventually to the brain and somatosensory cortex within the brain, where the severity and meaning of the pain is analysed. The ascending pain pathway consists of the following three neurones:

- First order neurones
- Second order neurones
- Third order neurones.

First order neurones transmit pain messages from the nociceptors to the spinal cord. **Second order** neurones carry the pain signal upwards through the spinal cord towards the diencephalon region of the brain. **Third order** neurones then convey the pain signals further into the brain towards the somatosensory cortex (Figure 23.2). The line of communication between the first, second and third order neurones is maintained by a number of neurotransmitters, such as substance P and serotonin (MacLellan 2006).

First and second order neurones

Several neurones are responsible for the transmission of sensations towards the spinal cord. However, the following two key neurones are responsible for transporting pain sensation from the site of injury.

- A-delta (Aδ) fibres
- C fibres.

The velocity of transmission is dependent on a number of factors. The wider the diameter of the neurone, the faster the nerve signals will travel. Also important is the presence of myelin on the

491

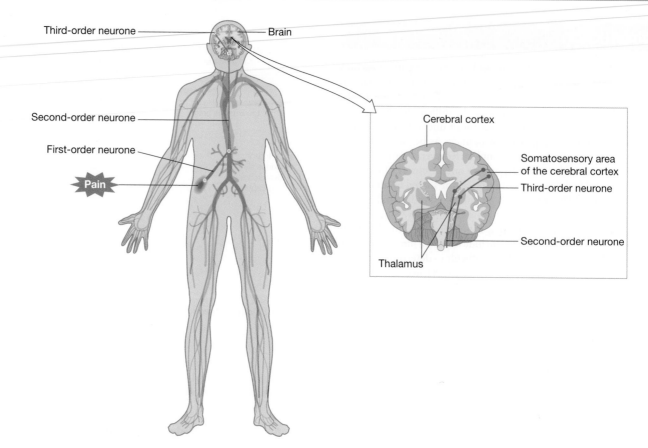

Figure 23.2 The ascending pain pathway.

axon portion of the neurone. Myelin is a multi-layered lipid and protein covering, which is often referred to as a myelin sheath (Figure 23.3). Neurones with a myelin sheath are said to be 'myelinated'. Myelinated neurones are able to transmit nerve signals at a faster rate because myelin electrically insulates and increases the speed of nerve conduction. **Aδ fibres** are myelinated, whereas **C fibres** are not. Aδ fibres are also wider in diameter (1–5 µm) than C fibres (0.2–1.5 µm) (Table 23.1). Aδ fibres therefore can transmit pain impulses much faster than the thinner and non-myelinated C fibres.

First order neurones enter the spinal cord at a location called the 'dorsal horn' (Figure 23.4). At this point, they synapse with a second order neurone, of which there are two distinct types:

- Nociceptive-specific (NS) neurones
- Wide dynamic range (WDR) neurones.

Second order neurones cross over into the white matter of the spinal cord. The white matter consists mainly of neurones with myelinated axons and are, therefore, able to transmit the pain signals upwards towards the brain at great velocity. This pathway, which travels upwards through the white matter to the brain, is called the spinothalamic tract (Figure 23.5).

First and second pain sensation

When pain is first encountered, it is often described as having two distinct phases or *first* and *second pain*. First pain sensation is a sharp or pricking pain, while second pain is the dull, burning or aching feeling that follows. First pain is generated by mechanoreceptors and is transmitted by Aδ fibres. Second pain on the other hand, is thought to be stimulated by polymodal nociceptors and transmitted by the slower C fibres. First and second pain impulses follow the same neurone pathway as sensation of touch, mild heat and cold. The sensory fibres responsible for the transmission of cutaneous sensation of touch, mild heat and cold are A-beta (**Aβ**) **fibres**. A-beta (Aβ) fibres are myelinated and wider in diameter than Aδ fibres and C fibres (see Table 23.1). They can, therefore, transmit signals of touch, mild heat and cold faster than Aδ fibres and C fibres can transmit pain sensation. While both nociceptor-specific (NS) and wide dynamic range (WDR) second order neurones react to noxious stimuli, WDR neurones also respond to the non-noxious stimuli transmitted by Aβ fibres. Therefore, stimulation of Aβ fibres, by rubbing a mild injury, for example, could help alleviate mild first and second pain.

Jot This Down

Spend a little time considering how many temperature-based non-pharmacological pain management interventions, such as heat patches or cold compresses, may help alleviate mild to moderate pain.

Third order neurones – pain interpretation

Pain is not sensed until nociceptor communication reaches the brain. Third order neurones receive pain sensation from second order neurones as the pain signal enters the brain. Pain transmission then continues through structures, such as the reticular

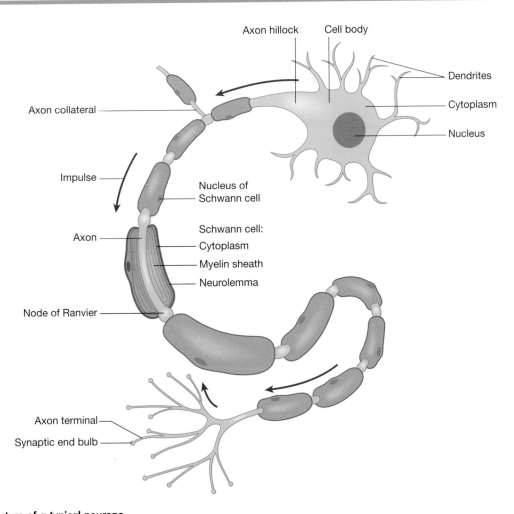

Figure 23.3 Structure of a typical neurone.

Table 23.1 Size and velocity of first-order sensory fibres.

SENSORY FIBRE	DIAMETER	MYELINATED	SPEED OF CONDUCTION
A-beta (Aβ) fibres	6–12 μm	Yes	35–75 m/s
A-delta (Aδ) fibres	1–5 μm	Yes	5–35 m/s
C fibres	0.2–1.5 μm	No	0.5–2 m/s

formation, the hypothalamus and the thalamus before moving towards the somatosensory cortex. The reticular formation, the thalamus and hypothalamus are responsible for the autonomic stress response to pain, i.e. tachycardia, diaphoresis, hypertension. Pain transmission then continues through the brain towards the somatosensory cortex, which allows the individual to locate and describe the pain. In addition to the location of pain, the brain will also generate an emotional response, be it anger or distress or mild irritation. The area of the brain thought to influence this emotional response is the limbic system (Figure 23.6). The limbic system is often referred to as the 'emotional brain', as it processes feelings of pain, pleasure, affection and anger. In addition to an emotional

response, the limbic system also establishes the seriousness of the pain; however the significance attributed to pain is dependent on the individual and their circumstances. The limbic system also helps the individual to remember why the pain occurred and over time people may learn to avoid painful stimuli, such as sharp objects and broken glass, thus protecting themselves from injury (Godfrey 2005a). However, this protective element has its limits, for example individuals may deliberately expose themselves to potential injury and pain if it means rescuing a loved one from a perilous situation, i.e. from a house fire (Johnson 2005).

Reflex Arcs

As pain is not interpreted until pain messages stimulated by nociceptors reach the brain, there is a minute fraction of time between the initial injury and pain sensation. Reflex arcs are a mechanism that aims to reduce the amount of potential tissue damage by forcing the body to move quickly away from the source of injury in that fraction of a second between nociceptor stimulation and pain sensation. A good example of a reflex arc in action is an individual's reaction to stepping on a pin. On stepping onto the sharp pin reflex arcs ensure that the foot will involuntarily move upwards and away from the pin before pain is sensed thus reducing the amount of potential tissue damage. This phenomenon

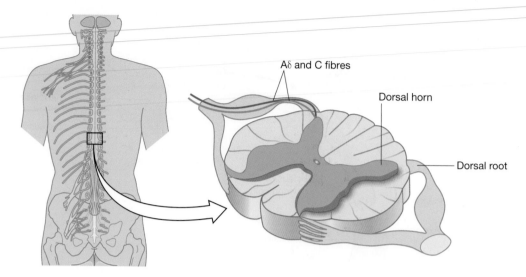

Figure 23.4 Cross-section of the spinal cord. Note that both sides are identical.

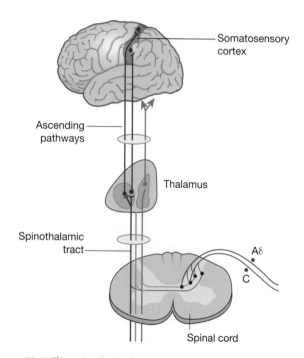

Figure 23.5 The spinothalamic tract.

analgesic properties. Because of their analgesic effect, these neuropeptides are often referred to as endogenous or natural opiates. The three major groups of endogenous opiate are:

- Endorphins
- Enkephalins
- Dynorphins.

Throughout the central nervous system, there are opiate receptors, which when stimulated can block the transmission of the neurotransmitter substance P. There are four major classifications of opiate receptor:

- mu (μ)
- kappa (κ)
- sigma (σ)
- delta (δ).

When released, endogenous opiates, such as endorphins, bind with opiate receptors in an attempt reduce pain sensation. Levels of **endorphins, enkephalins and dynorphins** increase not only during periods of stress and pain. Stimulation of opiate receptors can also promote feelings of euphoria and well-being and therefore endogenous opiate release can occur in many situations associated with pleasure, such as excitement, sexual activity and even exercise (Stranc 2002).

The Classification of Pain

Pain is classified according to its duration and is categorised as being either:

- Transient
- Acute
- Chronic.

Transient pain is a short episode of pain, which occurs as a result of a minor injury. Although the pain could be intense and even cause the individual to become momentarily upset it will eventually be considered to be pain of no significance. Transient pain is short lived and the individual is unlikely to seek medical attention. **Acute and chronic** pain are the major reasons for

occurs because special neurones called interneurons connect sensory and motor neurones within the spinal cord. This allows motor neurones leading to skeletal muscle and second order neurones to be innervated simultaneously, resulting in a reflex action that moves the foot away from the painful stimulus (Figure 23.7). A similar event occurs when individuals accidently touch very hot surfaces.

The Descending Pain Pathway

Descending pain pathways seek to inhibit the sensation of pain. This involves the release of special neuropeptides, which have

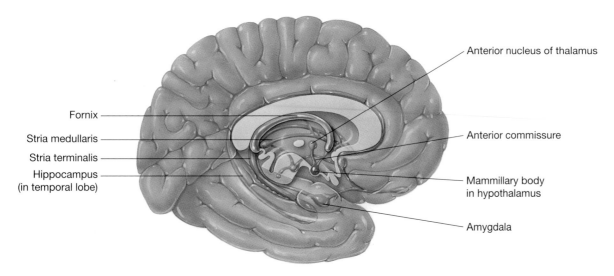

Figure 23.6 The limbic system.

Anterior nucleus of thalamus

Fornix

Stria medullaris

Stria terminalis

Hippocampus
(in temporal lobe)

Anterior commissure

Mammillary body
in hypothalamus

Amygdala

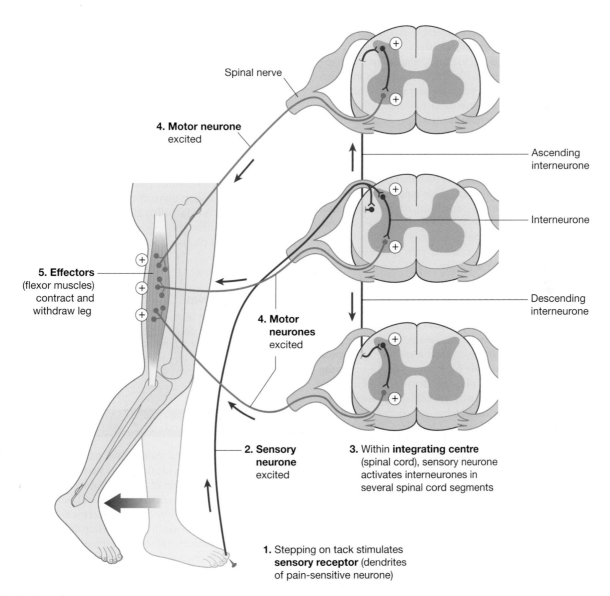

Spinal nerve

4. Motor neurone
excited

Ascending
interneurone

Interneurone

Descending
interneurone

5. Effectors
(flexor muscles)
contract and
withdraw leg

**4. Motor
neurones**
excited

**2. Sensory
neurone**
excited

3. Within **integrating centre**
(spinal cord), sensory neurone
activates interneurones in
several spinal cord segments

1. Stepping on tack stimulates
sensory receptor (dendrites
of pain-sensitive neurone)

Figure 23.7 The reflex arc.

Table 23.2 Differences between acute and chronic pain. Adapted from Gould (2006).

	DESCRIPTION	NEURONES RESPONSIBLE	NATURE OF PAIN
Acute pain	Fast, intense, localised	Fast wide diameter, myelinated Aδ fibres	Sudden, short term Present until healing starts Associated with stress response
Chronic pain	Slow, diffuse, prolonged	Slow, thin diameter, non-myelinated C-fibres	Long term, disabling Associated with fatigue, irritability and loss of hope Difficult to manage

individuals seeking medical attention. There are distinct differences between acute and chronic pain and it is essential that the nurse recognises and fully understands the major differences between these two pain states if they are to provide holistic care to their patients with pain (Table 23.2).

Acute Pain

Acute pain is associated with a severe sudden onset of intense pain, which continues until healing begins. The purpose of acute pain is to indicate tissue damage which may be localised or generalised. Acute pain is intense and can be an intolerable experience and in response individuals suffer an autonomic stress response, which manifests itself as hypertension, tachycardia, diaphoresis, tachypnoea and increased muscle tension. Patients in acute pain may also appear cool to touch and pale, and vomiting may occur. Acute pain is also associated with a strong emotional response, which may present with altered facial expressions, verbal expression, guarding and high levels of anxiety.

Chronic Pain

The term **chronic pain** is used to describe pain that continues even though healing is complete. Acute pain is a symptom of an associated medical condition or injury. Chronic pain, on the other hand, exists after the injury or disease has ceased. For this reason, chronic pain is often considered as a syndrome – a medical condition in its own right (Melzack & Wall 1988). Chronic pain is more likely to be perceived as generalised by the patient, which means that they will often found it difficult to inform practitioners of the exact location of their pain. Due to its long-term nature chronic pain is usually more difficult manage than acute pain. Stress responses are difficult to maintain over sustained periods of time and therefore despite experiencing pain that may remain as intense as acute pain, there is often little or no autonomic stress response. This could result in patients in tremendous pain presenting without any of the cardinal signs of pain, i.e. tachycardia, hypertension and diaphoresis. Often chronic pain does not have a specific or apparent cause, which results in a long term debilitating experience that has a number of psychological and physical side-effects. Patients with chronic pain complain of a range of psychosocial disorders such as disturbed sleep, reduced appetite, reduced libido, social isolation, depression and a loss of hope.

Care, Dignity and Compassion

Patients with chronic pain may present with no visible symptoms of pain – tachycardia, hypertension or diaphoresis, for example. However, the intensity of their pain may be as severe as that experienced in an episode of acute pain. Such patients will require as much comfort and reassurance as individuals in acute pain.

Superficial and Deep Pain

Pain can be classified according to its location. Pain is often described as being either **deep** or **superficial**. Superficial pain results from tissue situated towards the surface of the body, whereas deep pain comes from within the tissues deeper within the body. Deep pain can be either *somatic* or *visceral*. Visceral pain is caused by the stimulation of nociceptors in organs, kidneys, stomach, gall bladder and intestines. Somatic pain arises from structures such as bones, muscles, joints and tendons. Superficial pain is often described as a sharp, pricking sensation, whereas deep pain is a more dull and prolonged ache.

Understanding the nature of deep and superficial pain aids pain assessment. Although nociceptors are present in almost all body tissues (except for the brain), they are more abundant in tissue that is found in the outer regions of the body. Deep in the human body there are fewer nociceptors, which are spaced further apart. As a result the deeper within tissue the cause of pain is the harder it is to locate. Injuries that occur closer to the surface of the skin are often easily located, and therefore more readily diagnosed. Pain that emanates from deep tissue is often very difficult to locate; a good example is abdominal pain. Patients with acute abdominal pain often find it very difficult to verbalise and describe exactly where their pain is (MacLellan 2006). Given the number of organs and structures within the abdomen, it is often difficult for practitioners to make a diagnosis.

Jot This Down

Make a list of all the anatomical structures found in the abdomen and pelvic regions of the body. Then take some time to think of all the possible disorders that may present with acute abdominal pain.

The Pain Experience

While pain is an integral part of life, pain expression will differ from individual to individual. This is because pain expression is dependent on a multitude of influencing factors. Pain is an individual and personal experience, which will be influenced by life history, culture or psychosocial circumstances. In addition each individual will ascribe meaning to their pain that is often influenced by circumstances rather than intensity. A broken arm for instance may be excruciating but may be less worrying than sudden unexplained abdominal pain. The deep somatic pain from the injured bone will cause intense pain. However, while the sudden unexplained abdominal pain may be less intense, the affected individual's pain experience may exacerbated further due to the anxiety generated by the fact that it has no discernible cause. Past experiences are also a contributing factor. Patients who have been exposed to severe pain during a prior medical procedure may become anxious about future treatments and ultimately sense greater levels of pain. People also learn how to express and react to pain by observing those around them. A patient's attitude towards their pain may be influenced by the experiences of family members or their ethnicity and culture (Briggs 2010; Bell & Duffy 2009). An individual's circumstances can also influence the pain expression; sports people have been known to 'play' through intense pain and individuals can be known to dismiss pain when dealing with particularly stressful situations, escaping from violent conflict for instance.

Pain expression could also differ between sufferers of acute and chronic pain. The acute pain experience is associated with the presence of an autonomic nervous system response (sweating, tachycardia, hypertension, etc.), whereas individuals with chronic pain may present in the absence of those classic signs of pain. The pain experience of an individual with chronic pain, however may be as intense and debilitating as the person in acute pain.

We should conclude therefore that the management of pain is a significant nursing challenge and that nurses must accept that the pain experience is completely subjective and requires a holistic and individualised plan of care. Nevertheless, many misconceptions about the nature of pain and its management still remain (Table 23.3). It is perhaps for this reason that the most noteworthy and notorious explanation of pain is McCaffery's 1979 definition, which states that, 'Pain is whatever the experiencing patient says it is, existing when he says it does'. McCaffery (1979, p. 11).

Table 23.3 Common misconceptions about pain. Adapted from McGann (2007).

MISCONCEPTION	REALITY
You can teach patients to tolerate pain; the longer they have pain the more used to it they become	Tolerance to pain is an individual experience Individuals with prolonged pain tend to develop hypersensitivity to pain
Nurses and allied health professionals are the authority on pain and the nature of pain	Only the patient experiencing the pain fully understands how it feels and its impact on their life
Lying about the existence of pain or malingering is commonplace	Very few people lie about the existence of pain and fabrication of pain is very rare
Visible symptoms of pain can be used to verify its severity	Lack of pain expression does not equal lack of pain Patients with chronic pain may have the ability to carry on as normal
Patients should not be given analgesia until a reason for their pain is diagnosed	Pain should be treated even when there is no discernible cause. People seeking assistance for pain have the right to have their pain assessed, accepted and acted upon

Professional and Legal Issues

 Comprehensive pain assessment is closely aligned to the nurse's responsibilities, as stipulated in the NMC Code of Professional Conduct (NMC 2008).

Treat people as individuals	Pain control is a basic human right. If a pain control intervention does not work, or is inappropriate try another
Collaborate with those in your care	Patients need to be involved in decision-making
Ensure you gain consent	Ensure your patient understands any pain assessment or management intervention and why you recommend its use
Share information with your colleagues	It is vital that other members of the multidisciplinary team are fully aware of patient preferences and any successful pain interventions
Maintain professional knowledge and competence	Ensure that you are sufficiently knowledgeable to undertake pain assessment. If you are not, seek guidance from a more experienced member of staff
Keep accurate records	You must continually assess and re-evaluate the individual with pain. This is a legal requirement

Influence of Emotion

The limbic system within the brain (see Figure 23.6) processes our emotional response to pain. Pain expression is therefore influenced by our personality and state of mind. The limbic system interacts closely with the frontal lobes of the cerebral cortex, which are responsible for cognitive thought. This explains why people may at times act and behave irrationally, when in pain. Conversely, individuals are often able to control their emotions when pain occurs, when it is socially unacceptable to cry out or complain (Marieb & Hoehn 2007). An individual's state of mind has a significant influence on pain intensity and the pain experience. Low mood, anxiety and depression can all increase pain intensity (Carr *et al.* 2005), whereas relaxed and positive frames of mind can reduce pain to acceptable levels (Lin & Wang 2005).

The Meaning of Pain

The individual will ascribe meaning to their pain experience. This perceived meaning or reason for their pain affects its level and intensity. For example patients recovering from surgery may report less pain than people that have suffered sudden traumatic accidents. The patient recovering from surgery may view their pain as a symptom of surgery and therefore possibly something positive (Skevington 1995). Their post-surgical pain could be intense, but they may require less analgesia and be more able to cope because, from their perspective, their pain means 'healing' or 'getting better' and possibly relief. In situations when it is difficult to explain why pain has occurred, anxiety and stress can increase and heighten pain sensation. The individual with sudden acute abdominal pain, for example may not be able to explain the cause. From the individual's perspective, their pain means 'something is seriously wrong'. Circumstances and outside influences may alter the individual's pain perception and change the meaning of their pain. For instance, slight abdominal pain may be dismissed as a mild 'tummy bug' until the individual discovers that is may be something serious, in which case the pain may become severe and intense. Similarly, pain levels may reduce when the patient learns that the cause of their pain is trivial and/or easily resolved.

Care, Dignity and Compassion

Acute pain can be very distressing and patients may describe their pain as intolerable. Pain relief should be prioritised and patients will require constant comfort and reassurance.

Pain Threshold

The term **pain threshold** is often used to describe an individual's ability to cope with pain. It is common, for instance, to hear people being described as possessing a 'high or low' pain threshold. Often, social stereotypes and popular culture reinforce this theory with the popular misconception that women possess higher pain thresholds than men, being a good example. This interpretation of pain threshold is misleading and unhelpful to nurses aiming to provide optimum care for the patient living with pain. Pain threshold is the point at which an individual will report pain and it is generally accepted that all humans have a similar pain threshold. Where individuals differ, is the manner in which they express their pain. Nurses should conclude therefore that the expression of pain is influenced by emotional state, personality, life experience, culture, social status and current circumstances, rather than a personal pain threshold that is determined by sex or social stereotypes (Large et al. 2002).

Pain Theory

The nature of pain is a complex and intricate phenomenon, which involves both psychological and physiological changes. Many pain theories have been developed, which attempt to conceptualise the influence of both mind and body on the pain experience. The **specificity theory**, for example, hypothesises that pain is sensed when specific neurones are stimulated. Pain sensation is then transmitted to a specific pain centre within the brain. However, rather than the brain interpreting pain it is the characteristics of the original stimulus that determines the intensity of the pain. Another pain theory, **Pattern theory**, postulates that there is no separate system dedicated to pain transmission and sensation, instead pain is sensed and interpreted by the brain when intense peripheral nerve stimulation occurs (Gould & Thomas 1997). However, such theories leave many important aspects of pain unexplained. For example, theories like specificity theory and pattern theory, cannot explain why pain can occur in response to gentle stimuli, neuralgia for instance. Neither do they explain why pain can occur in the absence of tissue damage or why two individuals with the same injury may experience different levels of pain. Melzack and Wall's (1965) Gate Control Theory of Pain attempts to explain such anomalies and as a result, has become widely accepted as the most important pain theory (Main & Spanswick 2000).

Gate Control Theory of Pain

The **Gate Control Theory of Pain** was originally hypothesised by Melzack and Wall in 1965. Its popularity stems from its recognition

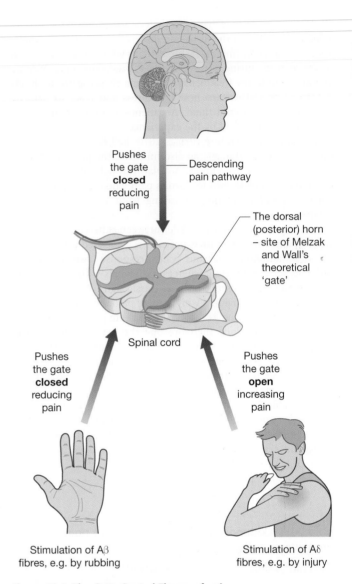

Figure 23.8 The Gate Control Theory of pain.

of the strong relationship between psychology and physiology and their influence on the individual pain experience. For this reason, it is a useful tool for clinicians who are caring for individuals in both acute and chronic pain.

The Gate Control Theory of Pain postulates that pain messages passing from first order neurones to second order neurones must first pass through a theoretical 'gate' situated at the dorsal horn of the spinal cord. If allowed to pass through the 'gate', the pain signal will ascend upwards along second order neurones towards the brain (Figure 23.8). However, if the 'gate' is closed, pain signals are blocked and because the brain does not receive pain communication no pain will be sensed. The 'gate' may also remain partially open, and depending on how ajar it is, will determine the intensity of the pain. The factors that influence the opening and closing of the 'gate' can be afferent, moving towards the brain or efferent, moving away from the brain. Examples include:

- Afferent influences – neurones such as Aδ, C and Aβ fibres
- Efferent influences – descending brain activity.

The intensity of an individual's pain, therefore, is determined by a balance between the levels of noxious stimuli sensed by nociceptors and transmitted along first order neurones and the actions of Aβ fibres or descending brain activity (McCaffery *et al.* 2003).

Afferent influences on the 'gate' include first order neurones and Aβ fibres. Pain messages from Aδ and C first order neurones will push open the gate, whereas the actions of the much faster Aβ fibres, which carry sensations of heat and touch, will push the gate closed. In other words, the stimulation of the larger Aβ fibres with touch and heat can inhibit pain transmission by Aδ and C fibres. This helps explain why rubbing mild injuries, acupuncture and transcutaneous electrical nerve stimulation (TENS) may reduce pain intensity.

Efferent factors include increased descending pain pathway activity. Melzack and Wall (1988) suggest that increased descending brain activity can either widen or close the 'gate' to pain sensation. This may explain why a person's emotional state, personality and culture may determine how their pain is expressed. The Gate Control Theory proposes that pain intensity is directly influenced by the action of transmission cells and substantia gelatinosa cells, which are found within the dorsal horn of the spinal cord. Transmission, or T, cells aid the transmission of the pain messages being sent towards the brain. Substantia gelatinosa or SG cells, on the other hand, inhibit T-cell activity and thus seek to close the 'gate' to pain sensation. The activity of both T cells and SG cells are enhanced by the descending pain pathway and therefore the individual's state of mind. In depressive and anxious states, T-cell activity is enhanced, pushing the gate open and increasing pain intensity. However, in relaxed and contented states, SG cell action is increased, pushing the gate closed and decreasing pain levels (Melzack & Wall 1988; Figure 23.9). This theory, therefore, helps explain the behaviour of individuals in pain or with injury. Sports people, for example are often able to cope with intense levels of pain when striving to win a contest or sporting event. Other instances include reports of people ignoring or remaining unaware of injury when in perilous circumstances or sustaining injury when rescuing children from a burning house, for example. Melzack and Wall would argue that in such circumstances, the desire to win or rescue a loved one would stimulate high descending brain activity, which would close the 'gate' to pain, even when faced with intense pain signals generated by injury. Conversely, low mood states, anxiety, depression and worry will cause the gate to remain open and even widen, heightening pain sensation and intensifying the pain experience. In terms of clinical application, nurses and other healthcare professionals should utilise interventions that seek to reduce anxiety and also recognise that the individual's mood and perception of their current situation will have a marked influence on their pain experience.

Pain Assessment

Pain is a complex multifaceted phenomenon and its assessment poses a significant nursing challenge. Nevertheless, effective pain management is essential if the nurse is to plan and implement an appropriate range of both pharmacological and non-pharmacological interventions. The pain experience involves four interlinked dimensions (Figure 23.10). Nursing assessment must pay attention to physiological, psychological, emotional and social aspects of pain, if effective holistic care is to be achieved (Manias 2003). Accurate nursing assessment can also be hampered by the subjective nature of the pain experience. Nurses must often rely

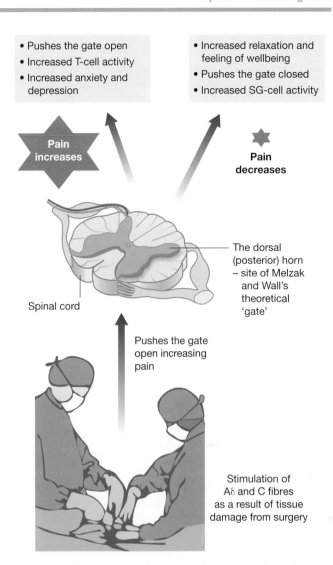

Figure 23.9 **The Gate Control Theory and influence of T and SG cell activity.**

499

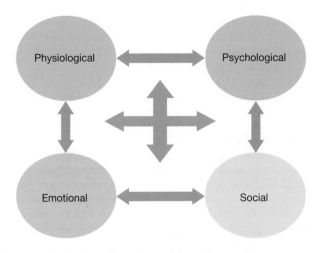

Figure 23.10 **The four dimensions of the pain experience.**

upon the patient's description of their pain. Many patients, however, are unable to verbalise or describe their pain and in such instances, nurses must look for visual non-verbal cues. However, a description of pain is rarely enough to determine appropriate treatment. Further information on the location, duration and onset of pain can assist nurses and other healthcare professionals when establishing the extent, nature and impact of an individual's pain. Every pain assessment must include the following:

- The location of the pain – i.e. where is the pain, does it move or radiate elsewhere?
- The duration of the pain – how long has the patient been in pain?
- Onset – when did the pain start and what was the patient doing at the time?
- Frequency – is the pain constant or spasmodic, if spasmodic how often does the pain occur and for how long does it last?
- Intensity – how painful is it, does the level of pain ever change?
- Aggravating factors – does anything make the pain worse?
- Relieving factors – does anything make the pain feel better?
- Sleep – does the pain disturb sleep; does it keep the patient awake at night?
- Other symptoms – does the pain cause other associated symptoms, i.e. dizziness, nausea, vomiting, shortness of breath, loss of appetite, diaphoresis.

(Adapted from Godfrey 2005b and MacLellan 2006)

Pain assessment must also address the patient's psychological and emotional response to their pain. Therefore, every pain assessment must gather information on the following:

- The individual's expectations of any potential treatments
- The individual's concerns about the cause of their pain
- Does the individual have any personal or spiritual beliefs
- What level of pain would the individual find acceptable
- What level of pain would allow the individual to return to work
- Does the individual have any feelings of stress or anxiety
- Does the individual use any coping strategies
- What are the individual's preferences regarding treatment options.

(MacLellan 2006)

Acute pain will produce an autonomic response and often, patients will present with the signs and symptoms of stress, therefore the following would also need to be recorded:

- Blood pressure – many patients in pain can experience hypertension
- Pulse – to check for tachycardia
- Respiratory rate – pain often produces changes in respiratory rate. Tachypnoea may suggest stress. Shallow respiratory effort is indicative of thoracic pain. Patients in acute pain may also have a tendency to periodically hold their breath.

Chronic pain, however, may not have an adverse effect on these vital signs; therefore the individual's description of the pain should remain the principle indicator of pain intensity (Lynch 2001).

Pain Assessment Tools

Formal structured pain assessment tools can facilitate and enhance the nurse's pain assessment. There are a wide variety of pain assessment tools at the nurse's disposal, ranging from simple single-dimension scales to comprehensive pain questionnaires. The verbal rating scale, the visual analogue rating scale and the numerical rating scale are the three most commonly used single-dimension scales. The verbal rating scale (Figure 23.11) asks the patient to select an adjective, from a pre-determined list, which best describes

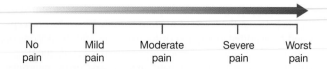

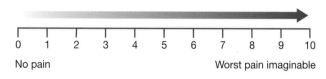

Figure 23.11 The verbal rating scale.

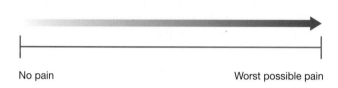

Figure 23.12 The verbal analogue scale.

Figure 23.13 The visual analogue scale.

their pain. The verbal analogue scale uses a numerical scale, 0–10 or 0–3 for example from which the patient selects the number that most accurately represents their pain. Numbers at the lower end of the scale signify low or no pain, whereas the higher numbers represent intolerable or worst pain imaginable (Figure 23.12). The visual analogue scale has a more basic format. The scale consists simply of a rudimentary continuum, which runs from no pain to the worst pain imaginable. The patient can point or state where on the continuum their pain is (Figure 23.13). The main advantage of simple scales such as these is their ease of use. They can be utilised swiftly and do not over-burden an individual in acute pain. However, it should be remembered that these scales only assess one aspect of pain, its intensity, and there is an assumption that the patient will be literate (MacLellan 2006).

A common example of a multidimensional pain assessment tool is the McGill Pain Questionnaire (Figure 23.14). The McGill Pain Questionnaire is a comprehensive assessment tool that comprises a series of descriptive terms from which the patient select the most appropriate to describe their pain. The adjectives are separated into the three classes: sensory, affective and evaluative. The assessment tool also utilises a simple rating scale, which runs from 0 (no pain) to 5 (excruciating). The assessment of pain is based on three separate measures: the pain rating index (PRI), which is based on numerical values assigned to each number, the number of words selected and the rating scale or present pain index (PPI). The McGill Pain Questionnaire also utilises line drawings of the human body that can facilitate the identification of the location of the pain. The McGill Pain Questionnaire is now widely used to assess chronic pain and has been shown to be very effective when assessing pain in patients with arthritis (Grafton et al. 2005).

Pain Management

Pain management is associated with the use of pain relieving medications. However, there are also a number of pain management

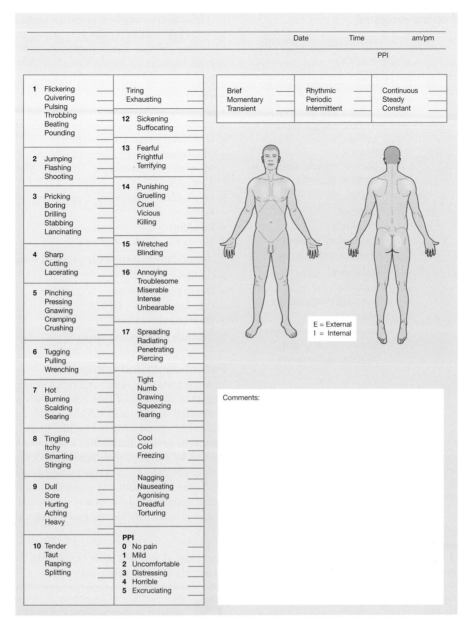

Date _____ Time _____ am/pm

PPI _____

1	Flickering Quivering Pulsing Throbbing Beating Pounding	___
	Tiring Exhausting	___
12	Sickening Suffocating	___
13	Fearful Frightful Terrifying	___
2	Jumping Flashing Shooting	___
14	Punishing Gruelling Cruel Vicious Killing	___
3	Pricking Boring Drilling Stabbing Lancinating	___
15	Wretched Blinding	___
4	Sharp Cutting Lacerating	___
16	Annoying Troublesome Miserable Intense Unbearable	___
5	Pinching Pressing Gnawing Cramping Crushing	___
17	Spreading Radiating Penetrating Piercing	___
6	Tugging Pulling Wrenching	___
	Tight Numb Drawing Squeezing Tearing	___
7	Hot Burning Scalding Searing	___
8	Tingling Itchy Smarting Stinging	___
	Cool Cold Freezing	___
9	Dull Sore Hurting Aching Heavy	___
	Nagging Nauseating Agonising Dreadful Torturing	___
10	Tender Taut Rasping Splitting	___

Brief — Momentary — Transient | Rhythmic — Periodic — Intermittent | Continuous — Steady — Constant

E = External
I = Internal

Comments:

PPI
0 No pain
1 Mild
2 Uncomfortable
3 Distressing
4 Horrible
5 Excruciating

Figure 23.14 The McGill Pain Questionnaire. Source: Melzack & Torgerson (1971). Reproduced with permission of LWW.

501

interventions that are non-pharmacological. As the name suggests, 'non-pharmacological pain management' does not involve any drugs. As pain is a total experience, effective pain control is often achieved through a combination of both approaches (Hader & Guy 2004).

Pharmacological Interventions

Pharmacological preparations that are administered for the relief of pain are referred to as **analgesia** or **analgesics**. There are two main types of analgesia:

- Opioids (or opiates)
- Non-opioids.

Opioids (or opiates)

Opioids should be prescribed for moderate to severe pain. Opioids mimic the body's own endogenous opiates (endorphins, enkephalins, and dynorphins) and bind to opiate receptors within the central nervous system. Opiate receptors such as mu (μ), kappa (κ), sigma (σ) and delta (δ) if stimulated, block the action of substance P, the neurotransmitter responsible for the transmission of pain. However, opioids differ from endogenous opiates in that are not rapidly broken down by the body (Stranc 2002). As a result, their analgesic properties are powerful and long-lasting.

Stimulation of the central nervous system's opiate receptors not only produces pain relief it can also produce other, often unwanted, side-effects (Table 23.4).

Table 23.4 Actions of opiate receptors.

RECEPTOR	PHYSIOLOGICAL EFFECTS
Mu (μ)	Analgesia Euphoria Respiratory depression Bradycardia Nausea and vomiting Inhibition of gut motility Miosis Pruritus Smooth muscle spasm Physical dependence
Kappa (κ)	Analgesia Sedation Dysphoria Respiratory depression Physical dependence
Delta (δ)	Analgesia Euphoria Respiratory depression Miosis Inhibition of gut motility Smooth muscle spasm Physical dependence

Jot This Down

Have a look at the list of side-effects noted in Table 23.4 and take some time to think about the effects opiates may have on those that are addicted to their use.

Red Flag

Opiate analgesia has many unwanted side-effects (see Table 23.4). Nurses should continually assess for the presence of side-effects as left untreated could be detrimental to their patient's well-being. Important side-effects to look out for are:

- Respiratory depression
- Nausea and vomiting
- Constipation
- Bradycardia and hypotension.

The administration of opioids is governed by the Misuse of Drugs Act (HMSO 1971) and are therefore subject to strict regulation.

Link To/Go To

Controlled Drugs (Supervision, Management and Use) Regulations 2013:

https://www.gov.uk/government/uploads/system/uploads/attachment_data/file/214915/15-02-2013-controlled-drugs-regulation-information.pdf

Opioids are classified as either weak or strong. Despite their name, weak opioids remain very strong analgesic agents.

Strong opioids used commonly within the National Health Service include:

- Buprenorphine – Temgesic, Transtec, Butrans, Subutex
- Diamorphine
- Dipipanone – Diconal
- Fentanyl – Durogesic, Matrifen, Effentora, Abstral
- Hydromorphone – Palladone
- Methadone
- Morphine – Oromorph, Sevredol, Morphine sulphate tablets, Zomorph
- Oxycodone – Oxynorm, Oxycontin
- Pentacozine
- Pethidine
- Tramadol – Zydol, Zamadol

Weak opioids commonly prescribed include:

- Codeine
- Dextropropoxyphene
- Dihydrocodeine – DF118
- Meptazinol – Meptid.

(British Pain Society 2010)

Patient-controlled analgesia

In many instances, after surgery for example, patients can administer their own opioid pain relief via a system known as **patient-controlled analgesia** (PCA). A small syringe that contains the prescribed opioid drug is attached to the patient via a small subcutaneous needle. The syringe is operated by a button, which when pressed by the patient delivers a set dosage. After each dose, the syringe driver locks for a short time ensuring no drug can be delivered even if the button is pressed, therefore protecting the individual against overdose. Patient-controlled analgesia has been used routinely and safely for the past 30 years (Layzell 2008).

Red Flag A Patient with No Visible Signs of Pain Requests Opiate Analgesia

One concern in situations such as these is that the request is due to dependence rather than analgesia. Nurses must remember that pain is what the patient says it is and it would be unethical to leave a patient in pain. However, under the Misuse of Drugs Act (HMSO 1971), doctors should not prescribe diamorphine to an addict or suspected addict without a special home office licence. In such situations, it will be the prescriber's decision but the nurse must act as the patient's advocate and act in their best interests.

Non-opioid drugs

Non-opioid analgesia drugs are prescribed for mild to moderate pain. As such, they are rarely effective in acute or postoperative pain control. They are mainly associated with transient pain, such as muscle strains or headaches. In the main, nonopioid analgesic medications are either:

- Non-steroidal anti-inflammatory drugs (NSAIDs)
- Paracetamol (acetaminophen).

Paracetamol (acetaminophen) is the most common non-opioid drug. Its precise pharmacological action remains controversial;

however, it is widely accepted that it suppresses the production of prostaglandins. Prostaglandins are hormone-like substances that stimulate and maintain inflammatory processes. Prostaglandins also chemically stimulate nociceptors, which in turn innervate first order neurones and send pain signals towards the central nervous system and promote pain sensation (MacPherson 2000). Despite being an effective analgesic, paracetamol rarely maintains its analgesic effects for longer than 4 hours and as a result, may not be appropriate for prolonged pain. Although considered a relatively safe pharmacological preparation, paracetamol can cause liver failure, even in small doses (Heath 1997).

Medicines Management

Paracetamol, if used correctly, can be an effective and safe analgesic. However, liver failure can occur even in small overdoses. Care should be taken to ensure that the drug is administered as prescribed and its use in patients with liver disease should be avoided.

Non-steroidal anti-inflammatory drugs (NSAIDs) also suppress prostaglandin production. Prostaglandins are derived from arachidonic acid, which is released from damaged cells (as a result of trauma, inflammation, etc.). The production of prostaglandins from arachidonic acid is accelerated by the actions of an enzyme called cyclooxygenase 2 (COX-2) (Figure 23.15). Non-steroidal anti-inflammatory drugs (NSAIDs) inhibit the actions of cyclooxygenase-2 (COX-2) and therefore the production of prostaglandins is severely reduced. As a result, inflammation is condensed and pain signals are diminished. In addition to the suppression of cyclooxygenase 2 (COX-2), non-steroidal inflammatory drugs (NSAIDs) may also suppress a similar enzyme called **cyclooxygenase 1 (COX-1)**. Unlike cyclooxygenase 2 (COX-2), cyclooxygenase 1 (COX-1) promotes prostaglandin production in the stomach, where it plays an important role in the protection of the stomach wall from erosion by gastric acid. A major side-effect of NSAIDs therefore is the development of gastric irritation and ulcers (Gilron *et al.* 2003). Care should also be taken in patients with respiratory disease as non-steroidal anti-inflammatory drugs (NSAIDs) are also associated with hypersensitive reactions in people with asthma (Jenkins *et al.* 2004). There are many different NSAIDs used within the UK (Box 23.1). However, the major non-steroidal anti-inflammatory drugs used with the National Health Service are:

- Aspirin
- Ibuprofen
- Diclofenac – Volterol
- Indomethacin
- Naproxen.

Medicines Management

One of the most likely side-effects of non-steroidal anti-inflammatory drugs is gastric irritation and drugs, such as ibuprofen, Diclofenac, indomethacin and naproxen should be administered either with or just after food to minimise the risk.

In addition to analgesia, non-opioid drugs have other potentially therapeutic effects, i.e. temperature control and prophylaxis of heart disease. Because prostaglandins promote pyrexia in addition to inflammation, non-steroidal anti-inflammatory drugs

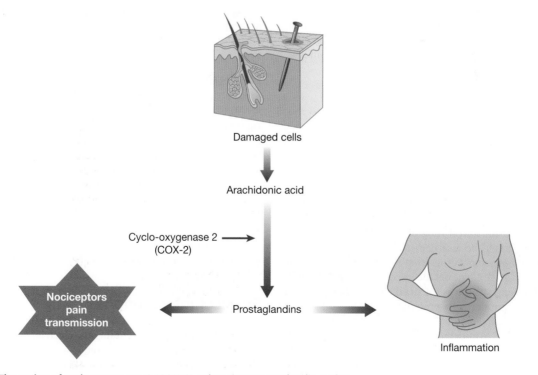

Figure 23.15 The action of cyclooxygenase-2 (COX-2) enhancing prostaglandin action.

Box 23.1 Common NSAIDs (Trade Names in Brackets)		
Aceclofenac (Preservex®)	Etodolac	Mefenamic acid (Ponstan®)
Acemetacin (Emflex®)	Etoricoxib (Arcoxia®)	Meloxican (Mobic®)
Aspirin (Caprin®)	Fenbufen (Fenbufen®)	Nabumetone (Relifex®)
Azapropazone (Rheumox®)	Fenoprofen (Fenopron®)	Naproxen (Arthroxen®)
Celecoxib (Celebrex®)	Flurbiprofen (Froben®)	Piroxicam (Brexidol®)
Dexibuprofen (Seractil®)	Ibuprofen (Brufen®)	Sulindac (Clinoril®)
Dexketoprofen (Keral®)	Indometacin (Rimacid®)	Tenoxicam (Mobiflex®)
Diclofenac (Volterol®)	Ketoprofen (Orudis®)	Tiaprofenic acid (Surgam®)

(NSAIDs) and paracetamol may reduce core body temperature and are often prescribed solely to counteract pyrexia. Aspirin, in addition to analgesia, has antiplatelet properties. When used in small doses, it has been shown to reduce the risk of cardiovascular disease; it is also used in large doses in patients with a suspected myocardial infarction (MI) (Fuster *et al.* 1993).

Opioid and non-opioid combinations

Some opioids are combined pharmacologically with non-opioid analgesic drugs, such as paracetamol and aspirin. Opioid drugs when used in combination with non-opioid drugs, can reduce opioid usage by 20–40% (Macintyre & Ready 2001). Such combinations are often prescription-only medications, rather than controlled drugs (HMSO 1968). Examples of common, weak opioid and non-opioid analgesic combinations are:

- Co-codamol – codeine phosphate combined with paracetamol
- Co-codaprin – codeine phosphate combined with aspirin
- Co-dydramol – dihydrocodeine combined with paracetamol
- Tramacet – tramadol combined with paracetamol

The analgesic ladder

The analgesic ladder was first produced by the World Health Organization (WHO) in 1986. The main aim of the ladder was to help health workers combat cancer pain; however it is now widely used to manage a wide variety of pain situations (Godfrey 2005b). The ladder postulates that there are three rungs or levels of treatment. On each rung, there is a recommended level of pharmacological treatment (Figure 23.16). The aim is for the patient to be on the lowest point on the ladder, which keeps them pain-free. Treatment should start on the lowest rung of the ladder and if unsuccessful, treatment should be escalated to the next step. Step one involved the use of non-opioid drugs, step two recommends a weak opioid and the final stage advocates the use of strong opioids. Each rung of the ladder suggests the use of an adjuvant. Adjuvants are a range of drugs that are normally prescribed for non-pain related conditions, but if used in conjunction with analgesia, can enhance their pain killer effect. Antidepressants, anticonvulsants, muscle relaxants, steroids and local anaesthetics have all been shown to reduce pain when used in conjunction with opioid and non-opioid drugs (MacPherson 2000).

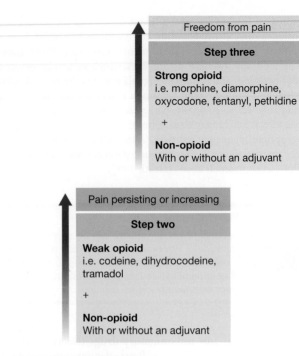

Figure 23.16 The World Health Organization analgesic ladder (WHO 1986).

Non-pharmacological Pain Management

A wide variety of **non-pharmacological** pain management interventions are available in the UK (Box 23.2). However, there is only rigid evidence of effectiveness for a small number of techniques; good examples include massage and cognitive behavioural therapy (Furlan *et al.* 2002; Eccleston *et al.* 2009). There is therefore much scepticism among healthcare providers regarding the effectiveness of non-pharmacological pain control choices, and their use remains controversial (Wigens 2006). Non-pharmacological pain control methods are divided into two distinct categories:

- Physical interventions – i.e. TENS machines, massage and acupuncture
- Psychological interventions – i.e. cognitive behavioural therapy, hypnotherapy.

Physical Interventions

Many non-pharmacological pain control techniques have a physiological basis. A **transcutaneous electric nerve stimulation (TENS)** machine, for example, sends a constant stream of small electrical impulses through the skin (Figure 23.17). These impulses are thought to reduce pain in two ways. In the first instance, they

Box 23.2 Popular Non-pharmacological Methods of Pain Management

- Cognitive behavioural therapy
- Transcutaneous electric nerve stimulation (TENS)
- Application of heat and cold substances
- Acupuncture
- Alexander technique
- Aromatherapy
- Massage
- Chiropractic
- Hypnosis
- Homeopathy
- Meditation
- Osteopathy
- Reflexology
- Relaxation
- Shiatsu

(*Source*: Adapted from Wigens 2006)

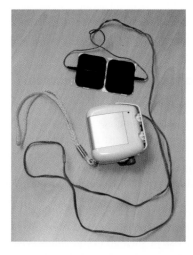

Figure 23.17 Transcutaneous electrical nerve stimulation (TENS) machine. Source: Nair & Peate (2013). Reproduced with permission of John Wiley & Sons Ltd.

are thought to stimulate the fast large diameter Aβ fibres that can transfer messages of touch, heat and cold quicker than pain and therefore interrupt the pain impulses travelling along the smaller and slower Aδ and C fibre first order neurones, in very much the same way as rubbing a mild injury can alleviate discomfort. Second, the continuous electrical stimulation could increase circulating levels of endogenous opiates, such as endorphins within the central nervous system (Sluka & Walsh 2003). Transcutaneous electric nerve stimulation (TENS) machines are widely used for the treatment of pain after surgery, chronic pain, lower back pain and pain during labour and childbirth. Despite this wide use and positive patient feedback, evidence of its effectiveness remains inconclusive (Nnoaham & Kumbang 2008).

Acupuncture entails the insertion of fine needles at a multitude of strategic anatomical points around the human body. Like the TENs machine, acupuncture is thought to stimulate the release of endogenous opiates (Lundeberg & Stener-Victorin 2002). Acupuncture is widely used throughout the world and is accepted as an effective analgesia in many countries. Nevertheless, despite its popularity, there is very little evidence to suggest that it is actually

effective and it remains a controversial treatment option (Lee & Ernst 2005).

The stimulation of large diameter Aβ fibres also helps explain the therapeutic effects of 'pressure and touch' based interventions, such as osteopathy, reflexology and shiatsu. However, the most widely used 'pressure and touch' based intervention is **massage**. Unlike many other physical non-pharmacological pain interventions, there is some evidence of its effectiveness. Massage has been shown to be potentially effective in patients with low back pain (Furlan *et al.* 2002).

In addition to sensing pressure and touch, Aβ fibres also respond to sensations of heat and cold. The provision of mild heat and cold in order to provide therapeutic relief from pain are widely used. Ice packs, for example are used on sports injuries and heat is also a popular method for the alleviation menstrual pain as well as joint and muscle strains. However, like many other non-pharmacological pain control methods, there is at present little evidence for the use of heat and cold substances in the clinical environment (French *et al.* 2005).

Psychological Interventions

Given that pain is an individual, personal and holistic experience, the psychological aspects of the pain experience are an integral element of the pain experience. The Gate Control Theory of Pain (see earlier) postulates that descending pain pathways from the brain have a direct influence on the level of pain intensity and therefore the pain experience. The most significant aspects of descending brain activity are the influence of anxiety, stress and low mood states on the pain experience. The Gate Control Theory of Pain suggests that anxiety, stress and low mood states are more likely to push open the gate to pain and increase pain intensity. Any non-pharmacological intervention, therefore, that aims to alleviate anxiety or stress, or is able to help the individual to cope with their pain could be beneficial. It is not surprising therefore that psychological-based non-pharmacological pain control methods are being increasingly utilised by chronic pain sufferers (Dopson 2010).

There are many simplistic and pragmatic psychological-based pain control interventions at the nurse's disposal. Relaxation, distraction and meditation for example can be used in many clinical settings to good effect. There are also other more alternative methods, such as the Alexandra Technique and hypnotherapy, which patients have utilised effectively. Overall, there is very little evidence of the effectiveness of psychological-based pain control interventions, other than the use of cognitive behavioural therapy or CBT, which has been proven to be effective in the treatment of chronic pain (Ecclestone *et al.* 2009).

Cognitive behavioural therapy (CBT) is an intense psychological approach that involves a series of structured, patient-focussed sessions, which aim to address the individual's psychological and emotional experience of their pain. The overarching aim of cognitive behavioural therapy (CBT) programmes is to enable chronic pain sufferers to self-manage and control their anxiety and therefore their pain.

Nursing Management of Acute Pain

Acute pain is an indicator of tissue damage. It is associated with sudden onset and is often described in terms, such as 'excruciating', 'unbearable' and 'intolerable'. Despite causing discomfort, acute pain has a limited lifespan and reduces, as healing progresses. Acute pain is not a diagnosis; it is a symptom (ICSI 2004). Nurses should tailor their assessments and interventions to suit the nature or cause of their patients acute pain, be it postoperative, abdominal pain, chest pain, burns or musculoskeletal.

Signs and Symptoms

Acute pain is associated with an autonomic nervous system response and individuals may present with signs and symptoms of stress. Acute pain is an emotional as well as physical experience and individuals may also verbalise their pain and may visually project their suffering. The major signs and symptoms of acute pain are:

- Tachycardia
- Hypertension
- Diaphoresis
- Altered respiratory rate
- Increased muscle tension
- Cool and clammy skin and peripheries
- Reduced peripheral blood flow
- Vomiting
- Anxiety, fear
- Altered facial expression, i.e. grimace
- Verbalisation of pain
- Agitation, restlessness, anger, irritability
- Guarding.

Investigations and Diagnosis

- Pain assessment
- *Remember pain is what the patient says it is.*

Nursing Care and Management

The main nursing aims for the patient in acute postoperative pain are to reduce discomfort and promote healing and recovery. The major treatment options are pharmacological and therefore nurses should also account for their potential side-effects. The major nursing objectives are:

- An accurate pain assessment (see earlier) – in order to best establish choice of interventions
- Safe administration of prescribed analgesia (see earlier)
- Monitor for evidence of the main side-effects of opioid therapy (Box 23.3)
- Use of psychological interventions, such as relaxation, distraction and imagery to complement pharmacological interventions
- Monitor patient for signs and symptoms of stress – to evaluate success of nursing strategies
- Regularly re-assess pain intensity – to evaluate success of pharmacological and psychological interventions.

Box 23.3 Major Side-Effects of Opioid Therapy

- Respiratory depression
- Bradycardia
- Nausea and vomiting
- Drowsiness
- Hypotension.

Consequences of Unresolved Acute Pain

Prolonged acute pain can result in pathophysiological changes that can have further detrimental effects on well-being. The individual suffering unresolved acute pain may also experience symptoms associated with respiration, cardiovascular function, mobility and gastric problems.

Acute pain and respiration

Pain in the thoracic region may result in an involuntary reduction in muscle contraction in the chest and abdominal area. Clinicians often refer to this phenomenon as 'muscle splinting', which means that muscles contract on either side of the injury in order to 'splint' the area and prevent movement. Closure of the glottis can also occur and individuals can present with a 'grunting', breathing sound. This response is a natural defence mechanism, which facilitates along with muscle spasms an increased intra-abdominal and intra-thoracic pressure that braces against an impending injury.

Respiratory changes if left untreated, will lead to reduced respiratory function and in-turn, regional atelectasis. The development of atelectasis results in reduced gaseous exchange and the development of hypoxaemia and hypoxia. Splinting can also result in an inability to cough and clear chest secretions, increasing the likelihood of chest infections.

Acute pain and cardiovascular function

The stress response associated with the acute pain experience increases cardiovascular workload. Stress responses increase heart rate, peripheral resistance, blood pressure and cardiac heart rate. The resultant escalation in cardiac effort will increase myocardial oxygen consumption. Simultaneously, intensification of heart rate also reduces diastolic filling time and oxygen delivery to the myocardium is reduced. In the patient with acute pain, there is the potential for a mismatch between myocardial oxygen demand and myocardial oxygen delivery and the potential for myocardial ischaemia and chest pain. Patients with pre-existing cardiac disease are at a greater risk of such an event. Unresolved acute pain and prolonged autonomic stress responses are also associated with reduced arterial flow and reduced venous emptying.

Acute pain and mobility

Acute muscular pain promotes muscle spasm and increased pain on movement. As a result, the patient becomes locked into a vicious circle: increased anxiety, increased pain and lack of mobility. A reduction of mobility is associated with reduced muscle metabolism, atrophy and a delayed return to normal muscle function.

Acute pain and gastric function

The stress response associated with acute pain increases intestinal secretions and smooth muscle sphincter tone but slows down intestinal motility. Gastric stasis and paralytic ileus may occur also occur. The reduced intestinal motility may be detrimental to the patient's nutritional status.

Postoperative Pain

The majority of patients undergoing surgery suffer acute pain in the aftermath, with up to 80% of patients reporting severe pain (Manias 2003). A significant contributory factor to postoperative pain is anxiety, which can increase pain intensity. Anxiety and depression prior to surgery, lead to high levels of anxiety postoperatively (Carr *et al.* 2005). In order to reduce postoperative pain, nurses and allied health professionals should select appropriate preoperative care interventions that counteract the impact of preoperative anxiety, patient education for example (Johansson *et al.* 2005). Nurses are ideally placed to minimise postoperative pain, as they are responsible for the administration and evaluation of prescribed analgesics.

The main nursing objective for the patient in acute pain postsurgery is the minimisation of the impact of their pain. This is because unresolved pain leads to a complicated postsurgical recovery. Pain in the chest or abdomen, for example can affect respiration. The resultant tendency to breathe shallowly and avoid coughing can cause retention of secretions and possibly chest infection. Painful movement can also render patients reluctant to mobilise, which when coupled with the reduced arterial inflow and venous emptying, leads to an increased risk of deep vein thrombosis and pulmonary emptying. Acute postoperative pain can reduce gastric emptying and reduce intestinal motility. The resultant reduced nutrition will reduce healing and lead to prolonged recovery. Protracted acute pain also increases anxiety, which can have a severe detrimental effect on the patient's postoperative recovery. Prolonged anxiety will lead to a stress response, as the body attempts to maintain homeostasis. During stress, numerous hormones released by the neuroendocrine system increase blood pressure, pulse and metabolism. Adrenaline, for example increases heart rate and aldosterone increases blood pressure. Cortisol and glucagon, on the other hand, liberate more glucose for the production of energy. Cortisol also decreases immune function (Macintyre & Ready 2001).

Acute Abdominal Pain

Abdominal pain is a very common symptom that occurs in all age groups from early childhood to the older person. In many cases, abdominal pain has no apparent physical cause and symptoms subside spontaneously. Nevertheless, acute abdominal pain has a number of causes and diagnosis and determination of the seriousness of the cause of pain can be problematic. To aid diagnosis the abdomen is divided into quadrants and the location of the pain informs clinicians of the most likely cause (Box 23.4).

Chest Pain

Acute onset of chest pain is a common presentation in many emergency departments. Chest pain is normally associated with myocardial pathology but there are many other causes of chest pain, which relate to other parts of the body – most notably the respiratory system (Table 23.5). However, it is noteworthy that the first-line treatment for myocardial chest pain is opioid analgesia, which is used for both pain relief and reduction of anxiety and therefore a reduced cardiac workload.

Burns

Pain control for burns victims presents a significant nursing challenging. This is due to a variety of different components that contribute to the severe pain people with burns experience (Choiniere 2003). These multiple components ensure that there is constant changing pattern to the patient's pain, resulting in complex analgesic prescription issues. It is vital that nurses caring for burns victims fully appreciate and recognise the factors that contribute to their pain experience. The contributing factors can be categorised as:

- Background pain
- Breakthrough pain

Box 23.4 Common Causes of Acute Abdominal Pain

Left Upper Quadrant	Right Upper Quadrant
Perisplenitis	Acute cholecystitis
Splenic infarct	Biliary colic
	Acute hepatic distension or inflammation
	Perforated duodenal ulcer

Left Lower Quadrant	Right Lower Quadrant
Acute diverticulitis	Acute appendicitis
Pyogenic sacroiliitis	Mesenteric lymphadenitis
	Infective distal ileitis
	Crohn's disease
	Acute pyelonephritis
	Acute cholecystitis
	Acute rheumatic fever
	Ectopic pregnancy
	Ruptured ovarian cyst

Central Abdominal Pain

Gastroenteritis
Small intestinal colic
Acute pancreatitis
(*Source*: Adapted from Blendis 2003)

Table 23.5 Main causes of chest pain. Adapted from MacLellan (2006)

Cardiovascular	Myocardial infarction
	Unstable angina
Pulmonary	Pleurisy
	Pulmonary embolism
	Pneumothorax
	Pneumonia
Musculoskeletal	Costochondritis
	Trauma
Gastrointestinal	Reflux
	Gastric ulcers
	Gallstones
	Pancreatitis
Psychological	Anxiety

- Procedural pain
- Pain associated with tissue regeneration.

Background pain is the pain that emanates from the burn wound sites and the surrounding areas. Pain may also be present in areas of normal skin that have been harvested for skin grafts (donor sites). This pain will be constant and at times excruciating. Movement, such as walking, changing position or in some instances breathing can cause **breakthrough pain,** which will exacerbate the patient's background pain. **Procedural pain** is caused by the numerous necessary procedures carried out by nurses and other healthcare workers, which form part of their therapeutic treatments. Good examples include wound cleansing, dressing changes and physiotherapy. Finally **pain associated with tissue**

regeneration concerns the pain associated with the healing process and the regeneration of nerve tissue. Patients often describe the pain of regeneration as being an itching or intense tingling sensation.

Nursing Management of Chronic Pain

Chronic pain is a term used to describe pain sensation that occurs in the absence of any obvious biological cause. In many instances, individuals develop chronic pain over time and it is associated with unresolved prolonged acute pain, which leaves the sufferer in chronic pain even though the injured tissue has fully healed. It is often considered and classified as a psychological phenomenon and often described as 'pain syndrome', suggesting that the pain sensation is a maladaptive psychological response to a protracted pain response. There are, however, a number of chronic health conditions that are associated with chronic pain. Chronic musculoskeletal disorders, such as back pain, neuropathies, arthritis and cancer pain are common examples of chronic conditions that cause chronic pain – but cardiovascular disease, gastrointestinal disease, diabetes, stroke and multiple sclerosis are also associated with chronic pain.

Signs and Symptoms

The stress responses associated with an acute pain response are difficult to maintain over sustained periods of time. People living with chronic pain therefore may not present with the some of the cardinal signs of pain, i.e. tachycardia, hypertension and diaphoresis. Chronic pain often results in long-term debilitating psychological effects and sufferers may measure their chronic pain by reporting the impact their pain has on their life. Factors the nurse must consider include:

- Sleep patterns – does the pain keep the patient awake
- Appetite – does the patient have reduced appetite
- Libido – does the patient's pain have a negative impact on their sex-life
- Social isolation – is the patient able to maintain social activities
- Depression.

Investigations and Diagnosis

- Pain assessment
- *Remember pain is what the patient says it is.*

Nursing Care and Management

The main nursing aims for the individual living with chronic pain are to reduce the impact of chronic pain on the quality of life. The major nursing objectives are:

- An accurate pain assessment (see earlier) – in order to best establish choice of interventions
- Safe administration of prescribed analgesia (see earlier)
- Monitor for evidence of the main side-effects of opioid therapy (see Box 23.3)
- Use of psychological interventions, such as relaxation, distraction and imagery
- Consider complimentary therapies, i.e. cognitive behavioural therapy
- Establish a pain management plan
- Monitor the individual's quality of care
- Refer to chronic pain services (Box 23.5).

> **Box 23.5 Functions of Chronic Pain Services**
> - Introduction of pain policies, protocols and guidelines
> - Education of staff and patients
> - Audit and evaluation of services
> - Alleviation of pain
> - Reduction of disability and restoration of function
> - Rationalisation of medication
> - Rationalisation of use of all health services
> - Attention to social, family and occupational issues
> - Ensuring a multidisciplinary approach to chronic pain.
>
> (MacLellan 2006)

> **Nursing Fields Mental Health: Pain and Depression**
> Almost every drug used in psychiatry can also serve as a pain medication. Relieving anxiety, fatigue, depression or insomnia with mood stabilisers, benzodiazepines or anticonvulsants will also ease any related pain. The most versatile of all psychiatric drugs, the antidepressants have an analgesic effect that may be at least partly independent of their effect on depression since it seems to occur at a lower dose.
>
> The two major types of antidepressants, **tricyclics** and **selective serotonin reuptake inhibitors (SSRIs)**, may have different roles in the treatment of pain. Amitriptyline (Elavil), a tricyclic, is one of the antidepressants most often recommended as an analgesic, partly because its sedative qualities can be helpful for people in pain. SSRIs such as fluoxetine (Prozac) and sertraline (Zoloft) may not be quite as effective as pain relievers, but their side-effects are usually better tolerated, and they are less risky than tricyclic drugs. Some physicians prescribe an SSRI during the day and amitriptyline at bedtime for pain patients.

Arthritis

Arthritis encompasses over more than 100 conditions, with **rheumatoid arthritis** and **osteoarthritis** being the two most predominant. The pain of arthritis can be caused by inflammation in the synovial membrane, tendons, ligaments and muscle strain. The majority of the different forms arthritis cause chronic pain, which could range from mild to severe and can last for weeks, months or even years. Pain due to arthritic inflammation is unpredictable, rendering pain management complex and challenging. The treatment of arthritis should include:

- *A comprehensive assessment of pain and function*
- *Paracetamol for mild to moderate pain*
- *Non-steroidal inflammatory drugs for moderate to severe pain*
- *Opioid drugs for severe pain not alleviated by paracetamol or non-steroidal anti-inflammatory drugs*
- *Consideration of surgery when analgesic therapy is ineffective*
- *Promotion of ideal body weight*
- *Referral to physiotherapy and occupational therapy.*

(MacLellan 2006)

Chronic Back Pain

Lower back pain remains one of the most common reasons for individuals to seek medical attention for pain. **Back pain** can be classified as follows:

- Transient back pain
- Acute back pain
- Persistent back pain.

Box 23.6 Causes of Neuropathy

Cause	Examples
Trauma	Painful scars Thoracotomy Amputation Damage through heat, cold, electricity, radiation
Ischaemia	
Toxins	Thallium Arsenic Clioquinol
Metabolic effects	Diabetes
Nutritional	Vitamin B$_{12}$ deficiency
Inflammation	Multiple sclerosis
Infection	Human immunodeficiency virus (HIV)
Cancer	Myeloma
Hereditary	Fabry's disease

From: Scadding (2003); Hanna et al. (2005)

Table 23.6 Types of cancer pain, their source, causes and descriptions. (Listed in order of prevalence. Most patients have a combination of somatic and visceral nociceptor pain.) Adapted from Kochhar (2002).

TYPE OF PAIN	STRUCTURES AFFECTED	CAUSES	PATIENT DESCRIPTION
Somatic nociceptor	Muscle and bone	Bone metastases	Aching, sharp, gnawing or dull
		Surgical incisions	Easily located
Neuropathic	Nerves	Chemotherapy	Burning, itching, numbness, tingling, shooting
		Tumour	
Visceral nociceptor	Organs of the abdomen, pelvis and thorax	Tumour	Crampy, colicky, aching, deep, squeezing, dull
			Less easily located

Transient back pain tends have a short lifespan and does not normally require medical attention, with the patient treating themselves. Often the cause of pain is unknown and does not have any long-term issues or any lasting significance to the patient.

Acute low back pain is a long-term manifestation of pain, which can be of a few days to a few months in duration. Treatments include analgesia and bed rest and surgery if associated with spinal injury/inflammation.

Persistent low back pain is back pain that persists for more than 6 months. Sufferers may become preoccupied with the pain and depression and anxiety may occur.

Neuropathy

Neuropathic pain arises from damaged nociceptors and neurones. The numerous conditions and situations that can lead to the development of neuropathic pain are summarised in Box 23.6. Patients with neuropathies describe their pain as being a burning, electric or tingling sensation that can be continuous or spasmodic. The nervous tissue in ascending pain pathways is described as being plastic, as it changes in response to different psychological and physical stimuli. Such changes include altered sensitivity of nociceptors, which then begin to generate pain impulses in response to ordinary feelings of touch. The patient may also complain of pain in response to slight pressure exerted on the site of injury, even after healing has occurred – a phenomenon called allodynia. Damaged nervous tissue also produces increased sensitivity to painful stimuli often individuals with neuropathy will verbalise pain that is out of proportion to the level of tissue damage. This increase in pain sensitivity is referred to as **hyperalgesia** (Scadding 2003).

Cancer Pain

There is a high prevalence of pain in patients with cancer. Indeed, up to 96% of patients with cancer experience pain, more than AIDS (80%), heart disease (77%), renal disease (77%) and chronic obstructive pulmonary disease (50%) (Solano et al. 2006). Cancer pain has numerous causes but the most likely contributing factor is bone metastases. Cancer pain can be classified as being either **nociceptive** or **neuropathic**. Table 23.6 summarises the main causes and descriptions of cancer pain.

The aim of palliative care is to minimise pain and its associated distressing symptoms (WHO 2002). Cancer pain is therefore classified according to when it occurs or if it becomes more intense and unmanageable. The three main classifications of cancer pain are:

- Breakthrough pain
- Incident pain
- End of dose failure pain.

Breakthrough pain occurs in addition to the underlying cancer pain. It is more intense than the patient's normal pain levels.

Incident pain is caused by incidental activities, i.e. walking, lifting, climbing stairs, washing and dressing.

End of dose failure pain occurs if the therapeutic effects of the patient's prescribed analgesia subside before the next dose is due. Breakthrough and incident pain are common even in patients whose pain is well-controlled. End of dose pain, however, is an indicator that the patient's current pain control may need reviewing (Hayden 2006).

What the Experts Say Pain Relief in Cancer Pain

Morphine is the most researched and most widely used opioid and is therefore the analgesia of choice for the patient in severe cancer pain. Morphine is a safe drug when used properly – the simplest method of dose titration is 4-hourly, with the same dose used for breakthrough pain. The total dose of morphine should then be reviewed daily and the regular dose then adjusted accordingly

(Deborah, Palliative Care Nurse)

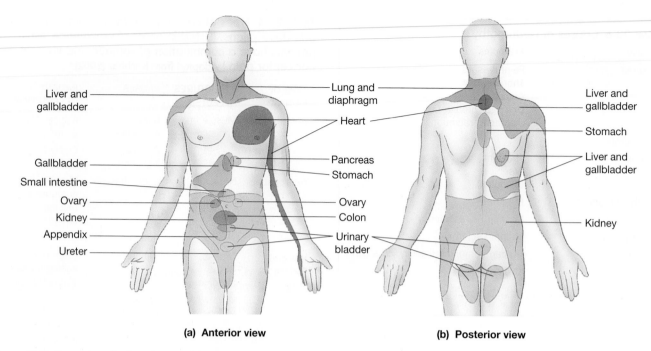

(a) Anterior view　　　　　　**(b) Posterior view**

Figure 23.18 Examples of referred pain and the origin of the tissue damage.

Referred and Phantom Limb Pain

Referred pain occurs when tissue damage in one area of the body manifests itself as pain elsewhere, for example pain as a result of angina that can be felt in the left arm. Although tissue damage occurs in the coronary arteries, pain is also felt radiating down the left arm and despite the intense pain present in the left arm, the tissue there remains perfectly healthy. Referred pain occurs because the damaged or inflamed organ and the area where the referred pain is felt are served by neurones from the same segment of the spinal cord. Another example is pain due to liver or gallbladder inflammation leading to intense pain in the right shoulder. Figure 23.18 highlights the main instances of referred pain (Tortora & Derrickson 2011).

The term **phantom limb pain** occurs when amputees verbalise pain sensed in the area where their removed limb once was. Patients describe the pain as being tingling, numb, itching or tickling in nature. Phantom limb pain has been reported by a significant number of trauma and surgical amputees (Richardson *et al.* 2006). The precise pathophysiology remains unexplained but the two most plausible explanations relate to brain interpretation. For instance when the brain interprets pain impulses from damaged fibres in and around the site of amputation (the stump), it processes the pain signals for the whole (now non-existent) limb. Another theory suggests that the brain contains neurones that provide awareness of body shape and that the neurones that processed information relating to the removed limb remain and continue to be active (Richardson 2008).

The Evidence

Back pain is a common problem that affects most people at some point in their life. It usually feels like an ache, tension or stiffness in your back.

The pain can be triggered by bad posture, while sitting or standing, bending awkwardly or lifting incorrectly.

Back pain is not generally caused by a serious condition and, in most cases, it gets better within 12 weeks. It can usually be successfully treated by taking painkillers and keeping mobile.

https://www.evidence.nhs.uk/topic/back-pain

Conclusion

Pain is an integral part of life. Each of us will experience pain from time to time. The pathophysiology of pain is complex and should be viewed as a physiological and psychological phenomenon. Pain is a personal and subjective experience and all pain care should be individualised, encompassing both physical damage and psychosocial circumstances. It is the nurse's aim that patients remain pain free or are able to live with and cope with their pain. While the main treatment options are analgesic in nature, many non-pharmacological interventions are at the nurse's disposal.

Key Points

- Pain is a universal phenomenon – everyone experiences pain at some point in their life.
- Nurses must always be non-judgemental in their assessment of the individual with pain – remember pain is what the patient says it is.
- Pain can be acute (short term) or chronic (pain which continues after healing is complete).
- Acute pain is often accompanied by visible and recordable symptoms, whereas chronic pain may not present with symptoms.
- Pain is both a physical and emotional experience and nurses need to pay equal attention to both if they are to provide effective holistic care.

- Unresolved pain has many unwanted physiological consequences which can exacerbate the patient's condition and affect well-being.
- Nurses must carry out a comprehensive pain assessment for all patients experiencing pain.
- Nurses must be able to explain, select and administer a range of both pharmacological and non-pharmacological pain control interventions.

Glossary

Adrenaline: hormone released during times of stress

Alexander technique: a method of teaching people to improve body posture and thereby avoiding muscle tension

Aldosterone: hormone that increases blood pressure by increased re-absorption of water and sodium by the kidneys

Allodynia: pain in response to stimuli that should not cause pain

Amputation: surgical removal of a limb

Analgesia: pain killer

Angina: central crushing chest pain that occurs as a result of reduced blood flow through the coronary arteries

Antiplatelet: substance that reduces the clotting action of platelets

Arachidonic acid: substance found in the cell membrane, which can produce prostaglandins

Aromatherapy: the use of odours and fragrances to alter an individual's mood

Autonomic: pertaining to the autonomic nervous system, associated with the maintenance of homeostasis

Axon: the long part of a nerve cell that carries nerve impulses

Bone metastases: cells from a tumour that have spread to bone tissue

Bradycardia: slow heart rate, less than 50 beats per minute

Central nervous system: the brain and spinal cord

Cerebral cortex: the outer surface of the brain

Chiropractic: the manipulation and realignment of the spine

Controlled drugs: therapeutic preparations governed by the Misuse of Drugs Act (HMSO 1971)

Coronary arteries: oxygenated blood supply to the heart

Cortisol: hormone released by the adrenal glands, which increases resistance to stress

Cyclooxygenase-2: enzyme which speeds up the production of prostaglandins from arachidonic acid

Deep vein thrombosis: formation of a blood clot in the veins of the legs

Diaphoresis: excessive sweating

Dorsal horn: the section of grey matter found on either side of a cross-section of the spinal cord

Dynorphin: neuropeptide found in the central nervous system

Dysphoria: low mood, opposite of euphoria

Endorphin: neuropeptide found in the central nervous system. Counteracts pain sensation by inhibiting substance P

Enkephalin: neuropeptide found in the central nervous system. Counteracts pain sensation by inhibiting substance P

Enzyme: a protein that speeds up chemical reactions

Frontal lobe: area of the cerebrum (outer part of the brain)

Glucagon: hormone released by pancreas, which increase blood sugar levels

Histamine: substance released during inflammation that causes vasodilation and increased capillary permeability

Homeopathy: treatment based on the principle that 'like can be cured with like'

Hyperalgesia: increased or heightened pain sensation

Hypertension: abnormally high blood pressure

Hypothalamus: small region of the brain found in the diencephalon; important regulatory organ of the nervous and endocrine systems

Hypoxaemia: reduced levels of oxygen in arterial blood

Hypoxia: reduced levels of oxygen in the tissues

Interneurons: short neurones that connect nearby neurones in the brain and spinal cord

Ischaemia: a reduction in blood supply to tissue

Kinins: substances released during inflammation that cause vasodilation and increased capillary permeability; also attracts phagocytes

Limbic system: part of the forebrain. Sometimes called the emotional brain, the limbic system controls feelings of emotion and behaviour

Miosis: contraction of the pupils

Motor nerves: a nerve that travels from the brain and spinal cord out to an organ, muscle or gland

Myelin: electrically insulating phospholipid

Myelinated: covered by a protected sheath of myelin

Neurone: a nerve cell

Neuropeptide: substance sound in the nervous system that counteracts the effects of neurotransmitters

Neurotransmitter: molecules that transmit messages from one nerve to another at a junction called the synapse

Nociceptors: special cells that detect damage and irritants that cause pain

Non-steroidal anti-inflammatory drugs (NSAIDS): group of non-opioid pain killers that reduce inflammation

Opiate: powerful analgesic agent that stimulates opiate receptors within the central nervous system

Opiate receptors: receptors found in the central nervous system, that are stimulated by neuropeptides and opiate drugs

Osteopathy: the manipulation of bones and joints to diagnose and treat illness

Patient-controlled analgesia: method of self-administration of intravenous analgesia

Peripheral nervous system: the nervous system outside of the central nervous system

Prostaglandins: substances released by damaged cells. Intensify the actions of histamine and kinins

Pruritus: itchy sensation on the skin

Pulmonary embolism: reduced blood flow through the lungs due to a blood clot

Pyrexia: raised body temperature or fever

Reflex arc: nervous pathway from sensory nerve to motor nerve via spinal cord

Reflexology: the manipulation of various areas of the feet and hands in order to promote well-being

Reticular formation: a network of neurones found in the central part of the brain stem

Sensory fibres: special nerve fibres that transmit sensations of pain, heat, cold and touch

Serotonin: neurotransmitter found in central nervous system; associated with pain sensation

Shiatsu: finger pressure applied to various areas of the body in order to stimulate the internal energy of the body and thus promote healing

Somatosensory cortex: region of the cerebral cortex that processes feelings of touch, pain, heat, cold and muscle and joint position

(Continued)

Spinothalamic tract: sensory pathway which transmits messages of pain, temperature, touch and pressure upwards along the spinal cord

Substance P: neurotransmitter found in sensory nerves, spinal cord and brain associated with the sensation of pain

Substantia gelatinosa: part of the spinal cord's grey matter; it is composed of large amounts of small nerve cells

Synapse: the junction where two neurones meet, or where a neurone meets tissue

Syndrome: a collection of symptoms that characterise a specific disorder

Tachycardia: pulse rate greater than 100 beats per minute

Tachypnoea: rapid and usually shallow respiration rate, greater than 20 breaths per minute

Thalamus: a pair of oval masses of grey matter which accounts for 80% of the diencephalon area of the brain

Thoracotomy: incision in the chest

Transcutaneous electrical nerve stimulation (TENS): method of pain control, which stimulates $A\beta$, $A\delta$ and C fibres, with small electrical currents

Ulceration: the erosion of skin or internal surface

White matter: tissue of spinal cord that surrounds the grey matter

References

Bell, L. & Duffy A. (2009) Pain assessment and management in surgical nursing: a literature review. *British Journal of Nursing*, 18(3), 153–156.

Blendis, L M. (2003) Abdominal pain. In: R. Melzack and P.D. Wall (eds) *Handbook of Pain Management: a clinical companion to Wall and Melzack's textbook of pain.* Churchill Livingstone, Edinburgh.

Briggs, E. (2010) Understanding the experience and physiology of pain. *Nursing Standard*, 25(3), 35–39.

British Pain Society (2010) The British Pain Society's Opioids for Persistent Pain: Good Practice: A Consensus Statement Prepared on Behalf of the British Pain Society, The Faculty of pain medicine of the Royal College of Anaesthetists, the Royal College of General Practitioners and the Faculty of Addictions of the Royal College of Psychiatrists. British Pain Society, London.

Carr, E.C.J., Thomas, V.N. & Wilson-Barnet, J. (2005) Patient experiences of anxiety, depression and acute pain after surgery: A longitudinal perspective. *International Journal of Nursing Studies*, 42, 521–530.

Choiniere, M. (2003) Pain of burns. In: R. Melzack and P.D. Wall (eds) *Handbook of Pain Management: a clinical companion to wall and Melzack's textbook of pain.* Churchill Livingstone, Edinburgh.

Dopson, L. (2010) Role of pain management programmes in chronic pain. *Nursing Standard*, 25(13), 35–40.

Ecclestone C, Williams A.C. & Morley, S (2009) Psychological therapies for the management of chronic pain (excluding headache) in adults (review), *Cochrane Database of Systematic Reviews*, (2):CD007407.

French, S.D., Cameron, M., Walker, B.F., Reggars, J.W. & Esterman, A.J. (2005) Superficial heat or cold for low back pain. *Cochrane Database of Systematic Reviews*, (1):CD004750.

Furlan, A.D., Brosseau, L., Imamura, M. & Irvin, E. (2002) Massage for low back pain. *The Cochrane Database of Systematic Reviews*, (2):CD001929.

Fuster, V., Dyken, M.L., Vokonas, P.S. & Hennekens, C. (1993) Aspirin as a therapeutic agent in cardiovascular disease. *Circulation*, 87(2), 659–675.

Gilron, I., Milne, B. & Hong, M. (2003). Cyclooxygenase-2 inhibitors in postoperative pain management. *Anaesthesiology*, 99(5), 1198–1208.

Godfrey, H. (2005a) Understanding pain, Part 1: Physiology of pain. *British Journal of Nursing*, 14(16), 846–852.

Godfrey, H. (2005b) Understanding pain, Part 2: Pain management. *British Journal of Nursing*, 14(17), 904–909.

Gould, B.E. (2006) *Pathophysiology for the Health Professions*, 3rd edn. Elsevier, Philadelphia.

Gould, D. & Thomas, V.N. (1997). Pain mechanisms: the neurophysiology and neuropsychology of pain perception. In: V.N. Thomas (ed.) *Pain: its nature and management.* Bailliere Tindall, London.

Grafton, K.V., Foster, N.E. & Wright, C.C. (2005) Test-retest reliability of the short-form McGill pain questionnaire. *Clinical Journal of Pain*, 21(1), 73–82.

Hader, C.F. & Guy, J. (2004). Your hand in pain management. *Nursing Management*, 35(11), 21–28.

Hanna, M., Holdcroft A. & Jaggar, S.I. (2005) Neuropathic pain. In: A. Holdcroft, & S. Jaggar (eds). *Core Topics In Pain.* Cambridge University Press, Cambridge.

Hayden, D. (2006) Pain management in palliative care. In: K. MacLellan (ed.) *Expanding Nursing and Health Care Practice: management of pain.* Nelson Thornes, Cheltenham.

Heath, M.L. (1997) The use of pharmacology in pain management. In: V.N. Thomas (ed.) *Pain: its nature and management.* Bailliere Tindall, London.

HMSO (1968) *The Medicine's Act.* Her Majesty's Stationery Office, London.

HMSO (1971) *The Misuse of Drugs Act.* Her Majesty's Stationery Office, London.

ICSI (2004) *Assessment and Management of Acute Pain.* Institute for Clinical System Improvement, London.

Jenkins, C., Costello, J. & Hodge, L. (2004) Systematic review of prevalence of aspirin induced asthma and its implications for clinical practice. *British Medical Journal*, 328, 434–440.

Johansson, K., Nuutila, L., Virtanen, H., Katajisto, J. & Salantera, S. (2005) Preoperative education for orthopaedic patients: Systematic review. *Journal of Advanced Nursing*, 50(2), 212–223.

Johnson, M. (2005) Physiology of chronic pain. In: C. Banks & K. Mackrodt (eds) *Chronic Pain Management.* Whurr Publishers, London.

Julius, D. & Basbaum, A.I. (2001) Molecular mechanisms of nociception. *Nature*, 413, 203–210.

Kochhar, S.C. (2002) Cancer pain. In: C.A. Warfield & H.J. Fausett (eds) *Manual of Pain Management*, 2nd edn. Lippincott Williams & Wilkins, Philadelphia.

Large, R.G., New, F., Strong, J. & Unruh, A.M. (2002) Chronic pain and psychiatric problems. In: J. Strong, A.M. Unruh, A. Wright & G.D. Baxter (eds) *Pain: a textbook for therapists.* Churchill Livingstone, Edinburgh.

Layzell, M. (2008) Current interventions and approaches to post-operative pain management. *British Journal of Nursing*, 17(7), 414–419.

Lee, H. & Ernst, E. (2005) Acupuncture analgesia during surgery: A systematic review. *Pain*, 114(3), 511–517.

Lin, L. & Wang, R. (2005) Abdominal surgery, pain and anxiety: Preoperative nursing intervention. *Journal of Advanced Nursing*, 51(3), 252–260.

Lundeberg, T. & Stener-Victorin, E. (2002) Is there a physiological basis for the use of acupuncture in pain? *International Congress Series*, 1238, 3–10.

Lynch, M. (2001) Pain as the fifth vital sign. *Journal of Intravenous Nursing*, 24(2), 85–94.

MacIntyre, P.E. & Ready, L.B. (2001) *Acute Pain Management: a practical guide*, 2nd edn. W.B. Saunders, London.

MacLellan, K. (2006) *Expanding Nursing and Health Care Practice: Management of Pain.* Nelson Thornes, Cheltenham.

MacPherson, R.D. (2000) The pharmacological basis of contemporary pain management. *Pharmacology and Therapeutics*, 88, 163–185.

Main, C.J. & Spanswick, C.C. (2000) *Pain Management: an interdisciplinary approach.* Churchill Livingstone, Edinburgh.

Manias, E. (2003) Pain and anxiety management in the postoperative gastro-surgical setting. *Journal of Advanced Nursing*, 41(6), 585–504.

Marieb, E. & Hoehn, K. (2007) *Human Anatomy and Physiology*, 7th edn. Pearson Benjamin Cummings, San Francisco.

McCaffery, M. (1979) *Nursing Management of the Patient with Pain*, 2nd edn. J.B. Lippincott, New York.

McCaffery, M. & Beebe, A. (1994) *Pain: clinical manual for nursing practice*. Mosby, Aylesbury.

McCaffery, R., Frock, T.L. & Garguilo, H. (2003) Understanding chronic pain and the mind–body connection. *Holistic Nursing Practice*, 17(6), 281–287.

McGann, K. (2007) *Fundamental Aspects of Pain Assessment and Management*. Quay Books, Gateshead.

Melzack, R. & Wall, P. (1988) *The Challenge of Pain*, 2nd edn. Penguin, London.

Melzack, R. & Wall, P.D. (1965) Pain mechanisms: A new theory. *Science* 9, 159–971.

NMC (2008) *The Code of Professional Conduct*. Nursing and Midwifery Council, London.

Nnoaham, K,E. & Kumbang J. (2008) Transcutaneous electrical nerve stimulation (TENS) for chronic pain (review). *Cochrane Database of Systematic Reviews*, (3):CD003222.

Richardson, C., Glenn, S,. Nurrmikko, T., Horgan, M. (2006) Incidence of phantom phenomena including phantom limb pain 6 months after major lower limb amputation in patients with peripheral vascular disease. *Clinical Journal of Pain*, 22(4), 353–358.

Richardson, C. (2008) Nursing aspects of phantom limb pain following amputation. *British Journal of Nursing*, 17(7), 422–426.

Scadding, J.W. (2003) Peripheral neuropathies. In: R. Melzack & P.D. Wall (eds) *Handbook of Pain Management: a clinical companion to Wall and Melzack's textbook of pain*. Churchill Livingstone, Edinburgh.

Skevington, S. (1995) *Psychology of Pain*. John Wiley and Sons, Chichester.

Sluka, K.A. & Walsh, D. (2003) Transcutaneous electrical nerve stimulation: Basic science mechanisms and clinical effectiveness. *Journal of Pain*, 4(3), 109–121.

Solano, J.P., Games, B. & Higginson, I.J. (2006) A comparison of symptom prevalence in far advanced cancer, AIDS, heart disease, chronic obstructive pulmonary disease (COPD) and renal disease. *Journal of Pain and Symptom Management*, 31(1), 58–69.

Stranc, D.S. (2002) Endogenous opioids. In: C.A. Warfield & H.J. Fausett (eds). *Manual of Pain Management*, 2nd edn. Lippincott Williams & Wilkins, Philadelphia.

Tortora, G.J. & Derrickson, B. (2011) *Principles of Anatomy and Physiology Organisation, Support and Movement, and Control Systems of the Human Body*, Vol. 1, 13th edn. John Wiley and Sons, New York.

Wigens, L. (2006) The role of complementary and alternative therapies in pain management. In: K. MacLellan (ed.) *Expanding Nursing and Health Care Practice: Management of Pain*. Nelson Thornes, Cheltenham.

WHO (1986) *Cancer Pain Relief*. World Health Organization, Geneva.

WHO (2002) *National Cancer Control Programmes: Policies and Management Guidelines*, 2nd edn. World Health Organization, Geneva.

Test Yourself

1. In the ascending pain pathway, which neurones travel upwards through the spinal column, towards the brain?
   (a) First order neurones
   (b) Second order neurones
   (c) Third order neurones
   (d) Interneurons

2. Which of the following statements is true?
   (a) C fibres are myelinated nerve fibres
   (b) A-delta (Aδ) fibres transmit sensation faster than both C fibres and A-beta (Aβ) fibres
   (c) A-beta (Aβ) fibres are non-myelinated and transmit sensation slower than C fibres
   (d) A-beta (Aβ) fibres transmit sensation faster than both C fibres and A-delta (Aδ) fibres

3. Which of the following is an endogenous opiate?
   (a) Endorphin
   (b) Substance P
   (c) Kappa
   (d) Morphine

4. Pain which continues even after healing is complete would be described as:
   (a) Visceral pain
   (b) Acute pain
   (c) Chronic pain
   (d) Transient pain

5. Which of the following statements on pain is true?
   (a) You can teach patients to tolerated pain
   (b) The longer people have pain the more used to it they become
   (c) Visible signs accompany pain and can be used to verify how severe it is
   (d) Pain is what the patient says it is

6. Which of the following is a strong opioid?
   (a) Codeine
   (b) Pethidine
   (c) Tramadol
   (d) Ibuprofen

7. Which of the following analgesics would inhibit the actions of prostaglandins?
   (a) Paracetamol
   (b) Morphine
   (c) Pethidine
   (d) Fentanyl

8. Which of the following systems are affected by unresolved pain?
   (a) Respiratory system
   (b) Cardiovascular system
   (c) Digestive system
   (d) All of the above

9. In cancer pain classification, what is pain that is caused by specific activities?
   (a) Breakthrough pain
   (b) Incident pain
   (c) Nociceptive pain
   (d) End of dose pain

10. Which of the following is recognised as an effective non-pharmacological pain control intervention for patients living with chronic pain?
    (a) Alexander Technique
    (b) Acupuncture
    (c) Cognitive behavioural therapy
    (d) Reflexology

Answers

1. b
2. d
3. a
4. c
5. d
6. b
7. a
8. d
9. b
10. c

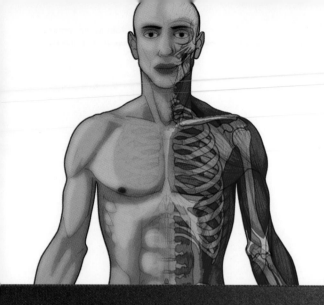

24

Fluid and Electrolyte Imbalance, and Shock

Muralitharan Nair

University of Hertfordshire, UK

Learning Outcomes

On completion of this chapter you will be able to:

* Describe the fluid compartments of the body
* Compare and contrast the causes, effects and care of the patient with fluid and electrolyte imbalance
* Explain the pathophysiology of fluid and electrolyte imbalance
* Discuss the risk factors, aetiologies and pathophysiologies of hypovolaemic, cardiogenic, obstructive and distributive shock
* Apply knowledge of fluid requirements needed for health and during illness and recovery, so that appropriate fluids can be provided
* Recognise and report reasons for poor fluid intake and output

Competencies

All nurses must:

1. Assess and monitor fluid and electrolyte balance
2. Determine the priorities of nursing care management of the patient based on the assessment data and to implement individualised nursing care
3. Provide information for the patient and their family regarding diet and medications used to maintain fluid and electrolyte balance
4. Assess physical and psychological needs of the patient
5. Advise the patient and their relatives of measures to maintain fluid and electrolyte balance
6. Evaluate nursing care of patients with fluid and electrolyte imbalance

 Visit the companion website at **www.wileynursingpractice.com** where you can test yourself using flashcards, multiple-choice questions and more.

Nursing Practice: Knowledge and Care, First Edition. Edited by Ian Peate, Karen Wild and Muralitharan Nair.
© 2014 John Wiley & Sons, Ltd. Published 2014 by John Wiley & Sons, Ltd. Companion website: www.wileynursingpractice.com

Introduction

In a healthy patient, the fluids they take balance the fluids they excrete. Fluid and electrolytes are essential for body function and to maintain homeostasis. Fluid loss via the skin and lungs will increase in a hot and dry environment or with increased respiration rate, fever or burns and even in injury. Fluid and electrolytes are not stationary in the body. There is constant movement of fluid and electrolytes between the intracellular and extracellular compartments. The movement of fluid and electrolytes ensures that the cells are constantly supplied with electrolytes such as sodium, chloride, potassium, magnesium, phosphates, bicarbonate and calcium for cellular function. In certain cases, subtle changes in the fluid and electrolyte balance can lead to death of the patient. Consequently, nurses must have a good understanding of fluid and electrolyte balance so that they can recognise or anticipate any changes and take the necessary steps to prevent harm to the patient. This chapter will consider fluid and electrolyte balance and some diseases resulting from fluid and electrolyte imbalance.

Body Fluid Compartments

Water is distributed between the two major compartments: intracellular and extracellular. The intracellular compartment is the space inside a cell and the fluid inside the cell is called intracellular fluid (ICF). The extracellular compartment is found outside the cell and the fluid outside the cell is called extracellular fluid (ECF) (Martini & Nath 2011). However, the extracellular compartment is further divided into the extravascular (interstitial) compartment, intravascular compartment (plasma) (Figure 24.1), lymph and transcellular fluid (e.g. cerebrospinal fluid, saliva). Two-thirds of body fluid is found inside the cell (40% of the total body weight) and one-third of the fluid outside the cell (20% of the total body weight). Some 80% of the ECF is found in the interstitial compartment and 20% in the intravascular compartment as plasma (Figure 24.1). The movement of fluid between the compartments is primarily controlled by two forces:

- Hydrostatic pressure – pressure exerted by the fluid
- Osmotic pressure – the pressure that must be exerted on a solution to prevent the passage of water through a selective permeable membrane.

Function of Water

Body fluid is composed of water, electrolytes such as sodium and potassium, gases (oxygen and carbon dioxide), nutrients, enzymes and hormones. Water is essential for the body as it:

- Acts as a lubricant and so makes swallowing easy
- Is a major component of the body's transport system for various substances, such as nutrients, gases, hormones, waste products of metabolism and electrolytes
- Regulates body temperature
- Provides an optimum environment for the cells to function and for chemical reactions
- Helps to break down food particles in the gastrointestinal (GI) tract
- Provides lubrication for joints.

Fluid Balance

Fluid balance is maintaining the correct amount of fluid in the body and this can vary with disease and illness. The amount of water varies with the individual, as it depends on the condition of the patient, the amount of physical exercise, and on the environment. Normally, water intake equals water loss and the body fluid remains constant. Most of the water essential for body function is obtained from drinking water, some from the food consumed and some from cellular metabolism. The organs, such as the kidneys play a vital role in fluid balance, as water is excreted in the urine and some water is lost in respiration, through the skin and in faeces. See Table 24.1 for a guide to fluid intake and output.

Osmosis

Osmosis is a process by which water moves from an area of high volume to an area of low volume, through a selective permeable membrane. The selective permeable membrane will allow water molecules to move across but is not permeable to solute molecules or ions (LeMone *et al.* 2011). Water movement through this selective membrane, into the compartments, occurs through a process called osmosis (Figure 24.2). The number of particles dissolved in a unit of water determines the concentration of that fluid. This concentration can be expressed as osmolality or osmolarity. Osmolality refers to the number of osmoles per kilogram of water, while osmolarity refers to the number of osmoles per litre of solution. When referring to body fluid the correct term to use is osmolality.

517

> ### Jot This Down
> The term *tonicity* is sometimes used instead of osmolality and solutions can be termed *isotonic, hypotonic and hypertonic*. Can you define these terms and give examples of each using intravenous fluids?

Table 24.1 Fluid intake and output. (Peate *et al.* 2012)

	INTAKE		OUTPUT
Drinking	1500–2000 mL	Urine	1500–2000 mL
Water from food	700–1000 mL	Faeces	100 mL
Cellular metabolism	300–400 mL	Expiration	600–800 mL
		Skin	300–600 mL
Total balance	2500–3400 mL		2500–3400 mL

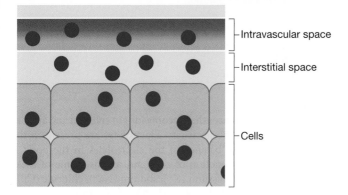

- Intravascular space
- Interstitial space
- Cells

Figure 24.1 Fluid compartments of the body.

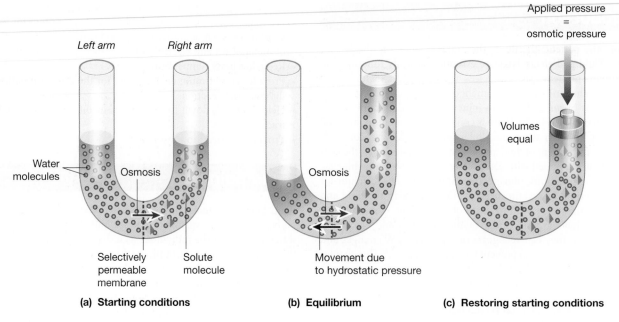

Figure 24.2 **Osmosis.**

(a) **Starting conditions** (b) **Equilibrium** (c) **Restoring starting conditions**

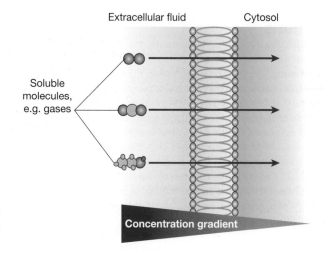

Figure 24.3 **Simple diffusion.**

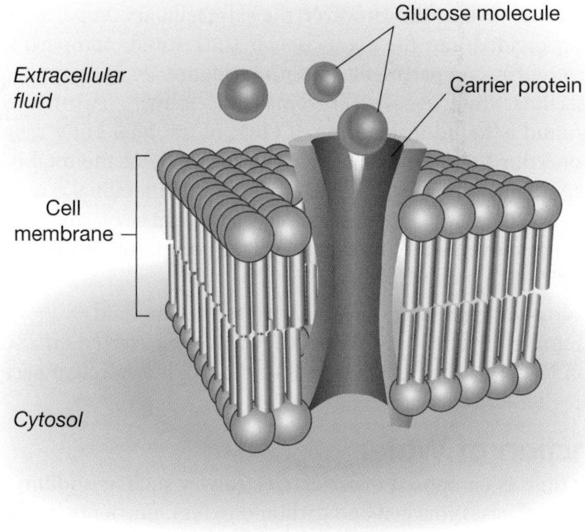

Figure 24.4 **Facilitated diffusion.**

Simple Diffusion

Diffusion describes the movement of solutes such as sodium, potassium, urea and uric acid from areas of higher concentration to areas of lower concentration (Figure 24.3). Diffusion is further subdivided into simple and facilitated diffusion. Liquid soluble molecules and gases move by a process of simple diffusion through a concentration gradient while larger molecules such as glucose and amino acids are transported across the cell membrane by facilitated diffusion (Figure 24.4). An example of simple diffusion is the exchange of oxygen and carbon dioxide between the alveoli and the lung capillaries. The rate of diffusion depends on several factors:

- Gases diffuse much more rapidly than liquids
- The temperature of the environment

- The size of the molecule (smaller molecules diffuse faster than larger molecules)
- Concentration gradient.

Electrolytes

Electrolytes are substances that become ions in solution and acquire the capacity to conduct electricity. Electrolytes are present in the human body, and the balance of the electrolytes in the body is essential for normal function of cells and organs. Some of these electrolytes include potassium (K^+), sodium (Na^+), chloride (Cl^-), magnesium (Mg^{2+}) and phosphate (HPO_4^{2-}). Electrolytes are positively (cations) or negatively (anions) charged, which allows them

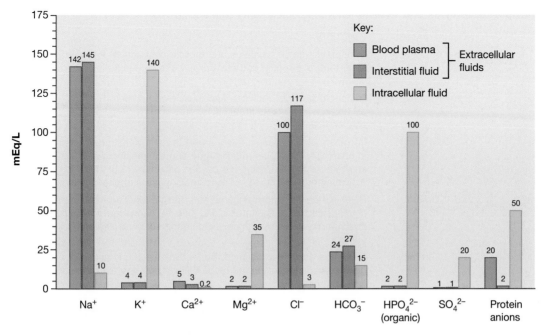

Figure 24.5 Electrolytes of intracellular and extracellular compartments.

to carry electrical impulses through nerves for certain physiological function. They also maintain fluid and acid–base balance of the body. The composition of electrolytes differs between the intracellular and the extracellular compartments (Figure 24.5).

Functions of the electrolytes

Electrolytes are important for:

- Regulating fluid movement between compartments, thus ensuring fluid levels inside and outside the cells are balanced
- Regulating blood pH levels
- Carrying electrical impulses across the cell and to neighbouring cells in order to promote muscle contractions and nerve impulses
- Enzyme reaction.

Table 24.2 gives a summary of the principal electrolytes and their functions.

Acid–Base Balance

Homeostasis and optimal cellular function require maintenance of the hydrogen ion (H^+) concentration of body fluids within a relatively narrow range. Hydrogen ions determine the relative acidity of body fluids. Acids release hydrogen ions in solution; bases (or alkalis) accept hydrogen ions in solution. The relative acidity or alkalinity of a fluid is measured as pH. The relationship between hydrogen ion concentration and pH is inverse; that is, as hydrogen ion concentration increases, the pH falls, and the solution becomes more acidic. As hydrogen ion concentration falls, the pH rises, and the solution becomes more alkaline (basic). The pH of body fluids is slightly alkaline, with the normal pH ranging from 7.35 to 7.45 (a pH of 7 is neutral). A pH outside this range, below 7.35 or above 7.45, can be fatal for the person. See Figure 24.6 for the pH scale.

A number of mechanisms work together to maintain the pH of the body within this normal range. Metabolic processes in the body continuously produce acids, which fall into two categories: volatile acids and non-volatile acids. Volatile acids can be eliminated from

the body as a gas. Carbonic acid (H_2CO_3) is the only volatile acid produced in the body. It dissociates (separates) into carbon dioxide (CO_2) and water (H_2O); the carbon dioxide is then eliminated from the body through the lungs. All other acids produced in the body are non-volatile acids that must be metabolised or excreted from the body in fluid. Lactic acid, hydrochloric acid and phosphoric acid are examples of non-volatile acids. Most acids and bases in the body are weak; that is, they neither release nor accept a significant amount of hydrogen ions (LeMone *et al.* 2011).

Investigations and diagnosis

In practice, analysis of arterial blood gases provides:

- *pH*: determines whether there is an overall acidosis or alkalosis in the blood
- *Carbon dioxide (CO₂) partial pressure (PaCO₂)*: if CO_2 is increased (in acidosis) or decreased (in alkalosis), it is a respiratory disorder
- *Standard bicarbonate*: analysis of blood gases provides a bicarbonate level, which is calculated from the $PaCO_2$ using the Henderson–Hasselbalch equation
- *Bicarbonate (HCO₃⁻)*: increased in metabolic alkalosis and decreased in metabolic acidosis. Otherwise, the change is compensatory (i.e. normal or raised in respiratory acidosis; normal or decreased in respiratory alkalosis).

Buffer systems

Buffers are substances that prevent major changes in pH by removing or releasing hydrogen ions. When excess acid is present in body fluid, buffers bind with hydrogen ions to minimise the change in pH. If body fluids become too basic or alkaline, buffers release hydrogen ions, restoring the pH. Although buffers act within a fraction of a second, their capacity to maintain pH is limited (LeMone *et al.* 2011). Several body systems, for example respiratory and renal systems, chemical buffers, such as bicarbonate–carbonic acid, catalysed by the enzyme carbonic anhydrase (Figure 24.7),

Table 24.2 Principal electrolytes and their functions. Adapted from Peate *et al.* (2012)

ELECTROLYTES	NORMAL VALUES	FUNCTION	MAINLY FOUND
Sodium (Na$^+$)	135–145 mmol/L	Transmitting nerve impulses and muscle contraction. Plays an important role in fluid and electrolyte balance. Maintains blood volume	Extracellular fluid
Potassium (K$^+$)	3.5–5 mmol/L	Transmitting nerve impulses and muscle contraction. Regulates pH balance, maintains intracellular fluid volume. Regulating cardiac impulses	Intracellular fluid
Calcium (Ca^{2+})	2.1–2.6 mmol/L	Important clotting factor. Plays a part in neurotransmitter release in neurones. Maintains muscle tone and excitability of nervous and muscle tissue. Maintains cardiac pacemaker automaticity. Activating enzymes such as pancreatic lipase and phospholipase	Extracellular fluid
Magnesium (Mg^{2+})	0.5–1.0 mmol/L	Helps to maintain normal nerve and muscle function; maintains regular heart rate, regulates blood glucose and blood pressure. Essential for protein synthesis. Operating sodium-potassium pump	Intracellular fluid
Chloride (Cl$^-$)	98–117 mmol/l	Regulates acid–base balance. Buffer for oxygen and carbon dioxide exchange in the red blood cells. Regulates extracellular fluid volume	Extracellular fluid
Bicarbonates (HCO$_3^-$)	22–30 mmol/L	Main buffer of hydrogen ions in plasma. Maintains a balance between cations and anions of intracellular and extracellular fluids	Extracellular fluid
Phosphate (PO$_4^-$)	0.8–1.1 mmol/L	Essential for the digestion of proteins, carbohydrates and fats and absorption of calcium. Essential for bone formation. Regulating pH balance	Intracellular fluid

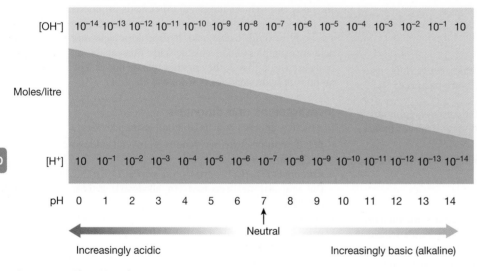

Figure 24.6 The pH scale.

phosphate buffer systems and protein buffers help to maintain pH balance in the body.

The lungs regulate acid–base balance by eliminating or retaining carbon dioxide. Carbon dioxide dissolved in water forms carbonic acid, a volatile acid. Increases in either carbon dioxide or hydrogen ions in the blood stimulate the respiratory centre in the brain. As a result, both the rate and depth of respiration increase and carbon dioxide is exhaled. The levels of carbon dioxide in the blood are measured as PCO$_2$. PCO$_2$ measures the pressure of carbon dioxide of the venous blood, whereas PaCO$_2$ measures the pressure of carbon dioxide in the arterial blood (Porth 2009). The normal

PaCO$_2$ is between 4.6 and 5.6 kPa (35–42 mmHg), PaO$_2$ (partial pressure of arterial oxygen) is between 11.3 and 14 kPa. Note that PACO$_2$ measures alveolar mean pressures (Alexander *et al.* 2006).

The renal system is responsible for the long-term regulation of acid–base balance in the body. Unlike the respiratory system, the kidneys are slower to respond to changes, requiring hours to days to correct any imbalance. Excess non-volatile acids produced during metabolism normally are eliminated by the kidneys. The kidneys also regulate bicarbonate levels in extracellular fluid by regenerating bicarbonate ions as well as reabsorbing them in the renal tubules. When excess hydrogen ion is present in the blood and the pH falls (acidosis), the kidneys reabsorb and regenerate bicarbonate ions. Conversely, in alkalosis the kidneys will excrete bicarbonate ions and retain hydrogen ions.

Acidosis and Alkalosis

Acidosis and alkalosis are terms used to describe the abnormal conditions when a patient's blood pH may not fall within the range of 7.35–7.45. Disorders of acid–base balance are primarily respiratory or metabolic in origin. Acidosis occurs when there is a high level of hydrogen ions, thus resulting in a low pH of below 7.35. Respiratory acidosis is caused by a build-up of carbon dioxide in the body as a result of primary disorders of the respiratory tract or

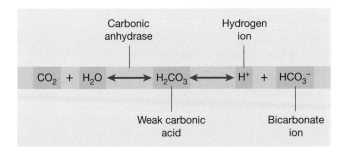

$$CO_2 + H_2O \longleftrightarrow H_2CO_3 \longleftrightarrow H^+ + HCO_3^-$$

Carbonic anhydrase | Hydrogen ion | Weak carbonic acid | Bicarbonate ion

Figure 24.7 Bicarbonate–carbonic acid buffer reversible reaction.

other conditions affecting the respiratory centre such as exacerbation of chronic obstructive pulmonary disease (COPD), muscular dystrophy, hypoventilation syndrome (Pickwickian syndrome), neuromuscular disorders and drugs that suppress breathing (including analgesics such as narcotics, and sedatives such as benzodiazepines), especially when combined with alcohol. Respiratory alkalosis (pH above 7.45), on the other hand, results from hyperventilation, e.g. anxiety, stroke, meningitis, liver diseases, salicylate poisoning and high altitude.

Metabolic acidosis occurs as a result of low pH and low levels of bicarbonate ions resulting from shock, hypoxia, diabetes and renal failure. Metabolic alkalosis, by contrast, occurs when there is an excess of bicarbonate ions, for example burns, vomiting and hypokalaemia. The management of these conditions depends on identifying and treating the underlying cause.

Antacids (alkaline) are prescribed for patients with gastric problems such as gastritis. Most antacids contain aluminium or magnesium hydroxides or derivatives of carbonates. When taken uncontrolled, they could cause metabolic alkalosis.

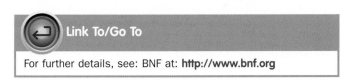

Link To/Go To

For further details, see: BNF at: **http://www.bnf.org**

When there is severe loss of fluid and electrolytes, all the organs of the body are affected. The heart is unable to pump enough blood to the organs, which can cause many organs to stop working because of inadequate tissue perfusion, resulting in the patient developing shock.

Fluid Volume Deficit (FVD)

FVD will arise when water loss exceeds water intake. This could result from many factors:

- Excessive fluid losses from the GI tract, such as diarrhoea and vomiting; profuse sweating
- Poor intake of fluid/dehydration
- Failure of regulatory mechanisms
- Diseases such as renal failure, diabetes, diabetes insipidus and acidosis
- Trauma, surgery, haemorrhage
- Medications such as diuretics or laxatives
- Pyrexia resulting in severe sweating
- Fluid loss into the third space.

FVD is a relatively common problem that may exist alone or in combination with other electrolyte or acid–base imbalances. The

term *dehydration* refers to loss of water alone, even though it often is used interchangeably with FVD.

Red Flag

Water loss of 1–2% can impair mental and physical performance. Loss of 7% of body fluid can lead to circulatory collapse. Nurses should report any changes in the patient's vital signs, such as low blood pressure, tachycardia or low urine output.

Pathophysiology of FVD

FVD may result from lack of fluid intake, inability to request or to drink fluids, oral infection, diarrhoea or certain diseases such as diabetes or diabetes insipidus. Elderly people are at particular risk for FVD (LeMone *et al.* 2011). FVD can develop slowly or rapidly, depending on the type of fluid loss. In certain cases, electrolytes are lost along with fluid, resulting in fluid and electrolyte imbalance. When both water and electrolytes are lost, the serum sodium level remains normal, although levels of other electrolytes such as potassium may fall. Fluid is drawn into the vascular compartment from the interstitial spaces as the body attempts to maintain tissue perfusion. As a result of the fluid loss from the interstitial space, fluid moves out from the intracellular compartment, thus depleting the intracellular volume.

Third fluid space Third spacing is a shift of fluid from the vascular space into an area where it is not available for normal fluid exchange. Examples of **third fluid space** are pleural, peritoneal, joint and pericardial cavities. The movement of fluid into these spaces may result from infection or burns or be idiopathic. The trapped fluid is not available for physiological function although the fluid is still in the body.

Signs and symptoms of fluid volume deficit

- Dry mucous membranes
- Weight loss
- Poor skin turgor (elasticity)
- Hypotension
- Flat neck veins, decreased central venous pressure
- Tachycardia
- Pale appearance
- Low urine output
- Sunken eyeballs.

Nursing care and management

Nurses are responsible for identifying patients at risk for FVD, initiating and carrying out measures to prevent and treat FVD, and monitoring the effects of therapy. The aim is to identify the cause of FVD and to replace the fluid loss. To achieve full fluid replacement, the volume that is infused must be three times the volume of fluid lost (Kozier *et al.* 2008). Nurses need to monitor the patient closely and:

- Weigh the patient daily and record outcome. *Weight helps to assess fluid loss or gain*
- Maintain accurate input and output record. *Accurate records are important in assessing the patient's fluid balance*
- Monitor vital signs every hour to 4 hours, including neurological observations. *Vital sign changes such as increased heart rate,*

decreased blood pressure and increased temperature indicate hypo-volaemia, seizures and irritability

- Administer fluids as prescribed. *Important to ensure that the patient is getting the correct amount of fluid*
- Provide frequent oral hygiene. *Oral mucous membranes become dry and sticky due to loss of fluid in the interstitial spaces*
- Regularly check blood pressure, temperature, pulse, respiration and mental state in patients receiving i.v. fluid therapy. *Observations are good indicators about the patient's response to treatment*
- Check patient's pressure areas every 4 hours to ensure that they are not developing pressure sores. *Patients with poor skin turgor are at risk of developing pressure sores*
- Assist with mobility when going for a walk or to the toilet. The patient may be unsteady when walking as a result of low blood pressure.

Jot This Down

During treatment, if the patient responds to your questions inappropriately and is confused, what do you think is happening with the patient?

Increasingly, there is a tendency to administer intravenous fluid subcutaneously to elderly patients over a 24-hour period.

Link To/Go To

The following link outlines the policy and guidelines with regards to subcutaneous infusion:

http://www.nht.nhs.uk/mediaFiles/downloads/85081641/
MMPr007%20Subcutaneous%20therapy%20protocol%20
Nov2013-Nov2014.pdf (accessed 8 March 2014).

What To Do If...

If a patient with FVD on i.v. therapy complains of breathlessness and has difficulty in breathing. Your actions may include...
 · Report immediately
· Taking and recording vital signs
· Reporting changes in patients immediately for prompt action

Health promotion and discharge

- Patients should be made aware of the importance of maintaining sufficient fluid and salt intake, particularly when exercising or if they develop diarrhoea and vomiting
- Inform the patient of the signs and symptoms of dehydration and the importance of replacing the fluid loss – approximately 2 litres of fluid per day
- Advise they always carry a bottle of water when exercising or going for walks so that they can replace any fluid lost through sweating
- Advise they weigh themselves weekly to ensure that they are not losing weight unnecessarily and to seek advice from the practice nurse if they are concerned.

Primary Care

Before discharging the patient, nurses need to ensure that the patient is well informed about their condition and the care they will have in their home. Discuss the increased risk for fluid volume deficit with adults and provide information about prevention. Discuss the importance of maintaining adequate fluid intake, particularly when exercising and during hot weather. Advise the patient to replace fluid lost during exercise and to take regular rest during exercise. Advise the patient (and their caregivers) that thirst decreases with ageing and urge the patient to maintain a regular fluid intake of about 1500 mL per day, regardless of whether they are feeling thirsty or not.

Jot This Down

If a large volume of fluid is trapped in the third space, such as the peritoneal or the pleural cavities, does this indicate that the patient is over- or dehydrated? Think about fluid compartments and fluid movement between compartments.

Care, Dignity and Compassion

Encouraging people to eat and drink is an important part of the nurse's role. Fear of incontinence resulting in the loss of dignity may lead to some patients not taking adequate fluid or nutrition. Nurses need to be sensitive in the delivery of care to older people both in the acute and community settings. Find out more about the guidelines of the Social Care Institute of Excellence by following the link below.

(http://www.scie.org.uk/publications/guides/guide15/factors/nutrition/index.asp accessed 21 August 2013). The guidelines state:

· Encourage people to drink regularly throughout the day. The Food Standards Agency recommends a daily intake of six to eight glasses of water or other fluids
· Provide education, training and information about the benefits of good hydration to staff, carers and people who use services, and encourage peer-to-peer learning
· Provide promotional materials to remind people who use services, staff and carers of the importance of hydration
· Ensure there is access to clean drinking water 24 hours a day
· If people are reluctant to drink water, think of other ways of increasing their fluid intake, for example with alternative drinks and foods that have a higher fluid content (e.g. breakfast cereals with milk, soup and fruit and vegetables)
· If people show reluctance to drink because they are worried about incontinence, reassure them that help will be provided with going to the toilet. It may help some people to avoid drinking before bedtime.

Fluid Volume Excess (FVE)

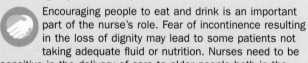

FVE is the abnormal retention of fluid and sodium in the extracellular space. This increase results from retention of serum sodium, which leads to retention of fluid. This could result from a patient having too much normal saline infusion or eating food containing a high amount of sodium.

Pathophysiology of FVE

FVE usually results from conditions that cause retention of both sodium and water. The risk of fluid overload is higher in elderly patients and if there is cardiac or renal impairment, sepsis, major injury or major surgery (Porth 2009). As individuals age, most of the systems (e.g. heart, liver, kidneys) will decline in their physiological functions, making the elderly more at risk of developing health-related illnesses such as fluid retention and electrolyte imbalance.

This retention of water and sodium could result from:

- Drinking large amounts of hypotonic fluid, for example water. Water moves from the intravascular space resulting in oedema
- Administration of an excessive amount of 0.9% normal saline infusion or Ringer's solution
- Excess intake of sodium chloride in the diet
- Diseases such as liver cirrhosis, renal failure and congestive heart failure
- Administration of drugs that cause sodium retention, blood transfusion, plasma volume expanders (gelofusine).

Red Flag

Critically ill patients are at risk of fluid and electrolyte imbalance. Careful monitoring of their vital signs is important.

Investigations and diagnosis

Initial investigations which will help make a diagnosis in most cases are:

- *Electrocardiogram* – this will detect any cardiac arrhythmias, infarction or hypertrophy
- *Chest X-ray* – may identify pulmonary oedema and looks for other chest pathology, e.g. pneumonia
- *Serum urea, creatinine and electrolytes* – for renal function; to check if electrolyte imbalance is contributing to problems. Excretion of excess sodium and water is impaired in injured or surgical patients (owing to various physiological responses to injury and surgery which affect renal function and fluid balance regulation)
- *Full blood count* – for anaemia and features of infection
- *Liver function tests* – albumin and protein levels.

Symptoms of FVE

FVE causes symptoms such as:

- Distended neck and peripheral veins
- Cough, dyspnoea (laboured breathing or difficulty in breathing)
- Orthopnoea (difficulty in breathing when supine)
- Moist crackles (rales) in the lungs
- Pulmonary oedema (excess fluid in pulmonary interstitial spaces and alveoli)
- Increased urine output (polyuria) with normal renal function
- Ascites (excess fluid in the peritoneal cavity)/weight gain
- Peripheral oedema
- Possible cerebral oedema (excess fluid in brain tissues)
- Confusion/headache/seizures/coma
- Full bounding pulse/hypertension.

Nursing care and management

Nursing care for the patient with excess fluid volume includes various interventions such as administering diuretics and maintaining sodium and fluid restriction, as well as monitoring the status and effects of the excess fluid volume. This is particularly critical in the elderly because of the age-related decline in cardiac and renal functions.

- Assessment of vital signs and heart sounds is important because hypervolaemia can cause hypertension and tachycardia. The patient should be assessed for peripheral oedema, particularly in the lower extremities, the back and the sacral region. With pulmonary oedema, gas exchange may be impaired by fluid in the alveolar sac. **Assessment of vital signs is important to detect any signs of deterioration so that prompt action can be taken.**
- Administer the oxygen as prescribed and monitor its effect on the patient's respiration rate. **Supplementary oxygen promotes gas exchange across the alveolar-capillary membrane, improving tissue oxygenation.**
- Weigh the patient daily and record the result. **Acute weight gain or loss represents fluid gain or loss. Weight gain of 2 kg is equivalent to 2 litres of fluid gain.**
- Advise the patient and their relatives on the importance of fluid regulation. All fluid intakes must be calculated, including water given to administer medications orally or intravenously. **Accurate fluid measurement is important to ensure that the patient is not in positive balance and developing complication of fluid retention.**
- Provide oral hygiene at least every 2 hours. *Oral hygiene may help prevent any oral infection and also promotes comfort for the patient.*
- Advise the patient and their relatives about the sodium-restricted diet, and emphasise the importance of checking with the nurse if any food is allowed to be brought from home. **Excess sodium promotes water retention; a sodium-restricted diet is advised to reduce water retention.**
- Monitor the patient's urine output hourly and maintain a strict input and output chart. *Fluid volume excreted is a good indicator of the patient's response to treatment.*
- Monitor the effects of diuretics, if prescribed, on urine output and electrolytes. Furosemide, chlorothiazide and amiloride are some of the diuretics that may be used to treat FVE (Table 24.3). **Diuretics can have undesirable side-effects such as excess fluid loss and loss of sodium and potassium chloride.**

Table 24.3 Three major group of diuretics and their site of action.

DRUG	GROUP	TARGET SITE IN THE KIDNEY
Furosemide	Loop diuretic	Thick ascending loop of Henle
Chlorothiazide	Thiazide-type	Distal tubule and collecting ducts
Amiloride	Potassium-sparing diuretic	Cortical collecting ducts

523

- Patients should be informed of the risk of fluid retention and high intake of sodium. Salt helps to retain fluid in the body resulting in fluid overload
- Patients suffering from heart or kidney diseases should be advised on fluid and electrolyte balance. If necessary, they should be referred to a dietician for advice on food containing high amounts of salt
- Encourage the patient to weigh themselves weekly and to inform the practice nurse of any gain in weight
- Advise the patient and their relatives to read food labels properly for salt additives in the food.

Medicines Management

Postural hypotension is common with both thiazides and loop diuretics and most likely in elderly patients. Advise the patient to stand up slowly and in stages. Compression support stockings may help venous return.

Medicines Management

Advise your patient not to take a potassium supplement or eat food high in potassium at the same time as potassium-sparing diuretics, unless recommended by the doctor.

Advise the patient to check with the practice nurse, doctor or pharmacist before taking any other medicines or herbal remedies at the same time as a diuretic.

- Problems can occur if the volume of interstitial fluid in the limb exceeds its capacity to retain it. This may be complicated if there is a breach in skin integrity or an infection. This can result in gross swelling, blistering and leakage of interstitial fluid on to the skin. Check pressure areas such as the sacrum, heels and shoulder blades regularly. **Skin breaks down rapidly in these areas as a result of lack of tissue.**

Red Flag

Do not use adhesive dressings on grossly oedematous legs because they may cause pain, tear the very fragile taut skin and require frequent changing.

Jot This Down

Following fluid therapy, the patient's circulation is in danger of becoming overloaded. Why might this occur?

What To Do If...

What would you do if the patient insists on adding salt to the food during their meal? As a nurse, you may want to find out why the patient wants to add extra salt and advise the patient on the importance of restricting salt intake.

The Evidence

Glasgow-based GP Margaret McCartney says that the NHS Choices website's advice that people should drink six to eight glasses a day is 'not only nonsense, but thoroughly debunked nonsense'. Dr McCartney wrote in the British Medical Journal that research shows that drinking when not thirsty can impair concentration, rather than boost it. Drinking excessive amounts can also lead to loss of sleep as people have to get up in the night to go to the toilet, and other studies show it can even cause kidney damage, instead of preventing it.

You can read more on this by following this link: **http://www.news-medical.net/news/20110713/Can-you-drink-too-much-water-Experts-say-yes.aspx**

Primary Care

Prior to discharge, the patient's nurses should offer health promotion advice related to fluid volume excess focused on teaching preventive measures to patients who are at risk (e.g. patients who have heart or kidney failure). Discuss the relationship between sodium intake and water retention. Provide guidelines for a low-sodium diet, and teach the patient to carefully read food labels to identify 'hidden' sodium, particularly in processed foods. Advise the patient to weigh themselves daily, using the same scale and wearing the same clothing, if possible. Inform the practice nurse if they gain more than 2 kg. Encourage the patient to monitor their urine output and note the volume of urine voided.

Electrolyte Imbalance

Levels of electrolytes in the body can become too low or too high. That can happen when the level of water in our body changes. The balance of electrolytes is constantly shifting due to fluctuating fluid levels in your body. For example, when you sweat as a result of exercise, hot weather or illness, the levels of some electrolytes such as sodium and potassium may be low (LeMone *et al.* 2011). Vomiting and diarrhoea are other causes of electrolyte imbalances, as they result in excessive fluid and electrolyte, for example sodium, potassium, calcium or chloride loss.

Where there is an imbalance in electrolytes, the aim is to restore the normal electrolyte levels in the patient as soon as possible; otherwise it could prove to be a serious health risk for the patient. See Table 24.4 for a summary of electrolytes: causes, signs and symptoms and nursing interventions.

Sodium Imbalance (Hyponatraemia)

Hyponatraemia refers to a lower-than-normal level of sodium in the blood, whereby the serum sodium is below 135 mmol/L. Sodium is the most abundant electrolyte in the extracellular fluid (ECF), with normal serum sodium levels ranging from 135 to 145 mmol/L. Sodium is the primary regulator of the fluid volume, blood pressure and osmolality of ECF. More than 95% of the sodium is in the ECF; in contrast the intracellular sodium is much smaller in quantity. The level of sodium is regulated by renin-angiotensin and aldosterone systems. The adrenal gland secretes aldosterone that stimulates the kidney to retain sodium by not excreting it into the urine. Addison's disease, which damages the adrenal gland, can therefore lead to low levels of sodium in the body.

Sodium is important to maintain neuromuscular activity. About 40% of the body's sodium is contained in bone, some is found within organs and cells and the remaining 55% is in blood plasma and other fluids outside the cell.

Sodium is essential:

- To regulate blood pressure
- To regulate blood volume
- For the proper function of nerves and muscles.

Pathophysiology

In hyponatraemia, there is excess sodium loss resulting from renal diseases, excessive exercise and sweating, through the GI tract by vomiting or diarrhoea, and excessive hypotonic fluid intake. Excessive sweating or loss of skin surface as a result of extensive burns can also result in hyponatraemia. Other reasons why hyponatraemia can develop include:

- Systemic diseases such as congestive heart failure, renal failure (diuretic phase of acute tubular necrosis) or cirrhosis of the liver
- Syndrome of inappropriate secretion of anti-diuretic hormone (SIADH), in which water excretion is impaired
- Excessive administration of hypotonic intravenous fluids
- Severe malnutrition
- Aldosterone deficiency
- Over hydration
- Compulsive water drinking.

> **Nursing Fields** Mental Health: Hyponatraemia
>
> In some people with mental health problems, excessive water intake may be relatively common. The syndrome is referred to as 'compulsive water drinking' in those with obsessive compulsive disorder or those with delusional psychosis. The syndrome of psychosis, intermittent hyponatraemia and polydipsia can be a challenge. Nurses caring for such patients need to be aware of this.

Investigation and diagnosis

Check:

- Serum sodium level.
- Serum potassium. If raised, consider Addison's disease.
- Urine sodium level. If this is >20 mmol/L, a renal function test is carried out to exclude any renal diseases.
- Serum thyroid-stimulating hormone and free thyroxine level. These are checked to exclude hypothyroidism.
- Random serum cortisol levels or adrenocorticotropic hormone (ACTH). These tests are carried out in patients with suspected adrenal suppression (e.g. patients who have recently taken oral steroids).
- CT scan. This may be contributory in some clinical situations. For example, a chest X-ray may be required in suspected congestive cardiac failure or a CT brain scan in patients with confusion or altered consciousness.

Symptoms of sodium imbalance

The symptoms of hyponatraemia are:

- Nausea and vomiting
- Abdominal cramp
- Anorexia
- Diarrhoea.

As sodium levels continue to decrease, the brain and nervous system are affected by cellular oedema.

- Headache
- Depression
- Personality changes
- Irritability
- Lethargy
- Hyperreflexia
- Muscle twitching
- Tremors.

If serum sodium falls to very low levels, convulsions and coma are likely to occur.

Nursing care and management

Nursing care of the patient with hyponatraemia focusses on identifying patients at risk and treating the underlying cause.

Fluid and dietary management

If hyponatraemia is less severe, increase the intake of foods high in sodium such as ham and add salt to the patient's diet. Fluids are often restricted to help reduce ECF volume and correct hyponatraemia. However, nurses need to ensure that the patient does not get dehydrated as a result of fluid restriction.

- When both sodium and water have been lost (hyponatraemia with hypovolaemia), sodium-containing fluids are administered to replace both fluid and sodium. These fluids may be given orally, subcutaneously or intravenously. Solutions such as isotonic Ringer's solution or isotonic saline (0.9% NaCl) solution may be administered to replace fluid and sodium
- Loop diuretics are administered to patients who have hyponatraemia with normal or excess ECF volume. Loop diuretics promote an isotonic diuresis and fluid volume loss without hyponatraemia, however thiazide diuretics are avoided because they cause a relatively greater sodium loss in relation to water loss
- Monitor urine output hourly to 2-hourly and maintain strict input and output charts. Any fluid loss through vomiting should also be recorded
- Check with the patient 2-hourly for symptoms such as stomach cramp or feelings of nausea as they are early signs of hyponatraemia
- Check serum sodium levels daily to ensure that the treatment is effective and to ensure a safe rate of correction of no more than 8–10 mmol/L per day (Craig 2010)
- Provide support in maintaining personal hygiene
- Monitor and record any CNS changes such as muscle twitching, confusion and restlessness. As a result of fluid movement, the patient with severe hyponatraemia may experience cerebral oedema, with increasing pressure within the brain
- Assess muscle strength and tone, and deep tendon reflexes. Increasing muscle weakness and decreased deep tendon reflexes are symptoms of increasing hyponatraemia.

Health promotion and discharge

- Hyponatraemia can result from excessive sweating, vomiting and diarrhoea. Nurses should advise the patient to replace the fluid loss. They should also be informed that drinking excessive amounts of water could result in hyponatraemia
- Advise the patient and their relatives on signs and symptoms such as abdominal cramps, irritability and muscle weakness and

to seek advice from their GP or the practice nurse if they are concerned
- Encourage the patient to drink varied fluid and not just water when feeling thirsty
- Encourage the patient to take fluid containing electrolytes when exercising
- Advise on salt supplement when cooking or eating food low in sodium content.

Red Flag

Nurses need to be aware that if potassium chloride is administered for concomitant hypokalaemia it will also raise the serum sodium by subsequent transcellular ion shifts of potassium, chloride and hydrogen ions.

Primary Care

Before discharging the patient, nurses should offer information:
  · Inform the patient on the causes of hyponatraemia
  · Advise the patient on the signs and symptoms of hyponatraemia
- Advise the patient and their relatives on the types of food and fluid that are rich in sodium content
- Encourage the patient to monitor their urine output
- Inform the patient of the importance of maintaining hydration during exercise and in hot weather
- Check with the practice nurse if diarrhoea and vomiting persists for more than a day
- If diuretics are prescribed on discharge, advise the patient on the importance of drinking oral fluid to balance fluid loss

Jot This Down

Can a postoperative patient following transurethral resection of the prostate develop 'water intoxication'? Consider the type of fluid that is being administered for bladder irrigation.

Hypernatraemia

Hypernatraemia is defined as a serum sodium concentration exceeding 145 mmol/L. Serum sodium concentration, and hence osmolality, is normally kept from rising significantly by the release of antidiuretic hormone (ADH) or vasopressin, which regulates water losses, and the stimulation of thirst, which increases water intake.

Pathophysiology

The fundamental problem of hypernatremia is hyperosmolality, resulting in an overall deficit of total body water. It may be a consequence of insufficient water intake due to severe nausea or vomiting, due to poor health or secondary to renal diseases. Hypernatraemia causes cellular dehydration by direct extraction of water by the osmotic load of sodium or by the body's free water deficit. The result is that cells shrink and transport electrolytes across the cell membrane to compensate for the osmotic force. Intracellular organic solutes are generated in an effort to restore cell volume and avoid structural damage.

Investigations and diagnosis

- Full urea and electrolyte check for serum sodium, potassium, urea, creatinine, calcium and plasma glucose.
- Urine and serum osmolality if diabetes insipidus is suspected; there would be a high serum osmolality (>300 mOsm/kg) combined with an inappropriately dilute urine (less than serum osmolality).

Signs and symptoms

- Polydipsia and polyuria
- Hyperosmolality of extracellular fluid
- Water is drawn out of cells, leading to cellular dehydration. The most serious effects of cellular dehydration are seen in the brain. As brain cells contract, neurological manifestations develop. The brain itself shrinks, causing mechanical traction on cerebral vessels
- Altered neurological function, such as lethargy, weakness and irritability can progress to seizures, coma, and death in severe hypernatraemia
- Orthostatic hypotension
- Tachycardia.

Nursing care and management

The aims are to:
- Treat any underlying disorder if possible. If diabetes insipidus or any other disease is present, then this should be addressed and appropriate treatment provided
- Correct dehydration by replacing free water losses
- Correct hypovolaemia, if present, by giving electrolytes in addition to free water.

Risk for injury As a result of hypernatraemia, the patient may present with CNS-related symptoms that could lead to harm to the patient. A full risk assessment of the patient and measures put in place to prevent injury to the patient are required.

- Administer any i.v. fluid as prescribed and monitor the outcome. Ensure that serum sodium levels and osmolality are checked daily and report rapid changes immediately. **Rapid water replacement or rapid changes in serum sodium or osmolality can cause fluid shifts within the brain, increasing the risk of cerebral oedema**
- Record neurological observations hourly and check with the patient if he/she has headaches or is feeling nauseous. **Careful monitoring of the patient is vital to detect changes in mental status that may indicate cerebral oedema**
- Monitor vital signs such as heart rate, blood pressure and respiration rate and report any changes immediately
- Administer medications prescribed, if any, and note the effects and report any side-effects immediately
- Maintain a strict input and output chart
- Weigh the patient daily to detect any rapid gain or loss in weight.

Health promotion and discharge

- Elderly patients are at risk of developing hypernatraemia as a result of dehydration or other illnesses. Advise the patient and their relatives of the importance of adequate fluid intake at regular intervals
- Advise the importance of restricting salt intake in their diet
- Advise the patient and their relatives on the signs and symptoms of hypernatraemia

- Advise them to see their GP or the practice nurse if symptoms of hypernatraemia persist.

Hypokalaemia

Hypokalaemia (low serum potassium levels) is a lower than normal amount of potassium in the blood. It is probably the most common electrolyte abnormality affecting hospitalised patients. Most cases are mild with a serum potassium in the range 3.0–3.5 mmol/L, but in 5% of cases it is <3.0 mmol/L, and in 0.03% cases very severe <2.5 mmol/L. Even mild hypokalaemia can increase the incidence of cardiac arrhythmias.

Pathophysiology

Hypokalaemia can result from the use of diuretics or occur via the GI tract as a result of nausea and vomiting. Large amounts of potassium could be lost as a result of inappropriate use of non-potassium-sparing diuretics or corticosteroids. Another cause is excessive secretion of aldosterone, which is a hormone that regulates electrolyte balance.

Patients who suffer from diabetes mellitus are also at risk of developing hypokalaemia, where large amounts of potassium could be lost as a result of glycosuria and osmotic diuresis. Poor dietary intake of potassium could be another factor. Hospitalised patients are at risk, especially those on extended parenteral fluid therapy with solutions that do not contain potassium.

Investigations and diagnosis

These include:

- Blood test: Urea and electrolyte checks
- Electrocardiogram (ECG): All patients with moderate or severe hypokalaemia should have an ECG to determine whether the hypokalaemia is affecting cardiac function. Typical ECG findings when potassium is lower than 3.0 mmol/L are:
  - Flat T waves
  - ST depression
  - Prominent U waves (Figure 24.8)
- Urine test: Low urinary potassium may suggest poor intake, shift into the intracellular space or GI loss. High levels may suggest renal loss. Low urinary sodium combined with high urinary potassium suggests secondary hypoaldosteronism.

Signs and symptoms

Some of the signs and symptoms are:

- Characteristic electrocardiogram (ECG) changes of hypokalaemia – flattened or inverted T waves and a depressed ST segment. The most serious cardiac effect is an increased risk of atrial and ventricular *dysrhythmias* (abnormal rhythms)

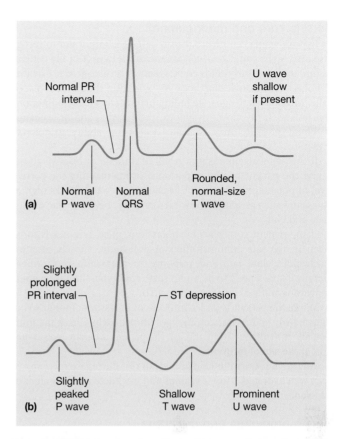

Figure 24.8 ECG showing the effects of (a) normokalaemia and (b) hypokalaemia.

- General malaise/muscle pain/constipation
- In severe cases, the patient may have severe muscle weakness and paralysis (beginning in the lower extremities, progressing to the upper extremities and torso)
- Respiratory failure (due to involvement of respiratory muscles)
- Paralytic ileus (due to involvement of GI muscles)
- Paraesthesia
- Tetany.

Red Flag Potassium Chloride

Potassium chloride must never be administered in a bolus as it can cause severe cardiac problems and can lead to the death of the patient. If the patient is to have i.v. potassium, then it must be mixed in intravenous fluid and given slowly to the patient via a volumetric infusion pump. Where possible, use a ready mixed solution rather than adding potassium to the i.v. infusion bag (if this is necessary, make sure that you mix the fluid in the bag thoroughly before administering it to the patient). Potassium has a higher density than water and therefore settles to the bottom of the bag.

The concentration of potassium for intravenous administration via a peripheral line should not exceed 40 mmol/L, as higher strengths can cause phlebitis and pain.

The infusion site must be checked 2–4-hourly for signs of inflammation.

Check with the patient that he/she is not in any pain as a result of the i.v. infusion.

Avoid giving i.v. potassium if the patient is dehydrated or has renal failure.

527

Nursing care and management

As hypokalaemia can be life-threatening, it is important to recognise early signs and take necessary measures to protect the patient. Failure to detect early signs could result in cardiac arrest. Any loss of potassium through diarrhoea and vomiting should be replaced daily. Monitor vital signs, including orthostatic vitals and peripheral pulses. Tachypnoea, dyspnoea, tachycardia, and/or a change in blood pressure may indicate decreasing ability to tolerate activities.

If the hypokalaemia is as a result of diuretic or laxative abuse, advise the patient on the importance of maintaining the correct level of potassium in the body. Encourage diet and drinks high in potassium such as spinach, raw carrots, pork, beef, banana, orange juice and cod.

If the patient is to have i.v. potassium, great care needs to be taken in the safe administration of potassium. Closely monitor intravenous flow rate and response to potassium replacement therapy. Nurses need to be aware that rapid potassium infusion is dangerous and can lead to cardiac arrest.

While the patient is on i.v. infusion of potassium, monitor vital signs hourly and report any changes immediately. Check the infusion site for inflammation and ask the patient if he/she feels irritation at the site of infusion.

Advise the patient to take periods of rest during exercise and to keep well hydrated. Muscle cramps and weakness are early signs of hypokalaemia.

Health promotion and discharge

- Identify patients who are risk of developing hypokalaemia and discuss the importance of a good intake of potassium
- If the patient is on a non-potassium-sparing diuretic, stress the importance of a potassium supplement in their diet
- Advise the patient to seek advice from their GP or practice nurse if signs and symptoms of hypokalaemia are evident
- Advise the patient that intense exercise and sweating can lower serum potassium and therefore advise caution in taking strenuous activities
- Encourage intake of fluid rich in potassium such as orange juice when excess fluid is lost through sweating, vomiting or diarrhoea.

528

Primary Care

Before discharge into the community, the patient and their relatives will need health promotion advice with regard to maintaining the potassium level in the body.

- Recommend diet and drinks rich in potassium, such as carrots, meat and fish
- Advise on the importance of taking any prescribed medications, including potassium supplements, and their unwanted effects
- Advise on using salt substitutes (if recommended) to increase potassium intake
- Advise them to report signs and symptoms of hypokalaemia and to see their GP or practice nurse at regular intervals
- If taking digitalis, advise the patient to see their GP if they experience any unwanted effects of the drug.

Hyperkalaemia

Hyperkalaemia is defined as plasma potassium in excess of 5 mmol/L and it is the most abundant intracellular cation. Approximately 98% of potassium is located inside the cell. Hyperkalaemia could occur as a result of:

- Renal causes, e.g. renal failure
- Increased intake of potassium in diet and medications
- A shift from the intracellular to the extracellular space
- Pseudohyperkalaemia – could occur as a result of:
  - Prolonged tourniquet time when taking a sample
  - Difficulty collecting the sample
  - The fist may have been clenched
  - Test tube haemolysis, e.g. blood may have been squirted through a needle into the bottle or shaking the tube
  - Use of the wrong anticoagulant, especially potassium ethylenediaminetetraacetic acid (EDTA)
  - Sample of blood stored for too long
  - Sample from limb receiving i.v. fluids containing potassium.

Pathophysiology

The major causes of hyperkalaemia are kidney disease, diseases of the adrenal gland, potassium leaking out of cells into the circulation, trauma and starvation and medications such as potassium supplement tablets. Potassium moving out of the cell could occur in acidosis – when hydrogen ions move into the cell, potassium moves out.

Cell membrane function is itself very susceptible to potassium levels. Even a small difference can affect cardiac muscle function, resulting in cardiac arrest. In diabetes, when patients are treated with insulin for hyperkalaemia, potassium moves into the cell with glucose via the co-transporter system, thus lowering the serum potassium level. If the treatment is not regulated properly, it could result in serious consequences for the patient. Porth (2009) reports that hyperkalaemia can also be managed by inducing diarrhoea or by using calcium polystyrene sulfonate resin (Calcium Resonium®) with regular lactulose, which will remove potassium via the gastrointestinal tract.

Investigations and diagnosis

- Blood test: Full blood count – looking for normocytic, normochromic anaemia (which may suggest acute haemolysis), thrombocytosis and/or leukocytosis. Bloods for urea and electrolytes
- ECG: In hyperkalaemia the ECG may show:
  - Tall T (tented) waves – can be difficult to determine
  - Prolongation of the PR interval
  - Widening and prolongation of the QRS (Figure 24.9)
  - Long PR interval.

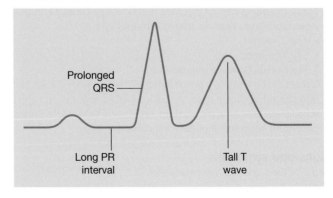

Figure 24.9 ECG pattern of hyperkalaemia, showing prolonged QRS and tall T wave.

Signs and symptoms

Symptoms are non-specific and include weakness and fatigue. Occasionally, a patient presents with muscular paralysis or shortness of breath. They also may complain of palpitations or chest pain.

Nursing care and management

Nursing care of the patient with hyperkalaemia focusses on identifying the problem and taking measures to return the potassium to within the normal range. Care should also include preventing fluid imbalance, cardiac problems (dysrhythmias) and the impact hyperkalaemia has on other systems of the body.

Fluid and dietary management Renal failure and Addison's disease are some of the causes of hyperkalaemia (Porth 2009). Patients are at risk for fluid retention and other electrolyte imbalances, which could affect other systems of the body. If the patient is in renal failure, then a strict fluid regimen needs to be adhered to as per Trust policy and regulation.

- Daily checks on serum urea and electrolytes should be done to ensure that the treatment is effective
- Weigh the patient daily to ensure that he/she is not gaining weight as a result of fluid retention
- Maintain an accurate fluid input and output chart and advise the patient and their relatives of the importance of maintaining a strict fluid balance chart
- Monitor urine output hourly. Oliguria (scanty urine output) or anuria (no urine output) may indicate renal failure and an increased risk for hyperkalaemia and fluid volume excess
- Ensure that the patient is on a low potassium diet. It is imperative that while waiting for this diet the patient does not consume fruit juice, fruits, chocolate, fruit gums, biscuits, coffee or potatoes as these food stuffs contain high amounts of potassium
- Provide reassurance and support for the patient and their relatives.

What the Experts Say One of the Doctors States That Low-Sodium Salt 'Creates Hyperkalaemia Risk'

A man was admitted to the hospital for the treatment of complications of diabetes. The nurse and the doctors noticed that the man's potassium levels were high (6.9 mmol/L) and they treated his hyperkalaemia. They noticed that he was not responding to the treatment and the potassium levels remained high.

One day the doctor noticed that the man, aged in his 80s, was in the habit of adding three or four sachets of a reduced-sodium salt to his meals. He was informed to stop adding these non-prescribed supplements as it was doing more harm to him. The patient's blood levels fell back to 5.3 mmol/L, within the normal range, once the reduced-sodium salt was taken out of his diet.

This was supported by doctors at the Royal Lancaster Infirmary who claimed that this type of salt could significantly raise potassium levels in patients with reduced kidney function or those taking certain drugs.

Protecting the heart Hyperkalaemia can affect myocardial contraction, resulting in poor cardiac output and leading to cardiac arrest, as high levels of potassium can affect atrial and ventricular depolarisation.

- An ECG should be done to assess any changes in cardiac function and any other abnormalities

- Monitor vital signs hourly and report any changes in the heart or respiration rates immediately so that prompt action can be taken.

Medications Discontinue any medications that may increase potassium levels in the body. These include ACE inhibitors, angiotensin receptor blockers, potassium-retaining diuretics, e.g. spironolactone, amiloride, NSAIDs and potassium-containing laxatives.

Monitor the effects of calcium polystyrene sulphonate resin (calcium resonium) enema and lactulose administered to increase GI losses of potassium. When given rectally, the calcium resonium must be retained for 9 hours followed by irrigation to remove resin from the colon to prevent faecal impaction.

Dextrose/insulin therapy Intravenous insulin facilitates the shift of potassium into the cells. This treatment is administered with 50 mL of 50% glucose. It lowers the serum potassium within 15 min and therefore serum potassium levels need to be checked regularly.

Blood glucose should be measured 30 min after starting the infusion and then hourly up to 6 hours after completion of the infusion as delayed hypoglycaemia is commonly reported when less than 30 g of glucose is administered with insulin.

Health promotion and discharge

- Advise the patient on food high in potassium, such as bananas, milk, shellfish, nuts and chocolate
- Advise the patient to check food labels and over the counter prescriptions for their potassium content
- Discuss the importance of adequate fluid intake to promote renal excretion of potassium
- Advise the patient to avoid adding salt supplement in their diet
- Hyperkalaemia is a serious condition that can be fatal for the patient. Inform the patient of the signs and symptoms of hyperkalaemia and to inform the GP or the practice if they recognise these symptoms.

Primary Care

Offer advice to the patient and their relatives on the following, so that they can continue their management at home. Advise the patient:

- On food rich in potassium, such as tea, coffee, whole-grain bread, chocolate
- On food low in potassium, for example butter, margarine, honey, cranberry juice
- To avoid taking potassium supplements
- To weigh themselves daily and inform the practice nurse of any weight gain
- To carefully read food and dietary supplement labels
- On the importance of maintaining an adequate fluid intake (unless a fluid restriction has been prescribed) to maintain renal function to eliminate potassium from the body.

Link To/Go To

You can get more information at:

http://www.gain-ni.org/images/Uploads/Guidelines/hyperkalaemia_guidelines.pdf

Hypocalcaemia

Calcium is the fifth most abundant ion in the body. The normal adult total serum calcium concentration is 2.12–2.62 mmol/L. Of the total body calcium, 99% is found in the bones, 0.5% in the teeth and another 0.5% in soft tissues.

Pathophysiology

Hypocalcaemia can result from hypoparathyroidism from surgery (parathyroidectomy, thyroidectomy), radiotherapy, acute pancreatitis, systemic disease (e.g. amyloidosis, sarcoidosis), deficiency or abnormal metabolism of vitamin D, renal failure or hypomagnesaemia.

Calcium exists in two forms in the extracellular fluid: in plasma, as free ionised calcium, and as a complex bound to protein. It is the free ionised calcium that is important for muscle contraction and conducting nerve impulses. Hypocalcaemia decreases the contractility of cardiac muscle fibres, leading to decreased cardiac output.

Symptoms

The symptoms of hypocalcaemia include:

- Low blood calcium, <2.12 mmol/L
- Tetany (tonic muscular spasm)
- Painful muscle spasm of hands
- Painful muscle spasm of feet
- Facial muscle spasms/grimacing
- Lip paraesthesias (tingling, pricking, or numbness of the lip)
- Numbness or tingling around the mouth
- Finger paraesthesias
- Foot paraesthesias
- Muscle aches/bone pain
- Fracture/deformity.

Nursing care and management

In hypocalcaemia, treating the underlying cause is essential. Usually, hypocalcaemia is not a major problem in the adult, as there is large amount of calcium reserve in the bones. However, women are more at risk of calcium loss than men and of developing osteoporosis.

- Monitor cardiovascular status including heart rate and rhythm, blood pressure and peripheral pulses. Hypocalcaemia can lead to poor cardiac output and hypotension
- Frequently monitor airway and respiratory status. Report changes such as respiratory stridor (a high-pitched, harsh inspiratory sound indicative of upper airway obstruction) or increased respiratory rate or effort to the doctor. These changes may indicate laryngeal spasm due to tetany
- Advise women of all ages of the importance of maintaining adequate calcium intake through diet and, as needed, calcium supplements
- Discuss hormone replacement therapy and its potential benefits during and after menopause
- Stress the importance of a well balanced diet to maintain dietary intake of calcium
- Encourage women and men to take regular aerobic exercise.

Medications Cooper and Gittoes (2008) report that in acute hypocalcaemia the following treatment should be carried out:

- Administer 10 mL (2.25 mmol) of calcium gluconate 10% by slow intravenous (i.v.) injection. Repeat as necessary, or follow with infusion of calcium gluconate 10% – 40 mL (9 mmol)/24 hours
- Oral calcium preparations may need to be given as supplements to i.v. treatment or where i.v. access is difficult
- Monitor serum calcium concentrations regularly to judge response
- If hypocalcaemia is likely to be persistent, give vitamin D by mouth
- If a patient has low magnesium, it is necessary to correct the magnesium level before the hypocalcaemia will resolve
- To avoid hypocalcaemia in patients on total parenteral nutrition, ensure magnesium and calcium levels are checked at least weekly and more frequently if the patient is acutely unwell.

A diet high in calcium-rich foods may be recommended for patients with chronic hypocalcaemia or low total body stores of calcium. Calcium supplements may be combined with vitamin D, or vitamin D may be given alone to increase gastrointestinal absorption of calcium. If hypocalcaemia is caused by malabsorption, the underlying problem should be treated if possible. Patients with coeliac disease should receive calcium and vitamin D orally and should comply with a gluten-free diet.

Health promotion and discharge

- Discuss the risk factors of hypocalcaemia with the patient and the preventative measures
- Advise the patient on calcium supplements and the importance of maintaining good fluid intake
- Provide information on food sources high in calcium and vitamin D
- Advise the patient on recognising the signs and symptoms of hypocalcaemia and the importance of seeing the practice nurse or their GP when the signs and symptoms persist
- If necessary, discuss hormone replacement therapy for women during and after menopause.

Primary Care

In preparing the patient with hypocalcaemia for discharge and home care, the nurse should discuss the following with the patient and their relatives:

- Discuss risk factors for hypocalcaemia specific to the patient, and provide information about managing these risk factors to avoid future episodes of hypocalcaemia
- Advise about prescribed medications, including calcium supplements
- Provide a list of foods high in calcium, as well as sources of vitamin D if recommended
- Discuss symptoms to report to the practice nurse/GP, and stress the importance of follow-up care.

Hypercalcaemia

Hypercalcaemia is a condition in which the serum calcium value is greater than 2.62 mmol/L. Excess ionised calcium in the extracellular fluid (ECF) can have serious widespread effects.

Pathophysiology

Hypercalcaemia results when the serum calcium is >2.62 mmol/L and usually results from increased resorption of calcium from the bones. This may be due to cancer of the bones, prolonged immo-

530

bilisation and milk-alkaline syndrome (caused by taking too much milk and antacids (calcium carbonate) at the same time). It may develop as a result of destruction of bone tissue by a tumour. Primary hyperparathyroidism results from increased parathyroid hormone production, and malignancy is responsible for greater than 90% of all cases. Prolonged immobility and lack of weight-bearing also cause increased resorption of bone with calcium release into extracellular fluids.

Increased absorption of calcium from the GI tract can also lead to hypercalcaemia. This may result from excess vitamin D, overuse of calcium-containing antacids or excessive milk ingestion. Renal failure and some drugs, such as thiazide diuretics, vitamin D and vitamin A supplements, can interfere with elimination of calcium by the kidneys, causing high serum calcium levels. Endocrine conditions, for example thyrotoxicosis (a condition where the thyroid gland produces too much thyroid hormone), phaeochromocytoma (a tumour of the adrenal gland) and primary adrenal insufficiency can also lead to hypercalcaemia.

Investigations and diagnosis
- Thyroid function test
- Plain X-rays may show features indicative of bone abnormalities, such as demineralisation, bone cysts, pathological fractures or bony metastases
- Ultrasound scan, computerised tomography (CT) scan or intravenous pyelogram (IVP) may be required to detect abnormalities of the urogenital tract, such as calcification or stones
- Ultrasound or technetium scan of the parathyroid glands may be indicated if hypertrophy or adenoma is suspected.

Symptoms
- Polyuria
- Polydipsia
- Constipation
- Muscle weakness
- Anorexia
- Nausea and vomiting.

Hypercalcaemia can also cause more serious problems, such as depression, dehydration, bone fractures, kidney stones and sudden heart attacks.

Nursing care and management
This can be considered under the headings of the immediate management of acute hypercalcaemia and the longer-term management of the underlying condition.

Fluid and diet management Patients with hypercalcaemia are administered 0.9% saline to increase the circulating volume and increase urine excretion of calcium. A loop diuretic, e.g. furosemide, is given to enhance the effect by inhibiting the tubular reabsorption of calcium. Hydration is needed because many patients are dehydrated due to vomiting or renal defects in concentrating urine. In addition, loop diuretics tend to depress renal calcium reabsorption thereby helping to lower blood calcium levels.

Cardiovascular and renal function is carefully assessed prior to fluid therapy; the patient is carefully monitored for evidence of fluid overload during treatment.

Discourage excessive consumption of high calcium foods such as milk, cheese and leafy vegetables. Ensure that there is adequate roughage in the diet to prevent constipation. If necessary, seek advice from the dietician regarding low calcium food.

Encourage fluids such as blueberry or cranberry juice to help maintain acidic urine. Acidic, dilute urine reduces the risk of calcium salts precipitating out to form kidney stones. Fluids also help to prevent calcium renal stones and urinary tract infection.

Closely monitor and maintain an input and output chart.

Risk for injury Take necessary precautions when moving or transferring patients, as their bones are prone to fracture due to bone resorption.

If the patient is on digoxin, observe the patient for the symptoms of digoxin toxicity, including vision changes, anorexia and changes in heart rate and rhythm. Monitor serum digitalis levels. Hypercalcaemia increases the risk of digitalis toxicity.

Bed-bound patients should be encouraged to perform passive and active exercises.

Red Flag

Hypercalcaemia can cause bradycardia, heart block and cardiac arrest. Immediate treatment is needed to preserve life.

Frequently assess vital signs, respiratory status and heart sounds. Report any changes immediately to the person in charge. Vital signs may indicate if the patient is improving, stable or getting worse.

Medications Glucocorticoids (cortisone), which compete with vitamin D, and a low calcium diet may be prescribed to decrease gastrointestinal absorption of calcium, inhibit bone resorption, and increase urinary calcium excretion. Also, calcitonin may be prescribed to decrease skeletal mobilisation of calcium and phosphorus and to increase renal output of calcium and phosphorus.

Bisphosphonates, such as sodium clodronate and ibandronic acid, are very effective drugs for helping to get the calcium levels down. They can also help to reduce pain from bone secondaries and help to stop damaged bones breaking.

Health promotion and discharge
- Identify risk factors and advise the patient on avoidance techniques, for example promoting mobility and light exercise. Physical exercise has frequently been shown to induce bone mass gain and prevent osteoporosis. Weight-bearing exercises, such as walking, mainly affect the bones in the legs, hips and lower spine
- Advise the patient on the effect of smoking. Smoking has been shown to increase bone loss as well as dramatically increase the risk of a number of serious health problems
- Advise the patient to drink plenty of fluids, especially water. Drinking fluids can prevent dehydration and formation of kidney stones.

Primary Care

Nurses should offer advice on the following topics when preparing the patient for discharge into the community:
- Avoid excess intake of calcium-rich foods and antacids

(Continued)

- Ensure that the patient understands why they have to continue taking the prescribed medications
- Encourage the patient to increase dietary fibre and fluid intake to prevent constipation
- Maintain weight-bearing physical activity to prevent hypercalcaemia. Encourage a generous fluid intake of up to 3–4 litres per day

- Report early symptoms of hypercalcaemia to the practice nurse
- Promote mobility in patients when possible as it helps the uptake of calcium
- Advise the patient to recognise the signs and symptoms of hypercalcaemia and preventative measures.

Table 24.4 Summary of electrolytes – causes, signs and symptoms and nursing interventions. Adapted from Kozier *et al.* (2008) *Fundamentals of Nursing: Concepts, process and practice.* Pearson Education, Harlow.

ELECTROLYTES	CAUSES	SIGNS AND SYMPTOMS	NURSING INTERVENTIONS
Sodium (hyponatraemia) serum sodium below 135 mmol/L	Excessive sweating, diarrhoea and vomiting, excessive consumption of hypotonic fluids, diuretics Inappropriate secretion of anti-diuretic hormone and aldosterone. Liver, kidney and heart diseases Excessive infusion of hypotonic infusions	Confusion, irritability, abdominal cramps, muscle twitching, personality changes, coma and convulsion if sodium level is very low Depression Headaches	Monitor fluid intake. Maintain strict input and output chart. Monitor and record vital signs. If permitted, encourage high salt intake until level is within normal range Monitor effects of diuretics if prescribed
Sodium (hypernatraemia) serum sodium above 145 mmol/L	Diarrhoea, excessive infusion of hypertonic fluids, excessive intake of salt in diet Hyperventilation Fever	Feeling thirsty, dry mucous membrane, fatigue, seizures, coma, death	Monitor fluid intake. Maintain input and output chart. Obtain and record vital signs. Advise on restricted salt intake in diet
Potassium (hypokalaemia) serum potassium below 3.5 mmol/L	Diarrhoea and vomiting, non-potassium diuretics, excessive sweating	Muscle weakness, feeling tired, cardiac dysrhythmias (atrial and ventricular), poor tendon reflexes Alkalosis, T wave flattening and ST segment depression	Obtain and record vital signs. Administer potassium in i.v. infusion. Advise patient to eat food containing potassium, such as bananas
Potassium (hyperkalaemia) serum potassium above 5 mmol/L	Renal failure, excessive intake of salt with potassium. Under secretion of aldosterone, potassium-sparing diuretics	Confusion, cerebral agitation, cardiac arrest, muscle weakness	Obtain and record vital signs, especially heart rate. Administer non-potassium diuretics and monitor the effects Advise patient to avoid potassium-containing salts
Calcium (hypocalcaemia) serum calcium below 4.5 mmol/L	Hypoparathyroidism resulting from surgery Alkalosis Acute pancreatitis	Tetany (tonic muscular spasm) Painful muscle spasm of hands Painful muscle spasm of feet Facial muscle spasms Facial grimacing Lip paraesthesias (tingling, pricking, or numbness of the lip) Tongue, finger, foot paraesthesias	Monitor and record vital signs, especially respiration and pulse rates Encourage diet rich in calcium Administer calcium supplement tablets
Calcium (hypercalcaemia) serum calcium above 5.5 mmol/L	Prolonged bed rest Hyperparathyroidism Sarcoma of the bones, excessive intake of calcium-rich food such as cheese and milk Paget's disease Calcium supplement	Urinary calculi, weakness, polyuria, heart block, flank pain, nausea and vomiting	Encourage mobility. Advise patient to take diet with less calcium Encourage fluid intake to flush kidneys Advise the patient on the signs and symptoms of osteoporosis

Shock

Shock is a life-threatening condition that occurs when the vital organs, such as the brain and heart, are deprived of oxygen due to a problem affecting the circulatory system. Shock develops when oxygen supply to the cells is insufficient to meet the metabolic demands of the cells.

Pathophysiology

Shock is a state in which there is inadequate tissue perfusion to maintain oxygen supply which is necessary for normal cellular function (Alexander *et al.* 2006). Shock can be divided into:

- **Hypovolaemic**: due to reduced blood flow resulting from trauma, blood loss through surgery, dehydration
- **Cardiogenic**: due to heart diseases such myocardial infarction and heart failure
- **Obstructive**: due to obstruction of blood flow, for example pulmonary embolism (this is the result of a clot in the blood vessels of the lungs that hinders the return of blood to the heart)
- **Distributive**: due to impaired utilisation of oxygen and thus production of energy by the cell. Septic, neurogenic and anaphylactic shocks all come under this group.

Red Flag

If intervention is timely and effective, the physiological events that characterise shock may be stopped; if not, shock may lead to death.

Stages of Shock

Stage I: early, reversible and compensatory shock

In the early stages, the signs and symptoms are non-identifiable. The pulse rate may be slightly elevated. If the injury is minor or of short duration, arterial pressure is usually maintained and no further symptoms occur. However, cellular changes may occur in response to poor blood flow. At this stage, certain compensatory mechanisms are initiated:

- The release of epinephrine (adrenaline) and norepinephrine (noradrenaline) from the adrenal medulla
- The renin–angiotensin system causes narrowing of the peripheral blood vessels and raises blood pressure and release of aldosterone from the adrenal cortex, which stimulates the kidneys to reabsorb sodium and excrete potassium
- The release of ADH from the posterior pituitary gland, which increases renal reabsorption of water to increase intravascular volume
- Glucocorticoids raise blood glucose by a process called gluconeogenesis. In addition, glucocorticoids release amino acids from tissues and decrease protein synthesis.

Stage II: progressive shock

If the shock is not successfully treated, it will proceed to the progressive stage. Due to the decreased perfusion of the cells, sodium ions build up within the cell, while potassium ions leak out. This can result in hyperkalaemia, which may in turn cause cardiac arrest. Anaerobic metabolism as a result of inadequate oxygen supply increases the body's metabolic acidosis. The arteriolar smooth muscle and precapillary sphincters relax, such that blood remains in the capillaries. Due to this, the hydrostatic pressure will increase and, combined with histamine release, this will lead to leakage of fluid and protein into the surrounding tissues. As fluid is lost from the blood vessels, the blood concentration and viscosity increases.

Stage III: refractory shock

At this stage, the vital organs have failed and the shock can no longer be reversed. Brain damage and cell death are occurring, and death will occur imminently.

Hypovolaemic Shock

Hypovolaemic shock is the most common type of shock and is caused by insufficient circulating volume. Its primary cause is **haemorrhage** (internal and/or external), or loss of fluid from the circulation, for example dehydration. The aim is to correct the hypovolaemia and hypoperfusion of vital organs such as the heart and the kidneys before irreversible damage occurs. In the early stages of hypovolaemia, the compensatory mechanisms are initiated (see Stage I). However, if the fluid loss is great, the compensatory mechanism may not be successful and the patient's condition will deteriorate.

Investigations and diagnosis

Tests that may be done include:

- Blood chemistry, including kidney function tests
- Arterial blood gases/oxygen saturation
- Blood pressure measurements
- Full blood count (urea and electrolytes, haemoglobin, cross-match for blood transfusion)
- CT scan, ultrasound or X-ray of suspected areas
- Echocardiogram to identify any heart diseases such as myocardial infarction or heart failure
- Urinary catheterisation to measure urine output.

Signs and symptoms

- Tachycardia, as a result of low blood flow. The pulse will be weak and thready
- Tachypnoea in response to sympathetic nervous stimulation, hypoxia, acidosis
- The periphery will be cold from poor perfusion, and capillary refill time will be prolonged. However, this may be a poor indicator of hypovolaemia
- Fall in blood pressure (BP) or postural hypotension as a result of poor cardiac output
- Late features include confusion or even coma
- Anxiety, restlessness and confusion as a result of decreased brain oxygenation.

Cardiogenic Shock

Cardiogenic shock occurs when there is failure of the pumping action of the heart, resulting in reduced cardiac output and consequent hypoperfusion and hypoxia of the tissues and organs, despite the presence of an adequate intravascular volume. **Myocardial infarction** is the most common cause of cardiogenic shock. Others include myocarditis, heart failure and cardiomyopathy.

Signs and symptoms

- Chest pain
- Nausea and vomiting
- Dyspnoea

- Profuse sweating
- Confusion and disorientation
- Palpitations
- Pale, cold skin with slow capillary refill and poor peripheral pulses
- Hypotension
- Tachycardia or bradycardia
- Peripheral oedema
- Oliguria (scanty urine output).

Obstructive Shock

Obstructive shock occurs when there is inadequate perfusion of tissues with oxygenated blood resulting from **pulmonary embolism**, cardiac tamponade or tension pneumothorax.

Signs and symptoms
- Hypotension (low BP)
- Weak and rapid pulse
- Cool and clammy skin
- Rapid breathing
- Hypothermia (low body temperature)
- Confusion
- Dry mouth
- Fatigue (feeling of being unwell).

Red Flag

It is a serious and potentially life-threatening condition as it can prevent the blood from reaching the lungs.

The signs and symptoms of a pulmonary embolism can sometimes be difficult to recognise because they can vary between individuals. The symptoms include:

- Chest pain – a sharp, stabbing pain that may be worse when breathing in
- Shortness of breath – which can come on suddenly or develop gradually
- Coughing – usually dry, but may include coughing up blood or mucus that contains blood
- Feeling faint, dizzy or passing out.

If prompt action is not taken, it can be fatal.

Distributive (Septic Shock)

Septic shock is a life-threatening condition that happens when your blood pressure drops to a dangerously low level. The fall in blood pressure is a reaction to a serious infection that develops in the blood. This causes a response from the body known as sepsis. If sepsis is not treated, it will lead to septic shock. Patients at risk for developing infections leading to septic shock include those who are hospitalised and those who have debilitating chronic illnesses or poor nutritional status.

The condition is often associated with Gram-negative bacteria such as *Escherichia coli*, *Meningococcus*, *Klebsiella*, *Proteus* and *Pseudomonas*. Gram-positive bacteria, for example streptococci, staphylococci and *Pneumococcus*, can also cause sepsis.

Septic shock occurs in two distinct phases: hyperdynamic phase and hypodynamic phase. In the **hyperdynamic phase**, the patient may present with low cardiac output, low urine output, vasodilatation, tachycardia, confusion, agitation and fever with chills. The **hypodynamic phase** is characterised by hypovolaemia and hypotension, and activity of the compensatory mechanisms results in

typical shock manifestations, including cold, moist skin, oliguria and changes in mental status. Death may result from respiratory failure, cardiac failure or renal failure.

Nursing Fields Children

Sepsis is a problem that presents a management challenge to those who care for infants and children; however, early recognition and intervention clearly improve the outcome for infants and children with infections or intoxications that lead to sepsis. Most infants and children with sepsis require monitoring and treatment in an intensive care unit. The initial focus should be on stabilisation and correction of metabolic, circulatory and respiratory imbalances. Appropriate antibiotic therapy should be started as soon as possible after evaluation. Ongoing re-evaluation is paramount to ensure the child is improving.

Neurogenic Shock

Neurogenic shock is the result of an imbalance between **parasympathetic** and **sympathetic** stimulation of vascular smooth muscle. It occurs as a result of an illness, a drug or an injury blocking impulses from the sympathetic nerve and thus increasing parasympathetic activity.

Neurogenic shock causes a dramatic reduction in systemic vascular resistance as the size of the vascular compartment increases. As systemic vascular resistance decreases, pressure in the blood vessels becomes too low to drive nutrients across capillary membranes, and cellular metabolism is impaired.

Signs and symptoms
- *Blood pressure*: hypotension
- *Pulse*: slow and bounding
- *Respirations*: vary
- *Skin*: warm, dry
- *Mental status*: anxious, restless, lethargic progressing to comatose
- *Urine output*: oliguria to anuria
- *Other*: lowered body temperature.

Anaphylactic Shock

Anaphylaxis is a severe, potentially life-threatening, **allergic reaction** that can affect many of the systems of the body, including:

- Airways
- Breathing
- Circulation (of the blood)

There are numerous triggers and some of them are: food (peanuts, fish, egg, milk), venom (bee and wasp stings) and drugs (antibiotics, NSAIDs, opioids).

What the Experts Say Tanya's Experience

Tanya, a first year student nurse, on her first placement noticed a painful sensation on her hands as she was cleaning a patient. Tanya was wearing latex that was provided on the ward. Tanya quickly took the gloves off as she was in pain. She ran to the ward sister to show her swollen hands. 'Look my fists have swelled up, and I have rashes on my face and arms and I am finding it difficult to breathe', she said.

The ward sister sent Tanya to Accident and Emergency to be treated. It was concluded that Tanya developed an allergy to latex that caused her to have anaphylactic shock.

Tanya, who left the NHS 3 years ago, now has to use latex-free phones and shoes, and avoid anything that contains latex.

Signs and symptoms

Signs include itching of the palate or external auditory meatus, dyspnoea, laryngeal oedema (stridor) and wheezing (bronchospasm). General symptoms include palpitations and tachycardia (as opposed to bradycardia in a simple vasovagal episode at immunisation time), nausea, vomiting and abdominal pain, feeling faint with a sense of impending doom, and, ultimately, collapse and loss of consciousness.

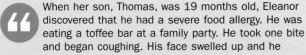

What the Experts Say Eleanor's Experience

When her son, Thomas, was 19 months old, Eleanor discovered that he had a severe food allergy. He was eating a toffee bar at a family party. He took one bite and began coughing. His face swelled up and he broke out in hives. Eleanor rushed Thomas to the hospital. He was experiencing a life-threatening allergic reaction called 'anaphylaxis', or 'anaphylactic shock'.

By the time medical personnel began treating him 'he was one huge hive', Eleanor recalls. 'They worked on him for 3 hours before he began to look like himself again'.

Eleanor's initial reaction was shock. 'I knew nothing about food allergies or anaphylaxis', she said. 'None of my friends or family members had food allergies'.

Link To/Go To

Refer to the following guidance on ananaphylaxis, by NICE:
http://guidance.nice.org.uk/CG134, (accessed August 2013) also

The Resuscitation Council (UK) for guidelines, medical information and reports

http://www.resus.org.uk/pages/medimain.htm

What To Do If...

If you know someone is prone to anaphylaxis, the advice you would give to prevent anaphylaxis would include:
- Seek advice if there is a sudden onset of symptoms, for example skin changes, such as swelling of the lips and tongue (angio-oedema), hives (urticaria) and flushing
- Avoid triggers that cause anaphylactic shock.

Nursing care and management

The nursing care of the patient in shock involves identifying patients at risk and taking appropriate measures to detect early signs of shock, to safeguard the patient. Currently, hospitals utilise various early warning tools such as the Medical Early Warning Systems (MEWS) or Acute Life Threatening Events Recognition

and Treatment (ALERT) to identify patients at risk of developing shock.

- Monitor vital signs (body temperature, pulse and respiration rate, blood pressure, oxygen saturation – using a pulse oximeter) half-hourly for patients at risk of developing shock and report any changes immediately so that prompt action can be taken. Continuous monitoring will provide information about the patient's respiratory status
- Ensure that the patient's airway is not obstructed; check their breathing. Administer oxygen as prescribed using a face mask or nasal cannula and monitor its effect. Nurses should be alert in detecting hyperventilation occurring in respiratory alkalosis leading to fatigue of the respiratory muscle. If this occurs, the patient may need ventilation to assist in breathing
- The patient may be connected to an ECG monitor to assess cardiac status. Nurses should be familiar with the normal ECG tracing of the heart so that they are able to detect and report any arrhythmias to the person in charge
- Communicate verbally with the patient when recording as it is vital to ensure that the patient is conscious and alert. If cerebral perfusion is low, leading to cerebral hypoxia, the patient will gradually become less responsive and eventually unconscious
- A urinary catheter may be inserted to measure and record hourly urine output. A decrease in circulating blood volume with hypotension and the effect of the compensatory mechanisms associated with shock can cause poor urine production. Urinary output of <0.5 1.0 mL/kg per hour may indicate reduced renal blood flow and early signs of renal failure. Measurement of urine osmolality and specific gravity may indicate renal function
- Monitor bowel sounds, abdominal distension and abdominal pain. Check with the patient if he/she is in any pain and administer any prescribed medication for pain regularly
- Check with the patient for any chest pain and observe for central (lips) and peripheral (finger nails) cyanosis, anxiety and restlessness
- Monitor the condition of the skin for colour and temperature, as they may indicate the severity of shock. If the skin is pale and clammy, this indicates overactive sympathetic activity
- Check for capillary refill. A slow capillary refill suggests that there is vasoconstriction, which would lead to poor delivery of oxygen to the tissues.

Medications In cardiogenic shock, the aim is to minimise the damage to the myocardium. Apart from oxygen therapy, inotropic (drugs modifying the force or speed of contraction of cardiac muscle) support with dopamine, dobutamine, epinephrine (adrenaline) and norepinephrine (noradrenaline) is administered to improve cardiac contraction and to elevate blood pressure. Nurses need to be aware that some of the side-effects include tachycardia, dysrhythmias, myocardial ischaemia, hyperglycaemia, lactic acidosis (which is usually transient) and excessive vasoconstriction and hypotension which may affect the progress of the patient.

Fluid replacement The most effective treatment for the patient in hypovolaemic shock is the administration of intravenous fluids or blood. Normal saline is the fluid of first choice in hypovolaemia. However, regular checks on urea and electrolytes (U&Es) should be done as saline contains a high amount of sodium and if the patient is in renal failure then the high levels of sodium could lead to hypernatraemia. Treatment of hypovolaemia depends upon its severity. When it is severe, intravenous fluids and possibly blood

535

transfusions may be necessary to rapidly raise blood volume. Medications may be used to increase blood pressure and stabilise heart rate and strength of heart contractions. Any underlying cause of hypovolaemia, such as injury, must also be treated to prevent ongoing fluid losses.

Nurses overseeing an infusion of fluids and monitoring of hypovolaemia should be aware of the potential complications and their related symptoms. Complications of infusing large volumes of fluids include hypothermia, acid–base imbalance, hyperkalaemia, hypocalcaemia, clotting problems and allergic reactions. Nurses need to check the patient's blood pressure, temperature, pulse, respiration and mental state hourly.

Blood and blood products If hypovolaemic shock is due to haemorrhage the transfusion of blood and blood products may be necessary. In certain cases, blood transfusion or plasma volume expanders may be used to treat hypovolaemia due to haemorrhage. When using blood and blood products, nurses need to check that they have been cross-matched and that they adhere to the guidelines in the correct administration of blood transfusion. Patient's temperature, heart and respiration rates and blood pressure should be obtained and recorded every 15 minutes for the first blood transfusion.

What To Do If...

A patient requires a blood transfusion: before commencing the blood transfusion, nurses should ensure that they are giving the blood to the correct patient.
Inform the patient well in advance that they will be getting a blood transfusion and the reason why they are having the blood transfusion. These are some of the action points:

- Always have a second nurse with you
- Positively identify the patient using an open question 'can you tell me your full name and date of birth?'
- Check these details against the patient's wristband for accuracy
- Check that the blood has been prescribed in the treatment chart
- Check that the blood group and the donation number on the compatibility label are identical to the blood group and donation number on the blood component
- Monitor the patient's vital signs every 15 minutes for the first unit of blood and then hourly
- Check with the patient if they are comfortable with the transfusion
- Ask the patient to report any reaction such as body rashes and fever immediately to the nurse.

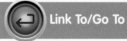 **Link To/Go To**

Serious Hazards of Transfusion: **http://www.shotuk.org**

Conclusion

This chapter has given you some information with regards to fluid and electrolyte imbalance and shock. It is essential for nurses to monitor the patients under their care for subtle changes resulting from these imbalances. The elderly and children are at risk from these subtle changes and therefore every measure should be taken to ensure safe recovery of the patient. Assisting patients suffering from these imbalances, whether in the hospital or community setting, presents the nurse with a major challenge. Patients and their relatives will need support and information with regard to these life-threatening situations.

Key Points

- The movement of fluid and electrolytes ensures that the cells are in constant supply of electrolytes, such as sodium, chloride, potassium, magnesium, phosphates, bicarbonate and calcium for cellular function.
- Fluid and electrolyte imbalance can affect all the body systems, especially the cardiovascular, respiratory, renal and the central nervous systems.
- The most common electrolyte imbalances relate to sodium, potassium and calcium.
- Both hyper- and hypokalaemia affect the conducting system of the heart. If not treated promptly they can prove fatal for the patient.
- Shock is a life-threatening condition that occurs when the vital organs, such as the brain and heart, are deprived of oxygen due to a problem affecting the circulatory system. Shock develops when oxygen supply to the cells is insufficient to meet the metabolic demands of the cells.
- Hypovolaemic shock is the most common type of shock and is caused by insufficient circulating volume. Its primary cause is haemorrhage (internal and/or external) or loss of fluid from the circulation, for example dehydration. The aim is to correct the hypovolaemia and hypoperfusion of vital organs such as the heart and the kidneys before irreversible damage occurs.
- Anaphylactic shock results in vasodilatation, pooling of blood in the periphery and hypovolaemia, which can affect cellular metabolism.

Glossary

Amines: organic compounds that contain nitrogen
Anions: negatively charged ions
Cations: positively charged ions
Compartments: spaces
Dehydration: excessive fluid loss from the body
Detoxification: removal of toxic substance from the body
Electrolytes: substances that dissociate in water to form ions
Epidemiology: the study of the distribution and determinants of health-related states or events (including disease), and the application of this study to the control of diseases and other health problems
Ethylenediaminetetraacetic acid (EDTA): a chemical that binds to metal atoms in a process known as chelation to inactivate the metal and limit vascular damage
Extracellular: space found outside the cell
Gluconeogenesis: the synthesis of glucose from molecules that are not carbohydrates, such as amino and fatty acids
Hypertonic: solution that has a large amount of solutes dissolved in it
Hypotonic: solution that has a low concentration of solutes
Iatrogenic: induced effects of treatment in hospital
Idiopathic: any disease that is of uncertain or unknown origin

Interstitial: space between cells

Intracellular: space inside the cell

Isotonic: solution that has same osmolality as the body fluids

Metabolism: chemical process of the cell

Nausea: an unpleasant sensation that produces a feeling of discomfort in the region of the stomach with a feeling of a need to vomit

Oedema: abnormal accumulation of fluid in the interstitial space

Osmosis: movement of water through a selective permeable membrane from an area of high volume to an area of low volume

Osmotic pressure: pressure created by water as it moves across through a selective permeable membrane

Plasma: fluid component of the blood

Pulse oximeter: equipment used to measure oxygen saturation

Resorption: the process by which osteoclasts break down bone and release the minerals

Tachypnoea: very rapid respiration

Tissue hypoxia: where tissues are deprived of oxygen

Tonicity: term used instead of osmolality

Vomiting: a disagreeable experience that occurs when the stomach contents are reflexly expelled through the mouth or nose

References

Alexander, M.F., Fawcett, J.N. & Runciman, P.J. (2006) *Nursing Practice – Hospital and Home: Adult*, 3rd edn. Churchill Livingstone, Edinburgh.

Cooper, M.S. & Gittoes, N.J. (2008) Diagnosis and management of hypocalcaemia. *British Medical Journal*, 336(7656), 1298–1302.

Craig, S. (2010) Hyponatremia in emergency medicine. *Medscape*, April, 767624.

Kozier, B., Erb, G., Berman, A., Snyder, S., Lake, R. & Harvey, S. (2008) *Fundamentals of Nursing: concepts, process and practice*. Pearson Education, Harlow.

LeMone, P., Burke, K. & Bauldoff, G. (2011) *Medical-Surgical Nursing: critical thinking in client care*, 4th edn. Pearson Education, New Jersey.

Martini, F.H. & Nath, J.L. (2011) *Fundamentals of Anatomy and Physiology*, 9th edn. Pearson Benjamin Cummings, San Francisco.

Peate, I., Nair, M., Hemming, L. & Wild, K. (2012) *Adult Nursing – Acute and Ongoing Care*. Pearson Education, Harlow.

Porth, C. M. (2009) *Pathophysiology: concepts of altered health states*, 9th edn. Lippincott, Philadelphia.

Test Yourself

1. The most abundant intracellular cation is:
   (a) Sodium
   (b) Potassium
   (c) Calcium
   (d) Magnesium

2. The most abundant extracellular cation is:
   (a) Sodium
   (b) Potassium
   (c) Magnesium
   (d) Calcium

3. Respiratory acidosis is caused by a build-up of:
   (a) Oxygen
   (b) Carbon dioxide
   (c) Helium
   (d) Neon

4. Fluid movement from compartment to compartment through a selective permeable membrane is by:
   (a) Diffusion
   (b) Active transport
   (c) Passive transport
   (d) Osmosis

5. The gland/s that regulate calcium in the body is/are the:
   (a) Lungs
   (b) Kidneys
   (c) Spleen
   (d) Parathyroid

6. Hyperkalaemia is defined as plasma potassium in excess of:
   (a) 5.5 mmol/L
   (b) 4.0 mmol/L
   (c) 3.5 mmol/L
   (d) 3.0 mmol/L

7. What type of shock causes widespread vasodilatation and decreased peripheral resistance?
   (a) Cardiogenic shock
   (b) Septic shock
   (c) Hypovolaemic shock
   (d) Obstructive shock

8. Distributive shock is caused by:
   (a) Blood loss
   (b) Widespread vasodilatation
   (c) Ineffective cardiac pumping action
   (d) Hypersensitivity reaction

9. Women are more at risk of osteoporosis than men because they lose more:
   (a) Calcium ions
   (b) Sodium ions
   (c) Potassium ions
   (d) Chloride ions

10. Furosemide is a:
    (a) Antibiotic
    (b) Analgesic
    (c) Steroid
    (d) Diuretic

Answers

1. b
2. a
3. b
4. d
5. d
6. a
7. b
8. b
9. a
10. d

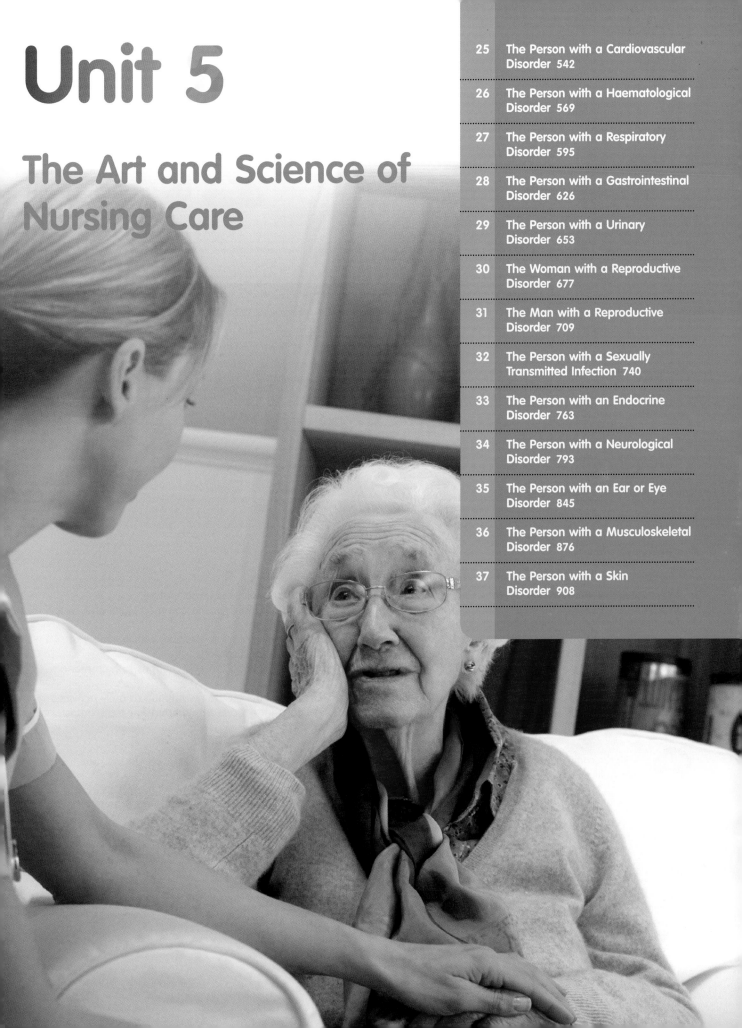

Unit 5

The Art and Science of Nursing Care

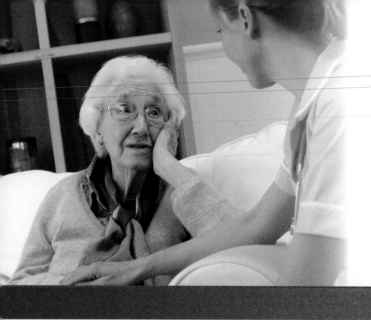

25

The Person with a Cardiovascular Disorder

Carl Clare

University of Hertfordshire, UK

Learning Outcomes

On completion of this chapter you will be able to:

- Describe the anatomy of the heart
- Explain the differences between arteries and veins
- Discuss the factors affecting blood pressure
- Explore the common components of health promotion in cardiovascular disease
- Describe the common sites of cardiac pain
- Explain the first-line treatment of a myocardial infarction

Competencies

All nurses must:

1. Identify and take the major pulses
2. Assess the patient for the common signs and symptoms of heart failure
3. Deliver nursing care to patients with a variety of cardiovascular disorders
4. Advise patients on lifestyle changes to help manage their pain
5. Advise patients on the resumption of daily activities
6. Categorise the stage of hypertension a patient is suffering from

 Visit the companion website at **www.wileynursingpractice.com** where you can test yourself using flashcards, multiple-choice questions and more.

Unit 5 image source: Monkeybusinessimages/iStock
Nursing Practice: Knowledge and Care, First Edition. Edited by Ian Peate, Karen Wild and Muralitharan Nair.
© 2014 John Wiley & Sons, Ltd. Published 2014 by John Wiley & Sons, Ltd. Companion website: www.wileynursingpractice.com

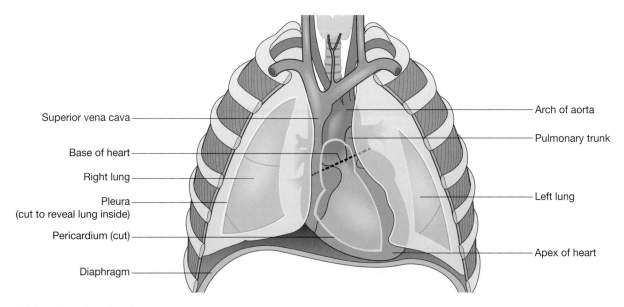

Figure 25.1 Location of the heart.

Labels on figure:
- Superior vena cava
- Base of heart
- Right lung
- Pleura (cut to reveal lung inside)
- Pericardium (cut)
- Diaphragm
- Arch of aorta
- Pulmonary trunk
- Left lung
- Apex of heart

Introduction

The cardiovascular system is made up of the heart, the arteries, the veins and the capillaries (the blood vessels) in a closed system. While the whole circulatory system is considered to be one unit, it is traditional and useful to review the heart and the blood vessels as separate entities. This chapter begins by reviewing the anatomy and physiology of the heart followed by the anatomy and physiology of the blood vessels. Following on from this is a review of some of the common conditions that affect the heart or the blood vessels.

Anatomy and Physiology of the Heart

The heart is a relatively small organ (about the size of your clenched fist) located in the thoracic cavity (chest) in the mediastinum (between the lungs), behind and to the left of the sternum (breast bone) (Figure 25.1). It is comprised of four muscular chambers surrounded by a membrane known as the pericardium. The pericardium is often referred to as a single sac surrounding the heart but it is actually made up of two membranes, the fibrous pericardium and the serous pericardium (Figure 25.2).

- The **fibrous pericardium** is a tough, inelastic, layer. The purpose of this layer is to prevent the overstretching of the heart. It also provides protection to the heart and anchors it in place
- The **serous pericardium** is a thinner, more delicate, layer that forms a double layer around the heart known as the parietal and visceral pericardium. Between the parietal and visceral pericardium is a very thin film of pericardial fluid (contained in the pericardial cavity) that reduces the friction between the membranes as the heart moves during its cycle of contraction and relaxation.

Underlying the pericardium is the **myocardium** (heart muscle), this constitutes the main bulk of the heart. The myocardium is a specialised muscle only found within the heart. The myocardium can be divided into two categories: the majority of the muscle fibres perform mechanical work (contraction); the remainder form the

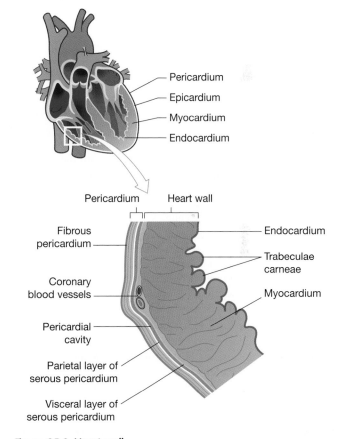

Labels on figure:
- Pericardium
- Epicardium
- Myocardium
- Endocardium
- Pericardium
- Heart wall
- Fibrous pericardium
- Coronary blood vessels
- Pericardial cavity
- Parietal layer of serous pericardium
- Visceral layer of serous pericardium
- Endocardium
- Trabeculae carneae
- Myocardium

Figure 25.2 Heart wall.

electrical system of the heart. The cardiac muscle cells (myocytes) are held together in spiral or circular bundles. Compared with skeletal muscle fibres, cardiac muscle fibres are shorter in length and have branches. The ends of the cardiac myocytes are attached to the adjacent cells in an end to end fashion allowing for the passage of electrical current rapidly between cells.

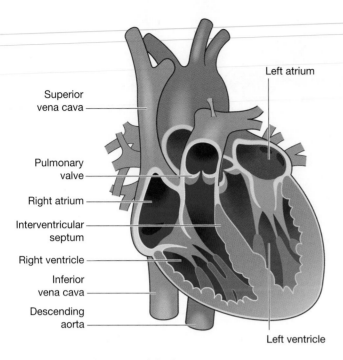

Figure 25.3 **The chambers of the heart.**

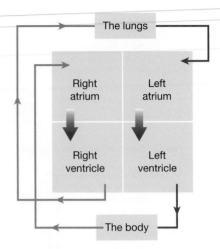

Figure 25.4 **A simplified diagram of the flow of blood through the heart.**

Myocytes differ from normal skeletal muscle, in that their mitochondria are both larger and there are more of them per cell. The benefit of this is that it makes cardiac muscle less prone to fatigue but it requires a large supply of oxygen and it is less able to cope with reductions in available oxygen.

Coating the inside of the myocardium is a smooth lining known as the endocardium. It is connected seamlessly with the lining of the large blood vessels that are connected to the heart.

The heart is divided into four chambers (Figure 25.3): two atria and two ventricles. Even though the heart is referred to as a pump, it is better to think of it as two pumps:

- The right heart pump receives deoxygenated blood (blood that has given up some of its oxygen to the cells) from the tissues and pumps it out into the pulmonary circulation (the lungs)
- The left heart pump receives oxygenated blood form the pulmonary circulation and pumps it out to the rest of the body (the systemic circulation).

The **atria** are the smaller chambers of the heart and are above the **ventricles**.

- The right atrium receives blood from the systemic circulation (blood returning form the majority of the body)
- The left atrium receives blood from the lungs (pulmonary circulation).

Between the atria, there is a thin dividing wall, the **interatrial septum**. The atria have thinner muscle walls compared with the ventricles, as they have lower pressures to overcome.

Between the atria and the ventricles are two valves (the **atrioventricular valves**):

- Tricuspid valve – lies between the right atrium and the right ventricle
- Bicuspid (mitral) valve – lies between the left atrium and the left ventricle.

The purpose of the atrioventricular valves is to prevent the backward flow of blood from the ventricles into the atria during the contraction of the ventricles.

- The right ventricle receives blood from the right atrium and pumps this blood out into the pulmonary circulation (the lungs). As the pressure in the pulmonary circulation is quite low the right ventricle has a thinner wall than the left ventricle.
- The left ventricle receives blood from the left atrium and pumps this blood out into the systemic circulation (the rest of the body) via the aorta. As the left ventricle has to pump against a higher pressure and over a greater distance it has a much thicker (more muscular) wall.

Between the ventricles is the interventricular septum. Thus, with the septum between the atria and the septum between the ventricles, there is no mixing of blood between the two sides.

At the outlet of each ventricle is a **valve**.

- The pulmonary valve is situated between the right ventricle and the pulmonary arteries (supplying the lungs) and prevents the backwards flow of blood into the right ventricle from the pulmonary arteries
- The aortic valve lies between the left ventricle and the aorta (the main artery leading to the systemic circulation) and prevents the backwards flow of blood into the left ventricle from the systemic circulation.

As noted earlier, although the heart is a single organ, it is best to think of it as two pumps, the right and the left heart pump. Each pump is made up of two chambers (atrium and ventricle).

- The right heart pump is composed of the right atrium and the right ventricle and receives blood from the systemic circulation (the body) and pumps it through the pulmonary circulation (the lungs)
- The left heart pump is composed of the left atrium and the left ventricle and receives blood from the pulmonary circulation and pumps it out around the systemic circulation.

Figure 25.4 gives a simplified explanation of the flow of blood through the heart. In this diagram deoxygenated blood is in blue and oxygenated blood is in red. It is important to note that 'deoxygenated blood' does not refer to blood that has no oxygen in it but blood that has given up some of its oxygen to the tissues. Typically deoxygenated blood contains 75% of the oxygen that oxygenated blood carries.

A more detailed and anatomical view can be seen in Figure 25.5. Blood enters the right atrium via the superior and inferior vena cava and leaves the right ventricle via the pulmonary arteries. Note that even though it is deoxygenated blood leaving the right ventricle, it is the vessels that the blood is carried in that makes it **arterial** or **venous**. Thus:

- Blood entering the atria is carried in veins and is therefore venous blood
- Blood leaving the ventricles is carried in arteries and is arterial blood.

Blood is transported through the pulmonary circulation and returned to the left atrium through the pulmonary veins; it is then pumped out by the left ventricle into the aorta.

Within the heart, there is a specialised network of myocardial cells dedicated to ensuring the rapid transmission of electrical impulses (Figure 25.6).

Normal electrical activity begins in the sinoatrial (SA) node and is rapidly transmitted across the atria by fast pathways, thus ensuring that the right and left atria beat as one unit. The electrical impulse travels to the atrioventricular (AV) node, where it is held for approximately 0.1 seconds before being transmitted to the ventricles via **the bundle of His** (otherwise known as the **AV bundle**). This ensures that the atria have completely contracted before ventricular contraction is initiated.

The cardiac cycle is a term used to refer to the changes in pressure that occur within the heart from the start on one heartbeat to

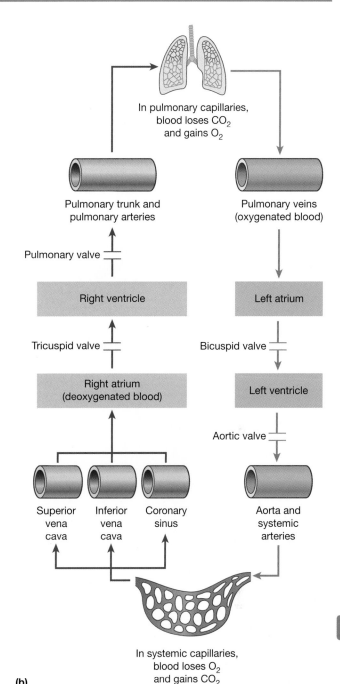

(b)

Figure 25.5 (Continued)

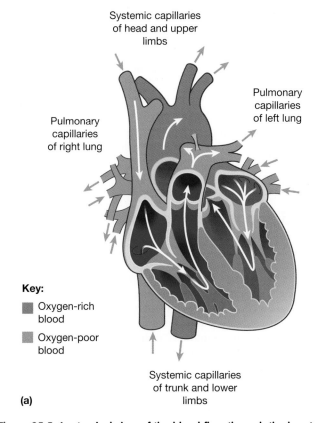

Key:

■ Oxygen-rich blood

■ Oxygen-poor blood

(a)

Figure 25.5 Anatomical view of the blood flow through the heart.

545

the next. A simple explanation of the cycle can be made by breaking the cycle into three parts (Figure 25.7):

1. **Atrial systole** (Figure 25.7, #1) – At this point, the atrioventricular valves (between the atria and the ventricles) are open but the valves between the ventricles and the arteries (aortic and pulmonary valves) are closed. The ventricles have been filling with blood that has been flowing freely from the veins. An impulse created in the sinoatrial node excites the atria and they contract (systole) pushing blood into the ventricles. This atrial contraction fills the ventricles with the final third of the total blood volume they receive before they contract.

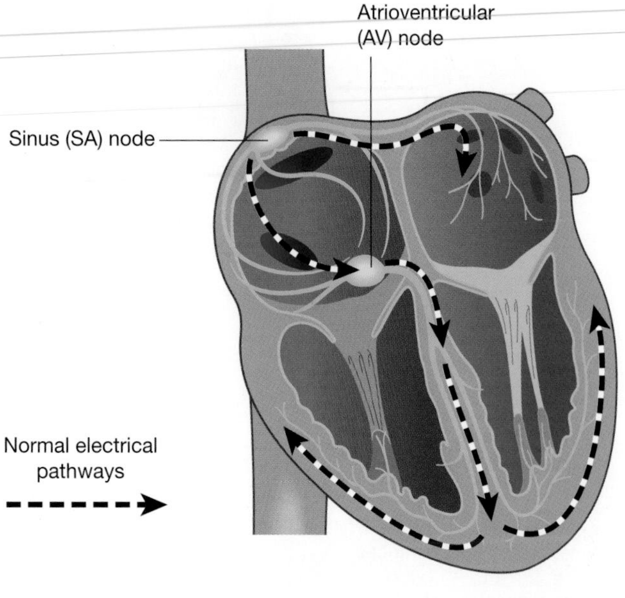

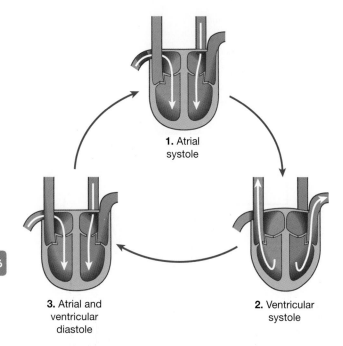

Figure 25.6 Conduction system of the heart (the white line shows the passage of the electrical impulses through the heart muscle).

Figure 25.7 The cardiac cycle.

2. **Ventricular systole** (Figure 25.7, #2) – The electrical impulse that has been held at the atrioventricular node is now passed through the bundle of His and ventricular contraction (systole) begins. The atrioventricular valves (between the atria and the ventricles) close and the aortic and pulmonary valves (to the arteries) open in response to the increased pressure. Blood is ejected from the ventricles into the pulmonary and systemic circulation.

3. **Atrial and ventricular diastole** (Figure 25.7, #3) – The atria and the ventricles have stopped contracting and are relaxing. The valves between the ventricles and the arteries are pushed closed by the pressure in the pulmonary arteries and the aorta. The atrioventricular valves (between the atria and the ventricles) are pushed open by the blood entering the atria from the veins and the ventricles begin to fill with blood.

The electrical impulse created in the SA node and transmitted through the heart muscle can be assessed using an electrocardiograph (ECG) and the pattern of this ECG trace can be matched to the mechanical activity of the atria and ventricles (see Figure 25.8). Note the terms **depolarisation** and **repolarisation**:

- **Depolarisation** leads to the contraction of cardiac muscle fibres
- **Repolarisation** leads to relaxation of the cardiac muscle fibres.

The amount of blood the heart pumps out in 1 minute is known as 'cardiac output' and is defined by the following formula.

$$\text{Cardiac output (CO)} = \text{stroke volume (SV)} \times \text{heart rate (HR)}$$

Thus, the amount of blood the heart pumps out in a minute is made up of the amount of blood pumped out of the ventricle in one beat (SV), measured in millilitres, times the heart rate (HR), measured in beats per minute. This gives a total volume. Therefore, if SV was 70 mL and the heart rate was 75, then cardiac output is 70 times 75, which equals 5250 mL (or 5.25 litres) per minute.

Stroke volume is affected by several factors:

- **Preload** – The strength of contraction of the ventricle is partly related to the amount of blood in the ventricle. This can be affected by increasing the return of blood from the veins to the heart by mechanisms such as exercise (where skeletal muscles squeeze the veins) or the release of hormones, such as adrenaline, leading to contraction of the veins. Alternatively, reduced blood volume in the ventricle will lead to reduction in stroke volume, for instance in hypovolaemia.
- **Force of contraction** – The contractility of the heart muscle can be affected by several factors. Hormones, such as adrenaline, can increase the force of contraction. Also sympathetic nervous system activity increases the force of contraction.
- **Afterload** – Afterload refers to the pressure in the arteries that the ventricle must overcome in order to pump out blood.

Heart rate is controlled by two main mechanisms:

- **Autonomic nervous system activity** – Sympathetic nervous system activity leads to an increase in heart rate and parasympathetic nervous system activity leads to decrease in heart rate
- **Hormone activity** – The release of adrenaline or large amounts of thyroxine leads to an increase in heart rate.

Blood Supply to the Heart

The muscles of the heart have a large and never ending demand for oxygen and nutrients and the removal of waste products. To supply this demand, the heart receives approximately 5% of the total cardiac output. The vast majority of the heart muscle is supplied with its blood by the coronary arteries (Figure 25.9).

The **main coronary arteries** (left and right) have their origins (ostia) in the wall of the aorta just after the aortic valve. These great arteries then subdivide into smaller and smaller branches that enter the heart wall and supply the cells deep in the myocardium, ensuring that the oxygen hungry myocardium is supplied throughout. Table 25.1 gives a brief description of the areas of the heart each major artery supplies and the names of its major branches.

As the arteries become smaller and become buried deeper in the myocardium they are subject to greater pressure during the contraction of the heart muscle. This leads to the situation whereby

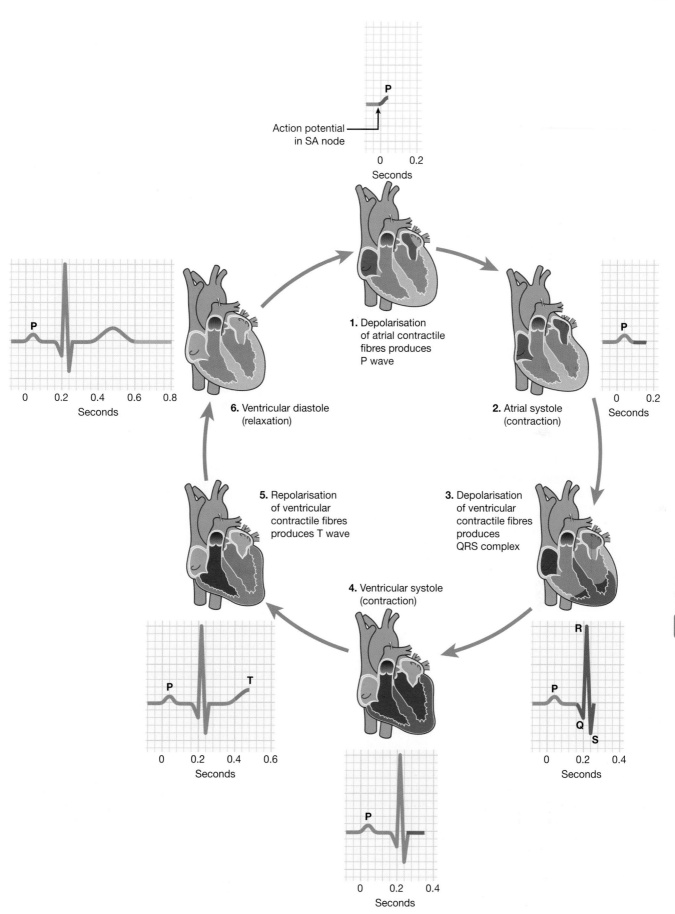

Figure 25.8 The cardiac cycle and the ECG.

Action potential in SA node

1. Depolarisation of atrial contractile fibres produces P wave

2. Atrial systole (contraction)

3. Depolarisation of ventricular contractile fibres produces QRS complex

4. Ventricular systole (contraction)

5. Repolarisation of ventricular contractile fibres produces T wave

6. Ventricular diastole (relaxation)

547

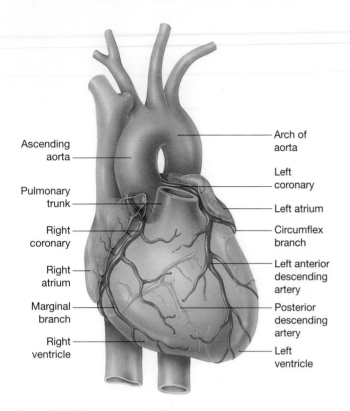

Figure 25.9 The coronary arteries.

Table 25.1 The coronary arteries, their major branches and the areas of the heart they supply.

ARTERY	AREA OF THE HEART SUPPLIED	MAJOR BRANCHES
Left anterior descending (LAD)	Front and side of the left ventricle, apex of the heart	Diagonals; septals
Circumflex artery	Back and side of the left ventricle	Oblique marginal
Right coronary artery (RCA)	Right ventricle, base of the heart and interventricular septum	Posterior descending artery

some of the arteries are 'obliterated' during systole, that is they are subject to such a pressure that all the blood is squeezed out of them. Blood flow is then restored as the heart enters diastole and the heart muscle relaxes. During the average cardiac cycle (one round of contraction and relaxation), the heart is in systole for approximately one-third of the total time and thus there are two-thirds of the cardiac cycle where the heart is in diastole and coronary artery blood flow can occur. However, as the heart rate increases, systole still takes the same amount of time even though the cardiac cycle is shorter and thus the time the heart is in diastole is reduced. This then leads to a reduction of the time the coronary arteries can supply the heart muscle.

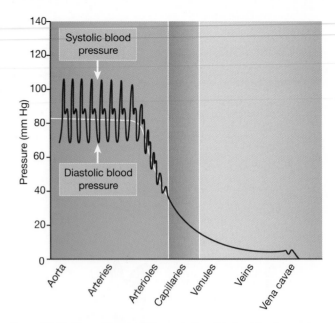

Figure 25.10 The pressure differences through the blood vessels.

Anatomy and Physiology of the Blood Vessels

This section will concentrate on the systemic blood vessels (those that serve the body other than the lungs). The pulmonary system works on the same principles as the systemic system but at a lower pressure. The blood vessels form a closed system that act as ducts for the distribution of blood throughout the systemic and pulmonary circulations. Blood travels through the blood vessels by following a pressure gradient. Thus, as water will flow from a point of high pressure to a point of low pressure, so blood flows from the heart through the arteries to the capillaries and then to the veins and back to the heart (Figure 25.10).

As can be seen from Figure 25.10, *the arterial system* is broken down into the aorta, the arteries and the arterioles.

- **Aorta**. This is the largest artery leading directly from the left ventricle
- **Arteries**. As the arteries get further away from the heart, their lumen becomes smaller but due to branching, the number of arteries become greater
- **Arterioles**. The arterioles are the smallest vessels of the arterial system.

The arteries all have a similar anatomy, shown in Figure 25.11a.

- Outer layer (tunica externa or tunica adventitia) – A tough protective layer of collagen and elastic fibres that serve to protect the artery and to prevent over stretching
- Thick middle layer (tunica media) – A layer of smooth muscle allowing for control of the size of the lumen of an artery
- Inner layer (tunica intima) – The main feature of the tunica intima is a covering of endothelium (on a basement membrane) that creates a smooth surface for blood flow.

The venous system is comprised of the venules, veins and vena cavae:

- **Venules**. The smallest of the veins, these collect the blood draining from the capillaries

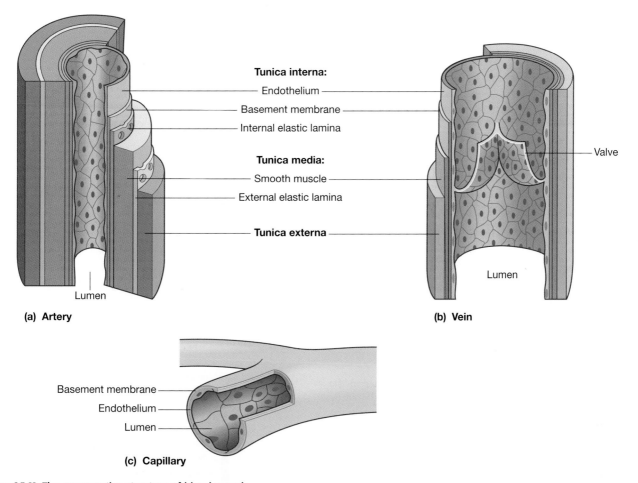

Tunica interna:
Endothelium
Basement membrane
Internal elastic lamina

Tunica media:
Smooth muscle
External elastic lamina

Tunica externa

Valve

Lumen

Lumen

(a) Artery

(b) Vein

Basement membrane
Endothelium
Lumen

(c) Capillary

Figure 25.11 The comparative structure of blood vessels.

- **Veins**. The veins converge into gradually larger and larger vessels
- **Vena cavae**. The two great veins that return the blood from the systemic circulation to the heart. The superior vena cava returns blood form the upper body and the inferior vena cava returns blood from the lower body.

While the anatomy of a vein is similar to that of an artery (see Figure 25.11b), there are some notable differences:

- The tunica media. This is thinner in veins as they do not have to overcome the same pressures as in an artery
- Valves. Veins and venules contain one-way valves that arise from the tunica intima preventing backwards blood flow away from the heart.

Once arterioles begin to enter into the tissues, the nature of the blood vessels change and multiple branches of tiny vessels called **capillaries** are found. The function of capillaries is the exchange of substances (such as oxygen, carbon dioxide and nutrients) and this exchange is possible due to the nature of the capillary wall (see Figure 25.11c). As the wall of the capillary is only made up of a single layer of cells on a basement membrane, substances can easily pass from the blood into the tissues and vice versa.

Blood Pressure

Blood pressure is composed of two components:

- **Systolic blood pressure** – The pressure in the arteries when the heart is in systole (contracting).

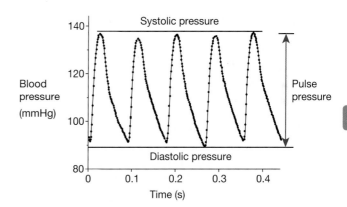

Figure 25.12 A diagram showing the relationship between systolic, diastolic and pulse pressures.

- **Diastolic blood pressure** – The pressure in the arteries when the heart is in diastole (relaxing).

The difference in pressure between the systolic and the diastolic pressures is known as the **pulse pressure** (Figure 25.12) and is a reflection of the pressure created by the ventricles of the heart when they contract.

549

The total systolic pressure is dependent on the baseline diastolic pressure plus the pressure created by the contracting ventricles of the heart (pulse pressure).

Thus, if the pressure created by the contracting ventricles is 60 mmHg and the diastolic pressure was 80 mmHg then the systolic pressure will be 140 mmHg (80 + 60 = 140), however if the diastolic pressure was 60 mmHg then the systolic pressure would be 120 mmHg (60 + 60 = 120).

Mean arterial blood pressure

Mean arterial blood pressure (MABP or MAP) is represented by the formula:

$$MABP = \text{Cardiac output (CO)} \times \text{Total peripheral resistance (TPR)}$$

Jot This Down

Total peripheral resistance (TPR) is also known as systemic vascular resistance (SVR).

Therefore, in order to increase blood pressure, there can be an increase in cardiac output or an increase in total peripheral resistance.

The factors affecting cardiac output were noted earlier in the chapter. Total peripheral resistance is most powerfully altered by changing the radius of the lumen of the arteries (particularly the arterioles), other factors that can alter TPR are the blood viscosity and the total blood vessel length. However, on a minute by minute basis, the alteration of TPR is regulated by the relaxation and constriction of the arterial walls thus affecting the diameter of the tube the blood must flow through.

The control of blood pressure

The control of blood pressure is carried out through the activities of two bodily systems:

- **Nervous system** regulation of blood pressure
- **Hormonal regulation** of blood pressure.

The control of blood pressure by both systems is mediated by a negative feedback loop involving monitoring receptors, known as **chemoreceptors** and **baroreceptors** (Figure 25.13).

- **Chemoreceptors** are sensory receptors that monitor the concentration of substances, such as oxygen, carbon dioxide and hydrogen ions in the blood. Increases in carbon dioxide and hydrogen ion concentrations, or decreased oxygen concentrations leads to the increased stimulation of the cardiovascular centre and thus an increase in sympathetic nervous system activity
- **Baroreceptors** are pressure receptors located in the aorta, the internal carotid arteries and large arteries in the chest and neck. When the baroreceptors are stretched less (reduced pressure in the arteries), this leads to a decreased rate of impulses form the baroreceptors to the cardiovascular centre. The reduction of the stimulus to the cardiovascular centre leads to an increase in sympathetic nervous system activation and therefore an increase in cardiac output and TPR (see Figure 25.13 for a summary of the effects of sympathetic nervous system activation on the heart and blood vessels).

Hormonal control of blood pressure is mediated through several mechanisms, these are summarised in Table 25.2.

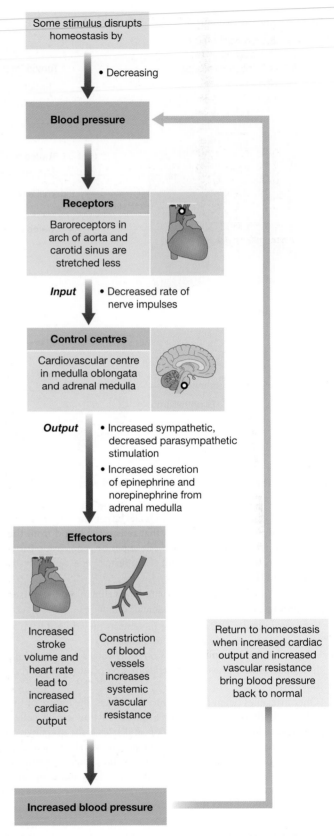

Figure 25.13 The negative feedback control of blood pressure through the baroreceptors.

Table 25.2 Blood pressure control by hormones.

HORMONE	PRINCIPAL ACTIONS	EFFECT ON ASPECTS OF THE MABP FORMULA	EFFECT ON BLOOD PRESSURE
Adrenaline	Vasoconstriction Increased heart rate	Increased TPR Increased CO	Increased
	Increased stroke volume	Increased CO	
Angiotensin II	Vasoconstriction	Increased TPR	Increase
Aldosterone	Increased reabsorption of water and sodium ions	Increased blood volume leading to increased CO	Increase
Antidiuretic hormone (ADH)	Increased reabsorption of water Vasoconstriction	Increased blood volume leading to increased CO Increased TPR	Increased

Further discussion of the endocrine system can be found in Chapter 33; further discussion of the role of angiotensin II in fluid maintenance can be found in Chapter 24.

Assessing the cardiovascular system

As with the assessment of any of the bodily systems, the nurse must always explain the procedures they are about to carry out and gain consent from the patient.

The first step in assessing the cardiovascular system is to obtain a medical history from the patient. Without this data, the nurse not only risks ignoring the patient experiences of their disorder and the effect it has on their lives but also this information can be useful in differentiating between different cardiovascular disorders, some of which can be intermittent.

History-taking for the patient with a potential cardiovascular disorder focusses on:

- Chest pain
- Shortness of breath
- Palpitations
- Syncope (fainting)
- Risk factors.

The physical assessment of the cardiovascular system requires the patient to have been resting quietly before examination, so that results such as pulse and blood pressure are not affected by exercise.

Radial pulse Pulses can be found at many points on the body (see Figure 25.14 showing the major pulse sites). When assessing the cardiovascular system, it is normal to start with the **radial pulse**. The radial pulse is found in the wrist on the same side as the thumb (Figure 25.15). To assess the radial pulse, place two fingers on the point of pulsation and using a watch with a second hand, count the number of beats in 60 seconds.

Once the pulse rate has been taken, then take time to assess the way the pulse feels:

- Is it thready and weak or strong and bounding?
- Is it regular or irregular?
- Is every pulsation the same strength?

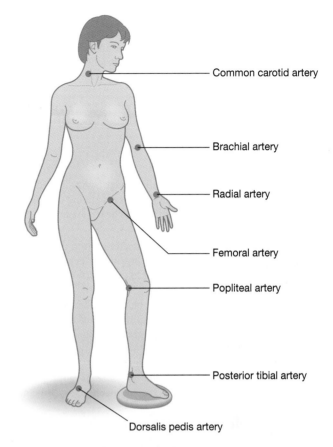

Common carotid artery

Brachial artery

Radial artery

Femoral artery

Popliteal artery

Posterior tibial artery

Dorsalis pedis artery

Figure 25.14 Pulse sites on the body.

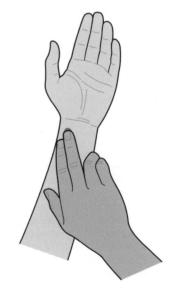

Figure 25.15 Assessing the radial pulse.

The normal **resting pulse** rate will vary from patient to patient and can be affected by many factors, including the physical fitness of the patient, the age of the patient and patient anxiety. The range considered to be normal for a patient's heart rate is 60–100 beats per minute but trained athletes may easily have a heart rate between

40 and 60 beats per minute. A weak and thread pulse may be suggestive of peripheral shut down in response to shock or a reduced pulse pressure. The regularity of the pulse and changes in pulse strength from beat to beat can be an important indicator of the presence of certain disturbances in heart rhythm such as atrial fibrillation.

Blood pressure In order to take a patient's blood pressure you will need a:

- Manual sphygmomanometer
- Stethoscope.

The patient should be seated and relaxed having rested for at least 5 minutes. Ensure no tight clothing is restricting the arm and have the arm supported at the level of the heart, for instance by a pillow.

1. Place the cuff of the sphygmomanometer around the arm with the centre of the bladder over the brachial artery. The bladder of the cuff should be large enough to circle 80% of the arm but not more than 100%
2. Estimate the systolic pressure by palpating the brachial pulse with two or three fingers and inflating the cuff until the pulse disappears. Remember to watch the reading on the sphygmomanometer so that you know at what point the pulse disappears. Release the pressure in the cuff
3. Inflate the cuff again until the pressure is approximately 30 mmHg above the point that you estimated the systolic pressure to be
4. Place the diaphragm of the stethoscope on the place where the brachial pulse was palpated. Some people place the diaphragm before inflating the cuff – this is acceptable so long as no part of the stethoscope is underneath any part of the cuff
5. Deflate the cuff at a rate of 2–3 mmHg per second until you hear a tapping sound (first Korotkoff sound). This is the *systolic pressure* – make a mental note of that number
6. Continue to deflate the cuff at a rate of 2–3 mmHg per second until the tapping sound disappears (fifth Korotkoff sound). This is the *diastolic pressure* – make a mental note of that number
7. Both the systolic and diastolic should be measured to the nearest 2 mmHg
8. Deflate the cuff fully and record the systolic and diastolic on the appropriate documentation.

What To Do If...the Tapping Sound Never Disappears

 This is often due to pressing too hard with the stethoscope. Reassess the blood pressure trying to be gentler with the stethoscope. If on repeat, the tapping noise does not disappear then use the point that the sounds change as the measurement of diastolic blood pressure and record in the documentation that the fourth Korotkoff sound was used to measure diastolic blood pressure.

If using an electronic blood pressure monitor:

The patient should be seated and relaxed having rested for at least 5 minutes. Ensure no tight clothing is restricting the arm and have the arm supported at the level of the heart, for instance by a pillow.

1. Place the cuff of the sphygmomanometer around the arm with the centre of the bladder over the brachial artery. The bladder

of the cuff should be large enough to circle 80% of the arm but not more than 100%
2. Read the systolic and diastolic blood pressures are displayed and record on the appropriate documentation.

 Link To/Go To

Guidelines on taking blood pressures (including in pregnancy) can be found on the British Hypertension Society website: **http://www.bhsoc.org/**

Normal blood pressure readings are considered to be between 90 and 140 mmHg systolic and 60–90 mmHg diastolic. However, patients should be reassured that one reading that is above these levels does not necessarily mean they have high blood pressure, as blood pressure varies widely throughout the day and unless they have symptoms (such as feeling dizzy), lower blood pressures are not necessarily an indication of a problem.

Assessing the peripheral vascular system in the legs

- Compare the colour and temperature of the two legs looking for colour changes (such as a blue or purple discolouration)
- Compare the temperature of the two legs using the back of the hand.

Jot This Down

Different parts of the hand are better for different types of assessment.

- The back of the hand is best for assessing temperature
- The palms are best for assessing vibration
- The fingertips are best for assessing pulsation.

- Press on the nail bed of the big toe, so that it blanches and then note how long it takes for the colour to return. Compare the time taken for both feet.
- Palpate the dorsalis pedis pulse (Figure 25.16) on both feet assessing strength and comparing the two. The dorsalis pedis pulse can be difficult to palpate and if you cannot find it, then it does not mean it is not present.

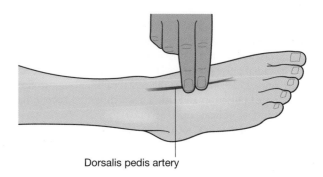

Dorsalis pedis artery

Figure 25.16 Palpating the dorsalis pedis pulse.

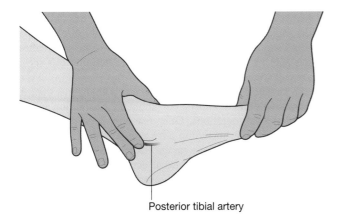

Figure 25.17 **Palpating the posterior tibial pulse.**

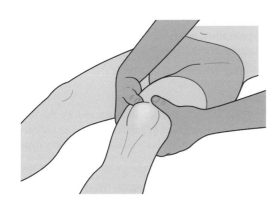

Figure 25.18 **Palpating the popliteal pulse.**

Jot This Down

Many nurses who work in areas such as cardiac catheter recovery areas or on vascular surgery wards mark the dorsalis pedis with a pen once it has been palpated (with the permission of the patient). This makes regular assessment easier.

- Palpate the posterior tibial pulse (Figure 25.17) in both ankles assessing strength and comparing the two. The posterior tibial pulse can be felt on the inside (big toe side) of your ankle. It is just below and behind the big bony part that sticks out (the medial malleolus)
- Palpate the popliteal pulse in both knees (Figure 25.18) assessing strength and comparing the two. The popliteal pulse is located in the fold behind the knee. The easiest way to find it is to have the patients leg slightly bent, place your thumbs on the knee cap and then curl your fingers round the knee into the fold behind the knee. This pulse is quite deep and may require some pressure to palpate but be careful not to be too firm.

Pulses should be equal on both sides of the body; any differences should be recorded and reported.

Disorders of the Cardiovascular System

Coronary Heart Disease

'Coronary heart disease' (CHD) is the label applied to a group of conditions based on the development of narrowing in the lumen of one or more of the coronary arteries. The group of conditions are:

- Stable angina
- Unstable angina
- Myocardial infarction.

Stable angina

Stable angina is one of a group of conditions known as coronary heart disease (CHD). It is characterised by chest pain/discomfort, jaw pain or pain in the arm (usually the left arm) that usually occurs when the patient is exercising or emotionally distressed.

Risk factors for coronary heart disease include:

- Smoking
- High fat diet
- Lack of exercise
- Family history of coronary heart disease
- High serum cholesterol
- High blood pressure
- Diabetes
- Obesity
- Ethnic origin.

Pathophysiology As noted previously in the chapter the heart muscle has a high oxygen requirement and the blood flow to the heart muscles is through the coronary arteries. In patients with any form of coronary heart disease, the pathophysiology of the early stages is based on the same processes. Cholesterol and other fatty substances are laid down into the artery wall into a structure known as a plaque. As the plaque are present between the tunica intima and tunica media the lumen of the artery becomes narrowed as the thick muscle layer of the tunica media creates a barrier that pushes the plaque into the lumen of the artery (see Figure 25.19).

The supply of oxygen to the heart muscle and the demand of the heart muscle for that oxygen are balanced by several factors. When we exercise (or increase our heart rates in other ways) the myocardium requires more oxygen as it is working harder. In people without significant narrowing of the coronary arteries this demand can be met by increasing blood flow. In the patient with significant atherosclerosis, leading to stable angina, the increased demand for oxygen by the heart muscle cannot be met due to the narrowing of the artery lumen and thus the patient experiences pain due to hypoxia of the myocardium.

Signs and symptoms The symptoms of stable angina include the experience of pain or discomfort in the chest, which may radiate into an arm (the left arm is usual), shoulder and jaw. Pain of cardiac origin is commonly described as tightness or heaviness and may be associated with shortness of breath. In stable angina, the pain is brief (usually no longer than 10 minutes), is associated with physical exertion or emotional distress and is normally relieved by rest or a GTN spray (which most patients with angina will have been prescribed). Some patients will experience more episodes of angina during the cold winter months. Entering the

553

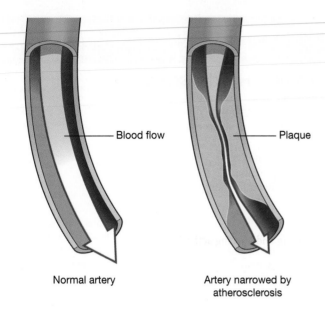

Figure 25.19 **Atherosclerosis.**

cold air from the house appears to be related to a sudden increase in blood pressure, leading to a greater work load for the heart and thus increased myocardial oxygen demand (Marchant *et al.* 1994).

Diagnosis and investigations The diagnosis of stable angina can usually be made with a good degree of certainty by taking a history from the patient. If they report typical chest pain occurring on exertion, lasting for a short period and relieved by rest, then the diagnosis is almost certainly stable angina. However, certain investigations and physical examination are still required to confirm the diagnosis and to assess the underlying coronary heart disease.

- Full blood count
- 12-lead ECG – this will often be normal but on occasion there may be indicators of previous myocardial damage or other factors related to the structure of the heart
- Exercise tolerance test (ETT) – this involves exercising the patient on a treadmill while they are attached to continuous ECG monitoring. This can give an indication of how much coronary artery disease is present (Hill & Timmis 2002). A significant result from the ETT may lead to the patient undergoing coronary angiography to assess the degree to which the coronary arteries are narrowed (often referred to as 'stenosis') and how many of the major arteries have narrowing in them
- Plasma glucose and cholesterol tests are also recommended to assess for two of the risk factors of coronary heart disease (DH 2000).

Nursing care and management Generally, patients with stable angina are managed by the GP or in the Outpatient Department (OPD) and hospitalisation is not required.

Often, episodes of pain can be managed by stopping the activity that has led to the pain and resting.

Patients with stable angina will be prescribed a nitrate spray for use when they have episodes of pain. The spray is administered under the tongue as required by the patient. However, it is best to warn patients who are new to the use of the nitrate spray that it is best to sit down before using the spray, as it can cause hypotension

and then the patient may faint. When using the nitrate spray to treat an angina attack, the patient should be taught that if the pain does not go after the first dose then to use the spray again after 5 minutes and if the pain has not gone 5 minutes after this second dose, to call an ambulance (NICE 2012).

If the patient has been newly diagnosed with angina, then it is important to give them information about their condition and give them time to ask questions. Offer reassurance and explore the concept of self-care, including advice on stopping exercise and resting and the use of nitrate sprays. Patients may wish to explore the possibility of continuing sexual activities and this must be explored with them, for instance discussing the need to pace themselves in any physical activity and recognising the signs of developing chest pain and to use their nitrate spray before any planned exertion. Partners especially can become worried about this aspect of their relationship, as they cannot see the pain the patient experiences and thus cannot judge it, furthermore the very concept of chest pain is worrying for many partners who may be worried about the risk of triggering a myocardial infarction (Dalteg *et al.* 2011).

As well as the nitrate spray for 'as required' use, patients will usually be prescribed two of the following regular medications for long-term control of their angina:

- Beta blocker
- Calcium channel blocker
- ACE inhibitor.

If the angina is not satisfactorily managed by the use of drug therapy, then the patient may be offered some form of revascularisation therapy, such as angioplasty or coronary artery bypass grafts (CABG).

Health promotion and discharge Health promotion for all patients with coronary heart disease (including angina) is based on risk factor reduction. Coronary heart disease is a progressive condition and health promotion can help to slow down its further development:

- Stopping smoking is one of the most important forms of health promotion in those with coronary heart disease (Jha *et al.* 2013)
- Weight reduction in those who are overweight
- Promoting a healthy balanced diet:
  - At least five portions fruit and vegetables a day
  - High fibre (at least 18 g per day)
  - Oily fish at least three times a week
  - Avoid fatty foods.

 Link To/Go To

Both the British Heart Foundation (**http://www.bhf.org.uk**) and the American Heart Association (**http://www.heart.org**) have excellent resources for patients regarding heart conditions and healthy living.

- Exercising at least 150 minutes per week (moderate intensity)

Red Flag

 Patients with coronary heart disease should not start a new exercise regime without consulting their doctor first.

- Patients with high blood cholesterol levels or high blood pressure will need treatment for these
- Patients with diabetes are especially at risk of heart disease and as well as the health promotion above stress must be placed on ensuring good control of their diabetes.

Unstable angina

Unstable angina is a severe form of angina that suggests a greater degree of coronary artery stenosis or instability of the plaques in the coronary arteries.

Pathophysiology The underlying pathophysiology of unstable angina is based on the same process of atherosclerosis but the plaque has become unstable and clots are developing on the top of the plaque leading to greater blockage of the artery. These clots will often partially dissolve and then reoccur with the associated pain waxing and waning as a result.

Signs and symptoms The signs and symptoms of unstable angina are:

- Chest pain similar to stable angina but can be more severe
- Often occurs while resting, sleeping or with little physical exertion
- May last longer than stable angina
- Rest or medicine usually do not help relieve it
- May get worse over time.

Diagnosis and investigations Diagnosis of unstable angina is based on:

- A 12-lead ECG
- Measurement of cardiac enzymes in the blood (such as CK(MB) and troponin I or troponin T)
- Coronary angiogram
- Plasma glucose and cholesterol tests are also recommended to assess for two of the risk factors of coronary heart disease (DH 2000).

Nursing care and management The nursing care of the patient with unstable angina will be based on the delivery of medical treatment according to prescription, including:

- Intravenous nitrates
- Antiplatelet therapy (such as aspirin or clopidogrel)
- Intravenous infusions of GpIIb/IIIa inhibitors
- Intravenous infusion of heparin or subcutaneous injections of low molecular weight heparin.

The initial nursing actions should be based around the acronym MONA (see later).

Specific nursing actions include:

- Provision of reassurance and a calm environment to minimise stress
- Implementation of bed rest
- Oxygen delivery as per prescription
- Cardiac monitoring
- Pain relief may be required (such as intravenous morphine).

Further treatment may involve angioplasty or CABG.

Health promotion and discharge Health promotion is the same as that for stable angina in promoting healthy lifestyles and reducing risk factors.

On discharge, the patient should be advised to call an ambulance if they have angina symptoms lasting for more than 10 minutes that are not relieved by rest or their usual medication. Patients should also be referred to the hospital cardiac rehabilitation programme. Cardiac rehabilitation is a structured programme of exercise and health promotion, carried out as a group activity under the supervision of a nurse or physiotherapist. The programme includes teaching sessions by dieticians and other health professionals.

Patients who have been diagnosed with unstable angina will require information on self-management, for instance some patients may benefit from attending an NHS Expert Patient Programme, which are now provided by a community interest company (**http://www.expertpatients.co.uk/** accessed 31/08/13); the Expert Patient Programme teaches patients skills, such as:

- Staging and spacing activities
- Taking appropriate rest
- Taking exercise
- Healthy diet
- Managing pain and fatigue
- Dealing with depression or anger
- Communicating with family, friends and healthcare professionals.

The Evidence

Stable angina usually occurs predictably with physical exertion or emotional stress, and is relieved within minutes of rest. Unstable angina is new-onset angina (usually within 24 hours) or abrupt deterioration in previously stable angina, often occurring at rest. Unstable angina usually requires immediate admission or referral to hospital.

Management of stable angina includes lifestyle advice:

- All people who smoke should be offered advice and assisted to stop
- A cardioprotective diet should be encouraged.

https://www.evidence.nhs.uk/topic/angina

Primary Care

Denial may involve forgetting to take prescribed medications. Nurses should advise on the importance of taking the prescribed medications.

Teach the patient of the side-effects of medications prescribed and the importance of not discontinuing medications abruptly.

Teach the patient how to take and store GTN and advise them to carry some GTN when they are going out, in case of emergency.

Advise the patient not to undertake strenuous exercise and to follow a programmed exercise as planned by their practice nurse.

Stress the importance of calling 999 (in the UK) when experiencing severe chest pain.

Myocardial infarction

Myocardial infarction (MI) or **acute myocardial infarction** (AMI), is the medical term for an event commonly known as a heart attack. It happens when blood stops flowing properly to part of the heart and the heart muscle is injured due to not getting enough oxygen. Usually, this is because one of the coronary arteries that supplies blood to the heart develops a blockage because of an unstable build-up of white blood cells, cholesterol and fat.

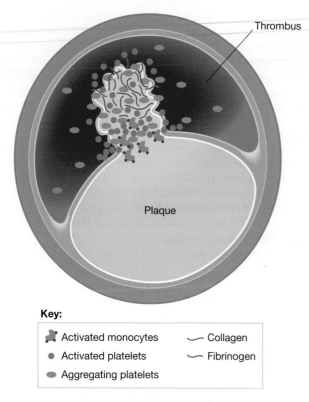

Key:

- 🧩 Activated monocytes   ⌣ Collagen
- ● Activated platelets   ⌣ Fibrinogen
- ⬭ Aggregating platelets

Figure 25.20 The ruptured atherosclerotic plaque.

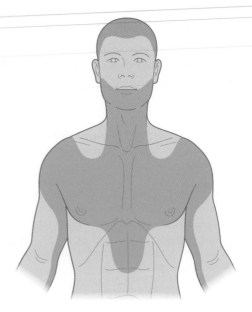

Figure 25.21 Typical areas where pain associated with myocardial infarction may be reported.

Pathophysiology The pathophysiology of MI is based on the same underlying development of atherosclerotic plaques as both forms of angina. However, in MI, the plaque in the arterial wall ruptures, exposing the mix of cholesterol, chemicals and fatty substances to the bloodstream activating platelets and blood cells (Figure 25.20). This leads to the development of a thrombus within the coronary artery that either completely or mostly blocks blood flow through the artery. This cessation of blood flow starves the part of the heart muscle supplied by the artery of oxygen and nutrients and leads to cell death.

Signs and symptoms

- Central crushing chest pain radiating into the arm, neck, jaw; may be epigastric. May be described as crushing, 'band like', 'like an elephant is sitting on my chest'. See Figure 25.21 for patterns of pain in myocardial infarction.
- Onset at rest or with exertion
- Persisting for longer than 15 minutes
- Sweating
- Pallor
- Shortness of breath
- Nausea and vomiting.

It is important to note that in certain patient groups, pain may be absent as a symptom. This is most likely in women, the elderly and patients with diabetes or hypertension.

Diagnosis and investigations A common phrase used with regards to acute myocardial infarction is 'time is myocardium'. The longer the diagnosis and subsequent treatment of the MI the more of the heart muscle dies and the greater the risk of death or long-term complications, such as heart failure. Therefore, the presenta-

tion of a patient with new chest pain is treated as a medical emergency and the patient is assumed to be suffering a myocardial infarction until proven otherwise.

The diagnosis is based on the taking an accurate patient history, including the patient's report of the current condition, past medical history and family history of heart disease. Specific investigations include:

- Cardiac enzymes – troponin I or troponin T and CK(MB). *Note*: Negative results from blood tests cannot be considered diagnostic for ruling out MI before 12 hours after the onset of pain
- Serial 12-lead ECGs. If the patient has presented very early after the onset of pain injury, patterns may not be obvious on the ECG and thus repeat ECGs are always taken if the first is not conclusive
- Plasma glucose and cholesterol tests are also recommended to assess for two of the risk factors of coronary heart disease (DH 2000).

Nursing care and management The initial management of the acute myocardial infarction is based on the acronym **MONA** (Resuscitation Council UK 2011):

M Monitor and morphine – Pain relief is paramount, current guidelines recommend the use of morphine (5–10 mg) or diamorphine (2.5–5 mg) titrated to pain. A popular method of titrating pain relief is to make a 10 mg dose of morphine in 10 mL of water for injection and administer the morphine in 1 mL (1 mg) increments until pain relief is achieved. The benefit of opiate pain relief is that it also acts to relieve anxiety in the patient. However, as opiates are associated with nausea and vomiting it is advisable to administer an anti-emetic at the same time (Steg *et al.* 2012). The patient is also attached to continuous cardiac monitoring as the risk of cardiac arrhythmias and even cardiac arrest are high.

O Oxygen – Oxygen should be given to patients who are short of breath, hypoxic or have heart failure. Whether oxygen should be administered to all patients suffering from acute myocardial infarction remains a matter of medical preference, as the evidence is not clear (Cabello *et al.* 2010).

N Nitrates – Some experts still recommend the use of sublingual nitrate spray in the patient suffering from myocardial infarction. If intravenous morphine is ineffective, then the recommendation is for the use of intravenous nitrates or beta-blocker drugs. Before the use of nitrates or beta blockers it is necessary to measure the patient's blood pressure as both nitrates and beta blockers can significantly reduce the blood pressure.

A Aspirin – Aspirin is an effective anti-platelet drug. In patients who are not already taking regular aspirin and are not allergic to aspirin, then the dose is 300 mg crushed and swallowed or chewed.

Patients suffering from an acute myocardial infarction will be maintained on bed rest to minimise cardiac work. Reassurance will be necessary for both the patient and relatives, as they will be anxious.

Definitive treatment of myocardial infarction is based on the restoration of blood flow to the myocardium. Previously, this was based on the use of thrombolytic therapy (otherwise known as fibrinolysis) to break up the blood clot. In the past 10+ years (since initial UK trials in 2003), there has been a growing use of primary angioplasty (also known as primary percutaneous coronary intervention – primary PCI). The patient has a catheter inserted through a hole made in the femoral artery and the catheter is manoeuvred to the artery, where the blockage is situated. A balloon is then passed through and inflated to push the thrombus into the walls of the artery and if necessary a metal cage (a stent) is inserted into the artery to keep the artery open (Figure 25.22).

Health promotion Health promotion is the same as that for angina in promoting healthy lifestyles and reducing risk factors for coronary heart disease. As with other patients suffering from cardiovascular diseases patients who are to begin exercise regimes should consult with their doctor.

Following myocardial infarction patients may need information and education to address misconceptions about cardiac disease (SIGN 2002).

Depending on the result of angiography or other testing if the patient has plaques in one or more arteries the patient may be referred for further angioplasty or CABG to help prevent further myocardial infarction and/or improve quality of life by improving myocardial oxygen supply and thus reducing symptoms of angina.

Discharge Patients should be referred to the hospital cardiac rehabilitation programme. Cardiac rehabilitation is a structured programme of exercise and health promotion carried out as a group activity under the supervision of a nurse or physiotherapist. The programme includes teaching sessions by dieticians and other health professionals.

Patients who have suffered a myocardial infarction will often have psychological needs (Mierzyńska *et al.* 2010) and may suffer from:

- Anxiety
- Sadness
- Depressed mood
- Anger
- Depression
- Exhaustion
- Social withdrawal.

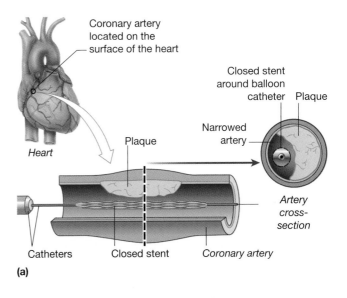

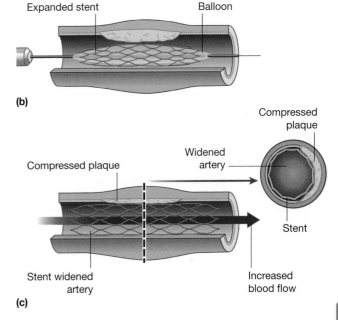

Figure 25.22 Coronary stent insertion.

Patients should be made aware of the availability of counselling therapies through their GP or may wish to access local support groups.

Return to work will be dependent on medical factors and the work that is undertaken and thus no single specific guideline can be formulated. In the majority of cases the patient may begin driving 4 weeks after the myocardial infarction so long as they have made a satisfactory recovery and they must inform their insurance company. Drivers of passenger carrying vehicles and light or heavy goods vehicles must contact the DVLA for further advice on returning to work. Patients wishing to travel on commercial airplanes as a passenger within four weeks of an MI should consult with their doctor and contact the airline and the travel insurance provider.

The Evidence

Antiplatelet treatment prevents the formation of blood clots (thrombi) by preventing platelet aggregation. Four main types of antiplatelet drugs are available:

- Aspirin – the most commonly used antiplatelet drug
- Clopidogrel and prasugrel
- Dipyridamole
- Glycoprotein IIb/IIIa inhibitors (abciximab, eptifibatide and tirofiban). They are given intravenously.

   The main indications for antiplatelet treatment are:

- To prevent further cardiovascular events in people who have had a myocardial infarction, ischaemic stroke or transient ischaemic attack.
- To prevent cardiovascular events: in people who are at high risk of ischaemic vascular disease; in people with established vascular disease (such as stable angina) who have not yet had a cardiovascular event; to prevent re-occlusion or re-stenosis after percutaneous interventions for coronary, carotid, or peripheral arterial disease.

   https://www.evidence.nhs.uk/topic/myocardial-infarction

Primary Care

When a patient has an MI, they report feelings of doom and boredom. Nurses need to take time to talk to their patient and relatives and alleviate the fears and anxieties they may have. Some of these fears and anxieties may include:

- Lack of self-confidence
- Frustration when unable to do what they previously managed
- Inability to return to normal life which they are accustomed to.

   Graduated physical activity should be encouraged to return to their normal ALs.

   Most patients should be able to resume driving 4–6 weeks after an uncomplicated MI and advise them to inform DVLA of their intentions.

   Occupational health and community nurses should be able to provide support for the patient and family throughout convalescence.

Pericarditis

Pericarditis is the inflammation of the pericardium and is a relatively common cause of chest pain.

Pathophysiology

Pericardial tissue damaged by bacteria or other mechanisms releases the chemical mediators of inflammation into the surrounding tissue, thus starting the inflammatory process. As inflammation becomes established, the pericardium will swell and friction occurs as the inflamed pericardial layers rub against each other.

Signs and symptoms

Chest pain is the primary presenting symptom:

- Progressive
- Frequently severe
- Sharp
- May radiate
- Worse when supine and relieved by sitting up/forward.

   Fever is possible but not always present.

Pericardial rub (a creaking or rustling sound that may be heard on auscultation of the heart) may be present but is relatively rarely heard as it is transient.

Diagnosis and investigations

- A 12-lead ECG – the ECG will often show changes similar to that of a myocardial infarction with some minor differences and are best reviewed by a cardiologist
- Troponin I or T may be raised
- Full blood count often shows an increased white cell count that is indicative of inflammation
- Raised serum CRP and ESR – indicative of inflammation
- Echocardiography may or may not be useful.

Nursing care and management

Most cases of pericarditis are self-limiting and respond quickly to non-steroidal anti-inflammatory drugs such as ibuprofen. Anxiety is often a problem and will increase the perception of pain and so the nurse should explain the diagnosis and give reassurance.

Health promotion and discharge

Patients who are being discharged following an episode of pericarditis usually require no specialist health promotion or discharge advice unless there is an underlying condition.

Disorders of the Cardiac Rhythm: Atrial Fibrillation

Atrial fibrillation is a common disorder of the cardiac rhythm.

Pathophysiology

Within the normal heart, the heart rhythm is regulated by the sino-atrial node, leading to a regular heartbeat. As noted earlier in the chapter, the impulse generated in the SA node is rapidly transmitted around the atria and both atria contract in an organised fashion. In atrial fibrillation there are multiple areas in the atrial wall creating electrical impulses and activating the cardiac muscle in their local area. Thus, the atrial myocardium no longer contracts in a coordinated fashion but 'fibrillates' – in essence viewed from the outside the atria look like jelly wobbling on a plate – and no coordinated contractions occur. This can lead to changes in blood pressure for several reasons:

- The loss of the 'atrial kick' means that the ventricles no longer receive that final third of the blood volume they would receive if the atria were working in a coordinated fashion. Thus the ventricles pump out less blood and cardiac output decreases
- The chaotic number of electrical impulses in the atria may mean that none are strong enough to activate the AV node and thus activate ventricular contraction. Cells lower in the conduction system of the heart will then take over but the rate of ventricular contraction will be lower (potentially falling as low as 20–30 beats per minute) and thus cardiac output falls
- In many cases of atrial fibrillation, the number of electrical impulses that are transmitted to the ventricles will be much higher than normal but also the transmission will be irregular leading to a rapid irregular heartbeat. If the heart beat is fast enough then the time the heart is in diastole will be shorter and thus ventricular filling will reduce and the volume of blood the ventricles will pump out will decrease thus reducing cardiac output.

The fact that the atria are fibrillating leads to blood pooling and mixing in the atria this can lead to the development of thrombi that may enter the circulation as emboli and being transported to the brain and causing a stroke.

There are several classifications of atrial fibrillation:

- Paroxysmal atrial fibrillation – this comes and goes and usually stops within 48 hours without any treatment but returns at varying intervals
- Persistent atrial fibrillation – this lasts for longer than 7 days (or less if it is treated)
- Long-standing persistent atrial fibrillation – this usually lasts for longer than a year despite treatment
- Permanent atrial fibrillation – this is present all the time and there are no more attempts made to treat it as it has proved to be resistant to treatment.

Signs and symptoms

The signs and symptoms of atrial fibrillation may include:

- Tiredness
- Shortness of breath
- Dizziness
- Fainting
- Palpitations
- Irregular pulse often with significant differences in pulse strength between beats (commonly this is rapid but may be very slow)
- Low blood pressure.

Diagnosis and investigations

- A 12-lead ECG – atrial fibrillation will show as an irregular ventricular activation (QRS wave) but there will be an absence of atrial waves (P wave). In patients with paroxysmal atrial fibrillation, it may be difficult to 'catch' the atrial fibrillation and therefore the patient may have a 24-hour ECG monitor attached in the outpatient department in an attempt to capture a recording of an episode of atrial fibrillation
- Echocardiography – transthoracic echocardiography (TTE) will be used to assess the function of the heart and the heart valves, this is a non-invasive test involving the use of a transducer placed on the chest wall

  Transoesophageal echocardiography (TOE) is a form of echocardiography where the transducer is passed down the patient's throat (in the same manner as endoscopy). The reason for TOE is to assess the atria for the presence of thrombi, which may not be seen by TTE.
- Chest X-ray – to assess for potential lung causes of atrial fibrillation
- Blood tests – especially to check for thyroid hormone levels and electrolyte levels in the blood.

Nursing care and management

Treatment of atrial fibrillation is based on three main components:

- **Rate control** – This is usually achieved by the use of medicines. The most common drug used in the treatment of atrial fibrillation is amiodarone. Traditionally, digoxin was prescribed but has increasingly fallen out of use. If patients are administered intravenous amiodarone then the prescription must be followed closely. The dose is administered in two separate infusions. The first infusion is given over 20–60 minutes and the second over 23 hours. **Under no circumstances should amiodarone be administered as a bolus or rapid infusion except to patients in cardiac arrest as rapid administration can cause cardiovascular collapse**. Patients receiving long-term amiodarone therapy (that is taking amiodarone tablets) should be warned that the drug can cause changes in skin colour and that they must avoid exposing their skin to the sun.

  Digoxin is less commonly used for atrial fibrillation but if it is prescribed, then it should not be administered to patients with a heart rate of less than 60 beats per minute. Patients should be warned to report episodes of vomiting and/or diarrhoea and episodes of dizziness or blurred vision, as these may be symptoms of digoxin toxicity.
- **Anticoagulation** – As noted, atrial fibrillation is a high risk for causing a stroke and thus patients with atrial fibrillation are prescribed warfarin. Patients prescribed warfarin will require education for the purpose of the anticoagulation and the importance of regular monitoring of their clotting by blood test. It is also vital that patients are educated to always take their warfarin at the same time every day, not to miss doses or adjust the dose except on medical advice, to avoid alcohol except in moderation and not to drink cranberry juice, as alcohol and cranberry juice can affect the anticoagulant effects of warfarin. Patients should be informed to report unusual levels of bruising or bleeding, blackened stools, rashes or hair loss to their doctor.
- **Cardioversion** – Cardioversion is the restoration of the heart rhythm to normal. It can be attempted by drug therapy (such as amiodarone) or by electrical shock under sedation. The majority of electrical cardioversions are undertaken as an elective procedure as a day case patient and the patient should be treated as a surgical patient, including being nil by mouth, according to protocol. Emergency cardioversion may be carried out on patients who are haemodynamically compromised (for instance a systolic blood pressure below 90 mmHg).

Health promotion and discharge

Health promotion and discharge advice will be dictated by the underlying cause of the atrial fibrillation (if known) and advice on medications, as detailed above.

 Link To/Go To

Patients with atrial fibrillation should be made aware of the support groups: the AF Association (**http://www.atrialfibrillation.org.uk/**) and the Arrhythmia Alliance (**http://www.heartrhythmcharity.org.uk/**).

Heart Failure

Heart failure is a syndrome characterised by an inability of the heart to pump blood around the body at a sufficient pressure. Heart failure can be acute or chronic and right-sided, left-sided or bilateral.

Heart failure is also known as:

- Congestive cardiac failure (CCF) – right-sided heart failure
- Congestive heart failure (CHF) – right-sided heart failure
- Left ventricular failure – left-sided heart failure

Risk factors for heart failure include:

- Age
- Sex

- Hypertension
- Coronary heart disease
- Diabetes
- Excess alcohol use.

Pathophysiology

The pathophysiology of heart failure is complex and remains the subject of much research.

Heart failure can be roughly categorised into three categories:

- Heart failure due to **left ventricular systolic dysfunction (LVSD)** – the part of the heart that pumps blood around the body (the left ventricle) becomes weak – most commonly caused by coronary heart disease, especially myocardial infarction
- Heart failure with **preserved ejection fraction (HFPEF)** – usually due to the left ventricle becoming stiff, leading to difficulty in filling with blood reducing the volume available to pump out and thus reducing the cardiac output
- Heart failure due to **valve disease**.

The cause of the heart failure is important, as it affects treatment choices.

As the heart begins to fail and cardiac output is reduced, there is a reduction in blood pressure; in compensation, several mechanisms become active:

- Sympathetic nervous system
- Hormonal outflow (such as adrenaline)
- Renin-angiotensin-aldosterone system.

This leads to an increase in total peripheral resistance, which has the short-term effect of increasing tissue perfusion but has the effect on increasing afterload and the work the failing ventricle has to do, thus exacerbating the original problem.

Signs and symptoms

Some of the signs and symptoms of heart failure can be seen in Figure 25.23 and include:

- **Shortness of breath** – As the failing left ventricle is unable to empty completely, there is an increase in the left ventricular pressure at the end of diastole (LVEDP). As this pressure increases the pressure within the pulmonary veins (supplying the left atrium) increases leading eventually to pulmonary oedema. The patient will be short of breath on exertion in the beginning but as the heart failure progresses shortness of breath at rest will also develop. Orthopnoea may also be present (usually first noted at night). As the patient lies down there is an increase in venous return thus leading to an increase in left ventricular pressure and an exacerbation of the symptoms.

Jot This Down

Orthopnoea is traditionally measured in 'pillows'. That is the doctor will ask (and record) how many pillows the patient requires to sleep at night. As the shortness of breath increases the patient will require more and more pillows to sleep at night, as they gradually have to lie more and more at an angle. Eventually, patients may end up sleeping upright in a chair.

As the pulmonary oedema progresses, the patient will develop a cough and produce white frothy sputum.

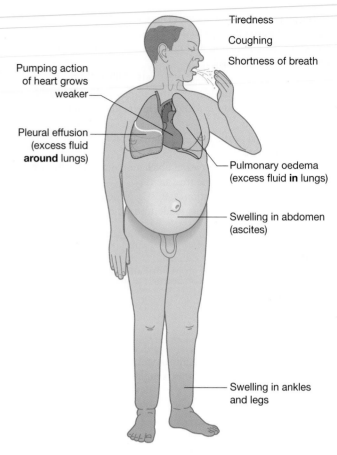

Figure 25.23 **Signs and symptoms of heart failure.**

- **Oedema** – Patients with right-sided heart failure (right ventricular failure) can develop oedema of the tissues supplied by the systemic circulation. These patients may show oedema of:
  - Legs – usually starting with foot or ankle oedema but potentially eventually leading to gross oedema of the legs
  - Sacrum
  - Abdomen (ascites)
  - Liver – oedema of the liver may lead to jaundice.

Red Flag

 Patients with oedema may have impaired drug metabolism and thus caution should be used in both the prescribing and administration of any medication that is metabolised by the liver as the half-life may be prolonged and blood levels may rise to toxic levels. Monitor patients with liver oedema closely for the known side-effects of any administered medication.

- **Anorexia** – Intestinal oedema may result from severe heart failure leading to reduced peristalsis and malabsorption of nutrients. Patients with liver failure may feel bloated and nauseas. Appetite and food intake decreases and muscle wastage occurs
- **Fatigue and lethargy** – A large proportion of patients with heart failure experience fatigue and lethargy. This may result from shortness of breath, poor tissue perfusion, muscle wasting, poor nutrition and a lack of sleep as a result of orthopnoea.

Diagnosis and investigations

Heart failure is diagnosed when:

- *There are symptoms of heart failure (at rest or on exertion)*
- *There is objective evidence of cardiac dysfunction*
- *There is a response to treatment for heart failure.*

(McMurray et al. 2012)

For heart failure to be diagnosed at least point one and point two must be met as the signs and symptoms of other disease processes (such as pulmonary disease) can be similar to the early stages of heart failure.

The severity of heart failure can be classified using several systems, however the most commonly used is the New York Heart Association (NYHA) Functional Classification:

- Class I (Mild): *No limitation of physical activity. Ordinary physical activity does not cause undue fatigue, palpitation, or dyspnoea (shortness of breath). Essentially well-treated heart failure*
- Class II (Mild): *Slight limitation of physical activity. Comfortable at rest, but ordinary physical activity results in fatigue, palpitation or dyspnoea*
- Class III (Moderate): *Marked limitation of physical activity. Comfortable at rest, but less than ordinary activity causes fatigue, palpitation or dyspnoea*
- Class IV (Severe): *Unable to carry out any physical activity without discomfort. Symptoms of cardiac failure at rest. Patient is essentially housebound.*

(Mosterd & Hoes 2007)

The tests and investigations undertaken include:

- Echocardiography, to assess the heart function and the heart valves
- Blood tests for:
  - Electrolytes
  - Albumin
  - Creatinine
  - BNP (B-type natriuretic peptide)
- A 12-lead ECG to assess for heart disease
- Cardiac catheterisation to assess for heart disease and to assess heart function
- Chest X-ray to assess the heart size and for signs of pulmonary oedema
- Exercise tolerance test to assess for heart disease and exercise ability.

Nursing care and management

Treatment of heart failure includes the administration of medications, such as diuretics, ACE inhibitors and beta blockers.

Patients who are hospitalised with severe heart failure may require treatment with inotropic sympathomimetics, such as dopamine or dobutamine. These drugs create the same response as sympathetic nervous system activation, thus increasing the force of contraction of the ventricles and increasing heart rate. Patients receiving these drugs should be nursed in a high dependency unit or CCU and will require continuous cardiac monitoring and hourly blood pressure measurement.

In addition, the patient will be administered diuretic therapy and may be placed on a fluid restriction. Strict fluid balance monitoring will be required.

Patients should be nursed upright or semi-recumbent (at the angle the patient finds most comfortable) and oxygen therapy administered, as prescribed. The combination of shortness of breath (including rapid mouth breathing) and oxygen therapy will result in a dry mouth and regular mouth care should be offered, as well as humidified oxygen.

Peripheral oedema along with shortness of breath and lethargy increase the risk of pressure sores and pressure area care is essential.

Referral to members of the multidisciplinary team will be required, such as the dietician, physiotherapist and occupational therapist.

Heart failure has a worse prognosis than most cancers and in end stage heart failure referral to palliative care should be made a priority (NICE 2010).

Health promotion

Patients with heart failure should be given advice on:

- Smoking cessation
- Abstaining from alcohol
- Reducing salt intake
- Having a yearly flu vaccination and pneumonia vaccination.
- Exercise and rehabilitation
- Medication compliance.

Discharge and community care

Patients with heart failure in the community cannot be asked to monitor their fluid balance. However, daily weights have proven to be an effective method of monitoring fluid retention in heart failure, as weight gain or loss on a daily basis is almost always a reflection of alterations of fluid levels in the body. Patients should be advised to:

- Always use the same scales
- Always wear the same things (or be naked)
- Weigh yourself first thing in a morning after going to the toilet but before having anything to eat or drink
- Record the weight in a diary for the doctor to review.

In some circumstances, patient's weight may be monitored remotely using telemonitoring. The scales are connected to the internet and the daily weight is recorded in a centralised database, monitored by healthcare staff (Riley & Cowie 2009).

Increasingly, evidence has shown that the use of specialist heart failure nurses in the community have improved the community management of heart failure and helped to prevent multiple readmissions (Grange 2005).

Hypertension

Hypertension (commonly known as high blood pressure) is often unnoticed by the patient but is a risk factor for many other cardiovascular conditions and for that reason, it is often referred to as the 'silent killer'.

Hypertension is a risk factor for:

- Coronary heart disease
- Stroke
- Renal disease
- Aortic aneurysm
- Heart failure.

Pathophysiology

Hypertension is categorised as either primary or secondary hypertension.

- **Primary** hypertension –is hypertension without a known medical cause and is the most common form of hypertension

- **Secondary** hypertension – is hypertension with a known medical cause, such as renal disease and certain types of tumour.

Current evidence for the pathophysiology of primary hypertension is complex and involves many physiological systems and processes, including the renin angiotensin aldosterone system, endothelial function and the autonomic nervous system.

Signs and symptoms

Hypertension rarely causes any symptoms, except in rare cases of extremely high blood pressure, which can cause headache, nose bleed and blurred or double vision.

Diagnosis and investigations

The diagnosis of hypertension is based on a series of blood pressure readings and is never based on a single reading. Current guidance suggests that a repeated blood pressure over 140/90 mmHg should be followed-up by ambulatory blood pressure monitoring (a 24-hour automated blood pressure monitor that allows the patient to continue with their everyday activities) to confirm the hypertension and rule out the possibility of 'white coat hypertension' (that is transient blood pressure elevation due to the anxiety of being in a healthcare facility). Alternatively, home blood pressure measurement may be used based on an accredited automated blood pressure monitor the patient can use twice a day for 7 days at home (NICE 2011).

Hypertension is graded into stages:
- *Stage 1 hypertension*: blood pressure of 140/90 mmHg or greater
- *Stage 2 hypertension*: blood pressure of 160/100 mmHg or greater
- *Severe hypertension*: systolic blood pressure of 180 mmHg or higher **or** a diastolic blood pressure of 110 mmHg or higher.

Further tests are undertaken to assess cardiovascular risk factors or secondary causes of hypertension:
- Urine dipstick for blood and protein
- Blood electrolytes and creatinine and eGFR (estimated glomerular filtration rate – a measure of renal function)
- Blood glucose
- Serum cholesterol
- 12-lead ECG.

Nursing care and management

Hypertension is managed almost exclusively in primary care and the outpatient department.

Treatment for hypertension is always based on health promotion (below) and normally, treatment with medication, such as calcium channel blockers, beta-blockers, diuretics or ACE inhibitors.

 Link To/Go To

The latest guidelines for medical treatment of hypertension can be found on the British Hypertension Society Website: http://www.bhsoc.org/

Health promotion

Health promotion for hypertensive patients includes:
- Losing weight if required
- Exercising regularly
- Eating a healthy diet

- Cutting down on alcohol
- Stopping smoking
- Cutting down on salt and caffeine.

Abdominal Aortic Aneurysm

An aneurysm is a localised dilation of a blood vessel; the most common place for an aneurysm to develop is in the abdominal aorta.

Aortic abdominal aneurysms (AAA) are much more common in men and the incidence increases with age (especially in patients with peripheral vascular disease).

Epidemiology

The risk factors for aortic aneurysm development are:
- Smoking
- Family history of aortic aneurysm
- High blood pressure
- High cholesterol
- Atherosclerosis
- Inherited conditions such as Marfan's syndrome
- Trauma.

Pathophysiology

The underlying pathophysiology for aortic aneurysm is unclear, while aneurysm formation is commonly associated with atherosclerotic disease, it appears that the underlying disease process may be different and atherosclerosis develops after other changes in the wall of the aorta or there may be a combination of atherosclerosis and other processes (Golledge & Norman 2010).

Regardless of the underlying processes, the result is a dilation of the aorta involving the entire aortic wall (Figure 25.24).

In most cases, the patient will not be aware of the aneurysm but in the event of the aneurysm rupturing, the mortality rate is over 80%.

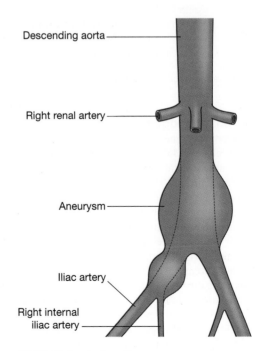

Descending aorta

Right renal artery

Aneurysm

Iliac artery

Right internal iliac artery

Figure 25.24 Abdominal aortic aneurysm.

Signs and symptoms

Most patients will not be aware of the fact they have an AAA, as there are often no sign or symptoms. If the aneurysm does become large enough to press on the nearby structures, the patient may be aware of mild abdominal and/or back pain but there are many causes of mild abdominal or back pain and therefore, help is rarely sought. In the event of a rupture, the patient will collapse with intense abdominal and/or back pain and will rapidly go into shock due to blood loss.

Diagnosis and investigations

Generally, AAAs are diagnosed during the assessment of the patient for other reasons, although there is now an NHS screening programme, which invites men for screening the year they turn 65 years of age.

Link To/Go To

For more information about AAA, go to: **http://aaa.screening.nhs.uk/**

Investigations for AAA include:

- Abdominal ultrasound
- CT scan.

Nursing care and management

Treatment of an AAA depends on its size; small AAAs tend to be managed medically with risk factor control and monitored regularly. Larger AAAs (those at a much higher risk of rupture) are treated surgically by:

- Open surgical approach – a traditional large incision is made into the abdomen, the dilated aorta removed and replaced with a synthetic graft. In most cases the graft will last the rest of the patient's life. The downside to this form of surgery is that it can be difficult in patients who have multiple risk factors, making surgery under general anaesthetic high risk.
- Endovascular graft placement. This is the placement of a tube-shaped graft within the aorta by using a similar method to angioplasty. The graft is mounted on a balloon and inserted into the aorta on a catheter via the large arteries. Once in place, the balloon is inflated and the graft is expanded into place. Not every patient is suitable for endovascular placement of their graft and the decision is based on factors, such as the size and location of the aneurysm.

Following traditional repair of an AAA, the patient should be nursed as per standard postoperative care (see Chapter 14), but most patients will be transferred to ICU immediately after theatre, as a period of support for the heart may be required after surgery (Bick 2000). Patients will require monitoring for shock (in the case of the graft leaking), a sudden reduction in renal output or limb ischaemia (due to the development of emboli) and paralytic ileus. Most patients will return to the general ward within 24–48 hours. Following endovascular repair, the puncture wound must be monitored for bleeding/haematoma formation. The potential risks include damage to the iliac arteries, stent migration within the aorta or bleeding around an undersized stent.

Health promotion and discharge

Health promotion and discharge advice for the patient following AAA repair includes:

- Healthy diet
- Exercise
- Lose weight
- Stop smoking
- If the patient has hypertension, diabetes or high cholesterol then advice should be given specific to those conditions
- May be required to take aspirin to prevent clot forming.

Peripheral Artery Disease

Peripheral artery disease can affect any of the limbs but is most common in the legs. For that reason, this section only discusses peripheral artery disease in the legs. It is also known as 'peripheral vascular disease'.

Pathophysiology

Peripheral artery disease is caused by the same underlying processes of atherosclerosis as coronary heart disease but affects the arteries of the legs. The risk factors for peripheral artery disease are the same as those for coronary artery disease.

Signs and symptoms

In many cases, peripheral artery disease will not create any symptoms but in others, it will lead to intermittent claudication. Intermittent claudication is a cramp-like pain felt in the calf, thigh or buttock during walking or other exercise. It is caused by lack of oxygen to the muscles because of a poor blood supply and is relieved by rest.

Diagnosis and investigations

Examination of the lower limbs:

- The affected leg may be pale and cold, with a loss of hair and with skin changes (for instance the skin may look 'shiny')
- The feet may be cold, pale or mottled and there may be evidence ulceration
- There may be poorly healing wounds of the extremities
- Patients with severe peripheral artery disease or critical lower-limb ischaemia may have ulceration or gangrene
- Palpation of the femoral, popliteal, dorsalis pedis and posterior tibial pulses may reveal weak or absent pulses.

Investigations include:

- Doppler ultrasound of the arteries
- Angiogram.

Nursing care and management

Treatment of peripheral artery disease can be:

- Medical – for less severe disease, treatment may rely on the reduction of risk factors and the use of medication to relieve symptoms (such as peripheral vasodilators)
- Angioplasty – the same treatment as used for coronary heart disease but in the peripheral arteries
- Bypass surgery. This involves the use of veins harvested from the patient's leg to use as conduits to bypass the narrowed section of arteries.

Nursing care will depend on the treatment option undertaken but after angioplasty or bypass surgery, great care must be made to assess and record limb colour, temperature and pulses, as thrombi and emboli are a risk to the patient's limb. The poor tissue viability of the leg presents a particular risk for the development of pressure sores.

Health promotion and discharge

The health promotion and discharge advice for patients who have peripheral vascular disease is the same as for all other conditions, based on underlying atherosclerosis with exercise being especially important.

Venous Insufficiency

Venous insufficiency is a condition in which the flow of blood through the veins is impaired. The most common manifestation of venous insufficiency is **varicose veins** but as the condition progresses venous ulcers may develop.

Pathophysiology

The pathophysiology of venous insufficiency is commonly based on venous hypertension due to two factors:

- **Incompetent valves** in the veins leading to increased pressure due to backwards flow of blood
- **Venous obstruction** due to thrombi (often developing on the valves).

The effect of obesity and lack of exercise on venous return have also been raised as potential contributing factors (Bergan *et al.* 2006).

Signs and symptoms

- Dull aching, heaviness or cramping in the legs
- Itching and tingling skin on the legs
- Aching, burning or throbbing sensations in the legs that gets worse when standing
- Pain that gets better when legs are raised
- Swelling of the legs

People with chronic venous insufficiency may also have:

- Redness of the legs and ankles
- Skin colour changes around the ankles
- Varicose veins on the surface (superficial)
- Thickening and hardening of the skin on the legs and ankles (lipodermatosclerosis)
- Ulcers on the legs and ankles.

If the venous insufficiency becomes chronic, then the patient may develop **venous eczema** (red, scaly, flaky and itchy skin) and finally **venous ulcers**.

Venous ulcers are the final stage of skin breakdown due to venous insufficiency, as the pressure in the veins increases fluid leaks into the tissue and the skin leading to swelling and eventually the skin breaking down.

Diagnosis and investigations

In most cases, history-taking and a physical examination are sufficient to diagnose venous insufficiency. Duplex scanning can be carried out to assess venous hypertension (and has mostly replaced the use of tourniquet tests) and ankle brachial pressure index (ABPI) using Doppler will help to rule out arterial disease.

Chronic venous insufficiency is categorised according to the CEAP classification system (Eberhardt & Raffetto 2005).

Investigations of a venous ulcer include:

- Measurement of ankle brachial pressure index (ABPI) using Doppler

- Measurement of the surface area of the ulcer – this helps in assessing healing
- Swabs for microbiology culture and sensitivity testing – only where there are signs of infection
- Biopsy – especially if the ulcer has an unusual appearance or fails to heal after 12 weeks.

Nursing care and management

The treatment for venous insufficiency will depend on the manifestations of the condition.

The most common form of treatment is compression stockings; patients may also be advised to elevate their legs when resting to aid venous return, to take daily exercise and to lose weight. If there is a background of thrombus development, then the patient may also be commenced on anticoagulants.

Varicose veins can be surgically removed (stripped) from the leg.

Venous eczema is treated with:

- Compression stockings to treat the underlying venous insufficiency
- Moisturising creams to rehydrate the dry, itchy, skin
- Corticosteroid creams are used to treat severe cases.

Venous leg ulcers Much of the care of venous leg ulcers is carried out in the primary care setting and includes:

- Graduated, multi-layer, compression – before this treatment is tried, diabetes, neuropathy and peripheral vascular disease should be excluded and any pre-existing swelling controlled by bed rest or elevation. The treatment involves applying bandages to the leg, maximising the pressure at the ankle and reducing the pressure as the bandages go higher up the leg.

Red Flag

 At 24–48 hours after the initiation of compression therapy, the patient's skin must be assessed for potential complications (SIGN 2010)

- Debridement and cleaning – adherent slough should be debrided and any trapped pus released
- Dressing – the treatment of choice for most vascular ulcers is a simple non-adherent dressing as there is insufficient evidence for the use of any other dressing (SIGN 2010)
- Antibiotics are only indicated in proven (clinically significant) infection
- Pain relief may be required.

Health promotion and discharge

Prior to discharge, nurses should encourage the patient to discuss any fears and anxieties he/she may have about coping in the community. Encourage the importance of taking all the medications prescribed and if they experience any unwanted side-effects to see their GP immediately.

- Use compression stockings during waking hours to decrease swelling. The stockings are available on prescription and a new pair will be required every 3–6 months
- Shower normally and use emollients to moisturise the skin

- Avoid long periods of sitting or standing. Even moving your legs slightly will help the blood in your veins return to your heart. Preferably begin some form of exercise
- Elevate the legs when resting to promote venous return
- Care for wounds if you have any open sores or infections
- Patients should be made aware of the Lindsay Leg Club Foundation (**http://www.legclub.org/**) if one is available in their area
- Stop smoking. Smoking damages the circulation.

Conclusion

This chapter has reviewed the anatomy and physiology of the cardiovascular system including:

- The heart
- The arterial system
- The venous system
- The special circulation for the heart muscle.

It then moved on to explore the examination of the cardiovascular system and address a few of the many conditions that may affect the heart or the vascular system.

The cardiovascular system is responsible for the transportation and delivery of oxygen and nutrients to the tissues via the blood and the removal of waste products from the tissues. The system relies on a central pump, the heart, which can be divided into two systems:

- Right heart pump, which circulates blood around the pulmonary circulation (the lungs)
- Left heart pump, which circulates blood around the systemic circulation (the rest of the body)

A disorder of either of these two pumps may be caused by conditions such as myocardial infarction and lead to the development of oedema in the lungs or the rest of the body.

The blood flow through the body is via tubes called arteries, arterioles veins and venules.

- Arteries and arterioles channel blood away from the heart to the lungs or the systemic circulation
- Veins and venules channel blood back to the heart.

Capillaries are the vessels that allow for the passage of oxygen and nutrients into the tissues.

Nursing patients with a cardiovascular disorder requires the nurse to be able to undertake a thorough physical assessment of the patient's circulatory system, to recognise the signs and symptoms of different disorders and to promote health by guided education.

Key Points

- The cardiovascular system is complex and interconnected and, particularly disorders of the heart will manifest in signs and symptoms in the circulatory system.
- Examination of the cardiovascular system requires both physical assessment skills and the ability to take a focussed history from the patient.
- In myocardial infarction. time is critical but the nurse should remain calm so as not to unduly distress the patient.
- Initial treatment for patients with acute cardiac pain is MONA.

- Patients with a disorder of the heart are often anxious and require psychological support and reassurance.
- Health promotion for patients with a cardiovascular disorder is often based on reducing modifiable risk factors, such as diet, exercise and smoking.
- There are many support groups available nationally for patients with a variety of cardiovascular disorders.

Glossary

Action potential: momentary change in the electrical status of a cell wall

Angiogram: a radiographic imaging test of part of a vascular system using radio-opaque dye

Angioplasty: mechanically widening a restriction in a blood vessel

Aorta: main artery leading from the left ventricle

Aortic valve: valve that lies between the left ventricle and the aorta

Arterial: pertaining to the arteries

Atria: upper chambers of the heart (singular = atrium)

Atrioventricular bundle: bundle of conductive nerve fibres that transmit action potentials from the AV node to the ventricular conduction system. Otherwise known as the bundle of His

Atrioventricular node: otherwise known as the AV node. Specialised area of cardiac cells located just above the point where the right atrium and right ventricle meets

Atrioventricular valve: collective name for the two valves that lie between the atria and the ventricles (bicuspid and tricuspid)

Bicuspid valve: the atrioventricular valve that lies between the left atrium and the left ventricle. Also known as the mitral valve

Bundle of his: see atrioventricular bundle

CABG: coronary artery bypass grafting. A surgical procedure using blood vessels harvested from the patient to bypass narrowing in their coronary arteries

Cardiac output: the amount of blood pumped out by a ventricle in mL per minute

Depolarisation: change in the electrical state across a cell membrane leading to the activation of that cell

Diastole: the relaxation of a heart chamber (atrium or ventricle)

Endocardium: innermost layer that lines the chambers of the heart and also lines the cardiac valves

Hormone: chemical substance that is released into the blood, by the endocrine system, and has a physiological control over the function of cells or organs other than those that created it

Inferior vena cava: large vein that returns blood to the right atrium from the lower parts of the body

LVEDP: left ventricular end diastolic pressure

Mitral valve: see bicuspid valve

Myocardium: muscle layer of the heart

Myocyte: cardiac muscle cell

Orthopnoea: shortness of breath when lying flat

PCI: percutaneous coronary intervention. Angioplasty of a coronary artery following insertion of a catheter through a major artery (usually in the leg) to access the coronary arterial system

Pericardium: double layer sac that surrounds the heart

(Continued)

Pulmonary circulation: circulatory system of the lungs

Pulmonary valve: valve that lies between the right ventricle and the pulmonary circulation

Purkinje fibres: specialised conductive fibres that rapidly transport action potentials through the ventricle walls

Repolarisation: a return of the electrical state across a cell membrane to the resting state

Semilunar valves: the valves that lie between the ventricles and the pulmonary or systemic circulation (aortic valve and pulmonary valve)

Septum: a dividing wall

Sinoatrial node: otherwise known as the SA node. Specialised area of cardiac cells located in the upper part of the right atrium – usually referred to as the pacemaker of the heart

Stenosis: abnormal narrowing of a tube

Stroke volume: the amount of blood ejected by a ventricle in one beat

Superior vena cava: the large vein that returns blood to the right atrium from the upper part of the body

Systemic circulation: the circulatory system of the body (excluding the lungs)

Systole: the contraction of a heart chamber (atrium or ventricle)

Tricuspid valve: the atrioventricular valve that lies between the right atrium and ventricle

Venous: pertaining to the veins

Ventricles: the large lower chambers of the heart

References

Bergan, J.J., Schmid-Schönbein, G.W., Smith, P.D.C., Nicolaides, A.N., Boisseau, M.R. & Eklof, B. (2006) Chronic venous disease. *New England Journal of Medicine*, 355(5), 488–498.

Bick, C. (2000) Abdominal aortic aneurysm repair. *Nursing Standard*, 15(3), 47–52.

Cabello, J.B., Burls, A., Emparanza, J.I., Bayliss, S. & Quinn, T. (2010) Oxygen therapy for acute myocardial infarction. *Cochrane Database Systematic Reviews*, (6):CD007160.

Dalteg, T., Benzein, E., Fridlund, B. & Malm, D. (2011) Cardiac disease and its consequences on the partner relationship: a systematic review. *European Journal of Cardiovascular Nursing*, 10(3), 140–149.

DH (2000) *National Service Framework for Coronary Heart Disease*. Department of Health, London.

Eberhardt, R.T. & Raffetto, J.D. (2005). Chronic venous insufficiency. *Circulation*, 111(18), 2398–2409.

Golledge, J. & Norman, P.E. (2010) Atherosclerosis and abdominal aortic aneurysm cause, response, or common risk factors? *Arteriosclerosis, Thrombosis, and Vascular Biology*, 30(6), 1075–1077.

Grange, J. (2005). The role of nurses in the management of heart failure. *Heart*, 91(Suppl 2), ii39–ii42.

Hill, J. & Timmis, H. (2002) ABC of clinical electrocardiography: Exercise tolerance testing. *British Medical Journal*, 324, 1084–1087.

Jha, P., Ramasundarahettige, C., Landsman, V. *et al.* (2013) 21st-century hazards of smoking and benefits of cessation in the United States. *New England Journal of Medicine*, 368(4), 341–350.

Marchant, B., Donaldson, G., Mridha, K., Scarborough, M. & Timmis, A.D. (1994) Mechanisms of cold intolerances in patients with angina. *Journal of the American College of Cardiology*, 23(3), 630–636.

McMurray, J.J., Adamopoulos, S., Anker, S.D. *et al.* (2012) ESC Guidelines for the diagnosis and treatment of acute and chronic heart failure 2012 The Task Force for the Diagnosis and Treatment of Acute and Chronic Heart Failure 2012 of the European Society of Cardiology. Developed in collaboration with the Heart Failure Association (HFA) of the ESC. *European Heart Journal*, 33(14), 1787–1847.

Mierzyńska, A., Kowalska, M., Stepnowska, M. & Piotrowicz, R. (2010) Psychological support for patients following myocardial infarction. *Cardiology Journal*, 17(3), 319–324.

Mosterd, A. & Hoes, A.W. (2007) Clinical epidemiology of heart failure. *Heart*, 93(9), 1137–1146.

NICE (2010) *Clinical Guideline 108: Chronic heart failure: management of chronic heart failure in adults in primary and secondary care*. National Institute for Health and Clinical Excellence, London.

NICE (2011) *Clinical Guideline 127. Hypertension: Clinical management of primary hypertension in adults*. National Institute for Health and Clinical Excellence, London.

NICE (2012) *Clinical Guideline 126. Management of Stable Angina*. National Institute for Health and Clinical Excellence, London.

Resuscitation Council (UK) (2011) *Advanced Life Support Manual*, 6th edn. Resuscitation Council (UK), London.

Riley, J.P. & Cowie, M.R. (2009) Telemonitoring in heart failure. *Heart*, 95(23), 1964–1968.

SIGN (2002) *SIGN Guideline 57. Cardiac Rehabilitation*. Scottish Intercollegiate Guideline Network, Edinburgh.

SIGN (2010) *SIGN Guideline 120. Management of Chronic Venous Leg Ulcers*. Scottish Intercollegiate Guidelines Network, Edinburgh.

Steg, P.G., James, S.K., Atar, D. *et al.* (2012) ESC Guidelines for the management of acute myocardial infarction in patients presenting with ST-segment elevation The Task Force on the management of ST-segment elevation acute myocardial infarction of the European Society of Cardiology (ESC). *European Heart Journal*, 33(20), 2569–2619.

Test Yourself

1. Normal electrical conduction in the heart begins with impulse generation in the:
   (a) Atrioventricular node
   (b) Sinoatrial node
   (c) Purkinje fibres
   (d) Bundle of His

2. The P wave on an ECG trace is related to:
   (a) Atrial contraction
   (b) Atrial repolarisation
   (c) Atrial depolarisation
   (d) Atrial relaxation

3. Afterload refers to:
   (a) The pressure in the arteries that the ventricles must overcome
   (b) The pressure in the veins that the arteries must overcome
   (c) The pressure in the atria that the veins must overcome
   (d) The pressure in the ventricles the atria must overcome

4. The difference in pressure between the systolic and diastolic pressure is known as:
   (a) Push pressure
   (b) Width pressure
   (c) Pulse pressure
   (d) Hydrostatic pressure

5. Syncope means:
   (a) Shortness of breath
   (b) Pounding feeling in the chest
   (c) Irregular heart beat
   (d) Fainting

6. When assessing the cardiovascular system it is normal to start with:
   (a) The femoral pulse
   (b) The brachial pulse
   (c) The carotid pulse
   (d) The radial pulse

7. When taking a blood pressure, the point where the tapping sound disappears is known as:
   (a) The third Korotkoff sound
   (b) The fourth Korotkoff sound
   (c) The fifth Korotkoff sound
   (d) The sixth Korotkoff sound

8. Patients with known angina should be advised to call an ambulance if the pain does not go away after rest, GTN and:
   (a) 10 minutes
   (b) 20 minutes
   (c) 30 minutes
   (d) 40 minutes

9. Atrial fibrillation that comes and goes is known as:
   (a) Permanent
   (b) Persistent
   (c) Paroxysmal
   (d) Long-standing

10. NHS screening for AAA in men is offered at the age of:
    (a) 55
    (b) 60
    (c) 65
    (d) 70

Answers

1. b
2. c
3. a
4. c

5. d
6. d
7. c
8. a
9. c
10. c

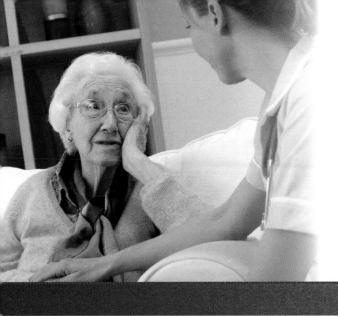

26

The Person with a Haematological Disorder

Louise McErlean

University of Hertfordshire, UK

Learning Outcomes

On completion of this chapter you will be able to:

- Describe the functions of blood
- Explore the pathophysiology of commonly occurring haematological conditions
- Discuss the red blood cell, white blood cells and platelet disorders
- Discuss the diagnostic investigations associated with these conditions
- Analyse the nursing care associated with each haematological condition
- Discuss the medication and treatment associated with each haematological condition

Competencies

All nurses must:

1. Assess, monitor, document and deliver care for patients with haematological disorders
2. Using evidence-based practice, identify and prioritise nursing care for the patient with haematological disorders
3. Safely administer treatment prescribed for patients with haematological disorders
4. Work in a collaborative way with the multidisciplinary team to plan and to provide coordinated effective care
5. Assess functional health status for patients with haematological disorders
6. Where necessary, provide health promotion to patients with haematological disorders

 Visit the companion website at **www.wileynursingpractice.com** where you can test yourself using flashcards, multiple-choice questions and more.

Nursing Practice: Knowledge and Care, First Edition. Edited by Ian Peate, Karen Wild and Muralitharan Nair.
© 2014 John Wiley & Sons, Ltd. Published 2014 by John Wiley & Sons, Ltd. Companion website: www.wileynursingpractice.com

Introduction

Blood is a fluid connective tissue. Its constant flow provides the cells of the body with a transport medium for many essential nutrients, gases, hormones and waste products. Its essential functions cannot be underestimated. Therefore conditions affecting the blood can have wide-reaching consequences with symptoms, which can range from being mild to extremely serious for the affected person.

Blood is more viscous than water; it is slightly warmer than body temperature at 38°Celcius and has a normal pH of 7.35–7.45 in health. There is approximately 5–6 litres of blood circulating in the average male and 4–5 litres in the average female (Marieb & Hoehn 2013).

Blood has three main functions:

1. **Protection** – the action of the white cells protects the body from invading pathogens; the action of the platelets protects the body from bleeding during trauma
2. **Distribution** – oxygen, nutrients and hormones are transported in the blood to where they are required. Waste products are transported to their destination for disposal
3. **Regulation** – the presence of the plasma proteins helps to maintain fluid balance, absorbing heat produced by the body and transporting it to the surface of the body for heat loss. Blood proteins and solutes dissolved in the blood act as buffers and therefore have a role in maintaining the pH of blood. (Marieb & Hoehn 2013)

Composition of Blood

Blood can be divided into the blood plasma and the formed elements (Figure 26.1).

Plasma is a straw coloured fluid that contains many dissolved substances, such as gases, hormones, waste products, nutrients, inorganic salts and enzymes. It also contains the plasma proteins. The plasma proteins have a role in maintaining the osmotic pressure of the blood and this is important as a reduced osmotic pressure will lead to fluid moving out of the blood and into the tissue presenting as oedema.

The formed elements are red blood cells (RBC), white blood cells (WBC) and cell fragments of thrombocytes called platelets. These blood cells are formed in the red bone marrow by a process known as haemopoiesis. All of the bloods cells originate from a stem cell called a haematopoietic stem cell. As these cells mature, the type of cell they will eventually mature into is determined by the body's specific needs at the time and is controlled by the action of hormones and other factors. Figure 26.2 shows the development of the blood cells from the haematopoietic stem cells through their differentiation into the formed elements.

Knowing the normal serum value of each of these elements in health and the function of each of the cell types allows health professionals to evaluate conditions that might affect the blood. Table 26.1 provides a summary of this information.

Red Blood Cells

Red blood cells are **erythrocytes**. They are circular, biconcave cells that do not contain a nucleus. They contain haemoglobin, which is responsible for binding with, and therefore transporting, the respiratory gases. Haemoglobin consists of the protein globin bound to iron containing haem molecules. Erythrocytes have a useful lifespan of approximately 100–120 days. They are constantly being replaced. The process of producing new red cells is called erythropoiesis (Marieb & Hoehn 2013).

Erythropoiesis is dependent upon a supply of iron, vitamin B_{12} and folic acid and the hormone erythropoietin (EPO). Erythropoiesis will increase when the body's demand for oxygen is not being met, for example in the presence of tissue hypoxia, when the number of erythrocytes decreases or there is an increased demand for oxygen (as seen in athletes). During these circumstances erythropoietin is produced in greater than normal quantities by the kidneys and released. Erythropoietin stimulates the erythrocytes to mature at a faster rate.

> ### Jot This Down
>
> Blood doping is the practice of boosting the number of red blood cells in the bloodstream in order to enhance athletic performance. Red blood cells carry oxygen from the lungs to the muscles, a higher concentration in the blood can improve an athlete's aerobic capacity and endurance. EPO doping is also illegal among athletes.

During erythropoiesis the haematopoietic stem cell undergoes a number of changes. It first transforms into a proerythroblast, which becomes an erythroblast and then a reticulocyte.

By the time the cell has become a reticulocyte, it has undergone dramatic change, including loss of its organelles and nucleus. It will be full of haemoglobin and have adopted its circular biconcave shape. Within approximately 2 days, the reticulocyte will become an erythrocyte (Marieb & Hoehn 2013). Reticulocytes are found in the blood of healthy people and account for 1–1.5% of the red cell count. Abnormal reticulocyte counts are indicator of abnormal rates of erythrocyte formation.

In health, the rate of erythrocyte production remains relatively constant, ensuring that its essential function of carrying oxygen to the body cells is maintained. An overproduction of erythrocytes will lead to increased blood viscosity and the potential for clot formation.

Destruction of Red Cells

The red blood cells are beginning to wear out after about 120 days (Nowak & Handford 2004). The red blood cells are broken down into their constituent parts, some of which are salvaged and reused by the body. The iron is reused in the bone marrow to form new haemoglobin and the remainder is reduced to bilirubin, which becomes a constituent of bile. Globin is broken down to amino acids, which are reused.

> ### Jot This Down
>
> Young red blood cells have a nucleus; however, mature red blood cells do not have a nucleus.

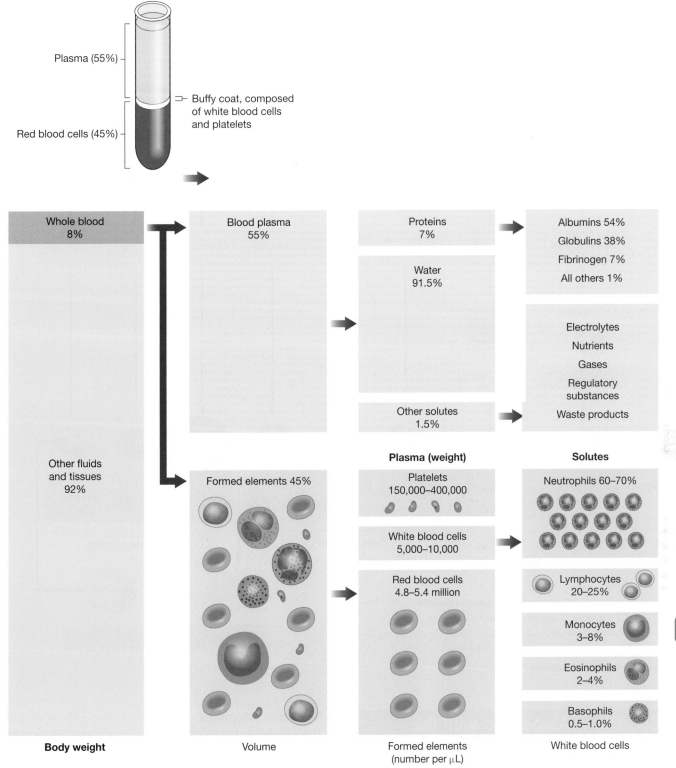

Figure 26.1 The constituents of blood.

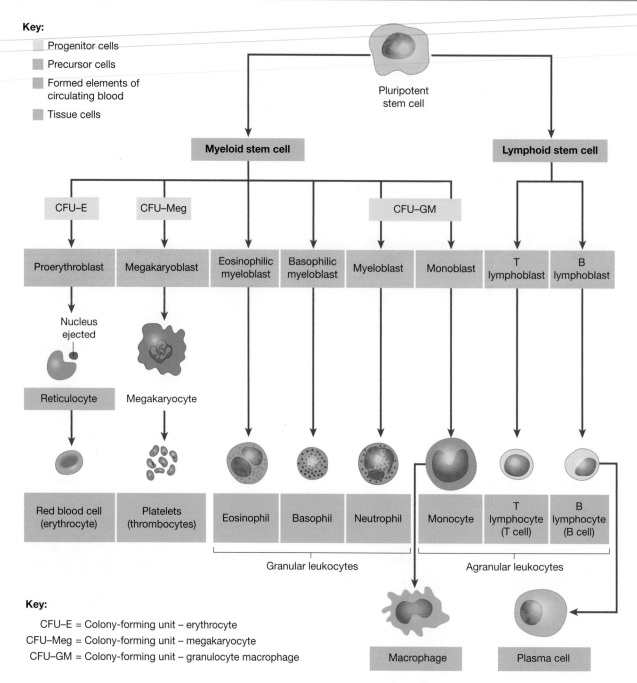

Figure 26.2. **Haematopoiesis.**

Conditions Associated with the Red Cells

Anaemia

The World Health Organization (WHO 2013) define anaemia as:

a condition in which the number of red blood cells or their oxygen carrying capacity is insufficient to meet physiologic needs, which may vary by age, sex, altitude, smoking and pregnancy status

It is characterised by an abnormally low number of circulating red cells or a low haemoglobin level or sometimes a combination of both.

Signs and symptoms

This leads to an oxygen deficit within the body and the patient with anaemia will have signs and symptoms associated with this deficit:

- Cells require oxygen for efficient cell metabolism. A reduction in oxygen will lead to a diminished cell metabolism. In order to compensate for this, there will be an increase in the respiratory rate and tachypnoea is a common symptom
- In order to compensate for a reduction in oxygen supply, peripheral blood vessels will constrict to conserve oxygen – pale peripheries are common
- Lack of oxygen-carrying capacity can make the simplest task appear arduous and extreme tiredness and fatigue are common

Table 26.1 The formed elements of the blood, how they are identified, the serum value in health, lifespan and function.

CELL NAME	IDENTIFICATION	NORMAL SERUM VALUE	LENGTH OF TIME TO DEVELOP	NORMAL LIFESPAN	FUNCTION
Erythrocyte (red blood cell RBC)	Nucleus absent, biconcave disc, pink colour, 7–8 μm in diameter	Man: $4.5–6.5 \times 10^{12}$ L Woman: $3.8–5 \times 10^{12}$/L	5–7 days	100–120 days	Transport of respiratory gases oxygen and carbon dioxide
Leukocytes (white blood cells, WBC)	Nucleus present, whole cells	Both: $4–11 \times 10^9$/L	See type of WBC	See type of WBC	Defence: see type of WBC
Neutrophil	Granulocyte, contains cytoplasmic granules; 10–12 μm in diameter	Both: $2.5–7.5 \times 10^9$/L	6–9 days	6 hours to a few days	Phagocytose bacteria
Eosinophil	Granulocyte, contains red cytoplasmic granules 10–14 μm in diameter	Both $0.04–0.44 \times 10^9$/L	6–9 days	8–12 days	Destroys antigen-antibody complexes; inactivates some of the allergy associated inflammatory chemicals; destroys parasitic worms
Basophil	Granulocyte, contains large blue-purple granules. 8–10 μm in diameter	Both: $0–0.1 \times 10^9$/L	3–7 days	A few hours to a few days	Contains the anticoagulant heparin, releases some inflammatory mediators such as histamine
Lymphocytes	Agranulocyte, pale blue cytoplasm, spherical nucleus, 5–17 μm in diameter	Both: $1.3–4 \times 10^9$/L	Days to weeks	Hours to years	Immune response, can attack cells directly or via antibodies
Monocytes	Agranulocyte, blue-grey cytoplasm, kidney-shaped nucleus, 14–24 μm in diameter	Both: $0.2–0.8$ 4×10^9/L	2–3 days	Months	Phagocytosis, can move into the tissue as a macrophage
Platelets	Cell fragments, deep purple, contain granules, 2–4 μm in diameter	Both: $150–440 \times 10^9$/L	4–5 days	5–10 days	Required for blood clotting, can seal small tears in blood vessels

- Tachycardia will occur to compensate for the diminished oxygen supply. Palpitations are common
- Decreased oxygen delivery to the skin and epithelium can lead to delayed healing and increased risk of ulcer formation
- Severe acute anaemia can lead to angina and severe anaemia over a long period of time can lead to congestive cardiac failure.

Anaemia can be due to the following pathophysiologies:

1. **Nutritional anaemia** – deficiency of a nutrient or nutrients required to produce red blood cells
2. **Haemolytic anaemia** – excessive destruction of red cells or red blood cell loss
3. **Aplastic anaemia** – impaired bone marrow function.

The signs and symptoms associated with anaemia are the same whatever the pathology.

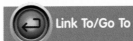 **Link To/Go To**

Use the following link to find out more about anaemia:
http://www.netdoctor.co.uk/diseases/facts/anaemiairon.htm
(accessed 11/10/2013)

Investigation and diagnosis

The following test may be carried out to confirm diagnosis.

Full blood count (FBC) shows a hypochromic microcytic anaemia (although there may be a mixed picture with co-existent B_{12} or folate deficiency).

- Hypochromia means that there is a low mean corpuscular hae-moglobin (MCH)
- Microcytosis means that there is as a low mean corpuscular volume (MCV)
- *Remember that a haemoglobinopathy will also cause a hypochromic microcytic anaemia.*

Nutritional anaemia
Iron deficiency anaemia

The most common type of anaemia is **iron deficiency anaemia**. It can occur for a variety of reasons. Iron is required in order to produce haemoglobin. If the supply of iron does not match the haemoglobin production requirement for iron, then iron deficiency anaemia will develop (McCance & Heuther 2010). This can lead to an insufficient number of red blood cells or the production of red cells that are malformed (poikilocytosis) or abnormally small (microcytic) or deficient in the red colour pigmentation associated with iron (hypochromic).

Causes It can occur as a result of a lack of dietary iron. Iron is found in green vegetables, liver, kidney, beef, egg yolks and wholemeal bread. Iron is especially required during pregnancy, and in adolescence during the growth spurt.

If there is a problem associated with the digestive tract, iron can be ingested in the correct quantity but malabsorption disorders, such as coeliac disease, prevent the iron from being absorbed.

Iron deficiency anaemia can also occur as a result of an excessive loss of iron through chronic bleeding. This is a common occurrence in women who suffer from heavy periods (menorrhagia). It can also be due to cancer, gastrointestinal bleeding from chronic and often undiagnosed gastric ulcers for example.

In addition to the signs and symptoms listed above, patients with iron deficiency anaemia often report cravings for unusual substances, known as pica (seen in pregnant women), brittle hair and nails, cracks at the corner of the mouth called angular stomatitis and a sore tongue.

Patients diagnosed with iron deficiency anaemia are required to increase the dietary intake of iron through eating iron rich foods or by taking an iron supplement. Parenteral iron can be prescribed if the patient cannot manage oral iron. Blood transfusion should not be the first-line of treatment, unless the anaemia is severe enough to lead to cardiovascular instability (Goddard *et al.* 2011). See Table 26.2 for iron rich foods and recommended daily allowance of iron. They should also seek help from their GP for identification and treatment of the cause. If the cause is not obvious, for example menorrhagia, the GP may consider GI investigations to rule out chronic bleeding or tests to rule out malabsorption disorders.

Signs and symptoms Many people with iron deficiency anaemia will only display a few signs or symptoms of the illness. The most common symptoms include:

- Tiredness
- Lethargy (lack of energy)
- Shortness of breath (dyspnoea).

Vitamin B$_{12}$ deficiency anaemia

Vitamin B$_{12}$ deficiency anaemia is also known as **pernicious anaemia**. It is the most common form of megaloblastic anaemia (McCance & Heuther 2010). Megaloblastic anaemia is characterised by very large erythrocytes. These erythrocytes are immature

and still contain a nucleus. Pernicious anaemia can occur as a result of a congenital deficiency of intrinsic factor, gastric mucosa atrophy associated with age or due to gastric surgery, where all or part of the stomach is removed. Gastric mucosa atrophy and gastric surgery lead to a reduction in the amount of intrinsic factor produced. Pernicious anaemia can also occur when intrinsic factor production is normal but there is a lack of vitamin B$_{12}$ in the diet.

Intrinsic factor is produced in the parietal cells of the gastric mucosa and is essential for the absorption of vitamin B$_{12}$. Ingested vitamin B$_{12}$ binds with intrinsic factor in the stomach and the resulting complex is absorbed via the ileum and transported to the bone marrow where it helps to promote the maturation of erythrocytes (Marieb & Hoehn 2013). Pernicious anaemia has a slow onset and may be diagnosed when the symptoms described previously occur.

Lack of dietary vitamin B$_{12}$ occurs in people who do not eat foods containing this vitamin such as those who adhere to a vegan diet. Vitamin B$_{12}$ is found in liver, milk and eggs. Vitamin B$_{12}$ can be given as a daily supplement. Table 26.2 shows vitamin B$_{12}$ rich foods and the recommended daily allowance of this vitamin.

Unfortunately, pernicious anaemia as a result of a lack of intrinsic factor, means that a dietary supplement of vitamin B$_{12}$ will not be absorbed by the stomach and will therefore have no effect. In this case, vitamin B$_{12}$ injections in the form of hydroxocobalamin are given every 3 months usually for life. (Hydroxocobalamin is the UK recommended treatment for pernicious anaemia associated with lack of intrinsic factor). Find out more about hydroxocobalamin by clicking on the link below.

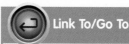

Link To/Go To

http://www.netdoctor.co.uk/diet-and-nutrition/medicines/hydroxocobalamin.html (accessed 11 October 2013)

Folic acid deficiency anaemia

Folic acid (or folate in its salt form) is essential for erythrocyte maturation and DNA synthesis (Marieb & Hoehn 2013). Folate is found in dark green vegetables, meat, eggs, fruits and cereals. Folate is metabolised in the liver to folic acid. Alcohol interferes with the metabolism of folate, and folic acid stores become depleted (McCance & Heuther 2010). Some malabsorption disorders and medications can also interfere with the ability to metabolise and store folic acid.

People diagnosed with **folic acid deficiency anaemia** are recommended to increase their dietary intake of folic acid containing foods or can be advised to take a folic acid supplement. Table 26.2 shows folic acid rich foods and the recommended daily allowance of folic acid.

Red Flag

Nurses should be aware not to administer folic acid instead of vitamin B$_{12}$ to any patient who is low on vitamin B$_{12}$ as this may lead to fulminant neurological deficit.

Oral iron therapy should be given before vitamin B$_{12}$ if iron deficiency is also present.

Table 26.2 Foods that contain vitamins and minerals associated with anaemia.

VITAMIN/MINERAL	FOODS	RECOMMENDED DAILY ALLOWANCE (RDA)	TOO MUCH	TOO LITTLE	NOTES
Iron	Liver, meat, nuts, dried fruit, wholegrains, beans, soya flour, fortified breakfast cereals, dark green leafy vegetables	**Men:** 8.7 mg **Women:** 14.8 mg	Constipation, nausea and vomiting, stomach pain. Very high doses can be fatal, particularly for children	Anaemia	Tea and coffee can make it more difficult to absorb iron. Liver should be avoided during pregnancy, spinach may be high in iron but it also contains a substance that makes it harder to absorb iron.
Vitamin B$_{12}$	Eggs, cheese, salmon, cod, meat, milk, some fortified breakfast cereals.	Adults: 0.0015 mg	Not known	Anaemia, degeneration of nerve fibres of the spinal cord	Vegan diets are usually vitamin B$_{12}$ poor
Folic acid	Fortified breakfast cereals, broccoli, Brussels sprouts. spinach, peas, asparagus, chickpeas, liver, brown rice	Adults: 0.2 mg	Can disguise vitamin B$_{12}$ deficiency and this could lead to nervous system damage.	Anaemia, increased incidence of spina bifida	Liver should be avoided during pregnancy. There are no stores of folic acid – it therefore needs to be part of the daily diet.

Anaemia is a condition that is usually managed in the community under the care of a GP. Hospital treatment in an acute care service is only required if the condition is severe or not being well managed.

Care, Dignity and Compassion

Advice for people requiring supplements to treat iron deficiency anaemia.

Iron tablets come in many formats. The most commonly used in the UK is ferrous sulphate (Provan 2005). It has to be continued for 3 months for iron haemoglobin and iron stores to return to normal values and the patient should be warned to expect monthly blood tests during this time. Iron is not recommended for children and adult patients should be advised to look out for the following side-effects:

· Nausea and vomiting
· Abdominal pain
· Heartburn
· Constipation
· Diarrhoea
· Black stools.

Taking the tablets with food may help and these symptoms may settle down with time. Alternatives can be prescribed if the patient is intolerant to ferrous sulphate, such as parenteral iron preparations.

Health promotion and discharge Tiredness and fatigue are problematic for those with anaemia. Some of the principles applied to cancer-related fatigue could be applied to the person with anaemia and they should be advised as follows (Kirshbaum 2010):

- Assess your activity; if it is not essential, then do not take part
- Delegate – those around you may want to help but do not know how, be specific, ask them to do the things that you cannot presently manage

- Sleep and rest need to be of good quality; set a routine, avoid stimulants such as caffeine and television before sleep and rest
- Manage symptoms which may be present such as pain by taking prescribed pain medication
- Organise the environment so that items that may be required are close by and do not require reaching or searching
- Tiredness can affect mood, discuss any mood changes with your GP
- Stop activity if there are signs of tachycardia, palpitations, pain or dizziness and get help.

Primary Care

It is important to encourage the person with anaemia to eat a healthy diet to rich in the vitamins and minerals they require. Anaemia can affect the oral mucosa, the tongue and the lips. A painful mouth may prevent the person from eating and therefore must be addressed (Dougherty & Lister 2011). The person with anaemia in the community should be encouraged to maintain good oral hygiene practices as follows:

· Assess the oral mucosa for pain, redness cracks, dryness, ulceration
· Brush the teeth and gums with a soft toothbrush and fluoride toothpaste twice a day
· Clean dentures and leave out overnight if possible
· Rinse the mouth after eating
· Apply a lubricant to the lips
· Avoid spicy foods or foods that irritate the mucosa
· Eat smaller amounts more frequently
· Analgesia may be required if there is pain present.

Seek advice from the GP if the condition of the mouth deteriorates.

Haemolytic Anaemia

In some instances, anaemia can be evident, despite the nutritional intake of the vitamins and minerals required for erythrocyte production being normal and the presence of a functioning bone marrow.

Erythrocyte numbers are maintained by a balance between erythrocyte production and destruction. If the destruction of the erythrocytes occurs before the normal lifespan (100–120 days), then this can also lead to anaemia. This anaemia is called **haemolytic anaemia**. Haemolytic anaemia can occur as a result of a problem associated with the erythrocyte (**intrinsic**) itself, such as sickle cell anaemia or as a result of disorders not necessarily associated with the erythrocyte (**extrinsic**) but which affect the erythrocyte such as infection or inflammation.

Intrinsic Haemolytic Anaemia
Sickle cell anaemia

Sickle cell anaemia is an inherited condition most commonly found in people of African descent but it can also be seen in Mediterranean areas, India and Saudi Arabia (Montague *et al.* 2005). In the UK, there are estimated to be 12 500 and 15 000 people living with sickle cell disease (NICE 2012a). It is a serious, chronic, long-term condition. It occurs as a result of a mutation on the β-chain of the haemoglobin molecule. The abnormal form of haemoglobin HbS can transport oxygen however the erythrocyte count is often low as evidenced by a low blood haemoglobin level.

This small structural change in the haemoglobin has a dramatic affect on function. Sickle haemoglobin (HbS) can lead to sickle trait or sickle cell disease. In sickle cell trait, 40% of the haemoglobin is HbS; in sickle cell disease, 80–95% of the haemoglobin is HbS (Porth 2005). A person who inherits the sickle cell gene from both parents (homozygous) will suffer from sickle cell disease. A person who inherits one normal and one sickle cell gene (heterozygous) has the sickle cell trait and may remain symptom free.

Those individuals with sickle cell trait are often asymptomatic. During episodes of severe hypoxia, there may be a tendency to sickle. When the HbS becomes deoxygenated, the HbS molecules form crystals and link together. This distorts the erythrocytes shape into a characteristic crescent or sickle shape (Figure 26.3). The erythrocyte can return to its normal shape when fully oxygenated again, however over time, if de-oxygenation persists, the erythrocyte will remain permanently in the sickle shape and be haemolysed more quickly. The lifespan of the erythrocyte can change from 120 days to 20 days (Gould & Dyer 2011). The breakdown of haemoglobin leads to hyperbilirubinaemia, which can present as jaundice and increases the incidence of the formation of gall stones in this group of patients. The bone marrow struggles to maintain the demand for erythrocytes and aplastic anaemia can develop.

Several conditions can precipitate sickling and include:

- Dehydration
- Infection
- Acidosis
- Hypoxia
- Low body temperature
- Low environment temperature
- Excessive exercise
- Anaesthesia.

Symptoms The symptoms of severe anaemia are often seen, such as pallor, fatigue, weakness, irritability, tachycardia and dyspnoea.

If the sickling is extensive, the microcirculation will be affected as the blood viscosity increases, blood flow is reduced and occlu-

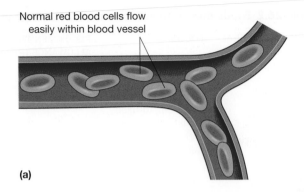

Normal red blood cells flow easily within blood vessel

(a)

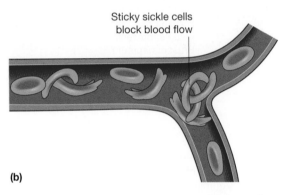

Sticky sickle cells block blood flow

(b)

Figure 26.3 The difference between normal red blood cells and sickled red blood cells, and the effects at the smaller blood vessels.

sion of blood vessels can occur. This is called sickle cell crisis. Sickle cell crisis typically last for 4–6 days. Vessel occlusion means that the tissue expecting to receive an oxygenated blood supply does not receive it and ischaemia, infarction and potentially necrosis can occur.

As the sickled cells stick to the blood vessel endothelium – activator substances are released which lead to hypercoagulation, platelet and thrombin activation and the formation of clot, vasoconstriction also occurs; all of which further occlude the vessel. Vessel occlusion may occur anywhere in the body, can occur suddenly and is accompanied by very severe pain. The most common sites are joints, bones, chest and abdomen (Gould & Dyer 2011).

Over time, the repeated infarcts associated with this condition can lead to damage to many major organs, including the heart, kidneys, liver and spleen. Cerebral vessel occlusion can lead to stroke and TIAs.

This life-threatening condition has no cure but supportive treatment has improved the life expectancy of those who suffer from this condition. Supportive treatment for sickle cell crisis should include oxygen therapy, analgesia, bed rest, hydration, good diet rich in erythrocyte requirements and vitamin and mineral supplements if required to help promote erythrocyte production.

Most people who have sickle cell disease are used to living with pain. This condition is managed in the community. Community care focusses on prevention of admission to hospital by good symptom management. Hospital admission is only required during vaso-oclusive episodes where the pain cannot be managed at home (Brown 2012).

Investigation and diagnosis The following tests may be untaken to diagnose sickle cell anaemia.

- Haemoglobin electrophoresis
- FBC to determine haemoglobin and serum iron levels.

Care, Dignity and Compassion

In this guidance, NICE (2012b) acknowledge the need to treat the patient as an expert in the management of this condition as many of the complaints received relate to length of time taken to administer analgesia, giving the wrong analgesia in the wrong quantity and labelling the patient as drug seeking. NICE recommendations include the following:

- Pain assessment using a tool appropriate to the patient:
  - Severity of the pain
  - Site of the pain
  - Character of the pain
  - How long has the pain been present?
  - Did anything aggravate the pain?
  - Does anything ease the pain?
  - Have you had this pain before?
- Analgesia within 30 minutes of arrival at hospital
- Discussion with the patient about pain, previous episodes and treatments, psychological and social support
- Nursing observations to include respiratory rate, oxygen saturation, pulse, blood pressure and temperature
- Assessment to rule out causes of pain not associated with sickle cell disease.

The choice of analgesia should include paracetamol and non-steroidal anti-inflammatory medication as well as a bolus of an opiate medication. Patient-controlled analgesia is also recommended if repeated boluses of opiate are required within 2 hours.

After administration of the analgesia, the patient should be re-assessed for pain, nursing observations and side-effects of the medication every 30 minutes until the pain is controlled, 2-hourly while on opiates and 4-hourly thereafter.

To prevent the complications of opiate analgesia occurring, naloxone should be available, the patient should be prescribed an anti-emetic for nausea and an aperient for constipation (Brown 2012).

Watching TV, reading, listening to music, having family present can distract the patient from the pain and should also be considered (Brown 2012).

The nurse should also be assessing for emergencies associated with sickle cell disease, such as acute chest syndrome, CVA and TIA. Therefore, respiratory rate, oxygen saturation, pulse and blood pressure and neurological assessment are undertaken and any deterioration should be reported. Rehydration with i.v. fluids should be prescribed in the acute stage and fluid balance should be monitored.

Rehydration, a warm environment, offering a nutritional diet and oxygen therapy if required should prevent the condition worsening and allow the patient to prepare for discharge home. On discharge pain management and rest will remain the focus of nursing care. Patients should be advised to avoid any triggers such as cold, dehydration or vigorous exercise.

Understanding that this patient is an expert in this condition demonstrates respect for the patient and allows the patient to keep some control of the disease.

Link To/Go To

NICE Guideline 143. Sickle Cell Acute Painful Episode: management of an acute painful sickle cell episode in hospital. **http://www.nice.org.uk/nicemedia/live/13772/59765/59765.pdf**

What the Experts Say

Inherited conditions, such as sickle cell disease can be difficult to manage, as people are not aware that they are carriers. Screening is offered routinely as part of antenatal care so that appropriate treatment and counselling can be provided (Laurent 2012). Genetic counselling should be considered by those who know that they are carriers or have the disorder (Nair & Peate 2013)

Nursing Fields Children's

When caring for a child with sickle cell anaemia, the nurse must ensure that the whole family is being cared for. This includes the child's siblings, parents and other family members. Provision must be made available to help support the family during acute phases of illness from a physical and psychological perspective. The nurse needs to be aware of the support mechanisms (statutory and non statutory) that are available making appropriate referral when required.

Thalassaemia

Thalassaemia is an inherited disorder that affects haemoglobin synthesis. Synthesis of the alpha (α) or beta (β) chains of adult haemoglobin can be affected. This can result in a reduction in the amount of haemoglobin being produced and a reduction in the number of red cells.

The α-thalassaemias are caused by the deletion of a gene and this leads to the production of defective α-chain synthesis. It is found to be prevalent in Asia.

The β-thalassaemias occur as a result of a mutation in the β-globin chain, which leads to a defect in β-chain synthesis. β-thalassaemia is sometimes called 'Mediterranean' or 'Cooley's anaemia'. It is found to be prevalent in the Mediterranean regions of southern Italy and Greece. α and β thalassaemia is common in the African and African-American community (Porth 2005).

α-Chain production requires the presence of four genes (two pairs). If all four genes are defective (α-thalassaemia major), then death usually occurs in utero or shortly after birth. If only one gene is defective, then that person may be asymptomatic. If two genes are defective, the symptoms of mild haemolytic anaemia will be present. Blood transfusions may be required.

β-thalassaemias – heterozygous individuals with one normal gene can usually produce enough haemoglobin to prevent severe anaemia (thalassaemia minor). Homozygous individuals cannot synthesise enough normal haemoglobin and present with severe anaemia (thalassaemia major). The condition is evident from a very young age (6–9 months old) and the patient becomes blood transfusion dependent.

Mild thalassaemia can lead to the following symptoms:
- Mild/moderate anaemia
- Bone marrow hyperplasia
- Mild splenomegaly.

Major thalassaemia is significantly more serious and can lead to the following symptoms:
- Severe anaemia – requiring repeated blood transfusions
- Liver and spleen enlargement (due to increased red cell destruction)
- Long bone fractures associated with bone marrow thinning due to increased haematopoiesis
- Repeated blood transfusions can lead to an accumulation of iron in the heart liver and pancreas and eventually lead to heart, liver and pancreas failure.

Acquired Haemolytic Anaemia

Factors extrinsic to the red blood cell production can also lead to haemolysis. Autoimmune disorders, infection (e.g. malaria), blood transfusion reactions and some drugs, are some examples of acquired haemolytic anaemia pathologies.

Mechanical destruction of red cells can occur secondary to trauma, prosthetic heart valves, vasculitis, radiation, haemodialysis or severe burns.

The severity and symptoms associated with this type of anaemia will depend on the underlying cause.

Haemolytic anaemia can be associated with the severe blood loss that can occur secondary to trauma. This is an emergency situation and attempts are made to stem the flow of blood and replace the lost blood volume through transfusion.

Link To/Go To

http://www.rcn.org.uk/__data/assets/pdf_file/0009/78615/002306.pdf

Blood transfusions and blood product transfusions may be required for the treatment of conditions associated with the haematological system. The administration of blood products is not without risk. The Royal College of Nursing (RCN 2013) has produced guidance for improving transfusion practice – right blood, right patient, right time.

Medicines Management

Nursing responsibilities for blood transfusion, including understanding the local policies for checking prior to administration are included in this guidance.

Once the correct product has been commenced for the correct patient the competent nurse must observe for transfusion reactions. These reactions can occur quite quickly hence the nurse is required to monitor respiratory rate, oxygen saturation, pulse, blood pressure and temperature 15 minutes after commencement. Transfusion reactions are serious and the patient may complain of feeling very anxious, loin pain, urticaria, back and loin pain, pain at the transfusion site, skin flushing and fever. If this does happen, then stop the transfusion and seek urgent medical help.

Aplastic anaemia – impaired bone marrow function

Impaired bone marrow function leads to aplastic anaemia, which is a rare condition. The failure of the bone marrow means that there is a reduction in stem cells and the production of all blood cells is inhibited. Blood analysis shows pancytopaenia – a reduction in the number of circulating erythrocytes, leukocytes and platelets. Normal bone marrow is replaced by fat (Porth 2005). The condition may be permanent but it is often temporary, depending on the cause.

Idiopathic aplastic anaemia accounts for approximately half of the cases (Gould & Dyer 2011). The cause is not known and it is more commonly seen in patients who are middle-aged.

Bone marrow damage can occur during viral illnesses such as HIV, hepatitis C and mononucleosis and this can lead to aplastic anaemia (Porth 2005).

Stem cells can be damaged by the action of some medications, such as antibiotics (chloramphenicol) or chemotherapy and radiation treatment for cancer. Patients may be advised to harvest some stem cells prior to commencing these treatments for transplant when required. Some autoimmune diseases, such as systemic lupus can affect the bone marrow.

Signs and symptoms Signs and symptoms of aplastic anaemia include weakness, fatigue, pallor, dyspnoea, headache, tachycardia and heart failure. If white cells are low, then infection can also occur and a reduction in the number of platelets can lead to bleeding problems. Stem cell or bone marrow transplant is the treatment for aplastic anaemia; immunosuppressive medications may also be prescribed (Porth 2005).

Investigation and diagnosis Diagnosis of anaemia is often made following a visit to the GP. The signs and symptoms described to the GP will usually result in blood tests being ordered. The most common of these is the full blood count (FBC). Please refer to Table 26.3 for the normal values of the red blood cell associated information obtained from the FBC test.

A full blood count will help the GP identify anaemia but further tests may be required to identify the type of anaemia. These tests include a blood film, which can identify abnormal or immature red blood cells. Irregularities may include red blood cells of variable sizes (anisocytosis). Normal mature red blood cells measure 7 μm. If the red blood cells are smaller than this (<7 μm), this is referred to as microcytosis and if they are larger than 7 μm, then this is macrocytosis.

The shape of the red blood cell is also important. It should be a biconcave disc shape. Abnormalities can lead to a change in this shape. If the cells are of different shapes, this is referred to as **poikilocytosis**. Sickle cells could be identified in this way as well as many other abnormally shaped red blood cells.

If iron deficiency anaemia is suspected, then three investigations can help diagnose this:
- Serum iron levels: normal values – 60–170 μg/dL
- Total iron binding capacity (TIBC): normal values – 240–450 μg/dL
- Ferritin: normal value 20–50%.

A low serum iron level and a raised total iron binding capacity level can be indicative of iron deficiency anaemia.

Ferritin is an iron storage protein. It is produced by the liver and its role is to mobilise iron stores when the body's demand for iron (for the production of haemoglobin) is not being met by the

Table 26.3 Normal red blood cell values from full blood count (FBC).

TEST	NORMAL RANGE	WHAT IS MEASURED
Red cell count (RCC)	Men: $4.5–6.5 \times 10^{12}$/L Women: $3.8–5 \times 10^{12}$/L	The number of red cells circulating per cubic millimetre of blood
Reticulocytes	$25–100 \times 10^{9}$/L	Reticulocytes are immature red blood cells. The number of red reticulocytes per cubic millimeter of blood
Haemoglobin (Hb)	Men: 13–18 g/dL Women: 11.5–16.5 g/dL	The amount of haemoglobin per 100 mL of blood
Haematocrit (Hct)	Men: 40.7–50.3% Women: 36.1–44.3%	The percentage of the volume of whole blood that is made up of red cells. The measurement is dependent on the number of red blood cells and the size of the red blood cells
Mean cell volume (MCV)	76–96 fL	The average volume of the individual red blood cells
Mean cell haemoglobin (MCH)	27–32 pg/cell	A calculation of the average weight of the haemoglobin per red cell
Mean cell haemoglobin concentration (MCHC)	30–36 pg/cell	The average concentration of haemoglobin per red cell

dietary intake of iron, when the iron reserves are depleted the serum level of ferritin is low.

Vitamin B_{12} deficiency anaemia can be caused by either a poor dietary intake of vitamin B_{12} or a lack of intrinsic factor. The Schilling test is used to identify which type of vitamin B_{12} deficiency is present. The test has two phases to it. Radioactive vitamin B_{12} is administered orally and then unlabelled vitamin B_{12} is given intramuscularly. A 24-hour urine collection is taken following this. The intramuscular B_{12} will saturate the liver receptors (briefly), while the radio B_{12} that was taken orally will be dealt with by the digestive system and as the liver receptors are full, it should be excreted via the kidneys. If less than 10% of the radioactive vitamin is found in the urine, then the test demonstrates impaired absorption of vitamin B_{12}. The test is repeated but this time with intrinsic factor also being administered orally. If the urine collection shows that there is more than 10% of the radioactive vitamin excreted, then this indicates pernicious anaemia. Lower than normal levels indicate malabsorption.

Sickle cell test looks at the haemoglobin in erythrocytes to identify HbS present in sickle cell trait or sickle cell disease.

Haemoglobin electrophoresis will differentiate between sickle cell trait from sickle cell disease. It is also used to identify other haemoglobin abnormalities such as thalassaemia or haemolytic anaemia.

Bone marrow aspirate can also be examined to identify abnormalities within the marrow itself.

Treatment Vitamin and mineral deficiency anaemias are best resolved by increasing the dietary intake of foods containing these vitamins or by taking prescribed supplements. Table 26.2 shows a list of vitamin/mineral rich foods and the recommended daily allowance. Pernicious anaemia is not able to be corrected using an oral supplement of vitamin B_{12} as the lack of intrinsic factor will prevent the oral vitamin from being absorbed. Monthly injections of Vitamin B_{12} are usually prescribed for life.

Nursing care and management The care required by the patient with anaemia will depend on the severity of the symptoms. Many patients with anaemia are managed at home under the care of the GP and community nurses. Nursing assessment should consider the patient's ability to manage the symptoms of anaemia at home and to assess for more serious symptoms such as pain where thrombosis may be affecting an area in sickle cell disease. Table 26.4 summarises the nursing interventions and goals required for managing anaemia.

All of the different types of anaemia will have symptoms in common. The most serious of which is an effect on the body's ability to provide oxygenated blood to the tissues. In its mildest form, this can lead to fatigue and shortness of breath on exertion as the body tries to increase oxygen intake. In its most severe form, where blood loss occurs, this can lead to circulatory collapse. The nursing care provided will depend on the severity of the symptoms.

Fatigue: Low haemoglobin levels lead to a decrease in circulating oxygen available to the cells of the body. Patients often feel too tired or weak to be able to manage the activities of living. Nursing care should be provided to manage this until the anaemia has responded to treatment.

Polycythaemia

An increase in the red cell concentration in the blood is known as **polycythaemia** or **erythrocytosis**. There are different mechanisms for developing polycythaemia. If there is an increase in red cells but the plasma volume is normal, then this is known as absolute 'polycythaemia'. If the plasma volume is reduced but the red cells are the normal in number, then this is 'relative polycythaemia'. Relative polycythaemia is often due to dehydration or secondary to the fluid loss associated with burns, excessive diuresis or excessive diarrhoea.

Absolute polycythaemia can be divided into two categories:

- Primary polycythaemia (polycythaemia vera)
- Secondary polycythaemia.

Primary polycythaemia or polycythaemia vera There is an increase in the production of red cells. White blood cells and platelets production are also increased but to a lesser extent. Originally, this was thought to be an idiopathic disorder, however recent

Table 26.4 Nursing care of anaemia.

ASSESSMENT	RATIONALE	INTERVENTION/HEALTH PROMOTION	EVALUATION
Respiratory system	Dyspnoea can occur as a result of a reduction in the oxygen carrying capacity of the red cells	If dyspnoea is severe the patient may have to be nursed in hospital where oxygen can be administered as prescribed. While the oxygen will assist with the dyspnoea the underlying cause will require to be treated. A blood transfusion may be required until the anaemia can be treated by diet or supplements	Eupnoea returns and oxygen therapy is no longer required
Nutritional intake	To ensure that the diet contains the vitamins and minerals required to overcome dietary anaemia	Health promotion: ensure the patient knows which foods will be required. ensure that the patient is able to manage administration of supplements if prescribed	Normal full blood count will show that the anaemia is adequately treated.
Activity tolerance	Inadequate tissue oxygenation leads to fatigue	Explain to the patient that anaemia can lead to fatigue. If possible, reduce activity level and rest more frequently to make and gradually increase activity as treatment improves this symptom. Assistance with the activities of living.	Patient is able to return to usual level of activity
Skin	A reduction in activity and a reduction in the oxygen supply to the tissues can lead to an increased risk of skin breakdown	Activity as tolerated. If on bed rest, then 2-hourly repositioning. Promote good skin hygiene practices.	Absence of pressure sores
Oral care	Oral mucosa, the tongue and lips become dry and cracked	Frequent oral assessment and hygiene	Intact oral mucosa

research suggests that it could be due to a mutation of a protein called JAK2. This signalling protein increases the production of red cells. JAK2 has been found in 95% of patients with this type of polycythaemia (Greenberg 2013). Polycythaemia vera affects more men than women and occurs in the 50–70 years age range. It is a progressive disease developing over 10–20 years and sufferers can go on to develop leukaemia. The high number of red cells increases the blood volume and viscosity, which leads to sluggish blood flow and congestion. Sluggish blood flow leads to clot formation within the blood vessels and the deprivation of nutrients and oxygen to the underlying tissue can lead to necrosis. Increased viscosity can also lead to hypertension (Porth 2005). This condition is often diagnosed following routine blood tests.

Signs and symptoms: include hypertension, full and bounding pulse, dyspnoea and headaches. Vision and hearing disturbances also occur. The sluggish blood flow can lead to cyanosis but the hands and faces can be very red in appearance (plethoric). Pruritis is common and accompanied by complaints of pain in the fingers and toes. Weight loss and drowsiness occur and delirium can develop.

Sluggish blood flow leads to congestion in the spleen and liver leading to hepatomegaly and splenomegaly. The patient can develop congestive heart failure.

The thrombosis associated with polycythaemia vera can affect the extremities as well as the organs, such as the brain, heart and liver, leading to deep vein thrombosis (DVT), transient ischaemic attacks (TIAs), angina and portal hypertension (Gould & Dyer 2011).

Diagnosis: serum erythropoietin levels are measured and are usually found to be low, while red cell count is high. Bone marrow aspiration would show an increase in proliferation of all of the blood cells. Haematocrit level is raised.

Nursing and management: Treatment will depend on the signs and symptoms the patient is presenting but could include the fol-

lowing: phlebotomy to remove 450–500 mL of blood and this will lower the haematocrit level; myelosuppressive therapy is used to slow down the production of red cells but it is used cautiously because of the risk of developing acute leukaemia; hydroxyurea can also be used to suppress bone marrow function but also carries a risk of developing leukaemia (Greenberg 2013). Antihistamine and steroid treatment have also been used. Aspirin may be prescribed to reduce the risk of thrombosis.

The nursing care is aimed at prevention, recognition and early intervention for management of the symptoms. Base line observation of blood pressure, pulse respiratory rate, oxygen saturation should be taken and these parameters should be measured regularly. Dyspnoea should be managed by encouraging the patient to sit up, physiotherapy and oxygen therapy if required. Cardiovascular assessment should include measures to prevent DVT, such as physiotherapy, elevating the legs and anti-thrombosis stockings (if prescribed). Smoking cessation and weight loss may also help reduce the risk of thrombus formation. Pain should be assessed and regular analgesia prescribed. If phlebotomy is prescribed, then the patient should be encouraged to increase their fluid intake before and after the treatment, to be aware of the orthostatic hypertension that can occur as a result of this treatment and to rise slowly from a sitting position. Hepatomegaly and splenomegaly can lead to the patient feeling full and not wishing to eat and therefore small frequent meals may be preferable (Greenberg 2013).

Secondary polycythaemia Secondary polycythaemia occurs when there is increased red cell production in response to increased erythropoietin (EPO) production by the kidneys. This occurs during hypoxia, as a result of renal tumours or renal disease, in people who smoke, secondary to lung or heart disease. It is the more common form of polycythaemia. With the exception of splenomegaly, the symptoms can be similar to that of polycythaemia vera.

Treatment will depend on the cause, so treatment of the renal and cardiac diseases should alleviate the symptoms. Smokers should try to stop smoking. Phlebotomy has been found to be useful for secondary polycythaemia.

White Blood Cells and Lymphoid Tissue Disorders

White cells are also called **leukocytes**. Unlike erythrocytes or platelets, they are whole cells complete with organelles and a nucleus (Marieb & Hoehn 2013). Leukocytes account for <1% of whole blood and are far fewer in quantity than erythrocytes. The function of leukocytes is to defend the body from invading pathogens, toxins and tumour cells.

Like erythrocytes, leukocytes are formed from the haematopoietic stem cell in the bone marrow. Hormones control the production of white cells or leukopoiesis. There are five different leukocytes and Figure 26.2 shows the stages in leukocyte development.

Unlike erythrocytes, which have to remain in the blood stream, leukocytes can migrate from the blood stream and into tissue, where they are able to contribute to the immune or inflammatory response (Marieb & Hoehn 2013). This process is called **diapedesis**. When the leukocytes respond to an attack or tissue damage, the body responds by increasing the production of white blood cells. Within a few hours the number of white blood cells in the blood can be seen to have increased. Table 26.1 summarises the function and normal serum values of the white blood cells. White blood cells can be divided into two types: the **granulocytes** and the **agranulocytes**.

The granulocytes are neutrophils, basophils and eosinophils and the agranulocytes are the lymphocytes and the monocytes. Granulocytes mature fully in the bone marrow. Agranulocytes leave the bone marrow not fully mature and enter the blood stream.

Neutrophils are the most abundant of the granulocytes. They account for 50–70% of the total number of white cells. They are attracted to the site of inflammation and are actively mobile. They are particularly affective against bacteria and some fungi. The neutrophil granules contain hydrolytic enzymes and some contain antibiotic-like proteins (defensins) (Marieb & Hoehn 2013). Neutrophils are efficient phagocytes. During bacterial infections the number of neutrophils in the blood can increase dramatically.

Eosinophils account for between 2% and 4% of the total number of white cells. Eosinophils are able to attack pathogens that are too large to be phagocytosed, such as parasitic worms. The worms enter the host via the digestive system on food or through the skin. They burrow into the respiratory or digestive mucosa. The eosinophils migrate to the loose connective tissue in the respiratory and digestive system. If they encounter a parasitic worm, they will release the digestive enzymes contained in their granules, killing and digesting the parasite. Eosinophils phagocytose antigen-antibody complexes involved in allergy responses thus lessening the severity of the reaction.

Basophils account for 0.5–1% of the total number of white cells. The granules of the basophil contain histamine and heparin. During inflammatory responses and in the presence of an allergen, the basophil releases the contents of its granules. Mast cells are very similar to basophils and are located in the tissues. Histamine is a vasodilator and its release produces a drop in blood pressure and in heart rate. Heparin is an anticoagulant, which inhibits the formation of blood clots.

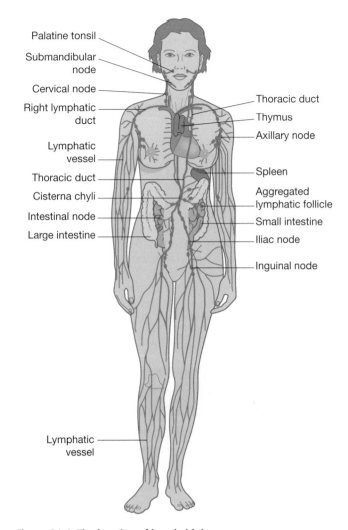

Figure 26.4 The location of lymphoid tissue.

Monocytes are agranulocytes that account for 3–8% of the total number of white cells. They leave the blood stream and enter the tissues where they mature into **macrophages**. They form part of the reticuloendothelial system in the spleen, liver, lymph nodes and bone marrow (Montague *et al.* 2005). Macrophages destroy bacteria, foreign material, dead cells and protozoa. They also participate in the immune response.

Lymphocytes are agranulocytes that account for 20–30% of the total number of white cells. Only a small proportion of small lymphocytes are found in the blood stream, the rest are found in lymphoid tissue (Figure 26.4). Lymphocytes mature in the lymph tissue and become one of two specialist cells:

- T lymphocytes (T cells) will defend the body against cells infected by viruses or tumour cells.
- B lymphocytes (B cells) are involved in the immune response and the production of antibodies.

The Lymphatic System

The lymphatic system consists of lymphatic vessel, lymphatic tissue and lymphatic organs which are located throughout the body (Figure 26.4). The **lymphatic vessels** return any fluid that has escaped from the vascular system back to the blood. When this fluid is located inside the lymphatic vessels it is known as lymph (lymphatic fluid). Lymphatic capillaries can allow pathogens, cancer cells and cell debris into the lymphatic system where they can travel throughout the body, threatening unaffected areas. The lymphatic fluid is filtered through the lymph nodes where the immune system can take action and some of the pathogens can be acted upon (Waugh & Grant 2010).

Lymphoid tissue is usually loose connective tissue (reticular connective tissue), with the exception of the thymus. Lymphoid tissue is the site for proliferation of lymphocytes and is found in many organ systems throughout the body.

Lymphoid organs include the spleen, the thymus and the tonsils. The spleen is the largest lymphoid organ and is a site for lymphocyte proliferation and the macrophages located here remove pathogens, foreign matter and debris from the blood passing through the spleen. It also has a role in the breakdown of red cells. The thymus is most active in early life. It secretes two hormones thymosin and thymopoietin which are responsible for ensuring that T lymphocytes become immunocompetent. The tonsils are located in the entrance to the pharynx. Trapped pathogens are dealt with here.

Conditions Associated with the White Blood Cells

Leukopenia and Neutropenia

Leukopenia – the total number of white cells is less than 4×10^9/L. As neutrophils make up the largest group of white cells often a reduction in the number of white cells is associated with a problem with neutrophils.

Neutropenia is decrease in the number of neutrophils to less than 2×10^9/L.

Moderate neutropenia is defined as a neutrophil count of $0.5–1.0 \times 10^9$/L. Severe neutropenia is defined as $<0.5 \times 10^9$/L.

In conditions such as severe sepsis, the production of new neutrophils is not meeting the body's demand for neutrophils. Neutropenia can also occur secondary to other conditions. Some haematological conditions such as aplastic anaemia or leukaemia can lead to poor or deranged neutrophil production. Autoimmune disorders such as systemic lupus or rheumatoid arthritis can result in neutrophils which do not survive as long as might be expected (see Table 26.1 for expected lifespan of the blood cells). Anorexia nervosa and starvation can lead to a pseudo-neutropenia where the neutrophils are not adequately distributed.

A drastic reduction in the neutrophil count (less than 500/mL) is known as **agranulocytosis** or **granulocytopenia**. This condition is seen when chemotherapy associated with cancer treatments interfere with the haematopoiesis in the bone marrow. Other drugs have been known to cause agranulocytosis through suppression of the bone marrow. This condition can also be caused by an increase in the destruction of the neutrophils in the circulating blood associated with haemodialysis, the immune response or infection (McCance & Heuther 2010).

Neutropenia predisposes the patient to infection as a major part of the body's protection is compromised. Commensals and opportunistic pathogens will invade usually via the respiratory, digestive or urinary tract. If the patient develops the more life-threatening agranulocytosis then hospital admission and treatment is required.

Nurses should be vigilant for the signs and symptoms associated with neutropenia. Infection is common, characterised by pyrexia, sepsis, tachycardia, and malaise.

Morbidity and mortality are increased by neutropenia related infections (Coughlan & Healy 2008), particularly if the neutropenia is secondary to cancer therapy (NICE 2012b).

Investigation and diagnosis

Diagnosis will be based on the result of the white cell count. Suspected sources of infection should be investigated through microbial analysis for example blood culture, sputum and swabs.

For neutropenia associated with cancer, NICE 2012 recommend teaching patients to recognise and get help if there are symptoms of sepsis. They also recommend that secondary and tertiary care professionals assess these patients promptly and manage suspected and actual sepsis using the appropriate therapy. Poor recognition and management of cancer patients and their susceptibility to developing sepsis can be better addressed by using a scoring system to identify those at risk of neutropenia with the aim of beginning the appropriate therapy earlier. Patients presenting with a pyrexia of $>38°C$ and/or clinical signs should have antibiotic therapy commenced within 1 hour (Higgins & Hill 2012). The psychosocial issues associated with neutropenia and resulting delay in chemotherapy treatment or potential reduction in chemotherapy treatment can affect the quality of life for the cancer patient and their families (Methven 2010).

Nursing care and management

Nursing care of the patient with neutropenia has three main goals:

1. To protect the patient from exposure to pathogenic agents
2. To observe for any signs of infection
3. To treat promptly any infection.

Many patients with neutropenia are nursed in community settings rather than acute care facilities. Health promotion and education about infection avoidance is important. It is also important that patients are able to recognise infection and know when and where to get help.

Nursing care delivered in all settings should take the following into consideration:

- Educate the patient, visitors and all staff on the benefits of good hand hygiene practices to avoid cross-infection
- Visitors should be asked not to visit if they know or suspect that they may have an infection to avoid cross-infection
- Skin care is important and the risk of infection through pressure ulcers or invasive procedures should be avoided by good hygiene and pressure area care practices. Opportunistic infections can be avoided by good hygiene practices
- Only essential invasive procedures should be permitted to reduce the risk of sepsis
- Oral hygiene should be carried out twice a day using a soft toothbrush
- If antibiotics have been prescribed, then there is an increase of fungal infections and this should be looked for and treated early if required
- Avoid spicy and unpasteurised foods
- Avoid damage to the rectal mucosa by preventing constipation. Offer stool softeners and aperients
- Avoid using urinary catheters to reduce the risk of urinary tract infection

- Neutropenic patients should be nursed in a side room to reduce the risk of cross-infection
- Nursing observations including temperature should be reported if abnormal and antibiotic therapy prescribed and commenced.

> **Primary Care**
>
> - Remember the importance of hand washing
> - Ensure eggs and meats are cooked well
> - Wash fruit and vegetables before eating
> - Do not use unpasteurised products
> - Avoid large crowded places where lots of people congregate
> - Limit visitors, particularly children
> - Pay attention to hygiene and oral hygiene
> - Be careful when dealing with pets and cleaning up after pets
> - Use gloves when cleaning the home or gardening
> - Be aware of the signs of infection and check body temperature daily
> - Contact the hospital or GP immediately if there are any concerns re-infection
> - Patients receiving chemotherapy should carry their chemotherapy alert card to alert healthcare practitioners they may meet (Higgins 2008)
> - Be aware that the inflammatory response is suppressed with a very low neutrophil count and fever may well not develop (Higgins 2008).

Leukaemia

Leukaemia is a malignant disorder of the white blood cells (Waugh & Grant 2010). The stem cells fail to mature and the bone marrow is replaced with proliferating, immature leukocytes. This leads to a decrease in the number of normal haematopoietic stem cells which do not function properly but which have a prolonged lifespan. This leaves little opportunity for the proliferation of normal blood cells such as erythrocytes and platelets (McCance & Heuther 2010). Immature malignant white blood cells will go on to infiltrate other organs such as the spleen, the liver and the lymph nodes. They do not function as white blood cells and therefore cannot protect the body from invading pathogens. This can lead to overwhelming sepsis, which can be fatal. There are several different types of leukaemia but they have many signs, symptoms, treatments and nursing care in common.

Signs and symptoms

Some signs and symptoms which are common for all types of leukaemia include:

- *Infection* – often the infection can be prolonged and difficult to get rid of. Infection can present in a number of sites such as oral mucosa, gastrointestinal tract, upper respiratory tract, urinary tract. Pyrexia and night sweats as a result of infection can also be present
- *Anaemia* – commonly present due to the inability to produce an adequate number of erythrocytes
- *Thrombocytopenia* – a relative decrease in the number of platelets leads to an increase in the tendency to bruise easily and to bleed. Bleeding gums and petechiae may be seen
- *Infiltration* of the liver, spleen and lymph nodes causes pain and swelling in these organs
- *Infiltration* of the meninges of the brain will lead to headache, raised intracranial pressure, altered levels of consciousness and nausea (Meenaghan *et al.* 2012)

- *Infiltration* of the kidneys leads to a decrease in the production of urine and an increase in urea and creatinine
- *Increased metabolism*
- *Fatigue.*

In the UK in 2010, there were 8257 new cases of leukaemia reported (Cancer Research UK 2013a).

The four main types of leukaemia are discussed in this chapter:

- Acute myeloid leukaemia (AML)
- Acute lymphoblastic leukaemia (ALL)
- Chronic myeloid leukaemia (CML)
- Chronic lymphocytic leukaemia (CLL).

Acute myeloid leukaemia (AML) is the most common type of leukaemia in adults, particularly those over 65 years old. The disease progresses quickly over days and weeks. There is uncontrolled proliferation of the precursor of the granulocytes called the myeloblast. Of those diagnosed with AML, 25% will survive for at least 5 years (Cancer Research UK 2012a). The outcome improves for those under 50 years old. For some people, there will be a cure or long-term remission but for the majority the disease will return (Porth 2005).

Exposure to high levels of radiation increases the risk of developing leukaemia. Undergoing radiotherapy treatment for cancer increases the risk of developing AML although this risk is small. Exposure to benzene increases the risk of developing AML, as does smoking and previous chemotherapy treatment. There is also a genetic link and children with Down's syndrome are more likely to develop AML.

Acute lymphoblastic leukaemia (ALL) is the most common type of acute leukaemia in children and young adults. It occurs more commonly in men than women. The risk factors are the same as those for AML but it is thought passive smoking can also increase the risk of developing this cancer (Cancer Research UK 2013b). It occurs due to a proliferation of lymphoblasts in the bone marrow inhibiting the growth of normal cells. This leads to the signs and symptoms described above.

ALL is diagnosed following a full blood count. The cells are analysed to identify any abnormalities. The white cell count will be high and the platelet and red cell count will be low. Bone marrow aspiration and biopsy will examine the maturity of the blood cells being produced; it is likely to show hyper-cellular marrow and an increase in the number T lymphocytes.

Complete remission is possible following combination chemotherapy treatment.

Chronic myeloid leukaemia (CML) also affects more men than women, however it is a rare form of leukaemia. In the UK, 610 people are diagnosed with this condition annually and the risk of developing the disease increases as age increases (Cancer Research UK 2013c). CML is associated with the Philadelphia chromosome. This is an abnormality involving translocation of chromosome 22 and chromosome 9. The onset of CML is slower and more insidious. The signs and symptoms can be present but often the disease is picked up during routine screening for something else. Abnormal proliferation of all of the bone marrow cells occurs with type of anaemia.

The disease pathway is characterised by three phases:

- *The chronic phase* – mild symptoms may be present such as tiredness and weight loss. Blood analysis usually shows a raised white cell and platelet count
- *The accelerated phase* – tiredness becomes fatigue, abdominal distension from an enlarged spleen leads to heavy uncomfortable

feeling under the ribs. An increasing number of blood cells in the bone marrow are immature

- *The blast phase* (blast crisis) – this presents like an acute leukaemia – large numbers of immature leukocytes are found in the blood. Leukaemic cells can spread and affect other organs. Deterioration in condition happens rapidly and even with treatment the prognosis is poor in this stage.

Treatment of CML with medicines such as imatinib and nilotinib can lead to remission. Stem cell transplant is also an option (Cancer Research UK 2013d).

Chronic lymphocytic leukaemia (CLL) is the most common type of leukaemia. CLL tends to affect older people over the age of 60 years. It affects more men than women. A total of 2800 people in the UK are diagnosed annually with CLL (Cancer Research UK 2013e). The B-lymphocyte is the cell involved. Large numbers are seen but they do not function, leaving the sufferer prone to bacterial infection (Nowak & Handford 2004).

CLL also has three stages. In the UK, the staging system used is the Binet staging system.

- *Stage A* – the patient may notice enlarged lymph nodes, a high white cell count is present and there has to be less than three groups of enlarged lymph nodes to fall into the stage A category
- *Stage B* – the patient may feel tired in addition to the enlarged lymph nodes. The high white cell count persists but there are more than three groups of enlarged lymph nodes
- *Stage C* – nose bleeds and bruising are common due to a low platelet count. The symptoms, such as tiredness and fatigue are present associated with anaemia. Weight loss and night sweats are common. The enlarged lymph nodes continue but the spleen may also be enlarged. Infection is common.

Investigations and diagnosis

Diagnosis of the leukaemias is achieved by the presenting symptoms, blood analysis and bone marrow analysis.

Full blood count looks not only at the number of cells (red, white and platelets) but the size and shape and therefore maturity of the white blood cells. Investigation of the bone marrow identifies erythropoiesis and leucopoiesis for abnormalities in the development of the red and white blood cells.

In all of the leukaemias, the red blood cell count, the haemoglobin and the haematocrit are low. The platelet count is also low.

Nursing care and management

Leukaemia is a life-threatening condition. Nurses must be skilled in managing the potential effects of treatments used to treat leukaemia patients.

Most leukaemias are treated using chemotherapy. The aim of the chemotherapy is to wipe out the leukaemia cells from within the bone marrow. Radiotherapy is also used, as it damages the cell DNA. The cell cannot divide and multiply but it can still function. Normal cells can also be damaged by radiation treatment but unlike the cancer cells, they can recover. Key areas of nursing include managing the risk of infection, haemorrhage, side-effects of chemotherapy and radiotherapy treatments and psychological support.

- The patient may be nursed in protective isolation (single room). Nurses need to follow the Trust policies and guidelines with regard to infection prevention

- Vital sign recording is critical for detecting early signs of infection. A low WBC means that the patient will not have the ability to fight any infections. Any complaints of chills, fever or coughs should be reported to the doctors promptly for immediate action
- The room should be cleaned daily with a damp cloth, bed linen changed and the mattress protected with suitable coverings.

Red Flag

A body temperature of 38°C for more than 1 hour should be treated immediately to prevent complications.

 Link To/Go To

Use the link to find out more about care of leukaemic patients.
http://www.nhs.uk/Conditions/leukaemia-chronic-lymphocytic/Pages/Treatment.aspx (accessed 12/10/2013)

Table 26.5 summarises the types of leukaemia.

Lymphomas

Solid tumours of the lymphatic tissue are called **lymphomas**. Lymphocytes and histiocytes (macrophages) proliferate. Although there are many types of lymphoma, the two most common lymphomas are Hodgkin's lymphoma (Hodgkin's disease) and non-Hodgkin's lymphoma.

Hodgkin's lymphoma

An abnormal cell called a Reed–Sternberg cell is seen in Hodgkin's lymphoma. This cell is a cancerous type of B lymphocyte. The symptoms first seen are enlargement of a single or a group of lymph nodes. This enlargement is not usually associated with any pain however it is usually progressive and because of the nature of the lymphatic system it can spread if left untreated. It commonly begins in the lymph nodes above the diaphragm (Porth 2005). It can also be seen in the spleen, the liver and the bone marrow. Hodgkin's lymphoma is a rare condition. In men it occurs in the age range 20–34 and again 75–79 years. In women it occurs between 20 and 24 and 70–74 years (Cancer Research UK 2013f).

People who have previously been treated for non-Hodgkin's lymphoma or who have a lowered immunity post-transplant, for example, have an increased risk of developing Hodgkin's lymphoma. Epstein–Barr virus is thought to be involved and there is also thought to be some genetic factors involved. Of the people in England and Wales diagnosed with this disease, 80% will live for 5 years.

The disease is staged according to the presenting symptoms.

- *Stage A* – no presenting signs and symptoms
- *Stage B* – significant weight loss; night sweats, pruritis; fever; malaise and anaemia.

As the disease progresses, organs such as the liver can become affected leading to jaundice. If the lungs are affected, breathlessness and a cough may be present. Pressure from enlarged lymph nodes can press on nerves and affect the nervous system.

Table 26.5 Summary of the types of leukaemia.

LEUKAEMIA	WHO DOES IT AFFECT	RISK FACTORS	SIGNS AND SYMPTOMS	TREATMENT (WILL DEPEND ON THE STAGE OF THE CANCER)
Acute myeloid leukaemia (AML)	Adults over 65 years old	Associated with exposure to radiation (radiotherapy) and previous chemotherapy smoking	Weakness and fatigue Fever Weight loss Frequent infections Bleeding and bruising easily Bone pain Breathlessness	Chemotherapy Growth factors to stimulate bone marrow Radiotherapy Bone marrow transplant or stem cell transplant
Acute lymphoblastic leukaemia (ALL)	Most common type of leukaemia to affect children and young adults. Can also affect adults	Associated with previous chemotherapy and some genetic conditions	Weakness and fatigue Fever Weight loss Frequent infections Bleeding and bruising easily Purpura Bone pain Breathlessness Swollen lymph nodes Swollen liver and spleen and the abdominal discomfort associated with this Can affect the central nervous system	Chemotherapy Radiotherapy Bone marrow transplant or stem cell transplant
Chronic myeloid leukaemia (CML)	A rare leukaemia more common in men than women	Philadelphia chromosome Previous radiotherapy	Frequent infections Poor appetite Weight loss Swollen lymph nodes Pale and tired appearance Easily bruises or bleeds Night sweats Headache Bone pain Large spleen	Chemotherapy Bone marrow transplant Stem cell transplant
Chronic lymphocytic leukaemia (CLL)	Adults over 60 years old. More men than women	Family history	May not have symptoms initially Swollen lymph nodes Abdominal discomfort Weight loss Infection Anaemia and tiredness Fever	Biological agents, such as Nilotinib to block the proteins responsible for stimulating the cancer cells to grow. Chemotherapy Interferon

Blood tests, lymph node biopsy and CT scan are usually required to produce a diagnosis as well as an evaluation of the presenting signs and symptoms.

Radiotherapy can be used to treat one or two small localised areas or lymph nodes where lymphoma is present. Chemotherapy is used to try and destroy the cancer cells and can be used in conjunction with radiotherapy and other treatments.

Biological agents are used to slow the progress of the cancer for some types of Hodgkin's lymphoma and stem cell or bone marrow transplant are considered where the lymphoma is unresponsive to other treatments.

Non-Hodgkin's lymphoma (NHL)

Malignant transformation of B cells or T cells in lymphoid tissue leads to the development of non-Hodgkin's lymphoma (NHL). B-cell lymphoma accounts for the majority of cases of non-Hodgkin's lymphoma. T-cell lymphoma affects young adults and teenagers. Annually, 12 200 people are diagnosed with non-Hodgkin's lymphoma in the UK; 60% of those diagnosed will be over 65 years old (Cancer Research UK 2013f).

The first symptom to present is a painless swelling in the lymph nodes (lymphadenopathy) of the neck, axilla or femoral region (Porth 2005). NHL can spread quickly to other lymphoid tissues and organs. Additional symptoms include frequent fevers, night sweats and significant weight loss. For some patients, pruritus will also be present. Not everyone with a diagnosis of NHL will have these symptoms.

If the lymphoma has spread to bone marrow, then there will be evidence of suppression of the other blood cells, leading to anaemia, bruising or bleeding easily and frequent infections. Other symptoms will be present if there is extra-nodal spread, such as enlarged tonsils, liver and spleen; breathlessness if the chest lymph nodes are involved and weight loss, nausea, vomiting and abdominal pain if gastrointestinal lymph nodes are involved. Extra-nodal involvement is more common in NHL than Hodgkin's lymphoma.

Full blood count is often normal until the late stages of the disease. Chest X-ray is used to identify lung involvement and may also show enlarged lymph nodes. Lymph node biopsy is undertaken to differentiate between NHL and Hodgkin's lymphoma. CT scan will also identify enlarged lymph nodes. The treatment will depend on the stage of NHL and will involve chemotherapy, radiotherapy, biological therapy and bone marrow/stem cell transplants.

Leukaemia and myeloma may be treated with chemotherapy and/or radiotherapy and stem cell/bone marrow transplant, as well as other medicines. Specific nursing care is required for patients undergoing these therapies.

Nursing care and management during chemotherapy

Chemotherapy is given in attempt to halt the growth of cancer cells. The cytotoxic medication interferes with cell division. Combination therapy (more than one drug) allows medications that act at different phases of cell division and this optimises the opportunity for disruption to cell division. Unfortunately, chemotherapy also interferes with the cell division of healthy cells, hence the side-effects experienced by patients. Chemotherapy can be given orally or intravenously. In some cases, a central line may be required.

The aim of chemotherapy is to make the cancer smaller, treat some of the symptoms of the cancer and for some cancers; chemotherapy can induce remission of the disease.

Psychosocial care: A cancer diagnosis and the prospect of chemotherapy are quite terrifying for patients and their relatives and it is important that expert staff are available to guide them through this process. Nurse-led pre-chemotherapy groups are advocated as a way of information giving to take some of the fear out of this process, improving patient education and the experience of chemotherapy (Sullivan 2013).

Patients having had the diagnosis of cancer and the need for chemotherapy feel a loss of control. They usually are highly anxious about the treatment and the future. The role of the nurse is to help reduce anxiety by clearly explaining what will happen, providing information leaflets about the treatment, going over the anticipated side-effects (see Table 26.6) and explaining what to do if patients have concerns. This will help the patient feel more in control and more able to manage the chemotherapy and treatments associated with the condition.

Before chemotherapy begins, patients must have blood tests to ensure that they are fit for the treatment. They should be warned that, on occasion, treatment may have to be postponed. This can be disconcerting for the patient who is relying on the treatment to overcome what is considered to be a life-threatening illness. By providing the patient with another appointment date for blood tests and/or treatment, some control can be returned to the patient. Side-effects of chemotherapy, such as hair loss should be explored.

Following the treatment, patients being discharged into the community should have a point of contact for when they have any concerns about their treatment or the side-effects. This is often a clinical nurse specialist, such as a McMillan nurse. If they are

Table 26.6 Chemotherapy advice for patients.

SIDE-EFFECTS ASSOCIATED WITH CHEMOTHERAPY	ADVICE/TREATMENT
Neutropenia leading to infection	Patients should be advised to look for signs of infection, such as pyrexia and report to A&E or a GP. Antibiotic therapy should be commenced within 1 hour of presenting at A&E
Anaemia	Blood transfusion may be prescribed if the haemoglobin <8g/dL. Look out for light headedness, fatigue, pallor, breathlessness or dyspnoea. Rest and sleep promotion should be discussed and planned
Thrombocytopenia	Low platelets can lead to bruising and bleeding. Take care to avoid bruising, report any bruising or bleeding
Hair loss	Hair loss can be an additional devastating blow to people newly diagnosed with cancer. The affect on self-esteem must not be under-estimated. Scalp cooling is contraindicated in patients with haematological cancers. Psychological support should be offered and referral to a wig-making service. Hospice services also offer a range of head coverings. Patients require advice on how long it will take for the hair to re-grow
Nausea and vomiting	The most commonly reported side-effect of chemotherapy is treated by commencing anti-emetics before treatment begins and continuing anti-emetic therapy for the duration of the treatment. Alternatives, such as acupressure bands may work for some patients
Loss of appetite/anorexia	Food can taste differently, with patients complaining of a metallic taste in their mouth. High calorie supplements can be prescribed. Patients should be encouraged to eat small amounts more frequently. Use plastic instead of metal cutlery may help (Dougherty & Lister 2011)
Diarrhoea and constipation	Both are side-effects of the cytotoxic medications and should be treated promptly to prevent additional discomfort
Fatigue	The fatigue associated with cancer and chemotherapy can surprise the patient in how overwhelming it can be. Patients are advised to conserve energy, include sleep and rest into their routine, limit visitors, participate in some activity followed by rest in order to carry out some of their daily activities
Psychological support	Chemotherapy can be an isolating time for patients. It is important that they have support of family and friends. If patients do not have this support, they should be referred to cancer support networks, such as McMillan, who can offer some support

having serious side-effects, they must be advised to seek support early by attending A&E or their GP.

Radiotherapy is often prescribed for patients with haematological cancers. The purpose of radiotherapy is to use X-rays to damage the DNA within the cancer cells. Radiotherapy can damage normal cells but these should be able to repair themselves. The radiotherapy can be applied externally or it can be implanted internally depending on the place and nature of the cancer being treated. Radiotherapy can be given as part of the treatment or for symptom management, when it is known as 'palliative radiotherapy'.

Like chemotherapy, patients have high levels of anxiety about radiotherapy and need a lot of support and information about the treatment. The nurse should advise the patient not to use lotions or perfumes prior to the radiotherapy and can advise how to look after the skin after the treatment. Radiotherapy is not without side-effects and nurses caring for patients undergoing radiotherapy should discuss the side-effects with the patient. These include:

- Tiredness
- Skin soreness
- Loss of hair at the site of the radiotherapy.

Bone Marrow Transplant and Stem Cell Transplant

Stem cell transplant occurs more commonly than bone marrow transplant. Both are used to treat some forms of cancer associated with the blood such as leukaemia, lymphoma or myeloma.

Bone marrow transplant begins with harvesting of haematopoietic stem cells from the bone marrow of the cancer patient when in remission (autologous) or from a donor (allergenic). The donor could be unknown or a relative with closely matched antigens. The procedure for bone marrow harvest is carried out in the operating theatre and is by aspiration from the posterior iliac crests. A volume of approx 1 litre is removed and stored to be given to the recipient.

The recipient is prepared for the bone marrow transplant. The aim of this preparation is to destroy the rogue leukaemic cells in the bone marrow. This is achieved by total body irradiation and high doses of chemotherapy via a central line. The donor cells are then filtered and transfused via a central line, to replace the leukaemic cells (Dougherty & Lister 2011).

Autologous bone marrow transplant is also known as 'bone marrow rescue'. The cells soon return to the bone marrow and the patient's bone marrow should return to functioning normally, as indicated by the patient's white cell counts.

Allogenic bone marrow transplant carries an additional risk of graft-versus-host disease, where the transplanted marrow cells see the recipient as foreign and attack the recipient tissue. Antibiotics, immunosuppressants and steroids are used to treat this condition.

Because of the high doses of chemotherapy and total body irradiation, the patient is susceptible to infections, which can be life-threatening. Particularly with allogenic bone transplant, there is a need to keep the patient in isolation to protect them from this risk. Isolation can last for 6 weeks and visitors are strictly limited in this time. It is important for the nurse to allow the patient access to technology so that they can remain in touch with friends and family and be protected from some of the affects of social isolation associated with being in protective isolation. Any signs of infection or rejection must be reported and treated quickly.

Stem cell transplants can also be allogenic or autologous. In autologous stem cell transplants, the patient is given growth factors to encourage the production of stem cells. When the blood levels of stem cells is deemed high enough the stem cells are removed and filtered and then stored to be returned to the patient following the high dose chemotherapy and total body irradiation treatment as per bone marrow transplant. Allogenic stem cells are harvested from a close match donor – often a sibling. Table 26.7 lists the side-effects and treatment associated with bone marrow or stem cell transplant.

Rehabilitation following stem cell or bone marrow transplant is crucial as the transplant process has a detrimental effect on the patient and this can lead to a longer recovery period. Exercise, support groups and complementary therapies may be useful in recovery (Bird *et al.* 2010).

Platelet and Haemostasis Disorders

Platelets (thrombocytes) are fragments of large cells called **megakaryocytes**. Platelets contain granules that contain many chemicals essential for blood clotting. Platelets originate from the haemapoietic stem cell and rely on the presence of thrombopoietin for their development. They have no nucleus and survive for 10 days if they are not required for blood clotting. **Haemostasis** is the term given to the stoppage of bleeding. Disorders of haemostasis occur because blood does not clot sufficiently or it clots inappropriately within the vascular system (Montague *et al.* 2005).

There are five stages to normal haemostasis:

1. *Vessel spasm*: endothelial injury results in vessel constriction reducing blood flow to the damaged area
2. *Platelet plug formation*: platelets aggregate to the area and form a plug to seal of the damaged vessel wall
3. *Blood coagulation*: blood is transformed from a liquid to a gel. The soluble plasma protein fibrinogen is converted to the insoluble fibrin which forms a mesh and eventually becomes a blood clot. Blood coagulation relies on activation of the Blood coagulation pathway, which includes the slower intrinsic pathway and the faster extrinsic pathway and the common pathway. Figure 26.5 illustrates the complexity of the blood clotting process and the many factors involved.
4. *Clot retraction*: the clot usually stabilises within 30 minutes. It then retracts as the trapped platelets contract. The platelets release growth factors which stimulates tissue repair at the site of the damaged vessel.
5. *Clot dissolution*: this stage allows a permanent repair to occur and blood flow to be re-established. The process of clot dissolution is called fibrinolysis. Plasminogen, an enzyme that promotes fibrinolysis, is converted to plasmin. Plasmin dissolves the fibrin strands that make up the clot.

There are many clotting factors involved in haemostasis and the clotting pathway (see Table 26.8). Any interruption to this pathway can lead to an inability to clot appropriately. A lack of any of the factors required for blood clotting also interferes with the normal coagulation pathway.

Some of the clotting factors are formed in the liver and rely on the presence of vitamin K for their formation. An absence of vitamin K can also disrupt the blood coagulation pathway.

A smooth and intact endothelium and naturally occurring anticoagulants such as heparin (secreted by the endothelial tissue) and antithrombin prevent platelets aggregating and clotting when it is

587

Table 26.7 Bone marrow/stem cell transplant advice.

SIDE-EFFECTS ASSOCIATED WITH BONE MARROW/STEM CELL TRANSPLANT	ADVICE/TREATMENT
Graft-versus-host disease (allogenic transplant only)	Can affect the liver, the digestive system or the skin. Ciclosporin can be given pre-transplant and antibiotics, immunosuppressants and steroids can be prescribed post-transplant
Infection	Antibiotics, protective isolation, daily cleaning of the room and changing linen, strict hand washing and limiting of visitors, daily shower and attention to mouth care, pasteurised and properly cooked foods, monitoring of vital signs – particularly temperature and monitoring of blood results. Potential infection sites should be swabbed for microscopy. The central line should be treated as a potential source of infection and strict aseptic no touch technique applied to its care
Anaemia	Due to a drop in the red cell count – blood transfusion may be required. The nurse must assess the patient for tiredness, light-headedness, fatigue and breathlessness
Bleeding	Due to a drop in the platelet count. Nose bleeds, bleeding gums and bruising may be observed. The patient may notice blood in the stools. A platelet transfusion may be required. careful monitoring of pulse and blood pressure are required
Stomatitis	The oral mucous membrane can be very fragile and painful following this procedure. Ice cubes can help care with oral hygiene using a soft toothbrush, analgesia and mouth washes may be required. Any oral infections should be treated
Nausea and vomiting	Nausea and vomiting are common secondary to chemotherapy. Anti-emetics should be prescribed prior to commencing the treatment and for the duration of the treatment
Loss of appetite/weight loss	Loss of appetite is not unusual due to the patient feeling extremely unwell, nausea and vomiting and a sore mouth. Patients should be encouraged to take small frequent meals. The dietician can provide some high calorie drinks and snacks and a suitable diet. In some circumstances parenteral nutrition may be prescribed as calories are essential for healing. The nurse should commence a fluid balance chart and a food intake chart to monitor the calorie intake. Daily weight is also a useful parameter
Diarrhoea	Diarrhoea is not uncommon as a side-effect of the many medications being taken. Toilet facilities and careful hygiene are required. A stool chart can be commenced and a stool sample sent for microscopy
Lethargy and fatigue	Rest is an important part of the post-transplant treatment. Establishing a routine of activity and rest will help demonstrate small improvements over the immediate post-transplant period. Tiredness and fatigue can continue for months following this procedure and the patient should be warned of this
Social isolation	While visitors may be limited – the use of social networking sites is a useful way of staying in touch with friends. Visitors have to be limited to prevent infection, however telephone contact is still possible. The nurse should monitor for signs of depression
Infertility	The high doses of chemotherapy required pre-transplant often lead to infertility and early menopause for women. Patients should discuss sperm banking, freezing eggs/embryos and hormone replacement therapy with their consultant prior to commencing this treatment

not required (McCance & Heuther 2010). Anticoagulants are products that inhibit blood clotting.

When patients present with bleeding with an unknown cause, blood is tested for its ability to clot and the presence of indicators of clotting (Table 26.9). Table 26.10 summarises the visual signs that may be present associated with blood clotting disorders.

What To Do If...

A patient tells you he has been having a frequent nose bleeds (epistaxis) lately, he brushes this off as a joke. Given this patient is receiving warfarin therapy, what will your next steps be?

The Haemophilias

These are the commonest of the clotting disorders Deficient or dysfunctional factor VIII is responsible for haemophilia A. This

disorder is a sex-linked recessive disorder that is passed from mother to son. The defect is on the X chromosome. Figure 26.6 demonstrates how this order occurs.

Haemophilia A is the commonest of the haemophilias. Bleeding is infrequent when the disease is classified as mild (5–33% of normal concentration of Factor VIII). In moderate disease, bleeding can occur secondary to trauma (1–5% of normal concentration of Factor VIII) and severe disease is characterised by less than 1% of the normal concentration of Factor VIII, and bleeding can be spontaneous and frequent. Treatment for this type of haemophilia is usually dependent on the severity of the condition and is considered preventative. Because of the risks associated with infected blood products, an engineered form of Factor VIII is now prescribed. It is usually administered by intravenous injection. The use of prophylactic treatment is also considered for severe forms of the disease.

The less commonly occurring **haemophilia B** occurs as a result of a deficiency in Factor IX. It is inherited in the same way as

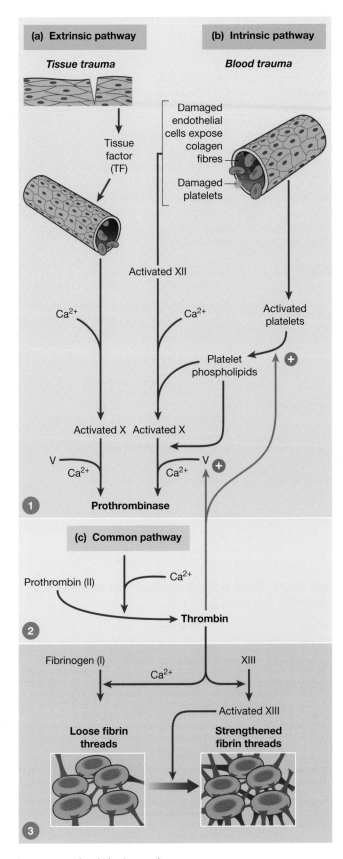

Figure 26.5 Blood clotting pathways.

haemophilia A and it is also known as 'Christmas disease'. Prophylactic treatment is injections of engineered Factor IX.

Von Willebrand's disease is an inherited bleeding disorder. People with Von Willebrand's disease have a deficiency of a protein made by the endothelial cells called 'Von Willebrand Factor'. The role of this protein is to promote platelet adhesion and to also to carry Factor VIII. Von Willebrand's disease is the most common of the inherited bleeding disorders (Montague *et al.* 2005). If Von Willebrand's disease is mild – little treatment may be required. Desmopressin (DDAVP-) can be given. This drug promotes the release of clotting factors and reduces the risk of bleeding. Tranexamic acid can also be given and if needed and clotting factor concentrate can be given intravenously.

Patients who are diagnosed with these conditions will bleed more easily than those who do not. This bleeding can be prolonged or appear extensive. It can happen spontaneously or in relation to an injury. They will bruise easily and there may be bleeding from the gums, gastrointestinal system (haematemesis or faecal occult blood), nose bleeds (epistaxis), bleeding into the central nervous system, joints and muscles. Bleeding into the joints is called 'haemarthrosis' and can eventually cause permanent joint deformity and disability.

Health promotion and discharge

Patients with these disorders are at significant risk from bleeding. It is easier to try and manage this risk than it will be to manage active bleeding. Health promotion advice is aimed at prevention of bleeding. Patients should be advised as follows:

- Learn about the condition – having an understanding of the implications of actions and activities allows the patient to take some control of the disease and make informed choices
- Learn about the medications that are required including how to take them and how to look for side-effects
- Be aware of the signs of internal bleeding, such as feeling light-headed and dizzy, weakness and disorientation, headache and pain – this is a medical emergency and requires urgent referral to the hospital
- Inform any medical practitioner, for example the dentist, prior to any treatment, as additional clotting support will have to be commenced before any invasive procedure such as surgery or a dental extraction
- Take care over personal hygiene. When cutting finger nails and toe nails try not to accidently nick the skin. Use an electric razor over wet shaving to prevent accidental nicks of the skin on the face and neck. Attend the dentist every 6 months and follow good oral hygiene practices to reduce the chances of having invasive dental procedures
- Avoid risks within the home from sharp objects or bumping into poorly placed objects or furniture
- Recognise the signs of haemarthrosis and rest any affected joint and use ice packs to alleviate swelling
- Analgesia can be taken for pain but aspirin has some anticoagulant properties, it should not be taken
- Consider sporting activities, non-contact sports are preferable to contact sports. Extreme sports should be avoided
- Consider carefully choice of career pathway. Some manual labour occupations will carry an additional risk of injury compared with white collar occupations
- Non-invasive procedures, such as tattooing should be avoided because of the associated risk of bleeding

Table 26.8 Blood clotting factors and their functions.

FACTOR NUMBER	FACTOR NAME	SITE OF FORMATION	FUNCTION
I	Fibrinogen	Synthesised by the liver (Plasma protein)	Converted to fibrin for clot formation
II	Prothrombin	Synthesised by the liver (Plasma protein) vitamin K is required to produce this plasma protein	Converted to thrombin required to convert fibrinogen to fibrin
III	Tissue factor (TF) (thromboplastin)	Released from damaged tissue (lipoprotein)	Required to activate the extrinsic pathway
IV	Calcium ions	Present in diet or released by the bone into the plasma	Essential for all of the stages of the clotting cascade
V	Platelet accelerator (proaccelerin/labile factor)	Synthesised by the liver (Plasma protein) also released by platelets	Required for the intrinsic and extrinsic pathways
VII	Serum prothrombin conversion accelerator	Synthesised by the liver (Plasma protein) vitamin K is required to produce this plasma protein	Required for the intrinsic and extrinsic pathways
VIII	Antihaemophilic factor A (AHF)	Synthesised by the liver – globulin	Required for the intrinsic pathway. A deficiency of AHF leads to haemophilia A
IX	Plasma thromboplastin component (PTC) or Christmas factor or antihaemophilic factor B	Synthesised by the liver (Plasma protein) vitamin K is required to produce this plasma protein.	Required for the intrinsic pathway A deficiency of PTC leads to haemophilia B
X	Stuart–Prower factor	Synthesised by the liver (plasma protein) vitamin K is required to produce this plasma protein	Required for the intrinsic and extrinsic pathways
XI	Plasma thromboplastin antecedent (PTA)or antihaemophilic factor C	Synthesised by the liver (plasma protein)	Required for the intrinsic pathway A deficiency of PTA leads to haemophilia C
XII	Hageman Factor	Synthesised by the liver (plasma protein; proteolytic enzyme)	Required for the intrinsic pathway Activates plasmin
XIII	Fibrin stabilising factor (FSF)	Synthesised by the liver (plasma protein) Also present in platelets	Promotes the insolubility of fibrin

Table 26.9 The blood test, normal range and explanation of what is being measured when assessing haemostasis.

TEST	NORMAL RANGE	USE
Platelets	$150–400 \times 10^9$/L	Number of platelets per 1 L of blood.
Prothrombin time (PT)	9–14 s	A measure of the extrinsic pathway which is vitamin K dependent
Activated partial thromboplastin time (APTT)	23–39 s	Measures the intrinsic pathway
Thrombin time	10–17 s	Time taken for fibrinogen to form fibrin
Fibrinogen	1.6–5.9 s	Amount of fibrinogen in the plasma
D dimer	<230 ng/mL	Predictor of recent clot formation

Table 26.10 Visual signs associated with bleeding disorders.

TERM	MEANING
Ecchymoses	Some areas of bleeding result in bruises. The red cells released into the tissue rupture and change colour through time going from dark blue to green to yellow before returning to normal tissue
Haematoma	Bleeding into the soft tissue – the blood becomes trapped and is called a haematoma
Petechiae	Tiny pinpoint haemorrhages seen in the skin
Purpura	Less regular large areas of bleeding seen in the skin

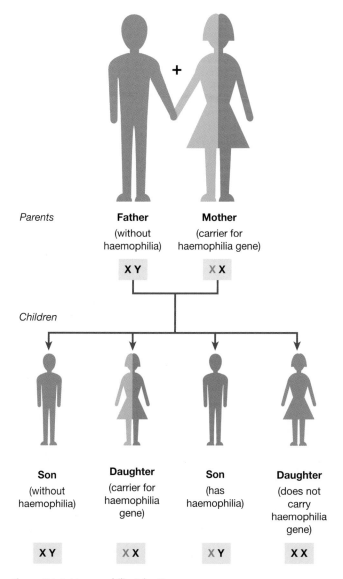

Parents

Father
(without
haemophilia)

Mother
(carrier for
haemophilia gene)

X Y   X X

Children

Son
(without
haemophilia)

Daughter
(carrier for
haemophilia
gene)

Son
(has
haemophilia)

Daughter
(does not
carry
haemophilia
gene)

X Y   X X   X Y   X X

Figure 26.6 **Haemophilia inheritance.**

- Be prepared to manage bleeding episodes by carrying a 'health alert card', bracelet or neck pendant
- Learn how to manage bleeding episodes by learning how to apply pressure to the bleeding point; the use of ice as a vasoconstrictor to reduce blood flow to the bleeding area; the use of haemostatic agents to stop bleeding and getting help if the bleeding is severe
- Be aware of medication regimes and the importance of complying with these to reduce the risk of severe bleeding episodes and bleeding into the tissues and joints
- Be vigilant in looking for signs of bleeding both externally and internally. Report any signs of bleeding, such as blood in the stool, to the GP
- When planning a family – genetic counselling should be considered in order to prepare for the future
- Haemophilia is a condition that impinges upon every activities and this can lead to social isolation and depression.

Link To/Go To

Some patients will find it useful to participate in patient forums associated with the haemophilia charities, such as haemophilia UK:

http://haemophiliacare.co.uk/index.html

Patients with the haemophilia clotting disorders are often well managed in the community but if they have a serious bleed they may require hospital treatment. The nurse will have to assess the patient to assess the significance of the bleed. Blood pressure may be low with tachycardia; the patient may be pale and disorientated. Examine the patient for obvious signs of bleeding.

Treatment and nursing care will focus on stopping the bleeding and administration of the necessary clotting factors required to treat the bleed. Oxygen therapy may be required and emotional and psychological support of the patient and his family.

Link To/Go To

Scottish Intercollegiate Guidelines Network (SIGN) have produced guidance concerning Antithrombotics: indications and management

http://www.sign.ac.uk/pdf/qrg129.pdf

These guidelines should be consulted when patients with haemophilia, for example are receiving antithrombotics.

Conclusion

This chapter has provided information regarding a variety of haematological disorders. Nurses need to have a good knowledge on the physiology of blood in order to understand the pathophysiology and to provide appropriate nursing care. It is essential for nurses to monitor the patients under their care, for any changes associated with haematological disorders. Vital sign monitoring is paramount in these patients, as any changes need to be identified as soon as possible for prompt action.

591

Key Points

- Anaemia is the most common disorder of the red blood cell. The signs and symptoms of anaemia relate to the functions of RBCs and gas transportation.
- An increase in the red concentration in the blood is known as polycythaemia or erythrocytosis.
- Leukaemia and lymphoma are haematological disorders of the white blood cells.
- Nursing care of the patient with leukaemia and lymphoma focusses on the risk of bleeding and managing the side-effects of chemo- and radiotherapies.
- Bleeding and clotting disorders can result from low platelet counts.
- Teaching self-care and safety to minimise bleeding in haemophilia is important.

Glossary

Agranulocytosis: an acute condition involving a severe and dangerous leukopenia (lowered white blood cell count)

Autoimmune disorder: a condition that occurs when the immune system mistakenly attacks and destroys healthy body tissue

Erythrocytes: red blood cells

Erythropoietin: a hormone produced by the kidneys that regulates RBC production

Haematopoiesis: the formation of RBC in the bone marrow

Haemolytic anaemia: when bone marrow activity cannot compensate for the increased loss of red blood cells (RBCs)

Heterozygous: refers to a pair of genes where one is dominant and one is recessive

Hormones: chemical messengers

Hypoxia: deficiency in the amount of oxygen reaching body tissues

Idiopathic: meaning arising spontaneously

Macrocytosis: means that the red blood cells are larger than normal

Microcytosis: means that the red blood cells are smaller than normal

Metabolism: chemical reaction that happens in living organisms to sustain life

Polycythaemia: having a high concentration of red blood cells in your blood

Reticulocytes: immature red blood cells

Tachypnoea: is the condition of rapid breathing

Vasculitis: group of disorders that destroy blood vessels by inflammation

References

Bird, L., Arthur, A., Niblock, T., Stone, R., Watson, L. & Cox, K. (2010) Rehabilitation programme after stem cell transplantation: randomized controlled trial. *Journal of Advanced Nursing*, 66(3), 607–615.

Brown, M. (2012) Managing the acutely ill adult with sickle cell disease. *British Journal of Nursing*, 21(2), 90–96.

Cancer Research UK (2013a) *Leukaemia Statistics*. http://www.cancerresearchuk.org/cancer-info/cancerstats/types/leukaemia/ (accessed October 2013).

Cancer Research UK (2013b) *Acute Lymphoblastic Leukaemia (ALL) Risks and Causes*. http://www.cancerresearchuk.org/cancer-help/type/all/about/acute-lymphoblastic-leukaemia-risks-and-causes (accessed October 2013).

Cancer Research UK (2013c) *Chronic Myeloid Leukaemia (CML) Risks and Causes*. http://www.cancerresearchuk.org/cancer-help/type/cml/about/chronic-myeloid-leukaemia-risks-and-causes (accessed October 2013).

Cancer Research UK (2013d) *Types of Treatment for Chronic Myeloid Leukaemia*. http://www.cancerresearchuk.org/cancer-help/type/cml/treatment/which-treatment-for-chronic-myeloid-leukaemia (accessed October 2013).

Cancer Research UK (2013e) *Chronic Lymphoblastic Leukaemia (CLL) Risks and Causes*. http://www.cancerresearchuk.org/cancer-help/type/cll/about/chronic-lymphocytic-leukaemia-risks-and-causes (accessed October 2013).

Cancer Research UK (2013f) *Hodgkin's Lymphoma Risks and Causes*. http://www.cancerresearchuk.org/cancer-help/type/hodgkins-lymphoma/about/risks-and-causes-of-hodgkins-lymphoma (accessed October 2013).

Cancer Research UK (2012a) *Statistics and Outlook for Acute Myeloid Leukaemia*. http://www.cancerresearchuk.org/cancer-help/type/aml/treatment/statistics-and-outlook-for-acute-myeloid-leukaemia (accessed October 2013).

Coughlan, M. & Healy, C. (2008) Nursing care, education and support for patients with neutropenia. *Nursing Standard*, 22(46), 35–41.

Dougherty, L. & Lister, S. (2011) *The Royal Marsden Manual of Clinical Nursing Procedures*, 8th edn. Wiley-Blackwell, Oxford.

Goddard, A.F., James, M.W., McIntyre, A.S. & Scott, B.B. (2011) Guidelines for the management of iron deficiency anaemia. *Gut*, 60(10), 1309–1316.

Gould, B.E. & Dyer, R.M. (2011) *Pathophysiology for the Health Professionals*, 4th edn. Saunders Elsevier, Philadelphia.

Greenberg, H. (2013) Polycythaemia Vera: an evidence-based examination from a nursing perspective. *Critical Care Nursing Quarterly*, 36(2), 228–232.

Higgins, A. (2008). Raising awareness of neutropenic sepsis risk in ambulatory patients. *Cancer Nursing Practice*, 7(9), 34–38.

Higgins, A. & Hill, A. (2012) Effectiveness of a neutropenic sepsis clinical pathway. *Cancer Nursing Practice*, 11(10), 20–22.

Kirshbaum, M. (2010) Cancer-related fatigue: a review of nursing interventions. *British Journal of Community Nursing*, 15(5), 214–219.

Laurent, C. (2012) Screening for sickle cell disease and thalassaemia in primary care. *Primary Health Care*, 22(7), 22–24.

Marieb, E.N. & Hoehn, K. (2013) *Human Anatomy & Physiology*, 9th edn. Pearson, Boston.

McCance, K.L. & Heuther, S.E. (2010) *Pathophysiology. The Biologic Basis for Disease in Adults and Children*, 6th edn. Mosby Elsevier, Missouri.

Meenaghan, T., Dowling, M. & Kelly, M. (2012) Acute leukaemia: making sense of a complex blood cancer. *British Journal of Nursing*, 21(2), 76–82.

Methven, C. (2010) Effects of chemotherapy-induced neutropenia on quality of life. *Cancer Nursing Practice*, 9(1), 30–33.

Montague, S.E., Watson, R. & Herbert, R.A. (2005) *Physiology for Nursing Practice*, 3rd edn. Elsevier, Edinburgh.

Nair, M. & Peate, I. (2013). *Fundamentals of Applied Pathophysiology. An essential guide for nursing and healthcare students*, 2nd edn. Wiley Blackwell, Chichester.

NICE (2012a) *CG143: Sickle Cell Acute Painful Episode*. National Institute for Health and Care Excellence, London. http://guidance.nice.org.uk/CG143 (accessed October 2013).

NICE (2012b) *CG151: Neutropenic Sepsis: prevention and management of neutropenic sepsis in cancer patients*. National Institute for Health and Care Excellence, London. http://guidance.nice.org.uk/CG151/Guidance/pdf/English (accessed October 2013).

Nowak, T.J. & Handford, A.G. (2004) *Pathophysiology. Concepts and applications for Health Care Professionals*, 3rd edn. McGraw Hill, Boston.

Porth, C.M. (2005) *Concepts of Altered Health States*, 7th edn. Lippincott Williams and Wilkins, Philadelphia.

Provan, D. (2005) Iron deficiency anaemia. *Independent Nurse*, pp. 23–24, 24 May.

RCN (2013) *Right Blood, Right Patient, Right Time*. RCN guidance for improving transfusion practice. Royal College of Nursing, London. http://www.rcn.org.uk/__data/assets/pdf_file/0009/78615/002306.pdf. (accessed October 2013).

Sullivan, T. (2013) Benefits of attending nurse-led pre-chemotherapy group sessions. *Cancer Nursing Practice*, 12(1), 27–31.

Waugh, A. & Grant, A. (2010) *Ross and Wilson. Anatomy and Physiology in Health and Illness*, 11th edn. Elsevier Churchill Livingstone, Edinburgh.

WHO (2013) *Health Topics. Anaemia*. World Health Organization, Geneva. http://www.who.int/topics/anaemia/en/ (accessed October 2013).

Test Yourself

1. Red blood cells' lifespan is approximately:
   (a) 1 month
   (b) 3–4 months
   (c) 72 hours
   (d) 3 days

2. The pH of blood is:
   (a) 7.35–7.45
   (b) 7.00–7.45
   (c) 6.00–7.00
   (d) 7.35–8.00

3. Mature red blood cells do not have:
   (a) Haemoglobin
   (b) Iron molecules
   (c) Haem
   (d) A nucleus

4. Haematopoiesis is the formation of RBC in the:
   (a) Spleen
   (b) Liver
   (c) Bone marrow
   (d) Kidneys

5. Thrombocytopenia is a term for:
   (a) Reduced white blood cells
   (b) Reduced platelets
   (c) Reduced lymphocytes
   (d) Reduced erythrocytes

6. Lymphocytes are:
   (a) Agranulocytes
   (b) Granulocytes
   (c) Manufactured in the kidneys
   (d) Chemical messengers

7. Leukaemia is a malignant disorder of the:
   (a) White blood cells
   (b) Red blood cells
   (c) Platelets
   (d) Lymphocytes

8. Chronic myeloid leukaemia (CML) affects:
   (a) More women than men
   (b) Both sexes equally
   (c) More men than women
   (d) None of the above

9. Solid tumours of the lymphatic tissue are called:
   (a) Lymphomas
   (b) Cartilages
   (c) Plaques
   (d) Scabs
   (e) Lymphatic stones

10. Bleeding and clotting disorders can result from low:
    (a) Erythrocytes
    (b) Neutrophils
    (c) Lymphocytes
    (d) Platelets

Answers

1. b
2. a
3. d
4. c
5. b
6. a
7. a
8. c
9. a
10. d

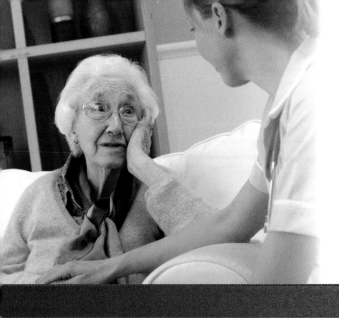

27

The Person with a Respiratory Disorder

Anthony Wheeldon

University of Hertfordshire, UK

Learning Outcomes

On completion of this chapter you will be able to:

- List the main anatomical structures of both the upper and lower respiratory tract
- Discuss the principles of pulmonary ventilation and external respiration
- Explain how the rate and depth of breathing is controlled
- Discuss the impact of infection on both the upper and lower respiratory tract
- Explain the difference between obstructive and restrictive lung disorders
- Explain the physiological principles of respiratory failure

Competencies

All nurses must:

1. Recognise the importance of respiratory rate and oxygen saturation as part of a comprehensive patient assessment
2. Demonstrate the ability to perform a comprehensive assessment of an individual's respiratory status
3. Recognise the cardinal signs and symptoms of acute deterioration in patients with severe and life-threatening respiratory diseases
4. Plan effective care strategies for individual's with respiratory disorders
5. Work with other members of the multidisciplinary team to ensure that patients receive care interventions that are based on the best available evidence
6. Promote self-management strategies in individuals living with chronic respiratory disease

 Visit the companion website at **www.wileynursingpractice.com** where you can test yourself using flashcards, multiple-choice questions and more.

Nursing Practice: Knowledge and Care, First Edition. Edited by Ian Peate, Karen Wild and Muralitharan Nair.
© 2014 John Wiley & Sons, Ltd. Published 2014 by John Wiley & Sons, Ltd. Companion website: www.wileynursingpractice.com

Introduction

Respiratory diseases place a hefty burden on patients, carers and healthcare services. According to the British Thoracic Society (BTS), respiratory illness is the second most common reason for hospital admission. Indeed, its impact on both Hospital and Primary Care resources is phenomenal. In Primary Care settings in the UK, around 24 million GP consultations for respiratory complaints occur each year. As a result, 51 million prescriptions for the prevention or treatment of respiratory conditions are being dispensed in England every year. In 2006, the total annual cost of respiratory disease to the National Health Service was estimated to be around £6.6 billion. Respiratory disease is also associated with a high mortality rate, with one in every five deaths in the UK occurring as a result of respiratory disease – more than ischaemic heart disease (BTS 2006). This chapter explores the pathophysiology, treatment and nursing care of respiratory disease.

Anatomy and Physiology

The functions of human cells are dependent upon the transfer of energy between molecules. The substance that provides the energy source is **adenosine triphosphate** (ATP). At any one time, a human cell will contain around 1 billion molecules of ATP, however each molecule will only survive around 1 minute before being used. Oxygen (O_2) is fundamental in the production of ATP and therefore cells only survive if they receive a continuous supply of oxygen. The manufacture of ATP also produces carbon dioxide (CO_2). If allowed to build up carbon dioxide can affect cellular activity and disrupt homeostasis. The principle function of the respiratory system therefore is to ensure that the body extracts enough oxygen from the atmosphere, while simultaneously eliminating excess carbon dioxide. In addition to the exchange of oxygen and carbon dioxide, the respiratory system also filters inspired air, excretes small amounts of water and heat, articulates vocal sounds, provides the sense of smell, as well as playing a major role in the regulation of arterial blood pH (Jenkins & Tortora 2013).

Respiratory Anatomy

The respiratory system is divided into the **upper and lower respiratory tract** (Figure 27.1). The lower respiratory tract consists of the all the structures found below the larynx. The respiratory tract also has distinct conduction and respiratory regions. The conduction region consists of the upper respiratory tract and the uppermost region of the lower respiratory tract. The air found within these regions of the lung is being conducted towards the lower respiratory regions. The respiratory region constitutes the functional part of the lungs, where oxygen diffuses into blood. The structures within the respiratory region are microscopic, very fragile and easily damaged by infection. For this reason, both the upper and lower respiratory tracts are designed to protect the respiratory region from invading air-borne pathogens.

The upper respiratory tract

As well as providing the sense of smell, the **upper respiratory tract** also ensures that the air entering the lower respiratory tract is warm, damp and clean. The nasal cavity is lined with course hairs that filter incoming air, ensuring that large dust particles do not enter the airways. The nasal cavity is also lined with a mucus mem-

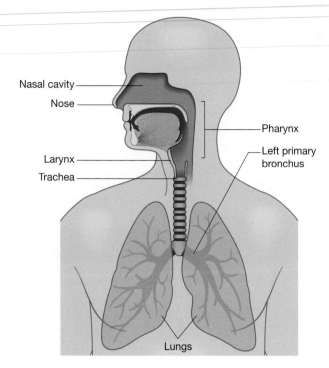

Figure 27.1 Upper and lower respiratory tract.

brane made from pseudostratified ciliated columnar epithelium, which contains a network of capillaries and a plentiful supply of mucus secreting goblet cells. The blood flowing through the capillaries warms the passing air, while the mucus moistens it. Mucus also traps and covers any passing dust particles, which are then propelled by the cilia towards the pharynx, where they can be swallowed or expectorated.

For further protection, the upper respiratory tract is lined with irritant receptors, which when stimulated by invading particles (dust or pollen for example) force a sneeze, ensuring the expulsion of the offending material through the nose or mouth. The pharynx also contains five tonsils (Figure 27.2). The two visible tonsils are the palatine tonsils; there are also two lingual tonsils, which are found under the tongue and a pharyngeal tonsil (adenoid), which sits on the upper back wall of the pharynx. The tonsils are lymph nodules and part of the immune system. The epithelial lining of their surface has deep folds, called 'crypts', which trap inhaled pathogens.

The nasal and oral cavities are connected by the pharynx. The pharynx is divided into three regions called the nasopharynx, the oropharynx and the laryngopharynx. The **nasopharynx** sits behind the nasal cavity and has two openings that lead to the auditory (Eustachian) tubes. The **oropharynx** and **laryngopharynx** sit underneath the nasopharynx and behind the oral cavity. The oropharynx and oral cavity are divided by the 'fauces' (throat) (see Figure 27.2).

Given its close proximity to the oesophagus the lower respiratory tract is also in danger of inhalation of solid or liquid food substances. On swallowing food, the **epiglottis**, a leaf-shaped piece of epithelial-covered elastic cartilage attached to the larynx, blocks the entrance to the lower respiratory tract and ensures that food and liquid is diverted towards the oesophagus.

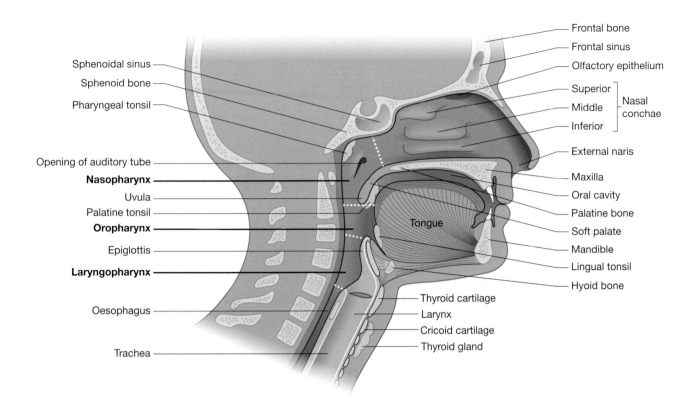

Figure 27.2 Structure of the upper airways.

Red Flag

Inhalation of solid or liquid substances can block the lower respiratory tract and cut-off the body's supply of oxygen – this medical emergency is referred to as aspiration and necessitates the swift removal of the offending substance.

Jot This Down

Take some time to think about the role of the speech and language therapist in the prevention of aspiration pneumonia.

The lower respiratory tract

The **lower respiratory tract** includes the larynx, the trachea, the right and left primary bronchi and all the constituents of both lungs (Figure 27.3). The larynx consists of nine pieces of cartilage tissue, three single pieces and three pairs. The single pieces of cartilage are the thyroid, epiglottis and cricoid cartilage. The thyroid cartilage is more commonly known as the 'Adam's apple' and together with the cricoid cartilage, protects the vocal cords. The three pairs of cartilage are the arytenoid, cuneiform and corniculate cartilages (Figure 27.4). The arytenoid cartilages are the most significant as they influence the movement of the mucus membranes (true vocal folds) that generate the voice. Speaking therefore is reliant upon a fully functioning respiratory system.

The lungs are two cone-shaped organs that almost fill the thorax. The lungs are protected by the thoracic cage, which consists of the ribs, sternum (breast bone) and vertebrae (spine). The tip of each lung, the apex, extends just above the clavicle (collar bone) and their wider bases sit just above a concave muscle called the diaphragm. The lungs are divided into distinct regions called lobes. There are three lobes in the right lung and two in the left. The heart, along with its major blood vessels, sits in a space between the two lungs. called the 'cardiac notch' (Figure 27.5). Each lung is surrounded by two thin protective membranes called the 'parietal and visceral pleura' (see Figure 27.3). The parietal pleura lines the wall of the thorax, whereas the visceral pleura lines the lungs themselves. The space between the two pleura, the pleural space, is minute and contains just a thin film of lubricating fluid. This reduces friction between the two pleura allowing both layers to slide over one another during breathing. The fluid also helps the visceral and parietal pleura to adhere to each other in the same way two pieces of glass stick together when wet.

The bronchial tree

The lungs consist of a massive network of airways of ever-decreasing size. For this reason, the structure of the lower respiratory tract is often referred to as the 'bronchial tree'. The first branch of the bronchial tree is the trachea (or 'windpipe'), which carries air from the larynx down towards the lungs. The trachea and the bronchi contain irritant receptors, which stimulate a cough, forcing large invading particles upwards towards the oesophagus and pharynx. The trachea is also lined with pseudostratified ciliated columnar epithelium, which traps smaller inhaled debris and propels them

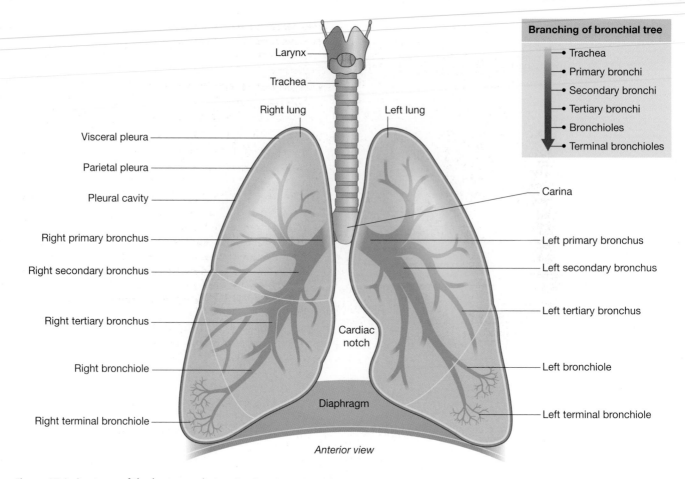

Branching of bronchial tree

- Trachea
- Primary bronchi
- Secondary bronchi
- Tertiary bronchi
- Bronchioles
- Terminal bronchioles

Larynx

Trachea

Right lung

Left lung

Visceral pleura

Parietal pleura

Pleural cavity

Carina

Right primary bronchus

Left primary bronchus

Right secondary bronchus

Left secondary bronchus

Right tertiary bronchus

Left tertiary bronchus

Cardiac notch

Right bronchiole

Left bronchiole

Diaphragm

Right terminal bronchiole

Left terminal bronchiole

Anterior view

Figure 27.3 Anatomy of the lower respiratory tract.

upwards into the upper respiratory tract, where they are swallowed and expectorated. The outermost layer of the trachea contains connective tissue that is reinforced by a series of 16–20 C-shaped cartilage rings. The rings prevent the trachea from collapsing, due to the pressure changes that occur during an active breathing cycle.

Before entering the lungs, the trachea divides into two primary bronchi at a point known as the 'carina'. Within the lungs, the primary bronchi divide into the secondary bronchi, each serving a lobe (three secondary bronchi on the right and two on the left). The secondary bronchi split into tertiary bronchi of which there are ten in each lung. Tertiary bronchi continue to divide into a smaller network of bronchioles, which eventually lead to a terminal bronchiole. The section of the lung supplied by a terminal bronchiole is referred to as a lobule and each lobule has its own arterial blood supply and lymph vessels. The bronchial tree continues to subdivide with the terminal bronchiole leading to a series of respiratory bronchioles, which in turn generate several alveolar ducts. The airways terminate with numerous sphere-like structures called alveoli, which are clustered together to form alveolar sacs (Figure 27.6). There are around 480 million alveoli in human lungs (Ochs *et al.* 2004). All of the airways from the trachea to the respiratory bronchioles form the conduction region of the lungs. As the air in this portion of the respiratory system does not supply the body with oxygen, it is often referred to as anatomical dead space. The transfer of oxygen from inhaled air into blood only occurs from

the respiratory bronchiole onwards, a region called 'the respiratory zone'. The respiratory zone accounts for two-thirds of the lungs' surface area (Tortora & Grabowski 2003).

Respiratory Physiology

The extraction of oxygen from the atmosphere and expulsion of excess carbon dioxide is referred to as respiration. Respiration involves the following four distinct physiological processes:

- *Pulmonary ventilation* – how air gets in and out of our lungs
- *External respiration* – how oxygen diffuses from the lungs to the blood stream and how carbon dioxide diffuses from blood to the lungs
- *Transport of gases* – how oxygen and carbon dioxide are transported between the lungs and body tissues
- *Internal respiration* – how oxygen is delivered to and carbon dioxide is collected from body cells.

Only pulmonary ventilation and external respiration are the sole responsibility of the respiratory system. As oxygen and carbon dioxide are transported around the body in blood, effective respiration is also reliant upon a fully functioning cardiovascular system. The understanding of all pulmonary ventilation, external respiration, transport of gases and internal respiration is reliant upon the appreciation of a series of gas laws, which are summarised in Table 27.1.

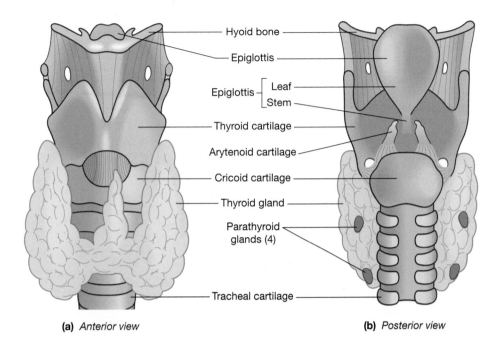

(a) *Anterior view*

(b) *Posterior view*

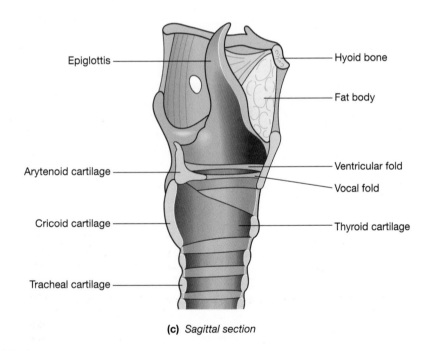

(c) *Sagittal section*

Figure 27.4 Structure of the larynx.

Pulmonary ventilation

Breathing In order for air to pass in and out of the lungs, a change in pressure needs to occur. Before inspiration, intrathoracic pressure is equal to atmospheric pressure. During inspiration, the thorax expands and intrathoracic pressure falls below atmospheric pressure, and air will naturally enter our lungs until the pressure difference no longer exists. This phenomenon is explained by Boyle's law, which states that the amount of pressure exerted is inversely proportional to the size of its container (Table 27.1). Dalton's law also explains that, in a mixture of gases, each gas exerts its own individual pressure that is proportional to its size. For example atmospheric air contains a mixture of gases. Each individual gas will exert its own pressure, dependent upon its quantity. Collectively, all the gases in the atmosphere exert a pressure, atmospheric pressure, which is 101.3 kilopascals (kPa) at sea level. On inhalation, the thorax expands and intrathoracic pressure falls

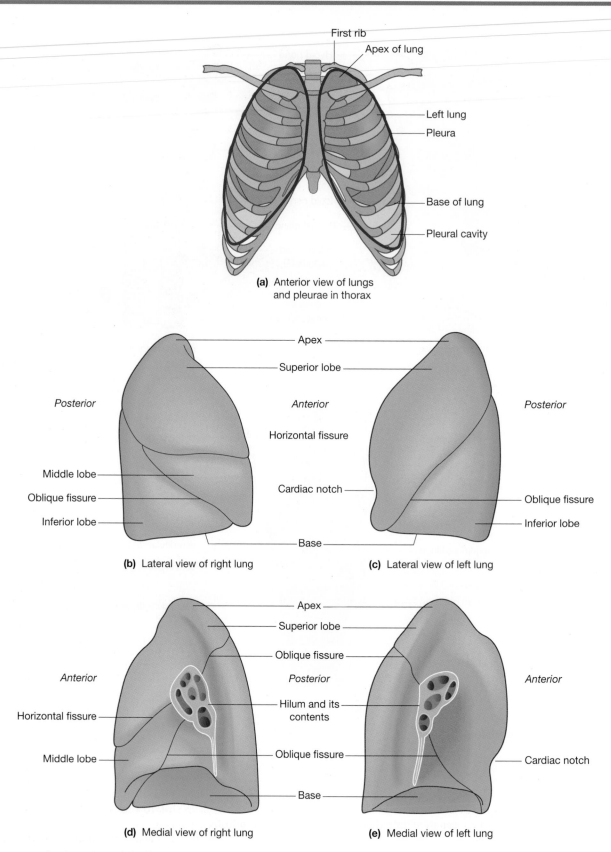

(a) Anterior view of lungs and pleurae in thorax

First rib
Apex of lung
Left lung
Pleura
Base of lung
Pleural cavity

(b) Lateral view of right lung

Apex
Superior lobe
Posterior
Anterior
Horizontal fissure
Middle lobe
Oblique fissure
Inferior lobe
Base

(c) Lateral view of left lung

Posterior
Cardiac notch
Oblique fissure
Inferior lobe

(d) Medial view of right lung

Apex
Superior lobe
Oblique fissure
Anterior
Posterior
Hilum and its contents
Horizontal fissure
Middle lobe
Oblique fissure
Base

(e) Medial view of left lung

Anterior
Cardiac notch

Figure 27.5 **Surface anatomy of the lungs.**

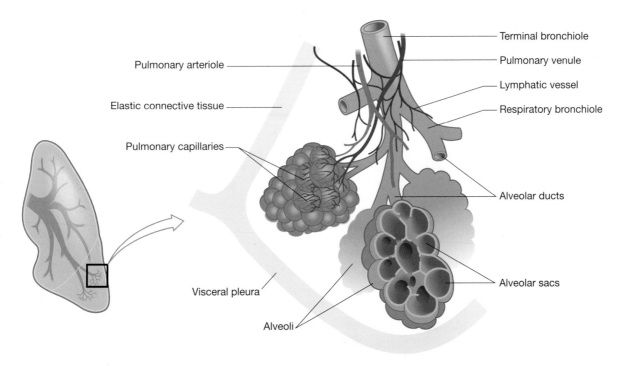

Terminal bronchiole
Pulmonary venule
Lymphatic vessel
Respiratory bronchiole
Pulmonary arteriole
Elastic connective tissue
Pulmonary capillaries
Alveolar ducts
Alveolar sacs
Visceral pleura
Alveoli

Figure 27.6 Anatomy of a lobule of the lungs.

Table 27.1 Summary of important gas laws. (Source: Davies & Moores 2003, reproduced with permission of Elsevier)

GAS LAW	SUMMARY	CLINICAL APPLICATION
Boyle's law	The pressure exerted by gas is inversely proportional to its volume	As the thorax expands intrapulmonary pressure falls below atmospheric pressure
Dalton's law	In a mixture of gases each gas will exert its own individual pressure, as if no other gases are present Gases move from areas of high concentration to low concentration	Differences in partial pressure govern the movement of oxygen and carbon dioxide between the atmosphere, the lungs and blood
Henry's law	The quantity of gas that will dissolve in a liquid is proportional to its pressure and its solubility	Oxygen and carbon dioxide are soluble in water and are transported in blood. Nitrogen is highly insoluble and despite accounting for 79% of the atmosphere very little is dissolved in blood
Fick's law	The rate a gas will diffuse across a permeable membrane will depend upon pressure difference, surface area, diffusion distance and molecular weight and solubility	Helps explain how altitude, exercise and respiratory disease can influence the amount of oxygen that is diffused into blood

below 101.3 kPa and air enters the lungs as a result (McGowan et al. 2003).

Thoracic expansion during inspiration is achieved by the contraction of respiratory muscles (Figure 27.7). Normal inspiration is achieved through the action of the diaphragm and 11 external intercostal muscles. The diaphragm is a dome-shaped sheet of skeletal muscle found beneath the lungs at the base of the thorax. The vast majority (75%) of the air that enters the lungs is as a result of diaphragmatic contraction. The external intercostal muscles sit in the intercostal spaces – the spaces between the ribs. On inspiration the diaphragm contracts in a downwards direction pulling the lungs with it. Simultaneously, the external intercostal muscles pull the rib cage outwards and upwards. As the thorax increases in size, intrapulmonary pressure becomes less than atmospheric pressure and air enters the lungs. Expiration is a more passive process. As the external intercostal muscles and diaphragm relax the natural elastic recoil of lung tissue forces the expulsion of air (Figure 27.8).

Other respiratory muscles can be also be utilised. The abdominal wall muscles and internal intercostal muscles for instance are utilised to force air out beyond a normal breath, when playing a musical instrument or blowing out candles on a birthday cake for example. The sternocleidomastoids, the scalenes and the pectoralis can also be used to produce a deep forceful inspiration. These muscles are referred to as accessory muscles, so-called because they are rarely used in normal quiet breathing (Simpson 2006).

Work of breathing During inspiration, respiratory muscles must overcome the elastic recoil of lung tissue and natural resistance to airflow through very small airways. The energy required by the

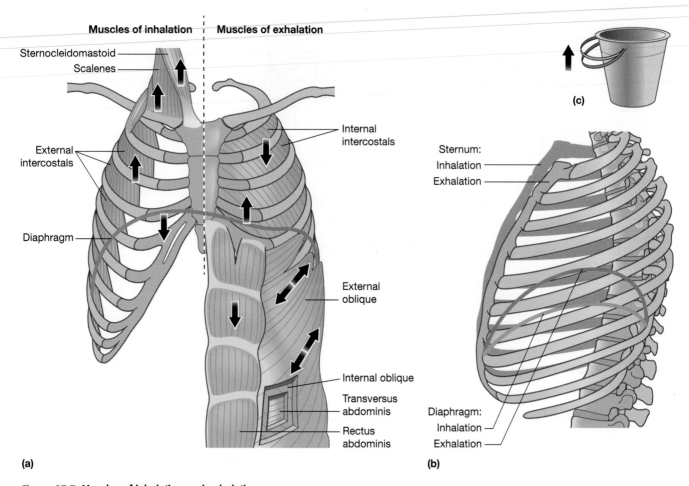

Muscles of inhalation | **Muscles of exhalation**

Sternocleidomastoid

Scalenes

External intercostals

Diaphragm

Internal intercostals

External oblique

Internal oblique

Transversus abdominis

Rectus abdominis

(a)

Sternum:
Inhalation
Exhalation

Diaphragm:
Inhalation
Exhalation

(b)

(c)

Figure 27.7 Muscles of inhalation and exhalation.

respiratory muscles to overcome these hindering forces is referred to as the **work of breathing**. The actual amount of energy expended is kept to a minimum by the ease with which lungs can expand. This ease of expansion is referred to as 'lung compliance'. Lung compliance is aided by the production of a detergent-like substance called 'surfactant', which is produced by type 2 alveolar cells found within the alveoli. Surfactant reduces the surface tension that occurs where alveoli meet pulmonary capillary blood flow in the lobule, thereby reducing the amount of energy required to inflate the alveoli. Despite these opposing forces, work of breathing accounts for less than 5% of total body energy expenditure. However, many lung diseases can affect lung compliance and airway resistance and therefore increase work of breathing. In acute respiratory failure, work of breathing could account for up to 30% of total body energy expenditure (Levitzky *et al.* 1990).

Volumes and capacities The total amount of air that an individual's lungs are capable of housing is referred to as **total lung capacity (TLC)**. Each individual's TLC will be dependent upon their age, sex and height but is often said to be around 6 litres of air in a person of average build. During normal, quiet pulmonary ventilation, however, only a small proportion of total lung capacity is utilised. In normal quiet breathing, only around 500 mL of air is inspired and expired. Air that is inhaled and exhaled in one respiratory cycle is called 'Tidal Volume' (V_T). Given that normal quiet breathing involves small volumes of air, the lungs have a great capacity of extra inhalation and exhalation if required. Humans can breathe in far beyond a normal inhalation and fill their lungs up with air. This capacity for inhalation is referred to as **inspiratory reserve volume (IRV)**. Likewise, after a normal, quiet breath, there remains the potential for a larger exhalation. This potential capacity of exhalation is referred to as **expiratory reserve volume (ERV)**. If tidal volume increases, due to exercise for example, IRV and ERV would be reduced. Tidal volume, inspiratory reserve volume and expiratory reserve volume can all be measured. However, because a small volume of air always remains in the lungs, total lung capacity can only be estimated, even after a maximal exhalation. This small volume of remaining air is called residual volume (RV). Because RV cannot be exhaled, the total amount of air that could possibly pass in and out of an individual's lungs is a combination of tidal volume, inspiratory reserve volume and expiratory reserve volume, collectively referred to as **vital capacity** (Figure 27.9).

Other important measures of lung volume include minute volume (V_E) and alveolar minute ventilation (V_A) (Table 27.2). Minute volume (V_E) is the amount of air breathed in each minute and is calculated by multiplying Tidal Volume (V_T) by respiratory rate. In health, minute volume is around 6–8 litres per minute. Alveolar minute ventilation (V_A) subtracts anatomical deadspace (V_D), from minute volume providing a better indication of the

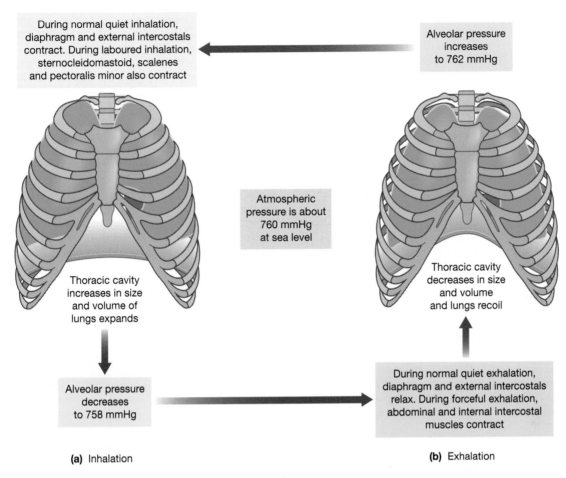

During normal quiet inhalation, diaphragm and external intercostals contract. During laboured inhalation, sternocleidomastoid, scalenes and pectoralis minor also contract

Alveolar pressure increases to 762 mmHg

Atmospheric pressure is about 760 mmHg at sea level

Thoracic cavity increases in size and volume of lungs expands

Thoracic cavity decreases in size and volume and lungs recoil

Alveolar pressure decreases to 758 mmHg

During normal quiet exhalation, diaphragm and external intercostals relax. During forceful exhalation, abdominal and internal intercostal muscles contract

(a) Inhalation

(b) Exhalation

Figure 27.8 **Events of inhalation and exhalation.**

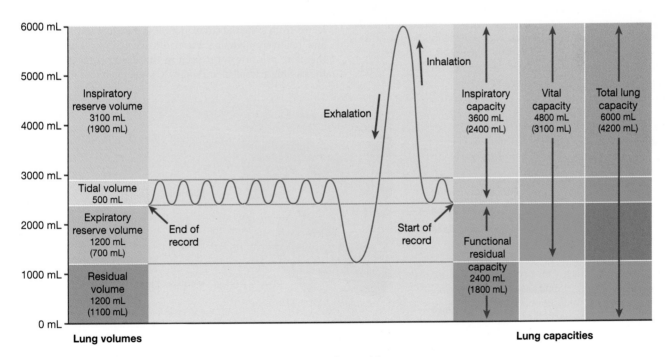

Inspiratory reserve volume 3100 mL (1900 mL)

Tidal volume 500 mL

Expiratory reserve volume 1200 mL (700 mL)

Residual volume 1200 mL (1100 mL)

Inhalation

Exhalation

End of record

Start of record

Inspiratory capacity 3600 mL (2400 mL)

Vital capacity 4800 mL (3100 mL)

Total lung capacity 6000 mL (4200 mL)

Functional residual capacity 2400 mL (1800 mL)

Lung volumes

Lung capacities

Figure 27.9 **Diagrammatic description of the major lung volumes and capacities.**

volumes of air available for gaseous exchange each minute, which in health is around 4–6 litres per minute (McGowan *et al.* 2003).

Control of breathing The rate and depth of breathing is controlled by respiratory centres within the medulla oblongata and pons in the brain stem. The main respiratory centres are the inspiratory, expiratory, pneumotaxic and apneustic centres (Figure 27.10). The **inspiratory centre** sets the respiratory rate, whereas the **expiratory centre** is thought to play a role in forced expiration. The **pneumotaxic** and **apneustic centres** refine the actions of breathing. The pneumotaxic centre achieves this by sending inhibitory signals to the medulla slowing breathing down, while the apneustic centre simultaneously stimulates the inspiratory centres, lengthening inspiration. Both these actions fine tune breathing and prevent the lungs from becoming over inflated. Also within the medulla oblongata, specialised chemoreceptors continually analyse carbon dioxide levels within cerebrospinal fluid (CSF). As levels of carbon dioxide (CO_2) rise, the phrenic and intercostal nerves are innervated and messages are sent to the diaphragm and intercostal muscles instructing them to contract. Rising levels of carbon dioxide detected by central chemoreceptors is the main stimulus for inspiration. As it relies solely on fluctuations in carbon dioxide, this stimulus for inhalation is often referred to as the *hypercapnic drive*. Another set of chemoreceptors referred to as the peripheral chemoreceptors are found in the aorta and carotid arteries. The peripheral chemoreceptors analyse levels of oxygen (O_2), as well as carbon dioxide (CO_2). If arterial levels of oxygen fall or arterial levels of carbon dioxide rise, the glossopharyngeal and vagus nerves are innervated, stimulating further contraction. As this stimulus for inhalation relies mostly on fluctuations of oxygen, it is referred to as the *hypoxic drive*.

Although breathing is essentially a subconscious activity, the rate and depth of breathing can be controlled voluntarily or even stopped all together, when swimming under water for example. Both the hypercapnic and hypoxic drives to breathe are very powerful; for this reason conscious control over breathing is somewhat constrained. When holding your breath, for example, the desire to breathe will become overpowering after only a short space of time. Breathing can also be influenced by state of mind. The inspiratory area of the respiratory centres can be stimulated by both the limbic system and hypothalamus, two areas of the brain responsible for processing emotion. Fear, anxiety or even the anticipation of stressful activities can cause an involuntary increase in the rate and depth of breathing. Other factors that can affect breathing include pyrexia and pain. Because breathing is largely beyond an individual's control any changes in respiration rate are clinically significant (Hogan 2006).

Jot This Down

Take some time to think about how anxiety may influence a patient's respiratory rate and consider what nursing interventions you could utilise in order to help reduce anxiety and breathlessness.

External respiration

External respiration is the diffusion of oxygen from the alveoli into pulmonary circulation and the diffusion of carbon dioxide from pulmonary circulation to the alveoli. This diffusion of oxygen and carbon dioxide occurs because gas molecules always move from areas of high concentration to low concentration. Each lobule of the lung has its own arterial blood supply, which originates from the pulmonary artery. The pulmonary artery originates from the right ventricle of the heart and the blood within it has been collected from systemic circulation. It is therefore low in oxygen (O_2) and relatively high in carbon dioxide (CO_2). The amount (and therefore pressure) of oxygen in the alveoli is far greater than in the passing arterial blood supply. Oxygen therefore moves passively

Table 27.2 Important lung volumes. (*Source:* **Martini & Nath 2009)**

VOLUME	CALCULATION
Minute volume (V_E)	Tidal volume (T_V) × Respiration rate e.g. 500 (T_V) × 12 = 6000 mL (V_E)
Alveolar minute ventilation (V_A)	(Tidal volume (T_V) − anatomical dead space (V_D)) × Respiration rate e.g. (500 (T_V) − 150 (V_D)) × 12 = 4000 mL (V_A)

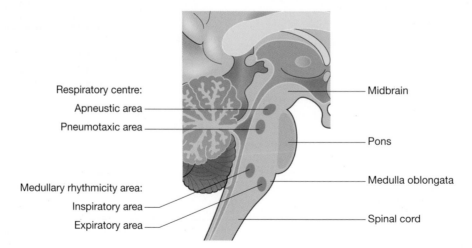

Respiratory centre:
Apneustic area
Pneumotaxic area

Medullary rhythmicity area:
Inspiratory area
Expiratory area

Midbrain

Pons

Medulla oblongata

Spinal cord

Figure 27.10 The respiratory centres of the brain.

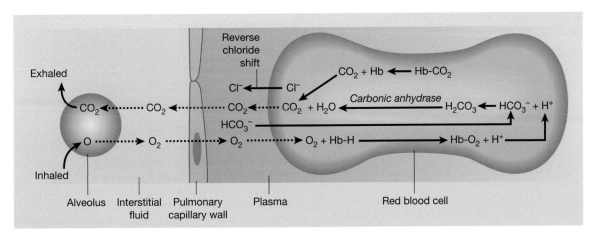

Figure 27.11 External respiration: the exchange of oxygen and carbon dioxide within the lungs.

through the wall of the alveoli, through interstitial fluid, through the capillary wall and into pulmonary circulation, a process which takes approximately 0.25 seconds. This swift process ensures that the blood flowing away from the lungs, through the pulmonary veins and towards the left atrium of the heart has been re-oxygenated. While oxygen is being transferred from the alveoli into blood, carbon dioxide makes the reverse journey. Because there is less carbon dioxide in the alveoli than in pulmonary circulation carbon dioxide diffuses through the capillary wall, across interstitial space and through the wall of the alveoli ready to be exhaled (Figure 27.11).

The rate at which oxygen and carbon dioxide diffuse between alveoli and pulmonary circulation, is influenced by a number of physiological factors. Fick's Law of Diffusion helps explain how these factors influence the rate of diffusion and therefore gaseous exchange. According to Fick's law, the rate of diffusion will be determined by gas solubility/molecular weight, surface area, concentration difference and membrane thickness (Box 27.1). The more soluble a gas is in water the easier it is for diffusion to occur. Oxygen (O_2) and carbon dioxide (CO_2) are both soluble in water and therefore easily diffused. Carbon dioxide (CO_2) is 20 times more soluble than oxygen (O_2). Nitrogen (N_2), the most abundant gas in the atmosphere, is highly insoluble in water and therefore very little diffuses into the bloodstream. The larger the surface area available for diffusion the greater the rate of diffusion will be. Large inhalations therefore will recruit more alveoli and more gaseous exchange will occur as a result. Conditions that reduce the surface are of the lung, a pneumothorax for example will result in less alveoli being recruited and a reduction in gaseous exchange. The greater the difference in concentrations of oxygen (O_2) and Carbon Dioxide (CO_2) in the alveoli and pulmonary circulation the faster both gases will diffuse. In health there always remains a large dif-

ference in concentration of oxygen between the alveoli and pulmonary circulation. However in respiratory failure the rate of diffusion can be enhanced if this concentration difference is increased, by administering prescribed oxygen therapy for example. The final factor considered by Fick's Law of Diffusion is membrane thickness. The further the distance gases have to travel, the slower diffusion will be. Conditions such as pulmonary oedema, in which fluid collects in the alveoli, result in an increased membrane thickness and distance and a reduced diffusion rate (Basset & Makin 2000).

Ventilation and perfusion Effective external respiration requires an adequate supply of both oxygen and blood. In order to ensure a good enough supply of oxygen, the alveoli have to be adequately ventilated. In health, an alveolar minute ventilation (V_A) of around 4 litres is required. In order to ensure that an adequate amount of blood is re-oxygenated a pulmonary blood flow of around 5 litres per minute needs to be maintained. This ideal delivery of adequate amounts of both air and blood is referred to as the ventilation V_A:perfusion Q ratio. A normal V_A: Q ratio would be 4:5 or 0.8. Any disruption to either ventilation or pulmonary blood flow leads to a V_A:Q mismatch and a reduced level of oxygen diffusion. During hypoventilation, V_A may fall below 4 litres and less oxygen would be available for gaseous exchange as a result. This situation would be described as a low V_A:Q ratio, i.e. 3:5 or 0.6. Another potential problem would be inadequate pulmonary blood flow, as a consequence of an embolism for example. Inadequate pulmonary blood flow results in less blood being re-oxygenated and a high V_A:Q ratio as a result, i.e. 4/3 or 1.34. In health, there are regional differences in V_A:Q ratio, due the individual's position (Margereson 2001).

Transport of gases

Both oxygen (O_2) and carbon dioxide (CO_2) are transported in blood plasma and attached to haemoglobin within erythrocytes (red blood cells). Key gas transport terminology is summarised in Table 27.3. The vast majority of oxygen, around 98.5%, is transported attached to haemoglobin in the erythrocyte (red blood cell). Each erythrocyte contains around 280 million haemoglobin and each haemoglobin has the potential to carry four oxygen (O_2) molecules. The remaining 1.5% of oxygen is dissolved in blood plasma, this volume of oxygen is measured in terms of the pressure it exerts (kilopascals – kPa). This measurement of oxygen is expressed as

Table 27.3 Definitions of important gas transport terminology.

GAS TRANSPORT TERM	DEFINITION
Oxygen saturation	SaO_2 – The percentage of arterial haemoglobin carrying oxygen molecules SpO_2 – SaO_2 measured by a pulse-oximeter
Partial pressure of arterial oxygen (PaO_2)	The amount of oxygen dissolved in arterial blood plasma measured in kilopascals (kPa)
Partial pressure of carbon dioxide ($PaCO_2$)	The amount of carbon dioxide dissolved in arterial blood plasma measured in kilopascals (kPa)
Oxygen capacity	The potential space for oxygen transport by haemoglobin (Hb) per 100 mL of blood Hb × 1.34 = oxygen capacity per 100 mL of blood
Arterial oxygen content (CaO_2)	The actual amount of oxygen in arterial blood by haemoglobin (Hb) per 100 mL of arterial blood Arterial oxygen saturation (SaO_2) × oxygen capacity = oxygen content per 100 mL of arterial blood
Oxygen delivery (DO_2)	The actual amount of oxygen being delivered to body tissues based on cardiac output Arterial oxygen content (CaO_2) × cardiac output = oxygen delivery (DO_2)
Oxygen consumption (VO_2)/Oxygen extraction ratio	The amount of oxygen utilised by body tissues each minute

partial pressure of arterial oxygen (PaO_2) and in health should be around 11–13.5 kPa.

Effective oxygen delivery is naturally reliant upon the presence of an adequate supply of erythrocytes and haemoglobin (Hb). In health the average male's circulation would contain between 15–18 g of haemoglobin (Hb) for every 100 mL of his blood. Each gram of haemoglobin can carry approximately 1.34 mL of oxygen. Therefore, a male patient with an Hb of 16 g/100 mL of blood would have the capacity to carry 21.44 mL of oxygen per every 100 mL of blood (16 × 1.34 = 21.44). This volume of oxygen is referred to as **oxygen capacity**. Even in health, it is rare for any individual's haemoglobin to be fully saturated with oxygen. To ascertain the actual amount of oxygen being transported by haemoglobin, oxygen saturation (SaO_2) needs to be taken into account. A male with an Hb of 16 g/100 mL of blood and an SaO_2 of 98%, for example would be carrying of 21 mL of oxygen (0.98 × 21.44) in every 100 mL of blood. The actual amount of oxygen being carried in arterial blood is referred to as 'oxygen content' (CaO_2). Multiplying CaO_2 by cardiac output will indicate the amount of oxygen being delivered to all body tissues each minute. This volume of oxygen is called **oxygen delivery** (DO_2) and assuming cardiac output is a steady 5000 mL of blood per minute the aforementioned individual would have an oxygen delivery (DO_2) of 1050 mL of oxygen per minute (21 × (5000/100) = 1050) (see Table 27.3).

Jot This Down

Take some time to think about how anaemia may affect distribution of oxygen throughout the body. How might a Hb level of 10 g per 100 mL of blood change a nurse's view of their oxygen saturation reading.

The relationship between oxygen attached to arterial haemoglobin (SaO_2) and oxygen dissolved in plasma (PaO_2) is described by the oxyhaemoglobin dissociation curve (Figure 27.12). As PaO_2 falls, SaO_2 decreases in an S-shaped curve. If PaO_2 falls as low as 8 kPa, SaO_2 will remain around 90%. Therefore, natural fluctuations in oxygenation, such as occur when singing, laughing and talking, will not result in dramatic reductions in oxygen saturations. The release of oxygen from haemoglobin can be increased by 2–3, diphosphoglycerate (2,3-DPG), which is released during hypoxia and high temperatures.

Just like oxygen (O_2), a small amount of carbon dioxide (CO_2), around 10%, is transported in plasma. The normal pressure levels of carbon dioxide in arterial plasma ($PaCO_2$) are between 4.5 and 6 kPa. Carbon dioxide is also transported attached to haemoglobin (Hb), although only around 20% is transported that way. Nevertheless, haemoglobin has a greater affinity for carbon dioxide than oxygen. Within the tissues, this facilitates the release of oxygen, as carbon dioxide is being created. However, as carbon dioxide levels increase (hypercapnia), the amount of oxygen binding to haemoglobin will be reduced. Any build-up of carbon dioxide will affect the oxyhaemoglobin dissociation curve by pulling the natural curve to the right, resulting in a greater risk of reduced arterial oxygen levels. Conversely, a fall in carbon dioxide (hypocapnia) has the opposite affect (see Figure 27.12). The remaining 70% of carbon dioxide combines with water to form carbonic acid. Carbonic acid then quickly dissociates into bicarbonate ions and hydrogen ions (see equation below).

$$CO_2 + H_2O \rightleftharpoons H_2CO_3 \rightleftharpoons H^+ + HCO_3^-$$

Where: CO_2 = carbon dioxide ions, H_2O = Water, H_2CO_3 = CARBONIC Acid, H^+ = hydrogen ions and HCO_3^- = bicarbonate ions.

Naturally, the carbon dioxide dissolved in plasma will also generate carbonic acid. However, the reaction which occurs within the erythrocyte is much faster due to the presence of the enzyme carbonic anhydrase. The production of hydrogen and bicarbonate helps to regulate arterial blood pH, which should rest between 7.35–7.45. As levels of hydrogen ion rise and pH starts to fall below 7.35, more hydrogen ions are combined with bicarbonate to form carbonic acid. As hydrogen ion levels fall and pH starts to rise, more carbonic acid dissociates. Effective respiration can, therefore help regulate hydrogen ion concentration (Clancy & McVicar 2007).

Internal respiration

Internal respiration describes the exchange of oxygen and carbon dioxide between blood and tissue cells; a phenomenon governed by the same principles as external respiration. Cells are continually using oxygen in the production of energy (ATP) and therefore, concentrations of oxygen within the tissues are always lower than within the capillaries. Similarly, the continual production of ATP ensures that the levels of carbon dioxide within tissue are always higher than within the capillaries. As blood flows through the capillaries, oxygen and carbon dioxide follow their pressure gradients and continually diffuse between blood and tissue (Figure

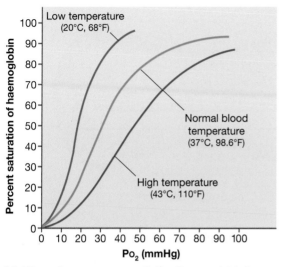

(a) Effect of temperature on affinity of haemoglobin for oxygen

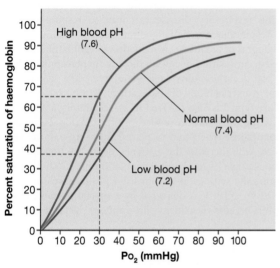

(b) Effect of pH on affinity of haemoglobin for oxygen

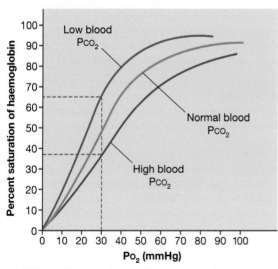

(c) Effect of Pco$_2$ on affinity of haemoglobin for oxygen

Figure 27.12 The oxyhaemoglobin dissociation curve.

27.13). The concentration of oxygen in the blood flowing away from the tissues in venous circulation is said to be de-oxygenated. In reality, if measured, the **oxygen saturation** of venous blood would probably be around 75% in health. This means that only around 25% of oxygen content (CaO$_2$) leaves the bloodstream, leaving a plentiful reserve. The actual amount of oxygen used by the tissues every minute is referred to as **oxygen consumption** (VO$_2$) or **oxygen extraction ratio** (OER) (Table 27.3).

Hypoxia and Hypoxaemia

Hypoxia is defined as a lack of oxygen within body tissues. **Hypoxaemia** meanwhile is defined as a lack of oxygen within arterial blood. Hypoxaemia is present when a patient's oxygen saturation is less than 90% or the partial pressure of oxygen dissolved in plasma is less than 8 kPa. Naturally, hypoxaemia will lead to hypoxia as the tissues are receiving less oxygen. However, as respiration also relies on a fully functioning cardiovascular system, hypoxia can also occur even when arterial blood is fully oxygenated (Table 27.4).

Respiratory Disease

The World Health Organization's (WHO) *International Statistical Classification of Disease and Health Problems* includes 10 sections on respiratory disease, which includes information on pneumonia, influenza, asthma, chronic obstructive pulmonary disease, pneumoconiosis and interstitial pulmonary disorders – all of which are addressed in this chapter (WHO 2010). When defining respiratory disease, The British Thoracic Society also includes illnesses that can affect lung function. This chapter therefore also includes a discussion on tuberculosis and lung cancer (BTS 2006). Respiratory disease has many causes. Some diseases, such as tuberculosis, pneumonia, influenza, are contracted via the inhalation of a pathogen. Others are associated with lifestyle or occupation. Chronic obstructive pulmonary disease and lung cancer for example, are caused by smoking and pneumoconioses develop due consistent exposure to harmful occupational agents. Whatever the cause of a patient's respiratory problem social class remains an influencing factor. People of lower social class are far more likely to develop and live with respiratory disease. This social inequality has an impact on mortality with adult males in unskilled work being 14 times more likely to die from a respiratory disease than adult males in professional roles (BTS 2006).

Link To/Go To

The NHS Atlas of Variation in Healthcare for people with Respiratory Disease – a presentation first made available in September 2012, outlines the importance of reducing variation in standards of care delivery for people with respiratory disease in the UK.

http://www.rightcare.nhs.uk/index.php/atlas/respiratorydisease/

Respiratory Failure

Respiratory failure occurs when respiration is unable to sustain the metabolic needs of the body (Schwartzstein & Parker 2006). Respiratory failure occurs when the individual's respiratory disease has altered lung function, to the extent that they are no longer able to

607

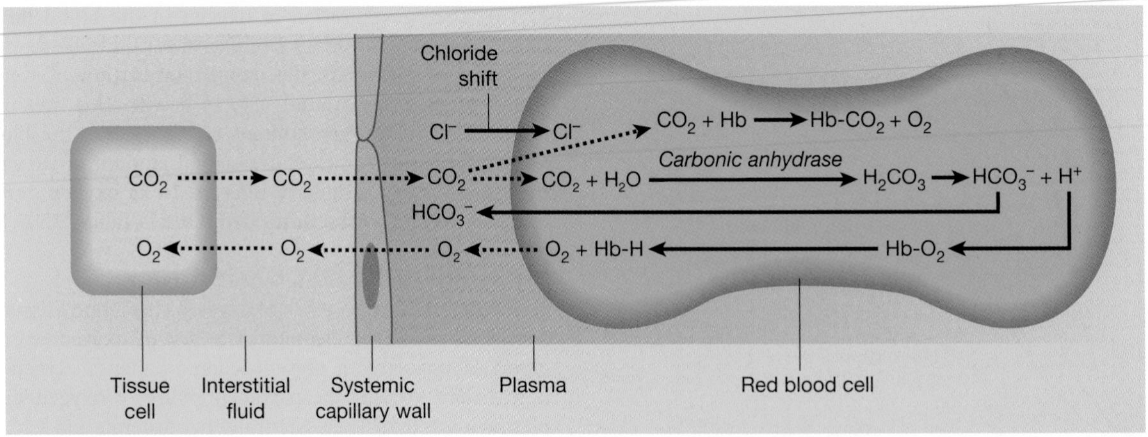

Figure 27.13 Internal respiration: the exchange of oxygen and carbon dioxide within the lungs.

Table 27.4 Table summarising the major types of hypoxia and their causes.

TYPE OF HYPOXIA	CAUSE
Stagnant or circulatory hypoxia	Heart failure, lack of cardiac output leads to hypoxia
Haemic hypoxia	Lack of blood or haemoglobin (haemorrhage, for example)
Histotoxic hypoxia	Poisoning, i.e. carbon monoxide inhalation
Demand hypoxia	May occur when the demand for oxygen is high, i.e. during fever
Hypoxic hypoxia	Hypoxia as a result of hypoxaemia

maintain adequate oxygen saturation levels and are at risk of developing hypoxaemia. In some instances, the individual's condition deteriorates to the extent that they are also no longer able to expel excess carbon dioxide. Respiratory failure therefore is categorised into two types, labelled type 1 and type 2. Individuals unable to maintain adequate oxygen levels are said to be in **respiratory failure type 1**, whereas those patients who deteriorate further and are unable to expel excess carbon dioxide are described as being in **respiratory failure type 2**.

Respiratory failure type 1

Hypoxaemic patients, with oxygen saturation readings lower than 90% or a partial pressure oxygen reading of less than 8 kPa will be in respiratory failure type 1. Ultimately, the management of patients in respiratory failure type 1 will focus on treating the underlying causative respiratory disease/disorder and the provision of oxygen to maintain oxygen saturations above 92% or 88% in patients with chronic carbon dioxide retention (O'Driscoll *et al.* 2008).

Red Flag

Individuals with chronic obstructive pulmonary disease (COPD) may have chronic carbon dioxide retention, which may desensitise their hypercapnic drive. As a result such patients may rely more on their hypoxic drive. Excess oxygen therefore may reduce respiratory effort and care should therefore be taken when administering oxygen to individuals with COPD.

Respiratory failure type 2

Respiratory disease often leads to increased respiratory effort ('work of breathing') and therefore acute exacerbation of any underlying respiratory disease can lead to respiratory muscle fatigue. Respiratory muscle fatigue may lead to shallow and weak rate and depths of breathing. A reduction in ventilation leads to an increased accumulation of carbon dioxide (hypercapnia). Elevated arterial blood carbon dioxide levels above 6 kPa will lead to a reduction in arterial blood pH (see earlier). For this reason, respiratory failure type 2 is also referred to as 'respiratory acidosis'. Ventilation is the only way to reduce carbon dioxide. Patients with respiratory failure type 2 may be placed onto a mechanical ventilator, which will increase the patient's depth of breathing. One common example of mechanical ventilation used in both hospital and community settings, is non-invasive positive pressure ventilation (NIPPV). NIPPV is delivered by a special portable machine that delivers breaths via a flexible hose and special facial mask (BTS 2002).

Respiratory Assessment

The nurse must ensure that they perform a thorough and systematic respiratory assessment in order to establish acute deterioration early, stabilise the patient's condition and avoid unnecessary transfer to intensive care units (Higginson & Jones 2009). A comprehensive respiratory assessment must include an initial assessment, to establish severity of condition and to detect early signs of acute deterioration and a patient history (Simpson 2006).

Respiratory rate

On initial assessment, the nurse must establish the severity of the patient's condition. Respiratory rate plays a pivotal role in the nurse's assessment. An adult's respiratory rate should remain between 12 and 16 respirations per minute at rest (Dougherty & Lister 2011). Any changes in respiratory rates are clinically significant. Respiration rates less than 12 respirations per minute at rest are associated with opiate overdose, respiratory fatigue, central nervous system depression and hypothermia. Raised respiratory rates greater than 24 respirations per minute (tachypnoea) at rest are a key indicator acute deterioration and are associated with high mortality rate. When assessing respiratory rate the nurse must also observe for signs of respiratory distress or dyspnoea (difficulty in breathing). Dyspnoea may be positional and patients may find relief if positioned appropriately. Table 27.5 details some common positional dyspnoeas.

Assessing respiratory rate alone will not provide all the necessary information for a comprehensive respiratory assessment. In order to fully establish a patient's respiratory status the nurse must check the following:

- Respiratory rate in respirations per minute
- Inspiration/expiration ratio
- Shape of chest expansion
- Added sounds.

In normal quiet breathing, exhalation should be approximately twice as long as inspiration, in other words, an inspiration : expira-

tion ratio of 1:2. This will ensure that minute volume (V_E) the volume of air inspired and expired in one minute (see Table 27.2) is adequate enough for both inhalation of oxygen and expulsion of carbon dioxide. Assessment of the inspiration: expiration ratio can detect signs of respiratory distress and inadequate lung function (Higginson & Jones 2009). Any changes in chest expansion are abnormal. Hypoventilation for example could lead to a reduction of gaseous exchange and therefore potentially hypoxaemia and asymmetrical breathing could suggest a flail chest or a pneumothorax. The nurse should also note the use of accessory muscles of breathing, such as scalenes or sternocleidomastoids (see Figure 27.7). The use of accessory muscles of breathing is regarded as a cardinal sign of respiratory distress (Cox 2001). Added sounds include wheeze, which occurs when increased airway resistance is present, as a result of airway inflammation in asthma for example, and stridor, a high pitched wheeze that occurs when the airway is obstructed. Many conditions can alter a patient's breathing pattern and if the nurse could identity such a change they are better placed to plan appropriate and effective care. Table 27.6 details some of the more common abnormal respiratory patters and their causes.

Table 27.5 Common positional dyspnoeas, their characteristics and causes.

POSITIONAL DYSPNOEA	CHARACTERISTICS	CAUSES
Orthopnoea	Difficulty in breathing when lying down	Severe asthma Congestive heart failure Chronic obstructive pulmonary disease Mitral valve disease
Trepopnoea	Patient is more comfortable lying on their side	Congestive heart failure
Platypnoea	Difficulty in breathing sitting up	Arterial hypoxaemia

Care, Dignity and Compassion

Patients often describe dyspnoea, difficulty in breathing, as breathlessness. Breathlessness can be very distressing and frightening. Breathless patients will therefore require comfort, reassurance and explanations of oxygen and prescribed respiratory medication.

Table 27.6 Abnormal respiratory patterns, their characteristics and their causes.

RESPIRATORY PATTERN	CHARACTERISTICS	CAUSES
Cheyne–Stokes respiration	Cyclic respiratory pattern which fluctuates between fast and slow respiratory rates interspersed with periods of apnoea	Increased intercranial pressure Severe heart failure Renal failure Drugs overdose Meningitis End of life
Tachypnoea	Rapid, shallow, respiratory rate greater than 24 respirations per minute	Exercise Fear and anxiety Respiratory failure Acidosis and alkalosis Brain stem lesions
Bradypnoea	Slow respiratory rate less than 10 respirations per minute	Drug overdose Brain stem lesions Coma
Hypoventilation	Slow, shallow respiration rate	Drug overdose Anaesthesia Chest or pleuritic pain
Hyperventilation Kussmaul's breathing (air hunger)	Increase in respiration rate and depth	Exercise Fear and anxiety Respiratory failure Acidosis and alkalosis Brain stem lesions
Biot's respiration	Irregular rate and depth interspersed with periods of apnoea	Head trauma Brain abscesses Heat stroke Spinal meningitis Encephalitis

What To Do If...The Patient Coughs When I'm Counting Respirations

It is important that your record of respiratory rate is accurate and if your patient does cough while you are counting respirations you should, once your patient has recovered, re-start your respiration count from the beginning – remember to count for a full minute.

Jot This Down

One of the signs of severe life-threatening asthma is an inability to speak in sentences. In terms of a comprehensive respiratory assessment, why is it so important for the nurse to establish whether their patient can speak in complete sentences.

Inspection

On initial assessment, the nurse must also observe for signs of cyanosis, a bluish or darkish hue, which could indicate hypoxaemia. Peripheral cyanosis, which is visible in the fingers and toes, is caused by deficient delivery of oxygenated blood to the peripheries. Because peripheral cyanosis is caused by deficient blood flow its presence does not necessarily indicate hypoxaemia. Heart failure, vascular occlusion or vasoconstriction (as occurs in extreme cold conditions, for example), could be the root cause of peripheral cyanosis. Central cyanosis, which is visible in the lips and mouth, occurs when haemoglobin are carrying reduced amounts of oxygen, often as a result of respiratory failure. Oxygen saturations usually have to fall below 90% (or plasma levels of $<8\,kPa$) before central cyanosis is visible. However, patients with anaemia may not display signs of cyanosis as their depleted levels of haemoglobin may still be fully saturated with oxygen. Central cyanosis may also be present in patients with polycythaemia, a condition which stimulates the over production of erythrocytes (red blood cells). Other useful assessments include the presence of finger clubbing, an indicator of respiratory disease and halitosis, which could be a sign of respiratory tract infection.

Peak flow and spirometry

Other essential assessments include **peak expiratory flow rate** (PEFR) or 'peak flow' and **spirometry**. PEFR is the force of expiration in litres per minute and as such, it measures the extent of airway resistance. An inability to meet a predicted value based on age, sex and height, could indicate increased airway resistance, as occurs during an asthma attack (Talley & O'Connor 2001). Spirometry is a measurement of expiration, which is used by the multidisciplinary team to measure the extent of airway obstruction. Spirometry measures the force and volume of a maximum expiration after a full inspiration, a volume referred to as forced vital capacity (FVC). The volume the patient expired after 1 second is called 'forced expiratory volume' in the 1st second (FEV_1). By comparing FEV_1 with FVC, the FEV_1: FVC ratio, the severity of airway obstruction can be ascertained. An FEV_1: FVC ratio of less than 80% is indicative of an obstructive airways disease (Sheldon 2005).

Red Flag

Peak expiratory flow rates provide a quick and simple assessment of the airways; however regular peak flow measurements are more revealing than single arbitrary readings and nurses should be mindful that peak expiratory flow rates are effort dependent.

Oxygen saturations

Pulse oximeters are used to gauge the percentage of arterial haemoglobin that carries oxygen. This reading is called **oxygen saturation** (SpO_2), which in health, should be between 97% and 99%. The pressure of oxygen dissolved in arterial plasma (PaO_2) provides practitioners with a more accurate reflection of oxygenation. Arterial blood gas readings are attained by placing a sample of the patient's arterial blood into a blood gas analyser. A printed or visual result is produced, which provides information on arterial blood pH, carbon dioxide, bicarbonate as well as oxygen. An oxygen saturation produced via blood gas analysis is referred to as SaO_2.

Red Flag

Certain factors affect the accuracy of pulse oximeter readings. Tremors, anaemia, polycythaemia, cold extremities and nail varnish can all jeopardise an accurate reading. For this reason, SpO_2 should only be used in conjunction with other nursing observations (Clark et al. 2006).

Cough and sputum

Ascertaining the nature of a patient's cough can aid diagnosis. A cough which is worse during the night for example, is an indicator of asthma, whereas a cough with a sudden onset suggests inhalation of a foreign object. If the patient has a productive cough, samples should be collected for microscopy and culture in order to determine the presence of infection. However, the colour and consistency of a patient's sputum could provide a clue as to the nature of the patient's respiratory problem (Table 27.7). The presence of blood is also significant, haemoptysis for example may indicate the presence of tuberculosis.

Table 27.7 Characteristics of sputum and possible diagnoses.

SPUTUM CHARACTERISTICS	POSSIBLE DIAGNOSIS
Mucoid: clear, grey or white	Asthma Chronic bronchitis
Serous: Watery or frothy	Pulmonary oedema
Mucopurulent: yellowish Purulent: dark green/yellow Foul smelling	Respiratory tract infection
Blood stained	Carcinoma Pulmonary embolism Trauma

Patient history

A patient history could help the multidisciplinary team to establish the nature and severity of a patient's respiratory complaint. Childhood respiratory disease could be a precursor to adult lung problems and a family history could determine potential congenital respiratory disease. Use of vaccines could rule out influenza and recent foreign travel may suggest tropical disease. The patient's age could also help determine diagnosis. Respiratory distress in individuals under the age of 30 would suggest asthma, pneumothorax or cystic fibrosis, whereas dyspnoea in those over 50 years are more likely to be suffering lung cancer, pneumoconiosis or chronic obstructive pulmonary disease. Information on appetite and weight changes can also be of significance. Reduced appetite and weight loss is indicative of lung cancer and tuberculosis, for example. It is also vital that the nurse establishes some of the patient's living conditions and lifestyle choices. Many respiratory infections are exacerbated by damp and over-crowded living conditions; they may also work in a profession that exposes them to irritant substances, such as paint fumes, dust and animal dander. The latter is also true of patients with pets, a common example is pneumoconiosis caused by the dander of birds – a condition called bird fancier's lung. Smoking is the major cause of chronic obstructive pulmonary disease and lung cancer and an accurate smoking history, in pack years, could aid diagnosis, as could the volume of alcohol the patient drinks. Alcoholism is a risk factor for the development of pneumonia. If the patient already uses respiratory medication, it is vital that the nurse establishes the patient's compliance and in some instances their inhaler technique. Medication misuse or omissions may exacerbate their respiratory problems.

> ### Medicines Management
>
>
> For patients with asthma, it is very important that they use their steroid inhaler regularly and that their inhaler technique is correct. The regular correct use of steroid inhalers is recognised as a major way of preventing/reducing the incidence of asthma attacks.

Respiratory Tract Infection

Influenza

Influenza is a highly infectious and very common viral respiratory infection. Although influenza can be contracted at any time of year, in the Northern Hemisphere, influenza is most predominantly active during the winter months. New strains of the influenza virus could lead to global outbreaks or pandemics.

Pathophysiology

The influenza virus is found within aerosol particles and droplets produced by infected individuals via coughs and sneezes. Others then inadvertently inhale droplets or self-contaminate by touching infected areas. The viruses that cause influenza are called **orthomyxoviruses**. Typically, there are three types of orthomyxovirus: type A, type B and type C. *Type A influenza* viruses are found in both animals and humans. The outer lipoprotein layer of the type A influenza virus normally displays three proteins: haemagglutinin, neuraminidase and M2. There are 16 identified subtypes of haemagglutinin and nine subtypes of neuraminidase and type A influenza viruses are classified according to which subtypes are

present. For example the most common variation of type A influenza is H1N1, which displays haemagglutinin subtype 1 and neuraminidase subtype 1 on its outer lipoprotein layer. As type A influenza viruses are found in both animals and humans, infections can occasionally transfer between species. Recent examples include 'swine flu', which is a variation of the H1N1 virus and 'avian' or 'bird flu', which is caused by a H5N5 influenza strain. *Type B influenza* viruses are considered less severe than type A and almost exclusively affect humans only. *Type C infections* are thought only to cause mild or even asymptomatic infections (Driver 2012).

Individuals most at risk

- Children under 5 years old
- The older person
- Immunocompromised individuals
- Women in the later stages of pregnancy
- People with chronic health conditions, such as diabetes, respiratory, heart and renal disease, cancer
- Young adults (in flu pandemics).

Signs and symptoms

- Fever (sudden onset)
- Headache
- Sore throat
- Muscle aches
- Dry cough
- Weakness and malaise
- Fatigue
- Loss of appetite.

Nursing care and management

Mild and uncomplicated cases of influenza can be treated with rest, antipyretic drugs (i.e. paracetamol and ibuprofen) and plenty of fluids. For those living with or caring for individuals with influenza, effective hand washing and appropriate use of tissues should be promoted. Anti-viral drugs, such as oseltamivir or zanamivir are usually only prescribed to vulnerable or 'at risk' individuals. Such drugs are also mainly reserved for prophylactic cover for people with 'risk factors' that have been exposed to contagious individuals. The most effective management strategy for the minimisation of the impact of influenza is vaccination.

Complications/prognosis

Infection with influenza viruses can lead to the development of lower respiratory tract infections such as bronchitis and pneumonia. Mortality rates for influenza are almost exclusively as a result of secondary lower respiratory tract infection. The development of lower respiratory tract infections are greater in individuals with suppressed immune systems or those living with chronic illnesses such as diabetes, respiratory disease, heart disease or renal disease.

Pulmonary Tuberculosis

Pulmonary tuberculosis (TB) is a lower respiratory tract infection, which is predominantly caused by *Mycobacterium tuberculosis*, an air-borne slow-growing bacillus. The disease typically follows two phases: a primary and secondary infection.

Pathophysiology

During the *primary infection*, lymphocytes and neutrophils congregate at the infection site, usually in the upper lobes. The bacilli are then trapped and walled off by fibrous tissue. During the primary infection phase of TB, the infected individual is often asymptomatic and unaware they have TB. Until secondary infection the bacilli remain latent and the individual is not infective. *Secondary infection* occurs at some point after primary infection and is caused by the re-exposure to TB or another form of bacteria. The bacilli are then reactivated and quickly multiply, as a result the patient soon becomes symptomatic and infectious. Bacilli are very arduous and can survive trapped in fibrous tissue for long periods. Individuals can remain unaware that they have TB for many years. Over recent years, many strains of TB have become resistant to the first-line pharmacological treatments (see below). TB that is resistant to one or more first-line drug is referred to as multi-drug resistant TB (MDR-TB). Some strains of TB have become resistant to almost all the second-line pharmacological treatments a condition called extensively drug resistant TB (XDR-TB).

Risk factors

- Close contact with infected individuals
- Travel to and from, or spending time with people from, areas of high TB prevalence
- Suppressed immune system (i.e. Human immunodeficiency virus, HIV)
- Age – infants and the older person are at greater risk of contracting TB
- Homelessness
- Drug abuse and alcoholism.

(NICE 2011a)

Signs and symptoms

- Chronic cough
- Haemoptysis
- Weight loss
- Pyrexia
- Fatigue
- Night sweats.

(NICE 2011a)

Investigations

TB is diagnosed by chest X-ray and a sputum acid-fast staining test, which determines the presence of the bacteria that cause TB. Further culture tests will determine whether the species of TB infection is – *Mycobacterium tuberculosis, Myobacterium bovis, and Myobacterium africanum.* The possible outcomes of both tests are:

Acid-fast bacillus positive/culture positive – these individuals are infective and will need to isolated

Acid-fast bacillus negative/culture positive – in the majority of cases these individuals may not be infective

Acid-fast bacillus negative/culture negative – although the test is negative. patients displaying symptoms may still get a positive diagnosis of TB from their X-ray.

(Gough & Kaufman 2011)

Nursing care and management

TB is treated with a 6-month medication regimen that consists of 2 months of rifampicin, isoniazid, pyrazinamide and ethambutol, followed by a further 4 months of rifampicin and isoniazid. Infective patients will remain infective for the first 2 weeks of treatment.

Generally, individuals with TB are cared for in the community, with the main nursing focus being infection prevention and com-

pliance with drug therapy. Only if there is a medical or socioeconomic reason should the patient be cared for in hospital.

In-hospital care (NICE 2011a):

- All patients with TB should be risk assessed for MDR-TB
- Individuals with MDR-TB or individuals being nursed in a ward area that also cares for immune-suppressed patients should be nursed in a negative pressure isolation room
- Non-MDR-TB patients should be nursed in a side room until they are no longer deemed infective
- Separate utensils and crockery and gloves and aprons are not required unless there is risk of exposure to body fluid or other contaminant bacteria
- Masks need only be worn by nursing patients with MDR-TB or if there is risk of contamination from coughing, i.e. bronchoscopy or sputum collection
- Patients should wear masks if infective (i.e. first 2 weeks of treatment) and/or if visiting different hospital departments – X-ray, for example.

Health promotion and discharge

Pulmonary TB remains very treatable if the individual complies with the 6-month drug regimen. Non-compliance could lead to the further development of MDR-TB or even XDR-TB. As XDR-TB is resistant to almost all pharmacological treatment options it has a high mortality rate. It is for this reason that support with drug compliance is the key to the control and prevention of TB (Karim 2011).

Primary Care

As most patients with TB are cared for in the community, the main focus of the Primary Care Nurse will be:

- Advice and support with treatment compliance
- Advice on the reduction of transmission
- Restriction on visitors, especially young children, in the first 2 weeks of treatment
- Remaining away from work or study for the first 2 weeks of treatment
- Avoiding public transport
- Cough etiquette – covering mouth when coughing or sneezing and disposing tissues safely. Maintaining good hand hygiene
- Maintaining good ventilation at home by opening windows.

(Karim 2011)

Jot This Down

Individuals with infective TB will be nursed in isolation. Take time to consider how this might impact on their psychological well-being.

Pneumonia

Pneumonia is a lower respiratory tract infection, which is caused by a variety of inhaled pathogens. Infected individuals mainly contract pneumonia by inhaling a bacterium, virus or fungus. Pneumonia can also be caused by the aspiration of secretions such vomitus or by transmission of blood-borne pathogens from an infection elsewhere in the body. Pneumonia is classified by its cause and location. Some pneumonia infections are localised in one or more lobes and are described as lobular while other pneumonia infections are spread or diffuse throughout the lungs. Pneumonia can also be categorised as community or hospital-acquired (noso-comial). Community acquired pneumonia can be caused by both viral and bacterial infections. Although individuals with chronic cardiorespiratory disorders are at risk, healthy individuals can also be affected, especially following an influenza infection. Hospital-acquired (nosocomial) infection affects patients with low immune resistance, the older person or an immunosuppressed individual for example. Such cases are normally caused by bacterial infections, such as *Klebsiella pneumoniae* or *Pseudomonas aeruginosa* (Gould 2006).

Pathophysiology

Lobular pneumonia – Pneumonia infections which are localised to one or more lobes, are referred to as lobular infections. Lobular pneumonia is normally caused by bacterial infections, such as *Streptococcus pneumoniae* or *Pneumococcus* and it is associated with a sudden and acute onset of symptoms. Once the invading bacteria reach the lower respiratory tract beyond the trachea they multiply quickly in the warm and moist confines of deep lung tissue. The resultant inflammatory response causes vasodi-lation of capillaries, which causes the alveoli to fill with debris and exudate. The exudate quickly fills with neutrophils, eryth-rocytes and fibrin and a solid mass called consolidation soon forms. Consolidation in the alveoli disturbs external respiration and less oxygen diffuses from the alveoli into pulmonary circulation.

Bronchopneumonia – Bronchopneumonia infections are character-ised by a diffuse affected areas, which are spread throughout both lungs. It is an insidious onset with symptoms developing over time. Many pathogens can cause bronchopneumonia but the infection normally starts in the bronchi before spreading to the alveoli. The resultant alveoli inflammation causes a build-up of exudate within the alveoli walls and gaseous exchange is reduced as a result.

Legionnaire's disease – Community and hospital-acquired pneumo-nias caused by *Legionella pneumophila*, a Gram-negative bacte-ria found in natural water sources, are called Legionnaire's disease. Contraction of Legionnaire's disease usually occurs when people come into contact with infected in-built water sources, i.e. cooling systems. Legionnaire's disease causes severe lung consolidation with lung necrosis and has a high risk of mortality.

Primary Atypical Pneumonia (PAP) – PAP is caused by bacterial or viral infection. Bacterial infections include *Chlamydia pneumo-niae* and *Mycoplasma pneumoniae,* a miniscule bacteria found within the upper respiratory tract. Viral pneumonia usually occurs as a result of influenza, when upper respiratory tract inflammation descends into the lower respiratory tract causing diffuse inflammation of interstitial tissue rather than the alveoli themselves.

Pneumocystis carinii pneumonia (PCP) – PCP is considered to be a fungal infection, which when inhaled, causes alveolar necrosis and diffuse interstitial tissue inflammation. The alveoli fill with exudate as a result. PCP is an opportunistic and often deadly infection, which preys on individuals with weakened immune systems (Gould 2006).

Risk factors

- Age – the very young and the older person are at greater risk
- Individuals living with chronic cardiorespiratory disease
- Immunocompromised individuals
- Smoking
- Alcoholism and drug abuse
- Intubation – unconscious patients have increased risk of devel-oping pneumonia
- Patients at risk of aspiration, i.e. patients with dysphagia, stroke, gastric reflux.

Signs and symptoms

- Hypoxaemia
- Tachypnoea and dyspnoea
- Tachycardia
- Pyrexia – in response to bacterial infection
- Dehydration – pyrexia causes fluid loss, also body loses humidi-fied air on expiration
- Reduced lung expansion – consolidation makes it hard to expand the lungs and breathing becomes difficult
- Pain – inflammation could spread to the pleura, causing pleuritic pain
- Productive cough – the exudate present in the alveoli often pro-duces rusty coloured sputum
- Lethargy.

Investigations

A diagnosis of pneumonia can be confirmed by sputum cultures that identify the causative agent. An X-ray can also establish the extent of lung tissue damage. In addition a white blood cell count of above 11×10^9 per litre can indicate inflammation, infection or an immune system response and raised urea levels of greater than 7 mmol/L are another indicator of severe infection (Hoare & Lim 2006).

Nursing care and management

Pneumonia is treated by the administration of antibiotics and the majority of cases will be nursed in the community. Nurses caring for individuals with pneumonia in hospital settings play a vital role in the early detection of deterioration. The main care goals include:

- Safe administration of prescribed antibiotics
- Safe administration of prescribed oxygen – to correct hypoxae-mia and maintain oxygen saturations above 90%
- Patient positioning – placing the patient in an upright position will promote diaphragm and intercostal muscle activity and enhance ventilation
- Establishing and minimising pain levels – to make the patient more comfortable and enhance respiratory effort
- Temperature management – safe administration of antipyretic agents, such as aspirin, paracetamol or ibuprofen, electric fans, reducing bed clothing
- Close monitoring of vital signs – respiration rate greater than 30 respirations per minute, new hypotension (systolic less than 90 mmHg or diastolic less than 60 mmHg) and new mental con-fusion could indicate life-threatening pneumonia (Lim *et al.* 2009). Vital signs should therefore be recorded hourly until patient's condition stabilises
- Fluid balance – as patient may be dehydrated. A minimum of 2.5 L every 24 hours is required. Fluids may be administered intravenously, if required (Dunn 2005)
- Communication – to reduce anxiety and promote comfort.

Health promotion and discharge

In the UK, prognosis for pneumonia managed in the community is good with a mortality rate just 1% of all cases. Mortality does, however, increase with severity and over time with mortality rates being significantly higher 5 years after diagnosis (Lim *et al.* 2009).

Primary Care

A sizeable proportion of patients with pneumonia will be cared for in the community and the main focus of primary care is ensuring a safe recovery. The nurse should ensure that the following occur:

· Regular assessment – nurses should be alert for the signs of acute deterioration
· Review patients well-being every 48 hours
· Refer any patients with signs of severe or life-threatening pneumonia to a hospital setting
· Advising patients to get plenty of rest
· Ensure patients increase fluid intake
· Advise patients to refrain from smoking
· Treat pleuritic pain with mild non-steroidal anti-inflammatory drugs, such as paracetamol.
· Consider nutritional supplements in prolonged cases.

(BTS 2001)

Obstructive Lung Disorders

Obstructive lung disorders disrupt airflow in and out of the lungs. In conditions such as asthma and chronic obstructive pulmonary disease (COPD), the obstruction to airflow occurs as a result of airway narrowing and an increased resistance to airflow, especially during expiration. In many patients, airway resistance can be overcome by increasing respiratory muscle work. However, normal passive expiration may not be enough to promote adequate alveoli emptying and resultant forced expiration may generate high intrathoracic pressures that force smaller airways to close, trapping air in the chest.

Asthma

Asthma is a chronic inflammatory airway disease. Individuals with asthma are said to have hypersensitive or hyper-responsive airways resulting in periods of reversible inflammation and constriction in the bronchi and bronchioles. Increased airway inflammation and constriction obstructs airflow resulting in a characteristic wheeze.

Pathophysiology

The pathophysiology of asthma is complicated and intricate. The walls of the bronchi and bronchioles contain smooth muscle and are lined with mucus-secreting glands and ciliated cells. Large quantities of mast cells are found adjacent to the airways' blood supply. Once stimulated the mast cells release a number of cytokines (chemical messengers), which cause physiological changes to the linings of the bronchi and bronchioles. The three main cytokines

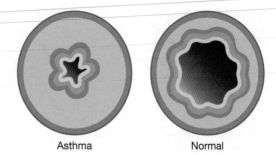

Figure 27.14 Airway pathophysiology, normal compared with asthmatic.

are histamine, kinin and prostaglandin, which cause smooth muscle contraction, increased mucus production and increased capillary permeability. As a result the airways soon narrow and become flooded with mucus and fluid leaking from blood vessels (Figure 27.14). As the airways become obstructed, it becomes increasingly difficult to breathe and to expectorate the mucus. If left unresolved, fatigue can occur resulting in a weak and inadequate respiratory effort, which may cause hypoxaemia and in severe cases hypercapnia (Sims 2006).

Risk factors

Individuals with asthma periodically react to triggers, substances or situations that would not normally cause airway inflammation and constriction. Traditionally individuals are divided into those who suffer with extrinsic asthma and those with intrinsic asthma. In individuals with extrinsic asthma, airway inflammation is thought to occur as a consequence of hypersensitive reactions associated with allergy, i.e. pollen, dust mites or foodstuffs. Whereas intrinsic asthma is linked to hyper-responsive reactions to other forms of stimuli, infection, sudden exposure to cold, exercise, stress or cigarette smoke, for example. In reality, many people have a combination of both intrinsic and extrinsic asthma and irrespective of the causative agents the pathophysiological changes, symptoms and treatments are the same.

Signs and symptoms

The main symptoms of asthma are:

• Cough, which may become productive with thick sticky mucus
• Dyspnoea and chest tightness
• Wheeze
• Peak flow less than predicted or best

  Signs and symptoms of acute-severe asthma:

• Peak flow 50% less than predicted or best
• Dyspnoea accompanied by an inability to complete sentences in one breath
• Tachypnoea
• Tachycardia

  Signs and symptoms of acute life-threatening asthma:

• Peak flow less than 33% of predicted or best
• Oxygen saturation (SpO$_2$) less than 92%
• Silent chest
• Weak and feeble respiratory effort
• Cyanosis
• Bradycardia or hypotension
• Confusion, exhaustion or coma.

  British Thoracic Society and Scottish Intercollegiate Guidelines Network (BTS & SIGN 2009).

Diagnosis/investigations

A diagnosis of asthma is complicated by the fact that many of its main symptoms are also indicators of other respiratory diseases. The British Thoracic Society and Scottish Intercollegiate Guidelines Network (BTS & SIGN 2009) consider the presence of one or more of the main symptoms to indicate a high probability of the presence of asthma if the symptoms are:

- Frequent and recurrent
- Worse during the night or in the early morning
- Occur in response to or are worse after exercise or contact with triggers
- Occur in the absence of a cold

A diagnosis of asthma is also likely in the presence of:

- Personal history of an atopic disorder
- Family history of atopic disorder or asthma
- Widespread wheeze on auscultation
- Improvement in lung function or symptoms after adequate therapy.

In addition, for adults, a diagnosis of asthma is likely if main symptoms of asthma occur after taking aspirin or beta-blockers, if they have an otherwise unexplained low peak flow or if they have unexplained peripheral blood eosinophilia.

Nursing care and management

Nurses must be aware of the signs of severe and life-threatening asthma (see earlier). Asthma is reversible and care should focus on close monitoring and health promotion. The main care goals are:

- Continuous monitoring of vital signs until patient has stabilised
- Safe administration of prescribed oxygen to maintain oxygen saturation above 92%
- Safe administration of prescribed bronchodilators and steroids – to alleviate dyspnoea (Table 27.8 and Table 27.9)
- Communication – as speaking requires a constant flow of air, patients experiencing acute breathlessness are only able to talk for very short periods before the need to breathe interrupts them.

Table 27.8 Summary of corticosteroids used in the treatment of respiratory disease. (Source: Adapted from Barnes 2008 and the Joint Formulary Committee 2011)

INDICATION	CORTICOSTEROIDS[a]	ROUTE	CARE CONSIDERATIONS
Prophylaxis and reduction of frequency of exacerbations	Beclomethasone Budesonide Fluticasone	Inhaler	Inhaled corticosteroids can cause hoarseness, loss of voice and candidiasis. Patients are advised to rinse out their mouths after taking these inhalers
Exacerbation	Prednisolone Hydrocortisone	Oral Intravenous	Patients taking prednisolone and hydrocortisone will need careful monitoring as steroids can cause the following side-effects: · Osteoporosis · Diabetes · Weight gain · Increased body hair · Altered mood

[a]Corticosteroids are potent anti-inflammatory agents. They are used to reduce bronchial hyperactivity in patients with asthma, chronic obstructive pulmonary disease and other respiratory diseases where reversibility is present. The table shows the main corticosteroids currently utilised.

Table 27.9 Summary of bronchodilator therapies given in asthma and chronic obstructive pulmonary disease. (Source: Adapted from Barnes 2008 and the Joint Formulary Committee 2011)

TYPE	ACTIONS	EXAMPLES	ROUTES	CARE CONSIDERATIONS
Beta-2 agonists	Mimics the actions of adrenaline. Beta-2 agonists stimulate beta-2 receptor sites in the airways promoting rapid bronchodilation within 15 minutes, with a duration of 4–8 hours – depending on dose	Salbutamol Terbutaline Fenoterol Salmeterol	Inhaler Nebuliser Oral Subcutaneous	Patient will need to be advised of the potential for tachycardia and hand tremor
Anticholinergics	Blocks the action of acetylcholine, a neurotransmitter released by the parasympathetic nervous system. Acetylcholine promotes bronchoconstriction and bronchial secretion. Peak bronchodilator effects occur within 1 hour, with a duration similar to beta-2 agonists	Ipratropium bromide	Inhaler Nebuliser	Patient may need frequent mouthwashes may cause dry mouth and a bitter taste
Methylxanthines	Increases concentration of intracellular cyclic adenosine monophosphate (cAMP). Increased cAMP causes bronchodilation	Theophylline	Oral Intravenous (as aminophylline)	Optimal effects occur when plasma theophylline levels are between 10 and 20 mg/L. Regular blood tests are required

The patient's inability to complete a sentence, therefore, provides a sensitive measure of the extent of a patient's respiratory distress (Higginson & Jones 2009)

- Regular peak flow (PEFR) measurement
- Comfort and reassurance – dyspnoea can be a traumatic experience and fear and anxiety also promote hyperventilation. Listen to the patient's anxieties and provide continuous explanations for the multidisciplinary team's actions
- Sputum collection – yellow or green sputum can indicate infection
- Health promotion – avoidance of triggers, compliance with prescribed pharmacological therapies, smoking cessation and weight reduction in obese patients may reduce the frequency of asthma attacks.

Red Flag

Singular or infrequent peak flows will not accurately reflect the patient's status. PEFR should be measured every 15–30 minutes after commencement of treatment until conditions stabilise. PEFR can also be used to measure the effectiveness of bronchodilator therapy; therefore, PEFR should be measured pre- and post-inhaled or nebulised beta-2 agonists at least 4 times a day throughout their stay in hospital.

Health promotion and discharge

Although each year around 1000–1200 people die as a result of an exacerbation of their asthma, the disease is reversible and it is estimated that 90% of asthma deaths are preventable. The natural history of wheeze suggests that the earlier the presentation the better the prognosis with infants developing symptoms of wheeze before the age of 2 years being more likely to be symptom free by mid-childhood. Males are more likely to develop asthma during childhood and are more likely to be asymptomatic after adolescence whereas females are more likely to develop symptoms during adolescence (BTS & SIGN 2009).

Primary Care

The major role of the Primary Care Nurse will be to promote self-management in patients with asthma. This should entail:

- A written personalised action plan
- Regular reviews by trained asthma clinicians
- Regular reviews of medication usage to optimise treatments
- Promotion of appropriate use of steroid inhalers
- Advice on smoking cessation.

Chronic Obstructive Pulmonary Disease

Chronic obstructive pulmonary disease (COPD) is often defined as airflow obstruction that is progressive, not fully reversible and does not change markedly over several months. Patients diagnosed with chronic bronchitis and emphysema are collectively regarded as having COPD. Chronic asthma sufferers are also at risk of developing fixed airway obstruction as their airways become re-modelled over time.

Pathophysiology

Emphysema **Emphysema** is the permanent enlargement of the airspaces beyond the terminal bronchiole and the destruction of the elastic recoil of the alveolar wall. This degeneration of lung tissue is thought to be related to the action of destructive enzymes called **proteases**. Proteases are released from neutrophils and macrophages during respiratory infections. To minimise the effects of proteases lung tissue produces a substance called (alpha) α-1 antitrypsin, which counteracts the destructive action of protease. Individuals with emphysema produce less effective α-1 antitrypsin and alveolar destruction is allowed to continue unabated. This reduction in the efficacy of α-1 antitrypsin is predominantly caused by smoking. The resultant damaged alveoli lack the elastic recoil that is required for exhalation often resulting in over-inflation and air trapping (Hogg & Senior 2002). Increased intrathoracic pressure pushes the diaphragm downwards, disturbing its natural concave shape and making breathing difficult. Respiratory infections can easily develop as individuals find it increasingly difficult to expectorate secretions. Also, further destruction of the alveolar walls and nearby capillaries will result in reduced surface area for external respiration rendering the patient at risk of hypoxaemia and hypoxia (Gould 2006).

Chronic bronchitis **Chronic bronchitis** is defined as the presence of a productive cough lasting for 3 months in each of two consecutive years when other pulmonary and cardiac causes of cough have been ruled out (Braman 2006). Chronic bronchitis is characterised by increased mucus production and damaged bronchial cilia in the bronchi. The increase in mucus stimulates airway irritant receptors, resulting in a chronic cough. Constant airway irritation produces inflammation and a thickening of the bronchial wall and the destruction of cilia makes mucus clearance difficult and mucus collects and blocks the smaller airways as a result. The individual is then susceptible to further infections which cause yet more irritation and inflammation. Over time, increasing numbers of airways become blocked reducing external respiration. The increased mucus production and cilia dysfunction found in chronic bronchitis occurs in response to a constant bombardment of inhaled pollutants such as cigarette smoke (MacNee 2006).

Risk factors

- Smoking
- Occupational pollutants
- Alpha(α)-1 anti-trypsin syndrome.

Signs and symptoms

- FEV_1 less than predicted
- Dyspnoea, due to airway obstruction and air trapping
- Productive cough
- Reduced exercise tolerance
- Cor pulmonale – chronic hypoxia causes hypertension within pulmonary circulation. Eventually, the right ventricle becomes enlarged and fails, ultimately leading to peripheral oedema.

Diagnosis/investigations

The symptoms of chronic asthma may be indistinguishable from COPD and many COPD patients may also have asthma. Accurate diagnosis therefore is often problematic (Devereux 2006; NICE 2010). However, the following investigations can help MDT members when a diagnosis of COPD is being considered.

- Spirometry – an FEV_1 of less than 80% of FVC indicates airway obstruction
- Chest X-ray (to exclude other respiratory disease, i.e. lung cancer)
- CT scan – can determine the presence of emphysema
- Arterial blood gas readings – to determine precise levels of arterial oxygen and carbon dioxide
- Sputum examination
- Lung function tests
- Exercise testing.

Nursing care and management

The main management goals for COPD are:

- Smoking cessation advice
- Education on prescribed oxygen and bronchodilator therapies – to maximise relief of breathlessness
- Immunisation – to minimise frequency of exacerbations
- Dietary advice – severe weight loss is a feature of both emphysema and chronic bronchitis
- Pulmonary rehabilitation
- Promotion of self-management techniques – COPD is associated with high levels of anxiety and depression.

Care, Dignity and Compassion

COPD is a diverse and varied condition and its management requires a holistic approach centred upon self-management and symptom control. Wherever possible the patient should be cared for in their own home.

Health promotion and discharge

COPD is a chronic irreversible respiratory disorder. Management should focus on holistic interventions that focus on self-management and symptom control. Patients with COPD can experience exacerbations of their condition and the following are factors that may lead to hospitalisation.

- Inability to cope at home
- Poor social circumstances
- Cyanosis
- Rapid onset of exacerbation
- Impaired levels of consciousness
- Need for long-term oxygen therapy
- Confusion or disorientation
- SpO_2 less than 90%
- Raised arterial carbon dioxide levels ($PaCO_2$) greater than 6 kPa
- Chest X-ray changes
- Comorbidities, i.e. associated heart disease, diabetes.

NICE (2010)

Primary Care

One of the major care concepts for patients living with chronic obstructive pulmonary disease is the maintenance of well-being through the active utilisation of coping strategies. This should entail:

- Regular reviews by trained respiratory clinicians
- Regular reviews of medication usage to optimise treatments
- Promotion of self-management and coping strategies
- Referral to pulmonary rehabilitation services
- Advice on smoking cessation.

Bronchiectasis

Bronchiectasis is chronic airway dilation caused by chronic inflammation. The inflammation is often caused by inadequate clearance of microorganisms or chronic/frequent lung infections. Patients with bronchiectasis have thickened bronchial walls and suffer frequent sputum production and chronic coughs.

Pathophysiology

In bronchiectasis, lung function deteriorates over many years. Patients become locked in a vicious cycle of infection, inflammation and damage. Once infected, the patient's inability to clear the pathogen leads to an inflammatory response. While inflammation protects against pathogens, in patients unable to clear microorganisms the inflammatory response may become chronic and counterproductive, leading to bronchial wall damage and irreversible dilatation of the airways (Goeminne & Dupont 2010).

Risk factors/causes

The most common causes of bronchiectasis are cystic fibrosis and childhood respiratory disease. Other risk factors include: viral, bacterial and fungal infections, aspiration, airway obstruction, inhalation of toxic substances and immunosuppression. Many lung conditions such as COPD, allergic bronchopulmonary aspergillosis (APBA) and bronchiolitis can lead to the development of bronchiectasis as can auto-immune or inflammatory disorders, such as coeliac disease, rheumatoid arthritis rheumatoid arthritis, systemic lupus erythematosus, ankylosing spondylitis, Sjögren's syndrome and inflammatory bowel disease. Patients with congenital conditions may also be at risk, especially cardiorespiratory disease such as Marfan's syndrome, tracheobronchomegaly, pulmonary ciliary dyskinesia or chest wall deformities such as scoliosis and pectus excavatum.

Signs and symptoms

- Chronic cough
- Increased sputum production
- Lethargy and malaise
- Haemoptysis
- Weight loss
- Dyspnoea
- Chest pain
- Bronchospasms
- Reduced exercise tolerance
- Reduced respiratory function.

Diagnosis/investigations

- Lung function test
- Spirometry
- Sputum cultures
- Chest X-ray
- CT scan.

Nursing care and management

Bronchiectasis is a chronic respiratory condition and, as with other chronic respiratory diseases such as COPD, its management requires a holistic approach centred upon clearance of secretions, self-management and symptom control. The main management goals are:

- Physiotherapy to assist the clearance of mucus and other respiratory secretions

- Pulmonary rehabilitation
- Antibiotic therapy
- Education on prescribed oxygen and bronchodilator therapies – to maximise relief of breathlessness
- Promotion of self-management techniques.

Primary Care

As with chronic obstructive pulmonary disease, people living with bronchiectasis will need care strategies that promote well-being through the use of coping strategies. This should include:

- Regular reviews by trained respiratory clinicians
- Regular reviews of medication usage to optimise treatments
- Promotion of self-management and coping strategies
- Referral to pulmonary rehabilitation services
- Advice on smoking cessation.

Restrictive Lung Disorders

Restrictive lung disorders impede lung expansion and therefore reduce ventilation. The causes of reduced lung expansion can be either anatomical or pathological. Anatomical causes include conditions such as kyphosis or scoliosis, in which malformations of the spine impact on the individual's ability to fully expand their thorax. Pathological reasons for reduced lung expansion include diseases which affect lung compliance, cause muscle paralysis or restrict lung function. Poliomyelitis, amyotrophic lateral sclerosis and botulism, for example can cause respiratory muscle paralysis, whereas muscular dystrophy causes muscle weakness. Respiratory diseases that restrict lung function are in the main chronic conditions caused by the inhalation of industrial or commercial pollutants. This group of respiratory diseases is called pneumoconioses. Chest expansion can also be restricted by acute problems such as adult respiratory distress syndrome, which occurs after lung trauma or pulmonary oedema.

Pneumoconiosis

Pneumoconiosis is a collection of respiratory diseases that restrict lung expansion. These chronic conditions are caused by long term exposure to industrial or commercial pollutants. The different types of pneumoconioses are often named after the job or pastime that generated them, for example coal worker's lung or bird fancier's lung (Gould 2006).

Pathophysiology

The constant exposure of lung tissue to pollutant particles through inhalation leads to repeated inflammation within the airways and as a consequence fibrous tissue develops. As the development of fibrous tissue spreads through the lungs large areas of the airways lose their functionality. As a result lung expansion becomes difficult and lung tissue loses much of its compliance. These pathological changes are chronic and irreversible.

Risk factors

The main risk factors for the development of pneumoconiosis are occupational, for example jobs which involve exposure to fine particles. However, exposure to animal dander can also lead to the development of the disease and people who keep animals, particu-

larly birds, are also at risk. Examples of pneumoconiosis and their causes include:

- *Coal worker's lung* – caused by coal dust
- *Farmer's lung* – caused by exposure to fungal spores present in hay
- *Silicosis* – caused by exposure to silica through stone cutting or sand blasting
- *Asbestosis* – caused by exposure to asbestos through construction, shipbuilding or working with insulation
- *Bird fancier's lung* – exposure to bird dander.

Signs and symptoms
- Progressive dyspnoea
- Increased respiratory effort
- Cough
- Recurrent chest infection.

Nursing care and management
Pneumoconioses are chronic respiratory conditions and like other chronic respiratory diseases, their management requires a holistic approach centred upon self-management and symptom control. The main management goals are:

- Pulmonary rehabilitation
- Antibiotic therapy for recurrent chest infections
- Oxygen
- Promotion of self-management techniques.

Health promotion and discharge
Exposure to asbestosis increases the risk of the development of lung cancer, especially in cigarette smokers.

What the Experts Say Smoking cessation

Smoking tobacco poses serious health risks to not only the individual who smokes but to those around them, through second hand smoke. Smoking is the most preventable cause of death and consequently smoking cessation, in which nurses help people to achieve abstinence from smoking is a key public health goal.

(Adelle, Community nurse)

Primary Care

People living with pneumoconioses need to develop self-care strategies that can help maintain well-being. This should include:

- Regular reviews by trained respiratory clinicians
- Regular reviews of medication usage to optimise treatments
- Promotion of self-management and coping strategies
- Referral to pulmonary rehabilitation services
- Advice on smoking cessation.

Lung Cancer

Lung cancer is the development of tumours within the lung tissue. The vast majority of lung cancers (95%) develop in bronchial tissue. There are two major types of bronchial carcinoma **non-small cell** and **small cell**. Non-small cell carcinomas account for 70% of all lung cancers. Non-small cell carcinomas can be subdivided again into: *squamous cell carcinomas* and *adenocarcinomas or large cell* *carcinomas*. Squamous cell carcinomas tend to develop within the larger bronchi, whereas other non-small cell carcinomas are found in the smaller airways making them much harder to detect. Small cell carcinomas tend to grow near the large bronchi and are the most aggressive bronchial carcinomas.

Pathophysiology
Smoking or other irritants (i.e. asbestos) damage the pseudostratified epithelium of lung tissue rendering them more susceptible to inflammation. Certain chemicals present within cigarette smoke are carcinogenic, and promote the development of tumours within the lung tissue.

Risk factors
- Smoking
- Passive smoking
- Exposure to occupational pollutants.

Signs and symptoms
The following signs and symptoms are considered indicative of lung cancer in patients who smoke tobacco:
- Cough
- Haemoptysis
- Dyspnoea
- Chest pain
- Wheeze
- Finger clubbing.

Diagnosis/investigations
- Biopsy
- CT Scan
- Chest X-ray.

Nursing care and management
- Safe administration of chemotherapy
- Minimisation of impact of the side-effects of chemotherapy
- Working with the patient and family to adjust to the diagnosis of cancer through good communication and teaching skills
- Providing practical information and support for patients and families

Care, Dignity and Compassion
The diagnosis of cancer is likely to be a traumatic event, not only for the person concerned but also for their family and friends. It is vital the nurse does not make assumptions about their patient and ensure that the plan and implement care on an individual basis.

Primary Care
For patients with a new diagnosis of lung cancer, primary care nurses must ensure that the following aspects of care are executed:
- Represent the patient's perspective – ensure that the patient's opinions and wishes are accounted for in all care decisions
- Ascertain whether or not the patient has any advance decisions relating to their care and treatment
- Refer all patients with a cancer diagnosis to a relevant clinical nurse specialist

---

- Promote self-care and coping strategies, i.e. coping with breathlessness
- Monitor patient for the following signs of deterioration or comorbidities:
  - Weight loss
  - Loss of appetite
  - Dysphagia
  - Depression
  - Increased breathlessness
- Ensure patient receives adequate pain relief
- Monitor and treat cough with opiate analgesia.

NICE (2011b)

Pleural Disorders

Any condition that causes air or fluid to collect in the pleural space can cause the lung to partially or fully collapse. Air within the pleural space is referred to as a **pneumothorax**. Fluid within the pleural space is called a **pleural effusion**, unless the fluid in question is blood, in which case the patient has a **haemothorax**.

Pathophysiology
The pleural space between parietal and visceral pleura only contains a thin film of fluid. Any air or extra fluid entering the pleural space will cause the lung to collapse resulting areas of underventilated lung, a phenomenon known as atelectasis. The surface area for external respiration is dramatically reduced and the patient may develop hypoxaemia (West 2003). Trauma is the major cause of a haemothorax; however cancer can also cause bleeding within lung tissue.

Pleural effusions can originate from within lung tissue or from pulmonary circulation. Exudate pleural effusions occur from within lung tissue as a result of respiratory disease. Diseases such as lung cancer, pneumonia or tuberculosis cause inflammation which can result in the generation of fluid that is rich in protein and white blood cells. Inflammation also increases pulmonary capillary permeability, allowing fluid to leak out of blood vessels and into the pleural space. Transudate pleural effusions occur as a result of a problem within circulation. Conditions such as left ventricular failure cause increases in capillary hydrostatic pressure, forcing fluid out of circulation and into the pleural space. A decrease in blood osmotic pressure will also force fluid from blood vessels into the pleural space. Causes of reduced blood osmotic pressure include hypoproteinaemia.

The presence of air in the pleural cavity is called a pneumothorax. Pneumothoraces are mainly caused by trauma or chronic respiratory disease. However, some individuals have a congenital defect or bleb within the alveolar wall, which can rupture spontaneously.

Risk factors
- Trauma
- Chronic respiratory disease
- Heart failure
- Tall young men are at particular risk of spontaneous pneumothorax as a result of a congenital defect or bleb. (Ryan 2005)

Signs and symptoms
Small pneumothoraces may not produce noticeable symptoms, however the larger the pneumothorax, the more severe the symptoms. Patients with a pneumothorax may present with the following:

619

- Sudden onset dyspnoea
- Sharp pleuritic pain, which is worse on inspiration
- Chest auscultation may reveal diminished or absence of breath sounds.

Diagnosis/investigations

The main investigation for pleural disorders is a chest X-ray; the critically ill patient, however, may require a computed tomographic (CT) scan. Oxygen saturations and arterial blood gas readings can also determine deterioration.

Nursing care and management

Chest drains are often used to assist the re-inflation of the affected lung. The main care responsibilities therefore, centre on the monitoring of both the patient and the drain and attention should be paid to the following (Sullivan 2008):

- Patient positioning – placing the patient in an upright position will encourage drainage and aid expansion of the thorax
- Position of the chest drain – the drainage bottle must be kept below the patient's chest level to prevent fluid re-entering the pleural space. Coiled and looped tubing should also be avoided as it can impede drainage flow and lead to a tension pneumothorax or surgical emphysema
- Continuous monitoring of vital signs until patient's condition stabilises
- Close monitoring of the chest drain
  - Swinging – the level of the fluid in the underwater seal of the drain should fluctuate between 5 and 10 cm when the patient breathes. Absence of swinging could indicate a kink or blockage in the tubing
  - Bubbling – bubbles often occur in the water seal bottle without suction when the patient exhales or coughs. Continuous bubbling indicates a problem with the drain or insertion site
- Administration of prescribed analgesics for pleuritic pain
- Accurate recording of drainage – the health professional should note the quantity, colour and consistency of the fluid being drained
- Infection control – the insertion site should be checked daily for signs of infection, i.e. redness, swelling, heat, pain and discharge.

Complications/prognosis

Patients with pleural disorders are at risk of developing an empyema, the formation of pus in the pleural effusion (Dobbin & Howard 2009).

Health promotion and discharge

Prior to discharge, patients should be taught how to clean and re-dress their chest insertion wound site. Patients should also be advised to continually assess the chest drain insertion site for signs of infection. If a suture is in place, arrangements must be made for removal by a community nurse.

Interstitial Lung Disease (Diffuse Parenchymal Lung Disease)

Interstitial lung disease and diffuse parenchymal lung disease are umbrella terms used to describe around 200 different acute and chronic lung conditions. They are characterised by both acute and chronic inflammation and progressive generation of fibrosis in the alveolar walls and interstitial lung tissue. Interstitial lung diseases are classified as follows (American Thoracic Society/European Respiratory Society, ATS/ERS 2002):

- Known cause – environmental causes, collagen vascular disease, drug induced
- Unknown cause – idiopathic interstitial pneumonias, for example
- Granulomatous – fibrosis as a result of disorders such as sarcoidosis
- Other rarer causes – lymphangioleiomyomatosis, histocytosis X, for example.

Pathophysiology

Although the exact cause of interstitial lung disease may not be known, the resultant damage to alveolar cells initiates an inflammatory response, which generates widespread fibrosis. Interstitial lung disease suggests that only the interstitium, the region of the alveolar wall which separates the alveoli from capillary circulation, is affected. However, the alveolar space and bronchioles are also at risk. Widespread regions of fibrosis lead to reduced capacity for gaseous exchange.

Signs and symptoms

- Progressive dyspnoea, often disabling
- Cough
- Abnormal breath sounds
- Finger clubbing in some instances.

Diagnosis/investigations

- Spirometry
- Chest X-ray
- CT scan.

Nursing care and management

- Pulmonary rehabilitation
- Oxygen
- Advice on smoking cessation
- Promotion of self-management techniques.

Complications/prognosis

Interstitial lung disease has a poor prognosis. At present, there are very few pharmacological treatments that have shown to be effective and life expectancy without a lung transplant is between 2–5 years.

Conclusion

Respiratory disease places a heavy burden on the National Health Service and its impact on services can be reduced by good quality, holistic nursing care. Whatever the cause, be it lifestyle choice, occupation or opportunistic infection, the main areas of care include clearance of secretions, enhancement of ventilation and oxygenation as well as more psychosocial factors such as self-management and coping mechanisms for those living with chronic respiratory illness and breathlessness. Patients living with or experiencing respiratory disorders are at risk of acute exacerbation and deterioration. The nurse must therefore be skilled in accurate comprehensive respiratory assessment.

Key Points

The absorption of oxygen and disposal of carbon dioxide follows four distinct processes: pulmonary ventilation, external respiration, transport of gases, and internal respiration. The rate and depth of breathing is dependent upon:

- Optimum oxygen and carbon dioxide levels
- Hydrogen ions
- Body temperature
- Cognitive well-being.

Changes in respiratory rate at rest are always clinically significant. An inability to maintain adequate oxygen levels constitutes respiratory failure, of which there are two types:

- Respiratory failure type 1 – inadequate oxygenation
- Respiratory failure type 2 – inadequate oxygenation and hypercapnia.

Nurses must be able to perform a comprehensive respiratory assessment, which must include the following:

- Respiratory rate
- Assessment of symmetry and depth of breathing
- Listening for added sounds
- Oxygen saturation.

Nurses must be able to recognise the cardinal signs of acute deterioration in patients with acute respiratory disorders, for example:

- Tachypnoea
- Tachycardia
- Hypoxia and hypoxaemia
- Cool clammy peripheries
- Confusion, disorientation, agitation
- Loss of consciousness.

Patients living with long-term respiratory disorders will require psychosocial care strategies that promote self-care and coping interventions.

Glossary

Amyotrophic lateral sclerosis: serious neurological disease in which motor neurones gradually deteriorate

Anaemia: a reduced number or function of erythrocytes (red blood cells) or haemoglobin

Antipyretic agents: drugs that can reduce high temperatures, i.e. paracetamol, aspirin, ibuprofen

Aorta: first major blood vessel of arterial circulation. Emerges from the left ventricle of the heart

Atelectasis: partial or complete collapse of lung tissue due to a blocked airway

Auscultation: the act of listening through a stethoscope

Bacillus: a form of bacteria. Bacilli are rod-shaped, Gram-positive and usually have motility

Botulism: a rare but serious bacterial infection which causes muscle weakness and paralysis

Carcinogenic: prone to promote the formation of carcinomas (tumours)

Carotid artery: major artery supplying the brain, stems from the aorta

Cartilage: type of connective tissue which contains collagen and elastic fibres. Cartilage can stand up to both tension and compression

Cerebrospinal fluid (CSF): Fluid found within the brain and spinal cord

Chemoreceptors: sensory cells sensitive to a specific chemical

Central cyanosis: a bluish hue or tingle visible in lips and mouth that occurs when arterial oxygen levels are abnormally low

Cilia: hair-like extensions to the plasma membrane

Cor pulmonale: right-sided heart failure caused by hypoxia

Diffusion: the passive movement of molecules or ions from a region of high concentration to low concentration until a state of equilibrium is achieved

Dyspnoea: difficult or laboured breathing

Elastic cartilage: cartilage that contains more elastin fibres, providing strength and stretchability

Enzyme: a protein that speeds up chemical reactions

Erythrocytes: red blood cells

Expectorate: to cough up and spit out mucus or sputum

External intercostal muscles: muscles that span the spaces between the ribs. As opposed to the internal intercostal muscles the external intercostal muscles sit closer to the outside of the thorax

External respiration: the transfer of oxygen from the alveoli in the lungs to the blood stream and the transfer of carbon dioxide from the blood stream into alveoli in the lungs

Extrinsic asthma: asthma caused by hypersensitive reactions to an allergy

Exudate: escaping fluid that spills from a space, contains cellular debris and pus

Fibrin: a protein essential for clotting

Fibrosis: the development of scar tissue

Fibrous: containing regenerated or scar tissue

Finger clubbing: alteration in the angle of finger and toe bases caused by chronic tissue hypoxia

Goblet cells: mucus-secreting cells found in epithelial tissue

Haemoglobin (Hb): Protein consisting of globin and four heme groups that is found within erythrocytes (red blood cells). Responsible for the transport of oxygen

Haemoptysis: coughing up of blood

Hydrostatic pressure: pressure exerted by a fluid

Hypercapnia: elevated levels of arterial carbon dioxide

Hypertension: abnormally high blood pressure

Hypoproteinaemia: a reduced level of plasma proteins

Hypotension: abnormally low blood pressure

Hypoxaemia: a reduced amount of oxygen within arterial blood

Hypoxia: a reduced amount of oxygen within the tissues

Immunocompromised/immunosuppressed: term used to describe a state of immunity that is impaired and incapable of an effective immune response

Intercostal nerves: nerves which link the respiratory centres in the brainstem with the intercostal muscles

Internal intercostal muscles: muscles that span the spaces between the ribs. As opposed to the external intercostal muscles the internal intercostal muscles sit closer to the inside of the thorax

Internal respiration: the transfer of oxygen from the blood stream into body cells and the transfer of carbon dioxide from body cells to the blood stream

Interstitial lung disease: disease that affects the region between the alveoli wall and pulmonary circulation

Intrinsic asthma: asthma caused by hyperresponsive reactions to non-allergic stimuli

Intubation: the insertion of a special tube into the pharynx and down into the trachea, in order to maintain a patent airway in an unconscious patient

Kyphosis: curvature of the thoracic spine

Lymph nodules: egg-shaped masses of lymph tissues that provide an immune response

(Continued)

Lymphocytes: specialist white blood cell involved in immune responses

Lymph vessel: a vessel that carries lymphatic fluid. Part of the lymphatic system which forms part of the immune system

Macrophages: a cell which ingests and destroys microbes, cell debris and foreign matter

Malaise: general weakness or discomfort

Mast cells: a cell found in connective tissue that releases histamine during inflammation

Medulla oblongata: lowest region of the brain stem

Muscular dystrophy: a group of diseases characterised by the progressive loss of muscle fibres. Almost all these diseases are hereditary

Neutrophils: a type of white blood cell

Non-invasive positive pressure ventilation (NIPPV): respiratory support technique that enhances the patient's rate and depth of breathing

Oedema: an abnormal collection of fluid

Osmotic pressure: pressure exerted by fluid flowing through a semipermeable membrane that separates two fluids with different levels of dissolved substances

Parenchymal: the functioning parts of an organ

Peak expiratory flow rate: the velocity at which a patient can expire their total lung volume

Pectus excavatum: a hollow in the thorax caused by a displacement of the xiphoid cartilage. Also called funnel breast

Phrenic nerve: nerve which links the diaphragm to the respiratory centre in the brain stem

Pleuritic: of or pertaining to the pleura

Poliomyelitis: an acute viral disease which affects the central nervous system

Polycythaemia: a condition in which there is an abnormally high number of erythrocytes (red blood cells)

Pons: upper region of the brainstem. Connects the midbrain to the medulla oblongata

Prophylactic/prophylaxis: a defensive or protective health measure

Pseudostratified ciliated columnar epithelium: covering or lining of internal body surface that contains cilia and mucus-secreting goblet cells

Pulmonary ventilation: breathing. The inspiration and expiration of air into and out of the lungs

Pulse oximeter: Device that provides an instant pulse and oxygen saturation (SpO_2)

Pyrexia: elevated temperature associated with fever

Respiratory acidosis: a blood pH of less than 7.35 caused by a rise in arterial carbon dioxide

Scoliosis: a sideways curvature of the thoracic spine

Spirometry: Diagnostic tool which measures a patient's forced vital capacity (FVC) and forced expiratory volume within the first second of expiration (FEV_1)

Surgical emphysema: air trapped in the tissues, usually as a result of a surgical or invasive procedure

Systemic circulation: arterial and venous blood flow through the body, except the lungs (pulmonary circulation) and the coronary arteries

Tachycardia: pulse rate greater than 100 beats per minute

Tachypnoea: rapid, shallow, respiratory rate greater than 24 respirations per minute

Thorax: the body trunk above the diaphragm and below the neck

Transport of gases: the movement of oxygen and carbon dioxide between the lungs and body cells

References

ATS/ERS (2002) International multidisciplinary consensus classification of the idiopathic interstitial pneumonias, *American Journal of Critical Care Medicine*, 165, 277–304.

Barnes, P.J. (2008) Drugs for airway disease. *Medicine*, 36(4), 181–190.

Bassett, C. & Makin, L. (2000) *Caring for the Seriously Ill Patient*. Arnold, London.

Braman, S.S. (2006) Chronic cough due to bronchitis: ACCP evidence-based clinical practice. *Chest*, 129, 104S–115S.

BTS & SIGN (2009) *British Guideline on the Management of Asthma: A National Clinical Guideline*. British Thoracic Society and Scottish Intercollegiate Guidelines Network, London.

BTS (2006) *The Burden of Lung Disease*. British Thoracic Society, London.

BTS Standards of Care Committee (2001) BTS guidelines for the management of community acquired pneumonia in adults. *Thorax*, 56 (Suppl 4), iv1–iv64.

BTS Standards of Care Committee (2002) Non-invasive ventilation in acute respiratory failure. *Thorax*, 57(3), 192–211.

Clancy, J. & McVicar, A. (2007) Immediate and long term regulation of acid-base homeostasis. *British Journal of Nursing*, 16(17), 1076–1079.

Clark, A.P., Giuliano, K. & Chen, H. (2006) Pulse oximetry revisited 'but his O_2 sat was normal!'. *Clinical Nurse Specialist*, 20(6), 268–272.

Cox, C.L. (2001) Respiratory assessment. In: G. Esmond (ed.) *Respiratory Nursing*. Bailliere Tindall, Edinburgh.

Davies, A. & Moores, C. (2003) *The Respiratory System Basic Science and Clinical Conditions*. Churchill Livingstone, Edinburgh.

Devereux, G. (2006) ABC of chronic obstructive disease definition, epidemiology and risk factors. *British Medical Journal*, 332, 1142–1144.

Dobbin, K.R. & Howard, V.M. (2009) Understanding empyema. *Nursing 2009*, 56, 1–5.

Dougherty, L. & Lister, S. (2011) *The Royal Marsden Hospital Manual of Clinical Nursing Procedures*, 8th edn. Wiley Blackwell, Chichester.

Driver, C. (2012) Pneumonia Part 3: Management and prevention of influenza virus. *British Journal of Nursing*, 21(6), 362–366.

Dunn, L. (2005) Pneumonia: classification, diagnosis and nursing management. *Nursing Standard*, 19(42), 50–54.

Goeminne, P. & Dupont, L. (2010) Non-cystic fibrosis bronchiectasis: diagnosis and management in the 21st century. *Postgraduate Medical Journal*, 86, 493–501.

Gough, A. & Kaufman, G. (2011) Pulmonary tuberculosis clinical features and patient management. *Nursing Standard*, 25(47), 48–56.

Gould, B.E. (2006) *Pathophysiology for the Health Professions*, 3rd edn. Saunders Elsevier, Philadelphia.

Higginson, R. & Jones, B. (2009) Respiratory assessment in critically ill patients: airway and breathing. *British Journal of Nursing*, 18(8), 456–461.

Hoare, Z. & Lim, W.S. (2006) Pneumonia: Update on diagnosis and management. *British Medical Journal*, 332, 1077–1079.

Hogan, J. (2006) Why don't nurses monitor the respiratory rates of patients? *British Journal of Nursing*, 15(9), 489–492.

Hogg, J.C. & Senior, R.M. (2002) Chronic obstructive pulmonary disease 2: Pathology and biochemistry of emphysema. *Thorax*, 57, 830–834.

Jenkins, G. & Tortora, G.J. (2013) *Anatomy and Physiology from Science to Life*, 3rd edn. John Wiley and Sons, New Jersey.

Joint Formulary Committee (2011) *British National Formulary*, 61st edn. Pharmaceutical Press, London.

Karim, K. (2011) Tuberculosis infection and control. *British Journal of Nursing*, 20(17), 1028–1133.

Levitzky, M.G., Cairo, J.M. & Hall, S.M. (1990) *Introduction to Respiratory Care*. WB Saunders, London.

Lim, W.S., Baudouin, S.V., George, R.C. *et al.*; Pneumonia Guidelines Committee of the BTS Standards of Care Committee (2009) Guidelines for the management of community acquired pneumonia in adults: update 2009. *Thorax*, 64(Suppl 3), iii1–iii55.

MacNee, W. (2006) ABC of chronic obstructive pulmonary disease pathology, pathogenesis and pathophysiology. *British Medical Journal*, 332, 1202–1204.

Margereson, C. (2001) Anatomy and physiology. In: G. Esmond (ed.) *Respiratory Nursing*. Bailliere Tindall, Edinburgh.

Martini, F.H. & Nath, J.L. (2009) *Fundamentals of Anatomy and Physiology*, 8th edn. Pearson Benjamin Cummings, San Francisco.

McGowan, P., Jeffries, A. & Turley, A. (2003) *Crash Course Respiratory System*, 2nd edn. Mosby, London.

NICE (2010) *Chronic Obstructive Pulmonary Disease. Management of Chronic Obstructive Pulmonary Disease in Primary and Secondary Care (Partial Update) Clinical Guideline 101*. National Institute for Health and Clinical Excellence, London.

NICE (2011a) *Tuberculosis: clinical diagnosis and management of tuberculosis, and measures for its prevention and control – Guideline 117*. National Institute for Health and Clinical Excellence, London.

NICE (2011b) *Lung Cancer: the diagnosis and treatment of lung cancer – Clinical Guideline 121*. National Institute for Health and Clinical Excellence, London.

O'Driscoll, B.R., Howard, L.S., Davison, A.G.; British Thoracic Society (2008) Guideline for emergency oxygen use in adult patients. *Thorax*, 63(Suppl 6), vi1–vi68.

Ochs, M., Nyengaard, A.J., Knudsen, L. *et al.* (2004) The number of alveoli in the human lung. *American Journal of Respiratory and Critical Care Medicine*, 169, 120–124.

Ryan, B. (2005) Pneumothorax assessment and diagnostic testing. *Journal of Cardiovascular Nursing*, 20(4), 251–253.

Schwartzstein, R.M. & Parker, M.J. (2006) *Respiratory Physiology: A Clinical Approach*. Lippincott Williams & Wilkins, Philadelphia.

Sheldon, R.L. (2005) Pulmonary function testing. In: R.L. Wilkins, R.L. Sheldon & S.J. Krider (eds) *Clinical Assessment in Respiratory Care*, 5th edn. Elsevier Mosby, St. Louis.

Simpson, H. (2006) Respiratory assessment. *British Journal of Nursing*, 15(9), 484–488.

Sims, J.M. (2006) An overview of asthma. *Dimensions of Critical Care Nursing*, 25(6), 264–268.

Sullivan, B. (2008) Nursing management of patients with a chest drain. *British Journal of Nursing*, 17(6), 388–393.

Talley, N.J. & O'Connor, S. (2001) *Clinical Examination: a systematic guide to physical diagnosis*, 4th edn. Blackwell Science, Oxford.

Tortora, G.J. & Grabowski, S.R. (2003) *Principles of Anatomy and Physiology*, 10th edn. John Wiley and Sons, New York.

West, J.B. (2003) *Pulmonary Pathophysiology: the essentials*, 6th edn. Lippincott Williams & Wilkins, Philadelphia.

WHO (2010) *International Statistical Classification of Diseases and Health Related Problems: ICD-10*, Version 2010. World Health Organization, Geneva. http://apps.who.int/classifications/icd10/browse/2010/en (accessed 14 June 2013).

Test Yourself

1. Which of the following statements about pulmonary ventilation is correct?
   (a) Air flow during breathing is due to a pressure gradient between the lungs and atmospheric air
   (b) Expiration during quiet breathing is an active process that utilises muscle contraction
   (c) Normal quiet inspiration is achieved by contraction of the sternocleidomastoids and scalenes
   (d) The diaphragm is an important muscle of expiration

2. Which of the following occurs during gaseous exchange?
   (a) Oxygen diffuses from the alveoli to erythrocytes in pulmonary circulation
   (b) Carbon dioxide diffuses from the alveoli to erythrocytes in pulmonary capillaries
   (c) Carbon dioxide remains in blood plasma
   (d) Oxygen diffuses from erythrocytes in pulmonary circulation to the alveoli

3. Which of the following statements is correct?
   (a) The central chemoreceptors respond to elevated levels of carbon dioxide
   (b) The peripheral chemoreceptors are found within the medulla oblongata and pons
   (c) The pneumotaxic and apneustic respiratory centres analyse levels of both oxygen and carbon dioxide
   (d) The central chemoreceptors in the aorta and carotid arteries respond to elevated levels of oxygen

4. What is the correct definition of apnoea?
   (a) A respiration rate of 10 respirations per minute or less
   (b) Difficulty in breathing while lying flat
   (c) Difficulty in breathing
   (d) The absence of breathing for more than 15 seconds

5. Which of the following would indicate that your patient was in respiratory failure type 2?
   (a) Hypoxia
   (b) Hypoxaemia and hypercapnia
   (c) Hypoxaemia
   (d) Hypocapnia

6. Which of the following statements on respiratory assessment is incorrect?
   (a) Peak flow measures velocity of expiration in litres per minute
   (b) Forced expiratory volume in the first second (FEV_1) should be at least 80% of the forced vital capacity (FVC)
   (c) In health oxygen saturation (SaO_2), rates should be between 90–94%
   (d) Dark green mucopurient sputum in indicative of a respiratory tract infection

7. What kind of medication is salbutamol?
   (a) Anticholinergic
   (b) Steroid
   (c) Methylxanthine
   (d) Beta-2 agonist

8. Which of the following statements regarding chronic obstructive pulmonary disease (COPD) is true?
   (a) COPD is an umbrella term for bronchiectasis and pneumoconiosis
   (b) An FEV_1 of 80% or more of FVC is an important diagnostic feature of COPD
   (c) The major cause of COPD is smoking
   (d) COPD is a restrictive respiratory disorder

9. Which of the following is a restrictive lung disorder?
   (a) Asthma
   (b) Pneumoconiosis
   (c) Bronchiectasis
   (d) Lung cancer

10. The presence of fluid in the pleural space is called:
    (a) Pneumothorax
    (b) Haemothorax
    (c) Empyema
    (d) Pleural effusion

Answers

1. a
2. a
3. a
4. d
5. b
6. c
7. d
8. c
9. b
10. d

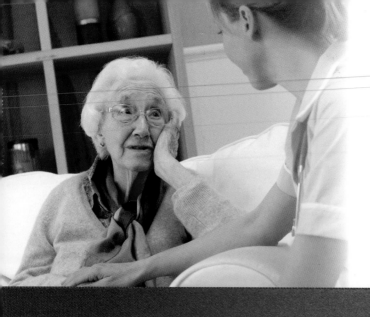

28

The Person with a Gastrointestinal Disorder

Muralitharan Nair

University of Hertfordshire, UK

Learning Outcomes

On completion of this chapter you will be able to:

- Describe the anatomy, physiology and functions of the gastrointestinal and hepatobiliary systems
- List the main functions of the gastrointestinal system and the accessory organs of digestion
- Describe the pathophysiology of commonly occurring disorders of the gastrointestinal system, liver and gallbladder
- Explain the differences between chemical and mechanical digestion
- Describe the assessment of bowel elimination
- Identify common causes and effects of conditions of the common digestive and accessory organ problems

Competencies

All nurses must:

1. Assess and document a health history for persons who have or are at risk of gastrointestinal dysfunctions
2. Use assessment data and tools to formulate individualised care
3. Assess physical and psychological care needs of the patient
4. Evaluate nursing care of patients with elimination disorders
5. Provide information for the patient and their family regarding care in the community
6. Work in partnership with the multidisciplinary team for the safe discharge of the patient into the community

 Visit the companion website at **www.wileynursingpractice.com** where you can test yourself using flashcards, multiple-choice questions and more.

Nursing Practice: Knowledge and Care, First Edition. Edited by Ian Peate, Karen Wild and Muralitharan Nair.
© 2014 John Wiley & Sons, Ltd. Published 2014 by John Wiley & Sons, Ltd. Companion website: www.wileynursingpractice.com

Introduction

The gastrointestinal (GI) system is also known as the digestive system or alimentary canal or tract. The principal structures of digestion are the mouth, pharynx, oesophagus, stomach and intestines. These structures are supported by the accessory organs of digestion: the salivary glands, liver, pancreas and gallbladder (Figure 28.1). The main function of the gastrointestinal system is to break down nutrients from the diet into the raw materials required by the cells of the body so that they can carry out their specific functions. The gastrointestinal system does this by digesting the dietary intake, absorbing the nutrients obtained from the process of digestion and eliminating any unwanted material. The chapter begins with a review of the anatomy and physiology of the GI tract and the accessory structures. The disorders covered in this chapter are some of the common conditions nurses will come across in practice.

Anatomy and Physiology

The GI system consists of the digestive tract – the mouth, pharynx, oesophagus, stomach, small intestine and the large intestine – and the accessory organs, which include the teeth, tongue, salivary glands, liver, gallbladder and the pancreas (Jenkins & Tortora 2013).

The GI tract is a continuous hollow tube, extending from the mouth to the anus. The length of the adult digestive tract is approximately 5–7 meters. Once foods are placed in the mouth, they are subjected to a variety of processes that move them and break them down into end-products that can be absorbed from the lumen of the small intestine into the blood or lymph. These digestive processes are as follows:

- *Ingestion of food* – the process of eating and drinking
- *Secretion of mucus, water, and enzymes* – approximately 7 litres is produced per day
- *Mixing and propulsion* – mixing of the food in the stomach by contracting and relaxing
- *Mechanical digestion of food* – the breakdown of foodstuff into smaller particles by the teeth and smooth muscles of the stomach and the small intestine
- *Chemical digestion of food* – digestive enzymes break the foodstuff down further for absorption
- *Absorption of digested food.*

The Layers of the GI Tract

There are four layers all along the GI tract; that is from the lower oesophagus to the anus. These are the:

- **Mucosa**: A mucous membrane composed of epithelium, connective tissue called the lamina propria and smooth muscle layer (muscularis mucosae)
- **Submucosa**: Contains connective tissue that binds the mucosa to the muscularis

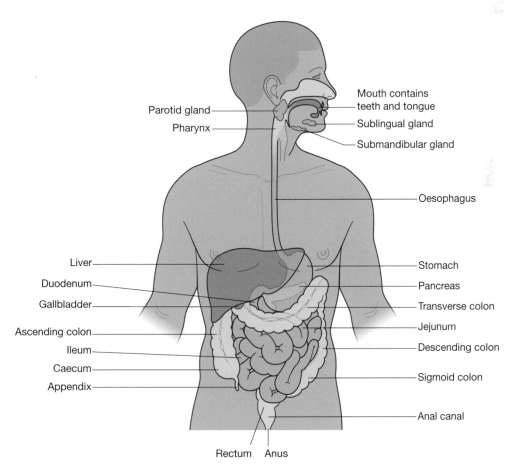

Parotid gland
Pharynx
Mouth contains teeth and tongue
Sublingual gland
Submandibular gland
Oesophagus
Liver
Duodenum
Gallbladder
Ascending colon
Ileum
Caecum
Appendix
Stomach
Pancreas
Transverse colon
Jejunum
Descending colon
Sigmoid colon
Anal canal
Rectum   Anus

Figure 28.1 Organs of the gastrointestinal tract.

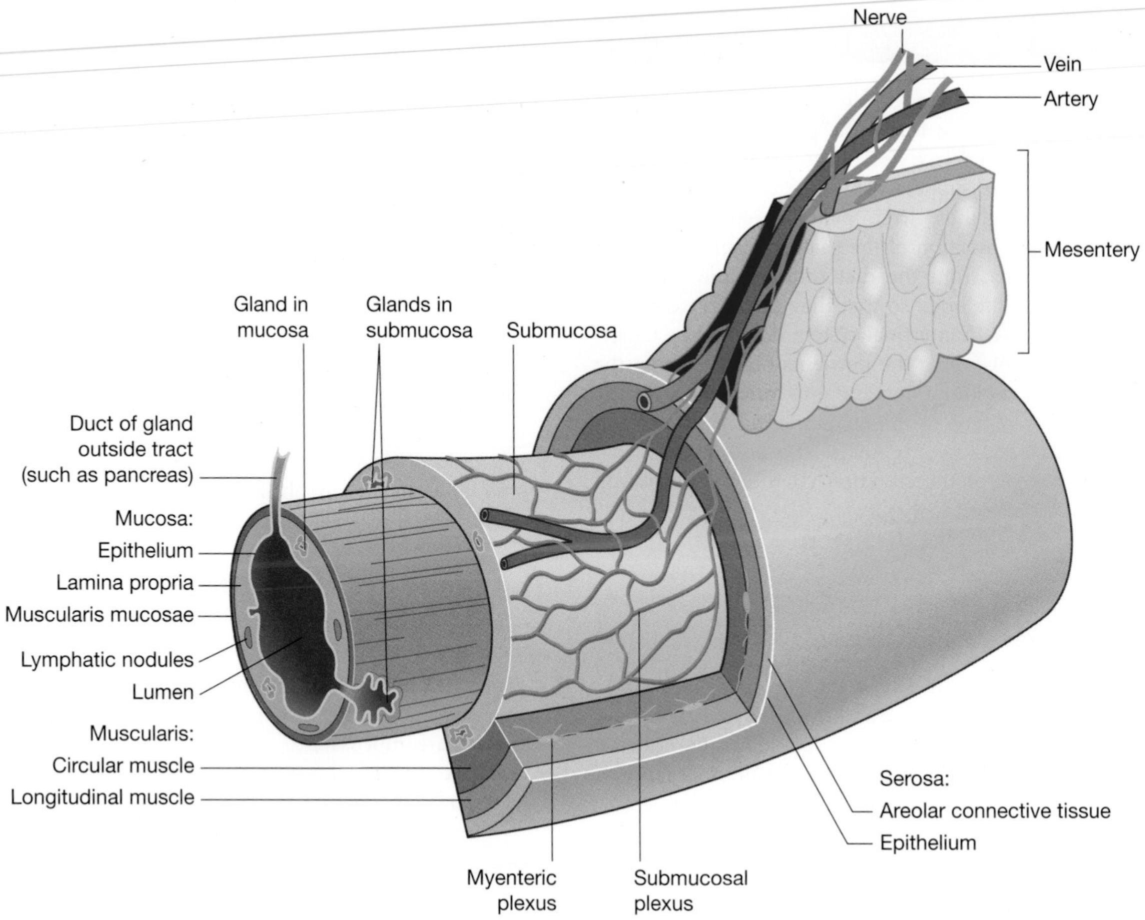

Figure 28.2 The four layers of the gastrointestinal tract.

- **Muscularis**: Consists of circular muscle and longitudinal muscle. The involuntary contractions of the muscularis help to break down foodstuff with the digestive juices and propel it down the tract
- **Serosa**: Containing connective tissue and epithelium. It secretes slippery watery fluid for lubrication.

See Figure 28.2 for the four layers of the gastrointestinal tract.

The Mouth

The mouth, also called the oral or buccal cavity, is lined with mucous membranes and is enclosed by the lips, cheeks, palate and tongue (Figure 28.3). It receives food and begins the mechanical breakdown of food by the action of chewing and grinding on the food. The chemical digestion of food also begins in the oral cavity.

The lips and cheeks are skeletal muscle, covered externally by skin. Their function is to keep food in the mouth during chewing. The palate consists of two regions: the hard palate and the soft palate. The hard palate covers bone in the roof of the mouth and provides a hard surface against which the tongue forces food. The soft palate, extending from the hard palate and ending at the back of the mouth as a fold called the uvula, is primarily muscle. When food is swallowed, the soft palate rises as a reflex to close off the oropharynx.

The tongue, composed of skeletal muscle and connective tissue, is located in the floor of the mouth. It contains mucous and serous glands, taste buds and papillae. The tongue mixes food with saliva during chewing, forms the food into a mass (called a *bolus*) and initiates swallowing (Marieb & Hoehn 2013). Some papillae provide surface roughness to facilitate licking and moving food; other papillae house the taste buds.

Saliva moistens food so it can be made into a bolus, dissolves food chemicals so they can be tasted, and provides enzymes (such as amylase) that begin the chemical breakdown of starches. Saliva is produced by salivary glands, most of which lie superior or inferior to the mouth and drain into it. The salivary glands include the parotid, the submaxillary and the sublingual glands.

The teeth chew (masticate) and grind food to break it down into smaller parts. As the food is masticated, it is mixed with saliva. Adults have 32 permanent teeth. The teeth are embedded in the gingiva (gums), with the crown of each tooth visible above the gingiva (Jenkins & Tortora 2013).

Lips

The lips form the opening into the mouth. They are fleshy folds that contain skeletal muscles and sensory receptors (Shier *et al.* 2009). These structures have a role in assessing the temperature and texture of foods and they direct food into the oral cavity. The lips have a rich blood supply, hence their usual ruby red colouring. The junction between the upper and the lower lips forms the angle of the mouth. These angles can become sore and dry during periods of ill health and this condition is known as angular cheilitis.

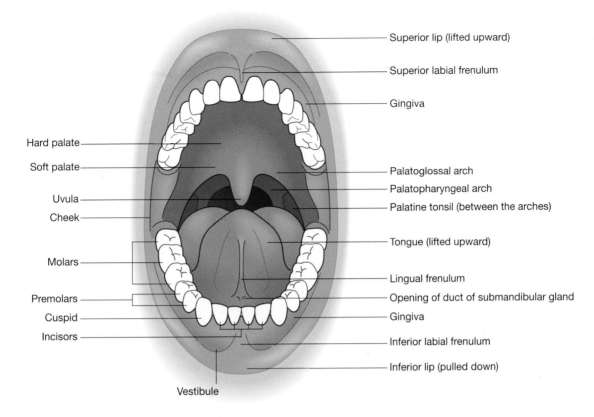

Figure 28.3 **Structures of the mouth.**

Cheeks

The cheeks, the sides of the mouth, are continuous with the lips and have a similar structure. A distinct fat pad is found in the subcutaneous tissue, muscles and mucous membranes. The cheeks assist in the chewing of food.

Palate

The palate is divided into the hard and the soft palates (see Figure 28.3); both form the roof of the mouth whereas the tongue lies at the bottom of the oral cavity and forms the floor of the mouth. The hard and the soft palates are covered by mucous membranes and participate in the mechanical breakdown of food.

Tongue

The tongue is a thick muscular organ composed of skeletal muscles and mucous membranes. It contains approximately 10 000 taste buds (Silverthorn 2009). It tells the person about the taste of food, for example whether the food is sweet or sour. Marieb and Hoehn (2013) state that the tongue detects four basic tastes: sweet, salt, bitter and sour. Silverthorn (2009) identified a fifth taste called *umami*. This word is derived from the Japanese word meaning 'deliciousness', and the taste is associated with glutamate and some nucleotides. Hence, in some Asian countries, monosodium glutamate (MSG) is sometimes used to enhance flavour when cooking.

The tongue is an accessory organ and forms the floor of the mouth; it helps to blend food when chewing and to push food particles to the back of the mouth when swallowing. Tongue movement can alter the volume of the oral cavity and also has an important role in speech, chewing, swallowing and taste.

Teeth

Humans develop two sets of teeth: milk teeth and permanent teeth. There are approximately 20 milk teeth which begin to develop usually from the age of 6 months. Often one pair of milk teeth grows per month and they usually fall out between the ages of 6 and 12 years (Figure 28.4). Once the milk teeth fall out, they are replaced by permanent teeth. Usually, there are 32 permanent teeth, which have the potential to last a lifetime. The first permanent molars appear at the age of 6 years, the second at the age of 12 years and the third may develop after the age of 13 years (Figure 28.5). The functions of the teeth include cutting, tearing and chewing food.

The Pharynx

The pharynx is the continuation of the digestive tract from the oral cavity. It consists of the oropharynx and the laryngopharynx (Figure 28.6). Both structures provide passageways for food, fluids and air. The pharynx is made of skeletal muscles and is lined with mucous membranes. The skeletal muscles move food to the oesophagus via the pharynx through peristalsis (alternating waves of contraction and relaxation of involuntary muscle). The mucosa of the pharynx contains mucus-producing glands that provide fluid to facilitate the passage of the bolus of food as it is swallowed.

The Oesophagus

The oesophagus is a muscular tube about 10 inches (25 cm) long that lies posterior to the trachea. It serves as a passageway for food from the pharynx to the stomach (Figure 28.7). The oesophagus is composed of three layers. The inner mucosal layer has an

629

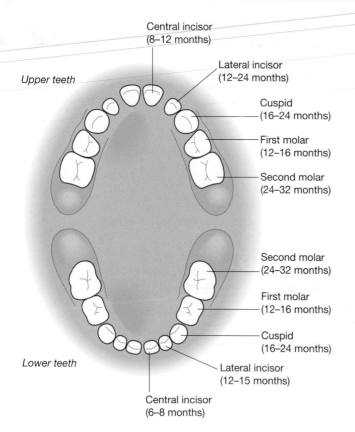

Upper teeth

Central incisor
(8–12 months)

Lateral incisor
(12–24 months)

Cuspid
(16–24 months)

First molar
(12–16 months)

Second molar
(24–32 months)

Second molar
(24–32 months)

First molar
(12–16 months)

Cuspid
(16–24 months)

Lower teeth

Lateral incisor
(12–15 months)

Central incisor
(6–8 months)

Figure 28.4 Milk teeth.

underlying submucosal layer that provides the nervous and blood supply. The mucosal layer contains glands that secrete mucus for lubricating food. There is a middle muscular layer, consisting of circular and longitudinal layers, and an outer connective tissue layer (Figure 28.8).

The function of the oesophagus is to move food down to the stomach by **peristalsis**. The peristalsis is entirely under involuntary control and the relaxation of the lower oesophageal sphincter allows food to enter the stomach.

The Stomach

The stomach is a muscular, hollow, dilated part of the digestive system. The stomach, located high on the left side of the abdominal cavity, is connected to the oesophagus at the upper end and to the small intestine at the lower end (Figure 28.9). It is approximately 25 cm (10 inches) long and is a J-shaped elastic sac that can expand to hold up to 4 L of food and fluid. The concave surface of the stomach is called the lesser curvature; the convex surface is called the greater curvature. The stomach may be divided into four regions extending from the distal end of the oesophagus to the opening into the small intestine. These regions are the cardiac region, fundus, body, and pylorus (Figure 28.9). The pyloric sphincter controls emptying of the stomach into the duodenum (portion of the small intestine). The stomach is a storage organ for food. It continues the mechanical breakdown of food, begins the process of protein digestion, and mixes the food with gastric juices into a thick fluid called chyme.

The stomach is composed of three layers; mucosal, submucosal and muscular. The surface of the mucosal layer is lined with simple columnar epithelial cells called surface mucosal cells (Figure 28.10).

The epithelial cells extend down into the lamina propria where they form columns of secretary cells called gastric glands. The gastric glands contain exocrine cells that secrete 2–3 litres of gastric juice into the stomach daily. The submucosal layer is lined with loose connective tissue. The muscular layer consists of three layers: an inner oblique layer of muscle tissue, a middle layer of circular tissue and an outer longitudinal layer (Figure 28.10).

The secretion of gastric juice is under both neural and endocrine control. Stimulation of the parasympathetic vagus nerve increases secretory activity; in contrast, stimulation of sympathetic nerves decreases secretions. There are three phases of secretory activity: the cephalic phase, the gastric phase and the intestinal phase.

1. The cephalic phase occurs even before food enters the stomach. It is triggered by the sight, odour, taste or thought of food. It originates from the cerebral cortex and the appetite centres of the amygdala and hypothalamus via the vagus nerve to the stomach.
2. In the gastric phase when food enters the stomach, gastrin secretion is stimulated, which in turn stimulates the gastric glands (especially the parietal cells) to produce more gastric juice. Histamine also stimulates hydrochloric acid secretion.
3. The intestinal phase is initiated when chyme enters the duodenum, which leads to inhibition of gastric secretion and release of hormones such as secretin, cholecystokinin and gastric inhibitory peptide.

The Small Intestine

The small intestine begins at the pyloric sphincter and ends at the ileocaecal valve. The average length of the small intestine in an adult human male is 6.9 m and in the adult female 7.1 m. It is approximately 2.5–3 cm in diameter. The small intestine has three regions: the duodenum, the jejunum and the ileum (Figure 28.11). The duodenum begins at the pyloric sphincter and extends around the head of the pancreas for about 25 cm. Both pancreatic enzymes and bile from the liver enter the small intestine at the duodenum. The jejunum, the middle region of the small intestine, extends for about 2.4 m. The ileum, the terminal end of the small intestine, is approximately 3.6 m long and meets the large intestine at the ileocaecal valve.

The Large Intestine

The large intestine, also known as the colon, commences at the ileocaecal valve and terminates at the rectum (Figure 28.12). It is approximately 1.5 m in length and 6 cm in diameter. The large intestine is made up of the caecum, ascending, transverse, descending and sigmoid colons, the rectum and the anus (Figure 28.12). The large intestine:

- Absorbs nutrients and water
- Produces vitamin K and some B complexes such as B_1, B_2 and folic acid
- Secretes mucus for lubrication of faeces
- Stores faeces for defaecation.

The Hepatobiliary System – Liver and Gallbladder

The liver weighs about 1.5 kg in the average-sized adult. It is located in the right side of the abdomen, inferior to the diaphragm and anterior to the stomach (Figure 28.13). The liver has four lobes:

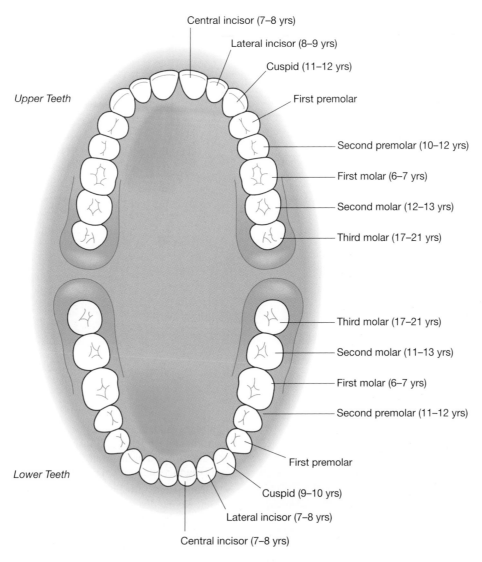

Figure 28.5 Permanent teeth.

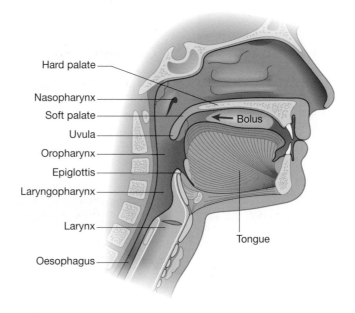

Figure 28.6 Nasopharynx and laryngopharynx.

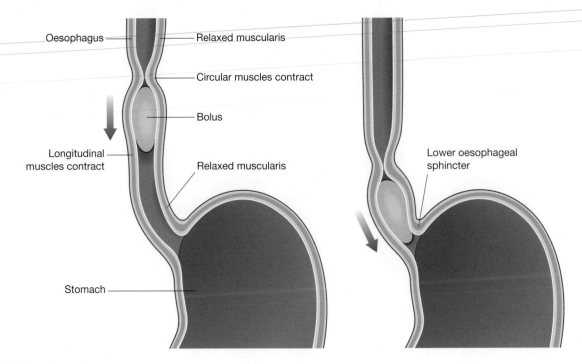

Figure 28.7 Oesophagus.

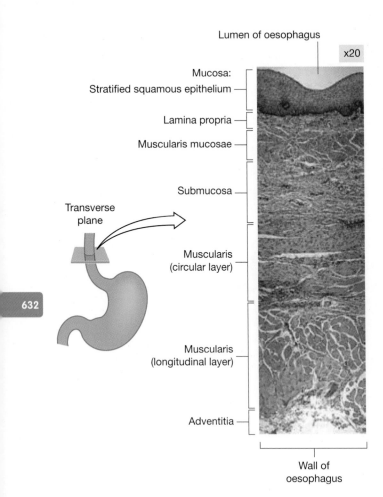

Figure 28.8 Histology of the oesophagus.

right, left, caudate and quadrate. A mesenteric ligament separates the right and left lobes and suspends the liver from the diaphragm and anterior abdominal wall. The liver has many diverse functions and they include:

- Carbohydrate, protein and fat metabolisms
- Detoxifying drugs and alcohol
- Production and secretion of bile
- Storage of vitamins (A, B_{12}, D, E and K)
- Activation of vitamin D
- Phagocytic action.

Lying beneath the liver is a sac called the **gallbladder**. The gallbladder is a pear-shaped organ approximately 7–10 cm in length (Figure 28.13). The gallbladder stores and concentrates bile, which is produced by the liver. Bile is a greenish, watery solution containing bile salts, cholesterol, bilirubin, electrolytes, water and phospholipids (Jenkins & Tortora 2013). These components of bile are essential for emulsification and absorption of fats. The liver cells produce approximately 1 L of bile daily which is stored in the gallbladder. When food containing fats enters the duodenum, hormones stimulate the gallbladder to secrete bile into the cystic duct. The cystic duct joins the hepatic duct to form the common bile duct, from which bile enters into the duodenum (Figure 28.13).

Peptic Ulcer

A peptic ulcer (PU) is an area of damage to the inner lining (the mucosa) of the stomach and/or the duodenum (Figure 28.14). A bacterium, *Helicobacter pylori* (*H. pylori*), is the main cause of ulcers in this area. PU can affect people of any age, including children, but the condition is most common in people who are 60 years of age or over. Both sexes are equally affected by PU.

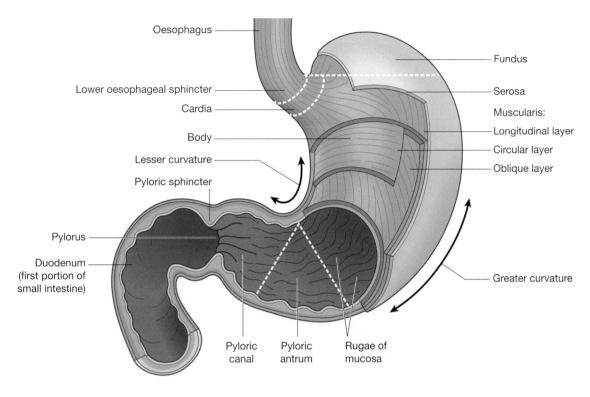

Oesophagus

Lower oesophageal sphincter

Cardia

Body

Lesser curvature

Pyloric sphincter

Pylorus

Duodenum
(first portion of
small intestine)

Fundus

Serosa

Muscularis:

Longitudinal layer

Circular layer

Oblique layer

Greater curvature

Pyloric
canal

Pyloric
antrum

Rugae of
mucosa

Figure 28.9 Anatomy of the stomach.

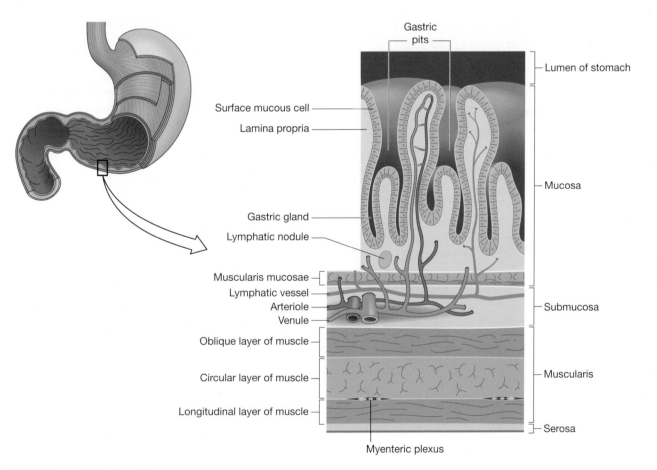

Gastric
pits

Lumen of stomach

Surface mucous cell

Lamina propria

Gastric gland

Lymphatic nodule

Muscularis mucosae

Lymphatic vessel

Arteriole

Venule

Oblique layer of muscle

Circular layer of muscle

Longitudinal layer of muscle

Mucosa

Submucosa

Muscularis

Serosa

Myenteric plexus

Figure 28.10 Layers of the stomach.

Jot This Down

List the 'risk factors' associated with peptic ulcer and discuss how the risk factors cause the peptic ulcer.

Pathophysiology

'PU' is a term used to define the formation of an ulcer in the stomach and the duodenum. Ulcers in the stomach (gastric ulcers) are found in any part of the stomach but are most commonly seen on the 'lesser curve' (Figure 28.14) and duodenal ulcers are found after the pyloric sphincter. The ulcers may be superficial or deep, affecting all layers of the mucosa. The possible causes of PU are:

- The most common cause is *H. pylori* infection. It is a Gram-negative spiral-shaped bacterium
- The second most common cause is excessive use of non-steroidal anti-inflammatory drugs (NSAIDs). Examples of these medicines are aspirin, ibuprofen, naproxen and diclofenac. Over a

period of time, these drugs can damage the mucous lining of the stomach and cause a peptic ulcer
- Cigarette smoking, excessive consumption of alcohol, caffeine and stress
- Familial history.

Red Flag

NSAIDs are associated with a small increase in the risk of a person experiencing a heart attack, stroke or heart failure.

Red Flag

Asthma attacks are triggered by aspirin or NSAIDs in some people.

Investigation and diagnosis

- Tests for *H. pylori,* which includes a ^{13}C urea breath test and a blood test to detect immunoglobulin G (IgG) antibodies
- Barium swallow may be used to identify any ulcer formation
- Endoscopy and biopsy of gastric lining to detect changes resulting from *H. pylori* infection
- Stool test for occult blood.

The Evidence

The National Institute for Health and Clinical Excellence (NICE 2004) guidelines state that endoscopy is *not required* unless the patient is presenting for the first time above the age of 55, or there are warning signs such as pernicious anaemia, excessive use of NSAIDs and/or a familial history of gastric carcinoma.

NICE (2004): **http://www.nice.org.uk/guidance/CG17** (accessed 18th September 2012)

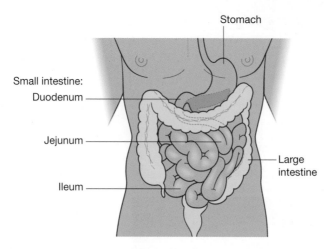

Figure 28.11 The small intestine.

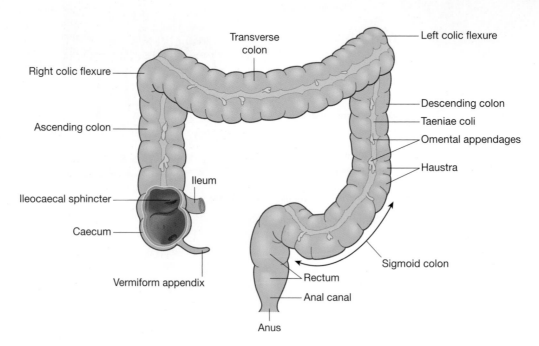

Figure 28.12 Large intestine.

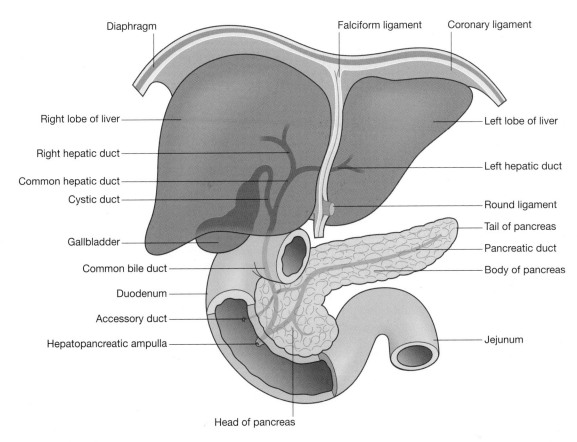

Figure 28.13 Hepatobiliary system.

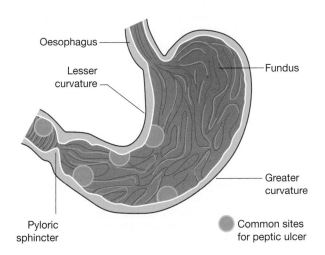

Figure 28.14 Common sites for peptic ulcer.

Signs and symptoms

Signs and symptoms of PU include:

- Epigastric pain usually 1–3 hours after eating a meal
- Heartburn as a result of gastro-oesophageal reflux
- Occult or obvious blood in the stool
- Haematemesis (vomiting blood) if the ulcer bleeds
- Fatigue, weakness, dizziness
- Dyspepsia (indigestion).

Nursing care and management

A full medical and nursing history should be obtained in order to formulate a care plan to meet the specific needs of the person. Following a thorough investigation, an accurate diagnosis is confirmed. Once peptic ulcer has been diagnosed, the healthcare provider should help the patient identify any lifestyle factors that may be associated with peptic ulcers, such as stress, heavy alcohol consumption, smoking or drinking a lot of coffee. The care should include dietary advice, altering lifestyle, avoiding stressful situations and adherence to the medications prescribed.

Nutrition Dietary advice should be offered to the patient. Small regular meals are encouraged (approximately five small meals per day) to prevent hunger pain. It is important to advise the patient that bland or restrictive diets are no longer necessary. Alcohol intake in moderation is not harmful; however binge drinking could lead to PU. Smoking should be discouraged because the ulcer may not heal or may take longer to heal.

635

What the Experts Say

 A freelance health writer advises people to: 'Eat 5 to 6 small meals a day instead of 3 larger meals. It is important that you avoid overeating. Frequent, smaller meals will be more comfortable and easier on the stomach than two or three large meals a day'.

Medications The medications used to treat PU include drugs to eradicate *H. pylori*, to decrease gastric acid content, and to protect the GI mucosa. Nurses should adhere to local and Nursing and Midwifery Council guidelines with regard to standards for medicine management and guidelines for record-keeping.

Medications may include:

- Proton-pump inhibitors (PPI) such as omeprazole and lansoprazole to inhibit the release of hydrochloric acid from the parietal cells
- Antacid for the relief of dyspepsia and alginates to protect the lining of the stomach
- Antibiotics such as amoxicillin, clarithromycin and metronidazole to treat *H. pylori* infection
- H_2-receptor antagonists. These work by blocking the actions of a protein called histamine, which is also responsible for stimulating the production of acid. Ranitidine is the most widely used H_2-receptor antagonist for treating stomach ulcers.

Nursing Fields Bulimia Nervosa: Mental Health

Self-induced vomiting damages the digestive system, resulting in peptic ulcer. The symptoms can vary, with some people not noticing anything out of the ordinary; others may vomit blood and experience abdomen or chest pains. The pain is usually increased when the individual eats or drinks.

Red Flag

Many people take an anti-inflammatory drug for arthritis, muscular pains, etc. Aspirin is also used by many people to protect against blood clots forming. However, these drugs sometimes affect the mucous barrier of the stomach and allow acid to cause an ulcer. About 2 in 10 stomach ulcers are caused by anti-inflammatory drugs.

Surgery Surgical procedures for peptic ulcer include vagotomy and pyloroplasty or distal subtotal gastrectomy (Duffy 2011). For general pre- and postoperative care, refer to Chapter 14. Many of the Trusts in the UK are using the Enhanced Recovery After Surgery (ERAS) protocol pathway for their care package.

 Link To/Go To

You can find out more on ERAS at:

http://www.nhs.uk/conditions/enhanced-recovery/Pages/Introduction.aspx

---

- The patient's vital signs are monitored hourly until the patient is haemodynamically stable
- If a nasogastric tube is inserted, ensure that it is draining freely and aspirate every 2–4-hourly. Note the colour and amount aspirated. Nurses should give regular nasal care and ensure that the nasogastric tube is comfortably positioned and secured
- The patient will be nil by mouth for the first 24 hours until bowel sounds return. Sips of water are introduced when bowel sounds

return and this is gradually increased to free fluids once the bowel sounds are normal
- Provide oral hygiene as required, by offering frequent mouth washes
- Check with the patient for pain and administer analgesia as prescribed.

What To Do If...

What would you do if you discovered that the patient you are looking after suddenly developed secondary haemorrhage postoperatively? Some of the nursing action should include:

- Check the wound site
- Report to the person in charge
- Repeat the observations ¼–½ hourly.

Health promotion and discharge

When the patient is ready to go home, advise the patient:

- Small, frequent meals may enable an adequate intake of nutrients and reduce dumping syndrome. Avoid simple sugars and reduce fluid intake with meals. Advise the patient to sit upright, especially after meals
- Iron and folic acid supplements may be required following subtotal gastrectomy and aspirin-containing drugs and NSAIDs should be avoided as they irritate the gastric mucosa. Ensure that the patient is concordant to the medications prescribed
- Advise the patient on stress avoidance, as stress is a risk factor for some patients
- Inform the patient to avoid highly seasoned foods, acidic drinks and heavy alcohol consumption
- If elderly, ensure that the patient has a relative with them and if necessary transport to go home
- Provide letters for the appropriate community healthcare providers, for example GP and district nurse, to explain the care given in the hospital and the follow-up care. Nurses should adhere to individual Trust policy with regards to discharging patients into the community.

Primary Care

Most of the patients with peptic ulcer are treated in the community by their GP and the care is provided by the community/practice nurse. Nurses should discuss all the relevant information with regards to the disease and the treatment the patient should adhere to. Nurses should discuss the:

- Prescribed medications, including desired and potential side-effects
- Importance of continuing their treatment even if they feel better
- Risk factors that contribute to PU formation
- Importance of taking regular small meals and avoiding any food that may increase the risk of developing PU
- Signs and symptoms of PU and encourage the patient to see their GP or the practice nurse if they feel unwell
- Resources available in the community for stress management, such as yoga classes, counselling, and formal or informal discussion groups.

Jot This Down

It is not certain how people contract *H. pylori*, but researchers think it may be through food or water. The organism is also found in the saliva of some infected people, so mouth to mouth contact can spread the bacteria.

What the Experts Say

Doctors suggest that the discomfort from an ulcer can be avoided by avoiding alcohol and spicy food, by not eating late in the evening, or by giving up smoking.

Care, Dignity and Compassion

You should read these Health Service Ombudsman case studies: Report of the Health Service Ombudsman on 10 investigations into NHS care of older people, at: http://www.ombudsman.org.uk/__data/assets/pdf_file/0016/7216/Care-and-Compassion-PHSO-0114web.pdf

Carcinoma of the Stomach

Stomach cancer is the second most common cause of cancer-related death in the world. It is a difficult disease to cure in Western countries, mainly because most patients present with advanced disease: 50% of cancers involve the pylorus, 25% the lesser curve and 10% the cardia.

Pathophysiology

Most stomach cancers (around 95%) are **adenocarcinomas** and 5% are lymphomas, sarcomas and carcinoids. Adenocarcinomas can spread along the stomach wall (Figure 28.15a) to the duodenum and to other organs in the abdominal cavity. If the tumour infiltrates the lymphatic system (Figure 28.15b) and blood vessels, then other organs, such as the liver (Figure 28.15c), lungs and ovaries, the bones and the peritoneum become affected. Lymphomas arise from the lymphatic tissue within the wall of the stomach, sarcomas arise from the muscle or connective tissue within the wall of the stomach and carcinoids arise from cells in the stomach lining that synthesise hormones.

It is generally assumed that food preservation by refrigeration and not by salting, reducing nitrate derivatives, is an important factor in the decline of the incidence of gastric adenocarcinoma.

Risk factors for stomach cancer

- Stomach cancer is more common in older people. Most cases are in people over the age of 55
- People who suffer from pernicious anaemia are at risk of developing stomach cancer
- There is a correlation between diet and stomach cancer. High intakes of salt, pickled and smoked foods have been associated with stomach cancer, while eating a lot of fruit and green vegetables can reduce the risk
- Smoking, alcohol and *H. pylori* infection may increase the risk of developing stomach cancer.

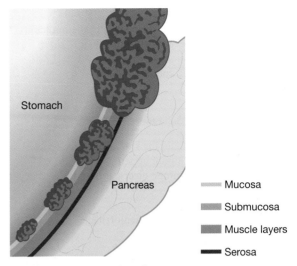

(a) Tumour growth in stomach wall

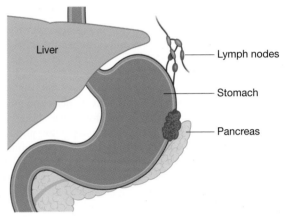

(b) Stomach cancer spreads to lymph nodes

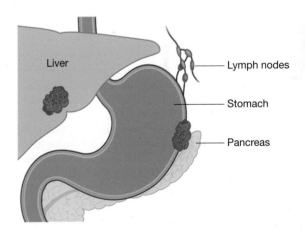

(c) Stomach cancer spreads to other organs (e.g. liver metastasis)

Figure 28.15 (a) Tumour affecting the layer of the stomach. (b) Tumour has spread into neighbouring lymph nodes. (c) Tumour has spread to the liver.

Investigation and diagnosis

- Medical history of eating and bowel elimination habits
- Physical and clinical examination
- CT scanning
- Fibreoptic gastroscopy and biopsy
- Barium meal.

Signs and symptoms

- Indigestion, acidity and burping
- Dysphagia if the cardia of the stomach is involved
- Anorexia as a result of poor appetite
- Epigastric pain (may mimic ulcer pain) and loss of appetite
- Difficulty in swallowing
- Nausea and vomiting
- If a blood vessel is involved, haemorrhage.

Nursing care and management

Surgery In most cases, stomach cancer is treated surgically. The removal of the stomach is called 'gastrectomy'. It could be either a partial gastrectomy (half of the stomach) or a total gastrectomy (all of the stomach). The type of operation needed depends on the size of the tumour and where it is location in the stomach.

For detailed principles of pre- and postoperative care, refer to Chapter 14.

Preoperative care

- Nurses should adhere to local and NMC policies and guidelines for the safe preparation of the person for gastric surgery
- Psychological care is paramount in the preoperative phase to give the patient confidence in the after care in the community. Visits from the Marie Curie or Macmillan nurses can be invaluable in giving the opportunity for the patient and the relatives to talk about their fears and worries.

Postoperative care When the patient returns to the ward, nursing care should be planned under these headings: airway, breathing, circulation, disability and the environment. Any changes should be reported to the nurse in charge in order to take prompt action.

The nasogastric tube (NG) is attached to intermittent suction to keep the stomach empty. If the entire stomach has been removed, the tube goes directly to the small intestine and remains in place until bowel function returns. This generally takes between 2 and 3 days and is determined by listening to the abdomen with a stethoscope for bowel sounds (the passage of gas). If repositioning or NG replacement is needed, nurses must inform the doctor immediately and not attempt it themselves. Note the amount and colour of the aspirate and ensure it is documented in the fluid balance chart.

Jot This Down

After a partial or total gastrectomy, nurses must not attempt to reposition or reinsert the nasogastric tube. They must always inform the doctor. Why it is not advised for the nurses to re-insert the NG tube?

When bowel sounds return, clear liquids are offered. If they are tolerated, the NG tube is removed and the diet is gradually advanced from liquids to soft foods, and then to more solid foods. Dietary adjustments may be necessary, as certain foods may now be difficult to digest. Diet may present a challenge after a total gastrectomy.

Food and liquids now enter the small intestine quickly, causing uncomfortable symptoms that can usually be relieved by eating several small meals, eating more protein and less sugar, and making other dietary changes. The dietary changes may be temporary, until the digestive system adjusts, or they may be permanent.

If inserted, the urinary catheter is removed in a day or two, depending on recovery. When food and liquid are tolerated, and urine output is normal, the catheter is removed. Maintain the input and output chart.

Administer analgesia as prescribed and check with the patient every 2–4 hours if he/she is pain free, using a pain assessment tool. Record all outcomes in the patient's care plan.

Vitamin B_{12} is absorbed in the stomach and must be supplemented with regular injections by patients who underwent a total gastrectomy. Absorption may be impaired in those who still have part of their stomach, so it is necessary to have B_{12} levels checked periodically. Supplementation with folate, iron and calcium may also be necessary to correct deficiencies caused by the surgery.

The Evidence Keyhole Surgery

Surgery for stomach cancer is usually done through a cut into the abdomen (laparotomy). Laparoscopy is already used to help stage stomach cancers and there is increasing interest in using it to treat stomach cancer. Laparoscopy looks into the stomach using a tube passed through a small cut. There is less scarring after laparoscopic surgery and time spent in hospital is generally shorter. Some studies show that patients feel better more quickly afterwards. However it is not suitable for people with larger cancers or advanced disease.

A new type of laparoscopic surgery combines an endoscopy with a laparoscopy. This is called *laparo-endogastric surgery* or laparoscopic resection. Because it is a new procedure, it is not yet known how good it is at removing cancer.

http://publications.nice.org.uk/laparo-endogastric-surgery-ipg25

Complications Dumping syndrome is a complication following gastric surgery that may occur 10–30 minutes after eating. The patient may experience epigastric fullness, discomfort, excessive sweating and feeling unwell. The patient should be encouraged to rest in a recumbent (reclining) or semi-recumbent position for approximately 30 minutes after meals.

Anaemia may be a chronic problem after gastric surgery. Iron is absorbed primarily in the duodenum and proximal jejunum; rapid gastric emptying may interfere with adequate absorption of iron from the diet.

Pernicious anaemia is another complication resulting from a deficiency of vitamin B_{12}. The absorption of vitamin B_{12} is dependent on the intrinsic factor produced by the stomach. These patients will need vitamin B_{12} injections for life. Other nutritional complications include poor absorption of calcium, folic acid and vitamin D.

Health promotion and discharge

Prior to discharge, nurses need to discuss some of the risk factors associated with stomach cancer. Advise the patient on:

- The relationship between gastric cancer and consumption of foods preserved with nitrates (such as bacon and other processed meats), and encourage limited consumption of these products
- Smoking is also a possible risk factor for stomach cancer. Advise the patient on cessation of smoking and provide information and leaflets to help stop smoking

- When eating fruits and vegetables, wash them thoroughly before eating
- Advise the patient to take regular small meals and to rest in a reclining position after each meal for approximately 30 minutes
- Ensure that the patient has all the necessary outpatient appointments before the patient is discharged home. Nurses should follow local and NMC policies in the safe discharge of the patient.

What the Experts Say

The World Cancer Research Fund reported that 14% of cases of stomach cancer could be avoided through reducing our salt intake. Kate, head of health information at WCRF, said, 'Stomach cancer is difficult to treat successfully because most cases are not caught until the disease is well established. This places even greater emphasis on making lifestyle choices to prevent the disease occurring in the first place – such as cutting down on salt intake and eating more fruit and vegetables'.

Primary Care

Nurses should ensure that the patient is fully prepared both physically and mentally, so that they and their relatives can maintain the care prescribed. Care in the community should include:

1. Information about the surgery
2. Information about fluid and diet intake. Preventing complications of surgery such as dumping syndrome
3. The patient may need analgesia and to contact their GP for repeat prescription
4. Provide referrals to cancer support groups as appropriate
5. Provide information about services available in the community, such as meals on wheels, voluntary groups, counselling services and other support groups
6. Palliative care services such as Macmillan nurses, cancer support groups.

Hepatitis

Hepatitis refers to liver inflammation, which is caused by a virus, alcohol, drugs and toxins and can be acute or chronic. It is characterised by the destruction of a number of liver cells and the presence of inflammatory cells in the liver tissue. There are different types of hepatitis, for example A, B, C and other rare ones (LeMone et al. 2011).

Pathophysiology

Viral hepatitis Viral hepatitis is the term given to infection of the liver by viruses, for example hepatitis A virus (HAV), hepatitis B virus (HBV), hepatitis C virus (HCV), hepatitis D virus (HDV) and hepatitis E virus (HEV). These viruses replicate in the liver and in the process cause severe damage to the liver cells. These viruses account for 95% of cases of acute viral hepatitis.

At 5–10 days after the onset of symptoms, the patient develops jaundice of the sclera, skin and mucous membranes. The jaundice results from inflammation of the liver and blockage of bile ducts which lead to bilirubin being absorbed into the blood stream. The serum bilirubin levels are elevated, causing yellowing of the skin and the sclera.

No symptoms are present during the incubation period after exposure to the virus. The prodromal phase may begin suddenly, with general malaise, anorexia, fatigue and muscle and body aches. These signs and symptoms of nausea, vomiting, diarrhoea or constipation may develop, as well as mild right upper quadrant abdominal pain. Chills and fever may be present.

The patients suffer from pruritus as a result of bile salts in the skin. The stools are light brown or clay-coloured because bile pigment is not excreted through the normal faecal pathway. Instead, the pigment is excreted by the kidneys, causing the urine to turn brown. Whereas persons with acute hepatitis A or B are likely to develop jaundice, many people with hepatitis C do not develop jaundice.

Hepatitis A Infection with hepatitis A, or infectious hepatitis, often occurs by the faecal–oral route via contaminated food, water, shellfish and direct contact with an infected person. It frequently occurs in crowded unsanitary conditions. It can also be transmitted sexually. Lifetime immunity probably results after the infection has run its course. Serum IgG may remain elevated for life.

Hepatitis B Hepatitis B, sometimes referred to as serum hepatitis, is transmitted by blood transfusion or a virus-contaminated needle, and also from mother to fetus via the placenta (Dougherty & Lister 2011). The HBV is found in the DNA and therefore is found throughout the body of the infected person. A person can be a carrier without suffering any symptoms and is capable of spreading it to others. Hepatitis B is a major risk factor for primary liver cancer. The HBV virus has been implicated in 60–90% of cases of liver carcinoma when the disease has reached its chronic phase.

Hepatitis C Hepatitis C, formerly known as non-A, non-B hepatitis, is the primary worldwide cause of chronic hepatitis, cirrhosis and liver cancer (LeMone et al. 2011). It is an RNA virus that may be transmitted through blood transfusion, needle-stick injury and body fluids. Many infected individuals develop chronic hepatitis. Acute hepatitis C usually is asymptomatic; if symptoms do develop, they often are mild and non-specific. Hepatitis C is unique in that it does not produce lasting immunity to re-infection. Only about 15% of acute infections completely resolve; most progress to chronic active hepatitis (LeMone et al. 2011).

Hepatitis D This is caused by a defective RNA virus distinct from all the others. The onset is sudden and the symptoms similar to those for HBV. Co-infection with HBV is necessary for the efficient replication of HDV. It is transmitted parenterally and often overlooked, as the person is infected with HBV infection.

Chronic hepatitis It is estimated that there are approximately 325 000 people in the UK with chronic hepatitis (Hepatitis B Foundation UK 2007). The exact cause of the disease is unknown but a number of different diseases are thought to be the cause, for example, infectious hepatitis, HBV, HCV and HDV, drug reactions, alcohol poisoning, autoimmune hepatitis and haemochromatosis (a disorder of the body's iron metabolism). Many patients have no symptoms, while some may experience malaise, fatigue and aching muscles and joints. Jaundice is a very late symptom of the disease and it is a sign that the liver is damaged. Liver enzymes, such as serum aminotransferase levels, are elevated. Chronic active hepatitis usually leads to cirrhosis of the liver and end-stage liver failure.

Investigations and diagnosis

Some of the investigations that may be carried out to confirm the diagnosis are:

- Full blood count and electrolyte levels
- Urinalysis for the presence of bilirubin and urobilinogen
- Renal function test
- Alpha(α)-1 antitrypsin
- Liver biopsy
- Ultrasound, CT or MRI scan of the liver.

Signs and symptoms

No symptoms are present during the incubation period after exposure to the virus. The prodromal phase may begin suddenly, with general malaise, anorexia, fatigue and muscle and body aches. These signs and symptoms of nausea, vomiting, diarrhoea or constipation may develop, as well as mild right upper quadrant abdominal pain. Chills and fever may be present.

The patients suffer from pruritus as a result of bile salts in the skin. The stools are light brown or clay-coloured because bile pigment is not excreted through the normal faecal pathway. Instead, the pigment is excreted by the kidneys, causing the urine to turn brown.

Nursing care and management

The nursing care of hepatitis is dependent on the type of infection. The care plan should reflect both physical and psychosocial care. Some of the nursing priorities include reducing demand on the liver, while promoting physical care, preventing complications and providing information about the disease, prognosis and the treatment. Most hepatitis patients do not need isolation unless they present a health risk to other patients.

Risk for infection An important goal when caring for persons with acute viral hepatitis is preventing spread of the infection.

- Use the local Trust and Health Protection Agency guidelines in the care of these patients. Wash hands before and after contact with the patient, as hepatitis viruses are spread by direct contact with faeces or blood and body fluids. Wear gloves when handling body fluids of the patient and always change gloves between patient contacts
- Always practise good hygiene, principally through hand washing after toilet use and before food preparation.

What To Do If...

When administering an intramuscular injection to a patient you sustained a needle-stick injury. What will you do and what steps need to be taken to prevent future needle-stick injury? Some of the precautions include:

- Follow the correct procedure for administering i.m. injections
- Follow the correct procedure for the disposal of used needles.

Fatigue Fatigue and anaemia are common in acute hepatitis. Always ensure that the patient is monitored during their normal activity. Assist the patient to identify essential activities, such as walking and having a bath, complete a risk assessment and inform the patient to rest between activities. As recovery progresses, increasing activity levels are tolerated with less fatigue.

Link To/Go To

You can find out more on infection prevention at:
http://guidance.nice.org.uk/CG139 (accessed 7 March 2014)

Medications The medications used to treat hepatitis depend on the viral infection. Some of the drugs include:

- Peginterferon alfa – used in the treatment of HBV and HCV. It is used with ribavirin.
- Ribavirin – inhibits a range of DNA and RNA viruses.
- Adefovir dipivoxil is used in the treatment of chronic hepatitis B. Patients should be informed about passing the disease on to others. Several different antiviral drugs, known as nucleoside analogues, are also now used to treat chronic hepatitis.

The majority of people with hepatitis B do not need treatment other than rest and they make a full recovery. However, careful monitoring of the person's recovery is essential to ensure that they are not developing chronic hepatitis B.

Link To/Go To

Use this link to find out more about the treatment:
http://www.nice.org.uk/TA106

Health promotion and discharge

Nurses play an important role in preventing the spread of hepatitis. Emphasis on personal hygiene measures, such as hand washing after toileting and before all food handling, is important.

Advise the patient to avoid alcohol to prevent further damage of the liver and encourage high calorie soft drinks as a high intake of calories is essential to promote healing. Advise the patient to eat regular small meals and to reduce their fat intake so that they do not feel sick after their meal.

Discuss recommendations for hepatitis A and hepatitis B vaccination with people in high or moderate risk groups for these infections. Ensure that nurses and other healthcare workers at risk for exposure to blood and body fluids are effectively vaccinated against hepatitis A and B.

Primary Care

Before the patient is discharged, nurses should ensure that the patient and their relatives are given the necessary information for home care. The following information should be provided:

- Advise the patient and their relatives in maintaining personal hygiene, strict hand washing when preparing food and not sharing eating utensils
- Advise the patient to rest when fatigue sets in
- Encourage good nutritious fluid intake
- Avoid alcohol consumption as alcohol is a risk factor for liver damage
- Offer advice on the medications they are discharged with, and the importance of continuing with the drug until further notice
- Inform the patient about any outpatient appointments and the importance of adhering to the time and date
- Always seek advice from the pharmacist or the GP when buying over-the-counter medications

    Offer counselling and information on support groups in the community.

Inflammatory Bowel Disease

Inflammatory bowel disease (IBD) is a term that includes **Crohn's disease (CD)** and **ulcerative colitis (UC)**. These are common diseases, occurring in the Western world and affecting young adults. CD can affect any part of the GI tract from the mouth to the anus, while UC mainly affects the colon and the rectum.

Pathophysiology

In CD, the inflammation occurs in segments along the GI tract, affecting all layers, while in UC the disease process mainly involves the mucosa and submucosa. In both disorders the damaged mucosa has a cobblestone appearance (to the affected areas) as fissures and ulcers surround islands of intact mucosa over oedematous submucosa. Fibrosis and narrowing of the tract can occur and lead to fistula formation.

In UC, the rectum is always inflamed (*proctitis*) and the colon variably along its length (Alexander *et al.* 2007). In the acute phase of UC, the inflammation affects the mucosal layer all along the colon so it becomes oedematous and usually secretions are absent. A small amount of haemorrhage may occur and small ulcerations. The ulcerations are confined to the mucosa and the submucosal layers. As the disease enters the chronic phase, the ulceration becomes fibrotic and the bowel wall shortens and thickens.

LeMone *et al.* (2011) state that the severity and extent of the disease could lead to malabsorption and malnutrition as the ulcers prevent absorption of nutrients. When the jejunum and ileum are affected, the absorption of multiple nutrients may be impaired, including carbohydrates, proteins, fats, vitamins and folate. Disease in the terminal ileum can lead to vitamin B_{12} malabsorption and bile salt reabsorption. The ulcerations can also lead to protein loss and chronic, slow blood loss, with consequent anaemia.

Investigations and diagnosis

- Sigmoidoscopy of the lower intestine and the taking of biopsy samples from the bowel wall. Since the lower bowel is involved in all those with ulcerative colitis and about half of those with Crohn's disease, this is a helpful investigation for inflammatory bowel disease
- Colonoscopy of the large intestine and terminal ileum using a flexible tube inserted through the anus. Colonoscopy has reduced the need for barium enema examinations. Colonoscopy can also be used to determine how much of the large intestine is involved

and the extent and severity of disease. It also has the advantage of allowing biopsies, tissue samples, to be taken from the bowel wall during the procedure
- Histopathology is the detailed microscopic examination by a pathologist of tissue samples, biopsies taken at the time of sigmoidoscopy and colonoscopy. Histopathology can be very helpful in confirming the diagnosis and indicating whether the inflammatory bowel disease is active or not.

Signs and symptoms

- Pain and discomfort. The duration of the pain can vary a great deal. Many patients with IBS describe the pain as a spasm or colic
- Bloating and swelling of the abdomen
- Diarrhoea or constipation. Sometimes the stools become small and pellet-like. Sometimes the stools become watery or ribbony. At times, mucus may be mixed with the stools
- Other symptoms include poor appetite, nausea, belching, headache, quick fullness after eating, heartburn
- CT or MRI scan of the abdomen
- Blood test for anaemia.

Complications

The two most common complications are:

- Bowel obstruction – severe inflammation that causes sections of your bowel to narrow and harden, causing your bowel contents to become stuck in the bowel
- Fistula – a channel that develops between the anus and the skin near the anus.

    For both these complications, surgery may be needed to prevent further complications, such as perforations and rupture of the colon.

 Link To/Go To

Use these links to learn more about inflammatory bowel disease:

https://arms.evidence.nhs.uk/resources/hub/36890/attachment

http://www.nhs.uk/conditions/Inflammatory-bowel-disease/Pages/Introduction.aspx

---

The Evidence Fish Oil and Inflammatory Bowel Disease

Eicosapentaenoic acid (EPA) is an essential fatty acid (EFA) found in fish and is also produced by the desaturation and chain lengthening linolenic acid, which is found in soya bean and rapeseed oil. EFAs are important in the production of prostaglandins, which play a role in inflammatory mediation.

 Link To/Go To

Use the link below to find out more about the evidence.

http://www.crohns.org.uk/Docs/3/Fish%20oils%20and%20Inflammatory%20Bowel%20Disease.html

Nursing care and management

Relieving pain is one of the primary goals. Some patients may complain of severe colicky pain, while others may have intermittent pain. Any analgesia administered needs to be individualised. Nurses need to check with the patient if they are pain free, using a pain assessment tool, after the administration of analgesia.

Nutritional risk assessment should be carried out using the Malnutrition Universal Screening Tool (MUST). The patient will need advice on the type of food they should eat and the ones to avoid.

The patient may also be receiving blood transfusions if they are anaemic. Nurses need to follow local and NMC guidelines in the monitoring of patients on blood transfusion. Report any adverse reactions to the person in charge immediately, so that prompt action can be taken to prevent any further complications. Ensure that the patient and their relatives are given time to express their worries and concerns.

The patient may be prescribed supplementary nutritional fluid in acute stages of the disease. Ensure that the patient does not get dehydrated as a result of the diarrhoea and vomiting. Record intake and output accurately on a fluid balance chart. Where necessary, maintain a stool chart and monitor the frequency and if there is any blood in the stool.

Medications Both Crohn's disease and ulcerative colitis are treated with medications such as corticosteroids, which help reduce inflammation, and immunosuppressants, which block the harmful activities of the immune system. Budesonide and prednisolone are steroids that are often used to treat Crohn's disease. Anti-inflammatory drugs such as sulfasalazine are also used to treat inflammation in the early stages of Crohn's disease. Immunosuppressants such as azathioprine and mercaptopurine may also be prescribed to reduce inflammation and suppress the immune system.

Medicines Management

Steroids come in different forms: injections, enteric-coated tablets, inhalers and ointments. Many people take glucocorticoids (steroids) and may not be aware that one of the side-effects is type 2 diabetes. Can you list the other side-effects of steroids?

Infliximab and adalimumab are recommended as treatment options for adults with severe active Crohn's disease whose disease has not responded to conventional therapy (including immuno-suppressive and/or corticosteroid treatments) or who are intolerant of or have contraindications to conventional therapy (NICE 2011).

Link To/Go To

You can read more on the guidelines for these drugs at:
http://www.nice.org.uk/nicemedia/live/12985/48552/48552.pdf

Nutrition During an acute attack, most patients find a diet lower in fibre and residue helps to relieve symptoms such as cramping and wind. It can also reduce the number of times the patient defaecates. A low residue diet aims to rest the bowel and allow it to heal. A low residue diet involves avoiding roughage (insoluble fibre) that the body cannot break down. Roughage is found in skins, pips, seeds, whole grain cereals, nuts and raw fruit and vegetables. Other food or drinks that can increase bowel motions are spices, greasy food, alcohol, caffeine and fizzy drinks. Often, these dietary changes are temporary and once the disease has resolved efforts should be made to reintroduce fibre gradually.

The Evidence

The rise of inflammatory bowel diseases could be down to our shifting diets, causing a 'boom in bad bacteria', according to US researchers. Mouse experiments detailed in the journal *Nature* linked certain fats, bacteria in the gut and the onset of inflammatory diseases. The researchers said the high-fat diet changed the way food was digested and encouraged harmful bacteria. Microbiologists said modifying gut bacteria might treat the disease.
http://www.bbc.co.uk/news/health-18432652

The Evidence

Blueberries are rich in cancer-preventing antioxidants and vitamins. Now researchers claim that the fibre in the fruit can help prevent a range of intestinal diseases such as ulcerative colitis. Experts say that the effect is even greater if eaten with probiotics – the good type of bacteria found in yoghurts.
http://www.fitday.com/fitness-articles/nutrition/healthy-eating/the-6-best-high-antioxidant-fruits.html

Surgery Surgery is often required when the symptoms of Crohn's disease cannot be controlled using medication alone. An estimated 80% of people with Crohn's disease require surgery at some point in their life. Surgery cannot cure Crohn's disease but it can provide long periods of remission, often lasting several years. During surgery, the inflamed section of the digestive system is removed and the remaining part is reattached.

Health promotion and discharge

Prior to discharge, nurses should advise the patient to:

- Minimise consumption of sugars and refined foods, as they tend exacerbate inflammation of the bowel, and avoid alcohol and caffeine
- Encourage the patient to drink approximately 2–3 L of fluid per day to prevent dehydration
- Eat a health-promoting diet. After identifying and removing any allergenic foods from the diet, choose a balanced diet composed of whole, unprocessed, preferably organic foods, especially plant foods (fruits, vegetables, whole grains, beans, nuts (especially walnuts), and seeds) and coldwater fish, such as salmon and mackerel. Fish are rich in omega 3 and fatty acids, which are a good source of anti-inflammatory substances
- Advise on vitamin and mineral supplements as they are essential for tissue healing; the absorption of the substances, especially vitamin B_{12}, may be affected by IBD
- Only use antibiotics when absolutely necessary
- Take regular exercise, as it helps tone muscles and improve bowel function

- Advise the patient to see their GP if the symptoms of IBD are affecting their physical and mental status
- Advise the patient to keep all outpatient appointments as organised, even if they feel better.

What the Experts Say

 Young women may have concerns about IBD and pregnancy. This is what a Consultant Gastroenterologist advises:
Generally, fertility is not affected by having IBD. However, it is important to keep the disease under control before and during pregnancy as it maximises the chance of conceiving and avoiding complications during pregnancy. If unduly worried, always discuss your plans with the gastroenterologist.

Primary Care

Inflammatory bowel disease is a chronic condition and the patient and their relatives will need advice on support services and on daily self-management. Advise the patient and their family on:

- The disease process and the signs and symptoms associated with the illness
- A significant number of patients who have IBD suffer from malnutrition. Therefore, nutritional intake and dietary advice are important when patients are discharged into the community
- Some patients may have had surgery and may have a colostomy/ileostomy and therefore they will need advice in the care of ostomies and the resources available in the community for stoma care. See the sections below on ileostomy and colostomy for detailed nursing care
- The adherence to prescribed medications, such as steroids, to control inflammation
- If necessary, encourage the intake of nutritional supplements such as 'Ensure' to maintain weight and nutritional status
- The importance of maintaining a fluid intake of at least 2–3 L/day, increasing fluid intake during warm weather, exercise or strenuous work.

Stomas

A stoma is a surgically created opening between the intestine and the abdominal wall that allows faecal material to flow out into a stoma bag (LeMone *et al.* 2011). There are two types of stoma: an ileostomy and a colostomy. Stomas may be required in patients with inflammatory bowel disease or cancer of the colon.

Pathophysiology

Ileostomies An ileostomy is formed when a portion of the ileum is brought out of the abdominal wall. In an ileostomy, the colon, rectum and anus are usually completely removed (Dougherty & Lister 2011). The surgery may be carried out in patients with Crohn's disease or carcinoma of the colon and the rectum. The anal canal is closed, and the end of the terminal ileum is brought to the body surface through the right abdominal wall to form the stoma (Figure 28.16). Ileostomies can either be temporary (loop ileosto-

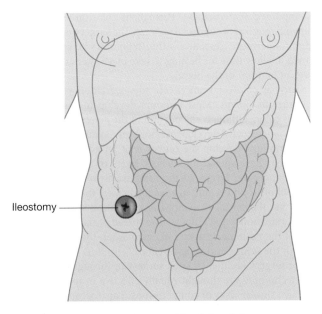

Figure 28.16 Ileostomy on the right side of the abdomen.

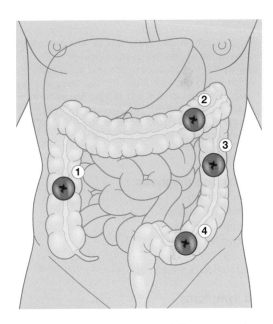

1. Ascending colostomy   3. Transverse colostomy
2. Descending colostomy   4. Sigmoid colostomy

Figure 28.17 Types of colostomy.

mies) or permanent. Permanent ileostomies are formed following total colectomy (total removal of the colon) and loop ileostomies are formed to allow time for healing to take place after an anastomosis (surgical joining) of the bowel.

Colostomies A colostomy can be formed along any section of the colon. Colostomies take the name of the portion of the colon from which they are formed: ascending, transverse, descending and sigmoid colostomies (Figure 28.17). The most common site for a colostomy is in the sigmoid colon. Colostomies can either be temporary or permanent. Permanent colostomies are formed following removal of colorectal cancers. The surgery is often termed abdominoperineal resection. The temporary colostomies are formed to allow time for healing to take place after an anastomosis (surgical joining) of the bowel.

Nearly all colorectal cancers are adenocarcinomas that begin as adenomatous polyps. Most tumours develop in the rectum and sigmoid colon, although any portion of the colon may be affected. The tumour usually develops without any symptoms and by the time symptoms develop the cancer is at an advanced stage. The cancer may have spread into deeper layers of the colon, the submucosa and outer layers. As the tumours grow they cause severe intestinal obstruction and, in advanced cases, they infiltrate other organs via the portal or lymphatic circulation such as the liver, lungs, brain, bones and kidneys. The spread of the tumour to other areas of the peritoneal cavity can occur when the tumour extends through the serosa or during surgery.

The surgery is either by open surgery or through a laparoscope. Both techniques are thought equally effective in removing cancer and have similar risks of complications. Laparoscopic colectomies have the advantage of a faster recovery time and less postoperative pain.

The Evidence

Scientists claim high levels of iron may be one reason why eating red meat raises the risk of bowel cancer.

Iron may switch on the disease process via a faulty gene in the gut, which would normally resist the disease. Red meat contains large amounts of iron and is also known to increase the likelihood of bowel cancer.

http://www.dailymail.co.uk/health/article-2186120/Red -meat-raise-risk-cancer-high-levels-iron.html

Investigations and diagnosis
- Physical examination
- Digital rectal examination
- Sigmoidoscopy and biopsies
- Colonoscopy and biopsies
- CT scan
- Ultrasound to detect metastases.

Signs and symptoms
- Rectal bleeding
- Change of bowel habits
- Diarrhoea or constipation
- Pain
- Anorexia
- Weight loss
- Anaemia from occult bleeding.

Staging of the cancer Staging of the cancer is based on the examination of the biopsies. For colorectal cancer, Duke's staging is most widely used and it identifies four stages:
- A = the tumour is in the mucosa and the submucosa
- B = the tumour has advanced to the serosa but not the lymph nodes
- C = the tumour has now infiltrated the lymph nodes
- C2 = the tumour has now spread to other organs and tissues resulting in metastasis.

The Evidence

Eating more cereals and whole grains could reduce the risk of developing colorectal cancer, a *BMJ* study says. Researchers from Imperial College, London found that for every 10 g a day increase in fibre intake, there was a 10% drop in the risk of bowel cancer.

http://www.bbc.co.uk/news/health-15674998

Nursing care and management
Enhanced recovery programme An enhanced recovery surgical programme should be used for most bowel cancer patients. In enhanced recovery, patients are involved in their own care. They choose what is best for them throughout their treatment with help and advice from their GP and healthcare team. This programme differs from traditional care by:
- Ensuring patients are in the best possible physical condition before surgery
- Minimising the trauma patients go through during surgery – for example, better pain control following surgery
- Ensuring patients experience the best possible rehabilitation after surgery.

For detailed principles of pre- and postoperative care, refer to Chapter 14. In planning and implementing care, consider both physical and psychosocial care needs of the patient. In the preoperative phase, there are some major considerations that should be taken into account. The formation of a stoma is stressful for the patient. They are worried about altered body image and other concerns. Psychological care needs should be considered with both the patient and their significant others in the preoperative phase.

Give the patient and their relatives time to express their concerns and worries. Nurses should give all the necessary information and build a trusting relationship with them. Some of their anxieties may include loss of control and normal bodily function and restrictions on current lifestyle and daily activities (Vujnovich 2008). Other concerns that should be considered include sexual activities, going out to socialise and travelling. All these worries should be addressed in the preoperative phase to ensure an uneventful recovery.

The Evidence

Research has shown that adequate counselling and education prior to surgery have a positive effect upon the individual's ability to cope following the stoma surgery.

(Alexander *et al.* 2007)

Preoperative care
- Nurses need to adhere to Trust policies and guidelines in the safe preparation of the person for a stoma
- Refer to a stoma specialist for teaching and counselling about the stoma and options for stoma appliances. It is important to begin teaching prior to surgery to facilitate learning and acceptance of the stoma postoperatively. This provides an ideal opportunity to discuss altered body image, grieving, family relationship, depression and anger
- Discuss the availability of support groups or associations, and provide a referral as necessary or desired. People from a support

group may help with information and support with regards to living with a stoma

- If necessary, refer the patient and their relatives to the dietician for dietary advice and to answer any questions they may have regarding food the patient can eat or should avoid
- Any verbal preoperative information given to the patient should be supported with written information for the patient to take away and read. Relatives and the patient should have contact details of various voluntary colostomy societies for advice and guidance and also know how to contact the stoma nurse.

Postoperative care The specific care for a stoma patient includes:

- Checking the stoma for bleeding, stoma viability and function. In the early postoperative period, small amounts of blood in the pouch are expected. A healthy stoma appears pink or red and moist as a result of mucus production
- After 4–5 days, the stoma may start to function. Teach the patient how to empty and change the stoma bag. Encourage the patient to participate in the cleaning of the stoma and changing of their stoma bag. If the patient agrees, involve their relatives when caring for the stoma. Preparation for discharge and the resources in the community should also be discussed.

What To Do If...

What will you do if the patient refuses to change the stoma bag and refers to their stoma as a foreign object? Some nursing considerations include:

- Talking to the patient about their anxieties
- Give time for the patient to come to terms with the altered body image
- Involve their relatives in stoma care.

What the Experts Say

Before I came into nursing, I thought nursing involved taking observations, helping the doctors and doing the ward round with them. If I knew then what I know now about nurses and their duties involved, I would not have considered this career.

(An 18-year-old student nurse)

- There may be changes to the amount and consistency of faeces. With ileostomies, faeces are produced approximately 4 hours after a main meal and are loose, whereas with a colostomy, faeces are produced the following morning and are formed. Ileostomies are associated with increased output (Hyland 2002). Often, patients have to change their diet to control wind and malodour, for example that caused by fizzy drinks and fish, respectively
- Ileostomies usually have a very high output and thus there is a risk of dehydration. Patients need to have a good intake of fluid and take an extra 1 L above the usual intake of fluid. However, advise the patient to avoid fizzy drinks and beer as these may cause flatulence
- During the first few weeks following the formation of a colostomy or ileostomy, patients may experience sudden urges to defecate. This is known as the 'phantom rectum' and can be very distressing for them. Nurses need to reassure and inform patients

that it is normal to have such a feeling and that over time this feeling will die down.

Jot This Down

List some of the complications associated with a stoma.

Red Flag

In abdominoperineal resection the anus is closed and sutured. Nurses should be aware that these patients cannot have rectal suppositories or any other medications, such as analgesia, rectally. Other routes of administration must be considered.

Acute pain In the early postoperative period an epidural infusion or patient-controlled analgesia (PCA) is often used to manage pain. Monitor for adequate pain relief. Use an appropriate pain assessment tool to check the intensity and character of the pain as well as non-verbal signs such as grimacing, muscle tension, apparent dozing, changes in pulse or blood pressure and rapid shallow respirations.

Monitor administered analgesic effectiveness 30 minutes after administration. Monitor for pain relief and adverse effects and document the level of pain in the care plan. The frequency, dosage or medication itself may need to be reviewed to provide adequate pain relief.

Diet Encourage the patient to eat a range of foods; over time they can adjust their diet to suit their needs. If necessary, discuss the foods that increase odour and gas, such as fish, cabbage, egg, cauliflower and beans. If the patient is worried about loose stools, advise the patient on foods that help to thicken stool, for example bananas and rice, and advise the patient that some food may be undigested, such as corn, skin of tomato and pips (Dougherty & Lister 2011). Encourage the patient to drink 2–3 L of water per day to avoid getting constipated.

Jot This Down

Why is it important to discuss dietary concerns with a person with a stoma, especially those to do with odour and gas-forming foods?

Altered body image Altered body image through stoma formation creates a lot of issues for the patient and their relatives. Nurses need to be sensitive when dealing with the patient's questions and worries. Opus (2010) state that the patient's worry about altered body image is often overlooked and that they struggle to come to terms with their condition. Thus, nurses need to be sensitive when answering questions about the stoma and the body image.

Care, Dignity and Compassion

Many people become self-conscious when undressed in front of others. Be sensitive to the situation and approach it in the way you think is most appropriate. The person you care for may feel isolated if you leave them alone. How you handle this depends on your relationship

(Continued)

645

with them. Have clothes and towels with you so you do not have to leave them alone in the bathroom if they do not want you to.

Use this link to find out more about dignity and care: http://www.scie.org.uk/publications/guides/guide15/files/guide15.pdf

---

Jot This Down

Think about a patient you have nursed following stoma surgery for bowel cancer. How did they react to their altered body image? Was there anything further you could have done to help the patient to come to terms with their condition?

Cultural and religious considerations These issues should be discussed with patients. Black (2004) states that, in Muslim cultures, the left hand is considered dirty and is used for cleaning and hygiene and the right hand for eating and touching clean items. The stoma nurse needs to consider this when discussing stoma care with the patient, choosing stoma equipment and the siting of the stoma.

Sexuality There are several issues that need to be addressed when offering advice to patients after stoma surgery. The impairment for both men and women depends on the complications during the procedure. Women who have their rectum removed may find having sex in the traditional 'missionary position' painful because the rectum is no longer available to support the vagina during sex. A different position may be one way to overcome this problem. Some women after surgery may find that their vagina is much dryer and therefore having sex may be uncomfortable. Advice on the use of lubrications should be offered to the patient (Black 2004).

Some men may find penile erection an issue, as a result of nerve and blood vessel damage to the penis during surgery. Some of the medications offered to these patients are tablets, such as sildenafil, tadalafil and vardenafil. These medications work on demand. They increase the blood flow to the penis (Kirby *et al.* 1999).

Work Once the bowel has returned to normal function there is no reason why the patient is not able to return to work. The stoma nurse should be able to advise on appliances that are suitable for the work they do. Stoma patients do not need to inform their work colleagues of their surgery unless they want to; some patients like to share their experience with others and this is perfectly normal.

Chemotherapy and radiotherapy Patients may need chemotherapy and/or radiotherapy treatment following stoma surgery. The tumour may have invaded other tissues and organs and this treatment is used to destroy any cancerous cells in these areas. Soreness of the skin and general tiredness are common side-effects of these treatments. Nurses should inform the patient that the skin around the genitals and the anus can be very sore following radiotherapy. Patients should be advised to refrain from any sexual activities until the skin around that region heals.

Chemotherapy drugs affect patients in different ways. No two patients experience the same side-effects with the same chemotherapy drugs. Some of the common side-effects include:

- Nausea and vomiting
- Diarrhoea
- Hair loss and thinning
- Fatigue
- Reduction in blood cells (red and white blood cells and platelets)
- Some drugs can affect the lining of the mouth and make it sore and temporarily alter the sense of taste. Some may even cause mouth ulcers.

Unfortunately, as well as causing short-term side-effects, radiotherapy to the rectum can cause some long-term side-effects. They include:

- Frequent bowel movements and sometimes diarrhoea
- Frequency as a result of shrinking of the bladder from radiotherapy
- Loss of fertility in both men and women
- Early menopause in women
- Erectile dysfunction in men.

Health education and discharge

Early detection of colorectal cancer is an important part of the nursing care, as the prognosis is much better if the cancer is detected early. Nurses are in the forefront to advise patients on diet that may be considered a risk factor in colorectal cancer. These foodstuffs include red meat, sugar and fat content in the food, and patients should be advised to increase fibre intake in their diet. Preventative measures should also include health screening and providing advice on all dietary intake.

Advise the patient to seek medical advice if they see blood in their stool and if they experience alterations in their bowel habit.

Discharge planning of the patient should be carried on the day the patient is admitted for surgery. Implementing the advanced recovery pathway, nurses should set a provisional discharge date and put into action the care needs of the patient in the community. As Borwell (2009) points out, effective communication between healthcare professionals, both in the acute and primary sectors, is key to psychological adaptation and successful rehabilitation of the patient. Some of the care needs include:

- Visits by the stoma nurse and their contact details
- Contact details of colostomy societies
- Stoma supplies and advice on further prescriptions
- Compliance on prescribed medications
- Advice on diet, fluid intake, exercise and work
- Contact details of counsellors in stoma care if necessary
- Refer to cancer support groups and social services as necessary
- Listen and give time for the patient and their relatives to express worries and concerns about living with a stoma.

What the Experts Say

When I came round from the operation, I was shocked to find that I now had a colostomy and was very apprehensive about how I would cope with it. I need not have worried because once the team of stoma nurse specialists became involved, I became a lot less concerned. They really put me at ease, taking me through care of my stoma, changing of my bag and so on, so that by the time I was discharged from hospital, I felt a lot more confident about things. However, any niggling doubts that I still had proved to be groundless, as the support I received from the stoma nurses was excellent, with regular home visits for the first few weeks, advice over the telephone if I called and seeing me at an outpatient clinic, if necessary.

This information is obtained from the RCN – Clinical Nurse Specialists – *Stoma Care Journal*, published in 2009. You can read more at:

http://www.rcn.org.uk/__data/assets/pdf_file/0010/272854/003520.pdf

Primary Care

Care in the community for a person with a stoma should include pain management. The patient should be provided with information on the type of analgesia they can purchase over the counter and when to take it. If the pain is severe, advise the patient to seek medical advice from their GP.

Emphasise the importance of adequate fluid and salt intake; the risk for dehydration and hyponatraemia is increased, particularly during hot weather when fluid is lost through perspiration as well as ileostomy drainage. Faecal output from the stoma should be monitored for colour, blood and consistency. If the patient complains of constipation, advise the patient on the medications they could take to prevent constipation.

Dietary advice should include the restriction of fat, salt and red meat intake, as they are all risk factors associated with colorectal cancer. Advise the patient on the importance of a high fibre diet and provide information on food that is high in fibre.

Offer the patient and their relatives information on services available in the community, such as colostomy societies, counselling (if necessary), meals on wheels and stoma nurses, to help them lead a normal life. Encourage the patient to discuss any worries or fears they might have about their body image, stoma, work or any other issues they might have regarding coping with a stoma in the community.

If the patient had chemo- and radiotherapies, nurses should provide information with regards to the side-effects of both treatments. If the tumour was at the advanced stage, discuss services available in the community such as Macmillan nurses and palliative care nurses and provide referral to these services.

Gallbladder Disorders

The most common disorders of the gallbladder include cholecystitis (inflammation of the gallbladder), cholelithiasis (stones in the gallbladder) and cancer of the gallbladder. In the past, the 5 'Fs' (fair, fertile, female, forty and fat) were used as a guide for cholecystitis, but this no longer applies as more younger people are diagnosed with the disease. Other risk factors include diabetes, oral contraceptives, pregnancy, oestrogen therapy and familial history.

Pathophysiology

Cholecystitis Cholecystitis is defined as inflammation of the gallbladder, which causes severe abdominal pain. It may result from bacterial infection or irritation from the stones in the gallbladder. Dietary factors, including high fat intake, have been associated with

cholecystitis. However, gallstones in the cystic duct have been identified as the main cause of acute cholecystitis resulting in biliary colic, which affects the shoulder, back and the right scapula (LeMone *et al.* 2011). If it is untreated and there are repeated attacks of acute cholecystitis, the person can develop chronic cholecystitis.

Cholelithiasis Cholelithiasis is a disorder resulting from stones in the gallbladder. The stones are found in the gallbladder and the biliary tract (cystic and the common bile ducts). The gallstones form primarily as a result of bile stasis in the gallbladder and also as a result of inflammation of the gallbladder. The gallstones differ in size, shape and composition. Approximately 80% of gallstones are composed of cholesterol with some calcium, 2–3% are pigmented stones and 10% consist of only cholesterol.

When the gallbladder fully empties the bile into the duodenum via the common bile duct, gallstones do not form. The stones form when the gallbladder fails to empty fully, leaving some of the bile in the gallbladder. Over time, the bile stasis results in the accumulation of cholesterol, which then forms into gallstones.

Cancer of the gallbladder The most common form of cancer of the gallbladder is adenocarcinoma. Although this cancer is rare, it is aggressive and if not treated can infiltrate neighbouring tissues such as the hepatic ducts, the liver (Figure 28.18) and the surrounding lymph nodes. This cancer is more common in females than males and the survival rates are poor as a result of the metastases.

Investigations and diagnosis

- Full blood count – the WCC is likely to be raised if there is an infection
- Liver enzymes for any abnormality

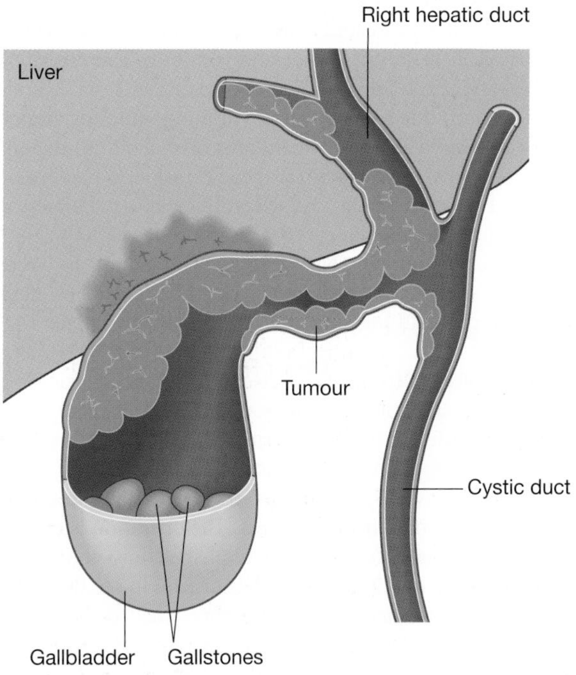

Figure 28.18 Carcinoma of the gallbladder. The tumour has spread into hepatic ducts and is partially blocking the right hepatic duct and the liver. Note some gallstones in the gallbladder.

647

- Ultrasound (US) of the gallbladder wall and for pericholecystic fluid and stones
- Endoscopic retrograde cholangiopancreatography (ERCP) is currently the only reliable and widely available investigation for common bile duct stones
- Computerised tomography (CT) may be useful when filling the bile duct is unsuccessful in ERCP, or when the procedure cannot be used for other reasons
- Cholecystograms if necessary but now US is more commonly carried out
- Urinalysis, chest X-ray and ECG to exclude other diseases
- A relatively new type of test, known as a 'hydroxy iminodiacetic acid (HIDA) scan', is the most effective method of diagnosing acute cholecystitis.

Signs and symptoms
Some of the signs and symptoms of gallbladder disorders include:

- Biliary colic
- Scleral jaundice (yellow colouration of the eye) and systemic jaundice (skin)
- Intolerance to fatty food, leading to nausea and vomiting, belching, pain after eating
- Abdominal distension after eating
- Strong, yellow coloured urine when the stones block the common bile duct
- Pyrexia (a high temperature), which is usually mild and no higher than 38°C.

Jot This Down
Explain why the urine is dark yellow in the patient with obstructive jaundice.

Nursing care and management
The patient with a gallbladder disorder is very ill and may be in shock as a result of severe nausea and vomiting. The priority is to admit the patient and administer appropriate analgesia, keep him/her nil by mouth due to nausea and vomiting, monitor vital signs hourly and observe signs and symptoms of shock until the condition stabilises; give fluids by intravenous infusion to prevent dehydration and monitor urea and electrolyte levels. Nurses must document and maintain all records in accordance with the Nursing and Midwifery Council (NMC 2009) Guidelines for record-keeping. The patient is then prepared for surgery. For detailed principles of pre- and postoperative care, refer to Chapter 14.

Surgery Cholecystectomy is carried out either laparoscopically or through open cholecystectomy. Unless the patient requires an open cholecystectomy, the preferred surgical procedure is laparoscopic cholecystectomy for gallbladder disorders. It is called keyhole surgery, as only small cuts are needed in the abdomen with small scars remaining afterwards. The operation is done with the aid of a special telescope that is pushed into the abdomen through one small cut. This allows the surgeon to see the gallbladder. Instruments pushed through another small cut are used to cut out and remove the gallbladder. The recovery of the patient following this procedure is much quicker than when open surgery is carried out.

An open cholecystectomy is an effective method of treating acute cholecystitis but has a longer recovery time than laparoscopic

cholecystectomy. Most people take approximately 6 weeks to recover from an open cholecystectomy. Open cholecystectomy is carried out for patients who:

- are in the last 3 months of pregnancy
- are obese (very overweight with a body mass index of 30 or more)
- have cirrhosis (scarring of the liver)
- have a condition that affects the blood's ability to clot, such as haemophilia.

Preoperative care For the principles of pre- and postoperative care, refer to Chapter 14.

- Patients are informed that following keyhole surgery they are allowed to drink and have a light meal on the same day if they do not have any complications from the anaesthetic. In the case of open surgery, fluid and diet may be introduced once bowel sounds return
- The nurse should discuss pain management and the type of analgesia that may be prescribed following surgery
- Allow the patient and their relatives time to discuss any fears or worries they might have about the surgery
- The length of stay in hospital varies. For laparoscopic cholecystectomy, the length of stay may be between 1 and 3 days, while for an open cholecystectomy it may be a couple of days longer.

Postoperative care Postoperative care for the patient who has had an open cholecystectomy involves monitoring of blood pressure, pulse, respiration and temperature. Breathing tends to be shallow as a result of the effect of anaesthesia and the patient's reluctance to breathe deeply due to the pain caused by the proximity of the incision to the muscles used for respiration. Advise the patient to support the operative site when breathing deeply and coughing, and give pain medication as necessary.

A small drain may be inserted for 24 hours and then removed as a precautionary measure to monitor excess fluid loss. Nurses must document all fluid loss on a fluid balance chart and should report any excess loss immediately for prompt action.

Fluid intake and urine output is measured and recorded and the operative site is observed for colour and amount of wound drainage. Fluids are given intravenously until the patient is allowed to take oral fluids, and when bowel sound returns, diet is introduced.

Pain management should commence with an assessment of the patient's pain at regular intervals. For pain assessment, nurses could use any of the pain assessment tools such as the visual analogue scale. The patient should be asked to indicate his or her personal level of pain and appropriate prescribed analgesia administered. The effect of the analgesia should be recorded in the patient's care plan.

To prevent postoperative complications, early mobility is encouraged. The patient should be encouraged to take active and passive exercises to prevent deep vein thrombosis and to improve circulation.

Measures to manage the patient's anxiety should be implemented preoperatively and continued throughout the postoperative recovery period, until discharge. This should include the provision of adequate levels of information for patients and their relatives.

Depending on the surgeon's preferences, some types of stitches will need to be removed by either the district nurse or the GP practice nurse; others will dissolve on their own over the course of the next few weeks. Patients should be informed exactly which type of stitch they have and when and if it needs to be removed, before they are discharged.

Alternative treatment

Extracorporeal shockwave lithotripsy (ECSL): Shock waves are used to break up or dissolve the stone, so that it can be passed via the GI tract.

Oral dissolution therapy: Gallstones that are made of cholesterol can sometimes be treated using a medication called ursodeoxycholic acid, which slowly dissolves gallstones. Ursodeoxycholic acid is also sometimes prescribed as a precaution against gallstones if it is thought that the patient has a high risk of developing them. Ursodeoxycholic acid is taken orally (in tablet form), and a course of treatment can last up to 2 years.

Contact dissolution therapy: Drugs to dissolve the stones are introduced into the gallbladder via a tube through the skin.

Diet After a cholecystectomy there is no need to follow a low fat diet. A low fat diet may result in weight loss. However, due to the role that cholesterol appears to play in the formation of gallstones, it is recommended to avoid eating fatty foods that have a high cholesterol content. Foods that are high in cholesterol include:

- Meat pies
- Sausages and fatty cuts of meat
- Butter and lard
- Cakes and biscuits.

A low fat, high fibre diet is recommended. This includes eating whole grains and at least five portions of fresh fruit and vegetables a day. A low fat diet is advisable for everyone to follow as a healthy option.

> ### The Evidence
> There is also evidence that regularly eating nuts, such as peanuts or cashew nuts, can help reduce the risk of developing gallstones, as can drinking alcohol in moderation (no more than 3–4 units a day for men and 2–3 units a day for women).
> http://www.nhsdirect.wales.nhs.uk/encyclopaedia/c/article/cholecystitis,acute/

Health promotion and discharge

Prior to discharge, nurses need to advise the patient on:

- Pain relief – the patient can take over-the-counter analgesics, such as paracetamol or ibuprofen. Advise the patient to read the patient information leaflet that comes with the medicine and if they have any questions, to ask the pharmacist for advice
- Regular exercise and lifting must be introduced slowly, to avoid any discomfort and to avoid complications such as secondary bleeding
- Driving – due to discomfort from the seatbelt, patients should be advised not to resume driving until approximately 2 weeks after the surgery. Some insurance companies may not insure drivers for a number of weeks after surgery, so it is best to check with the insurance company before starting to drive
- Outpatient appointments – advise the patient on the importance of attending the outpatient appointments as arranged
- If the patient has a dressing this can be removed after 2 days and no further dressing over the wound is necessary. They can have

a bath or shower daily to keep the wound clean. If there are sutures or clips to be removed, an appointment with the practice nurse is made to remove them.

> ### Primary Care
>
> Diet – most patients can continue to eat a healthy well-balanced diet after they have their gallbladder removed. However, if they get side-effects, such as mild diarrhoea, it may be advisable to eat more high fibre foods and avoid any foods that make the diarrhoea worse.
>
> If the patient is unduly worried about going back to work or doing physical activities, such as lifting, the nurse should advise the patient to seek advice from the GP or the practice nurse.
>
> If the patient is elderly, other services such as meals on wheels, a community social worker and the district nurse should be informed, so that they can monitor the patient's progress in the community.

Conclusion

This chapter has given you some insight into some of the common conditions associated with the gastrointestinal disorders. Nurses play an important role in supporting patients with physical, emotional and psychosocial issues surrounding gastrointestinal disorders. Nurses need to work with the patient, their relatives and other healthcare professionals to provide high quality care for the patient. Continuity of care, following discharge, is crucial for patients who have had altered body image as a result of the surgery. Effective communication and collaboration between healthcare professionals, both in the acute and primary sector, is important to a successful rehabilitation of the patient following discharge.

Key Points

- A bacterium, *Helicobacter pylori* (*H. pylori*), is the main cause of peptic ulcers. PU can affect people of any age, including children, but the condition is most common in people who are 60 years of age or over.
- The most common cause of PU is *H. pylori* infection. It is a Gram-negative, spiral-shaped bacterium. The next most common cause is excessive use of non-steroidal anti-inflammatory drugs (NSAIDs).
- Around 95% of stomach cancers are adenocarcinomas and 5% are lymphomas, sarcomas and carcinoids. Adenocarcinomas can spread along the stomach wall to the duodenum and can also spread to other organs in the abdominal cavity.
- There is a correlation between diet and stomach cancer. High intakes of salt, pickled and smoked foods have been associated with stomach cancer, while eating a lot of fruit and green vegetables can reduce the risk.
- Hepatitis is a viral disease and cannot be cured. Preventing the spread of hepatitis is an important nursing responsibility.
- The formation of a stoma results in altered body image and can affect both the patient and the relatives. Nurses should

(Continued)

give the patient and their relatives time to express their concerns and worries, and nurses should give all the necessary information and build a trusting relationship with them. Some of their anxieties may include loss of control of normal bodily functions, restrictions on current lifestyle and daily activities.

· During the first few weeks following the formation of a stoma, the patient may experience sudden urges to defecate. This is known as the 'phantom rectum' and can be very distressing for the patient. Nurses need to reassure and inform the patient that it is normal to have such a feeling and that over time this feeling will die down.

Glossary

Basal metabolic rate (BMR): the number of calories your body burns at rest

Bile: a bitter, yellowish, blue and green fluid secreted by hepatocytes from the liver

Buccal: pertaining to the cheek

Cheilitis: inflammation of the lips

Cheilosis: inflammatory lesion at the corner of the mouth

Chyme: semi-fluid substance of the stomach

Duct: tube

Dysphagia: difficulty in swallowing

Elimination: to get rid off, expel

Endocrine gland: ductless gland that secretes hormones into the bloodstream

Endoscopy: examination of the oesophagus and the stomach using a fibreoptic scope

Exocrine cells: cells that secrete their juices into ducts

Gallbladder: storage organ for bile

Gingivitis: inflammation of the gums

Glossitis: inflammation of the tongue

Leukoplakia: white plaques or patches on the mucous membranes of the oral cavity

Metabolism: chemical reaction in living organisms

Nutrition: relates to nutrients

Occult blood: unseen or invisible blood in the stool

Pancreatitis: inflammation of the pancreas

Parasympathetic: part of the autonomic nervous system

Peristalsis: symmetrical contraction of muscles which moves food down the intestine

Prolapsed stoma: outward telescoping of the stoma, that is, an abnormally long stoma

Pruritus: itching of the skin leading to scratching

Retraction: indentation or loss of the external portion of the stoma into the abdomen

Striae: stretch marks on the skin

Sympathetic: part of the autonomic nervous system

References

Alexander, M.F., Fawcett, J.N. & Runciman, P.J. (2007) *Nursing Practice – Hospital and Home. The Adult*, 3rd edn. Churchill Livingstone, Edinburgh.

Black, P.K. (2004) Psychological, sexual and cultural issues for patients with a stoma. *British Journal of Nursing*, 13(12), 692–697.

Borwell, B. (2009) Continuity of care for the stoma patient: psychological considerations. *British Journal of Community Nursing*, 14(8), 330–331.

Dougherty, L. & Lister, S. (2011) *The Royal Marsden Hospital Manual of Clinical Nursing Procedures*, 8th edn. Wiley-Blackwell, Oxford.

Duffy, K. (2011) *Medical-surgical Nursing Made Incredibly Easy*. Lippincott Williams & Williams, Philadelphia.

Hepatitis B Foundation UK (2007) *Rising Curve: chronic Hepatitis B infection in the UK*. http://www.hepb.org.uk/information/resources/rising_curve_chronic_hepatitis_b_infection_in_the_uk (accessed 14 August 2013).

Hyland, J. (2002) The basics of ostomies. *Gastroenterology Nursing*, 25(6), 241–245.

Jenkins, G. & Tortora, G.J. (2013) *Anatomy and Physiology*, 3rd edn. John Wiley and Sons, Singapore.

Kirby, R.S., Carson, C.C. & Goldstein, I. (1999) Erectile dysfunction: a clinical guide. In: L. Dougherty & S. Lister (2011) *The Royal Marsden Hospital Manual of Clinical Nursing Procedures*, 8th edn. Wiley-Blackwell, Oxford.

LeMone, P., Burke, K. & Bauldoff, G. (2011) *Medical-surgical Nursing: critical thinking in person care*, 4th edn. Prentice Hall, New Jersey.

Marieb, E.N. & Hoehn, K. (2013) *Human Anatomy and Physiology*, 9th edn. Pearson Benjamin Cummings, San Francisco.

NICE (2004) Technology Appraisal: Hepatitis C – pegylated interferons, ribavirin and alfa interferon. *Interferon Alfa and Ribavirin for the Treatment of Chronic Hepatitis C: part review of existing guidance no. 14*. National Institute for Clinical Excellence, London.

NICE (2011) *Infliximab (Review) and Adalimumab for the Treatment of Crohn's Disease*. [Includes a review of NICE technology appraisal guidance 40]. National Institute for Health and Clinical Excellence, London.

NMC (2009) *Record Keeping: guidance for nurses and midwives*. Nursing and Midwifery Council, London.

Opus (2010) Pre and post operative steps to improve body image. *Gastrointestinal Nursing* 8(2), 34.

Shier, D., Butler, J. & Lewis, R. (2009). *Holes Human Anatomy and Physiology*, 12th edn. McGraw Hill, London.

Silverthorn, D.U. (2009). *Human Physiology: an integrated approach*, 5th edn. Prentice Hall, Edgewood Cliffs, NJ.

Vujnovich, A. (2008) Pre and post-operative assessment of patients with a stoma. *Nursing Standard*, 22(19), 50–56.

Test Yourself

1. The mouth is also called the:
   (a) Pelvic cavity
   (b) Buccal cavity
   (c) Abdominal cavity
   (d) Thoracic cavity

2. The digestive function of the liver is to:
   (a) Secrete bile
   (b) Release glucose
   (c) Synthesise plasma proteins
   (d) Store iron as ferritin

3. The second most common cause of peptic ulcers is through excessive use of:
   (a) Antibiotics
   (b) Non-steroidal anti-inflammatory drugs
   (c) Antacids
   (d) Opioid drugs

4. A person has developed a paralytic ileus following a recent abdominal surgery. What is the most important nursing consideration when caring for this person?
   (a) Ensure that the person is able to eat a clear liquid diet
   (b) Maintain the person on strict bed rest
   (c) Monitor bowel sounds every hour
   (d) Ensure the nasogastric tube is functioning

5. Hepatitis B is sometimes referred to as:
   (a) Autoimmune hepatitis
   (b) Serum hepatitis
   (c) Non-specific
   (d) End-stage hepatitis

6. Inflammation of the rectum is called:
   (a) Proctitis
   (b) Cystitis
   (c) Colitis
   (d) Gastritis

7. The patient with obstructive jaundice may present with:
   (a) Blood in the stool
   (b) A clay-coloured stool
   (c) Parasites in the stool
   (d) Stones in the stool

8. Following cholecystectomy, patients are advised to eat:
   (a) Normal diet
   (b) Low protein diet
   (c) High fibre diet
   (d) High protein diet

9. UC mainly affects the:
   (a) Stomach and small intestine
   (b) Oesophagus and stomach
   (c) Colon and rectum
   (d) Mouth and stomach

10. Duke's staging is most widely used for colorectal cancer. Stage B is when:
    (a) The tumour has advanced to the serosa but not the lymph nodes
    (b) Has infiltrated the lymph nodes
    (c) The tumour is in the mucosa and the submucosa
    (d) The tumour has spread to other organs and tissues resulting in metastasis

Answers

1. b
2. a
3. b
4. d

5. b
6. a
7. b
8. a
9. c
10. a

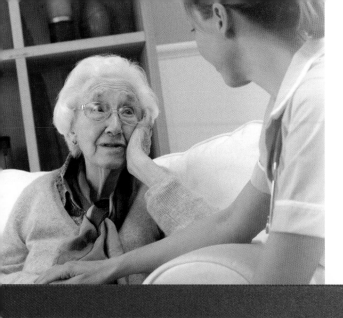

29

The Person with a Urinary Disorder

Muralitharan Nair

University of Hertfordshire, UK

Learning Outcomes

On completion of this chapter you will be able to:

- Describe the structure and functions of the urinary system
- Describe the microscopic structures of the urinary system
- Explain how the urinary system maintains homeostasis
- Explain urine production and its composition
- Discuss the pathophysiology of common urinary tract disorders encountered in practice
- Outline the nursing care, management and interventions of the disorders described

Competencies

All nurses must:

1. Take responsibility for collaborative assessment and planning care delivery for patients with urinary disorders, with the patient, relatives and their carers
2. Assess the health status of the patient with urinary tract disorders, using data collected to determine nursing diagnoses and interventions
3. Apply research-based evidence in implement nursing care for patient with urinary tract disorders
4. Provide effective nursing care for patients undergoing surgery of the urinary tract
5. Recognise and provide appropriate health promotion for prevention of and self-care of urinary disorders
6. Evaluate nursing care outcome, revising the care as needed to promote, maintain or restore the health of patient with urinary disorders

 Visit the companion website at **www.wileynursingpractice.com** where you can test yourself using flashcards, multiple-choice questions and more.

Nursing Practice: Knowledge and Care, First Edition. Edited by Ian Peate, Karen Wild and Muralitharan Nair.
© 2014 John Wiley & Sons, Ltd. Published 2014 by John Wiley & Sons, Ltd. Companion website: www.wileynursingpractice.com

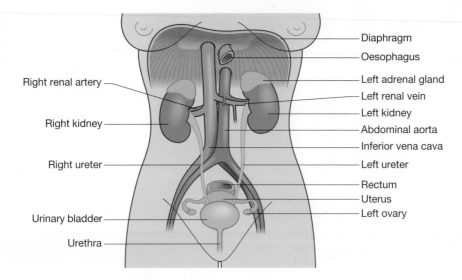

Figure 29.1 Organs of the urinary system in a female.

Introduction

The urinary system (also called the 'renal system') plays an important role in maintaining homeostasis by regulating body fluids, filtering metabolic wastes from the bloodstream, selectively reabsorbing substances and water into the bloodstream and eliminating metabolic wastes and water as urine. Therefore any disease relating to the urinary system affects the whole body. The kidneys (part of the urinary system) also have an endocrine function: production and release of hormones, such as renin and erythropoietin. This chapter discusses the structure and functions of the urinary system, nursing care management and interventions of some common disorders that nurses might come across in practice.

Anatomy and Physiology

The urinary system (renal system) consists of paired kidneys, the paired ureters, the urinary bladder and the urethra (Figure 29.1). These structures play a vital role in maintaining homeostasis in the body.

The Kidneys

The two kidneys are located in the abdominal cavity and lie at a slightly oblique angle on either side of the vertebral column at the levels of T12 to L3 (Figure 29.2). They are approximately 10–12 cm long, 5–7 cm wide and 3–4 cm thick (Jenkins & Tortora 2013). They are bean-shaped organs, where the outer surface is convex and the inner surface is concave in shape. Near the centre of the concave border is an indentation called the 'renal hilum' through which the ureter, renal artery, renal vein, lymphatic vessels and nerves enter and exit the kidney.

Jot This Down
Name the gland that sits on top of each kidney like a crown. What are some of its functions?

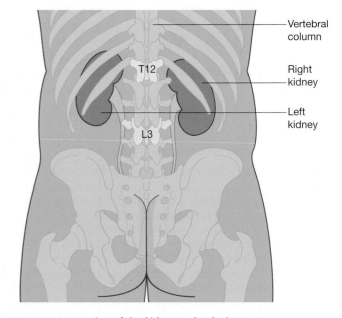

Figure 29.2 Location of the kidneys – back view.

The kidneys are surrounded by three layers of tissue:

- **The renal fascia:** A thin, outer layer of fibrous connective tissue that surrounds each kidney (and the attached adrenal gland) and fastens it to surrounding structures
- **The adipose capsule:** A middle layer of adipose (fat) tissue that cushions the kidneys
- **The renal capsule:** The inner fibrous membrane that prevents the entrance of infections.

Inside the kidney, there are three major sections. They are:

- **The renal cortex** along the convex side
- **The renal medulla** lying adjacent to the renal cortex. It consists of striated, cone-shaped regions called renal pyramids (medullary pyramids). The peaks, called 'renal papillae', face inward (Figure 29.3). The unstriated regions between the renal pyramids are called 'renal columns'.

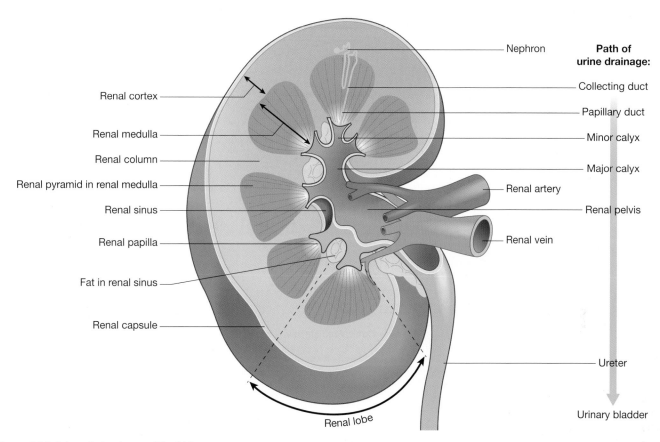

Path of urine drainage:

- Nephron
- Collecting duct
- Papillary duct
- Minor calyx
- Major calyx
- Renal artery
- Renal pelvis
- Renal vein
- Ureter
- Urinary bladder

Renal cortex

Renal medulla

Renal column

Renal pyramid in renal medulla

Renal sinus

Renal papilla

Fat in renal sinus

Renal capsule

Renal lobe

Figure 29.3 Internal structures of the kidney.

- **The renal sinus** – a cavity that lies adjacent to the renal medulla. The other side of the renal sinus, bordering the concave surface of the kidney, opens to the outside through the renal hilus. The renal pelvis is situated in the renal sinus, a funnel-shaped structure that merges with the ureter. Branches of the renal pelvis, known as the 'major and minor calyces' extend toward the medulla. They collect and convey urine to the pelvis of the kidney.

The renal pelvis is continuous with the ureter as it leaves the hilum. From the pelvis, urine is propelled, by peristalsis action, through the ureter and into the bladder for storage (see Figure 29.3).

Renal blood supply

The kidneys receive their blood supply directly from the aorta via the renal arteries and blood is returned to the inferior vena cava via the renal veins. The kidneys receive approximately 20% of the cardiac output. The blood supply to the kidneys arises from the paired renal arteries at the level of L2. Where the kidney curves inwards in a concave shape, the hilum is found, which is an opening where the renal artery enters. The renal veins return the blood from the kidneys and they lie anterior to the renal artery at the hilum (Figure 29.3). The left renal vein is longer than the right, as it crosses the midline to reach the inferior vena cava (IVC). For more detail on blood flow to the kidney see Figure 29.4.

Nephron

There are approximately 0.8–1 million 'nephrons' in each kidney and it is this structure that filters the blood to produce urine (Jenkins & Tortora 2013). The nephron consists of: a cup-shaped glomerular capsule (Bowman's capsule) and, immediately below the capsule, a twisted region called the 'proximal convoluted tubule'. This is followed by a long hair-pin like section called the 'loop of Henle', which runs deep into the medulla and then back into the cortex. This is followed by another twisted region, called the 'distal convoluted tubule' (Figure 29.5). The distal convoluted tubules of several nephrons empty into a single collecting duct in the medulla of the kidney that then converges to a renal papilla, which represents the apex of the renal pyramid. Urine then collects into 9–12 minor calyces, which then converge into approximately 3–4 major calyces (Jenkins & Tortora 2013). The major calyces then empty into the renal pelvis, which passes urine through the ureteropelvic junction (UPJ) and into the ureter, which then propels urine distally to the bladder through peristalsis. See Box 29.1 for the functions of the kidneys.

Formation of urine

The nephrons of the kidneys filter approximately 190 L of blood daily. Of this amount, only 1% is excreted as urine; the rest is returned to the circulation (Silverthorn 2009). Urine is formed from the filtered blood by: glomerular filtration, tubular reabsorption and tubular secretion.

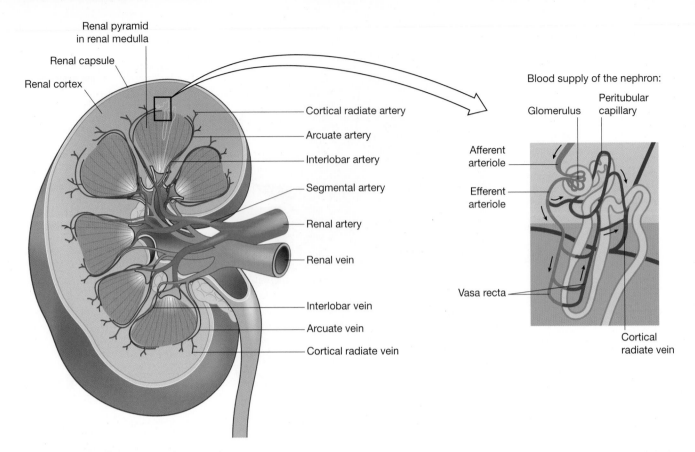

Figure 29.4 Blood flow through the kidney.

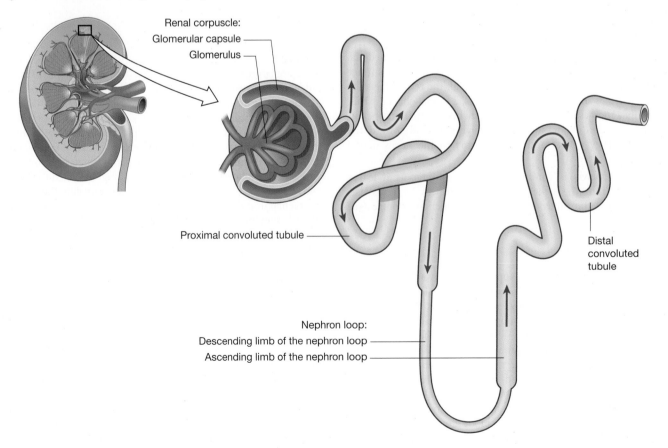

Figure 29.5 The nephron.

Box 29.1 Functions of the Kidneys

- Remove water and waste (such as urea and ammonium) from the body
- Regulate electrolyte balance in the body through the hormone aldosterone
- Release hormones: renin, which activates the renin–angiotensin system (which constricts blood vessels, increases the secretion of anti-diuretic hormone and aldosterone, and stimulates the hypothalamus to activate the thirst reflex), and erythropoietin (EPO; a hormone that stimulates red cell production in the bone marrow)
- Help maintain blood pressure through the renin–angiotensin system
- Regulate acid–base balance
- Play a role in the synthesis of calcitriol (vitamin D), which helps in the absorption of calcium from the diet.

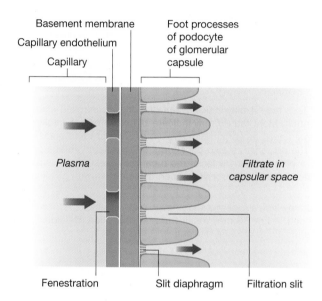

Figure 29.6 **Glomerular filtration.**

Glomerular filtration This is the first step in urine formation. The glomerular blood pressure pushes the water and most solutes, such urea, uric acid, electrolytes and other substances, from the blood into the capsular space through the basement membrane (Figure 29.6). The fluid in the capsular is now called 'the filtrate'.

Tubular selective reabsorption The filtrate flows along the nephron through the proximal convoluted tubule, loop of Henle, distal convoluted tubule and into the collecting duct. As the filtrate moves along the nephron, the cells lining the proximal and distal convoluted tubule selectively reabsorb useful solutes back into the circulation. These substances include: glucose, amino acids, lactate, vitamins and most ions. Of the filtered water, 99% is reabsorbed and only 1% is passed as urine.

Tubular secretion This is the final stage in the urine formation. As the filtrates move along the nephron, unwanted substances such as drugs, metabolic waste and excess ions are secreted into the tubule to be expelled in the urine. See Table 29.1 for the normal

and abnormal composition of urine. Through this process, the kidney helps to maintain homeostasis.

Red Flag

Always wear gloves and apron when handling body fluids. If precautions are not taken you can carry the bacteria to other patients or take it to your family.

The Ureters

The ureters are paired muscular tubes with narrow lumina that carry urine from the kidneys to the bladder. They are approximately 26–30 cm long. The ureter begins at the level of the renal artery and vein posterior to these structures (Figure 29.1). The ureter enters the pelvis, where it crosses anteriorly to the iliac vessels, which usually occurs at the bifurcation of the common iliac artery into the internal and external iliac arteries. Here, the ureters are within 5 cm of one another before they diverge laterally. The wall of the ureter is made up of an inner epithelial mucosa, a middle layer of smooth muscle, and an outer layer of fibrous connective tissue (LeMone *et al.* 2011).

Jot This Down

How does the urine in the ureter reach the urinary bladder?

The Urinary Bladder

The urinary bladder (Figure 29.7) is a musculomembranous sac that acts as a reservoir for the urine. Its size, position and relations vary according to the amount of fluid it contains. In males, the bladder lies immediately in front of the rectum; in females, the bladder is in relation behind with the uterus and the upper part of the vagina.

When the bladder is moderately full it contains about 500 mL and assumes an oval form; the long diameter of the oval measures about 12 cm and is directed upwards and forwards. However, in healthy adults the bladder holds about 300–500 mL of urine before internal pressure rises and signals the need to empty the bladder. The urinary bladder in the female is slightly smaller because the uterus occupies the space above the bladder.

In the floor of the bladder is a small triangular area called the 'trigone'. The trigone is formed by the two ureteral orifices and the internal urethral orifice (Figure 29.7). The area is very sensitive to expansion and once stretched to a certain degree, the urinary bladder signals the brain of its need to empty. The signals become stronger as the bladder continues to fill.

The Urethra

The urethra is a thin-walled muscular tube that channels urine to the outside of the body. It extends from the base of the bladder to the external urinary meatus. In males, the urethra travels through the penis and carries semen as well as urine (Figure 29.8). In males, the urethra is approximately 20 cm long. The prostate gland encircles the urethra at the base of the bladder in males. The male urinary meatus is located at the end of the glans penis. In females, the urethra is shorter and emerges above the vaginal opening

Table 29.1 The normal and abnormal findings in the urine.

URINALYSIS	NORMAL FINDINGS	ABNORMAL FINDINGS
Colour	Yellow to amber	This can vary depending on diet, medications and any diseases. Use the web link to learn more about different urine colours and urinary problems: **http://www.redurine.com/**
Odour	Aromatic smell	Early morning urine may smell a bit strong because it is concentrated. Use this link to find out more about urine odour: **http://www.netdoctor.co.uk/ate/liverandkidney/203657.html**
Leucocytes (white blood cells)	Negative	If present, it may indicate bladder or kidney infection, fever or kidney diseases
Urobilinogen	Normally found in urine	If elevated, it may indicate liver diseases or excessive destruction of red blood cells
Bilirubin	Negative	This may be positive in hepatic diseases
Glycosuria (glucose in the urine)	Negative	May be positive in diabetes mellitus, long-term steroid therapy and acute pancreatitis
Ketones	Negative	Found in patients with diabetes, high protein diet and in starvation
Haematuria (blood in the urine)	Negative	Positive in patients with urinary tract infection (UTI), kidney diseases and kidney trauma
Protein	A trace may be present	If present in larger amounts, it may be due to UTI, kidney diseases such as nephrotic syndrome, toxaemia of pregnancy, septicaemia, and side-effects of some drugs, such as neomycin, barbiturates and sulfonamides, and in patients receiving total parenteral nutrition
Nitrites	Negative	Positive when dietary nitrate is converted to nitrites by Gram-negative bacteria
pH	Normal range 4.5–8	A pH of less than 4 may indicate dehydration, uncontrolled diabetes or starvation. More than 8 may indicate UTI or be due to intake of some drugs such as kanamycin, sodium bicarbonate and potassium citrate. The pH range is also dependent on the dietary intake of the patient. A person eating a lot of red meat may present with strong acid urine, while a vegan or vegetarian may present with alkaline urine
Specific gravity (SG)	Normal range 1005–1030	High SG may indicate dehydration, fever, diabetes mellitus, vomiting or diarrhoea. A low SG may result from overingestion of fluid, diabetes insipidus or renal disease

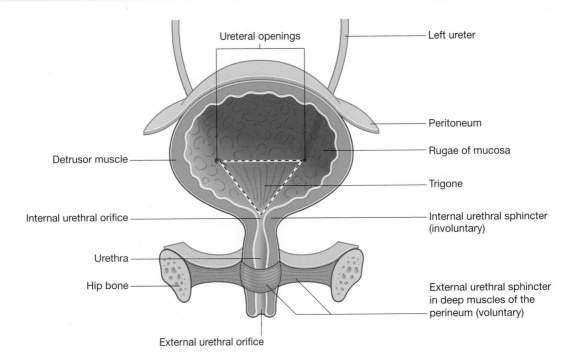

Figure 29.7 Urinary bladder in the female.

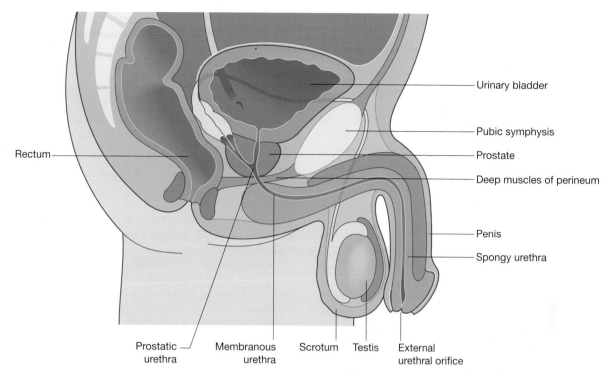

Rectum

Prostatic urethra

Membranous urethra

Scrotum

Testis

External urethral orifice

Urinary bladder

Pubic symphysis

Prostate

Deep muscles of perineum

Penis

Spongy urethra

Figure 29.8 The male urethra in relation to other pelvic organs.

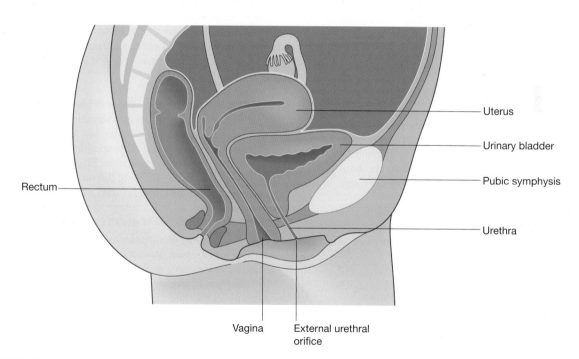

Rectum

Vagina

External urethral orifice

Uterus

Urinary bladder

Pubic symphysis

Urethra

Figure 29.9 The female urethra in relation to other pelvic organs.

(Figure 29.9). The female urethra is approximately 3–5 cm long, and the urinary meatus is anterior to the vaginal orifice.

Jot This Down

Between men and women, who is more prone to UTIs? Explain your answer.

Urinary Tract Infection

Urinary tract infection (UTI) is the presence and multiplication of microorganisms in one or more structures of the urinary tract with organisms invading the surrounding tissue (HPA 2012). The organisms that cause UTIs include *Escherichia coli*, common Gram-negative enteral bacteria, *Proteus, Klebsiella, Serratia* and

Pseudomonas. A UTI is normally described as either upper or lower infection. An upper UTI or 'pyelonephritis' is an infection in the kidneys. A lower UTI or 'cystitis' is an infection in the bladder.

Pathophysiology

The two main common UTIs are **cystitis** and **pyelonephritis**. Cystitis is more common in women, as women have a short urethra compared with men (Figure 29.8 and Figure 29.9). The urethra's opening is also located very close to the anus, which makes it easy for bacteria from the anal region to reach the bladder and cause an infection. Although men are less prone to cystitis, it could be more serious due to the fact that cystitis may be the result of prostatitis or other problems associated with an enlarged prostate. Cystitis can either be acute or chronic. In acute cystitis, the patient may experience painful frequency, urgency and suprapubic pain. In chronic cystitis, the patient may not have symptoms, except pyuria.

Pyelonephritis relates to inflammation of the parenchyma and the pelvis of the kidney and it is usually associated with bacterial infection. Pyelonephritis can either be acute or chronic. Acute pyelonephritis is a bacterial infection of the kidney, which may start from the lower urinary tract and ascend right to the kidney; chronic pyelonephritis is associated with non-bacterial infections and inflammatory processes that may be metabolic, chemical or immunological in origin (Porth 2009).

Chronic pyelonephritis involves chronic inflammation and scarring of the tubules and interstitial tissues of the kidney and can lead to chronic kidney disease (CKD). It can result from renal diseases, UTI, recurrent episodes of acute pyelonephritis or obstruction of the ureter. The kidney becomes scarred and irregular and the calyces and renal pelvis are deformed.

Investigations and diagnosis

Some investigations for UTI may include:

- History of any previous UTI
- Urinalysis – see Table 29.1 for some of the positive findings
- Urine culture – for high-risk patients, e.g. pregnant or immunosuppressed patients, or those who failed to respond to earlier antibiotic treatment. Urine culture should always be done in men with a history suggestive of UTI, regardless of the results of the urinalysis
- An ultrasound of the upper urinary tract should be carried out to rule out urinary obstruction or renal stone disease in acute uncomplicated pyelonephritis in premenopausal, non-pregnant women.

Signs and symptoms

- Dysuria
- Urgency
- Nocturia
- Pyuria
- Haematuria
- Fever (especially in pyelonephritis)
- Shaking chills (especially in pyelonephritis)
- Pyuria
- Flank pain (especially in pyelonephritis)
- Malaise (especially in pyelonephritis).

Nursing care and management

The main objective in UTI is to identify the cause and offer the appropriate treatment. The patient will need reassurance and psychological support and health education. The patient with acute pyelonephritis should be encouraged to be on bed rest until symptoms of pyrexia and severe groin pain subside. It is important for nurses to report signs of groin pain such as restlessness, sweating and tachycardia for prompt action.

Link To/Go To

You can read more about the management of suspected bacterial urinary tract infection in adults at: **http://www.sign.ac.uk/pdf/sign88.pdf**

Medications

Trimethoprim (e.g. Monotrim) is currently the first choice for lower UTI in the UK, because it is cost-effective, well tolerated and works in 80% of infections (EAU 2011).

Cephalosporins, nitrofurantoin and norfloxacin are reserved as second-line drugs in patients with lower UTI. However they are the first choices in patients with signs of upper UTI or kidney infection.

Antibiotics, such as amoxicillin, now have resistance levels of 50% in the community because of widespread use over many years, thus healthcare professionals are concerned about the possible overuse of the more powerful antibiotics as first-line therapy in the general community.

For the treatment of pyelonephritis, the Health Protection Agency recommends ciprofloxacin for 7 days (adult dose 250–500 mg, twice a day orally) or co-amoxiclav for 14 days (adult dose 500 mg twice a day orally or 250 mg orally 8-hourly). Cefalexin has a reduced spectrum of activity but is considered safer in pregnant women (EAU 2011).

Pain Pain is a common symptom of both lower and upper UTI. In cystitis, inflammation causes a sensation of fullness; dull, constant suprapubic pain; and possibly low back pain. The inflamed bladder wall and urethra cause dysuria (difficult or painful micturition), pain and burning on urination. Bladder spasms may develop, causing periodic severe, stabbing discomfort. Pain associated with pyelonephritis is often steady and dull, localised to the outer abdomen or flank region. Urologic disorders rarely cause central abdominal pain (LeMone *et al.* 2011). Nurses should:

- Assess the timing, quality, intensity, location and duration using an appropriate pain assessment tool. A change in the nature, location or intensity of the pain could indicate an extension of the infection or a related but separate problem
- Administer suitable analgesia or antispasmodic medication as prescribed and note its effect. Paracetamol and/or non-steroidal anti-inflammatory drugs (NSAIDs) are of use for symptomatic relief
- Advise the patient to see their GP if pain and discomfort persists after 24-hour treatment. Continued discomfort may indicate a complicated UTI or other urinary tract disorder.

Fluid and diet intake

- Encourage fluid intake of 2.5–3 litres unless contraindicated. Increased fluid dilutes urine, reduces irritation of the inflamed bladder and urethral mucosa and helps to flush out bacteria from the bladder
- Encourage the patient to drink cranberry and blueberry juice daily, take ascorbic acid (vitamin C), and avoid excess intake of

milk and milk products and other fruit juices (Jepson & Craig 2008). These fruits contain benzoic acid. Cranberry juice should be organic, undiluted and unsweetened. It should be diluted with water (50/50) due to its excess bitterness.

Cranberry fruits contain four beneficial natural acids, such as benzoic, citric, malic and quinic acids, which help to prevent UTI (**http://dherbs.com/articles/urinary-tract-infections-444 .html#ixzz2DQ8ObQjc**)

- Monitor hourly urine output and record the amount, colour, clarity and odour of urine. Urine should return to normal colour (light yellow or amber) after 48-hour treatment. If changes do not occur, report any findings immediately for prompt action
- Probiotic bacteria in foods such as yogurt and sauerkraut can help prevent UTIs by promoting the growth of beneficial bacteria and inhibiting overgrowth or infection by pathogens

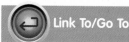

Link To/Go To

Use this link to find out more about different food sources that help to prevent UTI:

http://www.livestrong.com/article/506880-what-foods -promote-a-healthy-urinary-tract-system/#ixzz2DQFoMAVN

Health promotion and discharge

Prior to discharge, nurses should advise measures to prevent UTI. Encourage the patient to drink approximately 2.5–3 liters per day and advise them on the type of fluid to drink and which to avoid. Encourage the patient to empty their bladder every 3–4 hours and not to retain urine in their bladder over a longer period. Nurses should teach women to clean the perineal region from front to back after voiding and defecating. Voiding urine before and after sexual intercourse, to flush out bacteria, should be encouraged. Unless contraindicated, suggest measures to maintain acid urine by drinking low-sugar cranberry or blueberry juices daily; take ascorbic acid (vitamin C) and avoid excess intake of milk and milk products and other fruit juices (NICE 2006).

Primary Care

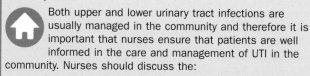

Both upper and lower urinary tract infections are usually managed in the community and therefore it is important that nurses ensure that patients are well informed in the care and management of UTI in the community. Nurses should discuss the:

- Risk factors for UTI and how to eliminate these factors through patient education
- The signs and symptoms of UTI and the need to seek advice when the preventative measure are not effective
- Appropriate fluid and diet intake and importance of monitoringurine output
- Importance of compliance to any prescribed medications and completing antibiotics as prescribed
- The importance of maintaining personal hygiene and the need to wash their hands before and after attending to the toilet needs.

Urinary Calculi

Urinary calculi are formed when the waste products accumulate in the renal tract as crystals and, over time, these crystals form hard stone-like lumps called 'stones'. These stones form from any of the following substances:

- Calcium
- Uric acid (a waste product of food metabolism)
- Cystine (an amino acid that helps build protein)
- Formation of struvite stones as a result of UTI.

Risk factors

- Family history of urinary calculi
- Dehydration
- Prolonged immobility as a result of illness or surgery
- Excess dietary intake of calcium, oxalate, proteins
- Gout (results in a chronically increased amount of uric acid in the blood and urine and can lead to the formation of uric acid stones)
- Hyperthyroidism
- Urinary stasis
- Urinary tract infection
- Carcinoma of the bone
- Some medications also raise the risk of kidney stones. These medications include some diuretics, calcium-containing antacids and the protease inhibitor indinavir (Crixivan), a drug used to treat HIV infection.

Pathophysiology

The formation of kidney stones is called 'supersaturation'. The kidneys filter and excrete salts, including calcium oxalate, uric acid, cystine and xanthine. These salts can become extremely concentrated if there is not enough urine production, or if unusually high amounts of crystal-forming salts are present. When salt concentration levels reach the point at which they no longer dissolve, these salts form crystals. These crystals eventually form kidney stones.

Often, the cause of *calcium stones* is not known. The condition is then called 'idiopathic nephrolithiasis'. Research suggests that nearly all stones result from problems in the breakdown and absorption of calcium and oxalate. Genetic factors may play a part in the formation of these stones. A number of medical conditions (dehydration) and drugs (calcium supplement tablets) can also affect digestion and intestinal absorption. Some drugs, for example loop diuretics and acetazolamide, increase the risk of calcium stones.

Human body tissues, and certain foods, contain substances called **purines**. Purine-containing foods include dried beans, peas and liver. When the body breaks down purines, it produces uric acid. The presence of a certain level of uric acid in the body is normal, but excess uric acid can lead to stones. Some drugs, such as allopurinol and salicylates, promote uric acid stone formation.

Struvite stones are almost always caused by UTI due to bacteria that produce certain enzymes. These enzymes raise the concentration of ammonia in the urine. Ammonia makes up the crystals that form struvite stones. The stone-promoting bacteria are usually *Proteus*, but may also include *Pseudomonas, Klebsiella, Providencia, Serratia* and staphylococci. Women are twice as likely to have struvite stones as men.

661

Cystine stones develop from genetic defects that cause abnormal transport of amino acids in the kidney and the gastrointestinal system, leading to a build-up of cystine, one of these amino acids. Researchers have identified two genes responsible for this condition and these are SLC3A1 and CLC7A9.

Investigations and diagnosis
- Abdominal X-ray to identify urinary obstruction
- Ultrasound
- Urinalysis to detect UTI
- Urea and electrolytes to detect imbalance.

Signs and symptoms
- Often asymptomatic
- Dull, aching flank pain
- Microscopic haematuria
- Renal colic
- Acute, severe flank pain on affected side, radiating to the suprapubic region, groin and external genitals
- Nausea, vomiting, pallor and cool, clammy skin.

What the Experts Say

Using the link below, read about the experience of patients in how they realised they had kidney stones and their experience.
http://www.medicinenet.com/kidney_stone/discussion-101.htm

Nursing care and management
Nursing care should include identification of the cause of renal stones and providing appropriate treatment and care. Initial management can either be done as an inpatient or on an urgent outpatient basis, usually depending on how severe the pain is and if the patient is presenting with complications such as retention of urine or excessive bleeding.

Medications
- Non-steroidal anti-inflammatory drugs (NSAIDs), for example, diclofenac, are administered intramuscularly or rectally. NSAIDs are more effective than opioids as NSAIDs have less tendency to cause nausea. If the pain is severe, then a suitable opioid analgesia should be prescribed and administered with a suitable antiemetic for nausea
- Nurses should document the outcome of the analgesia in the patient's notes. Reassess the patient's pain level 1–2-hourly using a suitable pain assessment tool such as the pain scale. Encourage the patient to lie in a comfortable position that brings relief.

Diet and fluid management
- Diet modifications may be necessary to prevent further episodes of renal calculi formation. This may include reduced intake of dietary calcium and vitamin D for calcium stones and limiting food intake high in purines such as sardines, kidneys and red meat
- Protein increases uric acid, calcium and oxalate levels in the urine, and reduces citrate levels. Diets high in protein, particularly meat protein, have been consistently connected with kidney stones. (Meat protein has higher sulphur content and produces more acid than vegetable protein.)

Link To/Go To

See

http://www.umm.edu/patiented/articles/dietary_factors
_lifestyle_measures_used_prevention_of_kidney_stones
_000081_8.htm

- Encourage the patient to drink 2.5–3 litres of fluid daily to promote urine production and to prevent the formation of kidney stones. Increasing urine volume decreases the concentration of minerals in the urine. This makes it less likely that a stone will form.

The Evidence

Drinking one-half cup of pure lemon juice (enough to make eight glasses of lemonade) every day raises citrate levels in the urine, which might protect against calcium stones. While orange juice also increases citrate levels, it does not lower calcium and it raises oxalate levels. Therefore, it is not recommended. Apple and cranberry juice contain oxalates, and both have been associated with a higher risk for calcium oxalate stones.
http://www.healthcentral.com/ency/408/guides/000081
_10_2.html

Invasive procedures Small calculi, 5 mm or less in diameter, will pass through the urinary tract without any intervention. Some stones become stuck in a kidney or the ureter and cause persistent symptoms or problems such as pain and a UTI. In these cases, the pain usually becomes severe and the patient may need to be admitted to hospital. There are various treatment options, which include the following:

- *Extracorporeal shock wave lithotripsy (ESWL).* This uses high-energy shock waves which are focussed onto the stones from a machine outside the body to break them up. The stone fragments are then passed in the urine
- *Percutaneous nephrolithotomy (PCNL)* is used when ESWL is not suitable. A nephroscope (a thin telescope-like instrument) is passed through the skin and into the kidney. The stone is broken up and the fragments of stone are removed via the nephroscope. This is usually carried out under general anaesthetic
- Ureteroscopy is another treatment that may be used. A telescope is passed up into the ureter via the urethra and bladder and a laser is used to break up the stone. This technique is used for most types of kidney stones.

Red Flag

A stone that completely obstructs the ureter can lead to hydronephrosis and damage to the affected kidney. As the other kidney continues to function normally, urine output may not fall significantly with the obstruction of one ureter.

Health promotion and discharge
Prior to discharge, the nurse should discuss:
- The importance of maintaining good fluid intake, for example 2.5–3 litres of fluid per day. This is to ensure that there is good

urine production and to prevent UTI. The patient should void urine into a container to catch any stones that may be passed. Advise the patient to drink cranberry juice as it increases citrate excretion and reduces oxalate and phosphate excretion

- Offer dietary advice on the importance of low salt intake. Reduce intake of oxalate-rich (e.g. chocolate, rhubarb and nuts) and urate-rich foods (e.g. offal and certain fish)
- The patient may be discharged home with medications to prevent further stone formation and these may include thiazide diuretics (for calcium stones), allopurinol (for uric acid stones) and calcium citrate (for oxalate stones). Stress the importance in taking the medication regularly.

Primary Care

Prior to discharge, nurses should discuss the following topics to prepare for self-care at home.
- The importance of maintaining adequate fluid intake of 2.5–3 L per day
- If the patient is discharged home with medications, the importance of taking the medications as prescribed
- Reduce salt intake to no more than 3 g (about half a teaspoonful) a day, as higher amounts may raise the level of calcium in the urine
- The signs and symptoms of UTI and the preventative measures to avoid reoccurrence
- The importance of keeping well hydrated during exercise.

Advise the patient to keep any outpatient appointments as booked and to see their GP if they are concerned or if they experience any severe pain as a result of stones blocking the urinary tract.

Bladder Cancer

Bladder cancer is a relatively common type of cancer in the elderly. Most cases are formed from the lining (known as the 'transitional cell lining') and this cancer is often referred to as 'transitional cell carcinoma' (SIGN 2005a). It is currently called **urothelial carcinoma**.

Other rarer types of bladder cancer include **adenocarcinomas** (2% of bladder cancers) and **squamous cell carcinomas** (1–2% of cases).

Causes of bladder cancer

Some of the possible risk factors include:
- Smokers are three to four times more likely to develop bladder cancer and passive smoking may also increase the risk
- Exposure to certain industrial chemicals (e.g. in the rubber, paint, dye, printing and textile industries, gas and tar manufacturing, iron and aluminium processing), radiation
- Three times more common in men than women and more common in white people than black people
- Bladder infection (schistosomiasis) caused by a parasite in certain hot countries increases the risk.
- Repeated bouts of other types of bladder infection may also slightly increase the risk.

Pathophysiology

Bladder cancer develops in the lining or the wall of the bladder. It is caused by the uncontrolled growth of cells. Bladder cancer mostly affects people over 50 and is more common in men than in women. Most cases of bladder cancer appear to be caused when the tissue of the bladder is exposed to harmful substances, which, over the course of many years, leads to abnormal biological changes in the bladder's cells. The most common harmful substance is tobacco smoke. It is estimated that half of all cases of bladder cancers are caused by smoking.

Carcinogenic breakdown products of certain chemicals and from cigarette smoke are excreted in the urine and stored in the bladder, possibly causing a local influence on abnormal cell development. Squamous cell carcinoma of the urinary tract occurs less frequently than transitional epithelial cell tumours.

Transitional cell carcinoma (TCC) is the most common bladder cancer and develops in the top layer of cells that line the bladder wall. These cells come into contact with waste products in the urine that may cause cancer. Squamous cell carcinoma develops in the flat cells that line the bladder wall. Adenocarcinoma is a rare type of bladder cancer that develops in the mucus-producing cells that line the bladder wall.

Bladder tumours are rated by their cell type and grade. Grade I tumours are highly differentiated and rarely progress to become invasive, whereas grade III tumours are poorly-differentiated and usually progress. The staging of bladder tumours is outlined in Table 29.2; for tissue involvement see Figure 29.10.

Table 29.2 Staging of bladder tumour.

STAGES	ORGANS AFFECTED
T_a	Affects the bladder mucosa
T_1	Bladder mucosa and submucosal layers
T_2	Superficial muscle of bladder wall
T_{3a}	Deep muscle affected
T_{3b}	Involvement of perivesicular fat
$T_{3-4}N_1$	Lymph node and adjacent organs affected

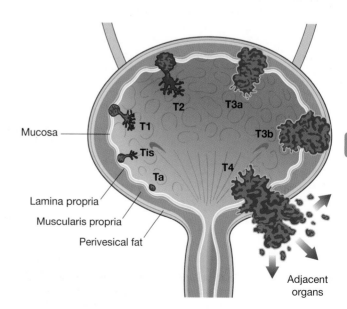

Figure 29.10 Stages of bladder cancer.

663

Investigations and diagnosis

- Cystoscopy – an invasive procedure using a cystoscope to look into the bladder
- Intravenous urogram (IVU): a special type of X-ray procedure used to look inside the bladder and urinary system
- Ultrasound, MRI scan or CT scan. These scans can help doctors to check the urinary system to see if the cancer has spread.

Signs and symptoms

- Painless haematuria is the presenting sign in 75% of urinary tract tumours
- Frequency
- Urgency
- Dysuria
- May cause UTI.

Nursing care and management

The most widely used type of surgery in bladder cancer is a 'radical cystectomy'. However, most superficial bladder tumours are removed via transurethral resection with the aid of a cystoscope. This could be followed by a course of radiotherapy or chemotherapy, which is directly instilled into the bladder to prevent reoccurrence. When the cancer has invaded into the muscle (Figure 29.10) then the whole bladder is removed (cystectomy) with a urinary diversion (Figure 29.11). For the principles of pre- and postoperative preparations, refer to Chapter 14, and for the care of the patient with a stoma, refer to Chapter 28.

Preoperative care

- *Psychological preparation.* Nurses should provide both verbal and written information about the surgery, pain management and contact numbers of whom the patient and their families can get in touch when in difficulties

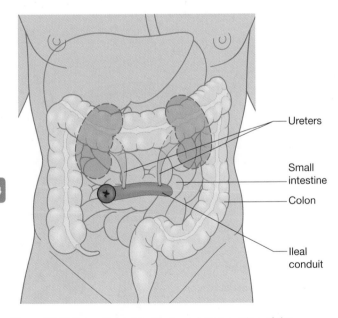

Figure 29.11 Formation of an ileal conduit. A section of the terminal ileum is used to form a stoma, where both ureters are implanted and for the urine to flow into. The stoma protrudes from the skin to minimise skin irritation from the urine.

Labels on figure: Ureters; Small intestine; Colon; Ileal conduit

- *Information about altered body image.* Nurses should allow the patient to discuss any concerns they may have about returning to usual activities, perceived relationship changes and resumption of sexual relations. Offer information about support groups or contact with someone who has successfully adjusted to a urinary diversion
- *Arrange visits by the stoma nurse* to discuss various appliances that are available and to advise and teach the patient on the care of the stoma and to answer any questions they may have regarding caring for the stoma at home
- *Physical preparation of the patient.* The nurse should adhere to local and professional guidelines in the safe preparation for urinary diversion.

Postoperative care

- Postoperative care should include monitoring vital signs, pain management, fluid management, risk assessment for deep vein thrombosis, pressure sores, personal hygiene, nutrition and other routine postoperative care.
- Maintain a closed drainage system if a catheter is attached to the urostomy bag and ensure that the bag is not blocked. Impaired urine flow can lead to urinary retention and distention of the bladder, a newly created reservoir, or the renal pelvis (hydronephrosis). Although urine is sterile, bacteria can multiply rapidly if the closed system is compromised, resulting in UTI
- When the patient is allowed to eat and drink normally, encourage the patient to increase fluid intake to approximately 2.5–3 L per day. Increased fluid intake results in good urine production and prevents UTI. Monitor urine output hourly for the first 24 hours postoperatively, then every 4–8 hours
- Empty the catheter bag or the urostomy bag every 2 hours. Overfilling of the collection may damage the seal, allowing leakage and contact of urine with skin
- Assess colour and consistency of urine. Urine may be cloudy due to mucus production by bowel mucosa. Bright red blood in the urine from a urinary diversion may indicate haemorrhage as a complication, and excessive cloudiness or malodorous urine may indicate UTI
- Check the stoma site and surrounding skin every 2 hours for the first 24 hours, then every 4 hours for 48–72 hours. Assess the skin for redness, excoriation or signs of breakdown, as impaired skin integrity may lead to local or systemic infection and impaired healing
- Advise the patient on the signs and symptoms of infection and the measures they could take to prevent UTI. Following cystectomy and formation of an ileal conduit, the patient is at risk of UTI for life because of impaired urinary defence mechanisms. Following strict protocols when providing urostomy care and increasing fluid may minimise the risk to a certain degree but do not eliminate it.

Radiation and chemotherapy treatment Radiation is another adjunctive therapy used in the treatment of urinary tumours. Although radiation alone is not curative, it can reduce tumour size prior to surgery and is used as palliative treatment for inoperable tumours and for persons who cannot tolerate surgery. Radiation therapy also is used in combination with systemic chemotherapy to improve local and distant relapse rates. If radiation or chemotherapy is planned as adjunctive therapy, the patient may experience hair loss, stomatitis, nausea and vomiting or other disturbing side-effects of therapy. Nurses should be sensitive to the patient's feelings, actively listening and responding to their concerns.

What the Experts Say One Person's Experience

I had my bladder removed in August this year for bladder cancer. I live with an ileal conduit and ostomy bag. I've also had a radical cystectomy. It's only been a few months since I had the surgery, I am unfortunately undergoing chemo at the moment so I kinda feel crap!! However, I dreaded living with a bag, but found it's not as bad as I thought, the surgery was hell and I'm still trying to come to terms with the fact that I no longer have a bladder, but I'm alive! Sometimes I find it hard to cope with the fact that I no longer have a bladder but a bag, which can sometimes leak!! I'm 46 years and a mother and wife, my love life is a no-no right now, but I guess that's due to the chemo, but it's been a positive experience, after all I'm alive.

Health promotion and discharge

Prior to discharge, nurses need to discuss the following with the patient and their family:

- Offer dietary advice and if necessary refer to a dietician
- Encourage 2.5–3 litres of fluid intake per day. Increased fluid intake promotes urine production and help to prevent UTI
- Encourage the patient not to smoke. Provide referral to smoking cessation programmes or clinics for people who wish to stop smoking
- Advise the patient of the importance of keeping the follow-up appointment as organised and the compliance to the medications prescribed
- Advise on the stoma nurse visit and care of the stoma.

Red Flag

Nurses must measure urine output hourly for the first 24 hours after the removal of urostomy catheter. Any obstruction could lead to hydronephrosis and kidney damage.

Primary Care

The need for individual and family teaching for the patient who has had surgery to treat a urinary diversion is important. They need to come to terms with altered body image and therefore nurses need to be sensitive when providing stoma care and answering any questions the patient or their family may have. The patient should be informed of the importance of being well-hydrated during exercise and in hot weather, as dehydration results in poor urine output and increases the chance of developing UTI (SIGN 2005b).

The patient who has had a urinary diversion needs teaching about care of the stoma and surrounding skin, prevention of urine reflux and infection, signs and symptoms of UTI and renal calculi, and, in some cases, self-catheterisation using the clean technique.

Provide information about the Urostomy Association and support groups. Joining a support group will provide the patient with the opportunity to form new friendships and explore what it is like to live with a stoma.

Renal Tumour

Most cases of kidney cancer develop in people over the age of 60, although it sometimes affects younger people. It can be either benign or malignant, primary or metastatic. Most primary renal tumours arise from renal cells; a primary tumour also may develop in the renal pelvis, although less frequently. Metastatic lesions to the kidney are associated with lung and breast cancer, melanoma and malignant lymphoma.

Pathophysiology of renal tumour

Most renal tumours are **renal cell carcinomas**. These tumours arise from tubular epithelium and can occur anywhere in the kidney. The affected kidney tends to become larger. In time, the tumour may grow through the wall of the kidney and invade nearby tissues and organs, such as the muscles around the spine, the liver and the renal blood vessels. The tumour, which can range in size up to several centimeters, has clearly defined margins and contains areas of ischaemia, necrosis and haemorrhage. Some cells may break off into the lymph circulation or the bloodstream. The cancer may then spread to nearby lymph nodes or to other areas of the body (metastasise). Some rare types of cancer arise from other types of cell within the kidney. For example, transitional cell (urothelial) cancers are cancers which arise from transitional cells. These are cells which line the renal pelvis, ureters and bladder. **Transitional cell cancer** is common in the bladder but, in some cases, it develops in the renal pelvis.

Risk factors

- Most cases develop in people over the age of 55 and kidney cancer is more common in men
- About one-third of kidney cancers are thought to be caused by smoking. Some of the chemicals from tobacco get into the body and are passed out in the urine. These chemicals in the urine can be carcinogenic to kidney tubule cells
- Industrial chemicals, such as asbestos, cadmium and some organic solvents, have been linked to an increased risk of kidney cancer
- Obesity is a risk factor for kidney cancer. About a quarter of kidney cancer cases are due to being overweight
- Genetic factors may play a role in some cases. People with some rare genetic disorders, such as von Hippel–Lindau syndrome and Birt–Hogg–Dubé syndrome have a higher risk of developing kidney cancer.

Investigations and diagnosis

- An ultrasound scan of the kidney can usually detect a kidney cancer. This is often one of the first tests carried out to diagnose kidney cancer
- A more sophisticated scan called a computed tomography (CT) scan may be used if there is doubt about the diagnosis
- Urinalysis to check the colour of urine and its contents, such as sugar, protein, red blood cells and white blood cells
- Biopsy to check for signs of cancer. To do a biopsy for renal cell cancer, a thin needle is inserted into the tumour and a sample of tissue is withdrawn.

Other tests may include a magnetic resonance imaging (MRI) scan of the abdomen and chest, a chest X-ray and blood tests.

Signs and symptoms

- Heavy haematuria
- Flank pain
- Palpable abdominal mass
- Fever without signs of infection
- Fatigue
- Weight loss
- Anaemia
- Loss of appetite.

Nursing care and management

Nephrectomy (removal of the kidney) is carried out for kidney tumours. In cases where the tumour is advanced, the adrenal gland, upper ureter, fat and fascia surrounding the kidney, as well as the entire kidney, are removed. Although laparotomy primarily is used for radical nephrectomy, NICE (2005) has issued guidance for laparoscopic nephrectomy.

Preoperative care For the principles of pre- and postoperative care, refer to Chapter 14.

- Nurses need to adhere to local policies and guidance of the Trust in the safe preoperative preparation of the patient for theatre, including giving information and identifying any special needs
- Discuss postoperative care including pain management with the patient. Preoperative teaching about postoperative expectations reduces anxiety for the person and family during the early postoperative period
- Although deep breathing and coughing may be painful due to the proximity of the incision to the diaphragm, breathing exercises are encouraged to prevent pneumonia
- Discuss operative and postoperative expectations as indicated, including the location of the incision and anticipated tubes, stents and drains.

Postoperative care

- Monitor vital signs such as temperature, blood pressure, heart rate and respiration rate hourly, until the condition of the patient is stable
- The location of the incision, combined with the respiratory depressant effects of narcotic analgesics, increases the risk for respiratory complications in the person who has had a nephrectomy. Change position frequently, and mobilise as soon as possible with the help of a physiotherapist. Encourage frequent (every 1–2 hours) deep breathing, spirometer use and coughing. Support the incision with a pillow when coughing, as it helps to reduce pain
- Monitor urine output and note the colour, amount and any haematuria, pyuria or sediment. Promptly report oliguria (scanty urine output) or anuria (absence of urine), as well as changes in urine colour or clarity. It is important to monitor the function of the remaining kidney. The urine output should be greater than 30 mL/hour
- Postoperative pain can be a problem due to the location and size of the surgical incision. Using a pain assessment tool, check with the patient every 2 hours for the severity, quality and duration of the pain. Observe other signs of pain, such as restlessness, facial expressions, guarding and changes in vital signs. It is helpful to complete this assessment before and after administration of analgesics, as well as non-pharmacological interventions

- Ensure all tubes and wound drains are clearly labelled and record all output on a fluid balance chart. Report any excess bleeding to the person in charge for prompt action. Maintaining drainage tube patency is vital to prevent potential hydronephrosis. Bright bleeding or unexpected drainage may indicate a surgical complication
- Fluid management is also crucial to postoperative management. The patient may be at risk for fluid deficit or excess. Close monitoring to ensure adequate renal and cardiac function can identify changes early and prevent or minimise complications. Accurate recording of all intake and output, daily weights, blood pressure and pulse assessments, and monitoring of serum creatinine and blood urea levels provide important information on renal status. The most accurate indicator of fluid loss or gain is daily weight (LeMone *et al.* 2011). Once the patient can tolerate oral fluid, slowly increase fluid intake of 2500 to 3000 mL per day. This helps prevent dehydration and maintain good urine flow
- Report signs and symptoms of UTI such as dysuria, frequency, urgency, nocturia or cloudy, malodorous urine to the person in charge. Prompt treatment of postoperative infection is vital to allow continued healing and prevent compromise of the remaining kidney.

Red Flag

Nurses should be aware that pneumothorax is a possible complication of nephrectomy. Hourly monitoring of the vital signs is needed during the early stages to detect any respiratory complications.

- Nurses should demonstrate respect for cultural, spiritual and religious values and beliefs. Values and belief systems can provide a structure and form for dealing with the grieving process as a result of altered body image
- Assist family members to share concerns with one another. Sharing of fears and concerns among family members promotes involvement and support of the entire family unit so that the individual is not left to cope alone
- Refer to cancer support groups, social services or counselling as appropriate. Support groups and counselling services provide additional resources for coping.

Health promotion and discharge

Prior to discharge, nurses should:

- Discuss any worries they may have regarding the surgery and after care. Allow the patient time to ask questions and respond in a sympathetic and empathetic manner
- Ensure that outpatient appointments are booked and advise the patient of the importance of keeping the appointment
- If necessary, arrange transport to and from the hospital after the outpatient appointment
- Advise the patient of the importance of taking medications that may be prescribed as part of the treatment
- Encourage the patient to drink approximately 2.5–3 litres of fluid daily and to monitor their urine output. Advise the patient on the signs and symptoms of UTI, such as frequency or burning sensation when voiding urine, and to see the GP if any of these symptoms occur.

Renal Failure

Acute kidney injury (AKI), has now replaced the term 'acute renal failure (ARF)' (KDIGO 2011). Clinically, AKI is a condition in which the kidneys are unable to remove accumulated metabolites from the blood, leading to altered fluid, electrolyte and acid–base balance. The cause may be a primary kidney disorder, or renal failure may be secondary to a systemic disease or other urologic defects. AKI may be either acute or chronic. AKI has an abrupt onset and, with prompt intervention, is often reversible. **Chronic kidney disease (CKD)** has now replaced the term 'chronic renal failure (CRF)'. It has a slow onset, with few symptoms until the kidneys are severely damaged and unable to meet the excretory needs of the body.

Acute Kidney Injury

AKI is a rapid decline in renal function with azotaemia and fluid and electrolyte imbalances. The most common causes of AKI are ischaemia and toxins in the blood. The kidney is particularly vulnerable to both because of the amount of blood that passes through it. A fall in blood pressure or volume can cause ischaemia of kidney tissues.

Risk factors of AKI

- Elderly
- Hypertension
- Vascular disease
- Pre-existing renal impairment
- Congestive cardiac failure
- Diabetes
- Myeloma
- Chronic infection
- Myeloproliferative disorder.

Causes

Pre-renal Pre-renal AKI results from conditions that affect renal blood flow and perfusion. Any disorder that significantly decreases vascular volume, cardiac output or systemic vascular resistance can affect renal blood flow. Pre-renal AKI is rapidly reversed when blood flow is restored, and the renal parenchyma remains undamaged. Some of these causes are:

- Volume depletion as a result of haemorrhage, severe vomiting or diarrhoea, burns, inappropriate diuresis
- Oedematous states resulting from cardiac failure, cirrhosis, nephrotic syndrome
- Hypotension
- Renal hypoperfusion from the use of non-steroidal anti-inflammatory drugs (NSAIDs) or selective cyclooxygenase-2 (COX-2) inhibitors, renal artery stenosis or occlusion, hepatorenal syndrome
- Septic shock.

Intrarenal Intrinsic or intrarenal failure is characterised by acute damage to the renal parenchyma and nephrons. Intrarenal causes include diseases of the kidney itself and acute tubular necrosis, the most common intrarenal cause of AKI.

- Glomerular disease, such as glomerulonephritis, thrombosis, haemolytic uraemic syndrome
- Vascular disease, such as renal artery stenosis, renal vein thrombosis, malignant hypertension.

Post-renal Any condition that prevents urine excretion can lead to post-renal AKI. This results in retention of urine, which could result in AKI. Some of these conditions include:

- Calculus
- Blood clot
- Papillary necrosis
- Urethral stricture
- Prostatic hypertrophy or malignancy
- Bladder tumour
- Radiation fibrosis
- Pelvic malignancy
- Retroperitoneal fibrosis.

Pathophysiology

The causes and pathophysiology of acute kidney injury are commonly categorised as pre-renal, intrinsic and post-renal AKI. Pre-renal AKI is the most common, accounting for about 55% of the total. In pre-renal AKI, hypoperfusion leads to acute kidney injury without directly affecting the integrity of kidney tissues. Intrinsic (or intrarenal) AKI, due to direct damage to functional kidney tissue, is responsible for another 40%. Urinary tract obstruction with resulting kidney damage is the precipitating factor for post-renal AKI, the least common form.

Investigations and diagnosis

- Urinalysis: blood and/or protein suggests a renal inflammatory process. Microscopy for cells, casts, crystals: red cell casts are diagnostic in glomerulonephritis; tubular cells or casts suggest acute tubular necrosis (ATN)
- Osmolality of urine is over 500 mmol/kg if the cause is pre-renal and 300 mmol/kg or less if it is renal; patients with ATN lose the ability to concentrate and dilute the urine and will pass a constant volume with inappropriate osmolality
- Serum urea, creatinine and electrolytes
- Full blood count
- Renal ultrasonography to determine renal size, symmetry, evidence of obstruction
- Chest X-ray (pulmonary oedema); abdominal X-ray if renal calculi are suspected
- Contrast studies, such as intravenous urogram (IVU) and renal angiography, should be avoided because of the risk of contrast nephropathy
- Doppler ultrasound of the renal artery and veins: assessment of possible occlusion of the renal artery and veins
- Magnetic resonance angiography: for more accurate assessment of renal vascular occlusion
- ECG: recent myocardial infarction, tented T waves in hyperkalaemia
- Renal biopsy.

Signs and symptoms

- Urine output: AKI is usually accompanied by oliguria or anuria, but polyuria may occur. Abrupt anuria suggests an acute obstruction, acute and severe glomerulonephritis, or acute renal artery occlusion. Gradual diminution of urine output may indicate a urethral stricture or bladder outlet obstruction, e.g. benign prostatic hyperplasia
- Nausea, vomiting
- Dehydration
- Confusion
- Hypertension
- Abdomen: may reveal a large, painless bladder typical of chronic urinary retention
- Dehydration with postural hypotension and no oedema
- Fluid overload with raised jugular venous pressure (JVP), pulmonary oedema and peripheral oedema
- Pallor, rash, bruising: petechiae, purpura and nosebleeds may suggest inflammatory or vascular disease, emboli or disseminated intravascular coagulation
- Pericardial rub.

Stages

668

The course of acute kidney injury due to ATN typically includes three phases: initiation, maintenance and recovery.

Initiation phase The initiation phase may last hours to days. During this period, the kidney function is suppressed. The patient may present with oliguria or anuria. Bleeding from the kidneys may be a problem if there is tubular damage. If AKI is recognised and the initiating event is effectively treated during this phase, the prognosis is good. The initiation phase of AKI has few symptoms; in fact, it is often identified only when symptoms of the maintenance phase develop.

Maintenance phase The maintenance phase of AKI is characterised by a significant fall in glomerular filtration rate (GFR) and tubular necrosis. This phase may last 1–2 weeks (Alexander *et al.* 2007). Oliguria may develop, although many persons continue to produce normal or near-normal amounts of urine (non-oliguric AKI). Even though urine may be produced, the kidney cannot efficiently eliminate metabolic wastes, water, electrolytes and acids from the body during the maintenance phase of AKI. Fluid and electrolyte imbalance occur during this phase and the specific gravity of urine is the same as plasma. Serum creatinine and blood urea and nitrogen (BUN) levels are elevated. The patient may present with oedema and hypertension, confusion, disorientation, agitation or lethargy, hyper-reflexia, and possible seizures or coma, due to azotaemia and electrolyte and acid–base imbalances.

Recovery phase The final phase is the recovery phase. Diuresis may occur as the nephrons and GFR recover, and retained salt, water and solutes are excreted. Serum creatinine, blood, urea and nitrogen (BUN), potassium and phosphate levels remain high and may continue to rise in spite of increasing urine output. Renal function improves rapidly during the first 5–25 days of the recovery phase, and continues to improve for up to 1 year. During this phase, the patient may pass approximately 4–6 L of urine per day depending on fluid retention. Dehydration is a problem, as a result of increased fluid loss and the inability of the kidneys to perform selective reabsorption.

Red Flag

If AKI is not treated promptly, it could lead to ischaemic acute tubular necrosis and intrarenal or intrinsic AKI. Restoration of blood pressure and blood flow to the kidneys reverses pre-renal AKI.

Nursing care and management

A full nursing assessment of vital signs, weight, fluid intake and output, nursing history and assessment of the patient's knowledge of the disease process should all be carried out in order to provide high-quality care. It is important to alleviate the patient's and relatives' worries and anxieties. Healthcare professionals should give the patient time to ask questions, and should respond appropriately. Psychological care is important in the care and management of the patient with AKI.

Medications The primary focus in drug management for acute kidney injury is to restore and maintain renal perfusion and to eliminate drugs that are nephrotoxic from the treatment regimen. The patient may be prescribed the following medications:

- Furosemide to induce diuresis
- Antihypertensives such as angiotensin converting enzyme (ACE) inhibitors to control hypertension
- Antacids to prevent gastric ulcers. The person in acute kidney injury has an increased risk of gastrointestinal bleeding, probably related to the stress response and impaired platelet function. Regular doses of antacids, histamine H_2-receptor antagonists (e.g. ranitidine) or a proton-pump inhibitorsuch

as omeprazole (Prilosec) are often prescribed to prevent GI haemorrhage

- A potassium-binding exchange resin, such as sodium polystyrene sulfonate (Kayexalate, SPS Suspension) may be given orally or by enema to treat hyperkalaemia. Dextrose (50%) and insulin may be given intravenously to reduce serum potassium levels by moving potassium into the cells.

Fluid management Adequate hydration is of paramount importance to the patient's management (*Northern Ireland Guidelines for Acute Kidney Injury*, GAIN 2010). Once vascular volume and renal perfusion are restored, fluid intake is usually restricted. Nurses need to follow local policy in the fluid management of a patient with AKI. Fluid balance is carefully monitored, using accurate weight measurements and the serum sodium as the primary indicators.

In AKI, the kidneys often cannot excrete adequate urine to maintain a normal extracellular fluid balance. Rapid weight gain and oedema indicate fluid retention and in addition, heart failure and pulmonary oedema may develop, which can present a significant management problem.

What To Do If...

The patient with AKI who you are looking after suddenly becomes breathless, is anuric and has distended neck veins. What should you do? Some of the nursing actions include:

- Inform the person in charge immediately
- Take and record his/her vital signs
- Check when they last passed urine and the amount.

- Prevention of infection
- Patients with AKI are susceptible to infection.
- Infection is a significant cause of mortality. Therefore, strict sepsis control is essential; avoidance of intravenous lines, bladder catheters and respirators is recommended.

Nutrition Strict nutritional status should be maintained. Protein intake should be limited to minimise the increase of nitrogenous wastes. Carbohydrates are increased to maintain adequate calorie intake and provide a protein-sparing effect. Where necessary, the dietician may be involved in the care of the patient with AKI. In some cases, parenteral nutrition is prescribed to provide essential amino acids, carbohydrates and fats when the patient cannot take an adequate diet as a result of nausea and vomiting. The disadvantages of parenteral nutrition in the patient with AKI are the risk of developing fluid overload and the risk for infection through the venous line.

Dialysis for AKI In oliguric or anuric patients the fluid intake required for maintaining hydration generally means that dialysis will be necessary. This may be offered as peritoneal dialysis or as haemofiltration. As excess fluid and solutes are removed more gradually in peritoneal dialysis it poses less risk; however, this slower rate of metabolite removal can be a disadvantage in AKI. However, in peritoneal dialysis there is an increased risk for developing peritonitis.

What To Do If...

Some of the tests carried out to determine kidney disease include: blood pressure measurement, measurement of albumin in the urine and a calculation of GFR based on a measurement of serum creatinine.

If these tests show a reduced kidney function, what other tests may be carried out to confirm the diagnosis?

Health promotion and discharge

Prior to discharge, nurses should advise the patient and relatives of the importance of maintaining adequate fluid intake. During exercise and hot weather, encourage the patient to keep well-hydrated. Inform the patient to adhere to the dietary advice offered by the dietician. Monitor the urine output and advise the patient to see the GP if symptoms of UTI, such as haematuria, frequency and a burning sensation when voiding urine, are present. If medications are prescribed to take home, inform the patient and their relatives of the importance of taking the medications as prescribed and to avoid over-dosing on any medications that are nephrotoxic.

Primary Care

AKI is a serious condition when it develops. The patient is often critically ill and it does put a lot of stress on their family. Nurses need to show empathy when dealing with the patient and the family. Include family members in teaching during the initial stages to promote understanding of what is happening and the reasons for specific treatment measures. Inclusion of the family reduces their anxiety and provides a valuable resource for reinforcing person teaching about care after discharge.

Patient teaching needs for home care include:

- Advise the patient and their relatives to avoid medications purchased over the counter that could lead to kidney damage
- Monitor their urine out to ensure that the patient does not develop a UTI. Encourage oral fluid, approximately 2.5–3 L per day
- Monitor weight, blood pressure and pulse
- Continue dietary restrictions as per advice by the dietician
- Advise them to contact their GP when necessary.

Chronic Kidney Disease (CKD)

Although the kidneys usually recover from AKI, many chronic conditions can lead to progressive renal damage, resulting in CKD. The functional units of the kidneys (nephrons) are lost and renal mass decreases, with progressive deterioration of glomerular filtration, selective reabsorption and tubular secretion. CKD can develop slowly for many years without any symptoms. It is often detected when the kidneys are in the final stage of CKD. The kidneys are unable to excrete metabolic wastes and regulate fluid and electrolyte balance adequately.

Table 29.3 Stages of CKD. (*Source*: Kathuria 2013)

STAGE	DESCRIPTION	GFR (mL/min/1.73 m²)
1	Slight kidney damage with normal or increased filtration	More than 90
2	Mild decrease in kidney function	60–89
3	Moderate decrease in kidney function	30–59
4	Severe decrease in kidney function	15–29
5	Kidney failure	Less than 15 (or dialysis)

Link To/Go To

You can watch short video clips on CKD and other kidney diseases at:

http://www.nhs.uk/Conditions/Kidney-disease-chronic/Pages/Introduction.aspx (accessed 3 April 2013)

Jot This Down

Diabetes is one of the leading possible causes of chronic kidney disease. Can you name any other conditions that cause CKD?

Pathophysiology of CKD

Any condition that destroys the renal function can lead to CKD. The pathophysiology of CKD involves a gradual loss of entire nephron units. Chronic kidney disease is divided into five stages of increasing severity (Table 29.3). In the early stages, as nephrons are slowly destroyed, remaining healthy nephrons take over their functions but become hypertrophied. The blood pressure and the filtration in the remaining healthy nephrons increase to compensate for the loss of nephrons, resulting in damage of the remaining healthy nephrons. This process of continued loss of nephron function may continue even after the initial disease process has resolved. See Table 29.4 for some of the common diseases leading to nephron destruction and end-stage renal disease.

As the number of sclerosed glomeruli increases, the symptoms of CKD can be observed. They include:

- Progressive fall in renal excretory function (assessed by excretory GFR)
- Proteinuria – detected by urine protein: creatinine ratio (PCR) or albumin : creatinine ratio (ACR)
- A tendency to hypertension
- Renal shrinkage – detected with renal ultrasound.

The course of CKD is variable, progressing over a period of months to many years. There are three phases of CKD (early, second and third phases). In the early phase, the blood, urea and nitrogen (BUN) levels are elevated (2–5 mg/mL) and the GFR is greatly reduced. During this phase, the unaffected nephrons compensate and the patient may be asymptomatic. In the second phase

Table 29.4 Pathophysiology of chronic kidney disease. (*Source*: Peate *et al.* 2012)

CAUSE	EXAMPLES
Diabetic nephropathy	Changes in the glomerular basement membrane, chronic pyelonephritis, and ischaemia lead to sclerosis of the glomerulus and gradual destruction of the nephron
Hypertensive nephrosclerosis	Long-standing hypertension leads to renal arteriosclerosis and ischaemia, resulting in glomerular destruction and tubular atrophy
Chronic glomerulonephritis	Bilateral inflammatory process of the glomeruli leads to ischaemia, nephron loss and shrinkage of the kidney
Chronic pyelonephritis	Chronic infection commonly associated with an obstructive or neurological process and vesicoureteral reflux leads to reflux nephropathy (renal scarring, atrophy and dilated calyces)
Polycystic kidney disease	Multiple bilateral cysts gradually destroy normal renal tissue by compression
Systemic lupus erythematosus	Basement membrane damage by circulating immune complexes leads to focal, local or diffuse glomerulonephritis

BUN levels are above 10 mg/mL and the creatinine is above 0.4 mg/mL. In the third phase, BUN levels are above 20 mg/mL and the creatinine is above 0.5 mg/mL. As CKD progresses, the patient presents with the symptoms of CKD (see below). Further damage to the kidneys at this stage, as a result of infection, dehydration or urinary tract obstruction, can precipitate the onset of renal failure.

Link To/Go To

NICE Clinical Guideline: Chronic kidney disease

http://publications.nice.org.uk/chronic-kidney-disease-cg73 (accessed 3 April 2013)

What the Experts Say Kalwant's Story

> *I became diabetic at the age of 18 and, although I knew there could be complications in 20 to 25 years, it didn't mean much to me at that age.*
> *When I began to put on weight, I thought it was connected to my thyroid, which had given me trouble since I'd had part of it removed at the age of 16. I thought my thyroid drugs needed adjusting. Then I started feeling breathless and very lethargic, and my feet and body started to retain water. My GP told me my kidney function was starting to deteriorate because of my diabetes.*

You can read other patients' stories at:
http://www.nhs.uk/Conditions/Kidney-disease-chronic/Pages/Kalwants-story.aspx (accessed 3 April 2013)

Risk factors

These include:

- Hypertension
- Diabetes (type 1 or type 2)
- A history of cardiovascular disease
- A family history of renal disease
- Structural abnormality of the renal tract
- A history of renal stone disease
- Prostatic hypertrophy
- Autoimmune disease (systemic lupus erythematosus, SLE).

Investigations and diagnosis

- Urinalysis to detect abnormalities and specific gravity
  - Haematuria may indicate glomerulonephritis
  - Glycosuria with normal blood glucose is common in CKD
- Blood urea and electrolyte levels to determine renal function
  - 24-hour urine creatinine is useful in assessing the severity of renal failure
- Ultrasound of the kidneys to determine the size of the kidneys
- Renal biopsy
- Urine cultures to detect UTI.

Signs and symptoms

In the early stages of CKD, the person may be asymptomatic. As the disease progresses, the patient may present with:

- Symptoms of anaemia
  - Pallor
  - Lethargy
  - Breathlessness
- Platelet abnormality
  - Epistaxis
  - Bruising
- Haematuria, polyuria
- Oliguria, anuria
- Polyneuropathy
- Confusion, coma
- Hypertension, heart failure
- Diarrhoea and vomiting
- Oedema due to salt and water retention and heart failure.

Complications of CKD

Anaemia Anaemia is one of the complications in CKD. Several factors have been identified and these include:

- Bone marrow fibrosis
- The kidneys produce erythropoietin (hormone). A deficiency in this hormone affects the production of red blood cells
- Increased red blood cell destruction
- Bleeding from GI tract or even blood loss during haemodialysis
- Nutritional deficiencies (iron and folate) and increased risk for blood loss from the GI tract also contribute to anaemia
- Anaemia contributes to symptoms such as fatigue, weakness, depression and impaired cognition
- Renal failure impairs platelet function, increasing the risk of bleeding disorders, such as epistaxis and GI bleeding. The mechanism of impaired platelet function associated with renal failure is poorly understood.

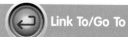

Link To/Go To

Use this link to find out about NICE guidance on the management of anaemia in patients with CKD: **http://guidance.nice.org.uk/CG114**

Fluid and electrolyte imbalance Loss of functional kidney tissue impairs its ability to regulate fluid, electrolyte and acid–base balance. In the early stages of CKD, impaired filtration and reabsorption lead to proteinuria, haematuria and decreased urine-concentrating ability. Salt and water are poorly conserved, and risk for dehydration increases. Polyuria, nocturia and a fixed specific gravity of 1.008–1.012 are common. As the GFR decreases and renal function deteriorates further, sodium and water retention are common, necessitating salt and water restrictions (Peate *et al.* 2012).

Cardiovascular disease Cardiovascular disease such as MI and heart failure is a common cause of death in CKD. Coronary artery calcification is common in patients with end-stage renal failure (ESRD). Hypertension, hyperlipidaemia and glucose intolerance all contribute to the process. Hypertension results from excess fluid volume, increased renin–angiotensin activity, increased peripheral vascular resistance and decreased prostaglandins. Increased extracellular fluid volume can also lead to oedema and heart failure. Pulmonary oedema may result from heart failure, resulting in blood pooling in the lung capillaries, which leads to fluid accumulation in the alveolar sac.

Immune system The immune system is affected as a result of high levels of urea and a build-up of metabolic wastes. This increases the risk of developing infection. The WBC count is low, humoral and cell-mediated immunity are impaired, and phagocyte function is defective. Both the acute inflammatory response and delayed hypersensitivity responses are affected.

Gastrointestinal tract Anorexia, nausea and vomiting are the most common early symptoms of uraemia. Hiccups also are commonly experienced. Gastroenteritis is frequent. Ulcerations may affect any level of the GI tract and contribute to an increased risk of GI bleeding. Peptic ulcer disease is particularly common in uraemic persons. Uraemic fetor (urine-like breath odour), often associated with a metallic taste in the mouth, may develop. Uraemic fetor can further contribute to anorexia.

Nervous system Severe uraemia causes depressed CNS function. CNS symptoms include difficulty in concentrating, fatigue, convulsions, seizures and insomnia. Asterixis, tremor and myoclonus are also features of severe uraemia. Peripheral neuropathy is also common in advanced uraemia. As uraemia progresses, motor function is impaired, causing muscle weakness, decreased deep tendon reflexes and gait disturbances.

Bone disease Hyperparathyroid bone disease, osteomalacia, osteoporosis and osteosclerosis are some of the diseases associated with CKD. Parathyroid hormone causes increased calcium resorption from bone. In addition, osteoblast (bone-forming) and osteoclast (bone-destructing) cell activity is affected. This bone resorption and remodelling, combined with decreased vitamin D synthesis and decreased calcium absorption from the GI tract, are all associated with bone diseases.

Endocrine abnormalities
These include:

- Hyperprolactinaemia, which could happen both in men and women
- Increased levels of luteinising hormone in men and women
- Decreased testosterone levels with decreased spermatogenesis
- Abnormal thyroid hormone levels
- Absence of the normal menstrual cycle.

Skin disease
Anaemia and retained pigmented metabolites cause pallor and a yellowish hue to the skin in uraemia. Dry skin with poor turgor, a result of dehydration and sweat gland atrophy, is common. Bruising and excoriations are frequently seen. Metabolic wastes not eliminated by the kidneys may be deposited in the skin, contributing to itching or pruritus. In advanced uraemia, high levels of urea in the sweat may result in *uraemic frost*, crystallised deposits of urea on the skin.

Nursing care and management
Nursing care requires careful planning to help the patient and relatives to come to terms with the condition. The aim is to ensure that the patient has good quality of life by developing ways to cope with the illness, the treatment and the complications that may occur as a result of CKD and treatment.

Palliative care
The patient may need referral, at some stage, to the palliative team for support, advice and coping strategies. The NICE Clinical Guidance (NICE 2004) on supportive and palliative care (CSG) advises those who develop and deliver cancer services for adults with cancer on what is needed to make sure that patients and their families and carers are well informed, cared for and supported. Some of the key recommendations include:

- Good communication and patients' and their relatives' involvement in decision-making
- The patient should be offered a range of physical, emotional, spiritual and social support
- Patients dying with cancer should have access to a range of services to improve their quality of life.

Pain management
- Nurses should assess each pain fully before administering analgesics. The use of a pain assessment tool is recommended
- Record a pain score and review the patient every 2 hours for the effect of analgesics
- Nurses should be aware that patients with pain may also have significant emotional, social or spiritual problems. These need to be considered when providing care. Agree goals for pain management with patient and family
- Morphine remains the first-line opioid for moderate to severe pain (NICE 2012)
- Administer prescribed analgesia for continuous pain on time and note its effect
- Most people taking regular opioids need a laxative, as one of the side-effects of opioids analgesia is constipation. Renal and hepatic impairment affect opioid metabolism and excretion (NICE 2012)
- Paracetamol is recommended as first-line for mild to moderate pain. The maximum 24-hour dose for adults is 4 g but this should be reduced in patients with a low body mass index or severe liver

impairment due to chronic alcohol dependence. Regular paracetamol may not improve analgesia in patients also receiving regular strong opioids.

Other medications
Diuretics such as furosemide or other loop diuretics may be prescribed to reduce extracellular fluid volume and oedema. This also helps to lower blood pressure, and also potassium levels. In some patients, antihypertensive drugs such as angiotensin converting enzyme (ACE) inhibitors are used to regulate blood pressure, slow the progress of renal failure and prevent complications of coronary heart disease and cerebral vascular disease. Most patients may require two or three drugs to control their hypertension. The choice of other antihypertensives used will depend on existing comorbidities. Following an ACE and angiotensin receptor blockers (ARB), a diuretic may be used (often a thiazide, but in CKD stages 4 and 5, a loop diuretic may be needed, such as furosemide, possibly at high doses if there is fluid overload). Next choice would be a calcium channel blocker (e.g. amlodipine), then a beta-blocker and then an alpha-blocker. Folic acid and iron supplements are given to combat anaemia associated with chronic renal failure.

Nutrition and fluid management
Where dietary intervention is agreed, this should occur within the context of education, detailed dietary assessment and supervision, to ensure malnutrition is prevented. In CKD, unlike carbohydrates and fats, the body is unable to store excess proteins. Any unused protein is broken down as urea and nitrogenous waste, which are normally excreted by the kidneys. In CKD, these waste products are retained by the body resulting in a toxic build-up, in turn causing uraemic symptoms. However, prolonged dietary protein restriction should be avoided. Once dialysis has commenced, a high protein diet is recommended. Water and sodium intake are regulated to maintain the extracellular fluid volume at normal levels. Strict water and sodium restrictions may be necessary as CKD progresses.

Dialysis
Patients with CKD usually require dialysis. This may be as peritoneal dialysis (PD) (NICE 2011), continuous ambulatory peritoneal dialysis (CAPD) or haemodialysis. Long-term dialysis has a higher risk for complications, for example fluid overload, electrolyte imbalance and the risk of death resulting from complications such as infection (peritonitis, *Staphylococcus aureus* infection) and cardiovascular disease (endocarditis, stroke and peripheral vascular disease). Kidney transplantation has become the treatment of choice for many persons with ESRD. It allows freedom from dietary and fluid restriction and complications of anaemia.

The Evidence Peritoneal Dialysis: Ongoing Research

NICE are conducting ongoing research with regard to PD. Use the link below to find out more.

http://www.evidence.nhs.uk/topic/peritoneal-dialysis

Nursing Fields Paediatric

Many children worry about what dialysis will feel like, whether it will hurt, and how they might look or feel after dialysis. It is normal to be scared of needles at first. They might be nervous about how they will get along with the other patients and the staff. The physicians, the nurses, the social worker and the child life specialists will be there for help and support while they are being treated. Nurses should be able to answer most questions.

Health promotion and discharge

Prior to discharge of the patient with CKD into the community, nurses need to focus on measures to reduce complications from CKD treatment and to provide information for the patient and the family to lead a healthy lifestyle.

- Discuss measures to reduce the risk for urinary tract infections, and stress the importance of prompt treatment to eradicate the infecting organism. Inform the patient that keeping well hydrated is important to ensure that they do not develop a UTI
- If dietary restrictions have been prescribed, ensure that the patient and family understand the need for these restrictions
- If the patient has been prescribed medications, ensure that the patient understands the need to take the medications as prescribed. Discuss any side-effects and what to do if these symptoms occur
- Encourage the patient to take regular programmed exercise.

The patient with CKD will require dialysis. It may be haemodialysis with an arteriovenous fistula or shunt or peritoneal dialysis with a permanent peritoneal catheter. Nurses should:

- Include the patient in decision-making and encourage self-care. Increased autonomy enhances the patient's sense of control, independence and confidence
- Help the patient develop and achieve realistic goals. Realistic goals allow the person to see progress
- Facilitate contact with a support group or other community members affected by renal failure. The person benefits by providing and receiving support in a group of people going through similar circumstances
- Refer for counselling as indicated or desired. Counselling can help the person develop effective coping and adaptation strategies
- Stress the importance of keeping the fistula sites clean, observing for any signs of infection, such as inflammation, swelling and pain, and reporting these signs and symptoms to the stoma nurse/GP/practice nurse immediately for prompt action.

Conclusion

Caring for patients with a urinary disorder is challenging and demanding. The disorders associated with the urinary system can be either acute or chronic. Treatment varies depending on the type of kidney or urinary disease present. In general, the earlier kidney or urinary disease is recognised, the more likely it is to be treatable.

IWith information on leading a healthy lifestyle and following the doctor's advice on treatment for high blood pressure and other conditions, it is possible to live without symptoms or further deterioration of the kidney function. At all stages of kidney disease, one can help reduce the chances of the kidneys getting worse and the risk of cardiovascular disease by living a healthier lifestyle.

Self-care is an integral part of daily life. It means the individual takes responsibility for their own health and well-being, with support from the people involved in their care, such as the GP, practice nurse and other support workers. Self-care includes daily activities to stay fit, maintain good physical and mental health, prevent illness or accidents and effectively deal with minor ailments and long-term conditions.

Patients and their relatives should be informed that in most cases, chronic kidney disease (CKD) cannot be completely prevented, although preventative measures can be taken to reduce the chances of the condition developing.

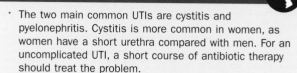

Key Points

- The two main common UTIs are cystitis and pyelonephritis. Cystitis is more common in women, as women have a short urethra compared with men. For an uncomplicated UTI, a short course of antibiotic therapy should treat the problem.
- Nurses should advise the patient on measures to prevent UTI. Encourage the patient to drink approximately 2.5–3 liters per day and advise on the type of fluid to drink and avoid.
- Kidney stones can obstruct any section of the urinary tract. Some of the obstructions may cause severe pain, such as renal colic, while others may be without any symptoms in the early stages, such the formation of stones in the kidney.
- In the UK, bladder cancer is the fourth most common cancer in males, and in females it is the eleventh most common cancer. Cigarette smoking is the most significant risk factor for bladder cancer.
- AKI is a frequent complication of critical illnesses, typically occurring in individuals with no prior history of kidney disorder. There may be no symptoms or signs, but oliguria (urine volume less than 400 mL/24 hours) is common. There is an accumulation of fluid and nitrogenous waste products demonstrated by a rise in blood urea and creatinine.
- People with any stage of CKD have an increased risk of developing heart disease or a stroke. This is why it is important to detect even mild CKD, as treatment may not only slow down the progression of the disease, but also reduce the risk of developing heart disease or stroke.

Glossary

Anterior: front
Anuria: absence of urine
Azotaemia: an elevation of blood urea nitrogen
Bifurcation: dividing into two branches
Calculi: stones
Calyces: small funnel-shaped cavities formed from the renal pelvis
Diuresis: excess urine production
Dysuria: painful urination
Erythropoietin: hormone produced by the kidneys that regulates red blood cell production
Excretion: the elimination of waste products of metabolism
Fibrosis: growth of fibrous connective tissue
Filtration: a passive transport system
Glomerulus: a network of capillaries found in the Bowman's capsule
Haematuria: blood in the urine
Hilus: a small indented part of the kidney
Hyperkalaemia: high potassium level in the blood
Hyponatraemia: low sodium level in the blood
Involuntary: cannot be controlled
Kidneys: organs situated in the posterior wall of the abdominal cavity
Micturition: the act of voiding urine.
Nephron: functional unit of the kidney

(Continued)

Nocturia: excessive urination at night
Oliguria: diminished urine output
Osmolarity: the osmotic pressure of a fluid
Parenchyma: soft tissue of the kidney involving the cortex and the medulla
Posterior: behind
Proteinuria: protein in the urine
Pyrexia: fever
Pyuria: presence of white blood cells in the urine
Renal artery: blood vessel that takes blood to the kidney
Renal cortex: the outer most part of the kidney
Renal medulla: the middle layer of the kidney
Renal pelvis: the funnel-shaped section of the kidney
Renal pyramids: cone-shaped structures of the medulla
Renal vein: blood vessel that returns filtered blood into circulation
Renin: a renal hormone that alters systemic blood pressure
Specific gravity: density
Sphincter: a ring like muscle fibre that can constrict
Ureters: membranous tubes that drain urine from the kidneys to the bladder
Urethra: muscular tube that drains urine from the bladder
Urgency: feeling of the need to void urine immediately
Voluntary: can be controlled

References

Alexander, M.F., Fawcett, J. & Runciman, P.J. (2007) *Nursing Practice – Hospitals and Home*, 3rd edn. Churchill Livingstone, Edinburgh.

EAU (2011) *Guidelines on Urological Infections*. European Association of Urology. http://www.uroweb.org/gls/pdf/15_Urological_Infections.pdf.

GAIN (2010) *Northern Ireland Guidelines for Acute Kidney Injury*. http://www.gain-ni.org/Guidelines/Chronic%20Kidney%20Disease.pdf (accessed March 2013).

HPA (2012) *Infectious Diseases: primary care guidance*. Health Protection Agency. http://www.hpa.org.uk/Topics/InfectiousDiseases/InfectionsAZ/PrimaryCareGuidance/ (accessed November 2012).

Jenkins, G.W. & Tortora, G.J. (2013) *Anatomy and Physiology*, 3rd edn. John Wiley and Sons, New Jersey.

Jepson, R.G. & Craig, J.C. (2008) Cranberries for preventing urinary tract infections. *Cochrane Database Systematic Reviews*, (1):CD001321.

Kathuria, P. (2013) Chronic Kidney Disease. *emedicinehealth*. http://www.emedicinehealth.com/chronic_kidney_disease/page2_em.htm (accessed 3 April 2013).

KDIGO (2011) *Clinical Practice Guidelines on AKI. Kidney Disease: Improving Global Outcomes*. http://kdigo.org/home/.

LeMone, P., Burke, K. & Bauldoff, G. (2011) *Medical-surgical Nursing: critical thinking in person care*, 4th edn. Prentice Hall, New Jersey.

NICE (2004) *Supportive and Palliative Care*. National Institute for Clinical Excellence, London. http://www.nice.org.uk/csgsp (accessed 6 April 2013).

NICE (2005) *Laparoscopic Nephrectomy (Including Nephroureterectomy) Guidance 136*. National Institute for Health and Clinical Excellence, London.

NICE (2006) *Urinary Incontinence: the management of urinary incontinence in women*. National Institute for Health and Clinical Excellence, London.

NICE (2011) *Peritoneal Dialysis. Peritoneal dialysis in the treatment of stage 5 chronic kidney disease*. National Institute for Health and Clinical Excellence, London. http://www.nice.org.uk/nicemedia/live/13524/58001/58001.pdf (accessed 9 April 2013).

NICE (2012) *Opioids in Palliative Care CG140*. National Institute for Health and Clinical Excellence, London. http://www.nice.org.uk/CG140 (accessed 6 April 2013).

Peate, I., Nair, M., Hemming, L. & Wild, K. (2012) *LeMone and Burke's Adult Nursing: acute and ongoing care*. Pearson Education, Harlow.

Porth, C. (2009) *Pathophysiology: concepts of altered health states*, 9th edn. Lippincott, Philadelphia.

SIGN (2005a) *Management of Transitional Cell Carcinoma of the Bladder*. Scottish Intercollegiate Guidelines Network, Edinburgh.

SIGN (2005b) *Management of Urinary Incontinence in Primary Care*. Scottish Intercollegiate Guidelines Network, Edinburgh.

Silverthorn, D.U. (2009). *Human Physiology: an integrated approach*, 5th edn. Prentice Hall, Englewood Cliffs, NJ.

Test Yourself

1. What part of the kidney filters the blood to produce urine?
   - (a) Ureter
   - (b) Medulla
   - (c) Pyramids
   - (d) Nephrons

2. Which hormone regulates fluid balance in the body?
   - (a) Thyroxine
   - (b) Renin
   - (c) Aldosterone
   - (d) ADH

3. What diagnostic test can be used to determine GFR, as well as glomerular damage?
   - (a) Routine urinalysis
   - (b) Renal scan
   - (c) Creatinine clearance
   - (d) Renal biopsy

4. What gland encircles the male urethra at the base of the bladder?
   - (a) Spleen
   - (b) Pancreas
   - (c) Prostate
   - (d) Adrenal

5. Which of the following terms indicates voiding urine several times in the night?
   - (a) Polyuria
   - (b) Nocturia
   - (c) Dysuria
   - (d) Haematuria

6. Struvite stones are almost always caused by:
   - (a) UTI
   - (b) Eating food containing a high amount of calcium
   - (c) A build-up of uric acid in the blood
   - (d) Taking in food that contains a high amount of cysteine

7. Before beginning the physical assessment of the urinary system, you should ask the person to:
   - (a) Empty the bladder
   - (b) Take several deep breaths
   - (c) Provide a urine specimen
   - (d) Drink several glasses of water.

8. If a patient does not pass urine for 12 hours after surgery, what would you do?
   - (a) Palpate for bladder distention
   - (b) Listen for bowel sounds
   - (c) Give the patient an enema
   - (d) Ask the patient to stand on the cold floor

9. Which is not normally a part of ageing of the urinary system?
   - (a) Increased risk for haematuria
   - (b) Decreased risk for infection
   - (c) Urine that is darker in colour
   - (d) Urinary incontinence

10. What assessment would you use to assess the hydration status of a person?
    - (a) Palpation of the abdomen
    - (b) Palpation for skin turgor
    - (c) Percussion for dullness over bladder
    - (d) Palpation of both kidneys

Answers

1. d
2. d
3. c
4. c
5. b
6. a
7. c
8. a
9. d
10. b

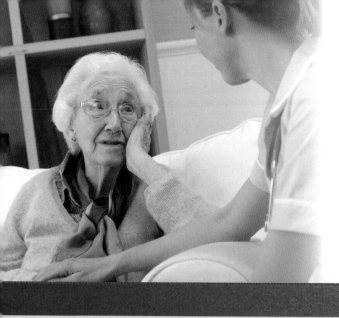

30

The Woman with a Reproductive Disorder

Ian Peate

School of Health Studies, Gibraltar

Learning Outcomes

On completion of this chapter you will be able to:

- Describe the overall functions of the female reproductive system
- Detail the female reproductive organs considering their key functions
- Provide an explanation for the normal and abnormal changes that can occur in the female reproductive system
- Use the nursing process as a framework for care provision
- Identify screening and diagnostic tests
- Understand risk factors for gynaecological cancers and conditions

Competencies

All nurses must:

1. Promote the rights, choices and wishes of all women
2. Work in partnership to address women's needs in all healthcare settings
3. Assess physical and psychological needs
4. Practise in a holistic manner
5. Respect individual choice
6. Support and promote the health, well-being, rights and dignity of women

Visit the companion website at **www.wileynursingpractice.com** where you can test yourself using flashcards, multiple-choice questions and more.

Nursing Practice: Knowledge and Care, First Edition. Edited by Ian Peate, Karen Wild and Muralitharan Nair.
© 2014 John Wiley & Sons, Ltd. Published 2014 by John Wiley & Sons, Ltd. Companion website: www.wileynursingpractice.com

Introduction

One of the unifying characteristics of all living things is the ability to reproduce. The reproductive system is made up of organs involved in the propagation of the species and, for some, the joy of sexual arousal and excitement.

One key aspect of reproductive health, often bound up in the person's attitudes as well as the nurse's attitudes, is the many ways individuals express themselves. Social norms and cultural upbringing can impact (positively and negatively) on a person's reproductive health; sexuality and sexual health are also very closely allied to reproductive health. The nurse must be aware of these issues and their ability to influence a person's reproductive knowledge and also the provision of health care; a sensitive and compassionate approach to care delivery must be employed at all times in all settings.

The physiological and anatomical aspects of the reproductive tract are predominantly associated with procreation; other important issues must also be considered, for example the psychological and social aspects of reproduction, as well as the pleasure often provided by the reproductive organs.

Understanding the anatomical and physiological aspects of this unique system can help you assess and undertake a detailed patient history and recognise normal and abnormal internal and external genitalia. Understanding, developing insight and applying the knowledge gained helps the nurse educate patients about their reproductive systems, provide care that is safe and effective, promote optimum health and function and reduce the transmission of sexually transmitted infections (STI) (see Chapter 32).

This chapter provides an overview of a variety of reproductive-related conditions and their associated nursing care is discussed.

Anatomy and Physiology

Hormones associated with female reproductive organs and the neuroendocrine system are important in biological development as well as sexual behaviour. There are aspects of the female reproductive organs that are related to the function of the urinary system; the urethra and urinary meatus are separated from the reproductive organs but being so close to each other increases health risk, with one often affecting the other.

The female reproductive system is diverse and remarkable:

- It manufactures ova
- It receives the penis and sperm during intercourse
- It is the location where conception occurs
- The embryo during growth is located and housed here, where it is protected and receives nourishment
- After birth, it nourishes the infant.

There are both external and internal structures. The breasts also form part of a women's reproductive organs.

External Genitalia

External structures collectively are called the **vulva**, including the mons pubis, labia, clitoris, vaginal and urethral openings and glands (Figure 30.1).

The *mons pubis* is a pad of adipose tissue covered with skin. The *labia* are divided into two structures:

1. The labia majora – folds of skin and adipose tissue covered with hair; these are outermost, beginning at the base of the mons pubis, ending at the anus
2. The labia minora – between the clitoris and the base of the vagina, enclosed by the labia majora, made of skin and adipose tissue, with some erectile tissue.

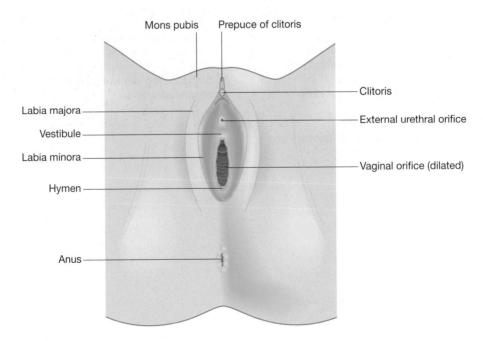

Figure 30.1 The external female genitalia.

Situated between the labia is the *vestibule*, containing the openings for the *vagina*, *urethra* and *Bartholin's glands*. Opening onto the vestibule are the *Skene's glands*. Lubricating fluid is secreted by these glands during sexual response and prior to menopause.

The *clitoris* (analogous to the penis) is an erectile organ, fashioned by the joining of the labia minora. It is highly sensitive, expanding during sexual arousal.

The *vaginal opening* (the introitus), opens between the internal and external genitalia. This is surrounded by the *hymen* (membranous tissue), which partially covers the external vagina.

Internal Organs

The internal structures:

- Vagina
- Cervix
- Uterus
- Fallopian tubes
- Ovaries.

(See Figure 30.2.)

The primary reproductive organs are the ovaries, producing sex hormones. Accessory ducts for the ovaries and developing fetus are the vagina, uterus and fallopian tubes.

Vagina and cervix

Located posterior to the urinary bladder and urethra and anterior to the rectum is the vagina, a fibromuscular tube 8–10 cm in length; the upper end contains the uterine cervix in the fornix. The walls are membranes that form folds (called *rugae*) composed of mucus-secreting stratified squamous epithelial cells. Vaginal secretions include leucorrhoea (white flow). It is odourless or has only a mild odour and is generally milky white in appearance. The vagina is an organ of sexual response and is the passage for the birth of an infant.

The walls are typically moist, maintaining a pH ranging from 3.8 to 4.2, inhibiting bacterial growth, sustained by oestrogen and normal vaginal flora.

The cervix extends into the vagina producing a pathway between the uterus and vagina. The uterine opening of the cervix is the internal os; the vaginal opening is the external os. The space between the endocervical canal provides a route for discharge of menstrual fluid, the entrance for sperm and infant delivery. The cervix is a firm structure, protected by mucus that changes consistency and quantity during the menstrual cycle and pregnancy.

Uterus

The uterus is located in the pelvic cavity. It is a hollow pear-shaped muscular organ with thick walls situated between the bladder and rectum, with three aspects:

1. Fundus
2. Body
3. Cervix.

It is supported in the abdominal cavity by:

- Broad ligaments
- Round ligaments
- Uterosacral ligaments
- Transverse cervical ligaments.

The uterus receives the fertilised ovum and provides a site for fetal growth and development. It has three layers:

1. Perimetrium (outer serous layer merging with the peritoneum)
2. Myometrium (middle layer making up most of the uterine wall)
3. Endometrium lines the uterus; its outermost layer is shed during menstruation.

Fallopian tubes

They are thin cylindrical structures 10 cm long and 1 cm in diameter, connected to the uterus at one end, supported by the broad ligaments. The lateral ends are open and constructed of projections called fimbriae draping over the ovary, picking up the ovum after discharge from the ovary.

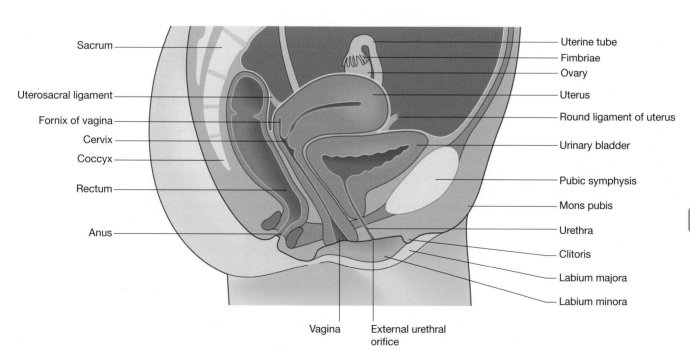

Sacrum

Uterosacral ligament

Fornix of vagina

Cervix

Coccyx

Rectum

Anus

Uterine tube

Fimbriae

Ovary

Uterus

Round ligament of uterus

Urinary bladder

Pubic symphysis

Mons pubis

Urethra

Clitoris

Labium majora

Labium minora

Vagina

External urethral orifice

Figure 30.2 The internal organs of the female reproductive system.

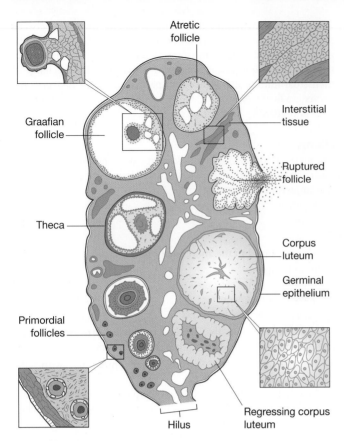

Figure 30.3 The ovaries. Source: Heffner & Schust (2014). Reproduced with permission of John Wiley & Sons Ltd.

The fallopian tubes are made up of smooth muscles lined with ciliated, mucus-producing epithelial cells. As cilia move along with contractions of the smooth muscle, the ovum moves through the tubes toward the uterus. Fertilisation by the sperm typically occurs in the outer portion of a fallopian tube.

Ovaries

These are flat, almond-shaped structures on both sides of the uterus below the ends of the fallopian tubes, connected to the uterus by ligaments. Ovaries store the germ cells, producing oestrogen and progesterone.

Ovarian follicles are contained in the ovaries, each with an immature ovum – *an oocyte*. Each month they are stimulated by follicle-stimulating hormone (FSH) and luteinising hormone (LH) to mature. The developing follicles are enclosed by graafian follicles, producing oestrogen, promoting the development of endometrium. Ovulation occurs monthly. The ruptured follicle becomes the corpus luteum, producing oestrogen and progesterone supporting the endometrium until conception occurs or the cycle recommences. As the corpus luteum degenerates, a scar is left on the outside of the ovary.

See Figure 30.3 for a macroscopic view of the ovaries.

Female Sex Hormones

The ovaries produce oestrogens, progesterone and androgens in a cyclic pattern. Oestrogens, steroid hormones, occur naturally in three forms:

1. Oestrone (E_1)
2. Oestradiol (E_2)
3. Oestriol (E_3).

Oestradiol is produced in the greatest amount. Oestrogens are secreted throughout the menstrual cycle but are highest during particular phases of the cycle.

For development and maintenance of secondary sex characteristics oestrogens are essential and with other hormones, stimulate the female reproductive organs to prepare for the growth of a fetus. Oestrogens are responsible for the structure of skin and blood vessels, decreasing the rate of bone break down, promoting increased high-density lipoproteins, reducing cholesterol levels and enhancing blood clotting. Oestrogens also promote retention of sodium and water.

Menopause is a normal physiological process, as a result of the steady decrease and final cessation of oestrogen. Tissues supported by oestrogen modify as menstruation ends. Oestrogen deficiency increases the danger of osteoporosis and cardiovascular disease.

Progesterone affects the growth of breast glandular tissue and endometrium. Throughout pregnancy, progesterone relaxes smooth muscle, reducing uterine contractions, increasing body temperature.

Oogenesis and the Ovarian Cycle

All of a woman's ova are present at birth as primary oocytes in ovarian follicles. Monthly, from puberty to menopause, the remaining events of oogenesis occur; this is the ovarian cycle. Three consecutive phases happen each 28 days (the cycle can be longer or shorter):

1. Follicular phase from the 1st to 10th day of the cycle
2. Ovulatory phase from the 11th to 14th day of the cycle concluding with ovulation
3. Luteal phase from the 14th to 28th day.

The follicle develops; oocyte maturation is controlled by the interaction of FSH and LH during the follicular phase. On day 1 of the cycle, gonadotropin-releasing hormone (GnRH) increases stimulating increased production of FSH and LH, which stimulates follicular growth and oocyte maturation. The structure, now called the 'primary follicle', becomes a multicellular mass, enclosed by a fibrous capsule, the 'theca folliculi'. As the follicle continues to grow, oestrogen is produced and a fluid-filled space forms inside the follicle. The oocyte is covered by a membrane, the 'zona pellucida'. At about day 10, the follicle is a mature graafian follicle bulging out from the surface of the ovary. Only one follicle becomes dominant and matures to ovulation, others disintegrate.

The ovulatory phase starts when there is enough oestrogen to stimulate the anterior pituitary gland; a rush of LH is produced. The LH stimulates meiosis in the developing oocyte; the first meiotic division happens. LH also stimulates enzymes working on the bulging ovarian wall, causing rupture and discharge. The oocyte is expelled from the mature ovarian follicle during ovulation.

In the luteal phase, the LH stimulates the ruptured follicle to alter into a corpus luteum, stimulating the corpus luteum to produce progesterone and oestrogen immediately. The increase of progesterone and oestrogen has a negative feedback effect on the production of LH, preventing further growth and development of other follicles.

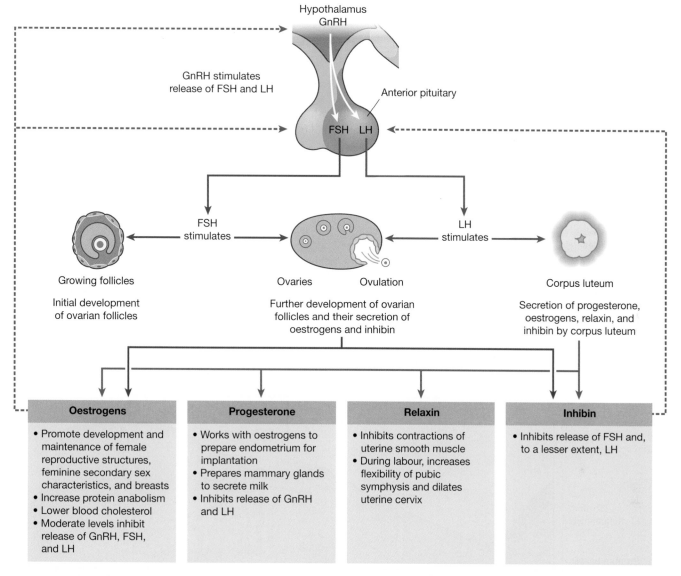

Figure 30.4 Secretion and physiological effects of oestrogen, progesterone, relaxin and inhibin in the female reproductive cycle. Dashed red lines indicate negative feedback inhibition.

If pregnancy does not occur, the corpus luteum degenerates and hormone production ends. The falling production of progesterone and oestrogen at the end of the cycle permits the secretion of LH and FSH to increase; a new cycle commences. See Figure 30.4 for an overview of the secretion and physiological effects of oestrogen, progesterone, relaxin and inhibin in the female reproductive cycle.

Menstrual Cycle
Sometimes called the 'uterine cycle', this describes changes in the endometrium as a result of ovarian hormones (see earlier). The endometrium responds to modification in oestrogen and progesterone during the ovarian cycle, preparing for implantation of the fertilised embryo. The endometrium is amenable to implantation of the embryo for a brief period monthly, coinciding with the time when the embryo would normally reach the uterus from the uterine tube (about 7 days) (Figure 30.5).

The menstrual cycle starts with the menstrual phase, lasting from days 1 to 5. The inner endometrial (functionalis) layer disconnects and is expelled as menstrual fluid for 3–5 days. As the maturing follicle begins to produce oestrogen (days 6–14), the proliferative phase starts. In response, the functionalis layer is repaired and thickens. Cervical mucus transforms to a thin substance, helping sperm travel up into the uterus.

The concluding phase, the secretory phase, lasts from days 14 to 28. As the corpus luteum produces progesterone, increasing levels act on the endometrium, causing increased vascularity, altering the inner layer to secretory mucosa, stimulating the secretion of glycogen into the uterine cavity, causing the cervical mucus to thicken again, blocking the internal os. If fertilisation fails, hormone levels decrease. The endometrial cells begin to disintegrate, sloughing off. The process begins again with the sloughing of the functionalis layer.

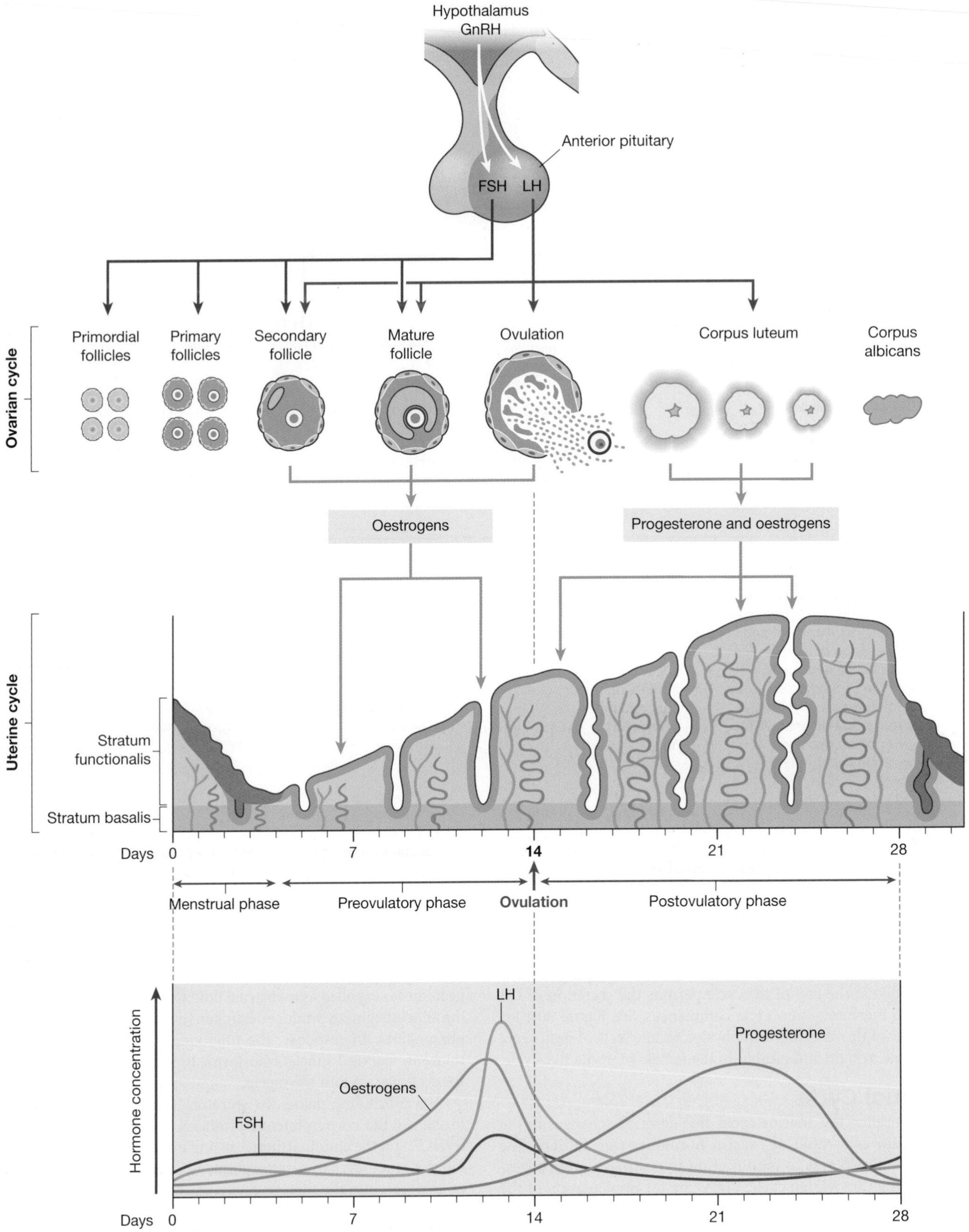

Figure 30.5 **The female reproductive cycle.**

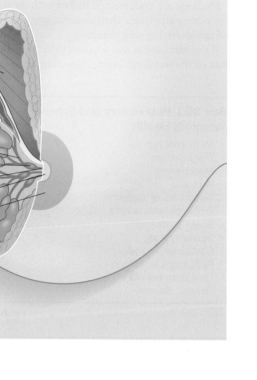

Suspensory ligaments of the breast

Rib

Fascia

Intercostal muscle

Pectoralis major

Lobule containing alveoli

Secondary tubule

Mammary duct

Lactiferous sinus

Lactiferous duct

Nipple

Areola

Adipose tissue in hypodermis

(a)

(b)

Figure 30.6 The breast: (a) sagittal and (b) anterior views.

Breasts

The breasts have an important role to play in sexual health in modern culture as they are visible, and their size and shape can sometimes be seen as a measure of sexuality, attractiveness and femininity. Breasts are a secondary characteristic, meaning reproduction can occur without them.

The breasts are situated between the third and seventh ribs on the anterior chest wall supported by pectoral muscles, supplied with nerves, blood and lymph (Figure 30.6). The areola is positioned underneath the centre of each breast, containing sebaceous glands and a nipple. Usually the nipple protrudes and becomes erect in response to cold and stimulation.

The breasts are composed of adipose tissue, fibrous connective tissue and glandular tissue. Bands of fibrous tissue support the breast and extend from the outer breast tissue to the nipple, separating into 15–25 lobes. Lobes are made of alveolar glands connected by ducts opening to the nipple.

The ability of the nurse to assess the reproductive system with compassion and sensitivity is important to the patient from both physical and psychological perspectives. Understanding the anatomy and physiology can help you provide care that is patient-centred, appropriate and safe.

Assessing the System

Skills of assessment are honed over years of practice; the nurse should demonstrate competence and confidence as well as employing a non-judgemental approach. Assessment is carried out in an environment that enhances patient comfort, cooperation and participation.

Gynaecological examination is not something many women look forward to, but it is a necessity. Some women may feel so intimidated by the prospect, they will delay the examination until something is obviously wrong or avoid the examination altogether, dreading physical discomfort, embarrassment, negative diagnosis or questions and queries about past sexual trauma. The woman should be assured that information provided and results of the examination will remain confidential.

A comprehensive health assessment of the female reproductive system will include gathering subjective and objective data (see Chapter 6). Physical assessment of the reproductive system begins with inspection and palpation of the external genitalia. A speculum is used to visualise the inner vagina and cervix and when collection of specimens is required. The uterus, fallopian tubes and ovaries are palpated during physical assessment.

In addition to gathering data about general health, the nurse needs to ask about past history and experiences specific to the woman's health (see Box 30.1).

What To Do If...

 During the examination the woman says she does not want a male student present? How will you deal with that?

Examination of the Breasts

The gynaecological examination (if appropriate) begins with an examination of the breasts. The aim is to assess breast health, including the breasts' lymphatic system and changes associated with puberty, pregnancy and menopause. The nurse can teach the woman how to breast self-examine if she does not already perform this monthly (see Box 30.2).

Findings are documented in line with local policy and procedure noting all masses, their location, size, shape, texture, mobility and any overlying skin changes.

If the woman has had a mastectomy, perform a routine assessment of the unaffected side, inspecting and palpating the scar as well as surrounding tissue, lymph nodes and axilla for lumps, redness, swelling, tenderness and lesions. For women who have had breast surgery, examine in the same sequence, paying specific attention to scars.

Examining the Genitalia

You may wish to show the woman the speculum or any other equipment to be used for the physical assessment; this may alleviate anxieties. Request she empties her bladder. This promotes comfort and makes the examination easier, as a full bladder can make palpation of the internal organs uncomfortable for the woman and difficult for the nurse; you may need to obtain a urine specimen as part of the total assessment. Ask her to wear a gown (provide privacy) and remove all clothing except for socks or shoes, which can be left on for comfort.

Equipment

The equipment depends on the purpose of the examination. This should be readily available and in the room, so that the examination can proceed smoothly, without unnecessary pauses or interruptions. The equipment cited in Box 30.3 should be available to examine the genitalia.

Position

The woman is usually asked to assume or is helped into the supine lithotomy position. It must be noted that other positions can be used if this is what the woman prefers or what her circumstances dictate.

Box 30.1 Past History and Experiences Specific to the Woman's Health

· Menstrual history
· Pregnancies
· Medications
· Pain with menses
· Symptoms of vaginitis
· Problems with urinary function
· Bowel problems
· Sexual history
· Contraceptive history
· Past surgical history
· Long-term conditions
· Genetic disorders.

Box 30.2 Breast Examination and Assessment

The woman is seated; inspect each breast visually, noting nipple retraction or deviation, skin dimpling, erythema, oedema, peau d'orange (oedema with skin pitting), induration or asymmetry. The woman raises her arms above her head, lowering them and shrugging her shoulders forward, this can bring an otherwise unnoticed abnormality into view. With the woman lying supine with one hand under her head (lifting the breast slightly), palpate the ipsilateral axilla and breast. Palpate in a smooth back-and-forth or circular motion with the palmar surfaces of your three middle fingers, using light and deep palpation. In a systematic manner, palpate first the axilla and then the entire breast lightly, using deeper palpation to assess full tissue thickness. Gently compress each nipple discovering any masses or discharges that are not attributable to pregnancy or postpartum changes (Figure 30.7).

Care, Dignity and Compassion

Intimate examinations can cause intense embarrassment. Being exposed with a variety of people observing can cause excessive stress and anxiety. You can demonstrate that you care, you are compassionate and that you are respecting the person's dignity by acting as advocate and by exposing only those aspects of the anatomy that need to be exposed. Ensure the woman is warm and comfortable and that she is given every opportunity to request that the examination stops if she is unhappy about any elements of it. Ensure privacy, i.e. doors are closed, screens and curtains are effective in providing dignity; only those people absolutely necessary for the examination should be present. Provide an opportunity to have a chaperone.

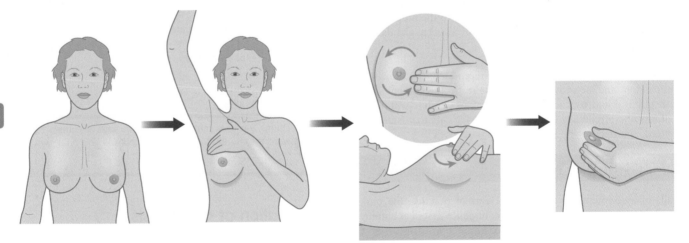

Figure 30.7 Breast self-examination.

Age-related changes

As a part of the normal ageing process, a number of age-related changes occur throughout the woman's body, specifically in response to a decrease in size of the reproductive organs. Reduced oestrogen affects the reproductive system, and neuroendocrinological, biochemical and metabolic changes occur throughout the body (Table 30.1).

Digital bimanual palpation

A bimanual examination completes the pelvic examination. External genitalia are observed noting lumps or ulcers, discolouration or discharge and signs of obvious prolapse. Standing, the nurse uses gloved fingers and a water-soluble lubricant, gently inserting the first two fingers of the dominant hand into the vagina; inside the introitus the fingers are advanced along the vaginal canal vertically and the vaginal wall is palpated. Place the other hand above the symphysis pubis, gently pushing down towards the pelvis. Examine the cervix, uterus and adnexa, noting irregularities, such as masses or abnormal tenderness.

Document all examinations and outcomes according to local policy and procedure. Give the woman clear explanations of any findings and the proposed next stages of care and treatment.

It is unwise to base treatment decisions on one diagnostic approach (i.e. digital bimanual examination). Abnormal findings should always be followed up using further assessment involving other assessment or screening techniques.

Primary Care Developing a High-Quality Hysterectomy Service

Delivering a hysterectomy service for the care of women with heavy menstrual bleeding (HMB) should be carried out in a number of different ways; mixed models of provision may be appropriate. There is an emphasis on integrated care, direct access to some procedures and consultant gynaecologists working in primary care.

Service specification needs to consider:
· Required competencies of and training for staff
· Expected number of patients
· Ease of access to all treatment options and service location within a geographical area
· Care and referral pathways to support patient choice of treatment and access
· Service monitoring criteria.

Nursing Field Learning disabilities

Women with learning disabilities are living longer and fuller lives and should have access to breast and cervical screening on the same basis as other women. Screening programmes have to ensure that women have access to information about screening, presented in a way which they can understand, and that staff in the screening programmes adopt good practice to enable women who choose to attend for screening to be screened successfully.

Link To/Go To

The move to care closer to home identifies innovative ways of delivering gynaecology services in primary care, while improving patient access.

http://webarchive.nationalarchives.gov.uk/+/www.dh.gov.uk/en/publicationsandstatistics/Publications/PublicationsPolicyandGuidance/DH_079728

Box 30.3 Equipment Required for Genital Examination

· Light source
· Vaginal speculae
· Alcoholic hand rub
· Disposable examination gloves
· Lubricant
· Various types of sampling devices (i.e. wooden, plastic spatula, cytobrush, cervix brush)
· Glass slides, slide container
· Pencil for labelling slides
· Fixative solution
· Specimen forms and bag
· Tissue paper
· Clinical waste container.

Table 30.1 Some changes associated with ageing and the reproductive system.

CHANGES TO STRUCTURE	CHANGES IN FUNCTION	PHYSICAL IMPACT
Ovarian function ceases	Decreased ovulation	Infertility increases
Decreased oestrogen production	Menopause begins	Ability to conceive decreases or is absent
Urinary and genital tracts become thinner	Hormonal fluctuation and vasomotor instability	Menses become erratic with eventual cessation
Pubic hair thins out	Bone formation decreases and disturbed homeostasis	Night sweats, hot flushes and flashes, sleep disturbance, fatigue, mood swings
Labia shrink	Vaginal secretion/lubrication decreases	Risk of osteoporosis as a result of bone loss, osteopathic fractures and height loss
Pelvic musculature relaxes	Vaginal pH alters (decreases)	Dyspareunia can result in loss of libido and lack of interest in sex
	Uterine prolapse	Increased risk for urinary tract infection
	Cystocele	Vaginitis, itching, discharge, vulval burning
	Rectocele	Dyspareunia
		Incontinence
		Feeling of pressure in perineal region

Table 30.2 Common menstrual terms and descriptions.

TERM/SYMPTOM	DEFINITION	DESCRIPTION
Menarche	Age when periods commenced	Average age 12 years, may be later if malnourished
Amenorrhoea	Absence of menses (usually 6 months or more)	Requires investigation
Primary amenorrhoea	No periods by age of 16 years	Requires investigation
Secondary amenorrhoea	No periods for 3 months or more in a woman who has regularly menstruated previously	Exclude pregnancy, sometimes resumes spontaneously, may require investigation
Oligomenorrhoea (or hypomenorrhoea)	Periods occurring at intervals longer than 35 days and/or being especially light	As above
Menorrhagia	Heavy menstrual bleeding at regular intervals	Investigate if impacting on quality of life
Metrorrhagia	Irregularly timed menstrual bleeding	As above
Hypermenorrhoea (or flooding)	Episodes of heavy menstrual bleeding	May cause acute embarrassment, soiling of bedding, chairs, clothing
Dysmenorrhoea	Painful menstrual bleeding prior to or during the period	Commonly experienced in lower abdomen, back or upper thighs
Perimenopause	Around menopause when periods become erratic with menopausal symptoms	Can last between 2 and 5 years
Postmenopausal bleeding	Spontaneous vaginal bleeding occurring more than 1 year after final menstrual period	Urgent investigation required

Abnormal Menstrual Bleeding

There are a number of causes of dysfunctional uterine bleeding and in order to understand abnormal menstrual bleeding, you must know about normal menstruation (discussed earlier). Table 30.2 provides an overview of common menstrual terms.

Pitkin (2007) defines dysfunctional uterine bleeding (DUB) as abnormal uterine bleeding in the absence of organic disease. Usually presenting as heavy menstrual bleeding (menorrhagia), the diagnosis can only be made when all other causes for abnormal or heavy uterine bleeding have been eliminated. The National Institute for Health and Clinical Excellence (NICE) (2007a) defines heavy menstrual bleeding as:

excessive menstrual blood loss which interferes with the woman's physical, emotional, social and material quality of life, and which can occur alone or in a combination with other symptoms.

Pathophysiology

The pathophysiology is largely unknown. Marjoribanks *et al.* (2006) reported that 80% of women treated for heavy menstrual bleeding have no anatomical pathology. Menorrhagia occurs when total menstrual blood loss is more than 80 mL per menstruation.

Other causes of heavy menstrual bleeding include:

- *Uterine pathology and lesions*: polyps, fibroids, carcinoma, infection – including pelvic inflammatory disease (PID), endometriosis
- *Systemic disease*: hypothyroidism, liver disease, obesity, polycystic ovarian syndrome (PCOS), haematological disorders
- *Iatrogenic causes*: intrauterine device, anticoagulant treatment, oral injectable steroids for contraception or hormone replacement, tranquillisers or other psychotropic drugs.

DUB is more common around the menarche and perimenopause. How heavy menstrual bleeding is perceived is subjective – 30% of women think their bleeding is excessive. Approximately 50% of women complaining of heavy menstrual bleeding match the clinical criterion (more than 80 mL blood loss per cycle). The nurse can help women provide a more objective assessment of blood loss by using a pictorial blood loss assessment chart.

It is estimated that of those women aged 30–49, one in 20 will consult her GP each year with menorrhagia (Pitkin 2007). Lethaby *et al.* (2008) suggest that heavy menstrual bleeding accounts for 12% of all gynaecology referrals in the UK. Approximately £7 million is spent each year in the UK on prescriptions in primary care settings to treat menorrhagia (Pitkin 2007).

Signs and symptoms

An in-depth history is taken in order to ascertain the signs and symptoms; the following should be considered:

- Menstrual history: cycle length, number of bleeding days, intermenstrual or post-coital bleeding, amount of blood loss, passage of clots; pain associated with bleeding
- Contraception: current method; need
- Symptoms suggesting an underlying pathology:
  - Metabolic disorders: symptoms suggesting PCOS and hypothyroidism.
  - Haematological disorders: excessive bleeding postpartum or tooth extraction, easy bruising
  - PID/infection: pelvic pain, dyspareunia, vaginal discharge
  - Endometriosis: pelvic pain, dysmenorrhoea
  - Post-coital and intermenstrual bleeding can suggest pelvic pathology.

Age is the most important factor in the assessment; the nurse should aim to rule out any pregnancy-related complications.

Examination

When carrying out an examination, look for the following:

- Signs of underlying pathology: bruising, typical hypothyroid features, features of PCOS (hirsutism, acne, overweight), pallor, koilonychias (spoon-shaped fingernails with longitudinal ridging)

- Abdominal examination: there may be tenderness, palpable masses (uterine, ovarian)
- Pelvic examination: vulval inspection, speculum examination, bimanual palpation for masses
- Cervical smear: if appropriate
- Infection screening: high vaginal and endocervical swabs as appropriate.

What To Do If...

 During the examination you notice an extensive amount of bruising to the woman's upper thighs and across her breasts. It looks as though she had been attacked. What should you do?

Investigations and diagnosis

The in-depth history helps make a definitive diagnosis. The nurse should enquire about the use of medications, ruling out their interference with normal menstruation. The physical examination may reveal an underlying systematic disorder. Genitourinary or gastrointestinal bleeding, for example from urinary tract infection or haemorrhoids, can be mistakenly interpreted by the woman as vaginal bleeding.

Manual pelvic examination can reveal an obviously abnormal structural irregularity, for example a cervical polyp.

NICE (2007a) suggests that every woman presenting with heavy menstrual bleeding should have a full blood count taken. Serum ferritin, female hormone testing and thyroid testing are not routinely recommended and should only be carried out if there is strong clinical suspicion of underlying pathology.

Endometrial biopsy (in non-pregnant women) or hysteroscopy can provide further information that helps make a detailed assessment of the uterus. If the cause of bleeding cannot be confirmed, a pelvic ultrasound may be required as this may help to diagnose structural abnormalities and endometrial thickness.

Nursing care and management

There are complications of dysfunctional uterine bleeding the nurse needs to be aware of, including:

- The presence of iron deficiency anaemia
- Psychological sequelae, e.g. depression, embarrassment
- Social implications: cost of pads and tampons, time off work.

Most women with abnormal vaginal bleeding can be successfully treated using a medical approach, especially when there is an absence of a structural lesion (Norwitz & Schorge 2010). Pitkin (2007) and Lethaby et al. (2008) suggest that treatments should be considered in the following order:

- First-line: levonorgestrel-releasing intrauterine system provides long-term use (at least 12 months is expected)
- Second-line: tranexamic acid or non-steroidal anti-inflammatory drugs (NSAIDs) or combined oral contraceptive pills (COCPs)
- Third-line: norethisterone (15 mg) daily from days 5 to 26 of the menstrual cycle, or injected long-acting progestogens.

If the hormonal treatments are unacceptable, either tranexamic acid or NSAIDs may be used.

1. *Levonorgestrel-releasing intrauterine system (LNG-IUS)* – Avoids endometrial proliferation, also acts as a contraceptive. LNG-IUS does not affect future fertility. There are some unwanted outcomes, including irregular bleeding that may continue for 6 months; amenorrhoea; progestogen-related problems, for example, breast tenderness, acne and headaches; uterine perforation at insertion (1 in 100 000 chance).

LNG-IUS is equally effective in improving quality of life and psychological well-being as hysterectomy (Hurskainen et al. 2001; Lethaby et al. 2008)

2. *Tranexamic acid* – An oral antifibrinolytic. If no improvement, stop after three cycles. Tranexamic acid can be used when the women is undergoing other investigations; it is not a contraceptive.

3. *NSAIDs* – Mefenamic acid is a commonly used NSAID. This is given orally, reducing the production of prostaglandin. If there is no improvement, stop after three cycles. It is preferred over tranexamic acid in dysmenorrhoea. The medication is not a contraceptive.

What To Do If...

 When about to administer the prescribed dose of mefenamic acid to the patient, she informs you that she vomited yesterday and it looked like there was blood in it. What should you do?

4. *COCPs* – Prevent proliferation of the endometrium, act as a contraceptive and do not impact on future fertility. There are some unwanted outcomes, for example mood change, headache, nausea, fluid retention, breast tenderness, deep vein thrombosis, myocardial infarction, cerebrovascular event

5. *Oral progestogen (norethisterone)* – Prevents proliferation of the endometrium and acts as a contraceptive, does not impact future fertility. Lethaby et al. (2008) demonstrated that progestogen results in a significant reduction in menstrual blood loss, however women find the treatment less acceptable than intrauterine levonorgestrel

6. *Injected progestogen (depot-medroxyprogesterone acetate)* – Prevents proliferation of the endometrium and acts as a contraceptive, will not impact on future fertility. Unwanted outcomes include weight gain, irregular bleeding, amenorrhoea, bloating, fluid retention, breast tenderness, bone density loss.

As there is a potential for bone density loss, depot-medroxyprogesterone acetate should only be used in adolescents if other treatments for heavy menstrual bleeding are unsuitable, ineffective or unacceptable. In all women, careful re-evaluation of the risks and benefits should be carried out at 2 years. If there are significant risk factors for osteoporosis, other treatment for heavy menstrual bleeding should be considered first.

Red Flag

 Symptoms develop suddenly in an upper gastrointestinal bleed. Some medications can cause a gastrointestinal bleed, with:

- Vomiting blood – can appear bright red or have a dark brown, grainy appearance similar to coffee grounds
- Passing black tar-like stools
- A sudden, sharp pain in the stomach getting steadily worse and not improving.

Surgical management of abnormal menstrual bleeding

Structural abnormalities often require surgical intervention to alleviate symptoms; this should only be considered if:

- Pharmacological management failed
- Severe impact on quality of life
- The woman has no desire to conceive
- The uterus is normal (or there are just small fibroids less than 3 cm).

Dilation and curettage Can help provide a diagnosis as well as being therapeutic, particularly in women with acute vaginal bleeding as a result of endometrial overgrowth.

Endometrial ablation Can dramatically reduce the amount of cyclic blood loss.

- Impedance-controlled bipolar radiofrequency ablation (bipolar radiofrequency electrode placed through the cervix and radiofrequency energy delivered to the uterus)
- Balloon thermal ablation (balloon is inserted through cervix to the endometrial cavity, inflated with a pressurised solution and heated to destroy the endometrium)
- Microwave ablation (microwave probe inserted into the uterine cavity heats the endometrium, moved side-to-side to destroy it)
- Free fluid thermal ablation (destroying endometrium by instilling heated saline solution into the uterus under hysteroscopic visualisation)
- Rollerball ablation (a current is passed through a rollerball electrode and moved around the endometrium)
- Transcervical resection of the endometrium (endometrial lining and small fibroids removed using a cutting loop).

  Some of the complications are:

- Vaginal discharge
- Increased period pain even if no further bleeding
- Need for additional surgery
- Infection, rarely perforation
- Rarely perforation.

  Contraception after endometrial ablation should still be advised even though fertility is usually not retained.

Hysterectomy Hysterectomy should not be used as first-line surgical management for DUB; this is usually reserved for women with structural lesions not responding to medical treatment.

- Should only be considered when:
  - Other treatments have failed, are contraindicated or the woman has declined them
  - There is a wish for amenorrhoea
  - The woman requests it
  - No desire to retain the uterus and fertility
- First-line is vaginal hysterectomy, second-line is abdominal hysterectomy
- Healthy ovaries should not be removed.

  There are potential adverse outcomes:

- Infection
- Intraoperative haemorrhage
- Damage to other organs (urinary tract and bowel)
- Urinary dysfunction
- Thrombosis
- Menopausal-like symptoms if ovaries are removed.

The Menopause

The menopause is defined as the cessation of menstruation for 12 months, usually occurring around the age of 50 years (Norwitz & Schorge 2010) and marking the end of a woman's reproductive capacity. With menopause the ovaries are no longer active and reproductive organs become smaller; this is not a pathological occurrence, it is part of the normal ageing process. Ovarian follicular development ceases, a finite number of ovarian follicles are depleted and gonadotrophin (follicle stimulating hormone, luteinising hormone) levels increase (Nelson 2008).

Climacteric (peri-menopause)

The climacteric, the menopausal transition stage, or peri-menopause, is the period of change leading up to the last period. It is a retrospective diagnosis from the time when menstruation stops permanently and can only be defined with confidence 12 months after spontaneous amenorrhoea.

Premature menopause (happening before 40 years) can occur in primary ovarian failure, surgically-induced menopause (hysterectomy with or without bilateral oophorectomy), radiation-induced menopause and chemotherapy-induced menopause.

The signs and symptoms of the menopause can begin as early as 35 years of age; however it usually occurs during the woman's late 40s. The duration of peri-menopause with obvious bodily effects can range from a few years to 10 years or longer. The final menstrual period usually occurs between the ages of 40 and 58. The average age of menopause is 52 years (Nelson 2008).

Smoking and low socioeconomic factors are identified as being linked with premature menopause. Hefler *et al.* (2006) have identified other factors affecting the age at which a woman can have her final period, including:

- Age at menarche
- Parity
- Previous oral contraceptive history
- Body mass index (BMI)
- Ethnicity
- Family history
- Breast surgery.

  Most women do not seek medical advice for menopausal symptoms. Differences in consultation patterns for menopause are dependent on several factors, including cultural and educational differences and also psychosocial difficulties.

Signs and symptoms

Nelson (2008) notes that epidemiological studies have identified only vasomotor dysfunction and vaginal dryness as being consistently linked with the menopausal phase. Other common symptoms:

- Mood changes
- Sleep disturbances
- Urinary incontinence
- Cognitive changes
- Somatic complaints
- Sexual dysfunction.

Menstrual irregularity Menstrual irregularity can last up to 4 years. The cycle can lengthen to many months or shorten to 2–3 weeks; a small increase in the amount of menstrual blood loss is usual. Three consecutive months of amenorrhoea, or mean cycle lengths longer than 42 days, are predictors of impending menopause (Nelson 2008).

Hot flushes and sweats The hallmarks of menopause are symptoms associated with hot flushes and sweats. Hot flushes usually affect the face, head, neck and chest, lasting a few minutes. Norwitz and Schorge (2010) suggest that 70% of peri-menopausal women experience hot flushes. Hot flushes can make the woman feel weak and break out in heavy sweating.

The Evidence

A meta-analysis suggested that in an average woman, vasomotor symptoms intensify from 2 years preceding the final menstrual period, peaking at 1 year after it and returning to normal after 8 years. There is much variation between individual women.

(Polit *et al.* 2008)

Urinary and vaginal symptoms These can include dyspareunia, vaginal discomfort and dryness, persistent lower urinary tract infection and urinary incontinence. It is the low oestrogen levels that cause vaginal discomfort but the connection with urinary incontinence has less of an evidence-base (Van Voorhis 2005).

Sleep disturbance Young *et al.* (2003) conducted a study concerning quality of sleep in menopausal women, noting that it is a common subjective symptom but not one established by polysomnography (a sleep test). Symptoms experienced may be secondary to vasomotor symptoms, are made worse by psychosocial factors and can contribute to depression, irritability and poor concentration.

Mood changes These include anxiety, nervousness, irritability, memory loss, depression and difficulty concentrating. DiDonato *et al.* (2005) suggest that the tendency to develop psychological symptoms have associations with level of education, high BMI and low physical activity.

Loss of libido This can be caused by a variety of hormonal factors with oestrogen, progesterone and testosterone all implicated. Vaginal dryness, performance of an ageing partner, loss of self-image and other psychosocial factors can also play a part.

Other changes As oestrogen levels fall, the following can occur:
- Nails become brittle
- Thinning of skin
- Hair loss
- Widespread aches and pains.

Investigations and diagnosis

A detailed history is required to make a definitive diagnosis; the age of the woman is also taken into account. A number of investigations will be required to help confirm diagnosis and rule out other potential causes.

There is no definitive test to diagnose the menopause; a blood test measuring the level of follicle-stimulating hormone (FSH) may sometimes be recommended. This measures levels of FSH. When oestrogen levels start dropping, the pituitary gland releases more

---

Box 30.4 Some Myths Associated with the Menopause

You cannot get pregnant after menopause – FALSE
- Pregnancy can and does happen. Contraception should still be used for 2 years after the last period if under 50 and for 1 year if over 50.

You are going to put on weight – FALSE
- There is no evidence that middle-age spread is the result of menopause. This is often linked to the hormonal changes at this time of life.

Your menopause will be difficult because your mum's was – FALSE
- The age at which the woman's mother experienced the menopause may predict when the woman is expected to experience symptoms. No evidence suggests that the mother's and daughter's menopause symptoms will be the same.

FSH, encouraging more oestrogen production in the ovaries. An elevated FSH may indicate menopause.

FSH levels vary during the perimenopause; a single measure is unreliable. FSH levels may be helpful in confirming the menopause in later stages. Those women with suspected premature menopause, for example those who have symptoms under the age of 40 years or those who have had a hysterectomy with conservation of the ovaries, should have serial FSH levels taken because of the implications of premature ovarian failure.

FSH levels should be tested when the woman is not taking oestrogen-based contraception or hormone replacement therapy (HRT).

FSH levels greater than 30 IU/L are considered to be in the postmenopausal range; estimates should be repeated in 4–8 weeks to confirm this. Levels above 12 IU/L are considered to be raised in women who are still having menstrual bleeds.

Thyroid function tests help in differentiating thyroid disease symptoms from menopausal symptoms.

Nursing care and management

The nurse should approach issues concerned with the menopause as part of a normal period of physiological adaptation, expressing this as a usual aspect of the ageing process. Offering reassurance and support is required and dispelling myths can help. Box 30.4 outlines some myths associated with the menopause.

Encourage a healthy lifestyle. Daley *et al.* (2009) suggests regular sustained aerobic exercise improves vasomotor and other menopausal symptoms, although the evidence is limited. Engaging in exercise can improve quality of life and symptoms such as mood and insomnia as well as providing cardiovascular and other benefits.

 Link To/Go To

Infrequent high-impact exercise can aggravate symptoms but low-intensity exercise, such as yoga, may help.

http://www.rcog.org.uk/files/rcog-corp/SAC%20Paper%20
6%20Alternatives%20to%20HRT.pdf

By identifying the woman's most troublesome symptoms, the nurse can discuss management options with her.

Vasomotor symptoms Hormone replacement therapy (HRT) is unquestionably the most effective form of treatment. Progestogens alone are not recommended as a substitute where combined HRT is contraindicated; progestogens may contribute to increased risk of breast cancer; the doses required to control vasomotor symptoms could increase risk of venous thromboembolism (RCOG 2010).

Red Flag

In some cases of deep vein thrombosis, there may be no symptoms but possible symptoms are:

- Pain, swelling, tenderness in one of the legs (usually the calf)
- Heavy ache in the affected area
- Warm skin in the area of the clot
- Redness of skin, particularly on the back of the leg, below the knee

Treatment for vasomotor symptoms with HRT is usually needed for 2–3 years. Some women require longer. Each woman is assessed individually. The nurse should inform the woman that for a short time after stopping HRT, symptoms might recur.

Sievert *et al.* (2006) suggests avoiding or reducing alcohol and caffeine can relieve vasomotor symptoms.

Urinary and vaginal symptoms Standard and topical HRT work well for menopausal atrophic vaginitis. Topical HRT should be used in the smallest effective dose to reduce systemic side-effects, in short courses, which may be repeated. This must be reviewed regularly (BMA & RPSGB 2012).

The nurse can suggest the use of lubricants (particularly during intercourse). Vaginal moisturisers (these have a longer duration of action) are available without prescription.

Sleep or mood disturbances HRT may be used if these symptoms are caused by hot flushes and night sweats. Selective serotonin reuptake inhibitors or serotonin norepinephrine reuptake inhibitors should be considered as an alternative or in addition to HRT.

Loss of libido The British Menopause Society (BMS 2008) suggests that where libido is reduced or lost, testosterone (patches and implants) helps to improve sexual desire.

Disorders of the Female Reproductive System

The following section provides an overview of some disorders of the female reproductive system. In association with this chapter, gynaecological texts should be consulted for further and detailed information.

Pelvic Organ Prolapse

Pelvic organ prolapse (genitourinary prolapse) occurs when one or more pelvic organs descends through the pelvic floor into the vaginal canal, for example:

- Uterus
- Rectum
- Bowel (small or large)
- Vaginal vault.

When pelvic organ prolapse occurs, this is often accompanied by urinary, bowel, sexual or local pelvic symptoms. The nurse needs to understand the pathophysiological and psychological issues that are at play.

Pathophysiology

The levator ani muscles and the endopelvic fascia (connective tissue network connecting organs to pelvic muscles and bones) provide most support to the pelvic organs (see Figure 30.8 for the muscles of the female pelvic floor).

Prolapse happens when the support structure is weakened; this may be due to direct muscle trauma, neuropathic injury, disruption or stretching. There are many potential causes.

The location and shape of the bones of the pelvis have also been connected to the pathogenesis of pelvic organ prolapse.

Known risk factors

- Age: risk doubles with each decade of life
- Vaginal delivery
- Increasing parity
- Overweight and obesity
- Spina bifida.

Potential risk factors

- Intrapartum variables
  - Fetal macrosomia (newborn with an excess birth weight)
  - Prolonged second stage of labour
  - Episiotomy
  - Anal sphincter injury
  - Epidural anaesthesia
  - Forceps delivery
  - Use of oxytocin
  - Younger than 25 years at first delivery
- Ethnicity
- Family history of prolapse
- Constipation
- Connective tissue disorders such as Marfan's syndrome
- Previous hysterectomy
- Menopause
- Occupations involving heavy lifting.

It is difficult to determine the incidence of genital prolapse, as a number of women choose not to seek medical advice. In most women, it is acknowledged there is some loss of uterovaginal support, but there is no consensus concerning the level of loss, what is normal and abnormal.

Types of pelvic organ prolapse

Prolapse can occur in the anterior, middle or posterior compartment of the pelvis (Table 30.3). Figure 30.9 provides a diagrammatic representation of the types of prolapse.

Cystourethrocele is the most common type of prolapse, followed by uterine prolapse and rectocele. Urethroceles are rare.

Classification of pelvic organ prolapse

Degree of uterine descent can be graded as:

- 1st degree: cervix observable when the perineum is depressed, prolapse contained within the vagina

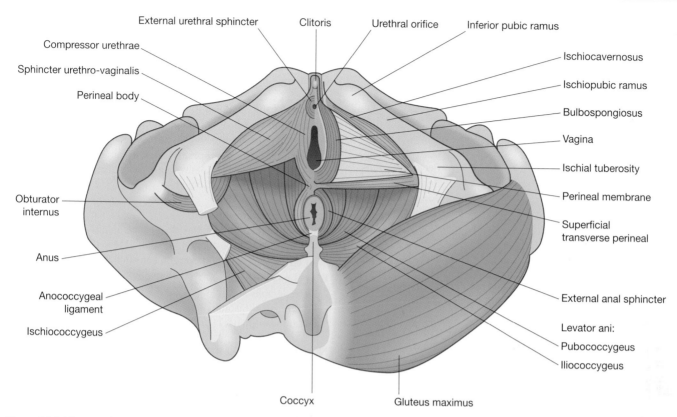

Figure 30.8 **The muscles of the female pelvic floor.**

Table 30.3 **Types of prolapse.** (*Source*: Adapted from Norwitz & Schorge 2010; Thakar & Stanton 2002)

ANTERIOR COMPARTMENT	MIDDLE COMPARTMENT	POSTERIOR COMPARTMENT
Urethrocele: prolapse of urethra into the vagina. Often associated with urinary stress incontinence.	**Uterine prolapse**: descent of uterus into the vagina.	**Rectocele**: prolapse of rectum into the vagina.
Cystocele: prolapse of bladder into the vagina. An isolated cystocele seldom causes incontinence and leads to few or no symptoms. A large cystocele may cause increased urinary frequency, frequent urinary infections and a pressure sensation or mass at the introitus.	**Vaginal vault prolapse**: descent of vaginal vault post-hysterectomy. Usually associated with cystocele, rectocele and enterocele. With complete inversion, the urethra, bladder, and distal ureters may be included.	
Cystourethrocele: prolapse of urethra and bladder.	**Enterocele**: herniation of the pouch of Douglas (including small intestine/omentum) into the vagina. Can occur following pelvic surgery.	

- 2nd degree: cervix prolapsed through the introitus with the fundus remaining in the pelvis
- 3rd degree: procidentia (complete prolapse). Entire uterus is outside the introitus.

Signs and symptoms

Genital prolapse may be an incidental finding as symptoms are generally asymptomatic, or may be mild. In some women, symptoms can have a severe impact on quality of life. The most troublesome symptom is bulging at the vaginal introitus. As a result of gravity, some women experience minimal symptoms in the morning but as the day goes on, symptoms may increase.

Symptoms are related to the site and type of prolapse. Vaginal/general symptoms can be common to all kinds of prolapse.

Vaginal/general symptoms
- Sensation of pressure, fullness or heaviness
- Sensation of a bulge/protrusion or 'something coming down'
- Noticing or feeling a bulge/protrusion
- Difficulty retaining tampons
- Spotting (when there is ulceration of the prolapse).

Urinary symptoms
- Incontinence
- Frequency

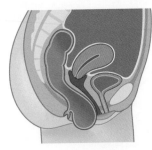

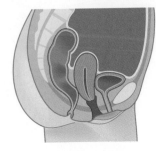

Cystocele

Rectocele

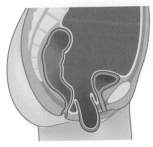

Vaginal vault
prolapse with
enterocele

Uterine prolapse

Figure 30.9 Types of prolapse.

- Urgency
- Feeling of incomplete bladder emptying
- Weak or prolonged urinary stream
- Need to reduce the prolapse manually before voiding
- Need to change position to start or complete voiding.

Sex difficulties
- Dyspareunia
- Loss of vaginal sensation
- Vaginal flatus.

Bowel symptoms
- Constipation/straining
- Urgency of stool
- Incontinence of stool, flatus
- Incomplete or feeling of incomplete evacuation
- Need to apply digital pressure to the perineum or posterior vaginal wall to enable defaecation (known as splinting)
- Digital evacuation to pass a stool.

Investigations and diagnosis
Every woman should be treated as an individual and assessed to determine the nature, severity and progression of symptoms and any current medical conditions, previous obstetric history and past and current medications.

Examination Taking a detailed holistic history is needed to ascertain the woman's main symptoms and the effect of these on her ability to perform the activities of living.

The woman should be examined in a standing position and also in the left lateral position. A speculum will be required so as to

assess the woman completely. She should be given clear explanations of what the examination entails. The nurse supports the women before, during and after the procedure.

A rectal examination can be helpful if there are bowel symptoms.

Investigations A diagnosis is made based upon the clinical examination and history. If the woman is experiencing urinary symptoms, consider the following:
- Urinalysis, and if appropriate a mid-stream specimen of urine
- Post-void residual urine volume testing using a catheter or bladder
- Ultrasound scan
- Urodynamic investigations
- Urea and creatinine
- Renal ultrasound scan.
  If bowel symptoms are present, consider the following:
- Anal manometry
- Defecography
- Endo-anal ultrasound scan (identifies anal sphincter defect if faecal incontinence).

Nursing care and management
Doshani *et al.* (2007) suggests that no treatment is necessary if incidental asymptomatic mild prolapse is found; Norwitz and Schorge (2010) advocate treatment is appropriate only when symptoms warrant it. Opinion concerning where or how to treat women with prolapse is varied, with no consensus (Doshani *et al.* 2007). The woman should be provided with as much information as she needs, in a format she understands to enable her to make an informed decision.

The current management options for women with symptomatic genitourinary prolapse include:

Watchful waiting If the woman reports little in the way of symptoms, watchful waiting may be the most appropriate approach. The woman should be observed for the development of new symptoms and provided with information as to what she needs to do should new symptoms develop.

> ### Jot This Down
> How do you think a woman may feel if she has been told that a part of her treatment will be to wait and see if any further symptoms develop? What impact might this have on her psychologically and physically? How might you help her?

Treatment may be needed if there is evidence of obstructed defaecation or urination, the presence of hydronephrosis or if vaginal erosions develop. All decisions will be made in conjunction with the woman's wishes and individual needs. Jelovsek *et al.* (2007) consider conservative treatment options including:
- Lifestyle modification: treatment of cough, smoking cessation, constipation, overweight and obesity
- Pelvic floor muscle exercises: Hagen *et al.* (2006) have concluded there is no definite evidence to support the benefit of pelvic floor muscle exercises in the management of uterine prolapse.

Vaginal pessary insertion Pessaries can be used as an alternative to surgery (Norwitz & Schorge 2010). Inserted into the vagina a pessary reduces the prolapse, provides support and relieves bladder and bowel pressure. Pessaries are made of silicone or plastic. A ring pessary is normally the first choice. There is little definite evidence supporting the use of pessaries; current opinion is that pessaries are effective for short-term relief of prolapse prior to surgery and in the long term if surgery is not wanted or contraindicated (Clemons *et al.* 2004).

Red Flag

When inserting a pessary:
- Bladder and bowel are emptied prior to fitting
- A bimanual examination is performed assessing the size of the vagina
- The largest possible pessary should be fitted
- If a finger can be swept between the pessary and the walls of the vagina, this is a good fit.

Surgery Surgery is indicated when a pessary is not effective, the woman requests definitive treatment or if the prolapse is combined with urinary or faecal incontinence.

The risks of surgery for some women, even for advanced prolapse, may not be warranted. Urinary incontinence can be caused by surgery and some procedures may result in a prolapse in another compartment. Choice of procedure depends on whether the woman is sexually active, the fitness of the patient and the surgeon's preference. If the prolapse remains corrected and the patient conceives, an elective caesarean section should be advised.

The nurse should advise women they should avoid heavy lifting after surgery and avoid sexual intercourse for 6–8 weeks (Thakar & Stanton 2002).

There are a number of surgical options for genitourinary prolapse, see Table 30.4.

Link To/Go To

The following websites provide more detail concerning genitourinary prolapse:

http://www.nice.org.uk/Guidance/IPG283

http://www.nice.org.uk/nicemedia/live/11002/30404/30404.pdf

Complications and prognosis

- Ulceration and infection of organs prolapsed outside the vaginal introitus
- Stress incontinence
- Chronic retention and overflow incontinence
- Recurrent urinary tract infections
- Bowel dysfunction (with rectocele).

Left untreated, uterine prolapse will gradually worsen. Younger women in good health and a body mass index within normal limits have a better prognosis. Poorer prognosis is associated with older

Table 30.4 Some surgical options for genitourinary prolapse. (*Source*: Adapted from Thakar & Stanton 2002; RCOG 2007; NICE 2007b)

Bladder/urethral prolapse	**Anterior colporrhaphy:** involves central plication (reducing the structure by taking in folds) of the fibromuscular layer of the anterior vaginal wall. Mesh reinforcement may be used. Performed transvaginally. **Colposuspension:** performed for urethral sphincter incontinence associated with a cystourethrocele.
Surgery for uterine prolapse	**Hysterectomy:** vaginal hysterectomy has the advantage that no abdominal incision is needed, pain and hospital stay are reduced. Can be combined with anterior or posterior colporrhaphy. **Open abdominal or laparoscopic sacrohysteropexy:** performed if the woman wishes to retain her uterus. The uterus is attached to the anterior longitudinal ligament over the sacrum. Mesh holds the uterus in place. **Sacrospinous fixation:** unilateral or bilateral fixation of the uterus to the sacrospinous ligament. Performed vaginally. Risk of injury to pudendal nerve and vessels and sciatic nerve.
Surgery for vault prolapse	**Sacrospinous fixation:** unilateral or bilateral fixation of the vault to the sacrospinous ligament. Performed vaginally. Risk of injury to the pudendal nerve and vessels and sciatic nerve. **Laparoscopic or open abdominal mesh sacrocolpopexy:** mesh is attached at one end to the longitudinal ligament of the sacrum and at the other to the top of the vagina and down the posterior and/or anterior vaginal walls
Surgery for rectocele/enterocele	**Posterior colporrhaphy:** involves levator ani muscle plication or repair of discrete fascial defects. Mesh can be used for additional support. Performed transvaginally.

age, poor physical heath, those with respiratory problems (e.g. asthma or chronic obstructive pulmonary disease) and obesity.

Preventive measures

There is scant evidence to support the possible preventative measures:

- Good intrapartum care includes avoiding unnecessary instrumental trauma and prolonged labour
- Pelvic floor exercises may prevent prolapse happening secondary to pelvic floor laxity, strongly advised after childbirth
- Smoking cessation reduces chronic cough
- Weight loss
- Avoidance of heavy lifting occupations
- Treatment of constipation throughout life.

Vulvodynia

A chronic disorder of vulval pain can be a distressing condition and impacts on interpersonal and psychological well-being. The cause is unknown but is usually multifactorial.

The International Society for the Study of Vulvovaginal Disease (ISSVD) recommends that the term 'vulvodynia' is used to describe any vulval pain – regardless of cause. It redefined vulvodynia as vulval discomfort in the absence of gross anatomical or neurological findings of pain (generalised versus localised, provoked, unprovoked or both).

A number of conditions can cause vulval burning and/or pain:

- Irritant dermatitis – irritants include:
  - Soap, panty-liners, synthetic underwear
  - Moistened wipes, deodorants, douches
  - Lubricants, spermicides
  - Topical medication
  - Urine, faeces, excessive vaginal discharge
- Allergic contact dermatitis, e.g. prescribed topical medication
- Other causes include:
  - Oestrogen-deficient vulvovaginal atrophy
  - Recurrent herpes simplex infection, herpes zoster and post-herpetic neuralgia, lichen sclerosus, erosive lichen planus
  - Behçet's syndrome, cicatricial pemphigoid, Sjögren's syndrome
  - Vulval intraepithelial neoplasia and carcinoma (Arnold *et al.* 2007).

Vulval pain is a common problem; a prevalence study in the USA suggested a rate of 3.8% of vulval pain of at least 6 months' duration in a random sample of women contacted by telephone. A study of patients at a gynaecology clinic found 15% had symptoms fulfilling the definition of vulval vestibulitis.

Vulvodynia occurs in any age group from the 20s to the 60s and older. The condition frequently starts early with the highest prevalence found in the under-25s, the average age of onset for primary cases being 19 years.

Signs and symptoms

Symptoms may have been present since childhood or the time of first intercourse. Onset is acute and attributed to:

- Vaginitis caused by yeast or bacterial infection
- A new sexual partner or increased sexual activity
- A medical procedure such as cryotherapy or laser.

If the condition continues unchecked, pain becomes chronic with severity ranging from mild to disabling; the nature of the pain is described as burning, stinging, irritating or raw. Allodynia (pain elicited by a non-painful stimulus) and hyperparaesthesia (a stimulus produces much greater pain than would be normally anticipated) are associated with neuropathic pain regularly found with vulvodynia. Pain may be constant or may come on suddenly when provoked by:

- Intercourse
- Tampon insertion
- Prolonged sitting
- Wearing tight clothes.

Little or nothing abnormal is apparent when examining the woman. A moist, cotton tip ped applicator can be used to touch the vestibulum lightly in order to 'pain map'.

Investigations and diagnosis

Diagnosis necessitates a thorough history and confirmatory physical examination. Investigation should exclude infective and inflammatory conditions. A biopsy may be required.

Nursing care and management

Vulvodynia has many possible treatments; there are very few controlled trials that can verify efficacy of treatments. A number of specialist clinics have been set up to treat and investigate the condition and best management (BASHH 2007).

Ovarian Cyst

The ovary is a common site for cysts (Smeltzer *et al.* 2010). The majority of women who still have a monthly period and one in five of those who have been through the menopause will have one or more ovarian cysts.

It is unusual for cysts to affect a woman's ability to conceive. Even if the cyst is large, requiring removal (through laparoscopy), this preserves fertility. Ovarian tumours are divided into three groups:

1. Functional (24%)
2. Benign (70%)
3. Malignant (6%).

These fluid filled sacs do not usually cause any symptoms, resolving spontaneously.

Ovarian cysts occur in 30% of women with regular menses and 50% of those with irregular menses. Benign ovarian tumours are unusual in premenarchal and postmenopausal women. Benign neoplastic cystic tumours of germ cell origin are most common in young females, accounting for 15–20% of all ovarian neoplasms.

There are two types of functional ovarian cyst:

- Follicular
- Luteal.

Follicular cysts

These are the most commonly seen ovarian cysts. The follicle enlarges and fills with fluid, becoming a follicular ovarian cyst, which usually disappears without treatment after a few weeks.

Luteal cysts

Less common than follicular cysts, luteal cysts develop when the tissue that is left behind after an egg has been released (the corpus luteum) fills with blood. These usually disappear on their own but can rupture causing internal bleeding and sudden pain.

Pathological cysts

The most common type of pathological cyst is a **dermoid cyst**, in women who are under 40 years. Over 40 years, the most common type is a **cystadenoma**.

Signs and symptoms

There may be a dull ache or pain in the lower abdomen and lower back. If there is torsion or rupture, this results in severe abdominal pain and pyrexia. The woman may experience:

- Dyspareunia
- Distended abdomen with palpable mass arising out of the pelvis
- Pressure effects on the bladder, causing urinary frequency

- Pressure effects on venous return, causing varicose veins, leg oedema.

  Torsion, infarction or haemorrhage can lead to:
- Severe pain
- Intermittent episodes of severe pain (as a result of intermittent torsion).

  Rupture can lead to:
- Peritonitis and shock
- Rupture of mucinous cystadenomas may disseminate cells, which continue to secrete mucin, causing death by binding the viscera (pseudomyxoma peritonei)
- Ascites
- Endocrine sequelae, for example hormone-secreting tumours, may cause virilisation (abnormal development of male sexual characteristics), menstrual irregularities, postmenopausal bleeding.

Conditions that cause ovarian cysts

Endometriosis – Women with endometriosis may be more at risk of developing ovarian cysts. Endometriosis happens when fragments of the endometrium are found outside the uterus, for example, in the:
- Fallopian tubes
- Ovaries
- Bladder
- Bowel
- Vagina
- Rectum.

  Blood filled cysts can sometimes form in this tissue.

Polycystic ovarian syndrome – Polycystic ovarian syndrome causes numerous small, harmless cysts to develop on the ovaries. The cysts develop as a result of ovarian hormonal imbalance.

Nursing care and management

Many women with simple ovarian cysts (below 50 mm) based on ultrasound findings do not require treatment or follow-up appointments, as most of these cysts resolve within three menstrual cycles (RCOG 2010).

Women with simple ovarian cysts 50–70 mm in diameter should have yearly ultrasound follow-up. Those with larger simple cysts should be considered for either further imaging (MRI) or surgical intervention. Monitoring with serial ultrasonography examinations may be required for a postmenopausal woman.

Surgical intervention for benign ovarian tumours is generally very effective, providing a cure with minimal effect on reproductive capacity for those who have been unsuccessful with conservative management.

Laparoscopic surgery for benign ovarian tumours is associated with reduced risk of any unfavourable effect of surgery, reduced pain and fewer days in hospital compared with laparotomy. Types of surgical intervention are based on type of cyst and include:
- Oophoropexy
- Salpingo-oophorectomy
- Surgical debulking (where there is *pseudomyxoma peritonei*).

Outcome is variable, depending on the type and size of the tumour, associated complications and age. Prognosis of surgically removed cysts will depend on the histology.

Gynaecological Oncology

Millions of women globally are diagnosed with cancer and this is a growing trend, year on year. The reasons are multifactorial, driven in part by the ageing population and other factors, including diet, obesity, genetics, economics and the availability and access to national screening programmes.

Cervical Cancer

In 2009, cervical cancer was the 19th most common cancer, accounting for 1% of all new cases. Cervical cancer is now the 11th most common cancer among women in the UK, responsible for around 2% of all new cases of cancer in females. A total of 3378 new cases of cervical cancer were reported in 2009. The crude incidence rate shows there are around 11 new cervical cancer cases for every 100 000 women (Cancer Research UK 2012a).

Risk factors associated with cervical cancer
Risk factors for cervical cancer include (among other things):
- Human papillomavirus (HPV)
- Smoking
- Socioeconomic status.

  Cervical cancers are theoretically 100% preventable, by preventing infection with HPV, which is present in all cervical cancers. Smoking plays a part in causing some cervical cancer, increasing the likelihood of infection with HPV or causing HPV infection to be more persistent.

Human papillomavirus (HPV) and cervical cancer risk Globally, HPV has been detected in virtually all cervical tumours. The highest risks are associated with HPV types 16 and 18. The majority of HPV infections will not progress to cervical intraepithelial neoplasia (CIN). However, it is understood that cervical cancer will not develop without the presence of persistent HPV DNA.

Genital HPV is generally sexually transmitted, occurring through contact with infected cervical, vaginal, vulvar, penile or anal epithelium. Genital HPV infection involves areas not easily covered by a condom; correct condom use therefore may not protect against infection.

HPV is more common in younger than older women. HPV is seldom detected in women who have had no previous sexual activity. There do not appear to be any geographical differences in HPV prevalence.

The main risk factors for CIN 3 among HPV-positive women are early age at first intercourse, long duration of the most recent sexual relationship and cigarette smoking.

> **Nursing Field** Children
>
> HPV vaccination for schoolgirls aged 12–13 was introduced in September 2008. The vaccine immunises against HPV types 16 and 18, the strains of the virus most commonly associated with cervical cancer. The vaccine was shown to offer 90% protection against CIN caused by either of these HPV types. Australia is the first country in the world to introduce HPV immunisation for boys and there is ongoing debate in the UK to determine if such a move is required here.

Smoking and cervical cancer risk The risk of squamous cell cervical cancer is increased by 50% in current smokers. Parkin *et al.* (2011) estimated around 7% of cervical cancer cases in 2010 (around 200 cases) were linked to smoking.

Reduction in early cervical lesion size in women who gave up smoking after diagnosis is evident. Acladious *et al.* (2002) have noted that smokers have been found to have a three-fold increased risk of treatment failure of CIN compared with non-smokers and require more intensive follow-up after treatment.

Socioeconomic status and cervical cancer risk Women who live in the most deprived areas have cervical cancer rates more than three times higher than those in the least deprived areas. A link has been demonstrated between social class and cervical cancer, indicating that cervical cancer incidence is considerably higher among women of working age in manual than in non-manual classes.

Other risk factors and cervical cancer

The association between oral contraceptive use and cervical cancer (as is the case with smoking) is complicated by the possible confounding sexual behaviour.

About 10% of cervical cancers in 2010 in the UK were linked to oral contraceptives. However, when the protective effect of the contraceptive pill on ovarian and uterine cancer was taken into account, oral contraceptives were estimated to have a net beneficial effect, reducing cancers in women by almost 1600 (Parkin 2011).

Women with HIV/AIDS have a six-fold increased risk of cervical cancer and those who have undergone organ transplant have more than double the risk, strongly suggesting immunosuppression plays a role.

Hussain *et al.* (2008) report the risk of cervical cancer is approximately doubled in women with a mother or sister who has been diagnosed with the disease.

Medicines Management The Oral Contraceptive Pill

Over 15 methods of contraception are available in the UK. The risk of thrombosis caused by the combined contraceptive pill is very low, despite news reports that using the pill is unsafe. These reports need to be put into context. It must be acknowledged that thrombosis can be a serious side-effect of taking combined oral contraceptives, but it is extremely rare.

For women who have concerns about taking the oral contraceptive pill, the nurse needs to offer them advice: they should not stop using it, they can make an appointment to discuss risks with their practice nurse or family planning clinic. There is a low incidence rate of thrombosis associated with the pill. The risk of thrombosis in women using the pill is much less than the risk of blood clots related to pregnancy.

It must be remembered that combined oral contraceptives are not suitable for every woman; risks differ depending on each woman's medical history. If a woman has any concerns about using the contraceptive pill, she might like to consider alternative options to best suit her individual needs and lifestyle.

Cervical screening in the UK Cervical screening aims to detect and treat abnormal changes in the cervix, which, if left untreated, may develop into invasive cervical cancer. There are a number of screening programmes in the UK.

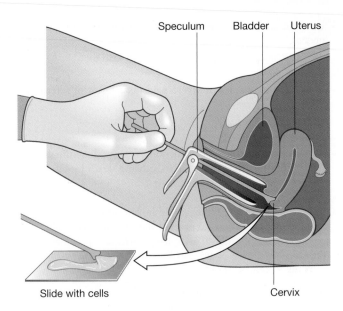

Figure 30.10 Taking a sample of cells.

Most cervical screening is conducted using the Papanicolaou (Pap) smear test (Figure 30.10). A sample of cells is scraped from the cervix at the junction between the endocervix (covered by columnar epithelium) and the ectocervix (covered by squamous epithelium), known as the transformation zone.

The cells collected are smeared onto a slide, fixed and sent to the laboratory for examination. Liquid-based cytology is another method. Cervical screening detects abnormalities ranging from borderline to severe.

The persistence and degree of severity of dyskaryosis determine whether the woman will need to undergo a further procedure, colposcopy, to provide a histological diagnosis of cervical intraepithelial neoplasia (CIN).

Pathophysiology

There are two main types of cervical cancers; both are treated in the same way. The most common type of cervical cancers (75–90%) are *squamous cell carcinomas*. *Adenocarcinomas* (developed from the glandular cells lining the endocervix) account for 20–25%; these are more difficult to detect and they are becoming more prevalent. Squamous cell carcinomas begin as neoplasia arising in the cervical epithelium. Other rare types of cervical cancer include *clear cell, small-cell undifferentiated, lymphomas* and *sarcomas*.

Cervical intraepithelial neoplasia (CIN) Systems of grading (four stages are used in cervical cancer) are used to determine the extent of dysplastic changes in the cervix. Knowing the stage of the cancer helps plan treatment. The stage of a cancer describes its size and whether it has spread beyond its original site. Cervical cancer is divided into four main stages (Table 30.5).

Squamous cell cancers spread by direct invasion of accessory structures, including the vaginal wall, pelvic wall, bladder and rectum. Metastatic spread is usually limited to the pelvic area; distant metastasis may occur through the lymphatic system.

Signs and symptoms

Many cases of cervical cancer are detected by screening. Early symptoms of established cervical carcinoma include:

Table 30.5 Staging, cancer of the cervix. (*Source*: Adapted from Norwitz & Schorge 2010)

STAGE	DESCRIPTION
Stage I	Cancer cells are within cervix only
Stage II	Cancer has spread into surrounding structures, i.e. upper part of the vagina or tissues adjacent to the cervix
Stage III	Cancer has spread to areas such as lower aspect of the vagina, or tissues at the sides of the pelvic area
Stage IV	Cancer has spread to the bladder or bowel or beyond the pelvic area

- Vaginal discharge – varies, can be intermittent or continuous
- Bleeding – can be spontaneous, post-coital, on micturition or defaecation. Occasionally, vaginal bleeding is severe
- Vaginal discomfort/urinary symptoms
- Examination can be relatively normal; there may be white or red patches on the cervix.

Later symptoms can include:

- Painless haematuria
- Chronic urinary frequency
- Painless fresh rectal bleeding
- Changed bowel habit
- Leg oedema, pain and hydronephrosis
- Pelvic discomfort or pain, poorly localised, described as dull or boring in the suprapubic or sacral regions, similar to menstrual discomfort, persistent or intermittent
- Rectal examination may reveal a mass or bleeding due to erosion
- Bimanual palpation may uncover pelvic bulkiness/masses due to pelvic spread
- Leg oedema may progress due to lymphatic or vascular obstruction
- Hepatomegaly may develop indicating liver metastases
- Pulmonary metastases are normally only detected if they cause pleural effusion or bronchial obstruction
- Abnormal appearance of the cervix and vagina, related to erosion, ulcer or tumour.

Investigations and diagnosis

Should be tailored to the unique needs of the woman. The nurse assists prior to, during and after procedures are carried out.

Those premenopausal women presenting with abnormal vaginal bleeding should be tested for *Chlamydia trachomatis*; many of the signs and symptoms suggestive of cervical cancer are common to genital *Chlamydia trachomatis* infection (Scottish Intercollegiate Guidelines Network, SIGN 2008). Postmenopausal women should be referred urgently to gynaecology services for assessment.

Colposcopy (Figure 30.11) allows for visualisation of the cervix, including the transformation zone (Figure 30.12). The cervix is cleaned with acetic acid, then inspected, biopsied and treated if necessary.

A cone biopsy may be performed (Figure 30.13). A full blood count (FBC) is undertaken to assess for anaemia; renal and liver function tests are carried out.

A chest X-ray determines metastatic spread and an intravenous urogram is performed. CT is used to stage disease, with appropriate

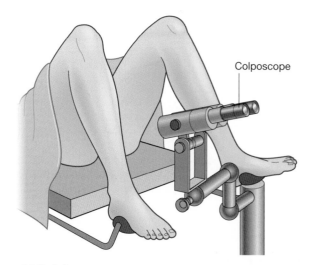

Figure 30.11 **Colposcope.**

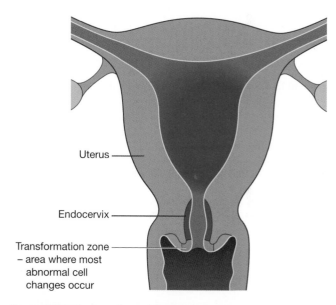

Figure 30.12 **The transformation zone.**

biopsies. Barium enema or proctoscopy is performed to assess rectal compression/invasion. Cystoscopy can assess bladder invasion. MRI provides images of a primary tumour, local invasion and nodal enlargement.

Nursing care and management

The woman must be consulted at each stage of her care programme. The nurse provides information in a way that allows the woman to make informed decisions. She should be given time to think about the decisions she will be making.

697

Jot This Down

What information might the woman need to make a decision? In what ways can this be presented to her? What are the potential issues she might face when presented with information? What is your role?

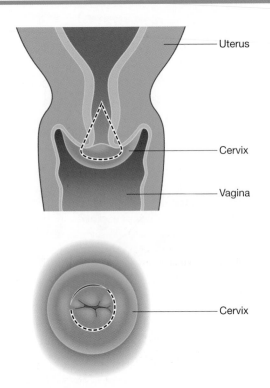

Figure 30.13 **Cone biopsy.**

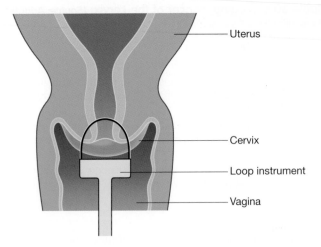

Figure 30.14 **Loop diathermy.**

If the woman is pregnant, treatment may be delayed until a viable fetus can be delivered (this is dependent on the delay being for a few weeks only) or a therapeutic abortion may be needed.

Surgery Surgery during early stage disease can conserve ovarian function, avoiding the effects of early menopause. Surgery is the preferred treatment option in young women, provided there are no contraindications. The outcome following surgery is associated with a variety of prognostic factors, including size of primary tumour (stage), age of the patient and comorbidities (SIGN 2008).

Excision of abnormal ectocervical epithelium performed during colposcopy is used for intraepithelial neoplasia confined to the visible ectocervix; loop diathermy (Figure 30.14) is considered the best approach (provides a specimen for histology) (NHSCSP 2010).

Removal of pelvic lymph nodes is not recommended during treatment for stage **1a1** disease. Pelvic lymph nodes should be removed if stage **1a2** disease is present; this is performed laparoscopically.

Histology may show the presence of more extensive disease than expected and the woman will be offered postoperative radiotherapy. There is a low risk of postoperative complications.

Radical (Wertheim's) hysterectomy provides definitive treatment for invasive, infiltrating and early metastatic carcinoma. This procedure involves excision of the primary tumour with a 1 cm margin of healthy tissue and *en bloc* resection of the main pelvic lymph node areas. It can also involve removal of the upper-third of the vagina and uterovesical and uterosacral ligaments.

Radiotherapy Concurrent chemoradiation (platinum-based chemotherapy) represents the standard treatment for stages **Ib2**–

IVb (Haie-Meder *et al.* 2010). Generally, a combination of external beam therapy and intracavity brachytherapy is used.

Pharmacotherapy Cisplatin-based chemotherapy has been used with some success. It can be given alongside radiotherapy with stage **Ib2-IVa** disease. Toxicity is high and it is only appropriate for high-risk women who are otherwise fit.

Chemoradiotherapy Adding cisplatin-based chemotherapy to radiotherapy significantly improves progression-free and overall survival for high-risk, early-stage women who undergo radical hysterectomy and pelvic lymphadenectomy for carcinoma of the cervix.

Chapter 15 of this text discusses the care of people with cancer. The nurse has a central role to play in helping people navigate and make sense of the different treatment options available, as well as providing impartial advice, which people can use to help them make decisions.

Ovarian Cancer

Ovarian cancer is the leading cause of death from gynaecological cancer in the UK; its incidence is rising. It is the 5th most common cancer in women, with a lifetime risk of about 2% in England and Wales (NICE 2011).

Most women who have ovarian cancer present with advanced disease and this important factor affects outcome. The woman's overall health at the time of presentation affects what treatments can be used. Most women have had symptoms for months prior to presentation, with delays between presentation and specialist referral. Nurses need to generate a greater awareness of the disease and to encourage women to present for initial investigations in primary and secondary care settings.

Ovarian cancer causes more deaths than any other female genital tract cancer. It has a lifetime risk of 2%. Median age at diagnosis is 61 years, peaking at 75–79 years but it can occur at any age. Elderly women are more likely than younger women to be in an advanced stage of disease at initial diagnosis.

Pathophysiology

Malignant ovarian tumours can be solid or cystic. They can contain solid areas, surface papillary protrusions, areas of necrosis and internal papillae.

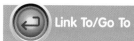

Link To/Go To

This website contains a wealth of useful information concerning some of the gynaecological cancers:

http://cancerhelp.cancerresearchuk.org/type/ovarian-cancer/treatment/stages-of-ovarian-cancer

---

Risk factors for ovarian cancer

Family history is a significant risk factor; there is a 50% risk of developing the disease if two or more 1st or 2nd degree relatives have site-specific ovarian cancer.

Risk factors include:

- Low parity
- Giving birth after age 35
- Exposure to talc or asbestos
- Endometriosis
- Pelvic inflammatory disease
- Diet: a high-fat diet may play a role in the aetiology of ovarian cancer.

Protective factors include:

- Multiparity
- Long-term contraceptive use
- Having a child before the age of 25
- Tubal ligation
- Breast-feeding
- Hysterectomy (Martin 2005).

No screening method has been shown to affect mortality significantly, even if high-risk women are screened. Screening may result in unnecessary surgery.

Signs and symptoms

The majority of women (75%) present with advanced disease. Onset of symptoms is insidious and early symptoms are frequently vague, including:

- Abdominal discomfort
- Abdominal distension or bloating
- Urinary frequency
- Dyspepsia.

The woman may also experience:

- Fatigue
- Weight loss
- Anorexia
- Depression (Bankhead *et al.* 2008).

Pelvic or abdominal masses are key presenting features associated with pain. Abdominal, pelvic or back pain is usually a late sign. There may be ascites and pleural effusion.

Investigations and diagnosis

A CA125 blood test is the most useful; if this is reported as raised (35 IU/mL or greater), then a pelvic and abdominal ultrasound scan should be arranged. Urgent referral is required if the scan is suggestive of ovarian cancer.

Just as cervical cancer has a staging system, so too does ovarian cancer The Fédération Internationale de Gynécologie et d'Obstétrique (FIGO) and the American Joint Committee on Cancer (AJCC) have designated staging (Box 30.5). There is also a substaging system available.

Box 30.5 FIGO Staging for Ovarian Cancer

Stage I is limited to the ovaries

Stage II is tumour involving one or both ovaries with pelvic extension and/or implants

Stage III is tumour involving one or both ovaries with microscopically confirmed peritoneal implants outside the pelvis. Superficial liver metastasis equals Stage III

Stage IV is tumour involving one or both ovaries with distant metastasis. Parenchymal liver metastasis equals Stage IV.

Nursing care and management

Nursing care for women with ovarian cancer is similar to the care for women with cervical cancer. Chapter 15 outlines the care required for people with cancer.

An exploratory laparotomy is undertaken if the physical examination and imaging suggests cancer. This provides histological confirmation, staging and tumour debulking. The standard comprehensive surgical staging approach consists of a total abdominal hysterectomy and bilateral salpingo-oophorectomy, along with examination of all peritoneal surfaces and biopsies of pelvic and para-aortic lymph nodes (Norwitz & Schorge 2010).

Adjuvant therapy to surgery varies according to the stage of the disease but, in most cases, will consist of chemotherapy. Because of late diagnosis, management is often directed towards palliative care. There is little evidence that radiotherapy is superior to chemotherapy for advanced Stage III and IV disease.

Female reproductive surgery

Type of surgical procedure depends on a number of factors, including the woman's wishes, extent of disease and overall well-being. Chapter 14 discusses the principles of care associated with the person undergoing surgery.

Dilation and curettage This procedure (D+C) is carried out for diagnostic purposes or for a number of pelvic conditions, such as abnormal uterine bleeding or when carcinoma of the endometrium is suspected.

There are two aspects to D+C:

- Dilatation – the cervix is dilated
- Curettage – the endometrium is removed using a sharp instrument.

D+C is often used in combination with a hysteroscopy (Figure 30.15), enabling the gynaecologist to assess for any abnormalities such as fibroids or polyps.

It is usually performed on an outpatient basis and under general anaesthetic. The procedure usually takes about 10 minutes and is performed through the vagina. The cervix is dilated using rods and a small scraping instrument – a curette is passed into the uterus to gently scrape off the endometrium. The removed tissue sample is sent to a laboratory to be tested, if this is a diagnostic procedure.

Postoperatively The woman will need to arrange for a friend, partner or relative to take her home and stay for 24 hours after the procedure. She should be able to return to work within 2–3 days.

There are a number of important issues associated with a D+C procedure postoperatively:

Cramps – The women may experience cramps similar to menstrual cramps. Within 24 hours they should have stopped. Painkillers such as paracetamol or ibuprofen help to relieve discomfort

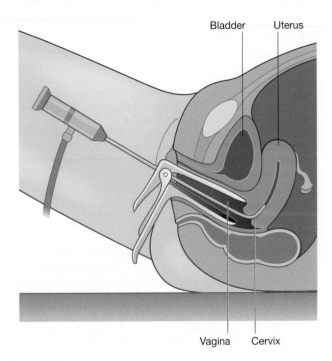

Figure 30.15 **Hysteroscope.**

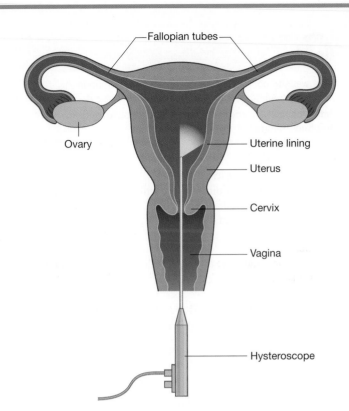

Figure 30.16 **Endometrial ablation. A heated wire loop or a rollerball (a ball on the end of a handle) is used to cut or burn away the lining of the uterus with the aid of a hysteroscope.**

Nausea – Nausea may be present and should only last for a few hours

Bleeding – It is likely that there will be some vaginal bleeding, appearing bright red at first, before fading to a brown stain.

Sanitary towels as opposed to tampons should be used to stem the bleeding (using tampons can increase the risk of developing an infection). Within 5–10 days of having the procedure, the bleeding should pass. During this time, the woman should be advised not to use any scented bath products or go swimming; this helps avoid infection.

Sexual intercourse – Penetrative sex should be avoided for several weeks. Exactly how long will depend on individual circumstances and the reason why the procedure was performed; on average this is around 10–14 days.

Endometrial ablation Endometrial ablation is a newer technique used to treat conditions such as heavy menstrual bleeding. This involves a small probe being inserted through the cervix into the uterus, after which lasers or microwaves are used to remove the endometrial lining (Figure 30.16).

This procedure is not suitable for all women, for example those who have an irregularly-shaped uterus and those who have had previous uterine surgery. In such cases, D+C may be recommended.

Hysterectomy

A surgical procedure in order to remove the uterus. This procedure ends menstruation and reproduction. There are approximately 60 000 hysterectomies performed in the UK annually; up to 20% of women will have the operation. It is most common for women aged between 40 and 50 years.

Hysterectomy may be performed when medical management of bleeding disorders is unsuccessful or malignancy is present. In premenopausal women, the ovaries are usually left in place; in postmenopausal women, a total hysterectomy or panhysterectomy, may be performed; involving removal of the uterus, fallopian tubes and ovaries. Hysterectomies are performed to treat:

- Menorrhagia
- Endometriosis
- Long-term pelvic pain
- Uterine leiomyoma
- Ovarian, uterine, cervical and fallopian cancers
- Genitourinary prolapse.

Hysterectomy is a major procedure, only considered after alternative, less invasive treatments have been tried.

> ### Jot This Down
> The nurse needs to offer the woman support in a number of areas, for example physically and psychologically. There are many decisions that need to be made about a hysterectomy and the decisions will be based upon the woman's personal feelings, medical history and any recommendations the gynaecologist may have.

Types of hysterectomy

The type will depend on why the operation is needed and how much of the uterus and surrounding reproductive organs can be safely left in place. Main types of hysterectomy:

- *Total hysterectomy*: uterus and cervix are removed; the most common procedure

- *Subtotal hysterectomy*: main body of the uterus is removed leaving the cervix in place
- *Total hysterectomy with bilateral salpingo-oophorectomy*: uterus, cervix, fallopian tubes and ovaries are removed
- *Radical hysterectomy*: uterus and surrounding tissues are removed, including fallopian tubes, part of the vagina, ovaries, lymph glands and fatty tissue.

Complications of a hysterectomy

There is a small risk of haemorrhage, thrombosis, infection, bladder or bowel damage or a serious reaction to the general anaesthetic.

Recovering from a hysterectomy

Postoperatively, analgesia is required and if the woman is feeling nauseous or is vomiting, anti-emetics are given.

The woman may have a urinary catheter *in situ* and an intravenous infusion. A wound drain is usually placed, remaining for 1–2 days.

Wounds will have dressings in place. A vaginal hysterectomy will have a gauze pack inserted into the vagina to reduce the risk of any bleeding after the operation and it usually stays in place for 24 hours.

The first day postoperatively, the woman is encouraged to mobilise, walking short distances. This aids venous return, reducing the risk of complications developing, such as venous thromboembolism.

Postoperative nursing care

- Assess and observe for signs of haemorrhage, low blood pressure, tachycardia, pallor
- Monitor vital signs as requested and as the woman's condition dictates, adhere to local policy and procedure, monitor and measure intake and output (intravenous infusion, catheter, drain, vomitus)
- If a urinary catheter is *in situ*, when it has been removed, note when urine was passed, measure and record amount
- Assess for potential complications, including infection, paralytic ileus, shock or haemorrhage, thrombophlebitis, pulmonary embolism
- Assess vaginal discharge; help with perineal care
- Assess incisional site, bowel sounds as policy and procedure
- Encourage mobilisation, turning, coughing, deep breathing
- Offer fluid and later diet as tolerated
- Teach how to splint the abdomen with pillows as the woman coughs and breathes deeply.

The length of time it will take before the woman is ready to leave hospital depends on a number of factors, including age and general level of health. Follow-up appointment will be arranged 6–12 weeks afterwards, to check on progress.

Hysterectomy is major procedure and the woman is usually hospitalised for up to 5 days. It can take 6–8 weeks to fully recover. Rest is advocated and the woman should not lift anything heavy, such as bags of shopping. Explain that she may feel tired for several days after the procedure and this is expected; she should rest periodically. Time is required for tissue healing to occur.

Douching, tampons and sexual intercourse should be avoided. A shower is preferable to having a bath, until bleeding has ceased.

Teach the woman to recognise signs of complications that should be reported to the doctor or nurse:

- Temperature more than 37.7°C
- Vaginal bleeding greater than a typical menstrual period or is bright red
- Urinary incontinence, urgency, burning or frequency
- Severe pain.

Encourage the woman to express feelings that may signal negative self-esteem. Provide an opportunity to voice concerns.

Provide information concerning risks and benefits of hormone replacement therapy, if appropriate.

The Evidence Information Needs of Hysterectomy Patients

A study carried out by the Hysterectomy Association:

- 78% of the information received was about hysterectomy and the majority was through the Internet, although 31% said their consultant had given them the most information
- 67% had most information before their operation yet over 10% said they weren't given any information at all
- Despite the amount of information they were given, less than 30% felt they knew exactly what to expect.
- The percentages of women who would like to receive more information about exercise post-hysterectomy and also sex after their surgery were 69.1% and 52.9%, respectively.

http://www.hysterectomy-association.org.uk/index.php/ hysterectomy-recovery/hysterectomy-research-interim-findings/

Breast Disease

Benign Breast Disease

Any lump in the breast can cause anxiety and instil fear, but not all lumps are breast cancer.

When the women presents with a history of breast lump(s) and after breast examination, differentiation is required.

A benign mass is often three-dimensional:

1. Mobile and smooth
2. Has regular borders
3. Is solid or cystic in consistency.

A malignant mass:

- Is firm in consistency
- Has irregular borders
- May be fixed to the underlying skin or soft tissue
- There may also be skin changes or nipple retraction.

Early breast growth in girls, or some growth of breast tissue in males, is common. At puberty, the breasts are the first of the secondary sexual characteristics to develop and there may be some early activity in quite young girls. Very early development may be asymmetrical and apparently unilateral. Examination will usually show some contralateral development.

Fibrocystic changes

Classification based on clinical and pathological findings includes:

- Physiological swelling and tenderness
- Nodularity
- Breast pain is not usually associated with malignancy
- Palpable breast lumps
- Nipple discharge including galactorrhoea
- Breast infection and inflammation – associated with lactation.

Physiological swelling and tenderness

The breasts are active organs changing throughout the menstrual cycle. Some degree of tenderness and nodularity in the premenstrual phase is so common that it is considered as normal, affecting approximately 50–60% of all menstruating women. As menstruation starts, it rapidly resolves. It is also called 'mammary dysplasia' and 'cystic mastopathy'.

- Affects women between 30 and 50
- Less frequent in association with combined oral contraceptive, rare after menopause
- Oral contraceptives reduce the risk of benign breast disease generally
- It can recur with HRT.

   Care and management may include:

- Reduction or avoidance of caffeine
- Vitamin E
- Pyridoxine
- Evening primrose oil.

Breast Cysts

Discrete cysts that are clearly palpable can be treated by needle aspiration (Figure 30.17).

Nodularity

Nodularity is a normal, hormonally-mediated change, with lumpiness of the breast and varying degrees of pain and tenderness. Symptoms are greatest about 1 week prior to menstruation, decreasing when it starts. Examination can reveal an area of nodularity or thickening, often in the upper outer quadrant of the breast. When changes are bilaterally symmetrical, rarely are they pathological.

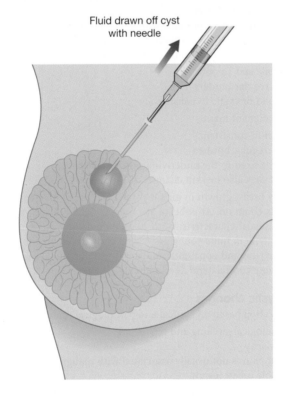

Fluid drawn off cyst with needle

Figure 30.17 Needle aspiration.

Mammography can be used in older patients; for younger women with denser breasts, ultrasound is preferred. Treatment is analgesia and a good bra.

Palpable breast lumps

Many breast lumps are benign, particularly in younger women. Most benign lumps will be cysts or fibroadenoma.

A fibroadenoma is a benign tumour common in young women under 40, composed of stromal and epithelial elements and is the result of increased sensitivity to oestrogens. Most stop growing at about 2–3 cm, but can enlarge further, with regression after the menopause. Mammography and ultrasound may be used to examine the lump; biopsy or excision may be required.

Duct ectasia and periductal mastitis affect women approaching menopause. Ducts behind the nipple become dilated and may become blocked with fluid, leading to discharge from the nipple; this may be bloody. The epithelium of the duct may become ulcerated leading to pain and infection.

A lump may develop with nipple retraction. Bloody discharge can suggest intraduct carcinoma; a retracted nipple may suggest malignancy and referral to a breast clinic is required.

Malignant Breast Disease

Breast cancer is by far most common cancer in women and the second most common cause of death from cancer in the UK. It is also an important cause of morbidity.

Women presenting with a lump in the breast will be aware of the possible diagnosis and will be very anxious. This should be taken into account when taking the history and discussing management.

In 2009, there were 48 788 new cases in the UK and, of those, 371 cases were in men (Cancer Research UK 2012b). Within the UK, rates are roughly similar for all countries except Northern Ireland, which has a slightly lower rate. For women, the lifetime risk of developing breast cancer is 1 in 8. The European age-standardised incidence rate is approximately 120/100 000 women.

Pathophysiology

Most breast cancers arise from:

- Epithelial lining of ducts (ductal)
- Epithelium of the terminal ducts of the lobules (lobular).

Cancer can be invasive or *in situ*. Cancers arise from intermediate ducts and are invasive. Paget's disease of the breast (an infiltrating carcinoma of nipple epithelium) represents about 1% of all breast cancers.

Inflammatory carcinoma occurs in less than 3% of all cases, with a rapidly growing, painful mass enlarging the breast, causing overlying skin to become red and warm. There may be diffuse infiltration of tumour.

Risk factors for malignancy

- Previous history of breast cancer
- As the woman ages, the risk increases; less than 5% of cases before age 35; less than 25% before 50
- Family history of breast cancer in a 1st-degree relative
- The BRCA1, BRCA2 and TP53 mutations carry very high risk but only 3–5% of women are likely to carry them on their chromosomes
- Never having borne a child, or first child after age 30
- Not having breast-fed

- Early menarche and late menopause
- Continuous combined HRT
- Radiation to chest (even small doses)
- High alcohol intake
- Breast augmentation is not generally associated with increased risk. Type of implant used may be important.

Signs and symptoms

There may be no signs and symptoms. Cancers are detected by mammography. Most women or their partner detect their breast cancer. In breast cancer:

- Most women will have felt a lump (20% as a painful lump)
- 10% present with nipple change
- 3% present with nipple discharge
- 5% present with skin contour changes
- Breast pain/mastalgia alone is uncommon
- Intraduct carcinoma may present as a bloody discharge from the nipple
- There may be a lump under the arm, lump in other regional lymph nodes
- A suspicious mass could have been found at routine mammography
- Metastases may cause pain in bones or pathological fractures
- Metastases at other sites – liver, lung or brain can cause symptoms
- Occasionally, some women present with a fungating mass that has been neglected for a long time.

Investigations and diagnosis

Aebi *et al.* (2011) have produced guidelines on the clinical assessment and techniques for accurate diagnosis.

Diagnostic radiography Mammography is more suited for less dense breasts (usually post-menopause). For more invasive tumours, a combination of ultrasound and mammography is more effective for detection. Ultrasound is useful when breast tissue is dense; in young women it can be diagnostically more useful than mammography. MRI is used in difficult cases:

- Dense breast tissue
- Cases of familial breast cancer associated with BRCA mutations
- Silicone gel implants
- Positive axillary lymph node status with occult primary tumour in the breast or where multiple tumour foci are suspected.

Diagnostic procedures Many diagnostic procedures are used; for non-palpable lesions:

- Core needle biopsy (image-guided)
- Open biopsy (needle localisation)

For palpable lesions:

- Fine-needle aspiration
- Core needle biopsy
- Excision biopsy (lesion removed)
- Incisional biopsy (part of lesion removed).

Nursing care and management

It is paramount that treatment is woman-centred, taking into account the woman's individual needs and preferences. All members of the multidisciplinary team have to employ effective communication skills, providing the woman with evidence-based support and information, allowing her to reach informed decisions about care. Any discussion and involvement of the woman's family must be facilitated with her consent.

Multidisciplinary treatment planning involving a breast nurse specialist/consultant, breast surgeon, radiologist, pathologist and medical and radiation oncologists should be convened to integrate local and systemic therapies and their sequence. Guidelines produced by Aebi *et al.* (2011) describe best practice and address treatment options, including surgery, chemotherapy, hormonal therapy and radiotherapy.

Supportive care services that comply with current best practice should be made available to the woman and her family. These should take account of physical, psychological, social, spiritual and financial needs and should be undertaken at key points, for example diagnosis and treatment commencement. A key worker should be nominated.

What the Experts Say Hair Loss

Many of the women I work with will lose either some or all of their hair due to treatment for breast cancer and this is often the most distressing side-effect of treatment. These are some of the practical tips I share with them, be careful – they may not suit all women but they can help you help them:

- Use a baby shampoo, un-perfumed shampoo and conditioner
- Try not to wash hair more than twice a week
- Use tepid water, not hot
- Use a soft hairbrush or wide-toothed plastic comb to brush or comb hair
- Avoid plaiting long hair; this may damage it
- Try not to use elastic bands to tie back long hair
- Hair colours and dyes, perms and other products containing strong chemicals should be avoided
- Avoid products containing alcohol, like hairspray, this can irritate the scalp
- Avoid excessive heat from hair straighteners, hairdryers, hot brushes and heated rollers
- On sunny days when you are not wearing a wig, be sure to wear a hat
- If there is eyebrow loss, recreate a natural appearance by using eyebrow make-up in a shade matching hair colour.

(Jenny, a breast cancer nurse for over 20 years)

Communicating effectively and working with other members of the multidisciplinary team when making decisions and leading care provision are included in the NMC's (NMC 2010) professional domains. Demonstrating competencies in these areas can help improve standards of nursing care.

Breast Surgery

The majority of surgical procedures on the breast are performed to establish a definitive diagnosis or to treat breast cancer (Pearsall 2011). Jones and Pomarico-Denino (2013) point out that the primary goal of breast surgery is to obtain local control of the disease by removing the cancer from the breast and to determine the extent and stage of the disease.

The extent and type of surgery depends on the type of cancer and an accurate diagnosis prior to the definitive surgical technique being chosen. As breast cancer is being diagnosed earlier, there are more options available to women that are of a less invasive nature.

Lumpectomy

This is the removal of the breast lump, with as little as possible of the normal surrounding tissue. Usually occurs after a fine wire needle localisation procedure has been performed, marking the tumour. Regional lymph nodes may be removed to determine if the cancer has spread beyond the breast.

Simple Mastectomy

In a simple or total mastectomy, the entire breast and nipple-areola are removed; there is no removal of the axillary lymph nodes. This may be performed for women who have non-invasive breast cancer or ductal carcinoma *in situ*; this does not have a tendency to spread to lymph nodes. In some cases, the procedure can be used prophylactically when women may be at high risk for breast cancer. A total mastectomy can be performed with sentinel lymph node biopsy for those with invasive breast cancer.

Sentinel Lymph Node Biopsy

This approach avoids compromising the lymphatic system. It is used to determine whether there is spread of cancer cells to the axillary lymph nodes; 1–3 sentinel lymph nodes are removed for pathological review, in this procedure those draining lymph closest to the breast (Figure 30.18). If analysis shows cancer cells, the woman will have to undergo formal axillary dissection.

Modified Radical Mastectomy

Used to treat invasive breast cancer, involves the removal of the entire breast tissue, including nipple-areola. A portion of the axillary lymph nodes is dissected. The pectoralis major and the pectoralis minor muscles are left intact.

Radical Mastectomy

Includes the removal of the entire breast and lymph nodes under the arms as well as removal of the pectoralis major and the pectoralis minor muscles. This approach is rarely used unless there is extensive local spread of the breast cancer; there are less aggressive procedures available. A long oblique scar remains. The chest wall may appear concave and the ribs are more prominent.

> ### What the Experts Say
>
> ❝ The nurses were smashing, they gave me loads of information before and after the boob job, sometimes too much. There were some little things they forgot to mention, for example, when the surgeon did the op she cut and must have damaged some of the nerves, not only in the chest area but also under my arm pit, it's impossible not to. So I had to learn to be aware of that and accept that there are bits of my chest that are numb or tingly. It wasn't only my chest, it was also under my arm pit, so I have to be careful when shaving there.
>
> (Diana 46, mastectomy a year ago)

Breast Conservation Therapy

The aim with this procedure, including lumpectomy, wide excision, partial or segmental mastectomy and quadrantectomy is to excise the tumour in the breasts totally, obtaining clear margins while achieving an acceptable aesthetic result. Lymph node removal is not needed if the procedure is being used to treat a non-invasive breast cancer; for invasive breast cancer, the lymph nodes are removed. Lymph nodes are removed through a separate semicircular opening in the axilla.

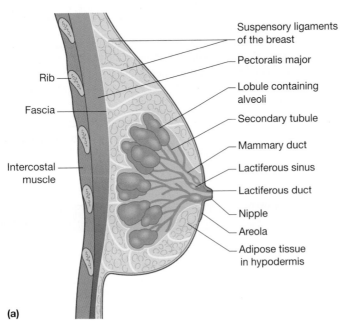

(a)

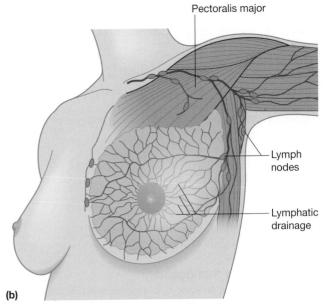

(b)

Figure 30.18 Lymph nodes and drainage – the breast.

Conclusion

This chapter has provided you with insight and understanding concerning the care that women who experience problems associated with the reproductive system will require. This care is complex and requires a skilled, sensitive and effective application. An understanding of the anatomy, physiology and pathophysiological changes is essential; it is also imperative that the nurse understands and respects the individual and holistic needs of the woman and her family.

Key Points

- The female reproductive system is essential for sexual reproduction as well as other important issues, which must be considered by the nurse when caring for women, for example, the psychological and social features of reproduction, as well as the pleasure often provided by the reproductive organs.
- This chapter has considered the female reproductive organs; it has outlined their key functions and given an explanation for the normal and abnormal changes that can occur in the female reproductive system.
- The nurse must use a framework, a systematic approach to guide assessment, planning, implementation and the evaluation of care provision. When applying a systematic approach, the physical, psychological and cultural needs of the woman should be taken into consideration.
- There are numerous screening and diagnostic tests available to help offer women care that is responsive and appropriate. The role of the nurse is multifaceted and will include acting as patient advocate. The nurse will also have to possess an understanding of risk factors for gynaecological cancers and other gynaecological conditions.
- Promoting the rights, choices and wishes of all women requires the nurse to be confident and competent as well as understanding the importance of working in partnership to address women's needs in all care settings.
- The nurse practises in a holistic manner, respecting individual choice, supporting and promoting the health, well-being and dignity of women.

Glossary

Amenorrhoea: absence of menstrual period
Anorgasmia: when a person is unable to reach orgasm during sexual intercourse
Dysfunctional uterine bleeding: the most common cause of abnormal vaginal bleeding
Dysmenorrhoea: severe pain during menstruation
Dyspareunia: painful sexual intercourse
Endometriosis: the condition where cells similar to those lining the uterus are found elsewhere in the body
Fibrocystic changes: when these changes occur in the breast, they can be felt as lumps
Fibroids: benign tumours that form in the muscular wall of the uterus
Laparoscopy: medical procedure that allows visualisation of the uterus and fallopian tubes
Leiomyoma: a benign change (often in the uterus) associated with the soft tissue
Lymphoedema: a collection of lymph fluid that does not drain away from the tissues
Menopause: cessation of female reproductive ability, the ending of menstruation
Menorrhagia: heavy menstrual blood loss
Menstrual cycle: a cycle of female reproductive changes
Metrorrhagia: irregular menstrual bleeding; bleeding between periods
Oestrogen: a general term for a female sex related hormone
Ovarian cycle: the normal cycle that includes the development of an ovarian follicle, rupture of the follicle and discharge of the ovum
Premenstrual syndrome: the name given to a set of physical, emotional and psychological symptoms that appear in the days preceding the woman's period
Progesterone: a hormone predominantly produced in the ovaries

References

Acladious, N.N., Sutton, C., Mandal, D., Hopkins, R., Zaklama, M. & Kitchener, H. (2002) Persistent human papillomavirus infection and smoking increase risk of failure of treatment of cervical intraepithelial neoplasia (CIN). *International Journal of Cancer*, 98(3), 435–439.

Aebi, S., Davidson, T., Gruber, G. & Càstiglione, M. (2011) Primary breast cancer: ESMO Clinical Practice Guidelines for diagnosis, treatment and follow-up. *Annals of Oncology*, 22(Suppl 6), vi12–vi24. http://annonc.oxfordjournals.org/content/22/suppl_6/vi12.full (accessed August 2012).

Arnold, L.D., Bachmann, G.A., Rosen, R. & Rhodes, G.G. (2007) Assessment of vulvodynia symptoms in a sample of US women: a prevalence survey with a nested case control study. *American Journal of Obstetrics and Gynecology*, 196(2), 128.e1–e6.

Bankhead, C.R., Collins, C., Stokes-Lampard, H., Rose, P., Wilson, P., Clementa, A. *et al.* (2008) Identifying symptoms of ovarian cancer: a qualitative and quantitative study. *British Journal of Obstetrics and Gynaecology*, 115(8), 1008–1014.

BASHH (2007) *Management of Vulval Conditions*. British Association Sexual Health and HIV, Macclesfield. http://www.bashh.org/documents/113/113.pdf (accessed August 2012).

BMA & RPSGB (2012) *British National Formulary*, 63rd edn. British Medical Association and Royal Pharmaceutical Society of Great Britain, London.

BMS (2008) *Non-estrogen Based Treatments for Menopausal Symptoms*. British Menopause Society, Marlow. http://www.thebms.org.uk/statementpreview.php?id=8 (accessed August 2012).

Cancer Research UK (2012a) *Cervical Cancer Statistics UK*. http://info.cancerresearchuk.org/cancerstats/types/cervix/ (accessed August 2012).

Cancer Research UK (2012b) *Cancer Incidence for Common Cancers*. http://info.cancerresearchuk.org/cancerstats/incidence/commoncancers/#Top3 (accessed August 2012).

Clemons, J.L., Aguilar, V.C., Tillinghurst, T.A., Jackson, N.D. & Myers, D.L. (2004) Patient satisfaction and changes in prolapse and urinary symptoms in women who were fitted successfully with a pessary for pelvic organ prolapse. *American Journal of Obstetrics and Gynecology*, 190(4), 1025–1029.

Daley, A.J., Sokes-Lampard, H.J. & MacArthur, C. (2009) Exercise to reduce vasomotor and other menopausal symptoms: a review. *Maturitas*, 6(3), 176–180.

DiDonato, P., Giulini, N.A., Bacchi Moderna, A. *et al.* (2005) Factors associated with climacteric symptoms in women around menopause attending menopause clinics in Italy. *Maturitas*, 52(3–4), 181–189.

Doshani, A., Teo, R.E., Mayne, C.J. & Tincello, D.G. (2007) Uterine Prolapse. *British Medical Journal*, 335(7624), 819–823.

Hagen, S., Stark, D., Maher, C. & Adams, E. (2006) Conservative management of pelvic organ prolapse in women. *Cochrane Database Systematic Reviews*, (4):CD003882.

Haie-Meder, C., Morice, P. & Castiglione, M. (2010) Cervical cancer: ESMO Clinical Practice Guidelines for diagnosis, treatment and follow-up. *Annals of Oncology*, 21(Suppl 5), v37–v40. http://annonc.oxfordjournals.org/content/21/suppl_5/v37.full (accessed August 2012).

Hefler, L.A., Grimm, C., Benz, E.K., Reinthaller, A., Heinze, G. & Tempfer, C.B. (2006) A model for predicting age at menopause in white women. *Fertility and Sterility*, 85(2), 451–454.

Hurskainen, R., Teperi, J., Rissanen, P. *et al.* (2001) Quality of life and cost-effectiveness of levonorgestrel-releasing intrauterine system versus hysterectomy for treatment of menorrhagia: a randomised trial. *Lancet*, 357(9252), 273–277.

Hussain, S.K., Sundquist, J. & Hemminki, K. (2008) Familial clustering of cancer at human papillomavirus-associated sites according to the Swedish family-cancer database. *International Journal of Cancer*, 122(8), 1873–1878.

Jelovsek, J.E., Maher, C. & Barber, M.D. (2007) Pelvic organ prolapse. *Lancet*, 369(9566), 1027–1038.

Jones, J.M. & Pomarico-Denino, V. (2013) Nursing management: patients with breast and female reproductive disorders. In: L. Honan-Pellico (ed.) *Focus on Adult Health. Medical Surgical Nursing*. Ch. 33, pp. 910–949. Wolters Kluwer, Philadelphia.

Lethaby, A., Irvine, G. & Canmeron, I. (2008) Cyclical progestogens for heavy menstrual bleeding. *Cochrane Database Systematic Reviews*, (1):CD001016.

Marjoribanks, J., Letharby, A. & Farquahr, C. (2006) Surgery versus medical therapy for heavy menstrual bleeding. *Cochrane Database Systematic Reviews*, (2):CD003855.

Martin, V. (2005) Straight talk about ovarian cancer. *Nursing*, 34 (4), 36–41.

Nelson, H. (2008) Menopause. *Lancet*, 371(9614), 760–770.

NHSCSP (2010) *Colposcopy and Programme Management: guidelines for the NHS cervical screening programme*, 2nd edn. NHS Cervical Screening Programme. http://www.cancerscreening.nhs.uk/cervical/publications/nhscsp20.html (accessed August 2012).

NICE (2007a) *Heavy Menstrual Bleeding. Clinical Guideline CG44*. National Institute for Health and Clinical Excellence, London.

NICE (2007b) *Mesh Sacrocolpopexy for Vaginal Vault Prolapse*. National Institute for Health and Clinical Excellence, London. http://www.truthinmedicine.us.com/images/nice2.pdf.

NICE (2011) *Ovarian Cancer. Recognitions and Initial Management of Ovarian Cancer. Clinical Guideline 122*. National Institute for Health and Clinical Excellence, London.

NMC (2010) *Standards for Pre registration Nursing Education*. Nursing and Midwifery Council, London. http://standards.nmc-uk.org/PublishedDocuments/Standards%20for%20pre-registration%20nursing%20education%2016082010.pdf (accessed August 2012).

Norwitz, E. & Schorge, J. (2010) *Obstetrics and Gynecology at a Glance*, 3rd edn. Wiley-Blackwell, Chichester.

Parkin, D.M. (2011) Cancers attributable to exposure to hormones in the UK in 2010. *British Journal Cancer*, 105(S2), S42–S48.

Parkin, D.M., Boyd, L. & Walker, L.C. (2011) The fraction of cancer attributable to lifestyle and environmental factors in the UK in 2010. Summary and conclusions. *British Journal of Cancer*, 105(S2), S77–S81.

Pearsall, E.B. (2011) Breast surgery. In: J.C. Rothrock (ed.) *Alexander's Care of the Patient in Surgery*, 14th edn., Ch. 16, pp. 588–609. Elsevier, St Louis.

Pitkin, J, (2007) Dysfunctional uterine bleeding. *British Medical Journal*, 334(7603), 1110–1111.

Polit, M.C., Schleinitz, M.D. & Col, N.F. (2008) Revisiting the duration of vasomotor symptoms of menopause: a meta-analysis. *Journal of General Internal Medicine*, 23(9), 1507–1513.

RCOG (2007) *The Management of Post Hysterectomy Vaginal Vault Prolapse. Green Top Guideline Number 46*. Royal College of Obstetricians and Gynaecologists, London. http://www.rcog.org.uk/files/rcog-corp/uploaded-files/GT46PosthysterectomyVaginalProlapse2007.pdf (accessed August 2012).

RCOG (2010) *Scientific Advisory Committee Opinion Paper 6*, 2nd edn. Alternatives to HRT for the Management of Symptoms of the Menopause. Royal College of Obstetricians and Gynaecologists, London. http://www.rcog.org.uk/files/rcog-corp/SAC%20Paper%206%20Alternatives%20to%20HRT.pdf.

Sievert, L.L., Obermeyer, C.M. & Prive, K. (2006) Determinants of hot flashes and night sweats. *Annals of Human Biology*, 33(1), 4–16.

SIGN (2008) *Management of Cervical Cancer. A National Clinical Guideline*. Scottish Intercollegiate Guidelines Network, Edinburgh.

Smeltzer, S.C., Bare, B.G., Hinkle, J.L. & Cheever, K.H. (2010) *Brunner and Suddarth's Textbook of Medical-Surgical Nursing*, 12th edn. Lippincott, Philadelphia.

Thakar, R. & Stanton, S. (2002) Management of genital prolapse. *British Medical Journal*, 324(7348), 1258–1262.

Van Voohris, B.J. (2005) Genitourinary symptoms in the menopausal transition. *American Journal of Medicine*, 118(12 Suppl 2), 47–53.

Young, T., Rabago, D., Zgierska, A., Austin, D., & Laurel, F. (2003) Objective and subjective sleep quality in premenopausal, perimenopausal, and postmenopausal women in the Wisconsin sleep cohort study. *Sleep*, 26(6), 667–672.

Test Yourself

1. What reproductive organ(s) of the female secretes fluid for vaginal lubrication during coitus?
   (a) Uterine tubes
   (b) Labia majora
   (c) Vestibular glands
   (d) Endometrium

2. What does dyspareunia mean?
   (a) Absence of menses
   (b) Pain during sexual intercourse
   (c) Anxiety about sexual performance
   (d) Pain when menstruating

3. Ovulation is triggered by:
   (a) Follicle stimulating hormone
   (b) Hormones from the follicular cells
   (c) Hormones from the theca interna
   (d) A mid-cycle rush of luteinising hormone

4. The _____ is a subcutaneous pad of adipose tissue covering the symphysis pubis.
   (a) Mons pubis
   (b) Perineum
   (c) Vulva
   (d) Clitoris

5. During the _____ phase of menstruation, the lining of the uterus rebuilds.
   (a) Menstrual
   (b) Proliferative
   (c) Secretory
   (d) Circulatory

6. Severe menstrual cramps accompany _____
   (a) Metrorrhagia
   (b) Menorrhagia
   (c) Dysmenorrhoea
   (d) Amenorrhoea

7. The opening to the uterus is called the:
   (a) Vagina
   (b) Clitoris
   (c) Cervix
   (d) Urethra

8. The primary female sex organs producing ova are:
   (a) The gametes
   (b) The hormones
   (c) The ovaries
   (d) The breasts

9. When menstruation ends in middle age, this is called:
   (a) Hysterectomy
   (b) Sterilisation
   (c) Gestation
   (d) Menopause

10. Periodic shedding of the endometrium is known as:
    (a) Ovulation
    (b) Oogenesis
    (c) The secretory phase
    (d) Menstruation

Answers

1. c
2. b
3. d
4. a
5. b
6. c
7. c
8. c
9. d
10. d

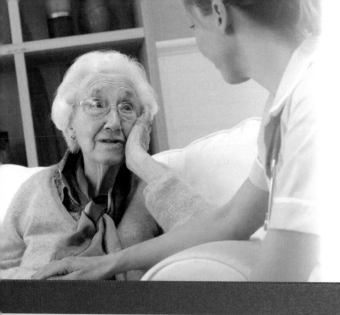

31

The Man with a Reproductive Disorder

Ian Peate

School of Health Studies, Gibraltar

Learning Outcomes

On completion of this chapter you will be able to:

- Describe the male reproductive system
- Detail the male reproductive organs considering their key functions
- Provide an explanation for the normal and abnormal changes that can occur in the male reproductive system
- Use the nursing process as a framework for care provision
- Identify screening and diagnostic tests
- Understand risk factors for male reproductive cancers and conditions

Competencies

All nurses must:

1. Promote the rights, choices and wishes of all men
2. Work in partnership to address men's needs in all healthcare settings
3. Assess physical and psychological needs
4. Practise in a holistic manner
5. Respect individual choice
6. Support and promote the health, well-being, rights and dignity of men

 Visit the companion website at **www.wileynursingpractice.com** where you can test yourself using flashcards, multiple-choice questions and more.

Nursing Practice: Knowledge and Care, First Edition. Edited by Ian Peate, Karen Wild and Muralitharan Nair.
© 2014 John Wiley & Sons, Ltd. Published 2014 by John Wiley & Sons, Ltd. Companion website: www.wileynursingpractice.com

Introduction

The male reproductive system, also called the genital system, is closely related to a man's notion of self-concept. The reproductive system is made up of the organs responsible for reproduction of the species; organs making up the reproductive system differ between the male and female. Key differences between the male and female are the presence of obvious external genitalia in the male and the internal location of the significant female reproductive organs which are located in the pelvic cavity.

The nurse must be aware that there are a number of values and beliefs (sometimes associated with culture and religion) that can influence a person's reproductive knowledge as well as ways in which reproductive health services are provided. Employing an approach that is respectful and sensitive, treating the man as an individual and using language that he can relate to and understand will help develop therapeutic nurse–patient relationship.

The NMC, in maintaining sexual boundaries with patients, states: Breaches of sexual boundaries between a nurse or midwife and the person in their care, or any other person involved with the person's care, include:

- Beginning a personal relationship during or after treatment
- Engaging in sexual activity
- Discussing sexual matters that are not relevant to treatment
- Using sexual humour or telling 'dirty jokes'

- Repeatedly engaging in prolonged conversation about personal matters unrelated to treatment.

The nurse must understand the anatomical and physiological aspects of this unique system in order to be able to explain the anatomy and physiology to the man, assess and undertake a detailed patient history and recognise normal and abnormal internal and external genitalia.

Anatomy and Physiology

The male reproductive tract produces spermatozoa; these are deposited inside the vagina, contributing to reproduction. The spermatozoa fertilise the female egg (ova). The male genitalia are found externally (Figure 31.1).

The male reproductive organs and the neuroendocrine system manufacture hormones required for biological development and sexual behaviour. These reproductive organs are closely associated with and are essential to the purpose of the urinary system. Assessment of the reproductive and urinary systems can be challenging for the man and the nurse and this activity must be undertaken with sensitivity when discussing personal issues. Tact and care is required when carrying out a physical assessment of the reproductive system: this is a part of the body that is often regarded as intimate and private.

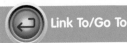 Link To/Go To

The NHS Constitution (interactive) can be found at:
http://www.nhs.uk/choiceintheNHS/Rightsandpledges/
NHSConstitution/Documents/2013/the-nhs-constitution-for
-england-2013.pdf (accessed 8 March 2014)

Link To/Go To

The NMC's website:
http://www.nmc-uk.org/Nurses-and-midwives/Regulation-in
-practice/Regulation-in-Practice-Topics/Maintaining
-Boundaries-/

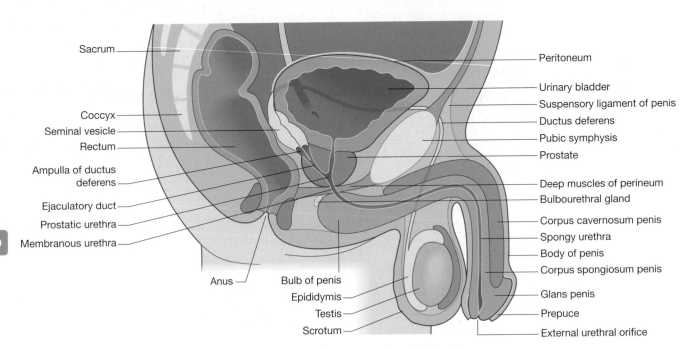

Figure 31.1 Male organs of reproduction and surrounding structures.

Labels: Sacrum, Coccyx, Seminal vesicle, Rectum, Ampulla of ductus deferens, Ejaculatory duct, Prostatic urethra, Membranous urethra, Anus, Bulb of penis, Epididymis, Testis, Scrotum, Peritoneum, Urinary bladder, Suspensory ligament of penis, Ductus deferens, Pubic symphysis, Prostate, Deep muscles of perineum, Bulbourethral gland, Corpus cavernosum penis, Spongy urethra, Body of penis, Corpus spongiosum penis, Glans penis, Prepuce, External urethral orifice

There are a number of disorders that can have an impact on a man's reproductive health and these include disorders of:

- The penis
- Scrotum
- Testes
- Prostate gland
- Breast.

Some of these disorders can threaten the man's fertility, sexual and urinary function and his life; these can be inflammatory, structural, benign or malignant. Testicular cancer is a bigger threat for younger men and conditions associated with the prostate gland are conditions impacting on the older man.

The Testes

Developmentally, the paired testes advance in the fetal abdominal cavity near the kidneys, descending through the inguinal canals into the scrotum usually at the 7th month of fetal development. They correspond to the female's ovaries. Each testicle is approximately 5 cm in length and around 2.5 cm in diameter. They are suspended in the scrotal sac by the spermatic cord. Two coverings surround each of them:

1. **An outer tunica vaginalis**
2. **An inner tunica albuginea.**

See Figure 31.2.

Each one is divided into 250 to 300 lobules, each contains one to four seminiferous tubules. The testes are responsible for the production of sperm (spermatogenesis) and testosterone (Figure 31.3).

The seminiferous tubules produce the sperm. Leydig's cells (sometimes called interstitial cells) are sited in the connective tissue that surrounds the seminiferous tubules and produce testosterone.

The seminiferous tubules contain two types of cells: spermatogenic cells (sperm forming cells) and Sertoli cells.

During spermatocytogenesis, the spermatogonia divide through forming two diploid cells (primary spermatocytes) (Figure 31.4). **Mitosis** is a type of cell division in which a parent cell grows,

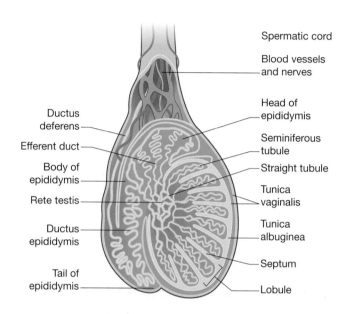

Figure 31.2 **The anatomy of a testis.**

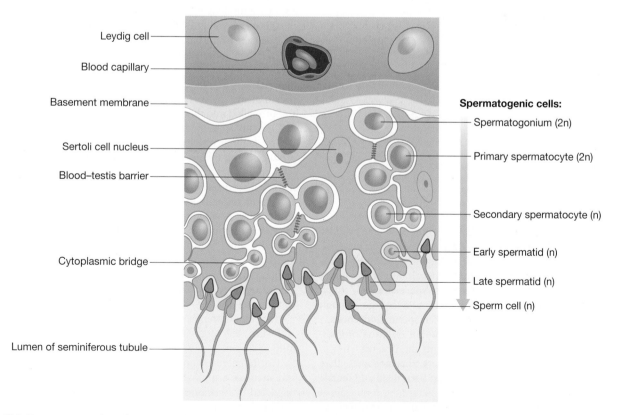

Figure 31.3 **Transverse section of a portion of seminiferous tubule. (n) and (2n) refer to haploid and diploid numbers and chromosomes.**

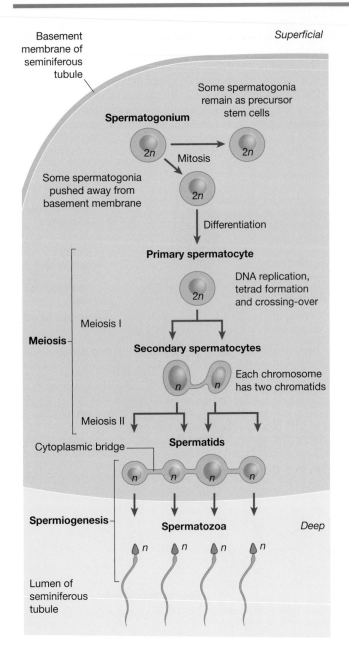

Figure 31.4 **Events in spermatogenesis.**

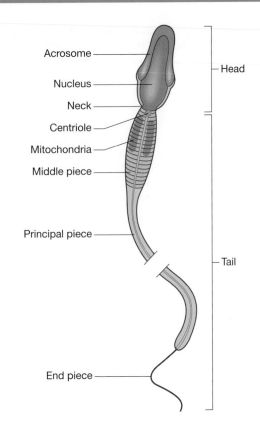

Figure 31.5 **Parts of a sperm cell.**

this process, the Golgi phase, the spermatids' genetic material is packed tightly together to form a nucleus and the spermatid undergoes structural change.

The sperm cell grows a tail that helps it to move. The sperm cell rotates itself around in the wall of the seminiferous tubules, so that its tail is facing towards the lumen, or inner space, of the tube. With the help of testosterone, the Sertoli cells consume the excess cellular materials in the maturation phase. In another process known as **spermiation**, the mature sperm cells are released into the lumen and propelled into the epididymis. Here the sperm becomes motile and is ready to be ejaculated into the female during sex.

The seminal vesicles located at the base of the urinary bladder produce about 60% of the volume of seminal fluid. Seminal fluid is composed of secretions from the accessory sex organs, the epididymis, the prostate gland, and Cowper's glands. Seminal fluid provides nourishment for the sperm, provides bulk, and increases alkalinity (it is essential to have alkaline pH in order to mobilise the sperm and ensure fertilisation of the ova). Sperm when mixed with this fluid is called semen. Each seminal vesicle joins its matching vas deferens to form an ejaculatory duct, entering the prostatic urethra. During ejaculation, seminal fluid combines with sperm at the ejaculatory duct entering the urethra for expulsion.

The total amount of semen ejaculated varies and is between 2 and 4 mL. The total ejaculate of a healthy male contains 100–400 million sperm.

Hormonal regulation and control of spermatogenesis is complex and involves a number of activities. The production of sperm is regulated by hormones (Figure 31.6).

The hypothalamus begins secreting gonadotropin releasing hormone (GnRH) at the onset of puberty. GnRH stimulates the

splitting in half to form two identical daughter cells. The primary spermatocytes, which have twice the amount of genetic material, undergo meiosis. In this type of division, the parent cell splits, forming two diploid daughter cells that have half the chromosomes of the parent cell. The resulting secondary spermatocytes, which have the normal amount of chromosomes, must then go through meiosis II, forming spermatids. This is called **spermatidogenesis**.

Spermatids have only half the total amount of chromosomes. This is because when the sperm joins with the ova, which also contains only half the amount of necessary chromosomes, they form a full set of chromosomes made from both male and female genes.

During the final phase of spermatogenesis, the sperm cell grows a tail and reaches full maturation (Figure 31.5). In the first stage of

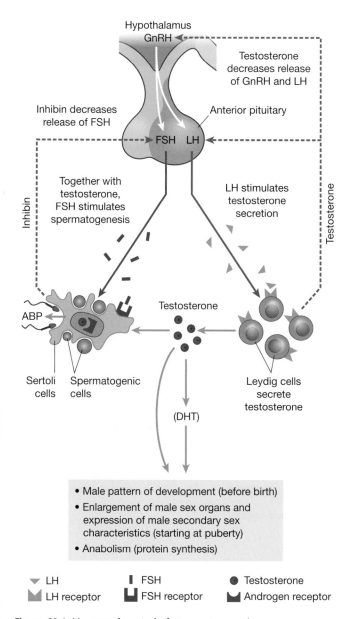

Figure 31.6 Hormonal control of spermatogenesis.

- Penile size increases
- Scrotum enlargement
- Growth of the testes
- Enlargement of larynx and deepening of the voice
- Muscle mass increases
- Basal metabolic rate increases
- Increase in sebaceous glands
- Thickening of the bones.

Levels of testosterone are regulated by a negative-feedback mechanism with the hypothalamus. When excessive amounts of testosterone are detected in the blood, it reduces the secretion of GnRH. The anterior pituitary responds, reducing its production of LH and FSH, resulting in a decrease in the production of testosterone by interstitial cells. GnRH secretion is further inhibited by inhibin, a hormone secreted by sustentacular cells in response to excessive levels of sperm production.

The Penis and Scrotum

The **penis** and **scrotum** comprise the male external genitalia.

The scrotum

The scrotum is a sac providing a supporting structure for the testes; it is composed of loose skin. Within the scrotal sac, a loose bag-like sac of skin, suspended by the spermatic cord in between the thighs, are the testes. The scrotum is separated into lateral portions by the median raphe; the dartos muscle is a smooth muscle that forms the scrotal septum. Associated with each testicle in the scrotum are the cremaster muscles. Contraction of the cremaster muscles brings the testes closer to the body, so as to absorb body heat. The dartos muscle when contracted causes the scrotum to become tight, conserving heat. When the man is exposed to heat these actions are reversed.

The penis

Within the penis is the urethra. The penis provides a route for the elimination of ejaculate and urine via the urethral orifice situated at the end of the penis; the enlarged aspect is called the **glans penis**. The glans penis corresponds to the female clitoris. The penis is cylindrical in shape and is made up of three columns of erectile tissue:

- Two corpora cavernosa
- One corpus spongiosum.

At the end of the corpus spongiosum is the bulbous glans penis, covered with a thin layer of skin that allows for erection and, in uncircumcised males, the skin at the glans folds over on itself forming the prepuce or foreskin; the area where the foreskin is attached, beneath the penis, is called the **frenulum**, which is homologous with the female clitoral hood. The urethra, the end of the urinary tract, lies at the tip of the glans and this is known as the **urethral meatus** (Figure 31.7).

Male Reproductive Physiology

Erection is a complex neurophysiological activity. The complex event occurs as blood rapidly flows into the penis becoming trapped in its spongy chambers. There are three systems directly involved in a penile erection:

1. The spongy corpora cavernosa
2. The autonomic innervation of the penis
3. The blood supply of the penis.

anterior pituitary gland to secrete follicle stimulating hormone (FSH) and luteinising hormone (LH). LH stimulates the interstitial cells in the testes to produce testosterone and other androgens. Testosterone produces the following effects:

- It stimulates the final stages of sperm development in the nearby seminiferous tubules, accumulating in these tissues because testosterone and FSH act together to stimulate sustentacular cells to release androgen-binding protein (ABP). ABP holds testosterone in these cells
- Testosterone entering the blood circulates throughout the body, stimulating activity in the prostate gland, seminal vesicles and various other target tissues.

Testosterone and other androgens stimulate the development of secondary sex characteristics, which are not directly involved in reproduction. The physical changes in the male related to testosterone are:

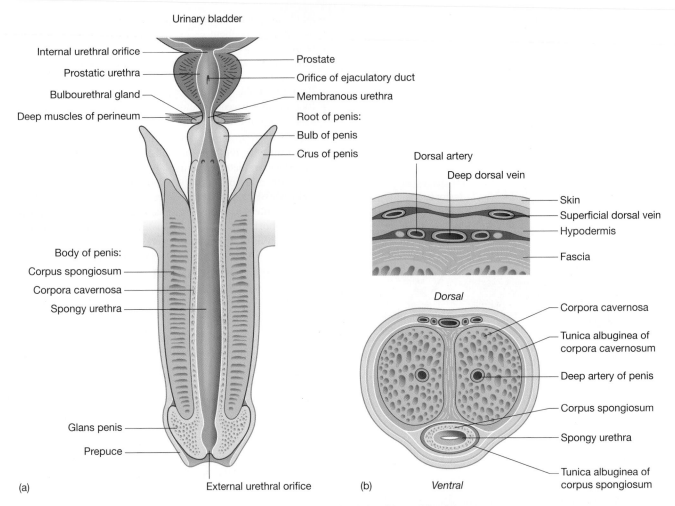

Figure 31.7 Internal structure of the penis. The inset in (b) shows details of the skin and fasciae.

There are sensory, peripheral and central nervous system pathways that integrate the response.

The two corpora cavernosa are primarily responsible for penile rigidity during an erection. The corpus spongiosum becomes tumescent during an erection and it does not become rigid. Its action is to redistribute the intraurethral pressure so that the urethra remains patent and an effective outlet for the ejaculate.

Small (helicine) arteries (with rigid muscular walls) transmit blood into the lacunar space, which is surrounded by smooth muscle inside the trabecular wall. Exiting from the lacunar space are small venules merging to become larger (subtunical) venules. The subtunical venules drain through the tunica albuginea forming the emissary veins. These veins have flexible walls and are easily compressed.

When the penis is flaccid, the smooth muscle in the lacunar walls is in a contracted state; noradrenergic sympathetic fibres provide this contraction. Noradrenergic tone is blocked upon activation of the parasympathetic system and the intralacunar smooth muscle relaxes.

Blood flows into the relaxed lacunar space via the helicine arteries. This causes distention in the lacunar space; the subtunical venules and emissary veins are physically compressed as the lacunae expand. Blood readily flows into the lacunar space but cannot exit via the penile venous system. Distension increases until the intralacunar pressure is the same as the mean arterial pressure (Figure 31.8).

Neural pathways also play an important part in penile erection. Regulation of cavernosal smooth muscle is essential in controlling an erection. Concurrent parasympathetic neural pathway activation and inhibition of sympathetic outflow are required for the smooth muscle relaxation that allows blood to flow into the sinusoidal spaces. The parasympathetic nervous innervation travels to the penis via the pelvic nerve and the sympathetic innervation travels via the hypogastric nerve. A number of neurotransmitters are involved in the parasympathetic modulation of cavernosal smooth muscle relaxation. Nitric oxide is the main pro-erectile neurotransmitter. It co-localises with acetylcholine and vasoactive intestinal peptide (VIP) in nerve fibres, terminating on the trabeculae of the corpora cavernosa and on the helicine arteries. Cavernosal smooth muscle contraction appears to be largely under noradrenergic control. The most important major anti-erectile agent is norepinephrine.

Reflex erection can be provoked by afferent signals from sensory nerve endings on the glans; this is mediated at the level of the spinal cord. The afferent limb of the reflex is carried by the internal pudendal nerves, which can also be activated by tactile stimulation

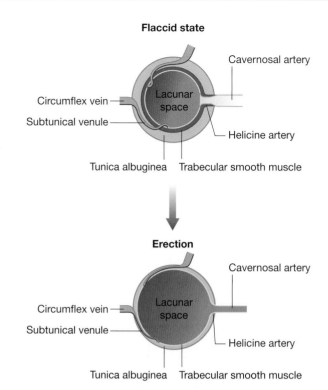

Figure 31.8 Model of vascular events controlling erection. Source: Heffner & Schust (2014). Reproduced with permission of John Wiley & Sons Ltd.

of the perineum close to the testes and scrotum. Erections can be modified by supraspinal influences in the central nervous system (Figure 31.9).

The significance of testosterone in erectile function is unknown. Nocturnal erections are testosterone dependent. Erections occurring in response to visual stimuli are non-testosterone dependent and occur in those men who are hypogonadal.

As ejaculation approaches, penile rigidity increases even more. Smooth muscles in the prostate, vas deferens and seminal vesicles contract repeatedly, expelling the seminal plasma and spermatozoa into the urethra. Emission is mediated by α-adrenergic sympathetic fibres travelling through the hypogastric nerve. Ejaculation is dependent upon the smooth muscles of the urethra and the action of the striated bulbocavernosus and ischiocavernosus muscles.

Jot This Down

A patient asks you to explain the function of the prostate gland. How would you explain this in a way that he understands?

The prostate gland

The function of the prostate gland is not well understood. The prostate is a glandular and muscular organ surrounding the beginning of the urethra, attached by a connective tissue sheath posterior to the symphysis pubis. Its measurements are about $2.5 \times 3.5 \times 4.5\,cm$.

The median lobe of the prostate is referred to histologically as the transition zone; it is wedge-shaped, directly surrounding the

urethra and separating it from the ejaculatory ducts. When hypertrophied (increased in size), the median lobe can cause an obstruction to urine flow; this occurs commonly in older men.

The anterior aspect of the prostate is composed chiefly of fibromuscular tissue. The glandular tissue of the prostate is situated at the sides of the urethra and immediately behind it. This glandular tissue is subdivided into a central and peripheral zone. The peripheral zone is larger than the central zone, made up of around 50 incomplete defined lobules. Each lobule contains tiny ducts emptying directly into the urethra just above the ejaculatory ducts.

The blood supply to the prostate most commonly arises from the common origin of the internal pudendal and inferior gluteal arteries off the internal iliac (hypogastric) arteries. The veins draining the prostate are wide and thin-walled. The prostatic plexus communicates with the vertebral venous plexuses; and as such, if a tumour arises in the prostate, this can give rise to secondary growth in the vertebral column. Lymphatic drainage follows that of the seminal vesicles and bladder neck into the iliac chain of nodes.

All the muscular tissues in the vas deferens, prostate, prostatic urethra and seminal vesicles are involved in ejaculation. Of the volume of the seminal fluid, 15% is made up of prostatic secretions. These secretions aid in semen liquefaction.

The breast

The male breast is comprised of fat with some glandular tissue, with an areola (circular pigmented area) and a small nipple lying over a thin disc of undeveloped breast tissue that may not be obviously dissimilar from nearby tissue.

The structure of the male breast is almost identical to that of the female breast, however the male breast tissue lacks the specialised lobules, as there is no physiological need for milk production by the male breast.

Red Flag

If the nurse notices or the man complains of:
- Unilateral eczematous skin or nipple change that does not respond to topical treatment
- Nipple distortion of recent onset
- Spontaneous unilateral bloody nipple discharge

then these should be reported **immediately** as they may be indications of breast cancer.

Assessing the System

Because of the dual role of some male reproductive organs (with the urinary system), this will result in data collection about reproductive and elimination functions. Many of the same diagnostic procedures will be used to evaluate both. The nurse will be required to carry out an assessment of the male reproductive system and an assessment of the man's needs in a number of clinical situations, with the intention of making a diagnosis, to plan care and evaluate interventions. Assessment of needs must be undertaken with the best interests of the man at heart, with compassion and respect at all times.

It should be remembered that assessment of the status and function of the reproductive system could reveal personal and private

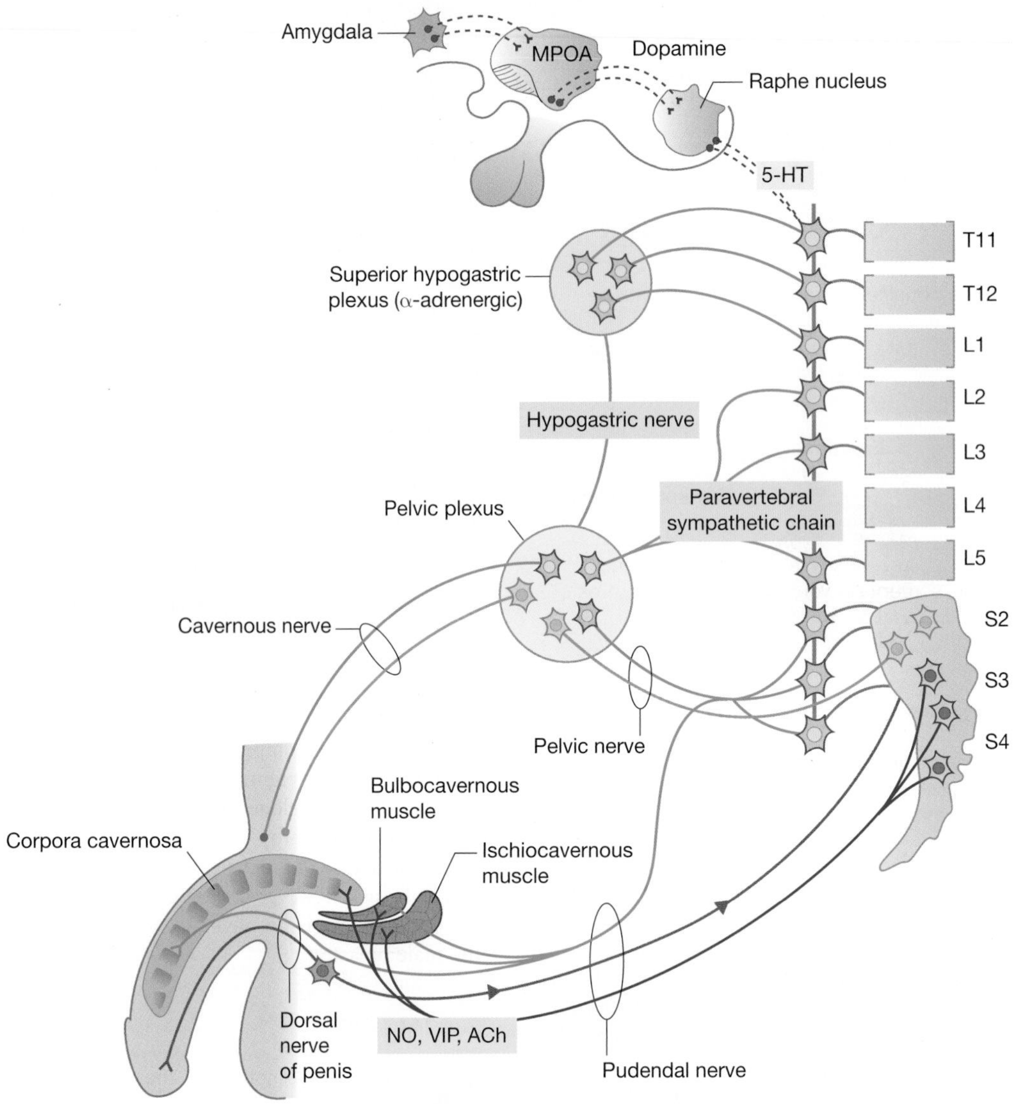

Figure 31.9 Neural pathways involved in penile erection. ACh – acetylcholine; MPOA – medial preoptic area; NO – nitric oxide; VIP – vasoactive intestinal peptide. Source: Heffner & Schust (2014). Reproduced with permission of John Wiley & Sons Ltd.

information. The man must be informed that the information gathered will remain confidential and if this information is to be shared with others, it will only be shared with his consent. The interview will focus on questions concerning:

- Illness
- Signs
- Symptoms
- Sexual health problems
- Sexual activity
- Fertility
- Sexually transmitted infections.

Subjective data includes information about hygiene, safe sex practices and habits that may create risks for reproductive system disorders.

The assessment phase of the nursing process is associated with the findings from diagnostic tests, a health history where subjective data is collected and a physical assessment enabling you to collect objective data. Chapter 6 of this text describes the nursing process in more detail.

The Health History

The health interview provides an additional method for assessing and determining problems. A number of situations arise whereby the interview may be undertaken, for example, during a health screening, or it may focus on a chief complaint (i.e. pain in the groin) or occur as part of an in-depth holistic health assessment. Using a holistic approach, you should take into account issues from a psychological, social and cultural perspective that can impact negatively and positively on sexuality and sexual activity. The choice of words used when carrying out the health interview should be given careful consideration; choose words that the man can understand, and try not to be offended or embarrassed by the words being used. Begin the interview with general questions about the man's overall health status and then move on to specific questions, using verbal and non-verbal cues that encourage him to explain behaviours, signs and symptoms.

Box 31.1 details issues to be considered when carrying out the interview. You should always ensure privacy. The questions asked will depend on the reason for the interview.

Box 31.1 Issues to Be Considered during the Health Interview

Ask the man about any health problems he is having, determine onset, characteristics and course, severity, exacerbating and relieving factors and any associated symptoms, noting timing and circumstances:

- When did you first notice you were having difficulty with your erection?
- Tell me about the changes that occurred in your urine stream after your prostatectomy.
- Have you ever had problems with your penis, testicles, prostate gland? Tell me more. How was the problem treated?
- Have you ever had surgery on your penis, testicles, prostate gland? What was this, when, and how are you now?
- Do you now or have you ever had a discharge from your penis? What was this?
- Have you noticed any changes when you urinate, such as a burning sensation, frequency when passing urine, a need to pass urine urgently, difficulty starting the stream, size of the stream, dribbling or getting up at night more often than usual?
- Describe any pain you have had in the groin area, testicles, penis or scrotum. Where is it? Do you experience it in other parts of your body? How long does it last? What makes it worse or relieves it?
- Has this condition affected your relationships with others?
- Has this condition interfered with your ability to work?
- Are you currently in a sexual relationship? Has this condition interfered with your usual sexual activity?
- Has this problem affected your relationship with your spouse or sexual partner?
- Do you use any medications to facilitate your sexual ability? If so what are these?

Ask about long-term illnesses, such as diabetes, chronic kidney disease, cardiovascular disease (including coronary heart disease, stroke), multiple sclerosis, trauma, thyroid disease (including autoimmune disease). These illnesses and treatments can result in erectile dysfunction.

- The following medications can cause problems with sexual functioning:
  - Antidepressants
  - Antihypertensives
  - Antispasmodics
  - Tranquillisers
  - Sedatives
  - H_2-receptor antagonists.
- Mental health problems, such as depression can contribute to erectile dysfunction
- Mumps as a child can, in later life, lead to infertility
- Those men who have had an undescended testis and those with a family history of testicular cancer are at greater risk for testicular cancer
- Enquire about lifestyle along with social history; ask about alcohol use, use of tobacco or street drugs, as these can impact or may affect sexual function
- Frequent sexual intercourse, particularly if sexual activity is high risk, will increase the risk for sexually transmitted infections

---

- Ask about sexual preference. High-risk sexual activity with same-sex partners increases risk for HIV infection.

  Other questions about sexuality should include:
- Number of sexual partners
- Kind of sexual activity
- History of premature ejaculation
- Erectile dysfunction (and other sexual problems)
- History of sexual trauma
- Condom use or other contraceptives
- Current level of sexual satisfaction.

Care, Dignity and Compassion

Respecting a person as an individual will mean that the nurse must also respect the choices that the person makes and this will include choices concerning sexuality and sexual activity. The nurse must act at all times in a non-judgemental way.

The Physical Examination

Ensure that the room where the examination is to take place is warm and private and free from distraction. 'Room in use' or 'Do not disturb' signs should be placed on the outside of the door; you should inform the man that you have done this. Have all the equipment that you are likely to need in the room; this prevents you having to go in and out to retrieve items of equipment, adding to the man's anxiety and extending the time taken to perform the examination.

Care, Dignity and Compassion

You must offer the man the use of a chaperone during the assessment, regardless of the gender of the examiner; adhere to local protocol, policy and procedure.

To reduce or lessen the man's anxiety, provide him with explanations for the procedures; do this in a matter-of-fact way as he may also feel less embarrassed if you do. You can provide the man with diagrammatic representations and the use of a model of the genitalia that demonstrates to him those parts that will be examined.

Offer the man the opportunity to empty his bladder before the examination and always check to see if a urine specimen is required prior to this. It is usual for a gown to be worn after the man has removed his clothing, or a drape cover for his genitals can be used; he may keep his underwear on until the examination is imminent. The man may be asked to sit or stand; reveal only those body parts that are being examined to respect the man and preserve dignity.

The nurse should adapt the method of assessment to the circumstances. Assessment may be undertaken as part of a holistic appraisal or this can be specifically focussed where the problem is known or suspected. If the examination is part of a total physical assessment, then it is usual for the reproductive system to be the last system to be assessed. Both reproductive and urinary systems are assessed.

Changes associated with an ageing male reproductive system can be found in Box 31.2.

Box 31.2 Age-Related Changes in the Male Reproductive Tract

Testes

Testicular mass reduces with a corresponding reduction in spermatogenesis and testosterone release. A reduced sperm count is an unavoidable effect of ageing, however, sperm are produced in such high numbers that some men in their 80s and 90s are able to father children.

Ducts

The vas deferens becomes progressively less elastic as a result of sclerosis (caused by an accumulation of collagen). The output of the seminal vesicles and prostate gland can decrease, with a resulting decrease in the volume of ejaculate.

Prostate gland

Many older men have some degree of age-related increase in the size of the prostate gland (benign prostatic hypertrophy). Generally, this is harmless; however, it can lead to the prostate compressing the urethra, making micturition difficult. Although ageing does not cause prostate cancer, incidence increases with age.

Penis

Penile arteries and veins may harden.

Changes in the vasculature of the penis can result in the man taking longer to achieve an erection and ejaculation.

Hormones

Most men do not experience the sudden physiological changes experienced by many women as they pass through the menopause. The changes experienced by men occur gradually; collectively, they are called the **andropause** (the male meno-pause). Little is known about these changes but it is believed that they are caused by a gradual decline in levels of circulating testosterone. Onset is slow and usually has little impact on general health.

The interstitial cells (testosterone-secreting cells of the testes) synthesise and release less testosterone. There is no consensus if this is caused by changes in the interstitial cells or in the secretions of the pituitary gland that control testoster-one output.

Reduced testosterone output may contribute to erectile dys-function, particularly if associated with blood vessel disease. Reduced levels of testosterone are associated with some impor-tant physiological changes, including:

· Increased body fat (usually central and visceral body fat)
· Reduced muscle mass
· Reduced bone mass
· Erectile dysfunction and reduced libido
· Increased risk of anaemia.

(*Source*: Adapted from Knight & Nigam 2008)

Box 31.3 Some Urinary Symptoms

Dysuria	Pain when passing urine
Urgency	Unable to put off micturition
Anuria	No urine produced
Oliguria	Reduced urinary output
Polyuria	Increased volume of urine
Frequency	Frequent passage of urine
Nocturia	Waking at night to pass urine
Haematuria	Blood in the urine
Strangury	Painful urge to pass urine
Urinary incontinence	Involuntary passage of urine. Urge incontinence occurs when the need to pass urine is felt. Stress incontinence – happens when sneezing, coughing or laughing
Prostatism	Hesitancy – having to wait for the urine stream to begin Slow stream – poor flow of urine Terminal dribbling – residual urine leaks from the urethra after micturition

(*Source*: Adapted from Douglas et al. 2009).

After taking a history, each symptom identified is assessed. It is advisable to use a permission type of questioning, for example, 'There are some men with diabetes who find it difficult to achieve an erection. Have you been experiencing any of these problems?' (Gleadle 2012). Time should be taken to ascertain if there have been any problems with the urinary stream. See Box 31.3 for an overview of urinary symptoms.

Put on gloves before beginning and wear them throughout the examination. Provide the man with an explanation for everything you do. Bear in mind that the man may be anxious and the exami-nation itself may cause discomfort. Table 31.1 provides an overview of the examination process.

Along with taking a detailed history and a physical examination other investigations may be required:

- Dipstick urine should always be undertaken and microscopy for blood, protein, white blood cells and casts
- Microbiology swabs should be taken if there is suspected infec-tion, e.g. *Candida* or any STI
- Laboratory tests may include:
  - Alpha-fetoprotein
  - Prostate specific antigen
  - Semen analysis
  - Plasma and serum testosterone levels
- Imaging studies can include:
  - Magnetic resonance imaging
  - Ultrasonography
- Other tests can include:
  - Prostate gland biopsy
  - Urinary flow test
  - Urodynamic studies.

A number of these tests will be used to help make a definitive diagnosis.

A skilled practitioner should undertake examination of the male reproductive system. The equipment required will depend on the extent of the examination but the following should be available:

- A good light source
- Disposable gloves
- Water-soluble lubricant.

Shah and DeSilva (2008) note that the examination should be carried out in a systematic manner. The penis, scrotum, pubis and groin should be inspected in turn. The nurse should use:

- Inspection
- Palpation
- Examination.

Table 31.1 An overview of the examination process.

	INSPECTION	PALPATION AND EXAMINATION
Penis	The skin of the penis should be slightly wrinkled, pink to light brown in white men and light brown to dark brown in black men. Inspect the penile shaft and glans for lesions, nodules, inflammation and oedema. When inspecting the urethral meatus, gently compress the tip of the glans to open. The urethral meatus should be located in the centre of the glans, pink and smooth with no discharge; if discharge is present, a specimen should be taken.	Gently use your thumb and forefinger to palpate the shaft of the penis. It should be firm and skin should move unrestricted and be smooth. Palpate to determine if there are any nodules or indurations.
Scrotum	With the man standing, hold the penis away from the scrotum so that you are able to clearly observe the size of the scrotum and its appearance. It is normal for one testis to hang lower (usually the left). The skin on the scrotum is often darker than the skin on the rest of the body. Gently spread the skin of the scrotum and inspect for swelling, nodules, redness, ulcerations and distended veins.	
Testes		When palpating the testes, they should be equal in size, move freely, and feel firm, smooth and rubbery. If there are any hard or irregular areas or lumps, then use a torch and transilluminate the scrotal sac by darkening the room and pressing the head of the torch against the scrotum, behind the lump. If there are any lumps, masses, warts or blood-filled sacs, they will appear as opaque shadows. The same test should be carried out on the other testis to make a comparison.
Epididymis		The epididymis is usually located in the posterolateral area of the testis. It should be gently palpated and appear smooth, easily identified, non-tender and free from swelling and induration.
Spermatic cords		Palpate both spermatic cords; located on top of the testes. Palpate them from the base of the epididymis to the inguinal canal. You can use transillumination should you feel any irregularity or the presence of nodules. If there is any serous fluid present, there will be no glow from transillumination.
Inguinal femoral areas	Ask the patient (still in the standing position) to perform the Valsalva manoeuvre (hold his breath and bear down) as you inspect the inguinal and femoral areas for any signs of bulging or hernia.	To palpate for a direct inguinal hernia, ask the man to perform the Valsalva manoeuvre and you will feel a bulge if he has a hernia. For an indirect inguinal hernia, examine the man in the standing position and then in the supine position with his knees flexed. In locating the presence of a femoral hernia, gently place your right index finger on the right femoral artery with your finger pointing towards the man's head. Keep your other fingers close together. The middle finger will rest on the femoral vein and your ring finger on the femoral canal. Be aware of any tenderness or masses. Use the left hand to check the left side.
Prostate gland		Explain to the man how you are going to examine the prostate gland. Help the man to lie on his left side with his right knee and hip flexed. Inspect the skin in the perineal, anal and posterior scrotal regions. The skin should be smooth and unbroken with no protrusions. Explain to the man that you are lubricating your index finger and you will insert this gently into the rectum. Ask him to relax, taking deep breaths, so as to ease the insertion of the finger. With the pad of the index finger, palpate the prostate gland on the anterior rectal wall past the anorectal ring. You should feel a smooth rubbery gland about the size of a walnut.

What To Do If...

 As you put on your gloves the man takes offence and accuses you of thinking he is dirty or infected. Do you continue with the procedure without the gloves on so as not to cause any offence? What would you do?

Reproductive Health Conditions

Testicular Disorders

There are a number of disorders of the testis and these include:

- Ectopic testis
- Cryptorchidism
- Testicular torsion
- Testicular cancer.

As the testes are the sites of spermatogenesis and androgen production, these disorders may have a potentially negative effect on fertility and secondary sex characteristics.

Cryptorchidism and ectopic testis

These are similar congenital conditions in which descent of the testis is incomplete (in cryptorchidism) or has taken an abnormal route (ectopic). In cryptorchidism, the descending testis stops in the pelvic cavity, inguinal canal or upper end of the scrotum. An ectopic testis ends up in the perineal or suprapubic region or just beneath the skin of the thigh.

Testicular torsion

Testicular torsion occurs with twisting of the testis on the spermatic cord. This can occur spontaneously or as a result of trauma or vigorous exercise. It occurs most often during puberty but may happen at any time of life. Twisting the testicular blood vessels causes testicular ischaemia and if left untreated, necrosis of the testis. Testicular torsion also results in scrotal swelling that is not eased by rest or support of the testis. The man complains of severe pain and nausea and may vomit. Pyrexia is common. Unless it is corrected within 4–6 hours, damage to the testis can permanently impair fertility.

Testicular Cancer

This is the most common malignancy in men in the 20–40-year age group accounting for less than 1% of male cancers. Germ-cell tumours (GCTs) are the most widespread type of testicular cancer; their incidence has risen over the past two decades, as has the most prevalent risk factor for GCT, an undescended testis (cryptorchidism). This, according to Heffner and Schust (2010), suggests that the number of men with testicular cancer will continue to rise.

Pathophysiology

The majority of primary testicular tumours arise from intratubular germ cells. There are six well-defined types of GCT. Five of these occur in young men; one is seen exclusively in older men (spermatocytic seminomas).

All GCTs of young men develop from spermatogonial cells. Prognosis and treatment depend upon whether GCTs are pure seminomas (SGCTs) or mixed cell tumours (non-seminomas, NSGCTs).

Approximately 80% of GCTs secrete tumour markers that can be detected in the serum. Tumours with yolk sac components typically secrete alpha-fetoprotein (AFP), an embryonic protein normally produced by the yolk sac during development. Other NSGCTs can also secrete AFP but seminomas do not. Human chorionic gonadotropin (hCG) is typically secreted by choriocarcinomas; however, small amounts of hCG production have been found in SGCTs as well as NSGCTs. Clinical models using serum levels of AFP and hCG have been developed to aid in the diagnosis and staging of GCT.

The majority of GCTs are diagnosed at an early tumour stage, when the tumour is confined to the testis. Serum screening, physical examination and testicular ultrasounds are valuable in identifying early tumours in men at high risk for GCT, such as men with cryptorchidism and intersex individuals who keep their gonads. When GCT metastasises, it usually spreads unilaterally to the para-aortic lymph nodes.

In 2009, approximately 2200 men were diagnosed with testicular cancer in the UK and the incidence is rising. While the cause of testicular cancer is unknown, there are some known risk factors. The highest incidence in England of testicular cancer occurs in men who are socially deprived. Geographically, the highest rates of testicular cancer occur in white Caucasian populations in industrialised countries, predominantly in western and northern Europe and Australia/New Zealand, while the cancer is generally rare in non-Caucasian populations, the New Zealand Maoris being the exception (Cancer Research UK 2012a). Box 31.4 summarises the key risk factors for testicular cancer.

Signs and symptoms

The most common sign is a lump, but not all testicular lumps are cancer. All testicular lumps or swellings should be reported to the practice nurse or general practitioner, they should not be ignored. The lump may be the size of a pea or larger.

The primary indication may be a slight enlargement of one testicle with accompanying discomfort. There can be an abdominal ache with a feeling of heaviness in the scrotum. Local spread of the cancer to the epididymis or spermatic cord does not usually occur. Lymphatic and vascular spread to other organs results in distant

---

Box 31.4 Some Risk Factors Associated with Testicular Cancer

- Cryptorchidism
- Hypospadias
- Family history
- Previous testicular cancer
- Some men with fertility problems
- Men with HIV/AIDS
- Ethnicity (white men are more prone to testicular cancer as opposed to black men or men from other ethnic groups in the UK)
- Microlithiasis (the presence of calcium specks in the testes)
- Height (taller than average men have an increased risk compared to shorter men)
- Testicular injury (this can mask the presence of a pre-existing testicular swelling)
- Maternal hormones and pregnancy factors.

(*Source*: Adapted from Cancer Research UK 2012b)

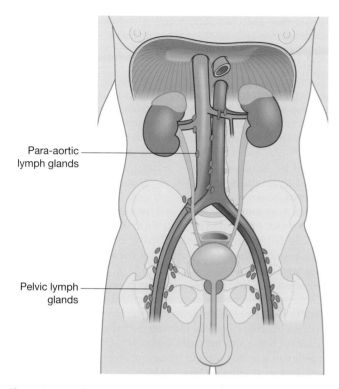

Para-aortic lymph glands

Pelvic lymph glands

Figure 31.10 Pelvic and para-aortic lymph nodes.

disease prior to large masses developing in the scrotum. Lymphatic distribution leads to disease in retroperitoneal lymph nodes, whereas vascular spread leads to involvement in the lungs, bone or liver (Figure 31.10). Cancer in both testes is uncommon. Human chorionic gonadotropin (hCG) producing tumours can lead to breast enlargement (gynaecomastia).

The following are signs of testicular cancer:

- Painless swelling on one testicle
- Dull ache in pelvis or scrotum that may come and go
- A feeling of heaviness in the scrotum
- Painless nodule on one testicle
- Acute pain in scrotum
- Infertility
- Gynaecomastia
- Malaise and fatigue

Signs and symptoms associated with metastatic spread:

- Neck mass
- Respiratory symptoms (including cough, dyspnoea, haemoptysis)
- Gastrointestinal disturbance
- Back pain
- Lower extremity oedema
- Back pain
- Dizziness.

Investigations and diagnosis

History and physical examination will be undertaken. The nurse may be required to act as chaperone to provide physical and emotional support before, during and after the procedures.

What To Do If...

A 16-year-old tells you he is very shy and would prefer it if his mother was not in the room while the examination is taking place. The mother says she wants to stay.
What would you do?

A number of laboratory investigations will be undertaken to make a definitive diagnosis. Analysis of blood will be undertaken to determine if there are any tumour markers present. Raised biochemical markers provide a strong indication of testicular cancer. Tumour markers are also assessed after surgery, helping establish the presence of residual disease. If these levels are persistently raised then this may indicate the need for further therapy. Serum LDH levels are increased in testicular cancer and if there is metastatic spread the level will be significantly elevated.

An ultrasound of both testes will be preformed. This can demonstrate if there is a solid lump, or a fluid filled cyst; the latter is less likely to be a cancer. A man with suspected urological cancer (when in the primary care setting) should be referred to urology or oncological services (NICE 2005).

Nursing care and management

The treatment offered reflects the man's individual needs and desires, and the stage of the cancer (Box 31.5). There are several treatment modalities including surgical intervention, radiation therapy and chemotherapy. The first-line of treatment is surgical removal of the testis (orchidectomy).

The man may be offered one type of treatment or several. The Scottish Intercollegiate Guidelines Network (SIGN 2011) provides national guidelines for the treatment of adults with testicular cancer. One of the recommendations is that a clinical specialist nurse should become involved as early as possible in the management of those men with testicular germ cell tumours. The nurse must be involved in treatment and follow-up. The outcome

---

Box 31.5 Testicular Cancer Staging Systems

There are two systems that can be used to stage testicular cancer.

The first is known as the *TNM staging* system:

- **T** – size of the **t**umour
- **N** – whether the cancer has spread to **n**earby lymph nodes
- **M** – whether the cancer has **m**etastasised.

The second approach is the Royal Marsden Hospital system:

Stage 1 – The cancer may be of any size and is only in the testes. These cancers are further divided depending on whether tumour markers remain elevated.

Stage 2 – The cancer has spread to local lymph nodes (retroperitoneal lymph nodes). These cancers are further divided depending on the size of the lymph nodes.

Stage 3 – The cancer has spread to lymph nodes in the chest or higher up, e.g. lymph nodes in the axillae or neck.

Stage 4 – The cancer has spread to other organs in the body, for example lungs or liver.

following treatment is positive; most men are completely cured, even if the cancer has spread beyond the testicles when it is diagnosed.

The stage of disease (see Box 31.5) usually determines the treatment options:

Stage 1 – The intervention at this stage is orchidectomy. If the cancer is a seminoma, radiotherapy may also be offered directed to the para-aortic lymph nodes. Chemotherapy can also be considered; this is often a dose of carboplatin. Regardless of the approach, the man will require close follow-up for several years.

Stage 2 – The treatment offered for stage 2 seminomas depends on the size of the cancer-containing lymph nodes: postoperatively, radiotherapy or chemotherapy will be offered.

In stage 2, non-seminomas (teratomas) are treated with chemotherapy, but this will depend on tumour markers. If tumour markers are normal, the person may be closely monitored with regular blood tests. Depending on the unique needs of the individual person, there may be a need to perform retroperitoneal lymph node dissection.

Stage 3 – After surgery, all stage 3 testicular cancers are treated with chemotherapy. If any lymph nodes have returned to their normal size after chemotherapy, surgical intervention may be needed with radiotherapy. If there is metastatic spread (e.g. to the lungs) and lung tumours do not reduce in size after chemotherapy, surgical removal may be needed.

Red Flag

Alopecia (hair loss) is a common side-effect of some chemotherapy. It usually begins 1–3 weeks after the first chemotherapy dose. Most people have significant hair loss after 1–2 months. Hair loss can occur on other parts of the body, including the arms, legs and face. For men, hair loss can be very traumatic. The nurse should prepare the man for this event just as they would a woman.

Care of the person with cancer and undergoing radiotherapy or chemotherapy is discussed in Chapter 15.

What To Do If...

As you are escorting the patient to theatre to undergo orchidectomy he confides in you that he is not sure that he wants to go through with the procedure but he doesn't want to cause anyone any trouble.
What do you do?

Nursing care – orchidectomy Preoperatively, the nurse has the opportunity to discuss the surgical procedure and allow the man time to express his fears and anxieties about forthcoming surgery and also about his future. Recognising needs at an early stage helps the nurse arrange support systems. The nurse must make referral to other health and social care agencies where needed. There may be a need to refer the man to a psychosexual counsellor, if he agrees with this.

The provision of information is important but care should be taken not to overload the patient with information. Remember that the man may understand and accept information provided but he may decide not to do anything about it (Caress 2003). Information giving has the potential to enhance recovery (Beddows 1997).

Care of a person postoperatively will include managing pain and observing and responding to the man's physiological and emotional needs (discussed in further detail in Chapter 14). The diagnosis will be confirmed postoperatively. A diagnosis of testicular cancer, regardless of how much preoperative preparation has been undertaken, will be devastating for the patient. The extent of the disease and the presence of any metastatic spread will be detected by increased levels of tumour markers and these will be used to aid diagnosis as well as the care and management of further treatment.

Many men worry that losing one testicle will affect their ability to have sexual intercourse or make them infertile; however a man with one healthy testicle can still have a normal erection and produce sperm. The man should be offered a prosthetic device. If this is what he requests it is usually provided when treatment is complete; it may help with his self-esteem and body image.

Surgery to remove the lymph nodes will not change a man's ability to have an erection or an orgasm; however the procedure can cause infertility as it can interfere with the nerves involved in ejaculation. Some men may have temporary stoppage, then recover the ability to ejaculate without treatment; others may be helped by pharmacological interventions (see later).

Radiation therapy does not change the ability to have sex; it may, however, interfere with sperm production. Usually the effect is temporary, and most men regain their fertility within a matter of months. There may be skin reactions in the area being treated and it is important to treat the skin gently; lotions and creams should not be used on these.

Most men who receive radiotherapy and chemotherapy for testicular cancer can continue to function sexually; some anticancer drugs, however, interfere with sperm production. Men about to have chemotherapy who are interested in having children can create their own sperm bank; specialist oncology nurses can provide advice about this.

Health promotion

Nurses play a central role in educating men about testicular cancer and self-examination. Nurses also have a duty to raise awareness about factors that put men at risk, as well as providing psychological support to the patient and his family. The nurse must be sufficiently informed about testicular cancer risk, symptoms, testicular self-examination (TSE) technique (Box 31.6), assessment procedures, treatment regimens and support services.

Discharge advice

It is essential that follow-up occurs as well as regular monitoring of the man's health and well-being. Information containing discharge and follow-up should be provided in written format. Provide the man with a written list of the medicines he is to take, the amounts, and when and why they are to be taken. Advise the man to call his practice nurse or the hospital if he thinks his medicines are not helping or if he feels he is having side-effects. If antibiotics are prescribed, explain the importance of taking the full dose.

Hormone antagonists may have been prescribed; explain what this medication is for and why it is given.

Explain about the analgesia that has been given, how to use it and how much to take. Encourage the man not to wait until the pain is severe before taking the medicine. Inform the practice nurse

Box 31.6 Advice to Men Concerning Testicular Self-Examination

In order to notice changes, you need to know what is normal for you.

- Hold your scrotum in the palms of your hands, so that you can use the fingers and thumb on both hands to examine your testicles
- Note the size and weight of the testicles. It is common to have one testicle slightly larger, or which hangs lower than the other, but any noticeable increase in size or weight may mean something is wrong
- Gently feel each testicle individually
- You should feel a soft tube at the top and back of the testicle. This is the epididymis. It may feel slightly tender. Do not confuse it with an abnormal lump
- You should be able to feel the firm, smooth tube of the spermatic cord, which runs up from the epididymis
- Feel the testicle itself
- It should be smooth with no lumps or swellings. It is unusual to develop cancer in both testicles at the same time, so if you are wondering whether a testicle is feeling normal or not, you can compare it with the other
- *Remember* – if you do find a swelling in your testicle, make an appointment and have it checked by your practice nurse as soon as possible.

Box 31.7 Discharge Advice

You should contact your general practice if:

- You are nauseous or vomiting
- You have a cough, feel weak and you are aching
- You have a fever or chills
- Your skin becomes itchy or swollen or you develop a rash after taking your medicines
- You have questions or concerns about your surgery, condition or care.

You should seek immediate advice (go to an accident and emergency department or call 999) if:

- You have chest pain, feel lightheaded, are having trouble breathing
- You have more pain when you take deep breaths or cough; you cough up blood
- You have severe pain in your legs or your legs become very swollen
- You have lower stomach or back pain that does not go away even after taking your medicines
- You have trouble passing urine or having a bowel movement
- Your incision is swollen, red, bleeding or pus is coming from it
- Your stitches come apart
- Your leg feels warm, tender and painful – it may look swollen and red.

or hospital if the pain is not being controlled. Let him know that some analgesia may make him dizzy or sleepy and he should not operate any machinery when taking these medicines.

Referral to the community nursing services may be required regarding wound care. Explain that he should not take off any dressings until the community nurse has made an assessment of his needs. He may be advised to wear a scrotal support to provide comfort. Box 31.7 provides a list of advice required after discharge.

Prostate Disease

The term 'prostate disease' addresses a number of prostate-related conditions. There are three main conditions that can affect the prostate gland:

1. Prostatic hypertrophy
2. Prostatitis
3. Cancer of the prostate.

Prostatic hypertrophy

Enlargement of the prostate gland, also called 'benign prostatic hypertrophy' (BPH) is a very common condition associated with ageing and is not usually a threat to the man's health.

The prostate gland becomes enlarged for a number of reasons – the exact cause is unknown. As some men age, the levels of dihydrotestosterone (DHT) increase, and it is thought that this hormone stimulates the growth of the prostate. Prostate enlargement may also be due to testosterone and oestrogen. Younger men produce high levels of testosterone and much lower levels of oestrogen. However, as men age, testosterone levels decrease, resulting in a higher proportion of oestrogen; the increase in oestrogen may be responsible for stimulating prostate growth. As the prostate gland enlarges, this can cause pressure on the urethra. This can affect how the man passes urine. It may cause:

- Hesitancy
- Frequency
- Difficulty emptying the bladder fully.

These symptoms range from mild to severe. Men with prostate enlargement do not have a higher risk of prostate cancer compared with men without an enlarged prostate. Treatment options include:

- Making lifestyle changes, such as reducing the amount of liquid the man drinks before going to bed; avoiding caffeinated drinks
- The use of alpha-blockers (medications used to help relax the muscles within the prostate gland), these include tamsulosin or alfuzosin
- Medications used to reduce the size of the prostate, making it easier to urinate (finasteride or dutasteride block the effects of DHT).

When lifestyle changes and the use of medicines fail, surgery can be used to remove the inner part of the gland. Transurethral resection of the prostate (TURP), transurethral incision of the prostrate (TUIP) and prostatectomy are surgical interventions used for moderate to severe symptoms that have not responded to medical treatment. For those men who may not be well enough to undergo surgery, laser treatment can be used where the prostate is moderately sized (NICE 2012).

Prostatitis

Prostatitis may occur in response to infection; however, in most cases of prostatitis, there is no evidence of infection. Prostatitis is a poorly understood condition where the tissues of the prostate gland become inflamed. Prostatitis can develop in men of all ages, in contrast to prostate cancer and BPH, which usually affect older men. Symptoms of prostatitis can include:

- Pelvic pain
- Testicular pain
- Strangury
- Pain when ejaculating
- Problems urinating
- Discomfort around the scrotum and at the tip of the penis
- Perineal pain.

Box 31.8 Types of Prostatitis

Chronic prostatitis	This is the most common type. Symptoms will have lasted for at least 3 months; they may come and go and vary in severity
Acute prostatitis	Symptoms are severe and develop rapidly. This is caused by a bacterial infection of the prostate gland

These symptoms come and go over a period of months, but can sometimes start suddenly and be a medical emergency. There are two main types of prostatitis: chronic and acute (Box 31.8).

Acute prostatitis is a medical emergency; prompt treatment with antibiotics is required. Failure to respond quickly to the condition can result in diffuse local infection. A combination of treatments can be used to treat prostatitis; analgesics and alpha-blockers can help to relieve the symptoms experienced.

Treating acute prostatitis Acute prostatitis is caused by a bacterial infection of the prostate gland and is treated with a long (4 week) course of antibiotics. The patient should notice that the symptoms are relieved after 2 weeks of antibiotic therapy; however, it is essential that the full course be taken. Pain can be managed by using paracetamol and/or ibuprofen; if pain is severe, a strong analgesic such as codeine may be prescribed.

What To Do If...

When carrying out the administration of medicines for a group of people you are looking after, you have administered one man his antibiotics. About 5 minutes after administration, the man has vomited. Do you administer the same dose of antibiotic again?

Treating chronic prostatitis If the cause of chronic prostatitis appears to be a bacterial infection, a long course of antibiotics will be prescribed. An alpha-blocker can be prescribed with the aim of relaxing the bladder muscles. If there is pain, paracetamol and/or ibuprofen can be used.

There are a number of other medications that have been used to treat non-bacterial chronic prostatitis:

- Finasteride – usually used to treat an enlarged prostate
- Fluoxetine – an antidepressant medication usually used to treat depression
- Mepartricin – a medication usually used to treat fungal infections.

Most men will make a full recovery within 2 weeks. Some, however, may find that the symptoms will return and require further treatment.

Prostate Cancer
Pathophysiology

In the UK, there are more than 200 different types of cancer. Four of them account for over half (54%) of all new cases:

Box 31.9 Risk Factors Associated with the Development of Prostate Cancer

Age – Age is the most significant risk factor of all. Prostate cancer is rare in men under 50 years.

A family history of cancer – If the man has a father or brother diagnosed with prostate cancer, he is 2–3 times more likely to get prostate cancer compared with the average man. The age at which the relative is diagnosed with prostate cancer may also be a factor; if diagnosed before the age of 60, risk increases more than if they were diagnosed after 60. If the man has one or more blood relatives affected – father or brother – the risk is about four times that of the general population.

Men who have relatives with breast cancer may also have a higher risk.

Genes and prostate cancer – There is an indication that other genetic factors may increase the risk.

Bowel cancer – There is an increased risk of prostate cancer in men who have had colorectal cancer.

Ethnicity – Prostate cancer is more common in black Caribbean and black African men than in white or Asian men.

Diabetes – Men with diabetes mellitus appear to have a lower risk of prostate cancer than the average man.

Diet and prostate cancer – Eating a healthy diet can lower the risk of many cancers. However, much of the research has not found any definite links between particular foods and the risk of prostate cancer.

Hormones and prostate cancer – Hormone levels may or may not play a part in the risk of developing prostate cancer; the evidence is inconclusive.

Aspirin and anti-inflammatory drugs – Taking aspirin regularly may reduce the risk of prostate cancer. There is some evidence to suggest that the use of other non-steroidal anti-inflammatory drugs (NSAIDs) reduces the risk of prostate cancer.

1. Lung
2. Breast
3. Colorectal
4. Prostate.

Prostate cancer is the most common cancer in men (not including non-melanoma skin cancer) in the UK. There are over 40 800 men diagnosed with prostate cancer annually, accounting for almost 25% of all cancers diagnosed in men (Cancer Research UK 2012c). There are a number of risks and causes that can affect the possibility of developing prostate cancer (Box 31.9).

The majority of prostate cancers are adenocarcinoma in origin (Varma & Chandra 2012) arising from one cell (Cash 2006).

Medicines Management Aspirin

All drugs have some side-effects. Common side-effects associated with aspirin include:

- Gastric irritation
- Indigestion
- Nausea.

Eating a bland diet and taking aspirin after a meal may relieve these side-effects.

Less common side-effects include:
- Bronchodilation and bronchospasm (caution should be used with asthmatic patients)
- Vomiting
- Gastric dilation
- Gastric bleeding in the stomach
- Bruising
- Allergy.

If any of these side-effects occur, inform the doctor immediately.

Signs and symptoms

Early prostate cancer is often asymptomatic (Weston *et al.* 2011). It is found in men who have an elevated serum prostate specific antigen (PSA) level (this is an enzyme only produced by the prostate gland) and an abnormal digital rectal examination (DRE). There is much debate about the use of PSA in men; however, this is a test that can help to determine the probability of prostate cancer. Table 31.2 outlines symptoms of advanced prostate cancer.

Link To/Go To

The NHS Cancer Screening Programmes website provides further information for the Prostate Cancer Risk Management Programme for England:

http://www.cancerscreening.nhs.uk/prostate/index.html

Bone is the most common site for metastatic spread, in particular the lower back, pelvis and hips.

Investigations and diagnosis

A history is taken from the man and a physical examination is performed. The nurse may be required to act as chaperone and to offer physical and emotional support to the man (and if appropriate his family) before, during and after the procedures.

Prostate specific antigen and digital rectal examination An estimation of PSA and a DRE are usually the first steps taken after the man has provided a medical history.

Table 31.2 Symptoms for prostate cancer. (*Source*: Adapted from LeMone *et al.* 2011; Weston *et al.* 2011)

LOCALLY ADVANCED	METASTASIS
Obstructed lower urinary tract symptoms (problems with storage and voiding urine) Haematuria Haemospermia Pain (penile, perineal) Obstructive uropathy (bladder outflow is impeded and a back up of urine leads to kidney injury) Erectile dysfunction	Bone pain Pathological fracture Anaemia Lower limb/inguinal oedema Hypercalcaemia

The Evidence

Prostate cancer screening guidelines vary widely between countries and between different medical organisations within individual countries, including the USA. Further, the evidence for and against prostate cancer screening remains highly controversial. Longitudinal follow-up of completed screening trials is ongoing and may yield additional findings as the time course of prostate cancer outcomes can be protracted. The literature controversy suggests that no standard of care exists for prostate cancer screening today. Until there is agreement in guidelines between major professional organisations that have weighed in on this topic, patients and nurses should be encouraged to consider engaging in a shared and informed decision process concerning screening for prostate cancer.

The researchers reviewed Medline for recent articles that discussed clinical trials, evidence based recommendations and guidelines from major medical organisations worldwide concerning prostate cancer screening.

This study calls for more work concerning prostate cancer screening.

(Gomella *et al.* 2011)

Prostate specific antigen (PSA) – Serum PSA is assessed and in normal male patients it is found in small quantities; in prostate cancer it is often elevated. It must be remembered that an elevated PSA is not specific to prostate cancer, there may be other causes of an elevated PSA including (but not exclusive to):
- Benign prostatic hyperplasia
- Urinary tract infection
- Inflammation
- Trauma (e.g. catheterisation).

It is not unusual to find an elevated PSA in older men who do not have underlying prostate cancer. About a quarter of those men with a level of 4–10 ng/mL will on biopsy be identified as having prostate cancer (Weston *et al.* 2011).

What the Experts Say

 I get my own PSA regularly tested because there is no better test for the early detection of prostate cancer and some of these cancers are life-threatening. Is PSA perfect? Not by any means. Is PSA the best we have today? Yes.

(A Consultant nurse urologist)

Digital rectal examination (DRE) – As prostate cancer normally occurs on the periphery of the prostate gland, so it is often palpable during the DRE. When the disease is localised and confined to the prostate gland, a hard nodule is felt. If the gland feels abnormal in shape with an irregular outline or distorted anatomy, the disease is often locally advanced. DRE should only be preformed by skilled practitioners (Brown 2011).

Prostate biopsy If the clinician has determined an elevated PSA and abnormal DRE, the man should be offered a biopsy to confirm diagnosis (Kirby & Patel 2012). Transrectal ultrasound (TRUS)-guided biopsy of the prostate is the most common method of obtaining a biopsy using a Tru-cut needle (Figure 31.11).

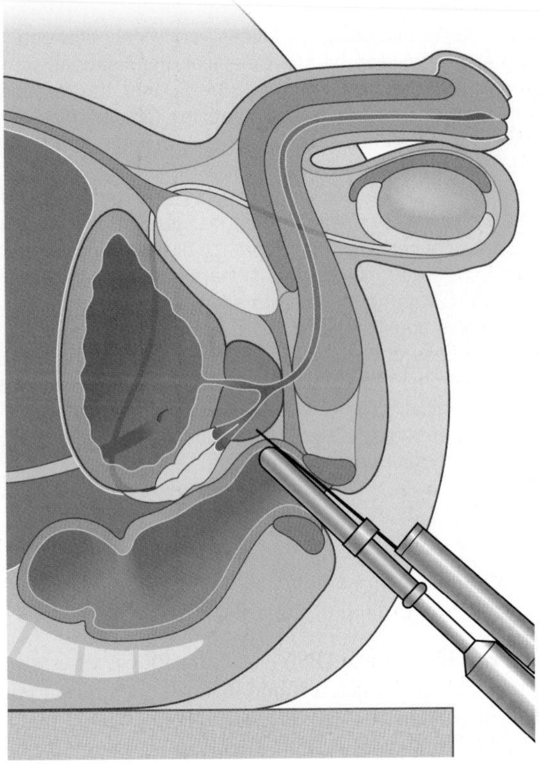

Figure 31.11 **Trans-rectal ultrasound-guided biopsy of the prostate.**

A local anaesthetic is administered and in some instances, sedation may be required. A 12 core biopsy approach is used (this reduces the possibility of a false-positive result). The biopsy not only helps the clinician establish a diagnosis but will also help to grade the tumour, assisting the man and the clinician to plan treatment interventions (see Box 31.10).

There are risks and complications associated with TRUS:

- Haematuria
- Haemospermia
- Rectal bleeding
- Infection
- Urinary retention
- Vaso-vagal syncope (fainting).

The use of prophylactic antibiotics provides some protection against infection.

Weston *et al.* (2011) discuss the increasing use of a transperineal template biopsy of the prostate. This approach is used with endorectal ultrasound guidance (Figure 31.12). The technique allows for a more accurate sampling of the entire prostate, providing better access to apical and transitional zone tissue. Approaching the gland in this manner can help to improve cancer detection rates.

The nurse's role is to make sure that the patient is safe, provide support and assist the person carrying out the test, offering physical and emotional support to the man and ensuring dignity is maintained. Explain that the test should not be painful, but it may be uncomfortable, helping the person as needed. Local policy may require the use of laxatives to ensure the rectum is empty. The procedure lasts for about 15–20 minutes and results are available within a week. After the procedure, the nurse assists the man in cleaning his anal area and helping him to dress if needed. Time

---

Box 31.10 The Gleason Grading System:

Grade 1 – Tumours consist of small, uniform glands with minimal nuclear changes.

Grade 2 – Tumours have medium-sized acini (a cluster of cells), still separated by stromal tissue but more closely arranged.

Grade 3 – Tumours show marked variation in glandular size and organisation and generally infiltration of stromal (a specific type of cells) and neighbouring tissues.

Grade 4 – Tumours demonstrate marked cytological atypia (an increase in cell production) with extensive infiltration (meaning that the cancer has infiltrated deeply).

Grade 5 – Tumours are characterised by sheets of undifferentiated cancer cells.

(*Source*: Gleason 1966)

---

should be provided for the man to ask questions. Provide the man with contact details of whom he can contact should he experience any of the complications discussed earlier.

Nursing care and management

Grading (see Box 31.10) and staging help to decide what the prognosis may be and to guide treatment. The pathologist examines the biopsy material and provides information concerning cancer cell differentiation. Treatment takes into account:

- Patient's age
- Comorbidity
- Patient choice.

As well as whether the cancer is:

- Localised (contained within the prostate gland)
- Locally advanced (has spread just outside of the prostate)
- Advanced (has spread to other parts of the body).

Box 31.11 outlines the choice of treatment.

Medicines Management

 Bisphosphonates have the potential to cause constipation or diarrhoea; this usually only lasts for a few days – it is important to encourage the patient to drink plenty of fluids (6–8 glasses a day).

Red Flag

Recommendations for the first 2 months after seed implantation (brachytherapy) may include:

· Avoiding sexual intercourse for 2 weeks
· Using a condom during sexual intercourse in case a seed is passed during ejaculation
· Limiting close contact with children and pregnant women
· Not allowing children to sit on your lap for extended periods of time.

Nursing care – transurethral resection of the prostate gland

This section of the chapter discusses the nursing care of the man who requires surgery as a result of benign prostatic hypertrophy. It must be remembered that not all men with BPH will require surgery.

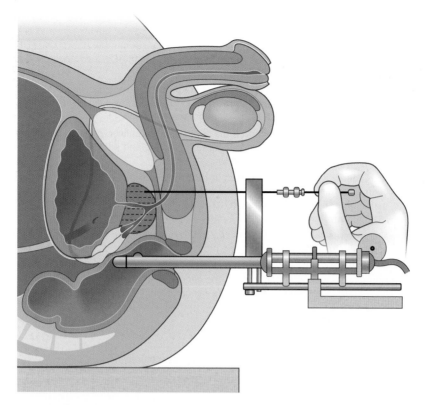

Figure 31.12 Trans-perineal template biopsy of the prostate.

Several surgical procedures are possible for the removal of the hypertrophic prostate gland. These are summarised in Table 31.3.

The aims of surgical intervention are to relieve the symptoms and improve quality of life by allowing the man to retain urinary control and normal sexual functioning.

The general anxiety and concerns people have about undergoing surgery are not uncommon, especially for the man who is to undergo TURP. He must be given a clear explanation of the surgery, its benefits and the consequences of having it done. This way he is making a truly informed decision. The nurse must answer any questions the man has with clarity and if there are issues he/she is unsure of, then appropriate referral must be made. There may be specific concerns about:

- The presence of an indwelling urinary catheter
- Urinary incontinence
- Infection
- The degree of pain
- Sexuality
- Sexual activity
- Fertility
- Erectile dysfunction.

Appropriate counselling is needed prior to surgery.

Care, Dignity and Compassion

To be a nurse is an extraordinary role. Nurses help people to recover from illness, sometimes when they are at their most vulnerable. They provide care and comfort when people's lives are coming to an end.

The Chief Nursing Officer has devised a vision for nursing and this includes the 6 Cs:

1. Care
2. Compassion
3. Competence
4. Communication
5. Courage
6. Commitment.

 Link To/Go To

Compassion in Practice can be found at:

http://www.commissioningboard.nhs.uk/files/2012/12/compassion-in-practice.pdf

Specific postoperative care After the patient has returned from the recovery room, the nurse conducts an initial assessment and continues to monitor for signs and symptoms of urinary compromise. Nursing interventions will involve assessing the urinary catheter for patency and blood loss every 1–2 hours. The nurse may observe red-tinged urine that fades to pink within 24 hours. Monitor for signs of excessive blood loss, including tachycardia and hypotension. A fluid balance chart is instigated and intake and output are checked and recorded. When calculating output, subtract the total amount of irrigation solution infused from the total amount of urine output emptied from the collection bag. If blood

Box 31.11 Treatment Options for Prostate Cancer

Active surveillance	This option provides a way of monitoring prostate cancer, aiming to avoid or delay avoidable treatment in those with less aggressive cancer. Prostate cancer can be slow growing. For many men, the disease may never progress or cause any symptoms. By monitoring the cancer, this can avoid or delay the side-effects associated with treatment
Watchful waiting	Watchful waiting is also associated with monitoring, especially when the cancer is not causing any symptoms or problems. The cancer is monitored over the long term; prostate cancer is usually slow growing and may not cause any symptoms or problems
Radical prostatectomy	This surgical procedure removes the gland and the cancer within it. This option is most successful when the cancer is contained within the prostate gland and the man has no other existing comorbidities (he is fit and healthy)
Radiotherapy	High energy X-ray beams are used in external beam radiotherapy to treat prostate cancer. The X-ray beams are directed at the prostate from outside the body. This is sometimes given in conjunction with permanent seed brachytherapy or temporary brachytherapy. If PSA levels rise postoperatively, then radiotherapy may be used after surgery if there is a possibility that not all the cancer was excised
Permanent seed brachytherapy	This involves the implantation of tiny radioactive seeds in the prostate. Radiation emitted from the seeds destroys cancer cells in the prostate. This treatment may be given by itself or in conjunction with external beam radiotherapy and/or hormone therapy
Hormone therapy	Hormone therapy can help control the cancer by interfering with the production of testosterone or preventing testosterone reaching the cancer cells. Hormone therapy is available in different forms: · Injections · An operation · Tablets · Implant There are side-effects associated with hormone therapy: · Hot flushes · Loss of sex drive · Tiredness
Temporary brachytherapy	Temporary brachytherapy (also known as high dose-rate (HDR) brachytherapy), requires the insertion of a source of high dose-rate radiation into the prostate gland for a few minutes at a time, destroying cancer cells. This can be given by itself or it may be given in conjunction with external beam radiotherapy and/or hormone therapy
High intensity focussed ultrasound (HIFU)	High frequency ultrasound waves are used to heat and destroy cancer cells. It is a fairly new treatment and efficacy is still being investigated. Not all centres in the UK offer this option
Cryotherapy	Sometimes this is also known as cryosurgery or cryoablation (Figure 31.13). The prostate cancer is frozen and then thawed with the intention of killing the cancer cells. This option is usually used for those men with recurrent prostate cancer (whose cancer has returned after treatment with radiotherapy or brachytherapy). This approach may be an option for men who are unable to have other treatments such as surgery or radiotherapy
Chemotherapy	Chemotherapy is used to help control symptoms and not to cure prostate cancer. There are a number of side-effects associated with chemotherapy. Chemotherapy may be used in conjunction with other treatments, such as: · Palliative radiotherapy · Bisphosphonates · Analgesics · Steroids
Abiraterone	This is a new hormone therapy used for men whose cancer has metastasised (advanced prostate cancer) and has stopped responding to other hormone therapy and chemotherapy treatments. It is used to help *control symptoms* and *not to cure* prostate cancer
Bisphosphonates	These drugs may help men with metastatic spread to the bones when their condition is no longer responding to hormone therapy. Bisphosphonates do not treat the cancer but they may help to relieve bone pain

(*Source*: Adapted from Kirby & Patel 2012; Acher & Popert 2012; Dickinson et al. 2012; Henderson & Davies 2012)

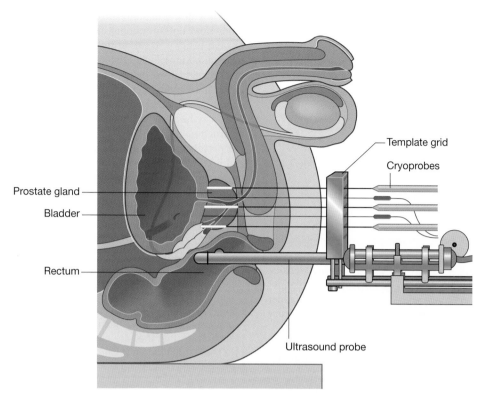

Template grid

Cryoprobes

Prostate gland

Bladder

Rectum

Ultrasound probe

Figure 31.13 Prostate cryotherapy.

Table 31.3 A summary of some potential surgical procedures that can be used to remove the enlarged prostate gland. (*Source*: Adapted from LeMone *et al.* 2011; Steggall 2011)

SURGICAL PROCEDURE	DESCRIPTION	COMMENTS
Transurethral resection of the prostate gland (TURP)	Involves insertion of a resectoscope through the urethra, using an electrically energised loop to excise hyperplastic lobes of the prostate	The surgical procedure of first choice. Requires an inpatient stay.
Transurethral incision of the prostate (TUIP)	Is similar to TURP, except the prostate capsule is cut in several places to reduce urethral stricture as opposed to more extensive tissue removal	Is limited to patients with prostates smaller than 30 g without extensive prostatic invasion of the urethral lumen.
Visual laser ablation of the prostate (VLAP)	A laser-scope is inserted through the cystoscope and vapourises the tissue beneath the epithelial layer causing coagulation necrosis of the prostatic tissue	Has less morbidity and blood loss than TURP. Has shorter total recovery than TURP. May be done in a day-care setting.
Transurethral microwave thermotherapy (TUMT)	A specially designed retention catheter with an internal microwave antenna is inserted into the urethra and a rectal probe with temperature sensors is placed along the anterior rectal wall. The hyperthermia treatment is multiphasic. Both urethral heating and cooling is used to cause tissue necrosis and shrinkage	The most common complication is urinary retention due to residual oedema from the treatment. Is considered cost-effective with good morbidity and mortality statistics. May be done in a day-care setting.
Prostatectomy	Excision of the prostate through suprapubic, retropubic or perineal incisions	The type of prostatectomy is determined by prostate size and whether any bladder abnormalities exist that can be treated conservatively. Requires a longer hospital stay than TURP.

clots prevent adequate catheter drainage, irrigation may be performed with a saline solution according to protocol.

After 72 hours, the urinary catheter is usually removed. The nurse must continue to monitor urinary output every 2–4 hours. The patient is encouraged to drink 2000–3000 mL (if there are no contraindications) of fluids daily to relieve initial dysuria and resolve haematuria.

Jot This Down

You are encouraging a patient to drink 2000 to 3000 mL of fluid a day:

1. How will you know if he has drunk this?
2. How would you encourage this?
3. How would you involve the patient and his family?

Discomfort after TURP is usually associated with bladder distention, irritation from the catheter or irrigation solution or bladder spasm. Smooth muscle relaxants may be prescribed if bladder spasms persist. Prescribed analgesia should be given and its efficacy noted.

TURP syndrome is an associated complication; nursing interventions focus on management and prevention of complications. TURP syndrome usually occurs within the first 24 hours. Abnormal vascular absorption of irrigating fluid during surgery causes severe dilutional hyponatraemia and hypervolaemia. The nurse carefully assesses the patient for symptoms of TURP syndrome, which can include:

- Dramatic increase in blood pressure
- Full, bounding pulse
- Bradycardia
- Tachypnoea
- Confusion
- Agitation
- Temporary blindness.

The nurse must seek help immediately should the patient be experiencing any of the above. Stay with the patient and provide reassurance.

Haemorrhage is the most common complication after TURP. Bladder spasms or movement may initiate bleeding. Nursing interventions include the monitoring of:

- Vital signs every hour (or as the patient's condition dictates)
- Urinary output for colour and consistency of bladder returns every hour
- Increasing the rate of bladder irrigation flow as needed to assure urine flows and prevent obstructions
- Instruct the patient to remain flat or at a slight incline immediately postoperatively; sitting may increase venous and bladder pressure, causing bleeding.

You must inform the nurse in charge if there is any increase in bleeding or change in vital signs that may indicate haemorrhage. Surgical intervention may be needed should the bleeding continue. Hypovolaemia may develop due to extensive bleeding; the patient may require intravenous fluids and a blood transfusion.

Urinary tract infection due to surgical intervention and the presence of an indwelling urinary catheter can lead to septic shock. Careful monitoring is required and the nurse must perform meticulous catheter care and maintain a closed urinary drainage system.

Clots or tissue debris can obstruct the urinary catheter. By assessing the colour and consistency of bladder returns, patency of inflow and outflow tubing and rate of irrigation, the nurse can prevent urinary retention postoperatively. A rapid irrigation may be required initially to flush out debris and clots. An adequate rate can be maintained by the nurse via gentle milking of the outflow tubing at frequent intervals (but at all times local policy, procedure and protocol must be adhered to).

It may be necessary to irrigate with a bladder syringe if a clot obstruction occurs but this must never be undertaken unless the person carrying out the procedure had assessed the patient and is competent in performing the procedure. The rate of irrigation is adjusted, so that a colourless or light pink (rose) output is maintained.

The surgeon must be notified if an obstruction cannot be resolved by hand irrigation or if the urine returns bright red.

Nursing Fields Learning Disabilities

Men with learning disabilities are living longer and fuller lives and should be provided with access to testicular and prostate cancer screening programmes. The information and options provided to men with a learning disability should be offered in such a way that they are able to make sense of it and use it to make informed decisions about choices available. Service provision should be adapted to meet their needs.

Health promotion

Nothing can prevent the development of BPH. Patient education and awareness of signs and symptoms of BPH should be provided to all men and targeting of at-risk groups should be considered. Nurses working in primary and secondary care settings are ideally placed to offer opportunistic or planned information giving sessions.

Primary Care

It has become apparent that the variance in life expectancy between the sexes reflects the fact that men look after themselves much less well than do women. For example, 40% of men will only go to see their GP if told to do so by their partner. Men have a greater susceptibility to heart disease. Most of the preventable risk factors for myocardial infarction or stroke, such as smoking, central obesity and hypertension, are considerably more common in men than in women. As men in the UK visit their doctor four times less often than women, they are less likely to have hypertension, diabetes or hyperlipidaemia diagnosed and treated.

Running a well-man clinic in primary care is just one of a number of ways of tackling these problems. There are major opportunities for improving the health of men in middle age by organising a well-man check in primary care. Providing a dedicated gender-specific service allows men the chance to spend time with experienced healthcare professionals.

It is important for men to know not to wait to seek treatment should they experience any of the signs and symptoms associated with BPH. Delay could result in severe obstruction of the urinary system and subsequent kidney damage.

Jot This Down

How would you go about providing specific services for the following groups of men:

- Men in the armed services
- Men in detention (prison)
- Men who are homeless
- Men who have sex with men
- Men from black and ethnic minority groups.

Discharge advice

Delayed bleeding caused by excessive physical exertion or straining for bowel movements may be experienced up to 2 weeks postoperatively. Advise the patient to drink at least 12 glasses of water per day and to avoid the use of alcohol, caffeinated beverages and spicy foods that can over stimulate the bladder. He should avoid strenuous activities, such as driving, for at least 2 weeks and notify the community nurse or general practitioner if the bleeding does not subside within 1 hour of resting and increasing fluid intake.

Explain to the man what the signs and symptoms of urinary tract infection might be and advise him to inform his GP should he experience any of them, as he may need antibiotic therapy.

If the man was sexually active prior to surgery, sexual activity (and this includes masturbation) can usually be resumed 2–4 weeks after surgery, as long as there is no bleeding in the urine (which indicates that the prostate still has some healing to do). Some men after a TURP have less or no semen after sexual intercourse. There may be retrograde ejaculation (dry climax). This should not impact on the man's desire for or the ability to have sex. Some men find their erection is poorer following TURP. If this is a problem, then encourage the man to speak to the community nurse or his GP.

Erectile Dysfunction

For most people, sex is an important aspect of everyday life. To attain and maintain an erection for many men demonstrates potency; failure to do this can be seen as impotency.

Erectile dysfunction (ED) is only one of a range of male sexual dysfunctions, but it is perhaps the most spoken about. The taboo that may have once been associated with this condition has almost gone, as a result of the advent of easily available and user friendly oral treatments. Despite the increase in understanding, coupled with advances in the field, the disorder is, however, still very distressing for men and their partners. The nurse can help to alleviate the distress caused; however in order to do this effectively, they must have an understanding of the condition and the possible options available to the men to help them manage their health and well-being.

Erectile dysfunction can affect men at any age. It is a psychophysiological disorder impacting on sexual arousal. Being aware of the psychological and physical consequences of ED for the patient (and partner) may help provide a service that meets the needs of a large number of men (Watson 2003).

Men can find it difficult to discuss with healthcare providers a number of issues that are related to their health; they are reticent about seeking help for their health problems (Kirby 2005). When it comes to talking about issues of a sexual nature, this becomes even more difficult. Many men do not find it easy to discuss ED with their own partners, let alone with the nurse. The nurse has to be proactive and provide ways in which the man will share his anxiety, fears and concerns.

Hall (2008) notes that practitioners must provide the man with accurate information and continue to demystify and challenge stereotypes associated with ED and those men who experience it. ED that is not diagnosed and treated can be a cause of morbidity, including low self-esteem, anxiety, depression and a diminished quality of life.

Definitions

There is no standardised definition for ED and estimations vary widely. Wespes *et al.* (2002) suggest that it is the persistent (present for at least 6 months) inability to attain and sustain an erection sufficient to permit satisfactory sexual performance. The American Psychiatric Association (APA 1994) add a psychological element to their definition, stating that the condition has to be characterised by an ability to attain and maintain an adequate erection but, they add, this is also accompanied by marked personal distress or interpersonal difficulties.

Pathophysiology

The prevalence of ED around the world is difficult to establish. As men are known to be reluctant to seek help or advice for ED, this makes it problematical when attempting to find data concerning prevalence; data cited are therefore under-representations of true numbers. Best estimates would suggest that ED affects approximately 5% of 40 year olds and increases to 10% in men in their 60s; this increases to 15% and 30–40%, respectively, in men in their 70s and 80s (Carson & McMahon 2008). ED is age-related but not an age-dependent disorder.

As a number of men may present with physical symptoms, they may also have feelings that impact on their emotions that are related to worries concerning inadequacy, as well as experiencing feelings of emasculation. The nurse should be aware of the pathophysiology of erection and how erections occur and are maintained sufficiently to permit satisfactory sexual performance.

Penile erection is a multifaceted physiological process occurring as a result of a coordinated arrangement of neurologic, vascular and hormonal events. There are complex interactions associated with erection and detumescence. These interactions involve several haemodynamic events resulting in muscle relaxation and vasoconstriction. These are integrated vascular processes that result in the accumulation of blood under pressure and the outcome is usually end-organ rigidity (see Figure 31.8 and Figure 31.9).

Erection happens as a result of an assortment of changes associated with:

- The vascular system
- The endocrine system
- Psychological changes.

If alteration in one of the above occurs, there is a potential for erectile failure. The vascular process can be divided into six phases:

1. Flaccidity
2. Filling phase
3. Tumescence
4. Full erection
5. Rigidity
6. Detumescence.

The male sexual response is shown in Figure 31.14.

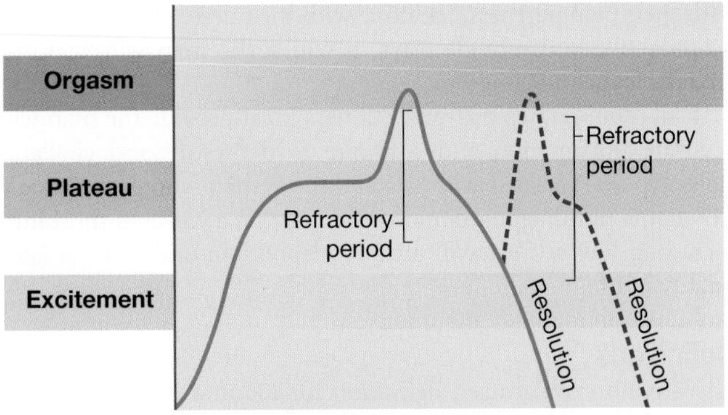

Figure 31.14 The male sexual response. Source: Heffner & Schust (2014). Reproduced with permission of John Wiley & Sons Ltd.

Risk factors associated with ED

ED is often multifactorial; the causes can be related to organic and/or inorganic disorders (a combination of both factors). Williams and Pickup (2004) suggest that organic causes are related to physiological disorders; inorganic causes are psychological in nature and may be more common in the younger person (see Table 31.4 for a list of factors).

What To Do If...

When working with a practice nurse in general practice, the man you are looking after confides in you that he has not told the nurse who has been assessing his needs that he uses cocaine on a regular basis and he wondered if he should tell her or keep it to himself?
What should you do?

Psychogenic factors are involved in the majority of all cases, in spite of the fact that in the majority of men with ED the dominant pathophysiology is organic.

Diagnosis and investigations

Patients are becoming more aware that simple, effective treatments are available and, as a result, are requesting more access to the treatments available (Carson & McMahon 2008).

Primary Care

Most cases of ED are treated in the primary care setting without the need to refer the patient to specialist secondary care.

A diagnosis will need to be made prior to offering treatment and providing the man with a choice concerning treatment options. Treatment options are based upon the underlying cause. Table 31.5 outlines the differences between psychogenic and organic origins of ED.

Table 31.4 Some potential organic causes of ED. (Source: Adapted from Dorey 2006; Paterson 2006)

FACTOR	POTENTIAL COMPONENTS
Vasculogenic	· Hypertension · Atherosclerosis · Venogenic · Ischaemia
Neurogenic	· Spinal injury · Multiple sclerosis · Dementia · Spinal tumour · Parkinson's disease · Cerebrovascular disease · Cauda equina compression · Prolapsed intravertebral disc

Endocrinologic	· Hormone deficiency
	  · Hypogonadism
	  · Thyroid disease
	· Hyperprolactinaemia

Drug-related	· Certain antihypertensives · Some psychotropics · Some hormonal agents
Systemic	· Diabetes mellitus · Malignancy · Chronic renal failure
Surgery	· Transurethral and radical prostatectomy · Cystectomy · Pelvic surgery (abdomino-perineal resection) · Radiotherapy
Lifestyle	· Smoking · Alcohol · Recreational drugs · Trauma to the perineum · Bicycling · Horse riding
Other	· Arthritis · Aetiology unknown

Nursing Fields Mental Health

Physical health and mental health are inextricably linked. There is a need to improve the physical health of people with mental health problems, and to make mental health a key public health priority. Nurses are required to ensure that men with mental health problems are also having their reproductive health needs considered.

Poor mental health is associated with an increased risk of diseases such as cardiovascular disease, cancer and diabetes; there are inequalities associated with these while good mental health is a known protective factor. Poor physical health also increases the risk of people developing mental health problems.

History-taking, physical examination and clinical investigation help to make a diagnosis. Investigations vary, depending on the findings from the history and the physical examination as well as the willingness of the patient. Clinical investigations can be divided

Table 31.5 Psychogenic and organic causes of ED.

PSYCHOGENIC ORIGIN	ORGANIC ORIGIN
Sudden onset	Gradual onset
Good quality or better spontaneous/self-stimulated/nocturnal erections/waking erections	Lack of tumescence
Premature ejaculation or inability to ejaculate	Normal libido (except in hypogonadal men) and ejaculation
Relationship problems or changes	Risk factor in current or past history in particular with reference to cardiovascular, endocrine and neurological systems
Major life events	Operations, radiotherapy or trauma to the pelvis or scrotum
Psychological problems	Use of medications recognised as being associated with erectile dysfunction
Specific situation	All circumstances
	Lifestyle factors, such as smoking, high use of alcohol, use of recreational drugs or body building drugs

into three sections: essential, possible and specialised. Investigations for ED will include:

- Testosterone
- Prolactin
- Glucose
- LH/FSH
- T_4 TSH
- Liver and renal function
- Neurological tests
- Vascular imaging.

Other investigations can include nocturnal penile tumescence and rigidity (NPTR) monitoring. This can differentiate between psychogenic and organic causes and the number and quality of erections occurring during REM sleep can be assessed. Cavernosometry and cavernosography are investigations that measure pressure and outline radiographically if there are any difficulties within the penile chambers; the aim is to assess arterial inflow and venous outflow of penile blood.

Nursing care and management

Treatments are provided on individual assessment; they vary and can include the increasingly popular oral pharmacological therapies. Other treatments are also available:

- Hormonal treatment
- Mechanical/physical devices, e.g. vacuum devices
- Surgical treatment
- Natural/homeopathic remedies.

All treatment options have the potential to harm; they all have advantages and disadvantages.

Red Flag

 Hormonal therapies, e.g. the use of testosterone, are incompatible with some cancers. Oral treatments are contraindicated when the person is using nitrates associated with cardiac medications.

The use of intercavernosal and transurethral medications, vacuum and ring devices have the potential to cause harm and discomfort and may be seen as unpleasant by some men and their partners. Surgical intervention, the insertion of penile implants, can also lead to complications such as infection.

Nursing care Some men with ED may not be aware of the cause; not knowing the cause can increase anxiety. The man may believe himself to be less than a man. A non-judgemental approach is essential; the cause may be blamed on unrelated factors, such as age, medications, illness or sexual partner.

Psychosexual approaches Popovic (2007) discusses some potential medical treatments. Gene therapy is being devised and stem therapy is also being considered. These pan-biological approaches, it could be suggested, may fail to address the humanistic aspects of sexuality.

Other therapeutic interventions such as psychological and behavioural interventions should be given consideration (sometimes referred to as talking therapies). Where the cause of ED is predominantly psychogenic in origin, a positive response to psychosexual therapy is often noted. The nurse needs to add these approaches to the repertoire of treatment options available. Counselling, psychotherapy, cognitive and behavioural therapy, group therapy and analytic therapy are methods that deserve consideration. Hall (2004) also includes online psychosexual therapy as another alternative to the biological approaches.

These non-invasive therapies can also have drawbacks. They require time investment; the length of time required to observe desired outcomes can be extensive. Their availability is variable: some healthcare providers do not have in-house therapists available and referral to an accredited sexual and relationship therapist will be needed. Sexual and relationship therapy is an important clinical discipline that requires specific training. Therapists have different ways of working and, as such, they may have different approaches to addressing the needs of the man (and partner).

Jot This Down

What do you think are the dangers of buying drugs such as Viagra (sildenafil) from the internet?

It is not expected that the nurse be an expert in the various psychosexual approaches, however; understanding is expected of the nurse in respect to the pharmacological and other potential interventions. It is also expected that he/she must have some understanding of the other non-biological approaches available to men. Knowing when and where to refer the patient is an important aspect of practice nursing. The Code of Professional Conduct

(NMC 2008) requires the nurse to make the care of people their first concern, treating them as individuals, protecting and promoting their health and well-being.

Modern treatment for ED, available worldwide in the form of PDE5 inhibitors (e.g. vardenafil, sildenafil and tadalafil), has transformed the way men with ED are treated. There are other forms of non-invasive, non-biological treatments that are also available. The nurse must ensure that the patient is provided with information about all treatment options prior to him making a final decision.

Erectile dysfunction treatment – NHS

NHS treatment for ED is only available for a limited list of medical conditions. Men whose ED is associated with any of the following conditions are eligible to receive treatment on an NHS prescription:

- Diabetes
- Kidney failure requiring dialysis
- Diabetes mellitus
- Kidney transplant
- Multiple sclerosis
- Parkinson's disease
- Polio
- Prostate cancer
- Prostatectomy, including men who have had a transurethral resection of the prostate
- Radical pelvic surgery
- Severe pelvic injury
- Single-gene neurological conditions
- Spinal cord injury
- Spina bifida.

If ED is judged to cause severe distress, the man can also receive treatment on the NHS – this will need to be assessed by a specialist. Men who were already receiving NHS treatment for erectile dysfunction on 14 September 1998 can continue to receive it on the NHS. All other men with erectile dysfunction will be prescribed treatment by their GP on a private prescription.

Circumcision

Circumcision is the oldest form of surgical procedure. There is also much controversy associated with its practice (Greenberg & Serlin 2008). Male circumcision is the surgical removal of the foreskin. The foreskin is a retractable fold of skin that covers the end of the penis.

> **Nursing Fields** Children's
>
> When a boy requires circumcision (for medical reasons) it is essential that the nurse plans his care with the family. Parents will be required to consent for the procedure but the child will also require information appropriate to his stage of development.
>
> Parents need to know why circumcision is required and can be told that the delicate bulb end (the glans) of the penis is protected by a sleeve of skin, the foreskin. Usually the front of the sleeve of skin progressively frees itself from the bulb. It will pull back over the bulb by the age of 3 or 4 years.
>
> There are times when this sleeve is too long or too tight to allow the sleeve to pull back. This can cause ballooning and pain in the foreskin when the child passes urine or it may cause infection, which makes the foreskin red, swollen and

---

> painful. It should be reiterated that it is not the fault of either parent.
>
> Parents need to know about alternatives. For example, inform them that if things stay as they are, generally there is an even chance that by the time the boy is 16, the foreskin will stretch up. If he gets repeated infections in the area of the foreskin, then the foreskin will get thicker and narrower and the problem will get worse and worse. This could lead to quite a lot of problems for him over the years, both physical and psychological. Simply peeling back the foreskin under an anaesthetic is worthwhile for a milder case.

Pathophysiology

It is estimated that there are currently 650 million males in the world who have been circumcised (Whitfield & Whitfield 2009). There are religious, cultural and medical reasons for circumcision. This aspect of the chapter only considers medical reasons for circumcision.

The only absolute indication why a man would need to have a circumcision (medically) is when a pathological condition called 'phimosis' occurs. This condition is due to balanitis xerotica obliterans – a skin condition resulting in scar tissue formation. Attempts to retract the foreskin fail.

Other conditions affecting the penis include 'balanoposthitis' (inflammation of the prepuce) and 'paraphimosis' (the foreskin is pulled back underneath the tip of the penis, becomes trapped and cannot be returned to its original position). Paraphimosis left untreated will result in death of the tissue of the penis.

Red Flag

> To prevent paraphimosis in the uncircumcised man with a urethral catheter *in situ*, never leave the foreskin behind the head of the penis (glans) for any longer than needed.
>
> If performing catheter care, check afterwards to be sure that the foreskin is covering the head of the penis.

Signs and symptoms

The sign of paraphimosis is a band of swelling around the penis. The man may complain of pain. The symptoms of balanoposthitis include:

- Pain when urinating
- A discharge of pus from the penis
- Inflammation of the shaft of the penis.

Investigations and diagnosis

Clinical examination and history confirm diagnosis.

Nursing care and management

The conditions described can often be managed by the administration of antibiotics and/or medications to reduce the swelling; the need for circumcision is avoided. However, when the condition continues to recur, circumcision can offer a permanent cure.

The operative procedure (circumcision) is similar for all age groups (Whitfield & Whitfield 2009). The procedure is usually carried out under general anaesthetic (local anaesthetic can be used) and is carried out as a day case. The foreskin is removed with a scalpel, scissors or a surgical clamp. Any bleeding is cauterised and the remaining edges of skin are stitched together with dissolvable stitches.

Nursing care

In boys and older men, it can take up to 3 weeks for healing to occur. Circumcision is a painful procedure and analgesia, such as paracetamol or ibuprofen, may be needed for at least the first 3 days postoperatively. A local anaesthetic such as lidocaine may be provided to apply topically.

Erection may occur after the procedure and a benzodiazepine may be required to limit the possibility of this happening (Cotton & Steggall 2011).

Exposure of the sensitive skin of the glans penis occurs when circumcision has been performed. Tight underpants can rub against the glans, making it sore. Therefore, the use of loose fitting boxer shorts or shorts may be better than tight underpants; some men, however, may prefer to wear tight underpants (or a scrotal support) to provide physical support.

Postoperatively, the penis will be red and swollen for a few days; petroleum ointment applied directly onto the area can help to reduce irritation. After circumcision, the man should not ride a bike until the swelling has completely gone down. The man can return to work about a week after the procedure.

There are a number of risks associated with circumcision, as is the case with all types of surgical procedure. These are rare but include:

- Pain
- Bleeding
- Oedema
- Infection (including septicaemia)
- A decrease in sensation in the penis, particularly during sex
- Impaired erection if too much penile skin is removed
- Urethral stricture.

Health promotion

It is safe to have a shower or sit in a bath. Keeping the penis clean and free from infection can help to avoid recurrent infections. The man should be advised to gently wash the penis with warm water each day when having a shower or bath. If he has a foreskin, he should pull it back gently and wash underneath.

If the man fails to wash underneath the foreskin correctly, a substance called 'smegma' may begin to gather. Smegma is a natural lubricant keeping the penis moist. It is found on the glans and under the foreskin. This can accumulate and become a breeding ground for bacteria, resulting in balanitis.

While regular personal hygiene is important, too much washing with soap and shower gels can cause soreness. If soap is used, the man should choose a mild or non-perfumed soap to reduce the risk of skin irritation. Men who have been circumcised also have to be careful about cleaning their penis. Gently washing the penis with warm water once a day is sufficient.

Discharge advice

The man should avoid any sexual activity (intercourse or masturbation) until the wound has fully healed. There may be occasions when nocturnal erection or nocturnal emissions occur beyond the control of the man and this may cause bleeding.

The man should seek advice from the practice nurse or GP following circumcision if:

- There is bleeding from the penis
- The penis remains swollen
- There is still pain and difficulty passing urine
- There is any discharge from the wound and the man has a temperature.

Conclusion

Caring for those men who may have problems associated with the male reproductive system, or even when offering men advice regarding the male reproductive system, demands that the nurse is sensitive in the approach taken. Caring, dignity and compassion must be at the heart of all that the nurse does.

Encouraging men to discuss their needs in respect of the male reproductive system can be a challenge for the man and the nurse. Health education and health promotion tools must reflect the community being targeted, for example, men in places of detention or younger men.

Early detection of some forms of cancer can mean that treatment can be instigated quickly and as a result, outcomes are more positive. Where treatment fails or is refused, the nurse can offer palliative care supporting the man and his family.

In order to offer evidence-based, safe and effective care, the nurse needs have an understanding of the anatomy and physiology of the male reproductive tract. This chapter has provided a general insight into the care required for men with reproductive disorders.

Key Points

- The male reproductive system and its function, along with normal and abnormal changes that may occur as a result of disease or injury, have been discussed.
- A systematic approach to care delivery is required to ensure the needs of the man have been fully explored and met, assessing his physical and psychological needs. The nurse should adopt a sensitive and caring approach when discussing intimate aspects of the man's health and well-being.
- A range of diagnostic tests are available to help make a diagnosis and to plan and implement subsequent care. The nurse is required to ensure that the man knows what is involved in these various tests, so that he is able to make an informed decision. Alternatives to planned treatments (where available) should be discussed.
- There are number of risk factors associated with male reproductive cancers and conditions. These have been outlined; there are some controversies surrounding some of these risk factors and the nurse must have an understanding of these.
- As an advocate, in all health and social care settings, the nurse should work in partnership with the man and, if appropriate, his family, to promote his rights, choices and wishes.
- Overall, the key aim of nursing care should be to practise in a holistic manner, respect individual choice and to offer support, promoting the health, well-being, rights and dignity of men.

Glossary

Androgens: male sex hormones

Benign: not malignant

Biopsy: the removal and examination of tissue, cells or fluids for analysis

Brachytherapy: radiotherapy in which the source of radiation is placed (as by implantation) in or close to the area being treated

Cauterise: to destroy tissue with heat, cold or caustic substances, usually to seal off blood vessels or ducts

Chemotherapy: the use of chemical agents in the treatment or control of disease

Cryosurgery: surgery in which diseased or abnormal tissue is destroyed or removed by freezing

Detumescence: subsidence or diminution of swelling or erection

Fertilisation: the process of combining the male gamete or sperm, with the female gamete or ovum

Gland: an organ or structure producing body fluids or hormones

Gonadotropin releasing hormone (GnRH): the hormone which controls the production and release of gonadotropins

Gonads: the testes

Hormone: a substance produced by an endocrine gland that travels through the bloodstream to a specific organ

Hyperplasia: an increase in the number of normal cells in a tissue or an organ can represent a precancerous condition.

Luteinising hormone (LH): gonads are stimulated by LH. LH is necessary in men for spermatogenesis and for the production of testosterone

Malignant: characterised by progressive and uncontrolled cell growth (especially of a tumour); cancerous

Meiosis: produces daughter cells that have one half of chromosomes as the parent cell

Mitosis: produces two daughter cells that are identical to the parent cell

Motility: the measurement of motion and forward progression of sperm

Orgasm: the climax of sexual excitement that is usually (but not always) accompanied by ejaculation of semen

Pituitary gland: the gland stimulated by the hypothalamus. Located at the base of the brain just below the hypothalamus

Pudendal nerve: a nerve that arises from the second, third, and fourth sacral nerves and that supplies the external genitalia, the skin of the perineum, and the anal sphincters

Radiotherapy: the use of high-energy X-rays beamed from a machine to kill cancer cells

Retrograde ejaculation: semen travels into the bladder instead of out through the urethra

Semen: the ejaculated fluid containing sperm and secretions from the testicles, prostate and seminal vesicles

Sperm: the male gamete or sex cell

Testosterone: responsible for the formation of secondary sex characteristics and for supporting the sex drive

736

References

Acher, P. & Popert, R. (2012) Prostate brachytherapy. In: P. Dasgupta & R.S. Kirby (eds) *ABC of Prostate Cancer*, Ch. 11, pp. 37–39. Wiley Blackwell, Oxford.

APA (1994) *Diagnostic and Statistical Manual of Mental Disorders*, 4th edn. DSM-IV. American Psychiatric Association, Washington.

Beddows, J. (1997) Alleviating preoperative anxiety in patients: a study. *Nursing Standard*, 11(37), 35–38.

Brown, H. (2011) Elimination. In: L. Dougherty & S. Lister (eds) *The Royal Marsden Hospital Manual of Clinical Nursing Procedures*, 8th edn, Ch. 6, pp. 239–320. Wiley-Blackwell, Oxford.

Cancer Research UK (2012a) *Testicular Cancer Incidence Statistics*. http://www.cancerresearchuk.org/cancer-info/cancerstats/types/testis/incidence/ last accessed December 2012.

Cancer Research UK (2012b) *Testicular Cancer Risks and Causes*. http://www.cancerresearchuk.org/cancer-help/type/testicular-cancer/about/testicular-cancer-risks-and-causes last accessed December 2012.

Cancer Research UK (2012c) *Cancer Incidence for Common Cancers*. http://www.cancerresearchuk.org/cancer-info/cancerstats/incidence/commoncancers/ last accessed December 2012.

Caress, A. (2003) Giving information to patients. *Nursing Standard*, 17(43), 47–54.

Carson, C.C. & McMahon, C.G. (2008) *Erectile Dysfunction*. Health Press. Abingdon.

Cash, J.C. (2006) Cellular characteristics, pathophysiology and disease manifestations. In: J. Held-Warmkessel (ed.) *Contemporary Issues in Prostate Cancer. A Nursing Perspective*, 2nd edn. Ch. 3, pp. 60–78. Jones and Bartlett, Boston.

Cotton, J. & Steggall, M. (2011) Nursing patients with disorders of the breast and reproductive systems. In: C. Brooker & M. Nicol (eds) *Alexander's Nursing Practice*, 4th edn. Ch. 7, pp. 193–272. Churchill Livingstone, Edinburgh.

Dickinson, L., Ahmed, H.U. & Emeberton, M. (2012) HIFU. In: P. Dasgupta & R.S. Kirby (eds) *ABC of Prostate Cancer*, Ch. 12, pp. 40–43. Wiley Blackwell, Oxford.

Dorey, G. (2006) *Pelvic Dysfunction in Men: Diagnosis and treatment of male incontinence and erectile dysfunction*. Wiley, Chichester.

Douglas, G., Nicol, F. & Robertson, C. (2009) *Macleod's Clinical Examination*, 12th edn. Elsevier, Edinburgh.

Gleadle, J. (2012) *History and Clinical Examination at a Glance*, 3rd edn. Wiley-Blackwell, Oxford.

Gleason, D. (1966) Classification of prostatic carcinoma. *Cancer Chemotherapy Reports*, 50, 125–128.

Gomella, L.G., Liu, X.S., Trabulsi, E.J., Kelly, W.K., Myers, R., Showalter, T. *et al.* (2011) Screening for prostate cancer: the current evidence and guidelines controversy. *Canadian Journal of Urology*, 18(5), 5875–5883.

Greenberg, G. & Serlin, D. (2008) The newborn/infant male. In: J.J. Heidelbaugh (ed.) *Clinical Men's Health. Evidence in Practice*. Saunders, Philadelphia, Ch. 5, pp. 47–54.

Hall, J. (2008) Psychosexual aspects of men's health. In: L. Serrant-Green & J. McLuskey (eds) *The Sexual Heath of Men*, Ch. 5, pp. 57–81. Radcliffe, Oxford.

Hall, P. (2004) Online psychosexual therapy: a summary of pilot study findings. *Sexual and Relationship Therapy*, 19(2), 167–178.

Heffner, L.J. & Schust, D.J. (2010) *The Reproductive System at a Glance*, 3rd edn. Wiley Blackwell, Oxford.

Henderson, A. & Davies, J. (2012) Cryotherapy for prostate cancer. In: P. Dasgupta & R.S. Kirby, (eds) *ABC of Prostate Cancer*, Ch. 13, pp. 44–47. Wiley Blackwell, Oxford.

Kirby, M. (2005) Look beneath the surface of ED. *Independent Nurse*, 9 May.

Kirby, R.S. & Patel, M.I. (2012) *Fast Facts: Prostate cancer*. Health Press Ltd., Abingdon.

Knight, J. & Nigam, Y. (2008) Exploring the anatomy and physiology of ageing. Part 8 – The reproductive system. *Nursing Times*, 104(46), 24–25.

LeMone, P., Burke, K.M. & Bauldoff, G. (2011) *Medical-surgical Nursing: Critical thinking in patient care*, 5th edn. Pearson, London.

NICE (2005) *Referral Guidelines for Suspected Cancer*. National Institute Clinical Excellence, London.

NICE (2012) *Lower Urinary Tract Symptoms: Evidence update March 2012*. National Institute for Health and Clinical Excellence, London.

NMC (2008) *The Code: Standards of conduct, performance and ethics for nurses and midwives.* Nursing and Midwifery Council, London.

Paterson, C. (2006) Erectile dysfunction in men with diabetes. *Practice Nurse*, 31(5), 41–48.

Popovic, M. (2007) Psychosexual treatment of erectile dysfunction in a man who had reluctance to couple therapy: a caser report. *Sexual and Relationship Therapy*, 22(3), 363–377.

Shah, M. & DeSilva, A. (2008) *The Male Genitalia: a clinician's guide to skin problems and sexually transmitted infections.* Radcliffe, Oxford.

SIGN (2011) *Management of Adult Testicular Germ Cell Tumours.* A National Clinical Guideline. Scottish Intercollegiate Guidelines Network, Edinburgh.

Steggall, M. (2011) Nursing patients with urinary disorders. In: C. Brooker & M. Nicol (eds) *Alexander's Nursing Practice*, 4th edn. Ch. 8, pp. 273–300. Churchill Livingstone, Edinburgh.

Varma, M. & Chandra, A. (2012) Pathology of prostate cancer. In: P. Dasgupta & R.S. Kirby (eds) *ABC of Prostate Cancer*, Ch. 2, pp 5–7. Wiley Blackwell, Oxford.

Watson, P. (2003) Primary care and sex: too close for comfort? *Journal of Family Planning and Reproductive Health Care*, 29(2), 43.

Wespes, E., Amar, E., Hatzichristou, D., Montorsi, F., Pryor, J. & Vardi, Y. (2002) Guidelines on erectile dysfunction. *European Urology*, 41, 1–5.

Weston, R., Costello, A.J. & Murphy, D.C. (2011) Prostate cancer diagnosis. In: P. Dasgupta & R.S. Kirby (eds) *ABC of Prostate Cancer*, Ch. 4, pp. 11–17. Wiley Blackwell, Oxford.

Whitfield, A.H. & Whitfield, H.N. (2009) Circumcision. In: R. Kirby, C.C. Carson, A. White & Kirby, M. (eds) *Men's Health*, 3rd edn. Ch. 22, pp. 280–287. Informa, London.

Williams, G. & Pickup, J.C. (2004) *Handbook of Diabetes*, 3rd edn. Blackwell, Oxford.

737

Test Yourself

1. Which of the following is considered the male primary sex organ?
   (a) The prostate gland
   (b) The penis
   (c) The vas deferens
   (d) The testes

2. Spermatogenesis is another name for:
   (a) The production of testosterone
   (b) The sequence of events associated with male climax
   (c) The process of sperm cell development
   (d) The fertilisation of the ova

3. The key function of prostatic fluid is:
   (a) To provide nourishment to the sperm
   (b) To secrete a slightly acidic fluid
   (c) To secrete a slightly alkaline fluid
   (d) To lubricate the glans penis

4. The total amount of semen produced is:
   (a) 2–4 mL
   (b) 4–6 mL
   (c) 2–4 cL
   (d) 4–6 cL

5. The total ejaculate of a healthy male contains:
   (a) 1–4 sperm
   (b) 1000–4000 sperm
   (c) 100–400 thousand sperm
   (d) 100–400 million sperm

6. A fluid containing sperm is called:
   (a) Saliva
   (b) Phlegm
   (c) Semen
   (d) Urine

7. The male sex hormone is:
   (a) The prostate gland
   (b) Oestrogen
   (c) Testosterone
   (d) Aldosterone

8. Release of sperm from the body is called:
   (a) Evisceration
   (b) Dissection
   (c) Ejaculation
   (d) Enucleation

9. The pituitary gland is located:
   (a) In the penis
   (b) In the brain
   (c) In the prostate
   (d) In the abdominal cavity

10. Surgical removal of the testes is called:
    (a) Orchidectomy
    (b) Oophorectomy
    (c) Vasectomy
    (d) Hysterectomy

Answers

1. b
2. c
3. b
4. a
5. d
6. c
7. c
8. c
9. b
10. a

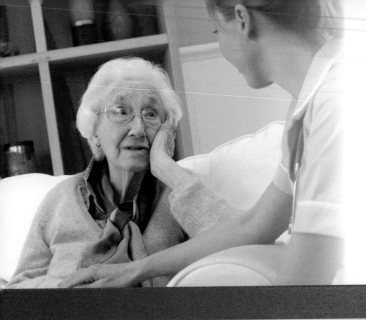

32

The Person with a Sexually Transmitted Infection

Ian Peate

School of Health Studies, Gibraltar

Learning Outcomes

On completion of this chapter you will be able to:

- Outline sexually transmitted infection prevention and control and prevention strategies and explain the epidemiology of sexually transmitted infections
- Describe the standards for the management of sexually transmitted infections
- Discuss the skills required to undertake an effective sexual history consultation
- Demonstrate an understanding of partner notification
- Describe the main presentations of sexually transmitted infections in men
- Describe the main presentations of sexually transmitted infections in women

Competencies

All nurses must:

1. Undertake a holistic assessment of a person with a sexually transmitted infection
2. Offer sexual health care in a non-judgemental way, demonstrating tact and empathy
3. Deliver sexual health care, based on best available evidence
4. Provide care tailored to meet the individual needs of vulnerable groups
5. Offer safer sex advice to specific communities
6. Refer for expert investigation and management

 Visit the companion website at **www.wileynursingpractice.com** where you can test yourself using flashcards, multiple-choice questions and more.

Nursing Practice: Knowledge and Care, First Edition. Edited by Ian Peate, Karen Wild and Muralitharan Nair.
© 2014 John Wiley & Sons, Ltd. Published 2014 by John Wiley & Sons, Ltd. Companion website: www.wileynursingpractice.com

Introduction

Untreated sexually transmitted infections (STIs) can lead to serious long-term health consequences for individuals, communities and nations. Nurses are at the forefront of promoting safer sex messages among the general population, young people and men who have sex with men (MSM).

In England, the sexual health of the nation has deteriorated over the last decade. Numbers of new diagnoses of STIs rose by 2% in 2011. There have been increases in the number of new diagnoses of gonorrhoea and syphilis. Large increases in STI diagnoses were seen in MSM (Health Protection Agency, HPA 2012a).

New diagnoses of genital chlamydia for the first time were stable rather than increased, despite a further increase in the number of chlamydia tests being performed. The impact of poor sexual health remains greatest in young heterosexual adults and in MSM and this is where the greatest burden falls.

Scotland has had a history of poor sexual health, with rising incidences of STIs (Healthcare Improvement Scotland, HIS 2011). Between 2000 and 2004, the number of chlamydia diagnoses in Scotland increased by 110%, from 7644 to 16 069. Two-thirds of cases were in people aged under 25 years. Diagnoses of gonorrhoea were higher in men; a high proportion of those were in MSM. Scotland has experienced challenges with the collection of data related to STIs and actions are in place to enhance data collection (ISD Scotland 2010).

Public Health, Wales (PHW 2011) report that the incidence of gonorrhoea in Wales has increased, with the rate of syphilis declining; genital chlamydia rates were similar to those seen in 2008.

In Northern Ireland in 2011 there was a slight decrease in annual numbers of new STI diagnoses made in genitourinary medicine (GUM) clinics (Public Health Agency, PHA 2011), with males accounting for just over half of new STI diagnoses. There are three types of infection that accounted for 84% of new STI diagnoses:

- Genital warts (first infections) (30%)
- Non-specific genital infection (29%)
- Chlamydia (25%).

MSM is the group most at risk of acquiring gonorrhoea and infectious syphilis. Some 55% of new STI diagnoses, for which age group information was available, occurred in young people under the age of 25 years during 2011.

Red Flag

Young people (aged 16–24 years old) are the age group most at risk of being diagnosed with an STI, accounting for 65% of all chlamydia, 50% of genital warts and 50% of gonorrhoea infections diagnosed in GUM clinics across the UK.

Geographically, there is considerable variation in the distribution of STIs; the highest rates are seen in urban areas, reflecting concentrations of the population who are at greatest risk. Prevention efforts, for example greater STI screening coverage and providing easier access to sexual health services, should be sustained and continue to focus on groups who are at the highest risk. Health promotion and education remain the foundations of STI and HIV prevention, providing improved public awareness of STIs and HIV and encouraging safer sexual behaviour including consistent condom use and reductions in both the numbers and concurrency of sexual partnerships.

The Evidence

Since the beginning of the HIV epidemic in the early 1980s, men who have sex with men (MSM) and transgender people have been disproportionately affected by the human immunodeficiency virus (HIV). The risk for infection remains high among them and there has been a resurgence of HIV infection among MSM, particularly in industrialised countries. Data are emerging of new or newly identified HIV epidemics among MSM in Africa, Asia, the Caribbean and Latin America.

A meta-analysis of surveillance data in low- and middle-income countries found that MSM are 19.3 times more likely to be HIV-infected than the general population. Reported HIV prevalence among MSM ranges from 0% to 32.9%, with rates surpassing 20% in countries as diverse as Bolivia, Jamaica, Mexico, Myanmar, Thailand, Trinidad and Zambia. HIV incidence among MSM ranges from 1.2 to 14.4 per 100 person-years. Recent studies from sub-Saharan Africa reported that HIV prevalence among MSM ranges from 6% to 31%. In Asia, the odds of MSM being infected with HIV are 18.7 times higher than in the general population, and the HIV prevalence ranges from 0% to 40%. In Latin America, it is estimated that half of all HIV infections in the region have resulted from unprotected anal intercourse between men.

(WHO 2011)

Across the UK, statistics on STIs are chiefly based on diagnoses made at GUM clinics. Chlamydia is also diagnosed in a variety of community settings. The governments of all four UK countries have or are producing strategies to help reduce the number of STIs and also to address the gender inequalities that are associated with STIs (Welsh Assembly Government, WAG 2010; Scottish Executive 2005; Department of Health, Social Services and Public Safety: Northern Ireland, DHSSPSNI 2008; DH 2001). The government is currently considering how to improve England's sexual health and has commissioned a review (HM Government 2010).

This chapter provides an overview of a number of STIs and provides readers with information that will help them offer services that are responsive to needs and are safe and effective. The Nursing and Midwifery Council (NMC) standards for pre-registration nurse education (NMC 2010) provide guidance on how programmes of nurse education are to be provided (they set the standards expected of educational institutions). One of the overriding principles of these standards is that the integration of public health principles and practice should be a central component of programmes of study. This chapter endeavours to ensure that this important public health topic – STIs – receives the attention it deserves. Those who are interested in developing their understanding and skill acquisition further should seek out health professionals who are practising in the field as well as accessing relevant texts on the subject.

 Link To/Go To

The British Association of Sexual Health and HIV (BASHH) provides a range of evidence-based guidelines with the intention of helping practitioners to provide safe and effective sexual health care:

http://www.bashh.org/guidelines

HIV is often considered alongside STIs; however, due to space constraints, this disorder of the immune system will not be discussed.

Assessing the System

Making an assessment of the person who has or may have an STI requires an understanding of the anatomy and physiology of the female and male reproductive systems, as well as the skills required to undertake a comprehensive assessment of them (see Chapters 30 and 31, respectively). The assessment aspects of this chapter build on the two previous chapters with an emphasis on assessment and STIs.

The Sexual Health Consultation

The sexual health consultation incorporates the taking of a sexual history and also a physical examination. A systematic approach to care is required, whereby the nurse makes an assessment, makes a diagnosis and, with the person, devises a plan of care, implements that care and then carries out an evaluation of the care delivered.

The relationship between the nurse and the patient has to be one where the person knows that the information given (and this is often intimate information that is shared) will remain confidential.

Confidentiality and sexual health

Confidentiality has been discussed in Chapter 5. To reiterate and with specific application to the person with an STI, all NHS employees are required to adhere to the Caldicott Principles for confidentiality and the guidance from the NMC (2009), emphasising the importance of confidentiality. It is a common duty of law to uphold confidentiality concerning a person's general health. This duty of confidentiality to the person is absolute, excluding very specific instances, such as when it is in the person's or public's interest. This could include child protection cases or cases where another individual is placed at risk of an infection. There are some infections that may be diagnosed in sexual health clinics (e.g. infectious hepatitis and infectious bloody diarrhoea) that may require statutory notification; this is the reporting of an infection to the appropriate authorities, i.e. a local authority.

The vulnerability of patients attending a clinic that offers tests for or treats STIs is considered in a number of statutory regulations. A duty of enforcement of confidentiality originates from The Public Health (Venereal Diseases) Regulations 1916 and has been updated in legislation: National Health Service (Venereal Diseases) Regulations 1974. The NHS Code of Confidentiality (DH 2010) is also applicable to those services managing STIs in England and Wales, with a further duty of enforcement of confidentiality required by the NHS Trusts and Primary Care Trusts (Sexually Transmitted Diseases) Directions 2000. Those services managing STIs have a duty (legally and professionally) to operate systems for clinical record management that will not allow disclosure and where identifying information is not shared, except for the purpose of treatment of STIs, or for the need to prevent infection.

In the UK, medical practitioners, for example the practice nurse or other healthcare workers, are not usually informed of a person's attendance for STI testing, unless the person has been initially referred by letter or the patient provides consent to such communication. It is seen as good practice to request consent to inform the practice nurse or GP of diagnoses or procedures that could have longer-term health implications (e.g. male or female sterilisation, skin biopsy and syphilis). If it is deemed in the patient's interest for another healthcare worker to be informed, then the person's consent to disclosure should be obtained. Caution should be taken to ensure that the results of tests that have been taken in a sexual health service are not viewable in a way that others can identify the person on an electronic results browser/viewer, unless specific consent to communication has been given.

The Sexual History

There are many situations where a consultation requires sexual history-taking. This aspect of the chapter concentrates primarily on settings such as genito-urinary medicine services or those offering sexual health services. The processes described can be adapted for use in other settings where STI assessments are required to be undertaken, for example facilities that integrate STI and contraceptive provision and other services, including general practice. The sexual history may be required when the person consults healthcare professionals:

- When they require care with symptoms that may be related to an STI
- If they have concerns about STIs
- If they require screening for STIs.

It must be understood that the content and detail of the sexual history is dependent on the setting in which it is taken, the role of the service and the needs of the individual person.

Kingsberg (2004) notes that whether you are a parent or a teenager, a patient or a physician, talking about sex is usually uncomfortable. There may be a number of reasons for this, for example you may not be equipped with the knowledge and skills needed to undertake this important activity or it could be that you feel uncomfortable or lack confidence when discussing matters associated with sex and sexuality (Tomlinson 2005).

The ability of the nurse to obtain an accurate sexual history is crucial to prevention and control efforts. How the nurse approaches issues surrounding sexual health can help to encourage the person to think about safer sex practices and other ways in which transmission can be reduced. The outcomes of the sexual history can help to ensure that people receive suitably targeted advice and guidance concerning the prevention of STIs, HIV or unintended pregnancies. When taking the sexual history and when assessing sexual health, you are concerned not just with gathering information to verify if a person has an STI, but also with the individual's sexual well-being, their entire being.

Brook et al. (2013) suggest that sexual issues are often difficult to discuss, even within a healthcare setting. Some people may feel ashamed, embarrassed or humiliated and the expectation is that the nurse will be non-judgemental and aim to put the person at ease. Questions about sexual health should be asked in a matter of fact manner but with sensitivity. Begin the consultation with the less intrusive questions before moving on to questions that may be more embarrassing.

Care, Dignity and Compassion

There has been growing concern that the fundamental elements of nursing care are lacking, leading to poor patient and care experience and poor clinical, social and emotional outcomes. When caring for people who seek help and advice regarding STIs the nurse must be non-judgemental and act in a moral and ethical way at all times.

Assumptions about people are unacceptable and must be avoided, and the nurse must make every effort to avoid doing this. When taking the history, you must not use terms that make assumptions about either the individual's sexual behaviour or their sexuality. If asking questions about sexual orientation, you are advised to use the term 'partner' as opposed to 'boyfriend' or 'girlfriend', 'husband' or 'wife'. It is better to ask the person how many partners they have instead of asking, 'Are you married and/or monogamous?'

Red Flag

 Gay men cite issues around confidentiality as a concern for them (Keogh *et al.* 2004).

The environment for sexual history-taking

A welcoming, comfortable, confidential physical environment is likely to encourage the person to be open and frank when providing details concerning sensitive issues, such as sexual behaviour (The Medical Foundation for AIDS, Sexual Health and HIV, MedFASH 2010).

Clearly displaying literature that stresses the way the service provides a confidential and non-judgemental approach to the nature of assessment can improve the consultation, as the person may feel safer in disclosing information. There should be a confidentiality policy and this should be made available for patients to consult, should they wish to.

The storage and visibility of files should be designed to ensure that confidentiality is maintained between patients. This approach reinforces the fact that the service takes confidentiality seriously. The service provider should decide on the most appropriate way of calling patients for consultations, for example using first name, full name or clinic number. The nurse must confirm that patient identification is correct.

The consultations must take place in private settings and in a sound-proofed room whenever possible. The consultation should be free from any interruptions: telephones diverted, pagers switched off and computer screens shut down, if needs be. A 'Do not disturb' sign should be placed on the door to avoid inadvertent interruptions. Student nurses or other students should only be present with the person's consent. If the person declines the presence of a student, this must be respected.

Seating arrangements should be given consideration. Attention to personal space must be taken into account; seats should be at the same height so that all participants are on the same level. If possible, arrange the seats side by side instead of behind a desk or table; in this way the nurse can clearly observe body language but you must remember that the person being cared for can also observe *your* body language.

Terminology and communication skills

When appropriate, the use of non-technical language should be encouraged. The type of language to be used must be given careful consideration because if the nurse uses a technical approach, for example using the terms 'cunnilingus' or 'urethral orifice', then this could lead to confusion, misunderstanding and also embarrassment. Just as using language that is non-technical, for example

'blow job' or 'pee', may be offensive to some people, so the nurse has to make a decision about what type of language is to be used, based on the interactions and knowledge of the person. This may be a challenge, as you may be embarrassed or even shocked about what you are hearing or what you think you are hearing. Human sexual behaviour is varied and you must never impose moral or religious judgements on people with regards to the sexual behaviour that they have chosen to engage in.

Care, Dignity and Compassion

 The choice of language used when communicating with patients should be given much thought. The aim should be to encourage the person to speak openly about issues that concern them. The nurse's body language may give away the fact they are feeing uncomfortable when the person is giving them details about their sexual history, and this is unacceptable.

If you do not understand, then you may need to say that to the person or ask for further clarification to confirm what you think you may have heard. Whatever approach is used, the nurse should endeavour to ensure that both parties are clear and being understood.

You should greet the person in a confident, competent and relaxed manner. Sometimes, it is a challenge to determine what exactly the problem is that the person is presenting with. Often, when discussing issues that cause embarrassment or shame, the person can be vague, use non-verbal communication as opposed to verbal communication and discuss the issue as if it is a 'friend' who is experiencing the problem. Be aware that people frequently use euphemisms when they are unsure or embarrassed about intimate matters. If this occurs, then you will have to listen very carefully and be aware of body language (both your own and the person's). Some may comment 'I have a discharge down below'; such a comment needs further investigation, as this could range from a minor irritation to a vaginal or rectal prolapse.

The ability to communicate effectively is required of all clinicians and can have both a positive and negative impact on health outcomes (Tsimtsiou *et al.* 2006). Attention should be paid to:

- The initial greeting
- Maintaining eye contact and using appropriate body language (beware of specific cultural nuances)
- Beginning the consultation with open questions, such as 'How can I help you?' or 'What has brought you to us today?' This can be followed by a consideration of the initial concerns. As the consultation progresses, use more closed type questions
- Providing the person with a rationale for some of the questions asked, for example 'I am about to ask some questions that are of a personal nature. I am asking these types of questions so that I can assess your needs fully and this will help you and me decide on the next steps of your care, so I need to ask more about your sex life'
- Mindfulness concerning signs of anxiety and distress from the patient
- Awareness of non-verbal cues from the patient.

Best practice in communication skills training, assessment of the quality of communication skills is complex and the nurse needs to be continually aware of how he or she is communicating (or not).

Link To/Go To

The Society for Sexual Health Advisors Manual provides information relevant to other professionals.

http://www.ssha.info/wp-content/uploads/ha_manual_2004 _complete.pdf

Communication challenges

There must be policies in place to address the communication needs of certain patient groups, including those people whose first language is not English, people with hearing or learning disabilities and people who cannot read. Strategies used to minimise communication challenges include:

- Sign language interpreters
- Foreign language interpreters
- Access to telephone interpretation services
- Use of communication aids, including websites
- Working with local support organisations
- Dedicated clinic times for those people with communication problems.

Nursing Fields Learning Disabilities

People with learning disabilities have the right to experience a full range of relationships, including friendships and community links, as well as personal relationships; they also have the same rights to develop personal relationships and express their sexuality as everyone else. This includes the right to consent to sexual relationships, including same sex relationships. These rights can only be denied on the basis of evidence of impaired capacity, as defined by the Adults with Incapacity (Scotland) Act 2000, or abuse.

Provision must be put in place for people with learning disabilities. The nurse should consider alternative modes of communication. What support and assistance is required will vary widely, depending upon the person's developmental age, communication levels, cognitive and conceptual abilities, interests, motivation and personal needs.

For the safe and effective care of people and communities, it is essential that a comprehensive sexual history be taken. The sexual history – usually obtained by a registered healthcare professional – allows the care team to offer care that is safe and appropriate.

The history provides the nurse with a clear and succinct clinical picture of the person's presenting problems and how to undertake a risk assessment. The nurse needs to understand the components of a sexual history and how it is taken.

The key features of a sexual history

When the nurse conducts the sexual history-taking as if they are asking questions from a questionnaire or from a list that has to be done as part of a paper exercise, this can take away all of its potential value. Asking a lot of questions will mean that the person will respond with a lot of answers. Using these approaches can be problematic. The nurse may have failed to identify the problems that the person is presenting with, as he/she might not hear what they

Box 32.1 Examples of Open, Closed and Judgemental Questions

Closed questions:

'Did you have safer sex?'
'Have you had this kind of pain before?'
'Does it hurt after you have had sex?'

Open questions:

'How can I help you?'
'What are your worries?'
'What do you think it is that may have caused the pain?'

Judgemental questions:

'You are a head teacher, don't you think you should know better?'
'Shouldn't you know better at your age?'

have to say. To provide the person with the opportunity to tell their story, effective communication skills are essential.

Sometimes it is easier for the nurse to avoid asking questions of a sensitive and intimate nature surrounding sex and sexuality. The nurse may choose to employ a closed questioning approach and this may limit the person's responses, instead of using open-ended questions that can invite the person to offer more. The nurse should make every effort to use open-ended questions where appropriate – those questions that do not require a yes/no response, with the aim of eliciting as much information as possible. Box 32.1 provides some examples of open, closed and judgemental questions.

The exact detail of what the sexual history should comprise varies between services but the following should be considered:

- A thorough assessment of symptoms to help guide the examination and testing
- An exposure history to identify which sites need to be sampled and the STIs to which the patient may be at risk
- An assessment of contraception use and risk of pregnancy
- Assessment of other sexual health issues (also allowing a discussion of any psychosexual problems)
- Assessing HIV, hepatitis B and C risk for offering both testing and prevention
- Assessment of risk behaviours; this will then facilitate health promotion activity, including partner notification and sexual health promotion.

Table 32.1 provides a summary of suggested sexual histories in various testing scenarios.

What the Experts Say

For me, working in the STI field is the best nursing I have ever done. The client is in charge and fully in control. They are responsible for their own decisions and behaviour changes. I like to think I provide them with options as opposed to directives. I like to focus on feelings as much as information. I am always aware that behaviour change is a process not a one off.

(Sean, staff nurse)

The Welsh government has made a number of recommendations to improve multiagency service delivery for victims of domestic abuse in Wales. The aim of the 10000 Safer Lives project is to

Table 32.1 Suggested sexual histories in various testing scenarios.

SCENARIO	ELEMENTS OF THE HISTORY
Minimum sexual history for asymptomatic patients attending for an STI screen	• Confirm lack of symptoms • Date of last sexual contact (LSC) and number of partners in the last 3 months • Gender of partner(s), anatomic sites of exposure, condom use and any suspected infection, infection risk or symptoms in partners • Previous STIs • For women: last menstrual period (LMP), contraceptive and cervical cytology history • Blood-borne virus risk assessment and vaccination history for those at risk • Agree the method of giving results • Establish competency, safeguarding children/vulnerable adults **Recommended** • Recognition of gender-based violence/intimate partner violence (**in Scotland and Wales, this is a requirement**) • Alcohol and recreational drug history
Minimum sexual history for symptomatic female patient attending for STI testing	• Symptoms/reason for attendance • Date of last sexual contact (LSC), partner's gender, anatomic sites of exposure, condom use and any suspected infection, infection risk or symptoms in this partner • Previous sexual partner details as for LSC for at least two partners and a note of total number of partners in last 3 months if more than two • Previous STIs • Last menstrual period (LMP) and menstrual pattern, contraceptive and cervical cytology history • Pregnancy and gynaecological history • Blood-borne virus risk assessment and vaccination history for those at risk • Past medical and surgical history • Medication history and history of drug allergies • Agree the method of giving results • Establish competency, safeguarding children/vulnerable adults **Recommended** • Recognition of gender-based violence/intimate partner violence (**in Scotland and Wales this is a requirement**) • Alcohol and recreational drug history
Minimum sexual history for symptomatic male patient attending for STI testing	• Symptoms/reason for attendance • Last sexual contact (LSC), partner's gender, anatomic sites of exposure and condom use, any suspected infection, infection risk or symptoms in this partner • Previous sexual partner details as for LSC for at least two partners and a note of total number of partners in last 3 months if more than two • Previous STIs • Blood-borne virus risk assessment and vaccination history for those at risk • Past medical and surgical history • Medication history and history of drug allergies • Agree method of giving results • Establish competency, safeguarding children/vulnerable adults **Recommended** • Recognition of gender-based violence/intimate partner violence (**in Scotland and Wales this is a requirement**) • Alcohol and recreational drug history
Additional history for a patient attending an integrated STI/contraception clinic	In addition to the items above, the following history may be taken in more detail if indicated. **For women** • Current contraception and any difficulties with the current method • Identify unmet contraception need and pregnancy risk • Abnormal vaginal bleeding • Menstrual pattern and changes in pattern • Mood changes with menstrual pattern • Identification of unmet need with regard to difficulties with sexual performance and satisfaction • Family history • Smoking history • HPV vaccination history **For men** • Contraception, including contraceptive use by female partners • Identification of unrecognised lower urinary tract symptoms • Identification of unmet need with regard to difficulties with sexual performance and satisfaction

make sure all relevant public service providers and organisations in Wales are able to identify and deal effectively with individuals experiencing domestic abuse (medium and standard risk), to ensure the safety of the individual and their family.

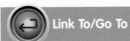

Link To/Go To

The Safer Lives Project full report can be found at:

http://wales.gov.uk/docs/dpsp/policy/12062010ksaferlivesrepenv1.pdf

Reviewing symptoms

Clinicians ask about specific genital symptoms, as this may reveal overlooked or ignored problems. For women, the following are usually asked about in relation to symptoms:

- Unusual vaginal discharge
- Vulval skin problems
- Lower abdominal pain/deep dyspareunia (painful sexual intercourse)
- Dysuria
- Unusual vaginal bleeding, including post-coital and intermenstrual bleeding.

For men, the following are usually asked about in relation to symptoms:

- Urethral discharge
- Dysuria
- Genital skin problems
- Testicular discomfort or swelling
- Peri-anal/anal symptoms (in MSM).

Look-back period

The look-back period concerns previous partners. The look-back period is the time during which the index case may have been infectious and transmitted infection and should be applied to all contacts, whether or not condoms were used. This look-back period also helps to establish which STIs the patient may be at risk of, to offer relevant vaccinations and to inform partner notification.

- The sexual history (as a minimum) should include the last two partners and a record of the number of other partners within the previous 3 months. Taking a 3-month risk history would identify risk behaviour not covered by a negative syphilis and third generation HIV antibody test on the day of the consultation. If no partners are reported during this time, the last time the patient had sexual contact should be noted
- Those people who recount no unprotected penetrative oral, vaginal or anal sex during this period should be asked the last time that these events took place
- All men should be asked if they have ever had sex with another man.

Previous STIs and other issues

All individuals should be asked about a history of STIs:

- You should record the diagnosis and approximate date of diagnosis
- Those with a history of previous syphilis should have the date of diagnosis, stage of syphilis, treatment given and clinic of treatment recorded

- Ask about past medical and surgical history in order to identify conditions that may be associated with or influence the management of STIs
- Drug history and history of allergies should be noted. Document current medication taken, including over-the-counter remedies, and ask about a history of previous allergies, particularly to antibiotics. This helps to determine if there are medications that may interfere with sexual function and to identify potential drug interactions and if drugs cannot be given safely
- An alcohol and recreational drug history must be taken. This may be indicated specifically in cases where disinhibition could be a factor in risk-taking behaviour and in young people taking risks. Alcohol and recreational drugs are a major factor in sexual risk taking (RCP & BASHH 2012).

Ellis *et al.* (2003) note that risky sexual behaviour may be influenced by a number of factors:

- Low self-esteem
- Lack of skills (e.g. in using condoms)
- Lack of negotiation skills (e.g. to say 'no' to sex without condoms)
- Lack of knowledge about the risks of different sexual behaviours
- Availability of resources, such as condoms or sexual health services
- Peer pressure
- Attitudes (and prejudices) of society, which may affect access to services.

Contraceptive and reproductive health history

The contraception and reproductive health history can therefore vary, related to whether the service primarily has an STI testing and treatment focus, or is providing a service that is integrated.

Contraceptive use and compliance:

- Last menstrual period and menstrual pattern. This helps to:
  - identify pregnancy or pregnancy risk
  - avoid drugs that are contraindicated in pregnancy
  - provide post-coital contraception if indicated
  - offer advice concerning contraception if required
  - eliminate contraceptive methods as a cause of irregular bleeding
  - prevent prescribing enzyme inducing drugs in conjunction with low-dose hormonal contraceptive methods
- Previous pregnancies including outcomes and complications
- When the last cervical cytology was taken (if aged 25 years or over in England, Northern Ireland and Republic of Ireland or 20 years or over in Scotland and Wales), the result and if ever abnormal. This will help to determine whether to offer cervical cytology.

Assessing for risk for blood-borne viruses

All individuals should be asked about the following:

- Current or past history of injecting drug misuse; sharing of needles, syringes or other drug preparation and injecting equipment – asking this identifies the need for hepatitis B, hepatitis C and HIV testing and hepatitis B vaccination (Rogstad *et al.* 2006)
- Sex with a partner from a country with a high HIV prevalence
- HIV-testing history, this will determine whether HIV testing is necessary
- Men should be asked if they have ever had sexual contact with another man

- Hepatitis B risk (including patient's country of birth, sex with sex workers, partners from high prevalence countries, MSM and injecting drug users) and hepatitis B vaccination history makes known the need for serological testing of hepatitis B and vaccination (BASHH 2008).

Where appropriate the following risks may also be asked about:

- Men and women may be asked whether they have ever exchanged money in return for sex. This allows for the appropriate health promotion and hepatitis B testing and vaccination.

Other risks are also assessed in order to identify specific behaviours associated with increased STI acquisition, that can provide opportunities for safer sex and substance use, information-giving and support and guide the offer of tests:

- Non-use of condoms associated with erectile dysfunction
- Recurrent condom breakage or slippage
- Taking part in group sex events
- Use of alcohol and non-injecting drug use
- Use of social networking websites to find sexual partners
- Use of high-risk venues
- Receptive fisting
- Traumatic sexual practice and use of sex toys
- Medical treatment/tattooing where sterility cannot be assured.

Concluding the sexual history

After the sexual history is completed, the clinician should:

- Ask the person if they have any other concerns that have not yet been considered. These could include psychosocial concerns, issues about 'coming out', safety in relationships and information about STI transmission
- Explain the need for how a clinical examination will be carried out and the tests that may be performed
- All patients must be given the option of a chaperone for the examination
- Discuss and agree with the person the method of communicating results.

Link To/Go To

The Family Planning Association (FPA) provides a range of resources for professionals working with young people. 'Talking with Young People About Sex and Relationships' can be used in conjunction with the FPA's booklets, such as 'Periods', 'Pregnancy', 'Love S.T.I.ngs'

http://www.fpa.org.uk/course/talking-young-people-about -sex-and-relationships (accessed 8 March 2014)

Documenting findings

Historically, sexual health clinics have maintained their own record sets and record systems. Regardless of this, they are still required to conform to national guidance and law concerning records retention, data protection and subject access requests (NMC 2010; Scottish Government Health Department, Scottish Government 2012). Specific care is required in sexual health service settings concerning the recording (and therefore possible disclosure) of third-party information (where a person who is not the patient discloses something about the patient). It is recommended (Mann & Williams 2003; NMC 2010) that:

- The record-keeping of a sexual history should be aligned with national standards of practice
- Services should agree minimum datasets, taking into account local and national health priorities and reporting requirements
- Sexual health records should be processed and stored in accordance with local and national guidance and law. Third-party data should be clearly indicated as such.

There are aspects of the sexual history that may also include the performance of a genital examination and the collection of specimens. The nurse may be required to assist in the collection of these specimens and provide physical and psychological support to the person being examined. Nurses who are deemed competent in specimen collection may undertake this activity only if they have the ability to do this safely and effectively.

When the history has been taken, and if appropriate the genitalia examined and specimens taken and analysed, a diagnosis can usually be made. After diagnosis, if required, treatment can then begin and health promotion activities commenced.

Sexual history summary

Box 32.2 provides a check-list to assist in carrying out the sexual history with confidence. As time goes by, the more sexual histories you take, the more confident and competent you will become. The approach that you use and the way in which you ask the questions along with the terminology chosen will be guided by the person you are caring for.

Nursing Fields Children's Nursing: Safeguarding Children

Where there are any concerns regarding a child's safety, serious consideration should always be given to liaison with the local safeguarding children team (DH 2010).

Answers to the following additional questions may flag up the need for further assessment and liaison with the local safeguarding children's team:

- Whether parents/carers are aware of the child's sexual activity
- Whether parents/carers are aware of the child's attendance at the clinic
- Whether the child has ever had non-consensual sexual contact
- Age of sexual partner(s)
- Vulnerability (e.g. self-harm, psychiatric illness, drug or alcohol misuse).

Where a child under 13 years of age reports sexual activity, this must be discussed with a senior nurse/colleague; it is expected that this will be discussed in confidence, with the local child protection lead. Although reporting to social services and the police may be indicated, it is not mandatory (Rogstad et al. 2010).

Medicines Management Storage of Vaccines

Immunisation is a highly effective way of protecting individuals and communities from infectious disease. However, to remain potent, vaccines must be stored within the temperature range recommended by manufacturers (+2°C to +8°C).

Incorrect storage of vaccines is not only wasteful and costly to the NHS; the failure to store vaccines correctly, particularly at temperatures below the manufacturer's recommendations, can reduce vaccine effectiveness and cause vaccine failures.

Box 32.2 Some Questions That May Help Guide and Inform the Sexual Health History

General issues:

- Do you engage in any sexual activity at the moment?
- Do you have any concerns about your sex life?
- With whom do you have sex, men, women or both?
- Tell me about your sexual activities, for example do you engage in oral/anal sex?
- Do you masturbate?
- Are you sexually satisfied?
- Is your sexual activity as frequent as you want it to be?
- Does your partner prefer more or less sexual activity than you do?
- Do you experience orgasms?
- Do you or your partner have any pain associated with sexual activity?
- Is there anything about your sexual activity that you would want to change?
- What other things about your sexual health and sexual practices should we discuss to help ensure your good health?
- What other concerns or questions concerning your sexual health or sexual practices would you like to discuss?

STIs:

- Have you ever had an STI?
- Have you ever been tested for an STI?
- Have you ever been tested for HIV? Would you like to be?
- Are you at risk, do you think, of contracting an STI?
- How many sexual partners have you had in the last 12 months?
- Have you ever experienced a burning sensation when you pass water?
- Have you ever noticed any discharge from your genitalia?
- Is there a rash or any lumps in the genital/groin area?

Hepatitis:

- Have you ever had a yellowing of the skin or eyes, or have you ever been told that you look yellow?
- Have you ever had:
  - Upper abdominal pain?
  - Light coloured stools?
  - Dark urine?
- Have you ever been told that you have a liver problem or hepatitis?
- Have you been immunised against hepatitis? Would you like to be?

(*Source*: Adapted from Wakley *et al*. 2003; Nusbaum & Hamilton 2002)

Box 32.3 The General Examination

Skin	Scabies – a rash that can be found at the wrists, the inter-digital web, the buttocks and the areolae
	Secondary syphilis and HIV seroconversion illness – generalised rash with typical lesions on the soles and palms
Lymph nodes	Secondary syphilis, HIV and primary herpes simplex – generalised lymphadenopathy
Mouth	Secondary syphilis – snail track ulceration and mucous patches
	HIV – ulceration in primary disease, oral hairy leukoplakia, oral candidiasis, Kaposi's sarcoma
	Herpes simplex – ulceration
	Warts

(*Source*: Adapted from Perez & Lee 2012)

The Physical Examination

Examination of the female and male genitalia has been discussed in Chapters 30 and 31, respectively. Some of the specific details concerning the examination in relation to STIs are discussed here.

The sexual history and examination will provide the nurse with direction concerning specific issues. While examination focusses upon the genitalia, the information obtained during history-taking may point to the need for a fuller examination. The general examination is outlined in Box 32.3.

The female patient

Inspect the pubic hair and the entire perineal region for evidence of pediculosis pubis, ulcers, warts, molluscum contagiosum and inflammation. Palpate the inguinal lymph nodes. Note any ulcers on the labia minora; observe for Bartholin's cysts and warts, ulcers or discharge.

Specimens can be taken during the examination. In the female, a urethral specimen for *Neisseria gonorrhoeae* can be taken, using a small cotton tip or a plastic loop. With the speculum *in situ*, the nurse should observe for abnormal discharge, inflammation and mucosal lesions. A specimen can be taken on the lateral vaginal walls if discharge is present. A narrow range pH paper should be used to test the vaginal pH. If the pH is elevated, a dry slide should be prepared and the specimen examined for bacterial vaginosis and *Candida*. Further specimens are obtained from the pool of vaginal secretions at the posterior fornix, a wet slide is prepared and the specimen examined for clue cells, *Candida* and *Trichomonas vaginalis*. In those women with abnormal discharge, a high vaginal swab can be taken for culture.

Specimens for cervical cytology can be taken at this stage. Use a large cotton mop to clean the cervix, then take an endocervical specimen to test for *N. gonorrhoeae* using a cotton swab or loop. At the endocervical canal, a second swab is taken for *C. trachomatis* and *N. gonorrhoeae*.

For those women who have abdominal symptoms or signs of pelvic inflammatory disease or a pelvic mass, a pelvic and abdominal examination should be undertaken.

If pregnancy is suspected, a urine specimen is requested or a mid-stream specimen of urine, if urinary tract infection is suspected. Observing ulcers would necessitate further examination of signs of syphilis. A swab should be taken for herpes simplex virus.

Pharyngeal specimens for *N. gonorrhoeae* can be taken. The specimen is taken by wiping a swab over the posterior pharynx, tonsil and tonsillar crypts.

If there are anal symptoms or the woman has a history of receptive anal sex, the perianal area should be examined for warts, inflammation and ulcers. A rectal swab can be taken for *N. gonorrhoeae*.

The male patient

Inspect the pubic hair for evidence of pediculosis pubis; examine the entire perineal region for ulcers, masses warts, molluscum contagiosum and inflammation. Palpate the inguinal lymph nodes.

Palpate the testes and epididymis, noting tenderness and swelling. Examine the shaft of the penis for lesions, including ulcers. Retract the foreskin (if present) and inspect the frenum. The urethral meatus is examined for discharge, inflammation, ulcers and warts.

If there is visible exudate, the man has a history of dysuria or discharge or has been in contact with a person with gonorrhoea, a urethral specimen is required using a swab or plastic loop gently inserted into the meatus. A urine specimen is taken to detect *N. gonorrhoea* and *C. trachomatis* (the man should not have passed urine for 4 hours).

If there are anal symptoms or the man has a history of receptive anal sex or receptive ano-oral sex, the perianal area is examined for warts, inflammation and ulcers. A proctoscopy may be performed to examine the anal and rectal mucosa for inflammation, pus and warts. The use of lubricating gel should be avoided, as this may interfere with the specimen analysis. A rectal swab is taken for *N. gonorrhoeae* and *C. trachomatis*. There may be a need to undertake a digital rectal examination of the prostate gland if there is inflammation.

Pharyngeal specimens can be taken for *N. gonorrhoeae* and *C. trachomatis*. The specimen is taken by wiping a swab over the posterior pharynx, tonsil and tonsillar crypts. These specimens are taken from MSM.

Blood tests

Local policy and procedure should be adhered to regarding the various blood specimens that are to be taken. BASHH (2006a) suggests that all patients should be offered HIV and syphilis assessment as a matter of routine and hepatitis B and C assessment should be offered where indicated.

Features of STIs

STIs, while caused by several organisms, have a number of common features:

- Many can be prevented by the use of condoms
- They can be spread through heterosexual and homosexual activities, including non-penetrating intimate exposure
- If treatment is to be effective, sexual partners of the infected person must also be treated to reduce onward transmission
- Often, two or more STIs co-exist in the same person.

Complications of STIs in women can include: pelvic inflammatory disease (this is a bacterial infection of the female upper genital tract, including the uterus, fallopian tubes and the ovaries); ectopic pregnancy (this occurs when a fertilised egg implants itself outside the uterus, usually in one of the fallopian tubes); infertility; chronic pelvic pain; neonatal illness and death; and genital cancer. There are some bacterial STIs that can be cured through early treatment with a course of antibiotics. Other STIs such as genital herpes (a viral infection) are chronic conditions that can be managed but, due to their viral aetiology, cannot be cured. The most serious STI is HIV; currently this is incurable. Treatment guidelines for STIs are updated on a regular basis, due to changing antimicrobial effectiveness and changes in technology and treatment options. Guidelines are available from a variety of organisations, including the British Association for Sexual Health and HIV (BASHH), Medical Foundation for AIDS and Sexual Health (Medfash) and the World Health Organization (WHO). Currently, there is no cure for some STIs and as such the focus has to be on prevention and control of transmission.

Medicines Management

When taking antibiotics, the person must be encouraged to ensure that they complete the treatment. If the person's symptoms disappear before they have finished their medication, they should continue to take the antibiotics until the end of the course. If they stop taking the medication early, the STI could still be prevalent and symptoms could return, which means the infection will last much longer and they may still be infectious.

Preventing STIs

Primary prevention of STIs aims to keep people uninfected while secondary prevention aims to prevent onward transmission of an STI from a person who is infected (Cowan & Bell 2012). The prevention and control of STIs are based on the principles of:

- Education
- Detection
- Effective diagnosis
- Treatment of infected persons
- Evaluation of treatment
- Counselling of sex partners of people who are infected.

The nurse's skills in obtaining an accurate sexual history are essential in prevention and control efforts. How the nurse manages issues surrounding sexual health can encourage the person to think about safer sex practices, as well as other ways in which onward transmission can be reduced.

Sexual abstinence is the most effective way to prevent sexual transmission of STIs and avoiding sexual intercourse with an infected partner (however, it must be recalled that there are a variety of other ways of transmitting infection, i.e. through intimate sexual contact). Condom use is advocated when a person chooses to have intercourse or to engage in other forms of sexual activity with a partner who has an infection or when that person's infection status is unknown; for each act of intercourse a new condom should be used.

Central to the control of STIs is the elimination of transmission and re-infection. This means that referral of sex partners for diagnosis, treatment and counselling is essential (partner notification).

Partner notification

Partner notification (also known as contact tracing) is the process of providing access to specific forms of health care to sexual contacts who may have been at risk of infection from an index case. This includes the provision of advice to contacts concerning potential infection and offering treatments for infection. The process includes:

- Identifying a look-back interval in which infection of contacts may have occurred
- Agreeing and recording contact actions with the index case
- Following up and recording the outcomes.

Only those healthcare workers who have obtained the required competencies appropriate to the care being provided should undertake partner notification.

Partner notification is an important activity. It is important for public health and is a central element in the prevention of sexually transmitted infections. Partner notification also provides an opportunity to address other sexual health needs, for example managing risk behaviour. The National Institute for Health and Clinical Excellence (NICE 2007) provides guidance on one-to-one interventions to reduce transmission of STIs.

McClean *et al.* (2012) suggest that when the first partner notification discussion takes place, a plan should be agreed with the index patient about which contacts to contact and, if so, how this should be done. Contacts include those believed not to be traceable, as well as those who had attended a service for management of the relevant infection before the index patient was first seen. In deciding whether a contact is traceable, consideration of all information sources should be undertaken.

No action is applicable when a contact is believed to be not traceable, or a contact has been confirmed as already seen. 'Not traceable' may include contacts who cannot be contacted by the patient, provider or contact methods because of a lack of information, or because of patient preference or welfare needs requiring not to involve a contact.

Red Flag

There may be situations requiring a best interest obligation to break confidentiality, for example when the health of another person is at risk. This is a complex area and legal advice may need to be sought.

The following aspects of this chapter provides an outline of some STIs. Those STIs that are discussed are not a full and complete list of STIs; there are many more and you are encouraged to delve deeper into the topic area.

Primary Care Community Care

In non-GUM (non-genitourinary medicine) settings (e.g. the primary care setting), referral into specialist STI clinics is recommended for appropriate treatment and partner notification and to complete a full STI screen, including HIV testing.

Genital Warts

The most common viral sexually acquired infection in the UK is genital warts (condylomata acuminata). In England and Wales, the number of genital warts cases (first episode, recurrent and re-registered) diagnosed in GUM clinics has gradually risen in both males and females.

Between 2000 and 2009 there was a 30% increase in diagnoses of first episode genital warts in males and females (70 414 and 91 202 diagnoses, respectively) in the UK. For the first time in 10 years, the number of diagnoses of first episode genital warts had decreased in the UK by 0.3% from 2008 (91 503) to 2009 (91 202). From 2000 to 2009 there was a 30% increase in recurrent and re-registered episodes (53 666 diagnoses in 2000 to 69 762 in 2009) and a 6.7% increase since 2008 (65 379 diagnoses) (HPA 2011).

Pathophysiology

Warts are caused by the human papilloma virus (HPV). Humans are the only known reservoir for HPV. HPV is not a single virus. There are over a 100 different genotypes; over 40 of these genotypes

are known to primarily infect genital epithelium. A small DNA virus causes the warts that infect cutaneous or mucosal epithelium. The majority of cases of infection with HPV cause no visible symptoms. Around 90% of all cases of genital warts are caused by two strains of the virus: type 6 and type 11 (Woodward & Robinson 2012). Other strains of HPV can cause cervical cancer.

What To Do If…

You are working on placement with a school nurse in a large inner city primary school and one of the teachers brings a pupil to the school nurse, as the pupil has multiple warts over her hands. The teacher tells the school nurse she thinks these may be sexually acquired warts. What might the next steps be?

Transmission and incubation period Genital warts are spread through direct skin contact (penetrative sex is not required to pass the virus on) with an infected person; they can be transmitted during vaginal or anal sex and also by sharing sex toys. Even using condoms cannot fully prevent the spread of warts, as condoms do not cover all of the genital skin.

It can take up to 1 year for warts to develop after infection with HPV (the incubation period). The median incubation period is 3 months with a range of 2–9 months but this may be longer. It has been suggested that many people who are infected with genital warts will never develop visible warts; however they are still capable of transmitting the virus (Woodward & Robinson 2012). As a result of this, it is not often possible to identify the source of the infection.

Investigations and diagnosis

Diagnosis is made primarily by clinical appearance; bright light is required to illuminate the area fully. An HPV DNA test is used to make a definitive diagnosis and this identifies the genotype. Making a definitive diagnosis means having laboratory confirmation; this can be carried out by screening. For the woman, this involves a cervical smear (BASHH 2006b). When diagnosis is uncertain, a biopsy may be taken if the warts are:

- Pigmented
- Indurated
- Fixed
- Not responding to treatment
- Persistently ulcerated or bleeding.

Signs and symptoms

Many people will discover lumps (lesions) around their genital area. These are usually asymptomatic, however they may be associated with itching or irritation and they may bleed. The lesions can be single or multiple (Box 32.4).

In women, genital warts can grow on the vulva, the walls of the vagina, the area between the external genitals and the anus and the cervix. Women are at a greater risk for HPV genital infections as they have a greater mucosal surface area exposed in the genital area. In men, they may occur on the urethral meatus, penile shaft, the scrotum or the anus. Genital warts can also develop in the mouth or throat of a person who has had oral sexual contact with an infected person.

Box 32.4 Genital Wart Appearance

Condylomata acuminata

- Cauliflower like appearance
- Skin-coloured pink, or hyperpigmented
- Generally not keratinised on mucosal surfaces; may be keratotic on skin.

Smooth papules

- Often dome-shaped and skin-coloured

Flat papules

- Macular to slightly raised
- Flesh-coloured with smooth surface
- Often found on the internal structures such as the cervix but can also appear on external genitalia.

Keratotic warts

- Thick, horny layer that can appear like common warts or seborrhoeic keratosis

(*Source*: Adapted from Woodward & Robinson 2012)

Jot This Down

As well as the impact that genital warts can have on a person physically, what do you think might be the psychological and emotional impact for the person and their partner(s)?

Complications

In men, apart from recurrences, it is unlikely that serious physical complications of genital warts will be experienced. However, women may experience an increased risk of cervical cancer. HPV DNA has been identified in almost all cervical cancers globally and in approximately 50–80% of vaginal, vulvar and anogenital cancers (Porth 2009).

Nursing care and management

The key aim of treatment is removal of the warts, relieving the symptoms experienced, along with the provision of health education with the intention of reducing the risk of recurrence and further transmission. People with genital warts should be offered a thorough explanation of their condition with specific stress on the long-term consequences for their health and the health of their partner(s). Clear and accurate written information, as well as allowing the person time to ask questions, can reinforce information giving.

A full STI screen should also be offered to exclude concurrent STIs. A variety of treatment modalities are available. Most warts are treated for aesthetic reasons or to provide relief from symptoms. The majority will recur and the person needs to be told this.

Treatment Treatment will depend on the structure, configuration (morphology), number and distribution of warts and the individual's preference. Treatment decisions are made after discussing the most suitable options with the person; this considers their preference and convenience.

Topical agents used to treat genital warts include podophyllotoxin and imiquimod or podophyllin and trichloroacetic acid. Podophyllin is contraindicated during pregnancy and can have side-effects, including nausea, diarrhoea and lethargy, paralysis and coma. Genital warts may also be removed by cryotherapy (use of

cold, freezing), electrocautery (use of heat, burning), laser vaporisation (the use of laser beams) or surgical excision. Table 32.2 provides an overview of topical treatment and physical ablation.

Response to treatment is often person-dependent, in that different people respond to treatments in different ways. Topical treatments are usually more effective when used for softer warts (non-keratinised); physical ablation is better suited to harder and rougher feeling warts (keratinised). A combination of topical treatment and physical ablation can be used. Regardless of the type of treatment, it may take several months to remove the warts.

Health education

Abstinence from any sexual activity greatly reduces the risk of genital HPV infection. For sexually active people, condoms reduce the risk of HPV infection, but they are not 100% effective. Nevertheless, condoms remain the safest option. If the person engages in oral sex, a condom should cover the penis. A dental dam (a latex or polyurethane square) can be used to cover the anal area or female genitals.

The person should avoid sharing sex toys. However, if they are shared, they should be washed or covered with a new condom before anyone else uses them.

Primary Care

A vaccine has been developed and is now available to prevent genital warts, pre-cancerous genital lesions and cervical cancer due to HPV. It is administered by three intramuscular injections, given over a 6-month period. As HPV is so closely associated with cervical cancer, the government has recommended that the vaccine be targeted at females aged 12–13. The vaccine (Gardasil) has now been included in the national immunisation programme (DH 2008). The vaccine does not protect against an existing HPV infection.

Jot This Down

Make a list of the potential side-effects associated with the vaccine Gardasil.

Gonorrhoea

The identification of people with gonorrhoea and testing to establish their infection status is a central component of good sexual health. The detection of gonorrhoea, along with the administration of effective antibiotic treatment, as well as notifying partners, will disrupt transmission and also prevent transmission of antimicrobial resistance.

In the general population the prevalence of gonorrhoea is very low, but it is significantly higher in certain defined subpopulations (e.g. men and younger people and those living in large cities). Sequelae (such as upper genital tract infection) caused by *N. gonorrhoeae* are infrequent but serious. Gonorrhoea is known to facilitate the transmission of HIV (HPA 2010).

Gonorrhoeal infection can be easily treated with the appropriate antimicrobials. Antimicrobial treatment should be expected to eradicate 95% of uncomplicated gonococcal infections within the

Table 32.2 Topical treatment and physical ablation methods used to treat warts. (*Source*: BASHH 2006b; American Cancer Society 2013)

TREATMENT	DESCRIPTION
Topical treatment There are several topical treatments that can be used to treat genital warts	**Podophyllotoxin** This is recommended to treat clusters of small warts. It comes in liquid form and works by having a toxic effect on the cells of the warts. A special application stick is used to draw up the correct dosage of the liquid, which is then dripped onto the wart. There may be some mild irritation when the liquid is applied to the wart. Treatment with podophyllotoxin is based on cycles: · The first treatment cycle involves applying the medication twice a day for 3 days · This is then followed by a rest cycle, where there are 4 days without treatment. Most people require four to five treatment cycles separated by rest cycles. **Imiquimod** Imiquimod is a cream usually used to treat larger warts and works by helping stimulate the immune system into attacking the warts. The cream is applied to the warts and then washed off after 6–10 hours. This should be done three times a week. It can often take several weeks of treatment before an improvement in symptoms is noted. Common side-effects of imiquimod include: · Hardening and flakiness of the skin · Swelling of the skin · A burning or itching sensation after applying the cream · Headache. These side-effects are mild and should pass within 2 weeks of stopping treatment with imiquimod. **Trichloroacetic acid (TCA)** Trichloroacetic acid (TCA) may be used to treat small warts that are very hard; it is also recommended for use by pregnant women, as it is thought to be the safest of all the topical treatments to use during pregnancy. TCA destroys the proteins inside the cells of the wart. However, if it is not applied correctly, it can damage healthy tissue. Therefore, the person will be asked to visit the local GUM clinic once a week for a nurse or doctor to apply the medication. After the treatment has been applied, some people experience an intense burning sensation for around 5–10 minutes.
Physical ablation There are four main methods used in the physical ablation of genital warts. All of these treatments are administered by a healthcare professional	**Cryotherapy** Cryotherapy is usually recommended to treat multiple, small warts, particularly those that develop on the shaft of the penis or on, or near, the vulva. Cryotherapy involves freezing the wart using liquid nitrogen, killing the cells of the wart by splitting their outer membranes. After being frozen, the wart is allowed to thaw out and, if necessary, it can be frozen and thawed again. During cryotherapy treatment, the person may experience a mild to moderate burning sensation. Once the treatment has finished, skin irritation is likely to develop and blistering and pain can occur at the site of the wart. The skin will take between 1 and 3 weeks to heal. The person should avoid having sex until the area of skin around the wart has fully healed. **Excision** Excision, in which warts are cut away, is sometimes undertaken to treat small, hardened warts, particularly where this is a mixture of smaller warts that have joined together to form a cauliflower shape. At the start of the procedure, a local anaesthetic is given to numb the area of skin around the wart. The wart is then cut away with a scalpel and the remaining incision sealed with stitches. Excision can cause scarring and as such this may not be suitable for very large warts. The area of skin from where the wart was removed will be sore and tender for around 1–3 weeks. The person should avoid having sex until the area of skin around the wart has fully healed. **Electrosurgery** Electrosurgery is usually combined with excision to treat large warts around the anus or vulva that have failed to respond to topical treatments. First, excision is used to remove the outer bulk of the wart. A metal loop is then pressed against the wart. An electric current is passed through the loop in order to burn away the remaining part of the wart. Removing a large number of warts in this way can be painful, so a regional anaesthetic (where everything below the spine is numbed, similar to an epidural) or a general anaesthetic is needed. **Laser surgery** This procedure may be recommended when there are large genital warts that cannot be treated using other methods of physical ablation, as they are difficult to access, such as deep inside the anus or urethra. Laser surgery may also be recommended for pregnant women who fail to respond to treatment with trichloroacetic acid (TCA). During the procedure, a laser is used to burn away the warts. Depending on the number and size of the warts, laser surgery can be performed under either a local or general anaesthetic. As with other types of ablation treatment, there will be soreness and irritation at the site where the warts were removed. This should heal within 2–4 weeks.

community. However, the effective treatment of gonorrhoea has been complicated by the ability of *N. gonorrhoeae* to develop resistance to the antimicrobial agents. Possible treatment failure, the likelihood of onward transmission of the organism within the community and the development of adverse clinical sequelae in the infected individual are considerably increased in the presence of resistance to first line antimicrobials.

Care pathways must be in place to ensure prompt and effective treatment of gonorrhoea and contact tracing in all settings. Referral should be made into specialist STI clinics for appropriate treatment and partner notification and to complete a full STI screen that includes HIV testing.

The annual HPA report for England (HPA 2012b) notes that gonorrhoea is up by 25% on 2010. The largest increase in new diagnoses between 2010 and 2011 was seen in MSM; gonorrhoea increased by 61%. Among heterosexuals, overall rates remained highest in young adults (15–24 years old), accounting for 57% of all new gonorrhoea diagnoses.

In Scotland in 2011, 1547 diagnoses of gonorrhoea were reported to Health Protection Scotland (HPS), representing a 12% increase on the 2010 total of 1378. When compared with 2010 data, the gender totals observed during 2011 reflect a 5% increase in the number of diagnoses among women (from 446 to 468) and a 16% increase in those among men (from 930 to 1077) (HPS 2012).

Pathophysiology

Gonorrhoea is the clinical disease resulting from infection with the Gram-negative diplococcus *Neisseria gonorrhoeae*. There are four types: T1, T2, T3 and T4. T1 and T2 are virulent, while T3 and T4 are not (Pareek 2012).

Transmission and incubation period Gonorrhoea can be transmitted through unprotected sexual contact, autoinoculation (e.g. sometimes from genitals to fingers to eyes, where it may cause conjunctivitis), the sharing of sex toys or from mother to fetus during vaginal delivery. The incubation period is 5–8 days.

Jot This Down

Do you think that people in prison should be provided with the same standard of health care as available to the rest of the population? Should prisoners be provided with condoms and sterile equipment for drug injection? What might be the implication for answering yes or no?

Signs and symptoms

Men Urethral infection usually causes urethral discharge (a mucopurulent or purulent urethral discharge) in the majority of cases; this can be accompanied by dysuria 2–5 days after the man has been exposed.

In some cases, urethral infection may be asymptomatic. Rectal infection is usually asymptomatic but it can cause anal discharge or perianal/anal pain or discomfort. Pharyngeal infection is usually asymptomatic.

Rarely, there may be epididymal tenderness/swelling or balanitis may be present. There may be conjunctivitis.

Women Infection at the endocervix is often asymptomatic. The commonest symptom is increased or altered vaginal discharge. The woman may complain of lower abdominal pain. Dysuria may be the result of urethral infection.

It is rare for gonorrhoea to cause intermenstrual bleeding or menorrhagia.

If there is rectal infection, this usually develops where there is transmucosal spread of infected genital secretions as opposed to anal intercourse. This is usually asymptomatic.

As in the male, pharyngeal infection is usually asymptomatic. *Neisseria gonorrhoeae* can co-exist with other genital mucosal pathogens, particularly *Chlamydia trachomatis*, *Trichomonas vaginalis* and *Candida albicans*. If symptoms are present, then these may be attributable to the co-infecting pathogen.

Mucopurulent endocervical discharge with easily induced endocervical bleeding may be noticed on examination or during intercourse. On examination, the woman may complain of pelvic/lower abdominal tenderness. Often, however, there are no abnormal findings present on examination. There may be conjunctivitis.

Investigations and diagnosis

Diagnosis should be based on an individual assessment that will include a detailed sexual history and physical examination. The HPA (2010) has produced guidance for gonorrhoea testing in England and Wales, and BASHH (2012) and Bignall and Fitzgerald (2011) have provided information related to testing and treatment for gonorrhoea.

The presence of *N. gonorrhoeae* at an infected site establishes the diagnosis of gonorrhoea. How the diagnosis is made is dependent upon the clinical setting, storage and transport system to the laboratory, local prevalence of infection and the range of tests available in the laboratory.

Microscopy of Gram-stained genital specimens provides direct visualisation of *N. gonorrhoeae*. Microscopy should be performed on men with rectal symptoms. In women, microscopy has poor sensitivity for the identification of gonococcal infection. For urethral smears in women or for detecting asymptomatic rectal infection because of low sensitivity, microscopy is not recommended. Microscopy is inappropriate for diagnosing gonorrhoea in pharyngeal specimens.

If there is discharge in the man, a swab of this is taken and examined (this provides immediate diagnosis). If the man is asymptomatic, a urine specimen is taken for analysis. There may be a need to obtain swabs from the throat, eyes and rectum.

Vaginal and endocervical swabs are taken from the woman for culture. It is usual for those undergoing testing for genital tract gonorrhoea to be tested for infection with *Chlamydia trachomatis*.

See Table 32.3 for an overview of specimen collection.

Screening for coincident STIs should routinely be performed in patients with or at risk of gonorrhoea.

Complications

The spread of *N. gonorrhoeae* may occur transluminally from the urethra or endocervix, causing epididymo-orchitis or prostatitis in men and, in women, pelvic inflammatory disease. Dissemination through the blood may also occur from infected mucous membranes, causing skin lesions, arthralgia, arthritis and tenosynovitis (disseminated gonococcal infection). Reporting from GUM clinics in the UK indicates that these conditions are uncommon (Bignall & FitzGerald 2011; Pareek 2012).

Table 32.3 Overview of specimen collection. (Source: Adapted from Bignall & FitzGerald 2011)

MEN	WOMEN
A first pass urine is the preferred sample for testing	Vaginal or endocervical swab specimens are sensitive for detecting *N. gonorrhoeae*
Microscopy and culture require a urethral/meatal swab specimen	Culture requires an endocervical and urethral swab specimen for maximum sensitivity
Sexual history and symptoms will dictate the collection and testing of rectal and pharyngeal swab specimens; this should also be considered in men who receive oral–anal or digital–anal contact	The collection and testing of rectal and pharyngeal swab specimens should be directed by sexual history; symptoms at these sites should be looked for in women who have had sexual contact with those with gonorrhoea

Nursing care and management

The nurse should provide patients with a detailed explanation of their condition and emphasise the long-term implications for their own health and the health of their partner(s). The information provided should be reinforced with clear and accurate written information.

The patient should be aware that some results for gonorrhoea may be available during the first visit. The nurse must inform the patient about how they are to receive their final results after the consultation and before leaving.

Treatment is recommended when the presence of intracellular Gram-negative diplococci on microscopy of a smear from the genital tract has been identified; a positive culture for *N. gonorrhoeae* from any site; a positive nucleic acid amplification test for *N. gonorrhoeae* from any site; or recent sexual partners(s) of confirmed cases of gonococcal infection.

In cases of adult uncomplicated anogenital infection, Bignall and FitzGerald (2011) recommend ceftriaxone 500 mg intramuscularly as a single dose with azithromycin 1 g orally as a single dose.

> **Medicines Management Administration of Ceftriaxone 500 mg**
>
> Ceftriaxone is supplied as a powder that needs to be reconstituted with lidocaine solution. In the UK, it is currently available as vials of 250 mg or 1 g.
> It should be given by deep intramuscular injection.

Alternative regimens for the treatment of gonorrhoea are available and all of the agents noted below should be accompanied by azithromycin 1 g orally as a single dose:

* Cefixime 400 mg orally as a single dose. This route should only be used if an intramuscular injection is contraindicated or refused by the patient
* Spectinomycin 2 g intramuscularly as a single dose
* Other single dose cephalosporin regimens, such as cefotaxime 500 mg intramuscularly as a single dose, cefoxitin 2 g intramuscularly as a single dose, plus probenecid 1 g orally
* Cefpodoxime as a single dose of 200 mg.

Complicated gonococcal infection

Gonococcal pelvic inflammatory disease – Ceftriaxone 500 mg intramuscularly immediately followed by oral doxycycline 100 mg twice daily plus metronidazole 400 mg twice daily for 14 days

Gonococcal epididymo-orchitis – Ceftriaxone 500 mg intramuscularly plus doxycycline 100 mg twice daily for 10–14 days

Gonococcal conjunctivitis – A 3-day systemic regimen is recommended as the cornea may be involved and is relatively avascular. The eye should be irrigated with saline/water and ceftriaxone 500 mg given intramuscularly daily for 3 days.

Disseminated gonococcal infection Ceftriaxone 1 g intramuscularly or intravenously every 24 hours or cefotaxime 1 g intravenously every 8 hours or ciprofloxacin 500 mg intravenously every 12 hours (if the infection is known to be sensitive) or spectinomycin 2 g intramuscularly every 12 hours. Therapy should continue for 7 days but may be changed 24–48 hours after symptoms improve to one of the following oral regimens:

* Cefixime 400 mg twice daily
* Ciprofloxacin 500 mg twice daily
* Ofloxacin 400 mg twice daily.

Allergy Contraindications to the administration of ceftriaxone are hypersensitivity to any cephalosporin or previous immediate and/or severe hypersensitivity reaction to penicillin or other beta-lactam drug. Recommended treatments for patients giving a history of such hypersensitivity are:

* Spectinomycin 2 g intramuscularly as a single dose with azithromycin 1 g orally as a single dose
* Azithromycin 2.0 g orally as a single dose
* Ciprofloxacin 500 mg orally as a single dose when the infection is known or anticipated to be quinolone sensitive.

Pregnancy and breast-feeding Pregnant and breast-feeding women should not be treated with quinolone or tetracycline antimicrobials. Pregnancy does not diminish treatment efficacy. Recommended regimens are:

* Ceftriaxone 500 mg intramuscularly as a single dose with azithromycin 1 g orally as a single dose
* Spectinomycin 2 g intramuscularly as a single dose with azithromycin 1 g orally as a single dose.

Pharyngeal infection Recommended treatments that must be prescribed:

* Ceftriaxone 500 mg intramuscularly as a single dose with azithromycin 1 g as a single dose
* Ciprofloxacin 500 mg orally as a single dose if *N. gonorrhoeae* is known to be quinolone-sensitive
* Ofloxacin 400 mg orally as a single dose if *N. gonorrhoeae* is known to be quinolone-sensitive.

Health promotion

Partner notification In all patients identified with gonococcal infection, partner notification should be pursued. Action and outcomes should be documented.

What To Do If...

The person you are providing information to with regards to a gonorrhoeal infection informs you that the only other person he has ever had sex with is his current male partner. You are discussing the need to notify his partner of his infection, with the intention of inviting the partner to the clinic for assessment and treatment. The man informs you that he cannot give you his partner's details as he is scared of him; he has physically abused him in the past. What might the next steps be?

Male patients with symptomatic urethral infection should notify all partners with whom they had sexual contact within the preceding 2 weeks or their last partner if longer ago. Patients with infection at other sites or those with asymptomatic infection should notify all partners within the preceding 3 months. Sexual partners should be offered testing and treatment for gonorrhoea.

Patients should be advised to refrain from sexual activity, including sexual intercourse with condoms, oral sex and masturbation, until they and their partner(s) have completed treatment.

The nurse should promote the use of condoms, encouraging the patient to protect themselves with new partners by ensuring a condom is used for all vaginal/anal/oral contact or ensuring that both the patient and a new partner have a sexual health screen before any unprotected sex. The person should avoid sharing sex toys. However, if they are shared, they should be washed or covered with a new condom before anyone else uses them.

What To Do If...

You are providing health promotion advice to a woman and during the consultation you suggest that one method of safer sex is to use a condom. The woman tells you her husband is Roman Catholic and their religion forbids the use of condoms. Can you think of other ways of engaging in safer sex that could be suggested?

Primary Care

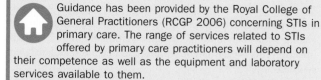

Guidance has been provided by the Royal College of General Practitioners (RCGP 2006) concerning STIs in primary care. The range of services related to STIs offered by primary care practitioners will depend on their competence as well as the equipment and laboratory services available to them.

Primary care providers can incorporate STI primary and secondary prevention as part of routine patient care by doing the following:

- Assessing and discussing STI risk
- Informing patients about signs and symptoms of STIs
- Helping patients recognise and minimise STI risk
- Offering patient-centred health education and promotion
- Offering hepatitis A (HAV) and B (HBV) immunisation, when indicated
- Offering STI screening and testing
- Appropriately treating, following up and counselling infected patients and their partners
- Making appropriate referrals to other agencies.

The Evidence

Sex industry laws in Australia and their impact on health promotion activities and service delivery were studied in Melbourne (licensed and legal), Perth (criminalised) and Sydney (decriminalised). It provided clear evidence that sex-work legislation significantly impacts on the delivery and result of health promotion services that target sex workers. It demonstrated that licensing, where police control unlicensed brothels and other illegal environments, such as street-based sex-work, excludes these workers from health promotion programmes, as they remain isolated from peer-education and support. Decriminalisation provides the best legislative framework. Community-based organisations have a higher capacity to provide advocacy services and hence achieve better health outcomes for sex-workers.

(Harcourt et al. 2010).

Syphilis

Syphilis is a contagious systemic disease and has a long history. It has been present for hundreds of years and was introduced into Europe around 1490 (Pareek 2012).

There has been an increase in the rates of syphilis. Epidemics are occurring in MSM and the over 25s and this STI is more prevalent in certain urban areas, e.g. London, Brighton and Manchester.

In the UK, 3762 diagnoses of infectious syphilis were made in 2007, more than in any other year since 1950. MSM account for nearly three-quarters (73%) of cases of infectious syphilis. HIV co-infection is common in those diagnosed with syphilis, reflecting the close relationships between the epidemics. The increased number of syphilis cases in women of reproductive age has resulted in an increase in cases of congenital infection (HPA 2011).

Pathophysiology

Syphilis is caused by the bacterium *Treponema pallidum* subsp. *pallidum*, a member of the *Spirochaetaceae* family. There are over 70 species and some of these are pathogenic to the human, causing:

- Syphilis
- Yaws
- Pinta
- Bejel.

T. pallidum is a thin spiral-shaped bacterium and is made up of 8–20 coils. The organism is 6 µm in length and 0.24 µm in width, making it invisible to the naked eye. The organism has a corkscrew-type movement.

Classification of syphilis Syphilis is classified as acquired or congenital (Table 32.4).

Transmission and incubation period The organism is transmitted from one person to another by direct contact with an infectious lesion (usually occurring during sexual contact), during pregnancy from mother to child, or via infected blood products. *T. pallidum* enters via abraded skin or intact mucous membrane and distributes via the bloodstream and lymphatics.

The incubation period is 9–90 days.

Table 32.4 Classification of syphilis. (*Source*: Adapted from Kingston *et al.* 2008)

ACQUIRED	CONGENITAL
Early · Primary · Secondary · Early latent (<2 years infection)	Early (diagnosed within the first 2 years of life)
Late · Late latent (>2 years infection) · Tertiary (including gummatous, cardiovascular, neurological)	Late (presenting after 2 years)

Diagnosis and investigations

A detailed history and examination are undertaken and this may reveal symptoms of early syphilis.

The nurse should ask for any details of previous treatment and also the woman's obstetric history and any potential complications of syphilis, e.g. miscarriages, stillbirths. Blood donation and antenatal screening history should be documented. The person should be asked about any other treponemal infections, such as yaws, pinta and a history of living in countries where these conditions are endemic.

In early infection, examination of the genitals, skin, mucosal surfaces and lymph nodes for signs of primary and secondary syphilis will be essential in making a diagnosis. In late and congenital syphilis, a thorough clinical examination should be undertaken for the clinical manifestations of syphilis.

Examination of an ulcerative lesion will identify *T. pallidum*. Blood is taken for reactive serology, including the following:

- Venereal disease research laboratory (VDRL) test
- Rapid plasma regain (RPR)
- Fluorescent treponemal antibody absorption (FTA-ABS)
- Immunoglobulin G (IgG) antibody test
- Immunoglobulin M (IgM) antibody test
- Enzyme immunoassay (EIA) test.

Other tests and investigations will be required depending on the person's individual needs, e.g.

- Chest X-ray
- Analysis of cerebrospinal fluid
- Liver function tests
- Neurological imaging
- Histological examination of a lesion.

Signs and symptoms

Primary syphilis is characterised by an ulcer (this is called the 'chancre') and regional lymphadenopathy. The chancre is typically in the anogenital region, single, painless and indurated with a clean base that discharges clear serum. However, chancres can be multiple, painful, purulent, destructive or extragenital (most frequently oral). Any anogenital ulcer should be considered to be due to syphilis unless this is proven otherwise.

Secondary syphilis is characterised by multisystem involvement within the first 2 years of infection. There is often a rash (typically generalised macular, papular or macular – papular usually on the palms and soles), condylomata lata, mucocutaneous lesions and generalised lymphadenopathy. The rash is classically

Table 32.5 A summary of the features of late syphilis.
(*Source*: Adapted from Kingston *et al.* 2008)

	TIMING AFTER INFECTION	SIGNS AND SYMPTOMS
Neurosyphilis		
Asymptomatic	Early/late	Abnormal cerebrospinal fluid (CSF) with no signs or symptoms
Meningovascular	2–7 years	Focal arteritis including infection/meningeal inflammation. There may be prodrome headache, emotional lability, insomnia
Parenchymatous		
General paresis	10–20 years	Gradual decline in memory and cognitive functions, emotional lability, personality change psychosis and dementia. There may be seizure and hemiparesis
Tabes dorsalis	15–25 years	Lightning pains, paraesthesia, sensory ataxia, Charcot's joints, optic atrophy, pupillary changes (e.g. Argyll Robertson pupils)
Cardiovascular	10–30 years	Aortitis, asymptomatic, substernal pain, aortic regurgitation, heart failure, coronary stenosis, angina, aneurysm
Gummatous	1–46 years (the average is 15 years)	Inflammatory granulomatous destructive lesions can occur in any organ but most commonly they affect bone and skin

non-itchy but may be itchy, particularly in people with dark skin.

Latent syphilis is *T. pallidum* infection diagnosed on serological testing with no symptoms or signs. Within the first 2 years of infection this is early latent syphilis and beyond that, late latent syphilis.

Symptomatic late syphilis can be categorised into (they may co-exist):

- Neurosyphilis
- Cardiovascular syphilis
- Gummatous syphilis.

Tertiary syphilis (a term that is often used synonymously with late symptomatic syphilis) usually excludes meningovascular syphilis (see Table 32.5 for the clinical features of symptomatic late syphilis).

Congenital syphilis:

- *Early* – includes a rash, condylomata lata, vesiculobullous lesions, snuffles, haemorrhagic rhinitis, osteochondritis, periostitis, pseudoparalysis, mucous patches, perioral fissures, hepatosplenomegaly, generalised lymphadenopathy, non-immune hydrops, glomerulonephritis, neurological or ocular involvement, haemolysis and thrombocytopenia

- *Late* (including stigmata) – interstitial keratitis, Clutton's joints, Hutchinson's incisors, mulberry molars, high palatal arch, rhagades, deafness, frontal bossing, short maxilla, protuberance of mandible, saddlenose deformity, sternoclavicular thickening, paroxysmal cold haemoglobinuria, neurological or gummatous involvement.

Complications

The sections above demonstrate the many complications that can be associated with syphilis. Those people with syphilis are three to five times more likely to become infected with HIV. This is because the genital ulcers caused by syphilis can bleed easily, making it easier for HIV to enter the blood. Being infected with both HIV and syphilis can be serious, as syphilis can progress much more rapidly than normal.

Nursing care and management

Those people with syphilis should receive their treatment in an STI clinic. Those who acquire syphilis are at considerable risk of reinfection and as such they should be regularly screened for syphilis and offered sexual health promotion. All patients should be offered screening for other STIs, including HIV.

What To Do If...

A patient you are looking after is confused and he unexpectedly bites you, drawing blood. He is known to have hepatitis C and is HIV-positive. What are the next steps that need to be taken?

The care of pregnant women and children requires specialist treatment and will not be discussed here. Management should be in close liaison with obstetric, midwifery and paediatric colleagues. Appropriate follow-up of babies is required.

Nursing Fields Children's Health: Fraser Competence. Young People and Sexual Health

Any competent young person in the UK can consent to medical, surgical or nursing treatment, including contraception and sexual and reproductive health. They are said to be competent if they are capable of fully understanding the nature and possible consequences of the treatment.

Consent from parents is not legally necessary, although the involvement of parents is encouraged. A parent is someone with legal parental responsibility. This is not always a biological parent.

Young people are owed the same duties of care and confidentiality as adults. Confidentiality may only be broken when the health, safety or welfare of the young person, or others, would otherwise be at grave risk.

Primary and secondary syphilis can be treated successfully with intramuscular antibiotic therapy – penicillin (Table 32.6).

Red Flag Jarisch–Herxheimer's Reaction

This systemic reaction is also known as the Herxheimer's reaction and was classically described in the treatment of people with syphilis. It is thought to be caused by the release of endotoxin-like substances when large numbers of *Treponema pallidum* are killed as a result of antibiotic therapy. Van Voorst Vader (1998) notes that the reaction can be expected in 50% of primary syphilis, 90% of secondary syphilis and in 25% of early latent infection, but is very rare in late syphilis. It has been suggested that people with HIV may experience a more severe reaction.

Clinical features

- The reaction usually starts between 1 and 12 hours after the first injection of antibiotics and lasts for a few hours or up to a day
- It is not seen with subsequent treatment
- There is malaise, slight-to-moderate pyrexia, a flush due to vasodilation, tachycardia and leukocytosis
- Any existing skin lesions appear more prominent
- Hyperventilation and tachycardia are accompanied by hypertension and then by a drop in blood pressure due to vasodilation and declining peripheral resistance
- In some people with early syphilis, a secondary rash may become visible, which was absent prior to treatment
- Pareek (2012) notes that there may be an exacerbation of alopecia due to the reaction.

A short course of steroids may be needed.

Health promotion

Patients diagnosed with syphilis should be given a detailed explanation of syphilis, including the long-term implications for their own health and the health of partners and families. This should be reinforced by providing them with clear and accurate written information.

The person should be advised to refrain from sexual contact of any kind until the lesions of early syphilis (if they were present) are fully healed or until after the results of the first follow-up serology are known.

Primary Care

It is essential that there are joint care pathways in place between the primary care setting and the secondary care provider, i.e. GUM clinic. The ability to screen people effectively in the primary care setting may be limited and as such, people with or suspected of having syphilis should be referred to the care providers in the secondary care setting.

What the Experts Say

The one thing I would say to a student who has been allocated to work with people who have sexual health needs is to treat them as you would like to be treated yourself. We are all human and we all have needs and lots of these are diverse and sometimes complex.

(Consultant Nurse)

Table 32.6 Recommended syphilis treatment regimens for adults (excluding pregnancy). (*Source*: Adapted from Kingston *et al.* 2008)

CLINICAL STAGE	RECOMMENDED REGIMENS	ALTERNATIVE REGIMENS	COMMENT
Incubating syphilis/ epidemiological treatment	Benzathine penicillin 2.4 mega units intramuscularly, single dose Doxycycline 100 mg orally twice daily for 14 days Azithromycin 1 g orally (stat)		
Early (primary/ secondary/early latent) syphilis	Benzathine penicillin 2.4 mega units intramuscularly, single dose Procaine penicillin G 600 000 units intramuscularly daily for 10 days	Doxycycline 100 mg orally twice a day for 14 days Azithromycin 2 g orally (stat) or azithromycin 500 mg daily for 10 days Erythromycin 500 mg orally for 14 days Ceftriaxone 500 mg intramuscularly daily for 10 days Amoxicillin 500 mg orally four times a day plus probenecid 500 mg orally	
Late latent, cardiovascular and gummatous syphilis	Benzathine penicillin 2.4 mega units intramuscularly weekly for 2 weeks (three doses) Procaine penicillin 600 000 units intramuscularly once a day for 17 days	Doxycycline 100 mg orally twice daily for 28 days Amoxicillin 2 g orally three times per day plus probenecid 500 mg four times a day for 28 days	Steroid cover should be given when treating cardiovascular syphilis
Neurosyphilis	Procaine penicillin 1.8–2.4 mega units intramuscularly once a day plus probenecid 500 mg orally, four times a day orally for 17 days Benzylpenicillin 18–24 mega units daily, given as 3–4 mega units intravenously every 4 hours for 17 days	Doxycycline 200 mg orally twice daily for 28 days Amoxicillin 2 g orally three times per day plus probenecid 500 mg orally four times a day for 28 days Ceftriaxone 2 g intramuscularly daily for 10–14 days	

Conclusion

Poor sexual health can have a negative impact on the health of the individual and the health of the nation. There has been an increase in sexually transmitted infections in the UK. The four UK governments have responded by introducing a number of infection control and prevention strategies. The nurse needs to ensure and take part in the implementation of the various strategies. Managing STIs requires a skilled, competent and confident approach in the primary and secondary care sectors. Central to these skills is the ability to undertake an effective sexual health history.

While STIs occur in all communities and both genders, there are some STIs that are more prevalent in some communities than in others. Understanding the anatomy and physiology of the male and female reproductive systems will help the nurse appreciate how STIs present and the impact they have on men and women.

Key Points

- Positive sexual health is a human right. Nurses are ideally placed to help people enjoy positive sexual health and they can do this in a number of ways using a sound evidence base.
- Identifying groups at risk, for example young people and MSM, and providing them with community specific health education and advice may help to reduce the incidence of STI in these groups.

- The incidence of STIs is increasing, despite a number of strategies in place locally, nationally and internationally.
- The ability to take comprehensive sexual history is paramount if the nurse is to offer care that is appropriate and effective. The skills required to do this effectively and with compassion can be honed as the nurse becomes more experienced.
- There is an increasing need to offer sexual health services in a variety of settings other than the sexual health clinic (the genitourinary medicine (GUM) clinic). Other primary, care settings, such as the general practice and the pharmacy, are important settings where the service can be offered closer to the patient.

Glossary

Abstinence: to stop or avoid – voluntary restraint from an activity, e.g. sex, alcohol or drugs

Antibiotic: a drug used to treat bacterial infection

Antibody: a special protein produced by the immune system, generally in response to infection or vaccination

Antigen: a substance (usually protein) recognised by the immune system as foreign (typically an infection, e.g. virus or bacteria) which stimulates the immune system to make antibodies

Asymptomatic: when a person has no signs or symptoms of a particular disease or infection they have, but may not be aware of

Autoinoculation: a secondary infection originating from an infection site already present in the body

Bacterial infections: infections caused by bacteria and which can be cured or treated with antibiotics

Balanitis: inflammation of the glans of the penis

Biopsy: taking of small sample to make diagnosis

Chancre: a painless ulceration formed during the primary stage of syphilis. Usually found in the genital area

Co-infection: infection with two or more infectious agents, e.g. HIV and hepatitis C (HCV)

Conjunctivitis: inflammation of the surfaces of the eye and eyelid; may be caused by a chlamydial or gonococcal infection

Dental dam: this is a square piece of thin latex (like a condom) that is used to prevent the spread of STIs when performing oral sex on an anal or vaginal opening. It is stretched across the anal opening or a woman's vagina to prevent the exchange of body fluids like blood, semen or vaginal fluids

Dyspareunia: painful sexual intercourse

Genotype: different genetic types or strains of an organism. Often used clinically in reference to chronic viral infections

Hepatitis: inflammation of the liver usually caused by one of the hepatitis viruses. Hepatitis B and C viruses are those with the potential to produce chronic infection and liver damage

Hepatitis B (HBV): hepatitis B is a virus that affects the liver and is very common worldwide. Approximately 95% of otherwise healthy adults will recover from acute HBV infection without progressing to chronic infection, but most babies and young children will develop chronic infection. Vaccine preventable and treatable

Hepatitis B vaccine: a series of injections which can immunise a person against HBV infection

Hepatitis C (HCV): hepatitis C is a virus that affects the liver. Approximately 75% of people who are infected will develop chronic HCV infection. Some people will clear the virus naturally or following antiviral treatment. No vaccine available

Human papilloma virus (HPV): a virus which infects the skin and mucous membranes. Some HPV are sexually transmitted. Causes genital and anal warts, and cervical cancer. A vaccine against HPV has recently become available

Incubation: the period of time between exposure to an infectious disease and the appearance of the first symptom or sign of disease

Lesion: a general term meaning an abnormal change or injury to any tissue or organ in the body

Lymphadenopathy: swelling of the lymph nodes in response to disease

MSM: a term used to describe 'men who have sex with men'. This includes bisexual men and men who do not identify or see themselves as homosexual

Mucosa: thin sheet of tissue that covers or lines various parts of the body – usually those areas that are 'wet', e.g. vagina, mouth, eyes, nose

Proctitis: inflammation of the rectal mucosa

Sex toy: an object or device used to facilitate sexual pleasure

Sign: something you can see or measure as an indicator of illness, e.g. rash, lesion

Symptoms: something a person experiences that may indicate illness, e.g. nausea, burning sensation when passing urine

Syndrome: a set of signs and symptoms that characterise a specific condition or illness

Vaccine: a medication given to produce immunity against infection. Usually given by injection but some are given orally

References

American Cancer Society (2013) *Human Papilloma Virus (HPV), Cancer, HPV Testing, and HPV Vaccines: Frequently Asked Questions.* http://www.cancer.org/acs/groups/cid/documents/webcontent/002780-pdf.pdf (accessed 8 March 2014).

BASHH (2006a) *Sexually Transmitted Infections: UK National Screening and Testing Guidelines.* British Association for Sexual Health and HIV, Macclesfield. http://www.bashh.org/documents/59/59.pdf (accessed January 2013).

BASHH (2006b) *United Kingdom National Guideline on the Management of Ano-genital Warts.* British Association for Sexual Health and HIV, Macclesfield. http://www.bashh.org/documents/86/86.pdf (accessed January 2013).

BASHH (2008) *National Guidelines on the Management of the Viral Hepatitides A, B and C.* British Association for Sexual Health and HIV, Macclesfield. http://www.bashh.org/documents/1927.pdf (accessed January 2013).

BASHH (2012) *Sexually Transmitted Infections. UK National Guideline for Gonorrhoea Testing.* British Association for Sexual Health and HIV, Macclesfield. http://www.bashh.org/documents/4490.pdf (accessed January 2013).

Bignall, C. & FitzGerald, M. (2011) UK National Guideline for the management of gonorrhoea in adults, 2011. *International Journal of STD and AIDS,* 22, 541–547.

Brook, G., Bacon, L., Evans, C. et al. (2013) *UK National Guideline for Consultations Requiring Sexual History Taking.* http://www.bashh.org/documents/Sexual%20History%20Taking%20guideline%202013.pdf (accessed 8 March 2014).

Cowan, F. & Bell, G. (2012) STI control and prevention. In: K.E. Rogstad (ed.) *ABC of Sexually Transmitted Infections,* 6th edn. Ch. 2, pp. 11–15. Wiley-Blackwell, Oxford.

DH (2001) *Better Prevention, Better Services, Better Sexual Health – The National Strategy for Sexual Health and HIV.* Department of Health, London.

DH (2008) *Statutory Directions for the Routine Human Papillomavirus Vaccination Programme.* Department of Health, London. http://www.immunisation.nhs.uk/publications/HPV_directions_2008.pdf (accessed January 2013).

DH (2010) *Working Together to Safeguard Children: A guide to interagency working to safeguard and promote the welfare of children.* Department of Health, London. https://www.education.gov.uk/publications/standard/publicationdetail/page1/DCSF-00305-2010 (accessed January 2013).

DHSSPSNI (2008) *Sexual Health Promotion: Strategy and Action Plan 2008–2013.* Department of Health, Social Services and Public Safety: Northern Ireland, Belfast, NI.

Harcourt, C., O'Connor, J., Egger, S., Fairley, C.K., Wand, H., Chen M.Y. et al. (2010). The decriminalisation of prostitution is associated with better coverage of health promotion programs for sex workers. *Australian and New Zealand Journal of Public Health,* 34, 482–486.

HIS (2011) *Improving Sexual Health Services in Scotland.* Healthcare Improvement Scotland, Edinburgh.

HM-Government (2010) *Department of Health Response to the Public's Comments on The Coalition: Our programme for government on public health.* HM Government, London.

HPA (2010) *Guidance for Gonorrhoea Testing in England and Wales.* Health Protection Agency, London. http://www.hpa.org.uk/webc/HPAwebFile/HPAweb_C/1267550166455 (accessed January 2013).

HPA (2011) *Trends in Genital Herpes and Genital Warts Infections, United Kingdom: 2000 to 2009,* Vol. 5, No. 17. http://www.hpa.org.uk/hpr./archives/2011/hpr1711.pdf (accessed 8 March 2014).

HPA (2012a) *Health Protection Report,* Vol. 6, No. 22. Health Protection Agency, London. http://www.hpa.org.uk/hpr/archives/2012/hpr2212.pdf (accessed January 2013).

HPA (2012b) *New Data Show Sexually Transmitted Infection Diagnoses on the Rise in England.* Health Protection Agency, London. http://www

.hpa.org.uk/NewsCentre/NationalPressReleases/2012PressReleases/ 120531newrisingSTInumbersreleased/ (accessed January 2013).

HPS (2012) *Genital Herpes Simplex, Genital Chlamydia and Gonorrhoea Infection in Scotland: laboratory diagnoses 2002–2010.* Health Protection Scotland, Edinburgh. http://www.hps.scot.nhs.uk/ewr/ subjectsummary.aspx?subjectid=136 (accessed 8 March 2014).

ISD Scotland (2010) *Sexually Transmitted Infections.* National Health Service Scotland. http://www.isdscotland.org/sti/ (accessed January 2013).

Keogh, P., Weatherburn, P., Henderson, L., Reed, D., Dodds, C. & Hickson, F. (2004) *Doctoring Gay Men: Exploring the contribution of general practice.* Sigma, London.

Kingsberg, S. (2004) Just Ask! Talking to patients about sexual function. *Sexuality, Reproduction and Menopause,* 2(4), 199–203.

Kingston, M., French, P., Goh, B., Goold, P., Higgins, S., Sukthankar, A. et al. (2008) UK National Guidelines on the management of syphilis. *International Journal of STD and AIDS,* 19, 729–740.

Mann, R. & Williams J. (2003) Standards in medical record keeping. *Clinical Medicine,* 3(4), 329–332.

McClean, H., Radcliffe, K., Sullivan, A. & Ahmed-Jushuf, I. (2012) BASHH Statement on partner notification for sexually transmissible infections. *International Journal of STD & AIDS,* 24(4), 253–261. http://www .bashh.org/documents/2012%20Partner%20Notification%20 Statement.pdf (accessed January 2013).

MedFASH (2010) *Standards for the Management of Sexually Transmitted Infections (STIs).* Medical Foundation for AIDS, Sexual Health and HIV, London.

NICE (2007) *One to One Interventions to Reduce the Transmission of Sexually Transmitted Infections (STIs) Including HIV, and to Reduce the Rate of Under 18 Conceptions, Especially among Vulnerable and at Risk Groups.* National Institute for Health and Clinical Excellence, London.

NMC (2009) *Confidentiality.* Nursing and Midwifery Council, London. http://www.nmc-uk.org/Nurses-and-midwives/Advice-by-topic/A/ Advice/Confidentiality/ (accessed January 2013).

NMC (2010) *Record Keeping. Guidance for Nurses and Midwives.* Nursing and Midwifery Council, London. http://www.nmc-uk.org/Documents/ NMC-Publications/NMC-Record-Keeping-Guidance.pdf (accessed January 2013).

Nusbaum, M.R. & Hamilton, C.D. (2002) The proactive sexual health history. *American Family Physician,* 66(9), 17051–17712.

Pareek, S.S. (2012) *Pictorial Atlas of Common Genito-urinary Medicine.* Radcliffe, London.

Perez, K. & Lee, V. (2012) Examination techniques and clinical sampling. In: K.E. Rogstad (ed.) *ABC of Sexually Transmitted Infections,* 6th edn. Ch. 5, pp. 26–28. Wiley-Blackwell, Oxford.

PHA (2011) *Sexually Transmitted Surveillance in Northern Ireland 2012. An Analysis of Data for the Calendar Year 2011.* Public Health Agency, Belfast.

PHW (2011) *HIV Trends in Wales. Surveillance Report.* Public Health Wales, Cardiff. http://www.wales.nhs.uk/sites3/Documents/895/HIV%20STI %20Trends%20March%202011.pdf (accessed January 2013).

Porth, C. M. (2009) *Pathophysiology: Concepts of Altered Health States,* 9th edn. Lippincott, Philadelphia.

RCGPs (2006) *STIs in Primary Care.* Royal College of General Practitioners, London.

RCP & BASHH (2012). *Alcohol and Sex: a Cocktail for Poor Sexual Health.* A report of the Alcohol and Sexual Health Working Party. Royal College of Physicians and British Society for Sexual Health and HIV. http://www.rcplondon.ac.uk/sites/default/files/rcp_and_bashh_-_alcohol _and_sex_a_cocktail_for_poor_sexual_health.pdf (accessed January 2013).

Rogstad, K., Palfreeman, A., Rooney, G., *et al.* (2006) UK National Guidelines on HIV Testing. *International Journal of STD and AIDS,* 17, 668–676.

Rogstad, K., Thomas, A., Williams, O. et al. (2010) *United Kingdom National Guideline on the Management of Sexually Transmitted Infections and Related Conditions in Children and Young People.* British Association for Sexual Health and HIV, Macclesfield. http://www .bashh.org/documents/2674.pdf (accessed January 2013).

Scottish Executive (2005) *Respect and Responsibility. Strategy and Action Plan for Improving Sexual Health.* Scottish Executive, Edinburgh.

Scottish Government (2012) *Records Management: NHS Code of Practice (Scotland).* Scottish Government, Edinburgh. http://www.scotland.gov .uk/Publications/2012/01/10143104/0 (accessed January 2013).

Tomlinson, J.M. (2005) Taking a sexual health history. In: J.M. Tomlinson (ed.) *ABC of Sexual Health,* 2nd edn. Ch. 4, pp. 13–16. British Medical Journal Books, London.

Tsimtsiou, Z., Hatzimouratidis, K., Nakopoulou, E., Kyrana, E., Salpigidis, G. & Hatzichristou, D. (2006) Predictors of physicians' involvement in addressing sexual health issues. *Journal of Sexual Medicine* 4(3), 583–588.

Van Voorst Vader, P.C. (1998) Syphilis management and treatment. *Dermatologic Clinics* 16(4), 699–711.

WAG (2010) *Sexual Health and Well-being Action Plan for Wales, 2010–2015.* Welsh Assembly Government, Cardiff.

Wakley, G., Cunnion, M. & Chambers, R. (2003) *Improving Sexual Health Advice.* Radcliffe, Oxford.

WHO (2011) *Prevention and Treatment of HIV and Other Sexually Transmitted Infections Among Men Who Have Sex With Men and Transgender People Recommendations for a Public Health Approach.* World Health Organization, Geneva.

Woodward, C.L. & Robinson, A.J. (2012) Genital growths and infestations. In: J.M. Tomlinson (ed.) *ABC of Sexual Health,* 2nd edn. Ch. 14, pp. 78–83. British Medical Journal Books, London.

Test Yourself

1. How many genotypes of the human papilloma virus have been identified?
   (a) 200
   (b) 50
   (c) Over 100
   (d) More than 1000

2. What is meant by prodrome?
   (a) The late manifestations of a disease
   (b) The early symptoms of a disease
   (c) The measurement used to assess vaginal discharge
   (d) The measurement used to measure penile discharge

3. Women are at greater risk for human papilloma virus because:
   (a) They menstruate
   (b) They use the contraceptive pill
   (c) They have a shorter urethra then men
   (d) They have greater mucosal area exposed in the genital area

4. Imiquimod is:
   (a) A cream used to help stimulate the immune system
   (b) A pessary used to help stimulate the immune system
   (c) A drug injected intravenously to help stimulate the immune system
   (d) A type of wart caused by a specific genotype

5. Balanitis is:
   (a) An infection of the clitoral head
   (b) An infection of the head of the penis and the foreskin
   (c) An infection of the anus
   (d) An infection of the vulva

6. In women, when gonorrhoea infection spreads transluminally this can cause:
   (a) Peritonitis
   (b) Pelvic inflammatory disease
   (c) Gastric ulceration
   (d) Uterine prolapse

7. What does the term 'gummatous' mean?
   (a) A rubbery-like lesion associated with syphilis
   (b) A rubbery-like lesion associated with orchitis
   (c) A rubbery-like lesion associated with conjunctivitis
   (d) A rubbery-like lesion associated with gonorrhoea

8. The incubation period for syphilis is:
   (a) 3 days
   (b) 9–90 days
   (c) It does not have one
   (d) 3 years

9. What is the most common cause of Argyll Robertson pupils?
   (a) Syphilis
   (b) Gonorrhoea
   (c) Lymphogranuloma venereum
   (d) Chlamydia

10. Proctitis refers to:
    (a) Inflammation of the fallopian tube
    (b) Inflammation of the vulval mucosa
    (c) Inflammation of the rectal mucosa
    (d) Inflammation of the peritoneal cavity

Answers

1. c
2. b
3. d
4. a
5. b
6. b
7. a
8. b
9. a
10. c

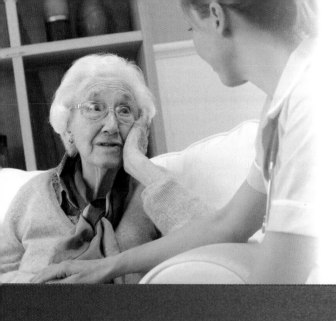

33

The Person with an Endocrine Disorder

Carl Clare

University of Hertfordshire, UK

Learning Outcomes

On completion of this chapter you will be able to:

- Describe the parts of the endocrine system
- Describe the negative feedback loop that controls many of the endocrine systems
- List the potential disorders of the endocrine system
- Discuss the role of self-care in the management of endocrine disorders
- Discuss the treatment of each of the endocrine disorders
- Explain the need for regular health checks for patients with diabetes

Competencies

All nurses must:

1. Carry out a basic physical survey for signs of an endocrine disorder
2. Ask focussed questions to aid in the diagnosis of a particular endocrine disorder
3. Provide advice to a patient about their endocrine disorder
4. Make referrals to the appropriate members of the multidisciplinary team
5. Promote health for patients with diabetes
6. Recognise and treat a hypoglycaemic episode

Visit the companion website at **www.wileynursingpractice.com** where you can test yourself using flashcards, multiple-choice questions and more.

Nursing Practice: Knowledge and Care, First Edition. Edited by Ian Peate, Karen Wild and Muralitharan Nair.
© 2014 John Wiley & Sons, Ltd. Published 2014 by John Wiley & Sons, Ltd. Companion website: www.wileynursingpractice.com

Introduction

The endocrine system is a diffusely distributed system of glands and organs (Figure 33.1). The endocrine system is a relatively, slow-acting, and yet very powerful system that acts in concert with the nervous system to maintain homeostasis. In human physiology, **homeostasis** refers to the regulation of the internal environment to maintain normal physiological balance and functioning within the body. In attempting to maintain homeostasis, the endocrine and nervous systems act together to regulate several different aspects of the internal environment, such as fluid balance and blood pressure. The nervous system reacts rapidly to stimuli and effects its changes over a period of seconds or minutes, thus it is involved in the immediate and short-term maintenance of homeostasis. Due to its rapid onset of action, the nervous system is responsible for the control of rapid bodily processes, such as breathing and movement. The endocrine system is mostly involved

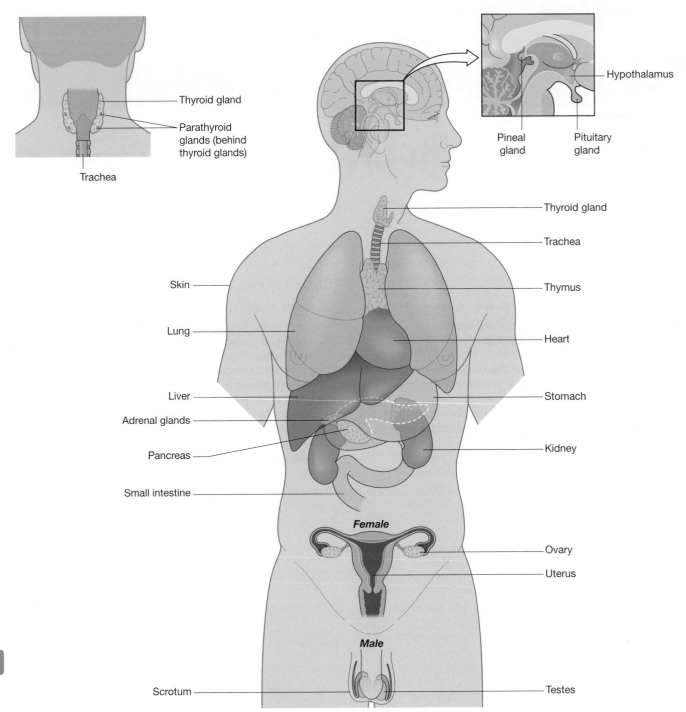

Figure 33.1 The location of the endocrine glands and the organs that secrete hormones.

in the longer-term regulation of homeostasis, some of the hormones released can exert an effect within seconds but mostly the effects are slower in onset but have a longer-term effect.

Anatomy and Physiology of the Endocrine System

The structures of the endocrine system can be split into three main types:

- **Endocrine glands** – These are organs whose only function is the production and release of hormones. These include:
  - The pituitary gland
  - The thyroid gland
  - The parathyroid gland
  - The adrenal gland
- **Organs that are not pure glands** (as they have other functions as well as the production of hormones) but contain relatively large areas of hormone producing tissue. These include:
  - The hypothalamus
  - The pancreas
- **Other tissues and organs that produce hormones** – areas of hormone producing cells are found in the wall of the small intestine, the stomach, the heart, the liver and the skin.

The endocrine system has many effects within the human body and can affect processes in both the short term and over a much longer period of time. The major functions the endocrine system coordinates are:

- Homeostasis – helps to maintain the internal body environment
- Storage and metabolism of energy substrates (carbohydrates, proteins and fats)
- Regulation of growth and development
- Regulation of reproduction and the sexual functioning of the body (see Chapters 30 and 31)
- Control of the body's responses to external stimuli (particularly stress)
- Helps to establish circadian rhythms.

The Endocrine Glands

The endocrine glands will usually have a rich blood supply delivered by numerous blood vessels and the hormone producing cells within the glands will normally be arranged into branching networks around this supply. This arrangement of blood vessels and hormone producing cells in close proximity ensures that secreted hormones enter into the bloodstream rapidly and are then transported throughout the body to the target cells (Figure 33.2).

Hormones

Hormones are chemicals that are secreted into the blood or the extracellular fluid by one cell and have an effect on the functioning of other cells (or occasionally on the same cell). Unlike the nervous system, where the outflow (the message) is targeted to particular cells by the physical layout of the nervous system, the endocrine system generally relies on the transport of the hormones produced to all parts of the body. Despite this seemingly indiscriminate 'broadcast' of chemicals, each hormone does not have an effect on every cell in the body. Nervous system activity could be said to be like an e-mail, in that it is targeted at certain recipients, whereas the hormone is more like a 'tweet' – it is only 'read' by those cells

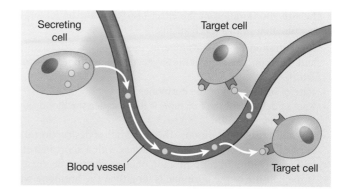

Figure 33.2 Transportation of hormones in the blood.

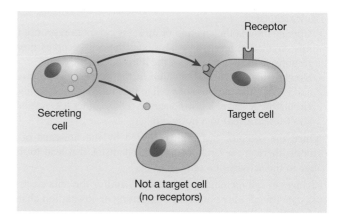

Figure 33.3 Target cell and non-target cell.

that are 'following' the endocrine gland but it is not sent specifically to those followers. Cells that are 'following' the gland have receptors specifically for the hormone released and are then known as 'target' cells. Without the particular receptor, the hormone will have no effect on the cell (Figure 33.3).

Depending on the underlying composition of the hormone that exerts the effect on the target cell, the receptor will either be contained within the cell or on the cell wall.

- The vast majority of hormones are amino acid-based hormones, which cannot cross the cell membrane and therefore their receptors are found on the cell wall. These hormones tend to exert their influence by activating enzymes and other molecules within the cell that then lead to a cascade of changes that ultimately affect the cell activity. Hormones in this class include: adrenaline, noradrenaline, parathyroid hormones and antidiuretic hormones
- The steroid-based hormones are derived from cholesterol and can cross the cell membrane because they are small and lipid soluble and therefore, their receptors are located within the target cell itself. These hormones usually exert their effect by stimulating the production of genes within the target cell, leading to the synthesis of new proteins. Examples of steroid hormones are: aldosterone and cortisol.
- Thyroxine is the exception to these rules, in that it is an amino-based hormone but it is lipid soluble and is able to cross the cell membrane. Thus, receptors for thyroxine are located within the cell.

The size and duration of the effect of a hormone on its target cell is a function of two mechanisms:

1. Concentration of the hormone in the blood or extracellular fluid. This concentration at the target cell is determined by three factors:
   - Rate of production of the hormone
   - Rate of delivery of the hormone – for instance the blood flow to the organ or cell
   - The half-life of the hormone. This is the rate of destruction and elimination of the hormone. Hormones with a short half-life will rapidly drop in concentration once production decreases. If the half-life of the hormone is long then the hormone will still be present in significant concentrations for some time after its production stops.

2. Changes in the number of receptors available for the hormone. The number of receptors can be upregulated or downregulated:
   - Upregulation is the creation of more receptors in response to low circulating levels of a hormone; the cell becomes more responsive to the presence of the hormone in the blood
   - Downregulation is the reduction in the number of receptors and is often the response of a cell to prolonged periods of high circulating levels of a hormone; the cell becomes less responsive (desensitised) to a hormone.

Once the receptor has been activated by the presence of a hormone, there are several potential mechanisms that lead to the change in the activity of a cell:

- Changes in cell membrane permeability and/or the cell's electrical state (membrane potential) by opening or closing ion channels in the cell membrane
- Synthesis of proteins or regulatory molecules (such as enzymes) within the cell
- Enzyme activation or deactivation
- Causing secretory activity
- Stimulation of mitosis.

Hormones can have a large effect at even low concentrations; it is therefore essential that active hormones are efficiently removed from the blood to prevent the constant stimulation of target cells. Some hormones are rapidly broken down within the cells; however most are inactivated by enzyme systems in the liver and kidneys and then excreted.

The control of hormone production and secretion

The creation and release of most hormones is preceded by a stimulus, which can be internal or external; for instance a rise in blood glucose levels or a cold environment. The further synthesis and release of hormones is then usually controlled by a negative feedback system, as detailed in Figure 33.4. An example of a simple negative feedback system can be seen in Figure 33.5. The influence of a stimulus, from inside or outside the body leads to the release of a hormone, which has an effect on the stimulus; following this, some aspect of the target organ function then inhibits further reaction to the stimulus and thus further release of the hormone by the organ. In the example noted in Figure 33.5, a rise in blood glucose levels (initial stimulus) stimulates the release of insulin. One of the effects of insulin is to cause the liver (the target organ) to store glucose from the blood, thus helping to reduce the blood glucose level (thus inhibiting further insulin release).

The initial stimulus for the release of a hormone is usually one of three types; though some organs respond to multiple stimuli.

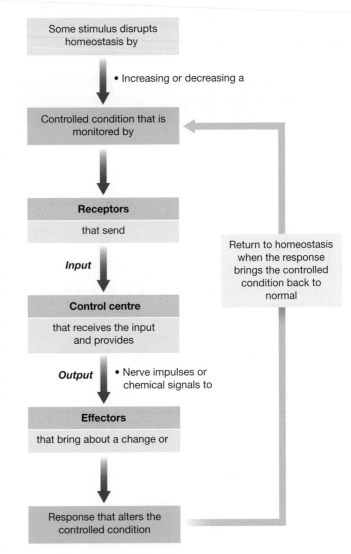

Figure 33.4 **Negative feedback loop.**

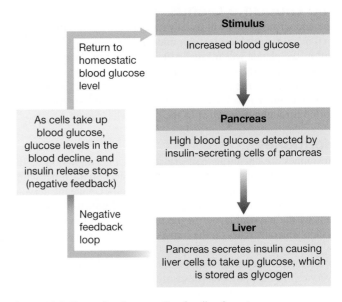

Figure 33.5 **Example of a negative feedback system.**

Humoral – A response to changing levels of certain ions and nutrients in the blood. For example parathyroid hormone is stimulated by falling blood levels of calcium ions.

Neural – A response to direct nervous stimulation. Very few endocrine organs are directly stimulated by the nervous system. An example would be increased activity in the sympathetic nervous system, which directly stimulates the release of catecholamines (adrenaline and noradrenaline) from the adrenal medulla.

Hormonal – A response to hormones released by other glands or organs. An example of hormonal control would be the release of thyroid stimulating hormone (TSH) from the anterior pituitary gland directly stimulates the production and release of thyroxine from the thyroid gland.

The anatomy and physiology of the individual endocrine glands

The **hypothalamus** is a small structure that is directly connected to the pituitary gland by the pituitary stalk (or infundibulum). One of the functions of the hypothalamus is to link the nervous system to the endocrine system via the pituitary gland. Almost all the secretion of hormones by the pituitary gland is controlled by either hormonal or electrical signals from the hypothalamus.

The hypothalamus receives signals from many sources within the nervous system and is also under negative feedback control by the hormones secreted by the pituitary gland.

The **pituitary gland** secretes at least nine major hormones and is the size and shape of a pea on a stalk. The pituitary gland is functionally and anatomically divided into two parts.

The **posterior lobe** (neurohypophysis) is made up mostly of nerve fibres which originate in the hypothalamus and terminate on the surface of capillaries in the posterior lobe (Figure 33.6). The posterior lobe receives two hormones directly from neurosecretory cells in the hypothalamus via the axons of the nerve bundles connecting them (the hypothalamic-hypophyseal tract). These hormones are then stored and, in response to a stimulus, these hormones are then released into the blood stream. Therefore, the posterior pituitary gland is in fact a storage area rather than a gland in the truest sense of the term.

The hormones that are secreted by the posterior pituitary are:

- *Oxytocin*. Oxytocin has an effect on uterine contraction in childbirth and is responsible for the 'let down' response in breast-feeding mothers. It also has a role in sexual arousal and orgasm
- Antidiuretic hormone (ADH). The effect of ADH is to increase water retention by the kidneys. The secretion of ADH is stimulated by:
  - Increased plasma osmolality – increased levels of certain substances in the plasma such as sodium
  - Decreased extracellular fluid volume
  - Pain and other stressed states
  - In response to certain drugs.

The **anterior lobe** of the pituitary gland (adenohypophysis) is much larger than the posterior lobe (Figure 33.7). The hypothalamus and the anterior pituitary have no direct nerve connections but do have a very rich vascular (blood vessel) connection known as the hypothalamo-hypophyseal portal system, whereby venous blood from the hypothalamus flows to the anterior lobe. Thus control of the anterior pituitary is by releasing and inhibiting factors (or hormones) secreted by the hypothalamus into this system.

There are five types of pituitary cell:

- *Somatotropes* – secrete growth hormones
- *Lactotropes* – secrete prolactin
- *Thyrotropes* – secrete thyroid stimulating hormone

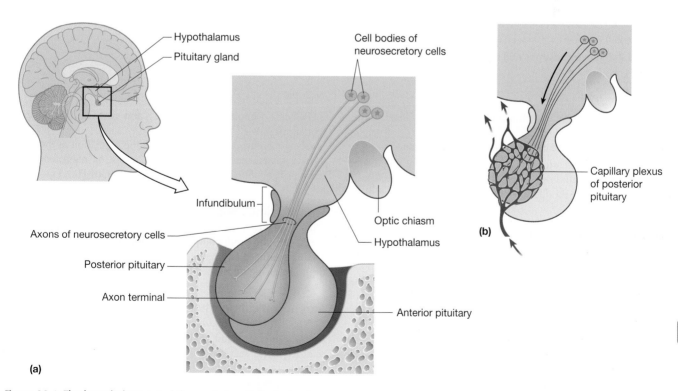

Figure 33.6 The hypothalamus and the posterior pituitary gland.

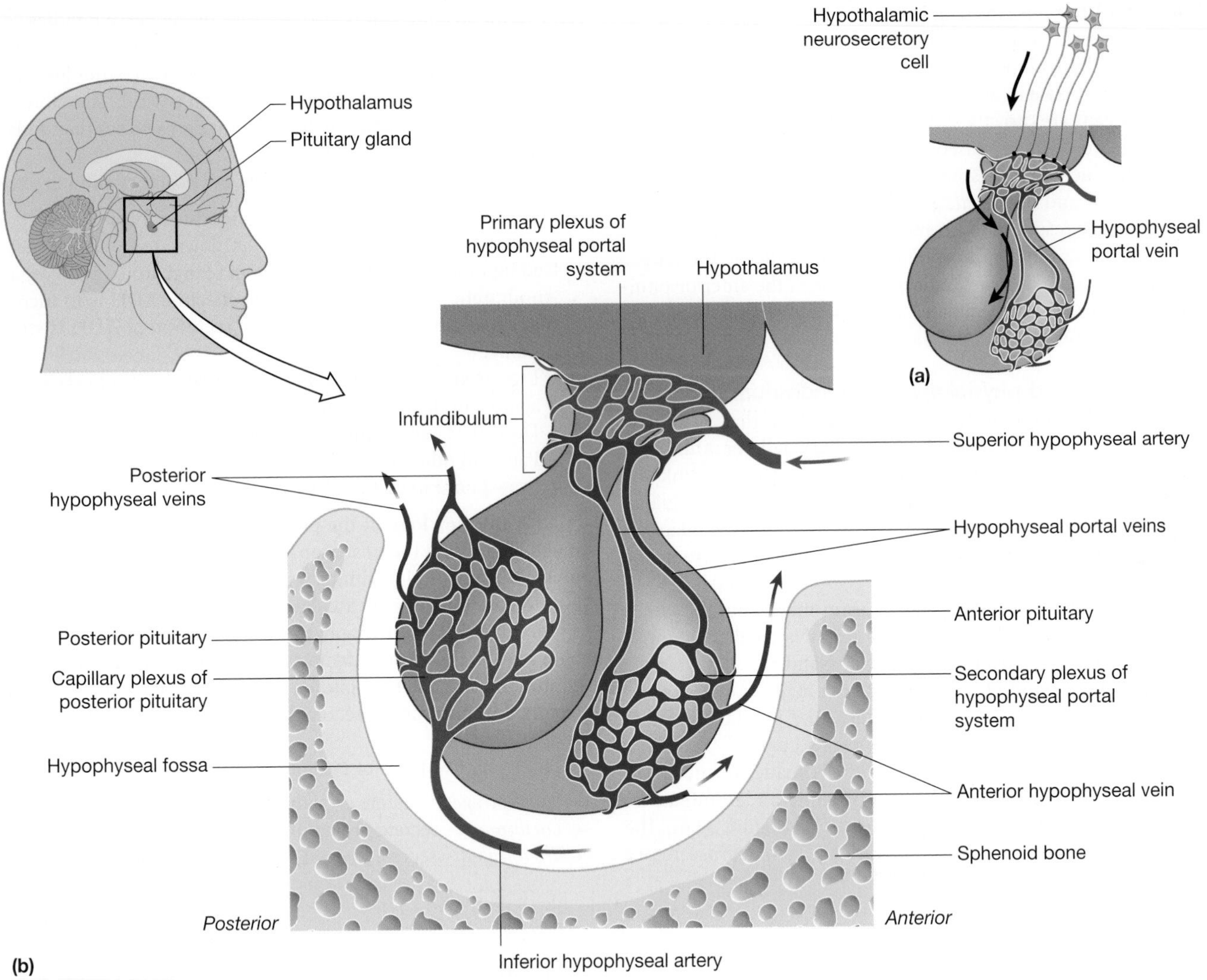

Figure 33.7 The hypothalamus and the anterior pituitary gland.

- *Gonadotropes* – secrete luteinising hormone and follicle stimulating hormone
- *Corticotropes* – secrete adrenocorticotropic hormone.

The hormones secreted by the anterior pituitary gland and the releasing or inhibiting hormones from the hypothalamus that influence their production and release, are summarised in Table 33.1.

Growth hormone

The secretion of growth hormone is controlled by the release of growth hormone releasing hormone (GHRH) and growth hormone release inhibiting hormone (GHRIH or somatostatin) by the hypothalamus. The effect of growth is to promote the growth of bone, cartilage and soft tissue by stimulating the production and release of insulin like growth factor (IGF-1).

Prolactin

Prolactin stimulates the secretion of milk in the breast. Regulation of the secretion of prolactin is by dopamine and prolactin releasing hormone from the hypothalamus.

Follicle stimulating hormone and luteinising hormone (gonadotropins).

The gonadotropins are involved in the regulation of the reproductive system and control of their release is regulated by the release of gonadotropin releasing hormone (GnRH).

Thyroid stimulating hormone (TSH)

TSH stimulates the activity of the cells of the thyroid gland leading to an increased production and secretion of the thyroid hormones. TSH is produced and released in response to the release of thyrotropin releasing hormone (TRH) from the hypothalamus.

Adrenocorticotropic hormone (ACTH)

ACTH stimulates the production of cortisol and androgens from the adrenal gland. It also leads to the production of aldosterone. ACTH is secreted from the anterior pituitary in response to the secretion of corticotropin releasing hormone (CRH). Excitation of the hypothalamus by any form of stress leads to the release of CRH.

Table 33.1 The hormone cascade from the hypothalamus to the anterior pituitary gland and target organs. (Source: Peate and Nair 2011. Reproduced with permission of John Wiley & Sons Ltd.)

HYPOTHALAMUS	ANTERIOR PITUITARY GLAND	TARGET ORGAN OR TISSUES	ACTION
Growth hormone releasing factor	Growth hormone	Many (especially bones)	Stimulates growth of body cells
Growth hormone release inhibiting factor	Growth hormone (inhibits release)	Many	
Thyroid releasing hormone (TRH)	Thyroid stimulating hormone (TSH)	Thyroid gland	Stimulates thyroid hormone release
Corticotropin releasing hormone (CRH)	Adrenocorticotropic hormone (ACTH)	Adrenal cortex	Stimulates corticosteroid release
Prolactin releasing hormone	Prolactin	Breasts	Stimulates milk production
Prolactin inhibiting hormone	Prolactin (inhibits release)	Breasts	
Gonadotropin releasing hormone	Follicle stimulating hormone Luteinising hormone	Gonads	Various reproductive functions

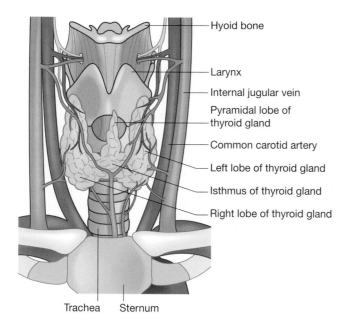

Figure labels:
- Hyoid bone
- Larynx
- Internal jugular vein
- Pyramidal lobe of thyroid gland
- Common carotid artery
- Left lobe of thyroid gland
- Isthmus of thyroid gland
- Right lobe of thyroid gland
- Trachea
- Sternum

Figure 33.8 The thyroid gland.

The Thyroid Gland

The thyroid gland is a butterfly-shaped gland located in the front of the neck on the trachea just below the larynx (Figure 33.8). It is made up of two lobes joined by a narrow strip known as an **isthmus**; some thyroid glands have a small third (central) lobe known as the 'pyramidal lobe'. Each lobe is made up of hollow, spherical, follicles surrounded by capillaries.

Inside the follicles are thyroglobulin molecules with attached iodine molecules; the thyroid hormones are created from this. The thyroid gland is unique in the endocrine system in that it can store the hormone it releases (up to approximately 100 days' supply). The thyroid gland releases two forms of thyroid hormones, both of which require iodine from dietary intake for their creation and are created in response to TSH release from the pituitary gland:

- *Thyroxine (T_4)*: the primary hormone released by the thyroid gland; it is converted into T_3 by the target cells
- *Triiodothyronine (T_3)*: created in smaller amounts than T_4 but has a more potent effect on receptors.

Thyroid hormone affects virtually every cell in the body, except:

- The adult brain
- Spleen
- Testes
- Uterus
- Thyroid gland.

In the target cells, thyroid hormone stimulates enzymes that are involved with glucose oxidation. This is known as the 'calorigenic effect' and its overall effects are:

- An increase in the basal metabolic rate
- An increase in oxygen consumption by the cell
- An increase in the production of body heat.

The basal metabolic rate is the amount of energy expended while at rest in a temperate environment. If the basal metabolic rate is increased, then oxygen consumption increases because oxygen is required in the production of energy. Thyroid hormone also has important role in the maintenance of blood pressure as it stimulates an increase in the number of receptors in the walls of the blood vessels.

Like most of the endocrine systems, the control of thyroid hormone release is regulated by a negative feedback system (Figure 33.9).

Blood levels of the thyroid hormones are monitored in the hypothalamus and by cells in the anterior lobe of the pituitary gland. When thyroid hormone levels in the blood are low, this is detected by the hypothalamus and it leads to the release of thyroid releasing hormone (TRH) and then the subsequent release of thyroid stimulating hormone (TSH) from the anterior pituitary gland. The target cells of TSH are the follicle cells of the thyroid gland. In response to stimulation by TSH, the follicle cells release T_3 and T_4 into the bloodstream. As the quantities of thyroid hormones increase, this is detected by the hypothalamus and anterior pituitary and there is gradual inhibition of the release of TRH and TSH in response to the gradual rise in thyroid hormones.

The half-life of T_4 is approximately 7 days and the half-life of T_3 is 1 day. Thyroid hormones are broken down in the liver and the skeletal muscle and while much of the iodine is recycled, some is lost in the urine and the faeces. Therefore, there is a need for daily replacement of iodine through dietary intake.

In addition to the thyroid follicles, there are C cells which are found between the follicles and secrete calcitonin. Calcitonin is involved in the metabolism of calcium and phosphorous within the body. It decreases calcium levels in the blood by reducing the

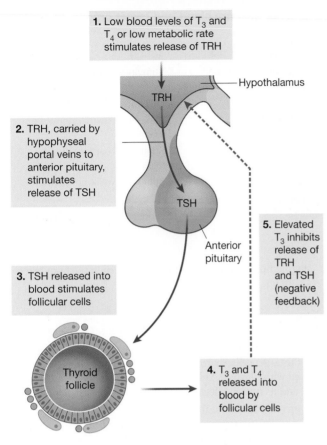

1. Low blood levels of T$_3$ and T$_4$ or low metabolic rate stimulates release of TRH

Hypothalamus

TRH

2. TRH, carried by hypophyseal portal veins to anterior pituitary, stimulates release of TSH

TSH

Anterior pituitary

3. TSH released into blood stimulates follicular cells

5. Elevated T$_3$ inhibits release of TRH and TSH (negative feedback)

Thyroid follicle

4. T$_3$ and T$_4$ released into blood by follicular cells

Figure 33.9 The negative feedback control of thyroid hormone release.

activity of osteoclasts (cells that 'digest' bone and thus release calcium and phosphorous into the blood). Calcitonin also inhibits the reabsorption of calcium from urine in the kidneys.

The parathyroid glands

The parathyroid glands are small glands located on the back (posterior) of the thyroid gland (Figure 33.10). There are usually two pairs of glands, but some patients have been reported to have up to four pairs. The cells that create and secrete parathyroid hormone (parathyroid chief cells) are arranged in cords or nests around dense capillary beds. Parathyroid hormone is the single most important hormone for the control of the calcium balance in the body. The target tissues and actions of parathyroid hormone are:

- Increasing intestinal calcium absorption
- Stimulating renal calcium absorption
- Stimulating osteoclast activity and therefore the release of calcium from the bones.

Calcium is important in the transmission of nerve impulses, is involved in muscle contraction and is also required in the creation of clotting factors in the blood. The regulation of parathyroid hormone synthesis and secretion is controlled by a negative feedback loop which is responsive to the levels of calcium in the blood. Calcium levels are monitored by cells in the parathyroid gland itself. A reduced blood calcium level leads to an increase in the synthesis and secretion of parathyroid hormone.

The control of blood calcium levels is also mediated through a hormone known as 'calcitriol' which is a hormone released by the kidneys in response to a decrease in calcium ions in the blood and the release of parathyroid hormone. Calcitriol it is known to have an effect on parathyroid hormone secretion and also inhibits the release of calcitonin from the thyroid gland. Parathyroid hormone

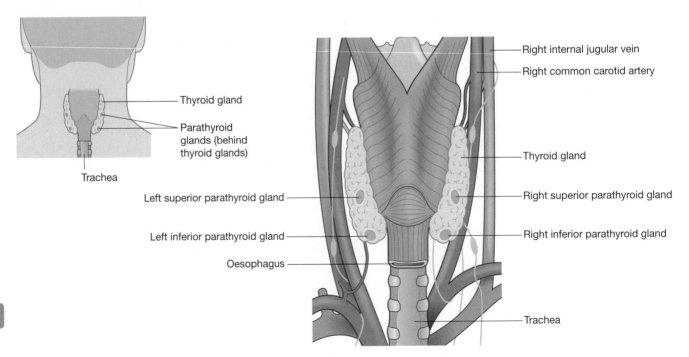

Thyroid gland

Parathyroid glands (behind thyroid glands)

Trachea

Left superior parathyroid gland

Left inferior parathyroid gland

Oesophagus

Right internal jugular vein

Right common carotid artery

Thyroid gland

Right superior parathyroid gland

Right inferior parathyroid gland

Trachea

Figure 33.10 The parathyroid glands.

is a known stimulus for the release of calcitriol but when calcitriol levels achieve a high enough level its effect changes to that of inhibiting the release of parathyroid hormone. This prevents an uncontrollable increase in calcium in the blood. A summary of the effects of parathyroid hormone, calcitriol and calcitonin on the calcium levels in the blood are summarised in Figure 33.11.

The adrenal glands

The adrenal glands are essential for the maintenance of homeostasis. The two adrenal glands are found on the top of each of the two kidneys (Figure 33.12), the right gland is roughly triangular in shape and the left is crescent shaped. Both the adrenal glands are covered in a capsule of connective tissue and surrounded by a layer of fat. In common with the other glands, adrenal glands have a rich vascular supply ensuring the rapid transportation of the hormones secreted to the target organs.

Functionally, each of the adrenal glands is comprised of two major regions (Figure 33.13):

- *Adrenal medulla*
- *Adrenal cortex*.

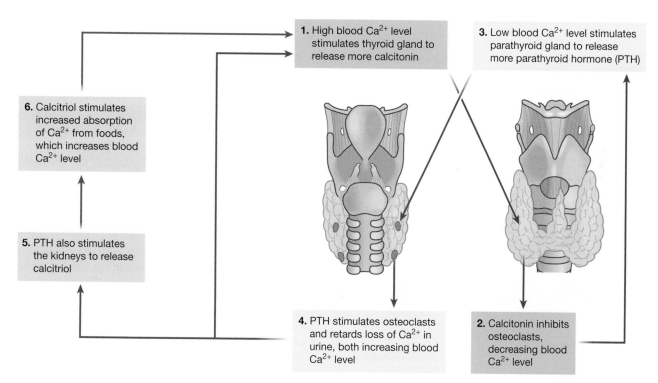

Figure 33.11 The effects of parathyroid hormone, calcitonin and calcitriol in the regulation of blood calcium levels. Purple arrows, calcitonin; blue arrows, parathyroid hormones; red arrows, calcitriol.

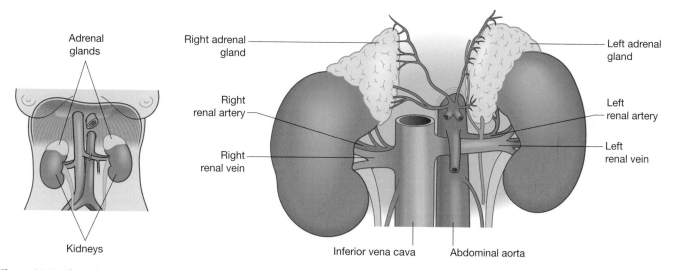

Figure 33.12 The adrenal glands.

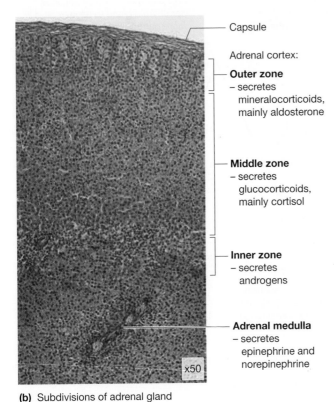

(a) Section through left adrenal gland

Capsule

Adrenal cortex:

Outer zone
– secretes mineralocorticoids, mainly aldosterone

Middle zone
– secretes glucocorticoids, mainly cortisol

Inner zone
– secretes androgens

Adrenal medulla
– secretes epinephrine and norepinephrine

x50

(b) Subdivisions of adrenal gland

Figure 33.13 Cross-section of an adrenal gland and its subdivisions.

Adrenal medulla The adrenal medulla is the innermost section of the adrenal gland. The function of the adrenal medulla is the secretion of the catecholamines:

- Adrenaline
- Noradrenaline.

The adrenal medulla is densely innervated, receiving sympathetic nervous system outflow, which means that hormone release can happen quickly in response to a stimulus such as:

- Pain
- Anxiety
- Excitement
- Hypovolaemia
- Hypoglycaemia.

The effects of the catecholamines are many and varied, they:

- Stimulate the nervous system
- Metabolic effects – for instance glycogenolysis in the liver and skeletal muscle
- Increase metabolic rate
- Increase heart rate
- Increase alertness – though adrenaline frequently evokes anxiety and fear
- Noradrenaline causes significant, widespread vasoconstriction
- Adrenaline causes vasoconstriction in the skin and viscera but vasodilation in skeletal muscles.

Although adrenaline and noradrenaline are essential for normal bodily functioning, the role of the adrenaline and the noradrenaline secreted by the adrenal medulla is not essential and serves only to intensify the effects of sympathetic nervous stimulation. Catecholamines have a very short half-life in the blood, as they are rapidly degraded by blood-borne enzymes.

Adrenal cortex The outer section of each adrenal gland is made up of three layers (Figure 33.13). Each layer is responsible for the production of one of the corticosteroid hormones:

- *Zona glomerulosa* – (outer zone) produces the mineralocorticoids
- *Zona fasciculata* – (middle zone) produces the glucocorticoids
- *Zona reticularis* – (inner zone) this zone is also involved in the production of glucocorticoids but also produces small amounts of adrenal sex hormones (androgens).

Mineralocorticoids – The role of the mineralocorticoids is the regulation of electrolyte concentrations in the blood. Aldosterone constitutes 95% of the mineralocorticoids synthesised and released from the adrenal glands. Aldosterone exerts its effect by increasing the reabsorption of sodium in the kidneys and thus increasing the blood levels of sodium. Aldosterone also has an effect on the levels of water in the body and several other ions (including potassium, bicarbonate and chloride) due to the fact that their regulation is coupled to the regulation of sodium in the body. The control of aldosterone secretion is primarily related to the blood concentrations of sodium (Na^+) and the mean arterial blood pressure (BP) and blood volume. Reduced blood concentrations of sodium and a reduction in blood pressure stimulate the release of aldosterone via the renin-angiotensin-aldosterone system (Figure 33.14).

Glucocorticoids – As far as researchers can tell, there appears to be no cell within the body that does not have receptors for the glucocorticoid hormones. The effect of the glucocorticoid hormones is important in several bodily systems. The main roles of the glucocorticoid hormones appear to be on metabolism and the inflammation and immune systems. Thus, the glucocorticoids are a necessary part of the bodily response to a stressor (such as an injury). The glucocorticoid hormones have several effects, they:

- Influence the metabolism of most body cells
  - Promote glycogen storage in the liver
  - During fasting they stimulate the generation of glucose
  - Increase blood glucose levels
- Involved in providing resistance to stressors
- Potentiate the vasoconstrictor effect of catecholamines
- Decrease the permeability of vascular endothelium
- Promote the repair of damaged tissues by promoting the breakdown of stored protein to create amino acids
- Suppress the immune system
- Suppress inflammatory processes.

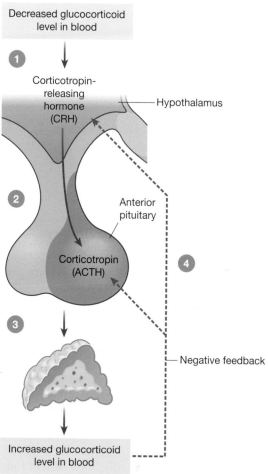

Figure 33.15 **The negative feedback control of cortisol production and secretion.**

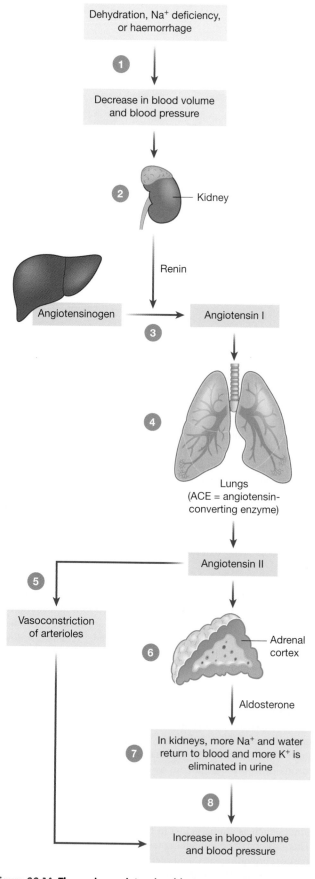

Figure 33.14 **The renin-angiotensin-aldosterone system.**

The glucocorticoid hormones include:

- Cortisol (hydrocortisone)
- Cortisone
- Corticosterone.

Only cortisol is secreted in any significant amounts. Cortisol is normally released in a diurnal pattern, with most being released shortly after the person gets up from sleep and the lowest amount being released just before, and shortly after, sleep commences.

Cortisol release is controlled by the negative feedback loop shown in Figure 33.15. A decreased level of cortisol in the blood leads to the release of corticotropin releasing hormone (CRH) from the hypothalamus. This stimulates the release of adrenocorticotropic hormone (ACTH) from the anterior pituitary gland. ACTH has the effect of increasing the production and secretion of cortisol. Increasing levels of cortisol have a negative feedback effect on both the hypothalamus and the pituitary gland inhibiting further release of both CRH and ACTH. However, this negative feedback system can be overridden by acute physiological stress (for instance trauma, infection or haemorrhage) and mental stress. The increase in sympathetic nervous system activity in response to an acute stress triggers greater CRH release regardless of blood concentrations of cortisol and thus there is a significant increase in subsequent cortisol production.

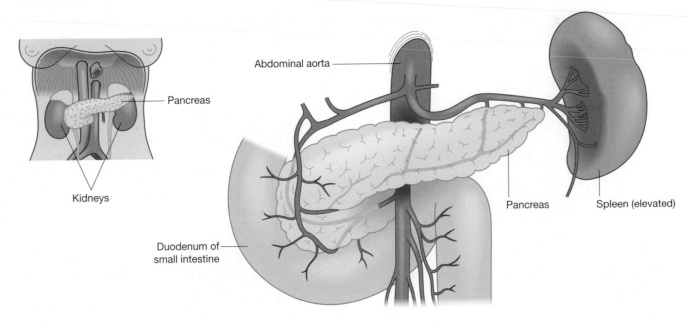

Figure 33.16 The pancreas.

Pancreas

The pancreas (Figure 33.16) is an elongated organ that is found next to the first part of the small intestine. It is composed of two different types of tissues. The majority of the pancreas is made up of exocrine tissue (acini) and their associated ducts. This tissue produces and secretes a fluid rich with digestive enzymes into the small intestine (see Chapter 28). Scattered throughout the exocrine tissue are many small clusters of cells called 'islets of Langerhans' (islets). These islets are the site of the endocrine cells of the pancreas. Each islet has three major cell types, each of which produces a different hormone.

- Alpha cells, which secrete glucagon
- Beta cells, the most abundant of the three cell types and which secrete insulin
- Delta cells, which secrete somatostatin.

The islets are highly vascularised ensuring rapid transit of the hormones into the blood stream. The pancreas is innervated by the parasympathetic and sympathetic nervous systems and it is clear that nervous stimulation influences the secretion of insulin and glucagon.

Insulin

The major action of insulin is well known, in that it reduces the blood glucose levels, and it does this by:

- Facilitating the entry of glucose into muscle, adipose tissue and several other tissues. It is interesting to note that the brain and the liver do not require insulin to facilitate the uptake of glucose
- Insulin stimulates the liver to store glucose in the form of glycogen.

However, insulin is also known to have an effect on protein and mineral metabolism. Furthermore, insulin has an effect on lipid metabolism, as glycogen accumulation in the liver rises to higher levels (5% of the total liver mass), further glycogen synthesis is suppressed. Glucose is then diverted into the production of fatty acids and insulin inhibits the breakdown of fat in adipose tissues

and facilitates the production of triglycerides from glucose for further storage in these tissues. From a whole body perspective insulin has a fat sparing effect in that it promotes the use of glucose rather than fatty acids and stimulates the storage of fat in the adipose tissue.

The main stimulus for insulin synthesis and secretion is a rise in blood glucose levels, but rises in the levels of amino acids and fatty acids in the blood also have the effect of stimulating insulin secretion. Some nervous system stimuli, for example the sight and smell of food, also appear to increase insulin secretion. As noted previously, the pancreas is innervated by the sympathetic and parasympathetic nervous systems and nervous system stimulation clearly influences the secretion of insulin (and glucagon). The half-life of insulin is approximately 5 minutes and it is destroyed in the liver.

The control of insulin production and secretion is via a negative feedback loop (Figure 33.17), therefore as blood glucose levels fall there is a corresponding fall in the production and secretion of insulin. When insulin levels in the blood are reduced glycogen synthesis in the liver also decreases. Enzymes that break down glycogen become active leading to an increase in the levels of glucose in the blood.

Glucagon

Glucagon has an important role in maintaining normal blood glucose levels in that it has the opposite effect to insulin (see Figure 33.17); this role is especially important as the brain and neurons can only use glucose as a fuel. The actions of glucagon are that it:

- Stimulates the breakdown of the glycogen stored in the liver
- Activates gluconeogenesis (the creation of glucose from substrates such as amino acids) in the liver
- Has a minor effect enhancing triglyceride breakdown in adipose tissue – providing fatty acid fuel for most cells and thus conserving glucose for the brain and neurons.

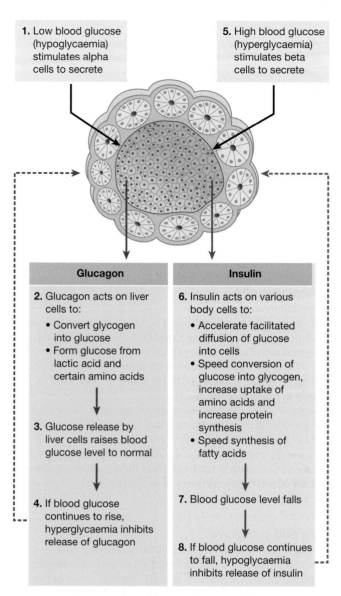

1. Low blood glucose (hypoglycaemia) stimulates alpha cells to secrete

5. High blood glucose (hyperglycaemia) stimulates beta cells to secrete

Glucagon	Insulin
2. Glucagon acts on liver cells to: • Convert glycogen into glucose • Form glucose from lactic acid and certain amino acids	**6.** Insulin acts on various body cells to: • Accelerate facilitated diffusion of glucose into cells • Speed conversion of glucose into glycogen, increase uptake of amino acids and increase protein synthesis • Speed synthesis of fatty acids
3. Glucose release by liver cells raises blood glucose level to normal	
4. If blood glucose continues to rise, hyperglycaemia inhibits release of glucagon	**7.** Blood glucose level falls
	8. If blood glucose continues to fall, hypoglycaemia inhibits release of insulin

Figure 33.17 The negative feedback control of insulin (red arrows) and glucagon (blue arrows) production.

The production and secretion of glucagon is stimulated in response to a reduction in blood glucose concentrations. Like most hormones, glucagon production and secretion appears to be controlled by a negative feedback loop related to rising blood sugar levels. However, it is unknown whether this is a direct effect of the blood glucose levels or a response to rising levels of insulin, as insulin is known to inhibit the release of glucagon. Furthermore, the sympathetic nervous system outflow associated with exercise stimulates the production and release of glucagon the benefit of which is to mobilise glucose stores for muscle use.

Assessing the endocrine system

Assessing the cardiovascular system is often based on a general interview of the patients' perceptions of their own health and symptoms, followed by a targeted, problem focussed, assessment based on an interpretation of the findings of the initial interview.

Therefore in assessing the endocrine system the initial history taking is essential.

The initial history is structured and includes the following steps:

1. Establish a rapport with the patient and his or her family, including preparation of oneself and the environment.
   - Ensure that you are presenting a professional, caring and attentive attitude. Show interest in the patient and what they have to say. There is little more off putting for a patient than an obviously disinterested health care worker. The patient is less likely to fully disclose to you either because they feel you do not care or because they feel inhibited by your attitude.
   - The environment should be comfortable and private with no interruptions. Patients are less likely to disclose personal information if they feel they may be overheard and constant interruptions disrupt the flow of the interview.

2. Gather information on:
   - *The patient's overall health status.* Ask open and general questions at this point, try not to focus too much on one symptom or concern, as this may narrow the discussion, at the same time allow the patient to talk about whatever they feel is important.
   - *The current concern.* Most patients will access health care with a particular concern/set of concerns that has led them to the hospital/clinic. Let the patient use their own words to explore their concerns. This will often be the point where the focus of the interview will be identified.
   - *The symptoms experienced and how they affect the patient.* Following on from the identification of the main concern (and often at the same time), the patient should be questioned on any symptoms they experience, what makes the symptoms worse, what makes them better and when do they occur? Often this will be the point that the history taker will begin to suspect the potential cause(s) of the symptoms and will wish to ask the patient about potential symptoms related to the suspected condition. For instance a patient who is reporting constantly feeling tired and lethargic may be suffering from hypothyroidism. The nurse may then wish to explore this by prompting the patient about their appetite and weight loss/gain, as these are also common symptoms of hypothyroidism. For a list of common clinical features that may aid diagnosis see Table 33.2.
   - *Medical history, emotional health and medication.* Relevant medical history and current medication should be ascertained and recorded to aid the maintenance of previous care. Emotional history is valuable as changes in emotional state can be a symptom of an endocrine disorder and/or can give an indication of how the disorder is affecting the patient's psychological state.
   - *Family history.* Many endocrine disorders have a genetic component and thus family history is a valuable aid in assessing the endocrine system.

3. Systematic enquiry using systems of the body and activities of daily living.
   - Systematically asking the patient about the various bodily systems and the activities of daily living may discover information that the patient did not regard as important or may attribute to other aspects of health (such as ageing).

4. The patient's perception of his or her well-being.
   - It is always important to discover what the patient's perspective is of both their concern/condition and what they hope the

Table 33.2 Common clinical features and the potential endocrine causes.

CLINICAL FEATURE	ASSOCIATED ENDOCRINE DISORDER(S)
Weight gain	Hypothyroidism Cushing's disease
Weight loss	Hyperthyroidism Diabetes mellitus Adrenal insufficiency
Menstrual disturbance	Thyroid disorders
Excessive thirst	Diabetes insipidus Diabetes mellitus
Sweating	Hyperthyroidism
Erectile dysfunction	Diabetes mellitus
Muscle weakness	Cushing's disease Hyperthyroidism

healthcare system can do for them. Only the patient can assess how much a symptom affects their life or which symptoms they feel are more important.

Following the history-taking, a physical examination can be undertaken. Aspects of physical assessment that may give particular indicators of an endocrine disorder are:

- General observations
  - *Demeanour and mental state.* Agitation may be a sign of hyperthyroidism, depression and apathy may be a sign of hypothyroidism
  - *Appearance.* For instance central obesity with thin arms and legs may be a sign of Cushing's disease
  - *Pallor.* Especially with a yellowish tinge, suggests hypopituitarism
  - *Hair distribution.* For instance absent axillary and pubic hair may be a sign of hypopituitarism
  - *Vitiligo.* Not normally a sign of an endocrine disorder but vitiligo is an autoimmune-based condition and it is more likely that the patient will develop an autoimmune-based endocrine disorder
  - *Hirsutism.* A potential sign of Cushing's syndrome.
- Hands
  - Skin crease pigmentation is a potential sign of Addison's disease
  - Tremor may be a sign of hyperthyroidism
  - Large fleshy hands are a potential sign of acromegaly
- Pulse and blood pressure
  - Tachycardia and/or atrial fibrillation may be a sign of hyperthyroidism
  - Hypertension may be a sign of Cushing's disease
  - Hypotension may be a sign of Addison's disease
- Eyes
  - Exophthalmos may be a sign of hyperthyroidism
- Face
  - A 'moon face' may be a sign of Cushing's disease
  - A large elongated face is associated with acromegaly
- Neck
  - A goitre (swollen neck) may be a sign of hyperthyroidism.

Disorders of the Endocrine System

 Link To/Go To

Endo Bible (**http://www.endobible.com/**) is a website of practical advice on endocrine diagnosis and management maintained by a consultant endocrinologist.

Hypopituitarism (Pituitary Insufficiency)

Hypopituitarism is a condition where the pituitary gland does not produce enough hormones for normal functioning (Schneider *et al.* 2007).

Pathophysiology

Hypopituitarism can be caused by disorders of the pituitary gland itself or the reduction of hypothalamic releasing hormones due to a disorder of the hypothalamus, thus reducing the stimuli for pituitary gland activity. The most common cause of hypopituitarism is a tumour of the hypothalamus or pituitary gland or a tumour in the region of the hypothalamus or pituitary gland that is large enough to cause pressure and prevent normal functioning. In the majority of cases these tumours are benign (non-cancerous) and pose no risk of spread to other parts of the body. However, the role of direct damage to the pituitary is increasingly being recognised. Causes of direct damage to the hypothalamus or the pituitary gland include stroke, surgery and radiation therapy. The incidence of pituitary insufficiency increases with age but it can be present in children.

Signs and symptoms

The signs and symptoms of hypopituitarism are related to the reduction of pituitary hormone production and will vary depending on the hormones affected and the speed of onset of the condition. A summary of potential signs and symptoms is given in Table 33.3.

Approximately 50% of patients with pituitary insufficiency will have deficits in 3–5 pituitary hormones (Prabhakar & Shalet 2006) and thus, patients presenting with possible hypopituitarism should be tested for deficits of all the pituitary hormones.

Investigations and diagnosis

The diagnosis of hypopituitarism is based on clinical examination, detailed history-taking, biochemical tests and investigations of the potential cause. Potential biochemical tests are summarised in Table 33.4.

Red Flag

 Insulin tolerance tests are potentially very dangerous and should only be carried out in strictly controlled circumstances. Patients with heart disease, stroke or epilepsy and elderly patients should not undergo an insulin tolerance test.

Table 33.3 Signs and symptoms of hypopituitarism categorised by hormone deficiency.

HORMONE DEFICIENCY	POTENTIAL SIGNS AND SYMPTOMS
Growth hormone	Reduced energy Reduced muscle mass and strength Increased central fat deposition Decreased sweating Reduced bone density In children, a reduction on growth hormone production leads to lack of growth (height), increased body fat and poor bone density
Adrenocorticotropic hormone	Fatigue Weakness Poor appetite Weight loss Nausea and vomiting Abdominal pain Acute circulatory collapse if sudden in onset Loss of pubic and axillary hair in women
Gonadotrophins	**Men:** Erectile dysfunction Reduced muscle mass Reduced energy **Women:** Menstrual changes Breast atrophy **Both:** Loss of libido Flushes Infertility
Thyroid stimulating hormone	Fatigue Apathy Cold intolerance Constipation Weight gain Slow reflexes and cognition
Antidiuretic hormone (Diabetes insipidus)	Polyuria Polydipsia Nocturia
Prolactin	Inability to breast-feed

Table 33.4 Potential biochemical tests and investigations for pituitary hormone insufficiency.

POTENTIAL HORMONE DEFICIENCY	BIOCHEMICAL TESTS
Growth hormone	Insulin tolerance test (growth hormone is secreted in response to the intentionally created hypoglycaemia)
ACTH	Insulin tolerance test or Synacthen test
Gonadotrophins	**Men:** testosterone levels and gonadotrophin levels **Women:** oestradiol levels and gonadotrophin levels
TSH	TSH levels and thyroid hormone levels
ADH	Normally based on 24-hour urine collection, blood sodium levels and urine osmolality. Occasionally, a water deprivation test may be carried out in hospital

Investigation of the potential cause of hypopituitarism is mostly based around the radiographical imaging of the hypothalamus and pituitary regions by magnetic resonance imaging (MRI) in order to detect and assess any potential tumour.

Nursing care and management

The treatment of hypopituitarism is based on treating the cause (where possible) and hormone replacement therapy for decreased hormone levels. Surgical removal of tumours may result in remission if the tumour is pressing on the hypothalamus or pituitary gland but not invading them. Medical or radiation therapy will also be considered to reduce tumour size.

Common to all the endocrine conditions, patients with hypopituitarism share a need for psychological support and information, as will their relatives and significant others (DH 2001a). Patients will require information on the particular disorders that they experience and the signs and symptoms that they can expect the condition to manifest. Providing the patient with a clear understanding will:

- Reduce anxiety as to what the future may hold
- Allow the patient to attribute signs and symptoms to their condition rather than enduring them
- Give the patient control of their health and illness
- Enable the patient to monitor their own condition and report deviations that may be attributed to a worsening state or poor control
- Encourage concordance with treatment regimens.

Nurses must be aware of the signs and symptoms of pituitary hormone insufficiencies in order to educate patients as to what signs and symptoms they should be monitoring for and reporting. It is possible for endocrine disorders to be poorly-controlled but no report is made to healthcare professionals because the patient did not know what aspects of bodily functioning may be related to their condition. Information giving and encouraging patients to be involved with their health care increases the sense of control patients have over their lives, creates a greater sense of well-being and reduces feelings of depression/anxiety and hopelessness.

Nurses must also be aware of the psychological impact of certain signs and symptoms on the patient. Body image may be altered by loss of hair, changes in body fat and the need to take lifelong medication. Depression may be related to loss of the previously healthy person (prior to the onset of the condition), loss of erections or the possibility of infertility. Couples may also require direction to relationship counselling due to changes in sexual relationships due to altered body image, loss of libido or depression.

Patients must be made aware of the need to take lifelong medication and to undergo regular blood tests. The importance of attending clinic appointments and ensuring compliance with medication must be reinforced.

Link To/Go To

Both patients and healthcare professionals may find the information on the Pituitary Foundation website useful and patients should be made aware of the existence of this support group:

http://www.pituitary.org.uk/

Red Flag

All patients with an endocrine disorder should be encouraged to register with the Medic Alert foundation and wear a medic alert talisman:
http://www.medicalert.org.uk/

Health promotion and discharge

Primary Care

Pituitary disorders are relatively rare and it is possible that a GP may only ever see one or two patients with a pituitary in their entire career. However, it is essential that both GPs and practice nurses are aware of the need for a multidisciplinary approach to pituitary disorder care.

Primary care professionals should also be aware of the signs and symptoms of inadequate hormone replacement and the potential side-effects of excess replacement.

Primary care practitioners have a significant role to play in reinforcing the need for treatment compliance and in the ordering and interpretation of blood tests.

Disorders of the Thyroid Gland

Disorders of the thyroid gland are categorised as either hypersecretion of thyroid hormones (excessive thyroid gland activity known as **hyperthyroidism**) or hyposecretion of thyroid hormones (reduced thyroid gland activity known as **hypothyroidism**). Thyroid disorders can be further categorised by the underlying mechanism leading to the change in thyroid hormone secretion:

- Primary – due to a disorder of the thyroid gland itself
- Secondary – alterations in thyroid function due to an increase or decrease in the production of either TRH from the hypothalamus or TSH from the pituitary gland.

This section will review the primary disorders of the thyroid gland.

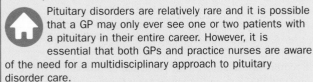

Link To/Go To

Both patients and healthcare professionals will find useful information on the following websites:

British Thyroid Foundation: **http://www.btf-thyroid.org/**
Thyroid UK: **http://www.thyroiduk.org.uk/tuk/index.html**

Hyperthyroidism

Excessive production and release of thyroid hormone.

Pathophysiology

Hyperthyroidism is commonly caused by an autoimmune disorder known as Graves' disease (Weetman 2013). This is a condition where antibodies mimic the effect of thyroid stimulating hormone (normally released from the pituitary gland) leading to excessive production of thyroid hormone. Grave's disease is often diagnosed alongside other autoimmune disorders, such as diabetes. The exact reasons for the development of the antibodies are unknown but the peak incidence appears to be between 20 and 40 years of age and there is strong evidence for a genetic cause (Weeks 2005). Other causes of hyperthyroidism include thyroid cancer, thyroid nodules (usually non-cancerous), viral thyroiditis (inflammation of the thyroid gland), postpartum thyroiditis and patients taking iodine containing drugs (such as amiodarone) (Medeiros-Neto *et al.* 2011).

Signs and symptoms

The signs and symptoms of hyperthyroidism are related to the activity of thyroid hormone and include:

- Nervousness, restlessness
- Tremors
- Fatigue
- Insomnia
- Tachycardia, palpitations (atrial fibrillation is common in the elderly)
- Shortness of breath
- Weight loss despite an increased appetite
- Frequency of passing stools
- Nausea and vomiting
- Muscle weakness, tremors
- Warm, moist flushed skin
- Fine hair
- Staring gaze, exophthalmos (bulging or protrusion of the eyes) – only related to Grave's disease
- Goitre (swelling of the neck – usually due to a swollen thyroid gland)
- Heat intolerance.

Jot This Down

Exophthalmos is often slow and insidious in onset, thus it may not be noted by the patient or their relatives. Photographing the patient on each clinic visit may be a useful method of assessing its development and progression.

Diagnosis and investigations

Diagnosis relies on patient and detailed history-taking, physical examination and diagnostic tests.

Blood will be taken to assess TSH and Free T_4 levels. As the thyroid gland is overproducing thyroid hormone, the negative feedback to the hypothalamus and pituitary gland will lead to a reduction in TSH production. A reduced TSH level in the blood is the most important biochemical result in diagnosing hyperthyroidism. Free T_4 levels may be normal or may be raised.

Isotope thyroid scans are commonly undertaken. The patient is asked to swallow small amounts of a radioactive substance as a capsule or liquid and then a scan is performed to assess how much of the isotope is taken absorbed by the thyroid gland. A high rate of absorption indicates Grave's disease or thyroid nodules, whereas low uptake may be related to inflammation, excess iodine in the diet or thyroid cancer. Potential cancer of the thyroid may require fine-needle aspiration cytology (taking cells from the swollen lump) to assess for the presence of cancerous cells.

What the Experts Say Missed a Tablet?

Everyone forgets to take their tablets from time to time. Don't worry, as it is not dangerous to miss the odd forgotten levothyroxine tablet. If you forget to take a dose, take it as soon as you remember, if this is within 2 or 3 hours of your usual time. If you do not remember until after this time, skip the forgotten dose and take the next dose at the usual time. Do not take two doses together to make up for a missed dose. However, you should try to take levothyroxine regularly each morning for maximum benefit.

http://www.patient.co.uk/health/hypothyroidism-underactive-thyroid

Nursing care and management

Treatment of hyperthyroidism is focussed on decreasing the excessive production of thyroid hormone. There are three main methods of treating hyperthyroidism:

Anti-thyroid drugs – Carbimazole is the most commonly used drug in the UK (Weetman 2013). Anti-thyroid drugs usually have a slow onset of action due to the storage of thyroid hormone, which is released despite the reduction in thyroid hormone production. All anti-thyroid drugs have significant side-effect profiles and patients must be made aware of these. Side-effects include:

- Pruritis
- Rash
- Joint pains
- Diarrhoea
- Altered taste.

Remission after stopping anti-thyroid drugs is very common with about 50–60% of patients relapsing within 3–6 months (Simmons 2010).

Red Flag

Patients taking anti-thyroid drugs should be advised that if they develop fever, chills and a sore throat to seek immediate medical assistance as they require a full blood count to assess for the potential development of agranulocytosis (suppression of white blood cell production).

Radioactive iodine – This treatment relies on the fact that the most active cells in the thyroid gland will take up the most iodine and thus be destroyed. In the first few weeks after treatment, there is often a need to take anti-thyroid drugs as there may be a sudden release of thyroid hormones and patients must be monitored for thyrotoxic crisis (thyroid storm). Following radioactive iodine treatment the patient may become hypothyroid as

there is little control over the amount of thyroid gland that is destroyed. Radioactive iodine is contraindicated in pregnancy.

Surgical removal of part, or all, of the thyroid gland – Thyroidectomy or partial thyroidectomy is the least used of the treatment options as it carries risks of damage to the parathyroid glands and the vocal cords and as the thyroid gland is very vascular there is also a risk of a major haemorrhage.

The Evidence

- Patients with severe symptoms and signs of hyperthyroidism (e.g. fever, agitation, heart failure, confusion or coma) should be admitted to hospital
- Refer all other patients for specialist management by an endocrinologist
- Pregnant women with hyperthyroidism require urgent referral to specialist care, as there is an increased risk of miscarriage

Link To/Go To

NICE Clinical Knowledge Summary (NICE CKS):

http://cks.nice.org.uk/hyperthyroidism#!topicsummary

Symptom relief may be required to treat certain symptoms or consequences of hyperthyroidism:

- Atrial fibrillation, tachycardia and heart failure should all be treated with appropriate medication
- Nutritional deficits may be present due to the excessive metabolism in hyperthyroidism. Frequent snacks should be encouraged to prevent weigh loss. High calorie, high protein diet should be encouraged until thyroid function is normalised and vitamin supplements (particularly A, thiamine, B_6 and C) should be advocated (Weeks 2005)
- Anxiety can be managed with the use of beta-blocking drugs, which may also be of use in the treatment of tremors. Provision of a quiet, calm environment will also be of value.

Exophthalmos will require monitoring by an ophthalmologist and may require treatment with steroids, radiotherapy or surgery. Patients may also benefit from:

- Raising the head of their bed – e.g. by using extra pillows – which could help reduce some of the puffiness around the eyes
- Stopping smoking because smoking can significantly increase the risk of the thyroid condition affecting the eyes
- Wearing sunglasses if they have photophobia (sensitivity to light)
- Using eye drops to help relieve soreness and to moisten their eyes if they have dry eyes
- Wearing a patch over one eye if they have double vision
- Taking selenium supplements, which may help people with mild thyroid eye disease that has recently started (selenium is a mineral found in Brazil nuts, meat and fish).

Further nursing care includes:

- Encouraging fluid intake in patients who are perspiring excessively
- Provision of fan therapy for comfort
- Light day-time clothes and bed clothes
- Providing a quiet comfortable environment to encourage rest and sleep

- Regular assessment of vital signs
- Regular assessment of mental state.

Nurses should also be aware of, and monitor for, the potential for thyrotoxic crisis (thyroid storm), as this is a medical emergency. Thyroid storm is due to the effect of high blood levels of thyroid hormone in association with increased sympathetic nervous system activity. There are several known causes of thyroid storm, including emotional or physical trauma and stress (Noble 2006). Patients with thyroid storm may present with the following signs/symptoms:

- Very high temperature (over 40°C)
- Very high heart rate (atrial fibrillation is common)
- Will be very agitated and confused
- Vomiting and diarrhoea

Management of this condition will require:

- Nursing in a critical care environment
- Beta-blockade for tachycardia
- Continuous heart monitoring
- Intravenous fluids for dehydration with strict fluid balance monitoring
- Active cooling therapies
- Control of thyroid hormone levels.

Health promotion and discharge

Primary Care

The role of primary care in the management of patients with hyperthyroidism involves the regular monitoring of thyroid hormone levels, education and advice regarding the treatment and control of hyperthyroidism.

Primary care providers will also need to monitor other bodily changes that can occur with hyperthyroidism such as high cholesterol levels, high blood glucose levels and electrolyte disturbances.

Hypothyroidism

Insufficient production and release of thyroid hormone for bodily functioning.

Pathophysiology

There are many causes of hypothyroidism including:

- Treatment for hyperthyroidism
- Radiation therapy of the neck
- Lack of iodine in the diet
- Viral infection of the thyroid gland
- Autoimmune disease.

The most common cause of hypothyroidism in the UK is autoimmune destruction of the thyroid gland, known as Hashimoto's thyroiditis (Biondi & Cooper 2008).

Jot This Down

An underactive thyroid can be caused by a problem with the immune system, the body's natural defence system, which can attack the body's own cells, including the thyroid.

Signs and symptoms

The signs and symptoms of hypothyroidism include:

- Confusion, memory loss, depression
- Lethargy
- Bradycardia, enlarged heart (cardiomegaly), pericardial effusions
- Constipation
- Weight gain
- Muscle cramps, myalgia (generalised muscle aches), stiffness
- Dry cool skin
- Brittle nails
- Coarse hair, hair loss
- Oedema of hands and eyelids
- Cold intolerance
- Vacant expression
- Hoarse voice.

The Evidence

Symptoms can develop slowly over several years, and are often nonspecific. The following symptoms have the greatest diagnostic value:

- Current or increased constipation
- Current or increasingly hoarse voice
- Current deep voice
- Feeling colder
- Puffy eyes
- Weaker muscles.

 Link To/Go To

NICE Clinical Knowledge Summary (NICE CKS):
http://cks.nice.org.uk/hypothyroidism#!topicsummary

Investigations and diagnosis

Diagnosis relies on patient and detailed history-taking, physical examination and diagnostic tests.

Blood will be taken to assess TSH and free T_4 levels. As the thyroid gland is no longer producing thyroid hormone, the negative feedback to the hypothalamus and pituitary gland will be absent and TSH levels will be increased. Free T_4 levels will be normal or reduced.

Red Flag

 TSH levels are elevated in patients with untreated primary adrenal insufficiency. Prescribing thyroxine in this situation may precipitate an adrenal crisis.

Nursing care and management

The treatment for hypothyroidism is replacement of the thyroid hormone with levothyroxine. Levothyroxine should be taken at the same time each day and about an hour before breakfast if possible (Weetman 2013). Patients should be warned that symptoms will not disappear immediately and weight loss will only occur when treatment is combined with a healthy dietary intake and exercise.

Patients must be advised that it may take months to find the correct dose of levothyroxine and frequent blood tests will be required in the first year. Over replacement of thyroid hormones is a common cause of hyperthyroidism and patients should be made aware of the possible symptoms of hyperthyroidism but warned not to titrate their own levothyroxine dose.

Red Flag

Elderly patients and those with heart disease will require a lower starting dose of levothyroxine (Papaleontiou & Haymart 2012).

Once the correct dose for the particular patient has been found patients will require yearly blood tests to ensure that their needs have not changed.

Monitoring of concordance with replacement therapy and the use of strategies to encourage and maintain concordance are essential as many patients are reluctant to take long-term thyroxine therapy (Crilly 2004). Patients should be informed of the possible side-effects of thyroid replacement therapy, including temporary hair loss (Roberts & Ladenson 2004), as this will affect concordance with treatment. Patients should be given information regarding the need for adherence to the replacement therapy and what to do in the event of prolonged gastrointestinal disturbance that prevents the taking of the daily levothyroxine dose. Acute illness or trauma may precipitate myxoedemic coma and patients must be made aware of the need to seek medical help.

Red Flag

Levothyroxine is known to interact with multivitamin preparations and should be taken 4 hours apart.
Antacids and proton pump inhibitors are known to reduce the absorption of levothyroxine and should be taken several hours apart.
Levothyroxine enhances the anticoagulant effect of warfarin.

Myxoedemic coma or crisis is an acute, life-threatening, emergency that can be brought on by acute events such as stroke, myocardial infarction, infection or trauma or by a lack of concordance with replacement therapy (Hampton 2013). Signs and symptoms include:

- Hypothermia (temperature less than 35.5°C)
- Bradycardia (slow heart rate)
- Bradypnoea (slow respiratory rate) and hypoventilation (shallow breathing) leading to hypoxia
- Potentially hypotension
- Deterioration in mental state
- Psychosis
- Swollen, puffy, face with oedema around the eyes
- Low sodium levels in the blood.

Treatment requires admission to a critical care area and:

- Intravenous thyroid hormone replacement
- Sodium replacement and fluid restriction
- Ambient warming and warm blankets (aggressive rewarming should be avoided)
- Vital signs monitoring and heart monitor
- Potentially respiratory support by intubation and ventilation.

Medicines Management Drugs: Drug Interactions

Drugs preventing absorption of levothyroxine:
- Calcium salts – calcium containing products
- Ferrous sulphate – iron containing products
- Aluminium hydroxide – antacids
- Cholestyramine – bile acid sequestrants

Health promotion and discharge

What the Experts Say

Hypothyroidism affects one in 50 British women. So why did Sarah O'Neil's debilitating condition take more than 6 years to diagnose? Use the link below to hear the story:

http://www.independent.co.uk/life-style/health-and -families/health-news/hypothyroidism-dont-suffer-in -silence-414738.html (accessed 11 September 2013)

Primary Care

Hypothyroidism is the most common endocrine disorder in primary care but it is often underdiagnosed as the symptoms are vague and diverse, and in the elderly many signs and symptoms may be attributed to age. Primary care practitioners should be alert for the possibility of hypothyroidism in patients with more than one potential symptom.

Most patients with hypothyroidism are managed in primary care and education and information giving are vital for ensuring concordance with treatment. Elderly patients may require regular community nursing follow-up to assess pill counts or to review dosset boxes and monitor concordance.

Patients should be referred to specialist care if they:
- are younger than 16
- are pregnant or trying to get pregnant (hypothyroidism in the mother can have significant effects on the fetus)
- have just given birth
- have another health condition, such as heart disease
- are taking amiodarone or lithium medication (both these drugs interfere with blood tests for TSH.

Disorders of the Parathyroid Glands

Disorders of the parathyroid glands are rare and include **hyperparathyroidism** and **hyperparathyroidism**.

Hyperparathyroidism
Excessive production of parathyroid hormone.

Pathophysiology
Hyperparathyroidism is usually caused by a benign tumour of the parathyroid gland.

Signs and symptoms

Hyperparathyroidism is often present without any symptoms, if symptoms do occur they are normally very mild and include:

- Depression
- Fatigue
- Increased thirst
- Polyuria
- Nausea
- Muscle weakness
- Constipation
- Abdominal pain
- Loss of concentration
- Mild confusion.

Investigations and diagnosis

Hyperparathyroidism is diagnosed by blood tests showing:

- High levels of parathyroid hormone
- High levels of blood calcium
- Low levels of blood phosphorus.

Treatment and management

Often, hyperparathyroidism does not require treatment but if required the current treatment is surgical removal of the overactive parathyroid gland(s) (Potts 2005).

Patients should be advised to avoid a high calcium diet (but not avoid calcium altogether) and to drink plenty of fluids to prevent dehydration.

Hypoparathyroidism

Reduced production of parathyroid hormone.

Pathophysiology

Causes of hypoparathyroidism include:

- Damage of the parathyroid glands during neck surgery
- Radiotherapy to the neck
- Autoimmune destruction of the parathyroid glands.

Signs and symptoms

The symptoms of hypoparathyroidism are partially dependent on the speed at which the disorder develops (Marx 2000):

- Sudden onset (for instance due to damage during surgery)
  - Tingling sensation around the mouth or in the hands or feet
  - Jerking, twitching or muscle spasms
  - Muscle cramps
  - Lethargy
  - Irritability
- Slow onset (for instance due to autoimmune destruction of the glands)
  - Eye problems (especially cataracts)
  - Dry, thick, skin
  - Coarse hair that may fall out
  - Brittle finger nails with horizontal ridges.

Diagnosis and investigations

Hypoparathyroidism is diagnosed by blood tests showing:

- Low blood calcium levels
- High blood phosphorus levels
- Low blood parathyroid hormone levels.

A urine sample is also tested for high levels of calcium.

Nursing care and management

Treatment is with oral calcium and vitamin D supplements. Patients should also be advised to eat a healthy diet including:

- High calcium
  - Milk, cheese and other dairy foods
  - Green leafy vegetables, such as broccoli, cabbage and okra, but not spinach
  - Soya beans
  - Tofu
  - Soya drinks with added calcium
  - Nuts
  - Bread and anything made with fortified flour
  - Fish where you eat the bones, such as sardines and pilchards
- Low phosphorous, phosphorous is found in:
  - Red meat
  - Dairy foods
  - Fish
  - Poultry
  - Bread
  - Rice
  - Oats.

Patients should be advised that if they develop muscle spasms to seek medical advice immediately as they may require intravenous calcium.

 Link To/Go To

Patients can be advised to go to Hypoparathyroidism UK: http://hpth.org.uk/home.php

Disorders of the Adrenal Glands

Disorders of the adrenal glands are classified as either **hypersecretion** or **hyposecretion** disorders. Disorders of the adrenal glands can be further categorised by the underlying mechanism leading to the change in hormone secretion:

- Primary – due to a disorder of the adrenal glands themselves.
- Secondary – alterations in adrenal gland function due to an increase or decrease in the production of either CRH from the hypothalamus or ACTH from the pituitary gland.

The effects on the body of primary or secondary disorders of the adrenal glands are different and these differences will be noted within this section.

Hypersecretion Disorders of the Adrenal Glands

Hypersecretion disorders of the adrenal glands are:

- Pheochromocytoma
- Conn's syndrome
- Cushing's syndrome
- Cushing's disease.

Both pheochromocytoma and Conn's syndrome are rare in the general setting and will not be discussed in this section. Both can be related to drug resistant hypertension and are potential diagnoses in the hypertension clinic.

Cushing's disease is a subset of the disorder known as Cushing's syndrome and the symptoms are almost the same; they are otherwise known as hypercortisolism. This section will review Cushing's syndrome, noting where Cushing's disease differs in pathophysiology.

Pathophysiology

The pathophysiology of Cushing's syndrome is generally classified as endogenous (caused by factors within the body) or exogenous (caused by factors outside the body).

- Endogenous causes of hypercortisolism are either primary or secondary (Prague *et al.* 2013):
  - *Primary hypercortisolism* is caused by a tumour of the adrenal gland, which leads to the hypersecretion of cortisol.
  - *Secondary hypercortisolism* is caused by a tumour of the pituitary gland leading to hypersecretion of ACTH and the subsequent production of high levels of cortisol from the adrenal glands. It is known as Cushing's disease. Cushing's disease is the leading cause of secondary hypercortisolism.
- Exogenous hypercortisolism is the most common cause of Cushing's syndrome and is caused by the administration of high doses of corticosteroids for conditions such as arthritis, asthma and other inflammatory conditions.

Signs and symptoms

The signs and symptoms of all the causes of hypercortisolism (Cushing's syndrome) are the same.

Common symptoms are:

- Weight gain
- High blood pressure
- Poor short-term memory
- Irritability
- Excess hair growth (women)
- Red, ruddy face
- Extra fat deposition at the neck and shoulders (buffalo hump)
- Round face (otherwise referred to as a 'moon face')
- Fatigue
- Poor concentration
- Menstrual irregularity
- Slow wound healing
- Depression and rapid mood swings.

Less common symptoms include:

- Insomnia
- Recurrent infections (especially fungal infections such as thrush)
- Thin skin and stretch marks (often showing as purple striations)
- Easily bruising skin
- Weak bones
- Acne
- Hair loss (women)
- Hip and shoulder weakness
- Swelling of feet/legs due to oedema
- Diabetes mellitus.

Diagnosis and investigations

The diagnosis of hypercortisolism is based on a detailed history-taking, a physical examination and a number of diagnostic investigations.

History-taking will focus on the development of symptoms and must include a full drug history to review the patient for the use of exogenous steroids. Signs and symptoms of hypercortisolism

without a history of steroid use, will lead on to the use of a number of potential investigations.

- Late night salivary cortisol: a sample of saliva is taken late at night (often around midnight) and tested for cortisol levels. As cortisol production is diurnal, cortisol levels at midnight should be very low. If they are high, then this suggests Cushing's syndrome.
- 24-hour urine collection that is then tested for cortisol levels
- Dexamethasone suppression test. The patient is administered a synthetic version of cortisol and the cortisol levels in the blood are measured after a suitable time period. The administration of dexamethasone should suppress the production of cortisol by the body. If cortisol levels do not fall then it is likely the patient is suffering from Cushing's syndrome.

If any one of these tests is negative, then Cushing's syndrome is unlikely. Positive results of a test often lead to the repeat of that test and the administration of at least one more of the other tests. Repeated positive results usually confirms a diagnosis of Cushing's syndrome and the patient will require a blood test for ACTH levels to assess for a pituitary cause (Cushing's disease). Further investigations will include scanning the pituitary and adrenal glands for tumours.

 Link To/Go To

The American Association of Endocrine Surgeons provides a flow diagram showing the process of diagnostic testing for Cushing's syndrome:

http://endocrinediseases.org/adrenal/cushings_diagnosis.shtml

Treatment and management

Treatment of hypercortisolism is dependent on the initial cause (Munir & Newell-Price 2009):

Reducing steroid use – For those patients who are taking high doses of steroids the treatment is to gradually reduce the steroid dose to lowest possible whilst still maintaining control of the disease the steroids were prescribed for. This must be done in conjunction with medical staff as the dose reduction must be tailored to the individual.

Red Flag

 Patients who have been taking steroids for more than a few days must never stop their steroids suddenly, as this may precipitate a hypoadrenal crisis. Patients who take steroids for more than 3 weeks must be issued with, and carry, a steroid treatment card.

Cortisol inhibiting medications – Often used for a short period before a more definitive treatment, cortisol inhibiting medications block the effects of cortisol in the body.

Radiotherapy and/or surgery – Definitive treatment of endogenous hypercortisolism is based on the removal of the affected gland or radiotherapy of the pituitary gland if surgery is not possible. Surgery to remove the pituitary gland will leave the patient with hypopituitarism which will require hormone replacement therapy. If the tumour is affecting the adrenal gland then often only one of the adrenal glands will need to be removed but removal of both may be necessary.

Nursing care and management

- Decrease the risk of injury by removing slip and trip hazards and helping unstable patients to mobilise
- Refer to the dietician for advice on diet to promote muscle mass and bone density
- Minimise the risk of infection. Advise the patient to avoid contact with people suffering from infectious diseases. Have a high suspicion for infection as the symptoms are often masked
- Promote moderate activity to prevent excessive muscle wasting
- Provide a quiet comfortable environment to promote sleep
- Maintain good skin care, avoid adhesive tapes, which may tear skin, monitor vulnerable areas of skin, such as the shins, for damage
- Explain to the patient and their family the reasons for their mood swings
- Provide information and support for issues, such as changes in body image
- Ensure patients who are reducing steroid doses understand the need to follow the reduction plan and not stop the steroids suddenly
- Ensure patients taking steroids have been given, and carry, the steroid treatment card.

The Evidence

Steroids that are targeted to particular part of the body they are intended for (such as inhaled steroids and steroid creams) are generally safe and have a much lower risk of side-effects.

Patients taking steroids should monitor for the potential signs of Cushing's syndrome but should always seek medical advice and not stop the medication if they suspect they have symptoms.

Patients taking steroids who have never had chickenpox should avoid anyone suffering from chicken pox or shingles. **http://www.mhra.gov.uk/home/groups/pl-p/documents/ websiteresources/con2032081.pdf**

Primary Care

Primary care practitioners have a vital role to play in the prevention of, and monitoring for, Cushing's syndrome.

Cushing's syndrome is often missed as a diagnosis, as it is slow in onset with a nonspecific set of symptoms that are easily confused with other conditions such as obesity and hypertension. The average time from the first symptom to diagnosis is 6 years (Prague et al. 2013). As the commonest cause of Cushing's syndrome is exogenous steroids, then primary care staff should be alert for the syndrome in any patient taking steroids.

Courses of steroid treatment may be prescribed in the hospital setting but are often continued in the community and primary care health professionals should be aware of the need to titrate steroid doses to the lowest effective dose.

Prolonged use of steroids can predispose patients to diabetes mellitus and thus patients should have a blood sugar taken once a year as urine dipsticks are not sufficiently accurate in non-diabetic patients (**http://bestbets.org/bets/ bet.php?id=311**).

Hyposecretion Disorders of the Adrenal Glands

Otherwise known as adrenal insufficiency.

Pathophysiology

Adrenal insufficiency (the reduced production and release of corticosteroids from the adrenal glands) is divided into two types (Arlt & Allolio 2003):

- *Primary adrenal insufficiency* (Addison's disease) due to a disorder of the adrenal glands. The leading cause of Addison's disease in the Western world is autoimmune adrenalitis, leading to destruction of the glands; other causes include tuberculosis, and fungal infection in immunosuppressed patients (such as HIV AIDS or therapeutic suppression of the immune system)
- *Secondary adrenal insufficiency*. This is most commonly due to the sudden cessation of steroid therapy; however disorders affecting the hypothalamus or the pituitary gland can also be a cause of secondary adrenal insufficiency.

In primary adrenal insufficiency, the adrenal glands no longer function and thus the production of adrenaline, glucocorticoids and mineralocorticoids is stopped.

In secondary adrenal insufficiency, either secretion of CRH from the hypothalamus or secretion of ACTH from the pituitary gland ceases. Either of these situations leads to a lack of ACTH production and thus, stimulation for the production and secretion of glucocorticoids by the adrenal glands is removed. However, as mineralocorticoid and adrenaline production is stimulated by factors other than ACTH, their production is preserved.

Patients who have been taking high dose steroid therapy are at risk of developing temporary adrenal gland atrophy. The steroid treatment leads to negative feedback to the hypothalamus and the pituitary gland, thus reducing stimulation for adrenal gland glucocorticoid production. The adrenal gland atrophies and sudden cessation of the steroid therapy leads to insufficient glucocorticoid levels in the blood as the adrenal glands require a gradual period of recovery. The patient can present with the signs and symptoms of adrenal insufficiency and even an acute adrenal crisis.

Signs and symptoms

The signs and symptoms of all forms of adrenal insufficiency are:

- Fatigue, lack of stamina, loss of energy
- Reduced muscle strength
- Increased irritability
- Nausea
- Weight loss
- Muscle and joint pain
- Abdominal pain
- Low blood pressure
- Women may report a reduction in or loss of libido due to the lack of adrenal sex hormones.

Due to loss of aldosterone production and high levels of ACTH in primary adrenal insufficiency these patients may also present with:

- Dehydration
- Hypovolaemia
- Postural hypotension
- Low levels of blood sodium
- High levels of blood potassium

- Hyper pigmentation of the skin – often a darkening in the skin creases (such as the palms, knuckles, inner elbow) or the waist (where clothes rub) but may be an all over sun tan.
- Vitiligo (pale patches of skin).

The loss of adrenaline and noradrenaline production from the adrenal medulla in primary adrenal insufficiency, does not create any symptoms as endocrine production of adrenaline and noradrenaline is complementary to the nervous system production of these chemicals.

Investigations and diagnosis

The signs and symptoms of Addison's disease are vague and may be slow and insidious in onset and patients may be showing signs and symptoms for up to a year before diagnosis. Occasionally, an acute adrenal crisis may be precipitated by trauma or infection and the patient will present with acute symptoms of severe hypotension, dehydration, hypovolaemic shock, acute abdominal pain and vomiting.

The definitive test for Addison's disease is a synacthen (artificial ACTH) test. Serum cortisol is measured before and after the administration of intramuscular synacthen. If the adrenal glands are working, there will be a rise in blood cortisol levels in response to the synacthen.

If secondary adrenal insufficiency is suspected, then blood ACTH and renin levels will be assessed. Both of these will be high in Addison's disease but in secondary insufficiency ACTH will be low and renin levels will be normal.

If tuberculosis or other infection is suspected as the cause of Addison's disease then CT or MRI scans will be used to image the adrenal glands.

Nursing care and management

Treatment of adrenal insufficiency is normally begun by an endocrinologist but continued in primary care with routine follow-up in the outpatient's clinic.

Treatment for Addison's disease is based on the replacement of glucocorticoid and mineralocorticoid hormones; androgen replacement is not usually prescribed in the UK. Replacement therapy in secondary adrenal insufficiency is only required for glucocorticoid hormones.

The Evidence

Replacement of the glucocorticoid hormones is based on the patient's body weight and varies between 15 mg and 30 mg of hydrocortisone taken orally in divided doses.

Doses are split to try and mimic normal cycles of glucocorticoid release but there is still debate as to which regime is best.

Patients working shifts (especially nights) should have a regime tailored to their daily routine not based on the clock. For instance the first dose is normally taken in the morning but patients on night shift should take their first dose when they get up after sleep.

Glucocorticoid replacement in children is difficult and requires frequent adjustment as they grow.

Mineralocorticoid replacement is between 150 μg(mcg) and 300 μg(mcg) of fludrocortisone once a day. Children's doses of fludrocortisone are much higher than the equivalent adult dose and children may need an additional salt supplement.

In hot weather, some endocrinologists recommend the mineralocorticoid dose is increased to compensate for the increase in sweating.

Link To/Go To

NICE Clinical Knowledge Summary (NICE CKS):
http://cks.nice.org.uk/addisons-disease#!scenariorecommendation

Replacement therapy is titrated by patient symptoms as there is no definitive test to assess correct replacement levels. Therefore, patients will need to be reviewed for the signs and symptoms of Cushing's disease (in the case of over replacement) and the signs and symptoms of Addison's disease (in the case of under replacement).

Alteration of the standard replacement regime must only be carried out by an endocrinologist but patients must be made aware of the need for glucocorticoid dose adjustment in certain circumstances (known as the 'sick day rules'):

- If the patient has a fever of 37.5°C, or higher, then the normal replacement dose should be doubled
- If the patient is taking antibiotics for an infection hydrocortisone doses should be doubled until the course of antibiotics is finished
- After vomiting the patient should take 20 mg hydrocortisone and an oral rehydration solution
- If the patient is injured they should take 20 mg hydrocortisone
- If vomiting persists the patient should be administered an emergency hydrocortisone injection and medical advice sought
- Advice regarding alterations of hydrocortisone doses in preparation for physical exercise vary and should be discussed with the endocrinologist.

Red Flag

 Patients should be educated as to the signs and symptoms of adrenal crisis and both they and family members must be taught how to administer emergency hydrocortisone injections.

The Addison's Disease Self Help Group has clear instructions for patients on how to administer emergency injections on their website:
http://www.addisons.org.uk/info/emergency/page3.html

Patients undergoing surgical or dental treatment may need to take extra hydrocortisone to cover the treatment period. Reports have made it clear that hospital doctors and nurses do not understand the need for hydrocortisone in Addison's disease leading to avoidable deaths (Wass & Arlt 2012).

Link To/Go To

For further guidance refer to the printable guide at:
http://www.addisons.org.uk/comms/publications/surgicalguidelines-colour.pdf (accessed 11 September 2013).

Patients with any form of adrenal insufficiency will require education and counselling on the need to take regular medication and to monitor for the signs of poor control.

Link To/Go To

Patients should be referred to the Addison's disease self-help group website, where there is a variety of resources for patients.

http://www.addisons.org.uk/

Link To/Go To

A full colour guide for nurses is available at:

http://www.addisons.org.uk/comms/publications/AD095A -nursesleaflet.pdf

Health promotion and discharge (if relevant)

Primary Care

The role of the primary care practitioner in the diagnosis and management of adrenal insufficiency is of great importance. Undiagnosed Addison's disease is universally fatal and deterioration can be rapid.

Primary care practitioners should have a suspicion of Addison's disease if the patient presents with being constantly fatigued, losing weight without dieting, has postural hypotension, unusual skin pigmentation and low blood sodium levels.

Patient reports have frequently highlighted the reluctance of primary care practitioners to prescribe more than the absolute minimum amount of oral hydrocortisone or an emergency injection kit leaving the patient with no ability to self-manage their dose when required or to deal with intermittent supply problems. Patients must be prescribed an extra month's supply of hydrocortisone as a 'back-up' and an emergency injection kit for the first line treatment of potential crisis.

Patients with adrenal insufficiency should be strongly advised to wear a medic alert talisman and carry a steroid card as emergency treatment in the event of a traumatic event must include intravenous steroids or the situation may become rapidly fatal.

Diabetes Mellitus

Diabetes mellitus is a disorder of the endocrine system characterised by high blood glucose levels.

Link To/Go To

The NICE diabetes pathway is a useful link to many of the current recommendations in diabetes care:

http://pathways.nice.org.uk/pathways/diabetes

Pathophysiology

There are two types of diabetes:

Type 1 diabetes – Type 1 diabetes develops most commonly in childhood or early adulthood and comprises about 15% of the total incidence of diabetes in the UK; however the rate of type 1 diabetes is increasing, particularly in children less than 5 years of age (DH 2001b). Type 1 diabetes is normally caused by autoimmune destruction of the beta cells of the pancreas and is therefore associated with a severe reduction in, or complete loss of, insulin production (Daneman 2006).

Type 2 diabetes – Type 2 diabetes is the most common form of diabetes and is generally considered to develop in patients over the age of 40, however the rates of juvenile onset type 2 diabetes appears to be rising (DH 2001b). Type 2 diabetes is normally characterised by the development of resistance to the effects of insulin in the tissues (especially body fat and skeletal muscles) and the continued production and release of glucose by the liver. These tissues are unable to respond effectively to insulin and absorb glucose from the blood. This leads to an increasing blood glucose level. There is an associated reduction in the ability of the beta cells to increase the production of insulin in response to this increased insulin resistance in the body (Stumvoll *et al.* 2005). The resulting high blood levels of glucose leads to toxic damage of the beta cells further reducing the production of insulin. Insulin production is rarely completely stopped in type 2 diabetes. Risk factors for type 2 diabetes include being overweight, lack of exercise, genetic inheritance and increasing age. Genetic predisposition to type 2 diabetes appears to be especially strong in patients from south Asian or Afro-Caribbean backgrounds.

Signs and symptoms

The signs and symptoms of diabetes are common to both forms of diabetes and are mostly related to the high blood glucose levels and include:

- Passing urine more often than usual, especially at night
- Increased thirst
- Extreme tiredness
- Unexplained weight loss (usually only in type 1 diabetes)
- Genital itching or regular episodes of thrush
- Slow healing of cuts and wounds
- Blurred vision
- Abdominal pain
- Increased blood glucose
- Glucose in the urine
- Ketones in the urine.

In both forms of diabetes, the increased blood glucose leads to excretion of glucose into the urine. The glucose has an osmotic effect drawing water into the renal tubules and increasing urine production. The increased excretion of urine in the urine leads to water depletion in the body and the increased thirst.

In type one diabetes, and occasionally in advanced type 2 diabetes, the inability of the cells to utilise glucose leads to the use of fats and amino acids as the primary fuel source in the cells leading to weight loss and the production of ketones as a by-product. Ketones are strong acids which are passed into the urine. As the ketones are negatively charged there is usually a simultaneous excretion of positively charged sodium and potassium ions leading to electrolyte imbalance and abdominal pain.

Diagnosis and investigations

The rapid onset of type 1 diabetes means that patients rarely remain undiagnosed for long. Many patients will present to their GP due to their symptoms, however in some cases, the onset is so rapid or is precipitated by an acute illness that the patient develops diabetic ketoacidosis (DKA) and is admitted to hospital as an emergency.

Type 2 diabetes is more insidious in onset and many patients will remain unaware of the fact they have diabetes for years before they are diagnosed (DH 2001), by which point they may have developed complications.

The diagnosis of type 1 diabetes is based on the presence of the classic symptoms of high blood glucose on finger prick test, weight loss, thirst and increased urine output. Formal diagnosis can then be confirmed by one laboratory blood glucose measurement.

Type 2 diabetes is often diagnosed after opportunistic screening or as a chance finding while being treated for another condition. Current guidance is focussed on identifying people at risk of developing type 2 diabetes and encouraging those patients to have a risk assessment and risk identification (NICE 2012).

The Evidence

NICE recommend the following strategy:

1. Identify those at risk and either administer a validated risk assessment tool or encourage those potentially at risk to self-administer a risk assessment tool such as the one found on the Diabetes UK website: **https://www.diabetes.org.uk/Riskscore/**
2. Those found to have high risk scores should be offered formal blood tests, such as HbA_{1c}, fasting blood glucose or glucose tolerance test
3. Those found to be at risk but who have not developed diabetes should be offered guidance on managing risk, such as healthy eating, losing weight and exercise.

   http://publications.nice.org.uk/preventing-type-2-diabetes-risk-identification-and-interventions-for-individuals-at-high-risk-ph38/recommendations#recommendation-3-risk-identification-stage-1

Nursing care and management

The treatment of type 1 diabetes is based on the replacement of insulin by the subcutaneous injection of insulin. There are several forms of insulin but they are all classified by:

- How soon it starts working (onset)
- When it works the hardest (peak time)
- How long it lasts in the body (duration).

The decision as to which insulin to choose is based on an individual's lifestyle, the physician's preference and experience and the person's blood sugar levels. Newly diagnosed patients will require education regarding self-injection and insulin doses. This should be reviewed and skills reassessed with the patient regularly. Patients should be advised regarding the storage of insulin and the rotation of injection sites.

Newly diagnosed type 1 diabetics should be offered a structured programme of education delivered by a qualified health professional and opportunity for education and information should be offered on a regular basis (NICE 2005).

Self-monitoring of blood glucose levels is essential using capillary blood glucose testing in the home environment. Education about testing should be offered at diagnosis and skills reassessed regularly.

Dietary advice for all type 1 diabetic patients should include:

- Discussion of the hyperglycaemic effects of different foods and ensuring adequate insulin to cover it.
- Types of, timing of and amount of snacks taken between meals and at bedtime
- Healthy eating to reduce arterial risk
- If the person wants it, information on:
  - Effects of alcohol-containing drinks on blood glucose and calorie intake
  - Use of high-calorie and high-sugar 'treats'
  - Use of foods with a high glycaemic index.

Patients with type 1 diabetes will also require education on the recognition and management of hypoglycaemia (often called 'hypos').

Red Flag

Hypoglycaemia is a potentially life-threatening condition characterised by a low blood sugar. The patient will present with:

- Hunger
- Nervousness and shakiness
- Perspiration
- Dizziness or light-headedness
- Sleepiness
- Confusion
- Difficulty speaking
- Feelings anxiety or weakness.

If possible, the patient should be encouraged to eat glucose (in the form of jam, chocolate, etc.) or glucose paste (such as glucogel) rubbed into the gums. The glucose will be short-acting and must be followed up with a longer-acting carbohydrate (such as brown bread) if the patient is able to eat safely. Semi-conscious and unconscious patients will require the administration of glucagon or intravenous glucose.

Treatment of type 2 diabetes will depend on the severity of the condition. Treatment will always include dietary adjustments (healthy diet with reduced fat and sugar) and lifestyle changes (such as exercising and losing weight if required) and in some patients with type 2 diabetes this will be enough to maintain normal blood glucose levels. Dietary advice for patients with type 2 diabetes includes:

- Include high-fibre, low-glycaemic-index sources of carbohydrate
- Include low-fat dairy products and oily fish
- Control the intake of foods containing saturated fats and trans-fatty acids
- Avoid the use of foods marketed specifically for people with diabetes as they often contain fructose as a substitute for sucrose. Fructose still affects blood glucose levels.

 Link To/Go To

The Diabetes UK website contains useful and up-to-date information on dietary advice for both types of diabetes:
http://www.diabetes.org.uk/

However, type 2 diabetes may require oral medication. Drugs for type 2 diabetes generally have one of three potential actions:

- Reducing the amount of glucose released by the liver
- Increasing the cells ability to utilise insulin (decreasing insulin resistance)
- Promoting the production of insulin by the pancreas.

Self-monitoring of type 2 diabetes is occasionally advised and the patient will need to be educated in the use of capillary blood measurement of glucose. More commonly, the primary care provider will monitor the HbA_{1C} (long-term blood glucose measurement) every 2–6 months.

Patients with both types of diabetes will require advice on:

- Regular physical activity, however strenuous exercise can reduce blood glucose levels and type 1 diabetics will need to monitor blood glucose levels and adjust insulin doses accordingly. Exercise regimes should be agreed with appropriate healthcare staff
- Stopping smoking. Smoking is a risk for anybody but diabetic patients have an increased risk of cardiovascular disease, which is compounded by smoking
- Monitoring cholesterol levels and managing cholesterol intake
- Reducing salt in the diet
- Weight loss, if required. Weight loss improves diabetic control in both types of diabetes.

Furthermore, patients will require regular (usually annual) checks and Diabetes UK have created a list of 15 healthcare essentials that patients should be receiving every year:

1. Blood glucose levels – HbA_{1C} should be measured at least once every year
2. Blood pressure recorded at least once a year
3. Cholesterol levels tested every year
4. Eye test for signs of retinopathy (damage to the retina of the eye)
5. Foot check. Diabetics have a higher risk of problems with the feet and therefore they should be checked by a professional at least once a year
6. Kidney function test – a urine test for protein and a blood test to measure kidney function
7. Weight check – regular weight checks as well as measurement of waist circumference to assess for the need for weight loss
8. Stop smoking support if required
9. Care planning. Diabetics should receive a yearly care plan from their diabetes healthcare team that includes their needs and health targets
10. Health courses – diabetics should be offered the opportunity to attend a course that could help them understand and manage their condition
11. Paediatric care. Children and young people with diabetes should receive care from specialist paediatric healthcare professionals
12. High-quality hospital care. Diabetics who need to stay in hospital should receive care from specialist diabetes healthcare professionals, whether or not they have been admitted because of their diabetes
13. Specialist pregnancy care. Diabetes has to be more highly controlled and monitored during pregnancy, so diabetics who are planning to have a baby should have the care they need from specialist healthcare professionals
14. Access to specialists. All diabetics need to see specialist diabetes healthcare professionals to help them manage their condition, including access to ophthalmologists, podiatrists and dieticians
15. Emotional support. Living with diabetes can have an effect on emotional and psychological health, so diabetics should be able to talk to specialist healthcare professionals about their concerns. Patients with both types of diabetes have an increased risk of depression and healthcare professionals can use two simple questions to screen for potential depression, e.g. During the last month, have you often been bothered by:
    - Feeling down, depressed or hopeless?
    - Having little interest or pleasure in doing things?

    If the answer to either of these questions is 'yes', then more detailed depression screening may be required.

Red Flag

Women of child-bearing age who are pregnant (or wish to become pregnant) will require close management of their diabetic control, as there is an increased risk of miscarriage and stillbirth.

Primary Care

As noted, primary care providers are at the forefront of risk assessment and screening for type 2 diabetes. The vast majority of type 2 diabetics are managed in primary care and the Department of Health have set a number of Quality and Outcomes Framework (QOF) indicators for diabetes care, including blood pressure measurement and control, foot examination, referral to a structured education programme and HbA_{1C} levels (**http://www.nice.org.uk/aboutnice/qof/indicators.jsp**)

Conclusion

This chapter has reviewed the physiology of the endocrine system and its related conditions. The major functions of the endocrine system are based around four main areas:

- The maintenance of homeostasis
- Metabolism and energy management
- Growth and development
- Reproduction.

The secretion of hormones can be stimulated by nervous impulses, hormones or changes in the body levels of ions and nutrients and further regulation of hormone release is then often controlled by negative feedback loops. Hormones can only have an effect on a cell if that cell has a receptor for the hormone; however there appears to be virtually no cell within the body that is not affected by the endocrine system. Any part of the endocrine system can become disordered but the effects of the disorder may be subtle and difficult to diagnose. Management of endocrine disorders requires the multidisciplinary team to work around the patient and with the patient to provide the best outcomes for health.

Key Points

- The nurse's role in the management of endocrine disorders requires knowledge of the normal functioning of the endocrine system.
- Endocrine disorders can be slow and insidious in onset with vague symptoms.
- Management of patients with an endocrine disorder requires skills in education and counselling.
- Most patients with an endocrine disorder will be required to carry out self-care activities in managing their disorder and many patients become experts in their own disorder.
- All patients with an endocrine disorder should be strongly advised to wear a MedicAlert talisman.
- Most endocrine disorders have an associated support group and patients should be made aware of any specific to their condition.
- Endocrine disorders are always managed in a shared care agreement between primary care and the hospital consultant.
- The care of patients with diabetes involves the management of risk for long-term complications as much as short-term hormone replacement.

Glossary

Adrenalitis: inflammatory condition of the adrenal glands

Amino acids: chemical compound that is the basic building blocks of proteins and enzymes

Bradycardia: a slow heart beat (usually defined as less than 60 beats per minute)

Carbohydrate: a group of compounds (including starches and sugars) that are a major food source

Catecholamines: a collective term for adrenaline, noradrenaline and dopamine

Concordance: current term for the patients' adherence to a prescribes treatment

Cortex: the outermost layer of an organ

Cytology: the medical speciality that deals with making diagnoses of diseases and conditions through the examination of tissue samples from the body

Electrolytes: a group of chemical elements or compounds that includes sodium, potassium, calcium, chloride and bicarbonate

Exocrine gland: a gland that secretes its products into an external space

Exophthalmos: excessive protrusion of the eyeballs

Fatty acids: dietary fats that have broken down into elements that can be absorbed into the blood

Free T$_4$: refers to thyroxine, in the blood, that is not bound to proteins

Gland: refers to any organ in the body that secretes substances not related to its own, internal, functioning.

Gluconeogenesis: creation of new glucose from non-carbohydrate substrates

Glycogen: a carbohydrate (complex sugar) made from glucose

Glycogenolysis: breakdown of glycogen to create glucose

Goitre: pronounced swelling of the neck

Hormone: chemical substance that is released into the blood, by the endocrine system, and has a physiological control over the function of cells or organs other than those that created it

Hyperglycaemia: high blood levels of glucose

Hypoglycaemia: low blood levels of glucose

Hypersecretion: high rate of secretion

Hyposecretion: low rate of secretion

Hypoventilation: shallow breathing

Hypovolaemia: low levels of fluid in the circulation

Insulin resistance: a condition where the usual body reaction to insulin is reduced

Libido: desire for sexual activity

Lipids: A group of organic compounds, including the fats, oils, waxes, sterols and triglycerides

Medulla: the most internal part of an organ

Neuropathy: inflammation and degeneration of the nerves

Nocturia: needing to get up at night to pass urine

Opportunistic screening: testing a patient for particular diseases or conditions, at a point in time they are accessing health care for other reasons

Osmolality: measure of solute concentration in a fluid

Osmotic: the movement of water through a semi permeable barrier from an area of low concentration of a chemical to an area of high concentration of a chemical

Osteoclasts: a type of cell that breaks down bone tissue and thus releases the calcium used to create bones

Osteoporosis: condition characterised by reduced bone density and an increased risk of fractures

Palpitations: a feeling of pounding or racing of the heart

Polydipsia: excessive thirst

Polyuria: excessive passing of urine

Portal system: normally blood flows from arteries to capillary beds to veins but in portal systems, blood flows from capillary beds to veins and then into another set of capillary beds

Postural hypotension: inability of the body to maintain an adequate blood pressure when the person rises from sitting or lying to standing too rapidly. Usually characterised by dizziness or fainting if the person rises too quickly to a standing position

Pruritis: itching

Radiotherapy: treatment that involves the use of high-energy radiation

Substrate: a molecule upon which an enzyme acts

Tachycardia: fast heart rate (typically over 100 beats per minute)

Tachypnoea: rapid respiratory rate

Thyroid nodule: growth of thyroid tissue or fluid filled cyst of the thyroid tissue

Triglycerides: a form of fatty acid having three fatty acid components

Vitiligo: long-term condition that causes pale, white patches to develop on the skin due to the lack of a chemical called melanin

References

Arlt, W. & Allolio, B. (2003) Adrenal insufficiency. *Lancet*, 361(9372), 1881–1893.

Biondi, B. & Cooper, D.S. (2008) The clinical significance of subclinical thyroid dysfunction. *Endocrine Reviews*, 29(1), 76–131.

Crilly, M. (2004) Correspondence: Thyroxine adherence in primary hypothyroidism. *Lancet*, 363(9420), 1558.

Daneman, D. (2006) Type 1 diabetes. *Lancet*, 367(9513), 847–858.

DH (2001a) *The Expert Patient: a new approach to chronic disease management in the 21st century.* Department of Health, London.

DH (2001b) *National Service Framework for Diabetes: Standards.* Department of Health. London.

Hampton, J. (2013) Thyroid gland disorder emergencies: thyroid storm and myxedema coma. *AACN Advanced Critical Care*, 24(3), 325–332.

Marx, S.J. (2000) Hyperparathyroid and hypoparathyroid disorders. *New England Journal of Medicine*, 343(25), 1863–1875.

Medeiros-Neto, G., Romaldini, J.H. & Abalovich, M. (2011) Highlights of the guidelines on the management of hyperthyroidism and other causes of thyrotoxicosis. *Thyroid*, 21(6), 581–584.

Munir, A. & Newell-Price, J. (2009) Cushing's syndrome. *Medicine*, 37(8), 403–406.

NICE (2005) *CG15 Type 1 diabetes: Diagnosis and management of type 1 diabetes in children, young people and adults*. National Institute for Health and Clinical Excellence, London.

NICE (2012) *PH38 Preventing type 2 diabetes: risk identification and interventions for individuals at high risk*. National Institute for Health and Clinical Excellence, London.

Noble, K.A. (2006) Thyroid storm. *Journal of PeriAnesthesia Nursing*, 21(2), 119–125.

Papaleontiou, M. & Haymart, M. R. (2012). Approach to and treatment of thyroid disorders in the elderly. *Medical Clinics of North America*, 96(2), 297.

Potts, J.T. (2005) Starling review: parathyroid hormone: past and present. *Journal of Endocrinology*, 187(3), 311–325.

Prabhakar, V.K.B. & Shalet, S.M. (2006) Aetiology, diagnosis and management of hypopituitarism in adult life. *Postgraduate Medical Journal*, 82(966), 259–266.

Prague, J. K., May, S. & Whitelaw, B.C. (2013) Cushing's syndrome. *British Medical Journal*, 346, 945.

Roberts, C.G.P. & Ladenson, P.W. (2004) Hypothyroidism. *Lancet*, 363(9411), 793–803.

Schneider, H.J., Aimaretti, G., Kreitschmann-Andermahr, I., Stalla, G. & Ghigo, E. (2007) Hypopituitarism. *Lancet*, 369(9571), 1461–1470.

Simmons, S. (2010) A delicate balance: detecting thyroid disease. *Nursing*, 40(7), 22–29.

Stumvoll, M., Goldstein, B.J. & van Haeften, T.W. (2005) Type 2 diabetes: principles of pathogenesis and therapy. *Lancet*, 365(9467), 1333–1346.

Wass, J. A. & Arlt, W. (2012) How to avoid precipitating an acute adrenal crisis. *British Medical Journal*, 345(7879), 9.

Weeks, B. H. (2005) Graves' disease: the importance of early diagnosis. *Nurse Practitioner*, 30(11), 34–45.

Weetman, A. (2013) Current choice of treatment for hypo- and hyperthyroidism. *Prescriber*, 24(13–16), 23–33.

Test Yourself

1. Pregnant women with hyperthyroidism cannot be treated with:
   (a) Antithyroid drugs
   (b) Surgery
   (c) Radiation
   (d) Iodine restriction

2. All patients with an endocrine disorder should be encouraged to:
   (a) Take plenty of rest
   (b) Wear a MedicAlert talisman
   (c) Carry a steroid card
   (d) Avoid alcohol

3. The majority of hormones are based on:
   (a) Cholesterol
   (b) Minerals
   (c) Phosphorous
   (d) Amino acids

4. A humoral stimulus for hormone release is:
   (a) A response to direct nervous stimulation
   (b) A response to changing levels of certain ions and nutrients
   (c) A response to hormones released by other glands or organs
   (d) A response to conscious thought

5. Thyrotropin releasing hormone is secreted from:
   (a) The parathyroid gland
   (b) The thyroid gland
   (c) The hypothalamus
   (d) The pituitary gland

6. A tremor may be a sign of:
   (a) Hyperadrenalism
   (b) Hyperthyroidism
   (c) Hypoadrenalism
   (d) Hypothyroidism

7. Many symptoms are common to both types of diabetes; which of the following is a symptom of type 1 diabetes only:
   (a) Increased thirst
   (b) Blurred vision
   (c) Ketones in the urine
   (d) Weight loss

8. Which of the following hormones is not released by the adrenal glands:
   (a) Androgens
   (b) Aldosterone
   (c) Somatotropes
   (d) Cortisol

9. Parathyroid hormone release stimulates the release of calcitriol from which organ:
   (a) Kidneys
   (b) Lungs
   (c) Heart
   (d) Intestines

10. Which of the following is not an action of the catecholamine hormones:
    (a) Increased heart rate
    (b) Increased alertness
    (c) Increased gut motility
    (d) Increased metabolic rate

Answers

1. c
2. b
3. d
4. b

5. c
6. b
7. d
8. c
9. a
10. c

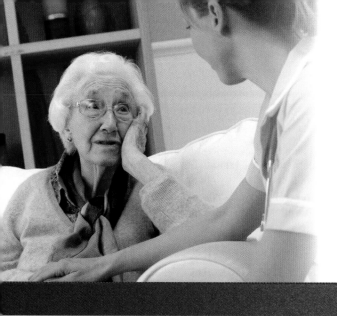

34

The Person with a Neurological Disorder

Mary E. Braine

University of Salford, UK

Learning Outcomes

On completion of this chapter you will be able to:

- Describe the overall functions of the neurological system, and detail the nervous system considering their key functions
- Provide an explanation for the normal and abnormal changes that can occur in the nervous system
- Gain an insight into some common neurological conditions
- Be aware of the various components of a neurological assessment
- List important investigations required to diagnose neurological conditions
- Outline the medical and nursing management of common neurological disorders

Competencies

All nurses must:

1. Conduct a health history and assessment of neurological function
2. Provide ongoing documentation following assessment of neurological function
3. Support and promote the health of the neuroscience patient and their family/carers
4. Monitor patients with neurological problems for expected and unexpected signs and symptoms
5. Determine priority nursing diagnoses, based on assessed data, to select and implement individualised nursing interventions for person with neurological disorders
6. Provide skilled care to patients with neurological conditions

 Visit the companion website at **www.wileynursingpractice.com** where you can test yourself using flashcards, multiple-choice questions and more.

Nursing Practice: Knowledge and Care, First Edition. Edited by Ian Peate, Karen Wild and Muralitharan Nair.
© 2014 John Wiley & Sons, Ltd. Published 2014 by John Wiley & Sons, Ltd. Companion website: www.wileynursingpractice.com

Introduction

The nervous system is one of the most complex body systems, regulating, controlling and integrating all other body systems and maintaining homeostasis. To accomplish these, the nervous system activities can be grouped into three basic functions: sensory, motor and integrative functions. Due to the nervous system's complexity, it is often difficult to understand and can be very challenging, however nurses will come into contact with patients with neurological disorders in a wide variety of situations. Thus, an understanding of this complex system is crucial in helping to assess and recognise normal and abnormal functions and underpins many aspects of patient care. Understanding is also critical in providing safe and effective care for this varied larger group of patients; with over 1000 neurological disorders affecting millions of people worldwide.

This chapter provides an overview of the function of the central and peripheral nervous system. Before a nurse can plan and give competent care to a patient with a neurological condition, assessment of nursing care needs must be made. This chapter provides an overview of the assessment processes to facilitate diagnosis, some common diagnostic interventions and related key nursing care considerations. General management and key nursing care provision for patients, their families and carers for a few commonly encountered neurological disorders are considered in this chapter.

Anatomy and Physiology

This system receives, processes and initiates actions through an intricate network of billions of specialised cells called **neurones** (nerves). It consists of two main subdivisions:

- **The central nervous system (CNS)**: brain and spinal cord
- **The peripheral nervous system (PNS)**: all nervous tissue outside the CNS.

(See Figure 34.1.)

Cells of the Nervous System

Nervous tissue consists of two major classes of cells, the **neurone** and **neuroglia** cells. The neurone is the basic anatomical and functional unit of the nervous system forming a complex processing network communicating with other neurones and cells within the brain and spinal cord. The neuroglia (also called 'glia') are the supporting cells in the CNS providing protection, support and nourishment to the neurones and maintaining homeostasis in the interstitial fluid that bathes them. Although smaller in size than neurones, they make up about half of the brain mass and outnumber the neurones 10-fold.

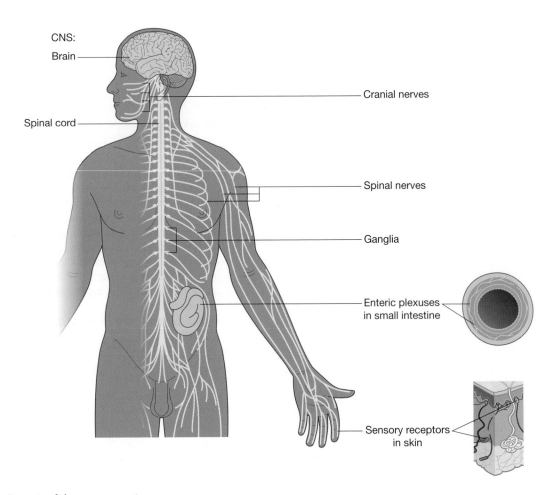

Figure 34.1 The main parts of the nervous system.

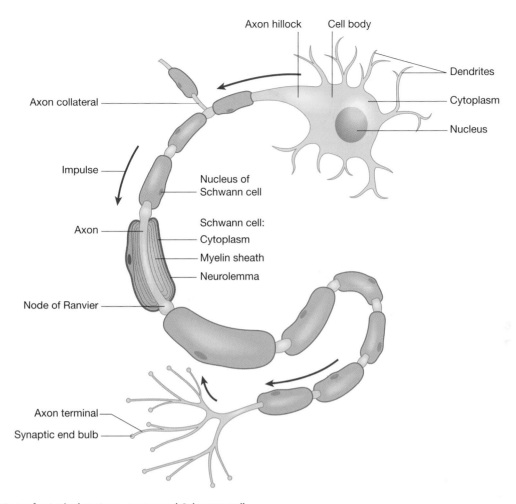

Figure 34.2 Structure of a typical motor neurone and Schwann cell.

Neurones

Most neurones consist of a soma (cell body), and two types of neuronal processes: dendrites and axon, see Figure 34.2. Neurones vary in shape and size, the longest extending from the brain to the toes. Cell bodies also vary in size and are found in clusters in the PNS known as 'ganglia', in the CNS these clusters are called 'a centre', and a centre with a discrete boundary is called a 'nucleus'. The dendrites emerge from the soma and conduct impulses towards (afferent) the cell body from the synapses at the end of the dendrites. Synapses are junctions where a neurone meets another cell; in the CNS, this is another neurone but in the PNS, this may be a muscle (neuromuscular junction), gland or organ. The axon (only one per neurone), a long process, conducts impulses away (efferent) from the cell body towards another neurone, muscle fibre or a gland cell (Figure 34.3).

Axons may be insulated by a white lipid sheath known as 'myelin' (myelinated) or not (unmyelinated). The myelin sheath is formed by Schwann cells in the PNS and oligodendrocytes in the CNS. The myelin sheath contains gaps (bare segments) called **nodes of Ranvier**, which allow movement of ions between the axon and the extracellular fluid and serves to increase the speed of nerve impulse conduction. The cell bodies and dendrites comprise what is often called the 'grey matter' of the CNS. Both functionally and structurally, features are used to classify neurones (Table 34.1 and Figure 34.4).

Neuroglia cells

A number of different neuroglia cells are to be found in the CNS and PNS. Table 34.2 summarises the main types and functions.

Glia (Greek for 'glue') cells once considered as just scaffolding for the neurones, are now known to play important roles in CNS functions, but they cannot conduct impulses (see Figure 34.5).

Communication within the CNS – synapses and neurotransmitters

Neurones are able to communicate with each other with precision known as 'synaptic transmission'. Stimulation of a neurone results in an electrical reaction that travels down the axon to the terminal, where it needs to pass the message onto another neurone the **synapse**. Two types of synaptic transmission may occur:

1. **Electrical transmission** in which the electrical charge is transmitted via small gap, the message can flow both ways across the synapse commonly found in the cardiac and smooth muscle for rapid transmission

2. **Chemical transmission** (majority of the synapses) requires chemicals to transmit the message, called 'neurotransmitters';

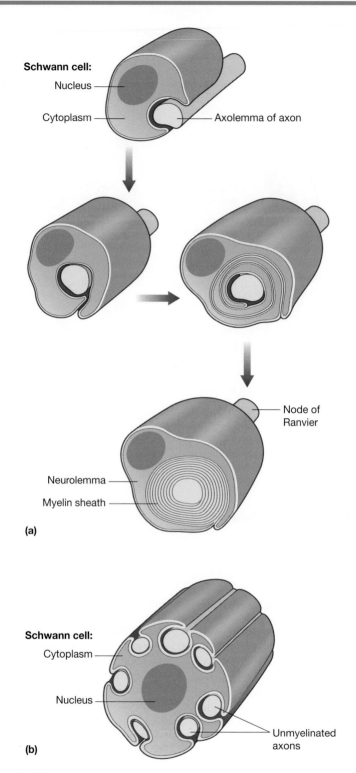

Schwann cell:

Nucleus

Cytoplasm

Axolemma of axon

Node of Ranvier

Neurolemma

Myelin sheath

(a)

Schwann cell:

Cytoplasm

Nucleus

Unmyelinated axons

(b)

Figure 34.3 **Myelinated and unmyelinated axons.**

Table 34.1 Structure, location and functions of the different neurones.

TYPE AND STRUCTURE	LOCATION IN NS	FUNCTION
Sensory (afferent) Unipolar (one axon and dendrites are in continuous process that emerge from the cell body)	PNS and CNS Originate in the sense organs	Once the sensory receptors at the distal ends (dendrites) are stimulated, impulses are conveyed to the CNS via cranial nerves or spinal nerves
Bipolar neurones (single axon and a single dendrite) 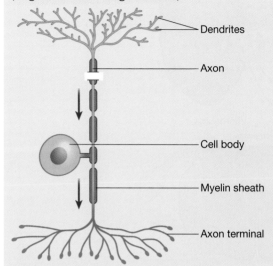	Rare, found in the sensory organ, e.g. retina of the eye, inner ear	
Motor (efferent) Multipolar (one axon and several dendrites) 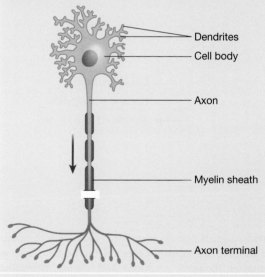	CNS Originate in the brain stem and the spinal cord	Transmits impulses from the CNS to the PNS through cranial and spinal nerves to the muscles and glands within the body
Interneurones Mostly multipolar	Mainly in the CNS Includes most large nerves, e.g. the brachial and spinal nerves	Integrate incoming sensory information from sensory neurones and then activate a motor response by activating the motor neurones

(Bipolar neurone diagram labels: Dendrites, Axon, Cell body, Myelin sheath, Axon terminal)

(Motor neurone diagram labels: Dendrites, Cell body, Axon, Myelin sheath, Axon terminal)

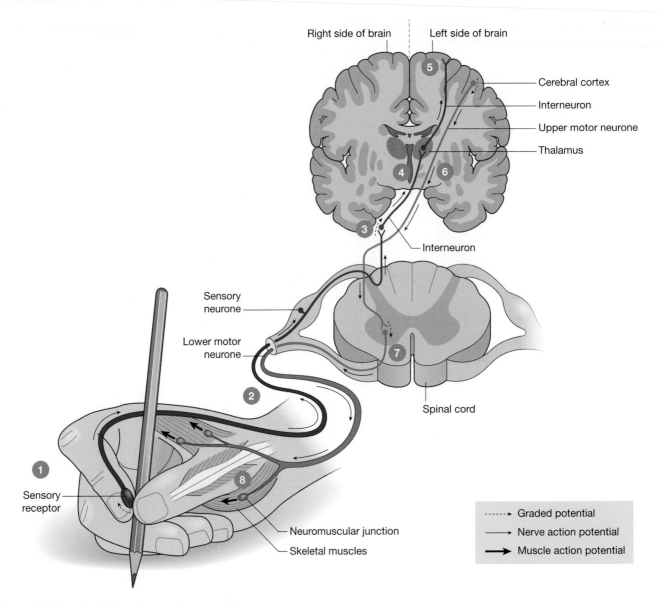

Figure 34.4 How the different types of neurones interact.

synthesised by the neurone and released into the gap between two neurones, called the 'synaptic cleft' and diffuse across the gap to activate the other neurone.

Some neurotransmitters modulate the effect of a particular neurotransmitter by prolonging, exciting, inhibiting or limiting their effect, known as 'neuromodulators'. There are over a 100 different neurotransmitters with different neurones in the brain releasing different neurotransmitters. A summary of the main types can be found in Table 34.3.

The Central Nervous System
Overview

The CNS controls and integrates the whole nervous system receiving information (input) about the changes in the internal and external environment and processes and interprets this informa-

tion and provides signals that are manifested in sensory or motor outputs. The **brain** is the control centre of the nervous system and also generates thoughts, emotions and speech. Averaging 1400 g in weight, the brain is a relatively small structure constituting about 2% of body weight in adults. The brain is protected from the external environment by three barriers: the skull, the meninges and the cerebral spinal fluid. The brain has four major parts: the cerebral cortex, the diencephalon (thalamus, hypothalamus and epithalamus), the brain stem and the cerebellum. The general functions of these regions are summarised in Table 34.4 and Figure 34.6.

Cerebral cortex (cerebrum)

The surface of the cerebral cortex (cerebrum) is folded into elevated ridges of tissue called 'gyri', which are separated by shallow grooves called 'sulci' or 'fissures' (deeper groves). Fissures further divide the

Table 34.2 Types of neuroglia, their description, function and location in the NS.

NEUROGLIA	DESCRIPTION		FUNCTION	LOCATION
Macroglia	Astrocytes: · Largest and most numerous neuroglia · Star-shaped cells with many processes · Contain specific glia fibrillary acidic protein · Known as astroglia when clumped together		Cling to and support neurones Regulate the extracellular chemicals and ions Transports glucose and other substances from the blood Reactive astrocytes, together with microglia are involved in repair of damaged neural tissue Form part of the blood–brain barrier Control the distribution of neurotransmitters released by neurones Involved in signalling	CNS
	Oligodendrocytes: · Second most abundant neuroglia cells · Large cells, cytoplasm and nucleus more dense than in astrocytes		Provides support to axons Electrical insulation of axons forming a fatty myelin sheath Involved in growth of damaged CNS axons	CNS
	Schwann cells: · Equivalent of oligodendrocytes in the PNS		Electrical insulation of single axons forming a fatty myelin sheath Facilitates neuronal regeneration of peripheral nerves following injury	PNS
Microglia	Small and the rarest glia cells: Round cells with numerous long spiny processes Resting or active/reactive		Phagocytic engulfing debris resulting from injury, infection or diseases Activated by the release of inflammatory modulators, such as cytokines	CNS
Polydendrocyte	2–9% of all cells in the central nervous system Stem cells of the CNS		Primary function is the generation of oligodendrocytes in the developing and mature CNS Primary source of remyelinating cells in demyelinating lesions Receive direct synaptic input from neurones	CNS
Aldynoglia	Collective group of specialist neuroglia cells Originate from different areas in the brain		Pituitary glia assist in the storage and release of hormones Retina (Müller) glia found in the retina support the neurones in the retina and act as a light filter	CNS
Ependymal cells	Cuboidal or columnar cells in single layers Lines the ventricles in the brain and the central canal of the spinal cord		Form part of the choroid plexus producing cerebral spinal fluid Involved with the directional flow of cerebrospinal fluid Facilitate transport of nutrients and removal of waste	CNS
Satellite cells	Flat cells with thin cellular sheaths that surround the individual neurones, in particular sensory, sympathetic, and parasympathetic ganglia		Structural support of the neurones Satellite cells also act as protective, cushioning cells Surround neurone cell bodies within ganglia regulating the environment and exchange of material between neuronal cell bodies and interstitial fluid The creation and persistence of chronic pain	PNS

surface of the cerebrum into the four lobes. The longitudinal fissure separates the two hemispheres, the transverse fissure separates the cerebrum from the cerebellum, and the lateral fissure separates the temporal lobe from the frontal and parietal lobes. The thick white matter is comprised of hundreds of millions of myelinated axons (fatty sheaths causing the white appearance) bundled into different tracts or pathways that run in three principal directions connecting the various grey matter areas (neurone cell bodies).

- Association fibres connect and transmit nerve impulses between one area and another in the same hemisphere
- Commissural fibres connect areas in one cerebral hemisphere to the corresponding area in the opposite hemisphere, the majority pass through the largest commissure, the **corpus callosum**
- Projection fibres form ascending and descending tracts that transmit impulses from the cerebrum to other parts of the brain and spinal cord, e.g. internal capsule.

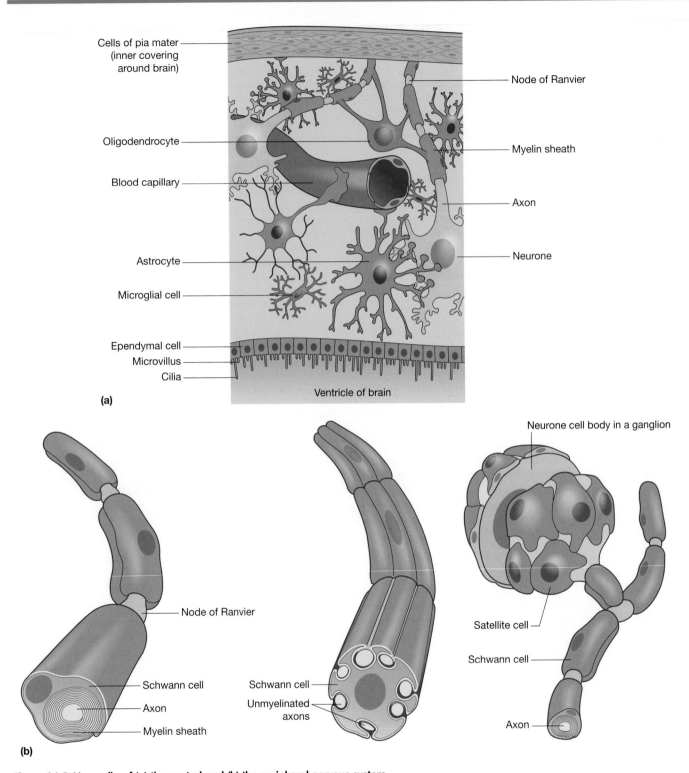

Figure 34.5 Neuroglia of (a) the central and (b) the peripheral nervous system.

Table 34.3 Main types of neurotransmitter, examples and main areas found in the CNS.

NEUROTRANSMITTER	MAIN AREAS IN THE CNS
Excitatory neurotransmitter	
Acetylcholine (ACh) released by cholinergic synapses	Throughout the brain, motor neurones that innervate muscles (neuromuscular junction), neurones in the para-sympathetic nervous system (PNS)
Norepinephrine (NE) (noradrenaline) released by adrenergic synapses (amine)	Brain stem, hypothalamus and neurones in the sympathetic nervous system (SNS)
Glutamate	Most CNS synapses
Inhibitory neurotransmitters	
Gamma aminobutyric acid (GABA)	Throughout the CNS
Dopamine (amine) (is also excitatory at other synapses)	Neurone in the brain stem, basal ganglia, CNS (5 types D_1–D_5); 7 subtypes in CNS and PNS
Serotonin (5-hydroxtryptamine; 5-HT)	Brain stem, hypothalamus

Table 34.4 General functions of the four main parts for the brain.

MAIN PART	FUNCTIONS
Cerebral cortex	
Largest part of the brain Divided into right and left hemisphere Both hemispheres are connected internally by the corpus callosum The right sends and receives information from the left side of the body and vice versa Each hemisphere is divided up into four lobes named after the bone that cover them Hemispheres are made up of outer cerebral cortex grey matter, internal white matter and nuclei, deep within the white matter	Receive sensory (afferent) impulses Initiate motor (efferent) impulses The seat of all – interprets sensory input Controls skeletal muscle activity Processes intellect and emotions Contains skills memory
Diencephalon	
Provides a structural connection between the cerebrum and the brain stem, in particular the midbrain Includes the following areas: · Thalamus consisting of small paired egg-shaped nuclei approximately 3 cm in length, constituting 80% of the diencephalon · Hypothalamus located below the thalamus and composed of several nuclei. A stalk-like infundibulum connects the pituitary gland to the hypothalamus · Epithalamus consists of the pineal gland · Subthalamus consists of two main cell groups the subthalamic nuclei and the zona incerta	Thalamus · Main synaptic relay centre, processes motor information · Receives and relays sensory information to and from the cerebral cortex Hypothalamus · Main visceral control and vital for overall homeostasis · Regulates autonomic nervous system · Senses change in body temperature and regulates core body temperature · Regulates and produces hormones · Mediates emotional responses · Regulates water balance and thirst · Regulation of appetite · Regulation of sleep–wake cycle (circadian rhythm) · Part of the arousal/alerting mechanism
Brain stem	
Consists of the: · Midbrain composed of the paired bundles of axons called 'cerebral peduncles', several nuclei including the red nuclei and the substantia nigra and is approximately 1 cm long · Medulla oblongata containing all ascending and descending motor and sensory tract and several nuclei and serves as site of crossing of nerve tracts (decussation)	Midbrain · Conducts impulse from the motor areas in the cerebral cortex to the brain stem · Reflex centre for some visual activities, e.g. eye movement, light reflex and accommodation and convergence reflex

801

(Continued)

Table 34.4 (Continued)

MAIN PART	FUNCTIONS
· Pons consists of bundles of ascending and descending fibres and nuclei Also extensive throughout the brain stem are a network of white and grey fibres called the 'reticular formation'	Medulla oblongata · Controls voluntary movement of lower limbs and trunk · Cardiovascular centre controls heart rate and force of heart beat · *Rhythmicity* area controls basis breathing rate · Controls reflexes for vomiting, coughing, swallowing, hiccupping, yawning and sneezing · Nuclei for several cranial nerves Pons · Coordinates voluntary movements · Pneumotaxic and apneustic area help control breathing · Nuclei for several cranial nerves
Cerebellum	
Second largest area and contains nearly half of all the neurones in the brain Consists of two hemispheres and a central area *vermis* and attached to the brain stem by three paired *peduncles* Consists of an outer cortex of grey matter and an inner white matter called the *arbour vitae* Incoming information is received from the cortex via the pons and outgoing information goes to the cortex via the thalamus	Balance Muscle tension Eye movement Equilibrium of the trunk Spinal nerve reflexes Provides information necessary for balance, posture and coordinated muscle movement

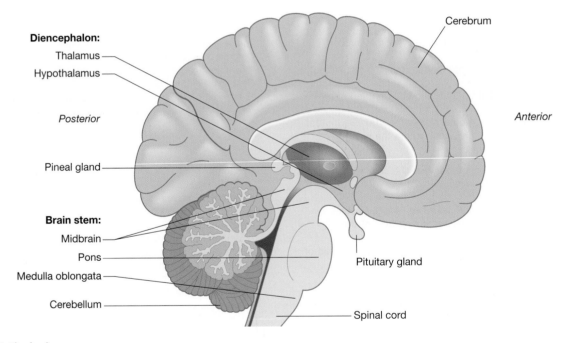

Figure 34.6 The brain.

Each cerebral hemisphere is divided into: frontal, parietal, temporal and occipital lobes see Figure 34.7. The cortex can be divided up into areas that serve a single function and these are called 'primary areas' (touch, vision, hearing, taste and smell and the production of movement). Clustered around these primary areas, and associated with them, are areas known as association areas (cortex). It is important to understand these functional areas of the cortex as selective damage to these regions can lead to discrete neurological deficits. A fifth area of the cerebrum buried in the cortex and separating the frontal and temporal lobes is called the **insula lobe**.

The right side of the body is controlled by the left hemisphere of the cerebral cortex and vice versa, known as **decussation**. However, the two hemispheres are not alike; each hemisphere has highly specialised regions that serve differing functions, *lateralisation* (see Table 34.5). For example for the majority of persons, 95%

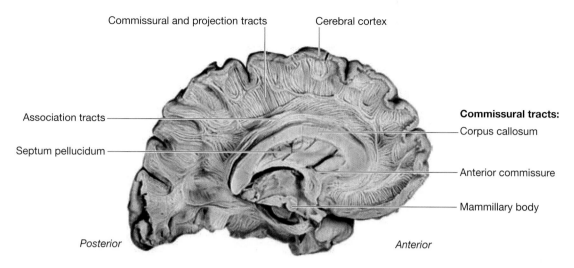

Commissural and projection tracts

Cerebral cortex

Association tracts

Septum pellucidum

Commissural tracts:

Corpus callosum

Anterior commissure

Mammillary body

Posterior

Anterior

Figure 34.7 Structure of the left cerebral hemisphere.

Table 34.5 Summary of the key-specific functions of each cerebral hemisphere.

LEFT-SIDE DOMINANCE	GENERAL FUNCTION	RIGHT-SIDE DOMINANCE
Words and letters	Vision	Geometric patterns Face recognition and facial emotional expression Visual imagery
Language sounds	Audition	Non-language sounds Music and artistic awareness
Complex movements	Touch	Tactile patterns (Braille)
Verbal memory	Movement	Spatial movement patterns
Speech (70–90%) Reading, writing Arithmetic and logical abilities	Language	Generating emotional content
	Spatial ability	Geometry Direction Distance Mental rotation of shapes

the left hemisphere contains two speech centres, one concerned with the expression of language, 'Broca's area' in the frontal lobe and 'Wernicke's area' concerned with understanding the spoken word located at the junction of the temporal, parietal and occipital lobes. Based on this specialisation location, *the left hemisphere is often referred to the dominant hemisphere.*

Handedness can be defined as the hand that performs faster or more precisely on manual tests, such as writing and the hand that one prefers to use, regardless of performance. Handedness, however, reveals a much more complex process with regard to dominance. Up to 90% of the population is right-handed and almost all right-handed persons (∼98%) have a left-hemispheric language specialisation. However, in the left-handed person, this is much less (∼70%) and many left-handed persons have bilateral hemispheric

control of language. See Table 34.5 for a summary of the key-specific functions of each cerebral hemisphere.

The limbic system

The limbic system is a highly complex system. It consists of the **limbic lobe**, although not a discrete lobe, consisting of a number of cortical structures that form a ring of cortex spanning the frontal, temporal and parietal lobes and subcortical areas that are interconnected with each other and with the hypothalamus, by multiple pathways. Major subcortical areas and their functions are summarised in Table 34.6.

Spinal cord

The spinal cord is a long cylindrical segmented structure, which begins at the foramen magnum, where the lower part of the brain stem ends, and terminates, in adults, at the first lumbar vertebra. It receives sensory information from the limbs, trunk and internal organs and somatic motor tracts that supply the skeletal muscles, visceral, smooth muscles and glands. The spinal cord gives rise to 31 spinal nerves (part of the PNS) corresponding to each segment and exits the spinal cord between the vertebral bones of the spinal cord. The spinal cord does not reach the end of the vertebral column; as a result, the lumbar and sacral nerve roots travel inferiorly through the vertebral canal for some distance before exiting the vertebral column through their associated intervertebral foramina. This collection of descending nerve roots is called the 'cauda equina' (Figure 34.8).

The coverings of the brain and spinal cord – meninges The
brain and spinal cord is covered by three layers of connective tissue (the meninges); the cranial and spinal meninges are continuous and bear the same structure (Figure 34.9):

- The *dura mater* (tough mother), a pain sensitive thick double outer fibrous membrane consisting of external periosteal layer and inner meningeal layer. These layers are fused together, except when they separate to form large venous sinuses in which cerebral veins drain
- The *arachnoid mater* (*arachn* = spider), a middle thin avascular membrane, which is attached tightly to the inner dural layer. The space between the arachnoid and pia is called the 'subarachnoid space'. In the region of the brain stem, the space increases to form

Table 34.6 Limbic system major subcortical areas and their functions.

LIMBIC SUBCORTICAL AREA	FUNCTION
Hippocampus – 5 cm long seahorse-shaped cortex located in the temporal lobe and forms part of the floor of the lateral ventricle	Formation of new memory Expression of emotions and emotional behaviour
Amygdala – almond-shaped structure lining the roof of the lateral ventricle	Drive related behaviour, e.g. motivation Emotional learning and memory Emotional behaviour, e.g. fear, sadness aggression, pleasure Sexuality
Septal nuclei – small group of nuclei located in the frontal lobe	Emotional behaviour, e.g. reward and pleasure

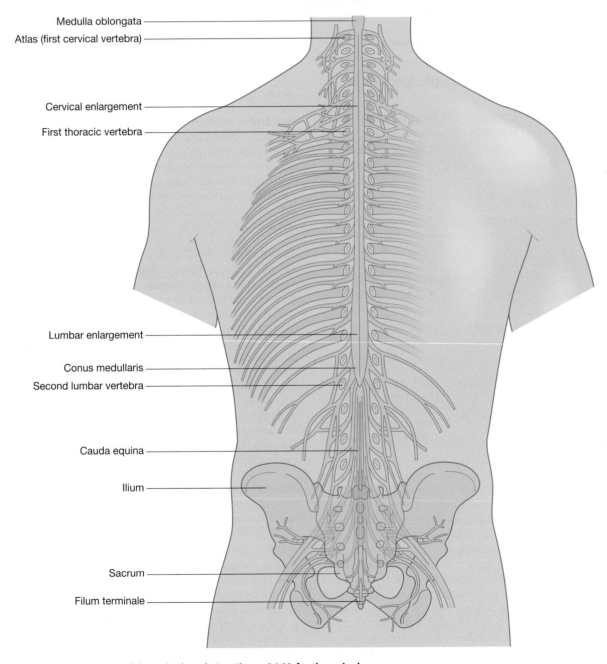

Figure 34.8 External anatomy of the spinal cord. See Figure 34.13 for the spinal nerves.

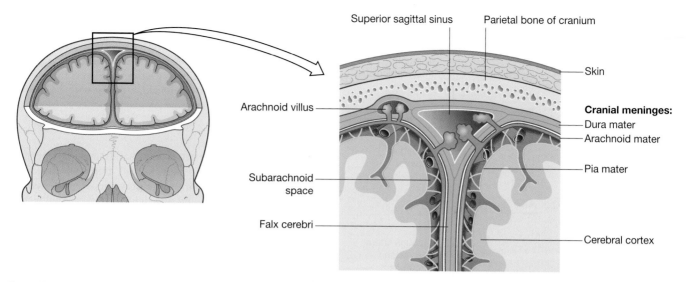

Figure 34.9 **The protective coverings of the brain.**

cisterns, e.g. cisterna magna found between the cerebellum and medulla. The arachnoid contains specialised parts that protrude into venous sinuses and are responsible for the reabsorption of cerebrospinal fluid (CSF), known as arachnoid villi or granulations
- The *pia mater* (*pia* = delicate) a thin inner transparent fibrous membrane, tightly attached to the surface of the brain parenchyma following the contours of the gyri and sulci and the spinal cord. It contains small groups of blood vessels embedded in the connective tissue.

Cerebrospinal fluid CSF is a clear, colourless liquid that flows in the subarachnoid space in a unidirectional flow. About 400–500 mL of CSF is produced per day, mostly by the specialised ependymal cells found in the choroid plexus in the brain ventricles. At any one time the total volume of CSF is 80–150 mL, approximately 30 mL is located in the chambers in the brain known as the 'ventricles', the remaining is in the subarachnoid space. It has three basic functions:

Mechanical protection – cushioning and protecting the delicate brain against impact, injury, the fluid acting as a buoyancy aid for the brain
Chemical protection – providing optimum chemical environment for accurate neuronal signalling
Circulation protection – medium for carrying nutrients from the blood to the adjacent brain tissue and removing waste and potentially noxious substances, such as drugs.

Circulation of CSF CSF circulates around the CNS and is often referred to as the *third circulation* (the first being the cardiovascular the second, the lymphatic system). CSF is normally produced and absorbed in equal amounts, with the entire volume being replaced roughly every 8 hours. The continuous production of new CSF is the main motor of CSF circulation, starting with the flow from the paired lateral ventricles (one in each hemisphere) to the third ventricle via two narrow openings: the **interventricular foramina** or foramina of Monro and then to the fourth ventricle via a duct, **aqueduct of Sylvius** or cerebral aqueduct. The outflow

from the fourth ventricle is through the three openings; two lateral **foramina of Luschka** and the medial **foramina of Magendie** into the subarachnoid space or the central canal of the spinal cord (Figure 34.10).

Blood–brain barrier

The blood–brain barrier (BBB) located at the interface between the capillary walls and the brain tissue acts to isolate the brain from the rest of the body. It regulates the exchange of substances entering the brain in order to maintain optimum levels of, e.g. glucose, proteins and electrolytes, for normal brain activities. In addition, the BBB acts to filter and restrict diffusion and permeation of molecules in order to protect against harmful toxins and metabolites. The BBB is able to do this via tight endothelial cells lining the capillary walls and astrocyte processes (end feet) pressing up against the capillaries from the brain tissue side forming a barrier to large molecules. However, there are several areas within the brain where there is an absence of the BBB; these are collectively called the **circumventricular organs**.

Clinically, the BBB is important as it limits most potential drugs that can be administered to treat brain disorders from penetrating the tight mesh off endothelial cells, and only allows the entry of small /fat (lipid) molecules, e.g. some viruses and toxins (carbon monoxide).

Overview of the blood supply to the CNS The CNS is one of the most metabolically active systems in the body and thus requires a blood system to meet these demands. A large amount of oxygen is necessary for the aerobic metabolism of glucose: the brain's sole source of energy. The brain receives about 700–750 mL/min of blood and consumes 20% (50 mL/min) of cardiac output and the total intracranial blood volume at any one time is 100–150 mL. Blood flow to the brain is maintained at a constant via cerebral autoregulation, which is closely related to the brain's metabolic needs: carbon dioxide (major stimulus for vasodilation), hydrogen ion and oxygen concentrations. Even a brief interruption of blood flow (seconds) can cause serious neurological disturbances and cell death in minutes.

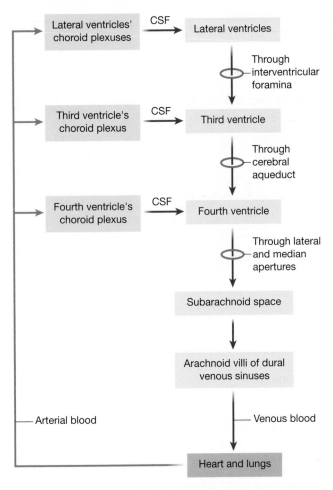

Figure 34.10 The formation and circulation and absorption of the CSF.

Blood supply to the brain comes from two main sources: two internal carotids (anterior or carotid system) arising from the common carotid artery, and two vertebral arteries (posterior or vertebral-basilar system), arising from the subclavian artery. Both sets of arteries give rise to pairs of arteries that supply the blood to both sides of the brain and are joined at the base of the brain to form the **Circle of Willis**, from which major arteries supplying the brain arise (Figure 34.11).

Venous drainage of the brain Cerebral drainage is dependent upon a system of valveless superficial and deep veins into three main dural sinuses (superior sagittal, cavernous and transverse sinuses), which then empty into the right and left internal jugular vein (Figure 34.12).

Blood supply of the spinal cord The blood supply of the spinal cord comes from the anterior spinal artery and paired posterior spinal arteries, arising from the vertebral artery.

The Peripheral Nervous System

The peripheral nervous system links the CNS with the rest of the body. It is responsible for receiving and transmitting information from and about the external environment. The PNS includes the neuromuscular structures outside the skull and vertebral column; spinal nerves and cranial nerves, neuromuscular junction and receptors. Spinal nerves emerge from the spinal cord while cranial nerves emerge from the brain (Figure 34.13).

The PNS provides input via the sensory neurones and output information via motor neurones to the CNS and can be further subdivided into: the somatic nervous systems (SNS) (nerves that transmit information from the skeletal muscles), autonomic nervous system (ANS) and the enteric nervous system (ENS) (Figure 34.14).

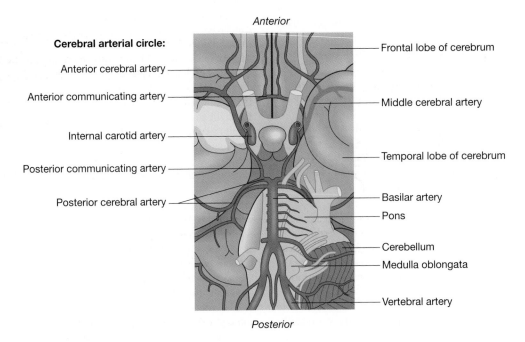

Figure 34.11 Inferior view of base of brain showing cerebral arterial circle.

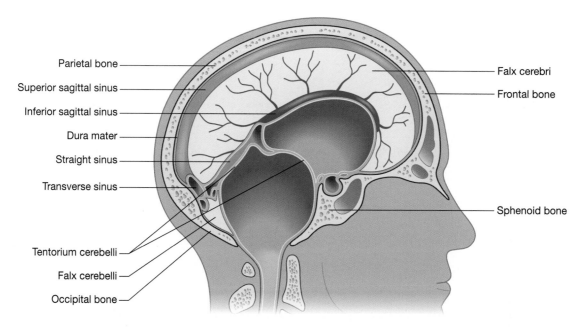

Figure 34.12 Sagittal view of extension of the dural mater.

The spinal (peripheral) nerves each contain motor and sensory fibres and can be myelinated or unmyelinated. Each spinal nerve innervates a specific skin area called a **dermatome**, and each spinal nerve further divides into branches called **rami**. Some of these branches form complex clusters of nerves called 'plexuses', of which there are four: cervical, brachial lumbar and sacral. Ganglia are small clusters of nervous tissue primarily neurone cell bodies outside the CNS (see Figure 34.13).

The nerves can be classified according to their size, which is related to speed of conduction and whether they are myelinated or unmyelinated. The PNS is divided into a sensory (afferent) division and a motor (efferent) division.

Autonomic Nervous System

The autonomic nervous system (ANS), a division of the PNS, is subdivided up into enteric, sympathetic (SNS) and parasympathetic nervous system (PNS) and functions to control the internal environment of the body and the exchange between the internal and external environment. Along with the endocrine system, the ANS regulates homeostasis and controls a range of functions and behaviours. The enteric nervous system found in the wall of the gut, is involved in coordinating the contractions of the gut musculature, resulting in gastrointestinal mobility (peristalsis).

The major sensory system consists of: somatic, visual, auditory, vestibular, taste and olfactory systems. The somatic sensory system includes: sensations for pain, tactile sensation (touch, pressure and vibration), temperature perception of the joint position and movement. The human body gathers information from the environment via peripheral sensory nerve receptors and specialised sensory cells. Sensory receptors are grouped into different classes, depending upon structure location and function (Table 34.7). Sensation is relayed via somatosensory pathways (spinothalamic), somatosensory area, via the brain stem and thalamus, to the primary in the cerebral cortex located in the parietal lobe and the cerebellum.

Each area receives sensory information from different parts of the body (Figure 34.15).

The cranial nerves

There are 12 pairs of cranial nerves (I–XII), which all emerge from the brain, except the IXth cranial nerve, which emerges from the spinal cord, and of the peripheral nervous system. The numbers indicate the order, anterior to posterior, in which the nerves arise from the brain. Table 34.8 describes the functions of each cranial nerve and see also Figure 34.16.

Nursing Assessment of the Neurological System

Neurological assessment requires a nurse who is both a competent and skilled practitioner to recognise changes. This assessment begins at first encounter, with the patient and includes gathering information about the past and current health state and a comprehensive physical assessment. Accurate assessment helps determine the extent of the cerebral dysfunction and improvement or deterioration of cerebral function. Assessment of the neurological system involves assessing the following five areas:

- Level of consciousness
- Vital signs respiration and pulse rate, temperature and blood pressure
- Pupil reactivity
- Motor function
- Sensory function.

Assessing Consciousness

The precise neurobiology of consciousness is unknown, however it can be viewed as having two main components: arousal and

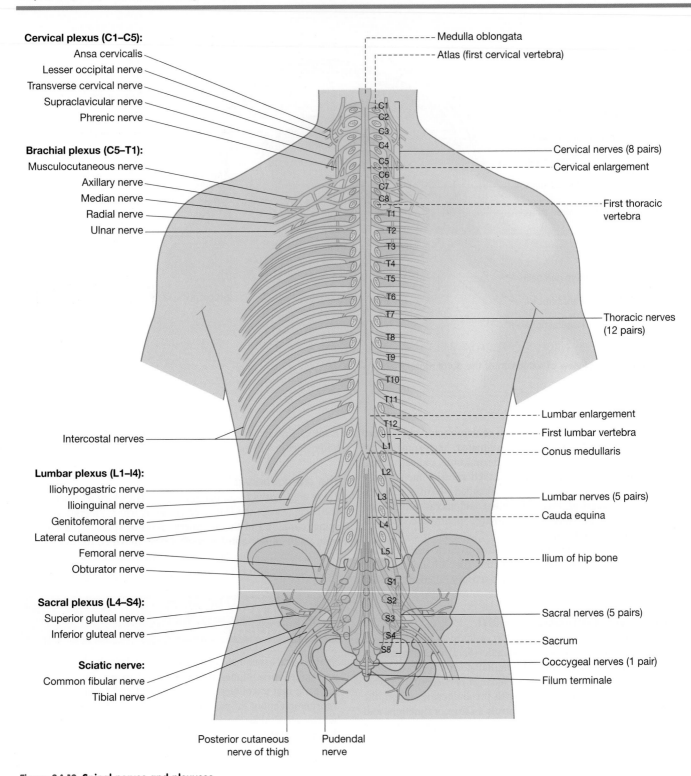

Cervical plexus (C1–C5):
Ansa cervicalis
Lesser occipital nerve
Transverse cervical nerve
Supraclavicular nerve
Phrenic nerve

Brachial plexus (C5–T1):
Musculocutaneous nerve
Axillary nerve
Median nerve
Radial nerve
Ulnar nerve

Intercostal nerves

Lumbar plexus (L1–I4):
Iliohypogastric nerve
Ilioinguinal nerve
Genitofemoral nerve
Lateral cutaneous nerve
Femoral nerve
Obturator nerve

Sacral plexus (L4–S4):
Superior gluteal nerve
Inferior gluteal nerve

Sciatic nerve:
Common fibular nerve
Tibial nerve

Medulla oblongata
Atlas (first cervical vertebra)

C1
C2
C3
C4
C5
C6
C7
C8
T1
T2
T3
T4
T5
T6
T7
T8
T9
T10
T11
T12
L1
L2
L3
L4
L5
S1
S2
S3
S4
S5

Cervical nerves (8 pairs)
Cervical enlargement

First thoracic vertebra

Thoracic nerves (12 pairs)

Lumbar enlargement
First lumbar vertebra
Conus medullaris

Lumbar nerves (5 pairs)
Cauda equina

Ilium of hip bone

Sacral nerves (5 pairs)

Sacrum
Coccygeal nerves (1 pair)
Filum terminale

Posterior cutaneous nerve of thigh
Pudendal nerve

Figure 34.13 Spinal nerves and plexuses.

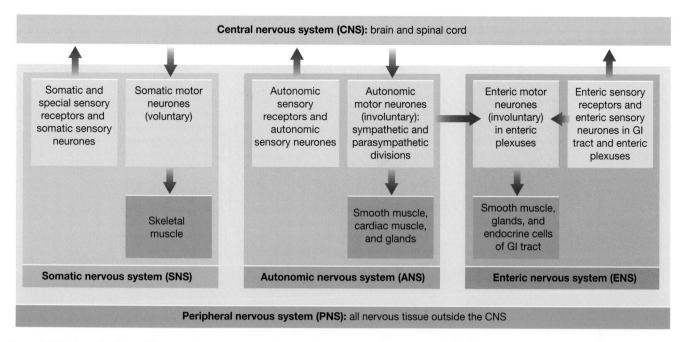

Figure 34.14 **Organisation of the nervous system. Grey boxes represent sensory components of the peripheral nervous system (PNS). Yellow boxes represent motor components of the PNS. Red boxes represent effectors (muscles and glands).**

Table 34.7 **A list of the different types of peripheral receptors, their location and function.**

TYPE OF RECEPTOR	LOCATION	FUNCTION
Mechanoreceptors – encapsulated nerve endings		
Merkel's receptors	Found in the skin dermis	Touch (pressure sensitive)
Muscles mechanoreceptors	Muscles	Limb position and movement
Ruffini's corpuscle	Skin	Magnitude and direction skin stretch
Meissner corpuscle	Skin	Touch and vibration
Hair cells	Organ of Corti in the inner ear	Hearing
Thermoreceptors – free nerve endings		
	Skin	Cold and hot temperature in the skin
Nociceptors – free nerve endings		
	Three types; mechanical, thermal and polymodal Throughout the body except the brain	Tissue damage and pain
Chemoreceptors – specialised receptor cells		
Olfactory receptor cells	Mucosa of the nasal cavity	Smell
Taste buds	Surface of the tongue	Taste
Photoreceptors	Retina – rods and cones	Cones day colour light vision Rods detect dim light

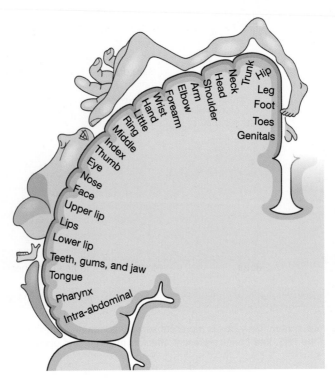

Figure 34.15 Somatic sensory map in the cerebral cortex.

Table 34.8 Cranial nerves: type and function.

NUMBER	NAME	CLASSIFICATION	MAJOR FUNCTION
I	Olfactory	Special sensory	Sense of smell
II	Optic	Special sensory	Conducts impulses for vision from retina on occipital cortex (acuity and field of vision)
III*	Occulomotor	Motor	Eye movements Eyelid elevation Pupillary constriction
IV*	Trochlear		Downward/inward eye movements
VI*	Abducens		Lateral eye movements
V	Trigeminal – three branches: · Ophthalmic · Maxillary · Mandibular	Mixed · Motor · Sensory	Sensory facial sensation of: · Cornea · Face · Mouth · Jaw Motor · Chewing
VII	Facial	Mixed · Motor · Sensory	Sensory · Sensation of the face · Lachrymal glands secretion of tears · Salivary glands secretion of saliva · Sensory-taste – anterior two-thirds of the tongue Motor · Control of facial expression
VIII	Known as: acoustic or vestibular-cochlear	Special sensory	Conducts impulses from the ear to the auditory temporal lobe – hearing Equilibrium

Table 34.8 (Continued)

NUMBER	NAME	CLASSIFICATION	MAJOR FUNCTION
IX	Glossopharyngeal	Mixed · Motor · Sensory	Sensory · Coordination of swallowing and gag reflex · Sensations to pharynx · Taste posterior third of the tongue · Regulation of blood pressure via chemo-receptors in the carotids sinus Motor · Salivation and assists in swallowing
X	Vagus	Mixed · Motor · Sensory	Sensory · Sensation to mucosa of pharynx, soft palate, tonsils, viscera of the thorax and abdomen Motor · Controls swallowing, phonation and movement of the soft palate and uvula · Motility and secretion of gastrointestinal organs · Decreased heart rate
XI	Spinal accessory	Motor	Movement of the head and neck via sternocleidomastoid muscles, upper trapezius
XII	Hypoglossal	Motor	Movement of the tongue facilitating speech, manipulation of food and swallowing

*These three cranial nerves are usually grouped together because they are concerned with eye movement.

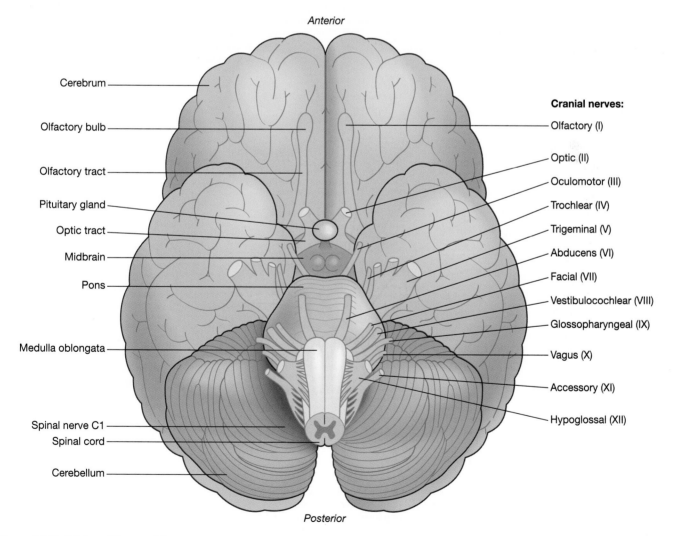

Figure 34.16 Origins of the cranial nerves.

awareness and both are dependent upon a complex network of activating pathways (Table 34.9 and Figure 34.17). Consciousness can be defined as a state of general awareness of oneself and the environment. Consciousness is the most sensitive indicator of neurological change and although it is difficult to measure by directly observing how a patient responds to certain stimuli, it can be estimated.

Altered states of consciousness exist due to the damage of these neural pathways and coma is caused by disordered arousal, rather than impairment of the content of consciousness. There some common terms used to describe the assessment of level of consciousness (LOC), these include: alert, drowsy, confused, stuporous and comatose (see Table 34.10 for patient characteristics and disorders of the consciousness). It is important that the terms used are

Table 34.9 Relationship of the component of consciousness and brain structures.

CONSCIOUSNESS FUNCTION	BRAIN STRUCTURES – PHYSIOLOGICAL AND ANATOMICAL	RELATED TO THE GLASGOW COMA SCALE (GCS)
Arousal (alert and awake) (level of consciousness or arousal)	Arousal depends on an intact ascending reticular activating system (RAS); a network of neurones and fibres arising from the brain stem stimulated by sensory pathways and proceeds through the thalamus to the cerebral cortex Reflects whole brain function rather than a specific region of the brain For arousal to occur, the RAS must be stimulated	Eye opening spontaneously provides an indication of the arousal mechanisms An absence of eye opening implies substantial impairment of the brain stem arousal mechanism Sensory stimuli can activate the RAS, e.g. painful stimuli detected by nociceptors, touch and pressure on the skin, movement of the limbs, bright lights
Awareness (content of consciousness)	Cognitive and affective mental function, dependent on an intact cerebral cortex and RAS	Verbal response is the highest level of response and implies awareness of self and environment Awareness can be evaluated by focussing on four main areas: orientation, attention span language and memory

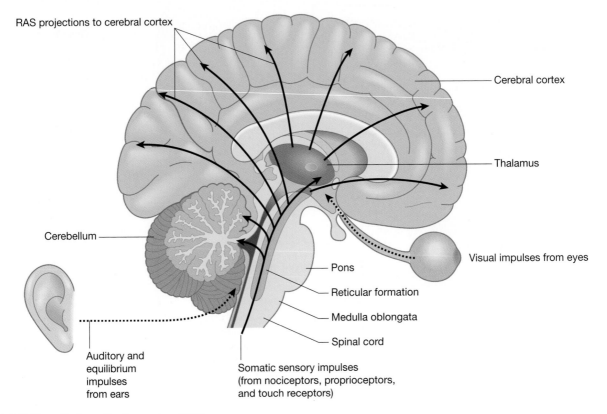

RAS projections to cerebral cortex

Cerebral cortex

Thalamus

Cerebellum

Visual impulses from eyes

Pons

Reticular formation

Medulla oblongata

Spinal cord

Auditory and equilibrium impulses from ears

Somatic sensory impulses (from nociceptors, proprioceptors, and touch receptors)

Figure 34.17 The reticular activating system (RAS).

Table 34.10 Terms used to describe varying levels and disorders of consciousness. Monti *et al.* (2010).

TERMINOLOGY	CHARACTERISTICS
Full consciousness	Alert; oriented to time, place, and person; comprehends spoken and written words
Confusion	Unable to think rapidly and clearly in a logical coherent way; easily bewildered, with poor memory and short attention span; misinterprets stimuli; judgement is impaired, responds to simple orders
Disorientation	Not aware of or not oriented to time, place or person
Obtundation	Lethargic, somnolent; responsive to verbal or tactile stimuli but quickly drifts back to sleep
Stupor	Generally unresponsive; may be briefly aroused by vigorous, repeated or painful stimuli
Semi-comatose	Does not move spontaneously; unresponsive to stimuli, although vigorous or painful stimuli may result in stirring, moaning or withdrawal from the stimuli but without arousal
Coma	Lack of arousal; will not stir or moan in response to any stimulus; may exhibit non-purposeful response (slight movement) of area stimulated, there is no eye opening and no verbal response
Deep coma	Complete lack of arousal and unresponsive to any kind of stimulus, including pain; absence reflexes
Vegetative state 1 month	Wakefulness without awareness of self or surroundings; eyes are open or closed and there is evidence of sleep–wake cycle on EEG. If the vegetative state duration is >1 month, it is termed persistent vegetative state (PVS)
Minimal consciousness state (MCS)	Awareness is partial and inconsistent; there may be purposeful movements; eyes may be open or closed and there is evidence of sleep–wake cycle on EEG. May also be referred to as post-coma unresponsiveness (PCU) or minimally responsive state (MRS)
Locked-in syndrome	Pseudocoma is not a disorder of consciousness, as the patient is fully conscious and has preserved cognitive function, but there is impairment of voluntary motor function. In complete locked in syndrome there are no motor movements

defined and used consistently. Regular neurological assessments identify trends and changes in LOC, and specific signs and neurological function are critical for early detection; even subtle changes may be clinically significant.

The Glasgow coma scale (GCS) (Teasdale & Jennett 1974) is a universal assessment instrument, and provides an indication of the initial severity of trauma to the brain and its subsequent changes over time. The GCS does not diagnose the cause of the altered state of consciousness, it is a rating score to grade the best possible central (brain) response.

The Evidence Glasgow Coma Scale

The Glasgow Coma Scale is the universal gold standard means of assessing consciousness. Initially developed to assess the head injury patient, it is now used to assess a range of patients with neurological problems.

Feature	Response	Score
Best eye response (record C if unable to open eyes, e.g. from orbital swelling or facial fractures)	Opens spontaneous	4
	Open to verbal commands	3
	Open to pain	2
	No eye opening	1
Best verbal response (Record 'ET' if the person has a endotracheal or 'T' for a tracheostomy tube in place and record 'D' if the person is dysphasic)	Orientated to questions	5
	Disorientated/confused	4
	Inappropriate words	3
	Incomprehensible sounds	2
	No verbal response	1
Best motor response (Record best upper arm response)	To verbal commands obeys	6
	To painful stimuli localises pain	5
	Withdrawal from pain	4
	Flexion to pain	3
	Extension to pain	2
	No response to pain	1

(Teasdale & Jennett 1974)

The GCS is also used as an indication of neurological status and to effectively monitor changes. Individual components of the assessment should be adequately described and communicated, both verbally and orally. The GCS comprises three scales, concerning eye opening, verbal response and motor response, for which a score is assigned for each scale, for example a patient with a total score of 12 (3 for eye-opening, 4 for verbal response, 5 for motor response) should be reported as E3, V4 and M5 (NICE 2007). The maximum score of 15 would indicate that patients are fully conscious, alert and responsive. The minimum score of 3 indicates comatose and unresponsive patients.

The nurse must first observe any spontaneous responses to these three scales and use an auditory stimulus if the patient is to be roused, for example speech. If this does elicit a response, then a noxious stimulus is applied. It is generally recommended that central pain is used as a stimuli and the source is either supraorbital pressure or trapezium pinch.

Box 34.1 The AVPU Scale

A = **A**lert	Are they alert?
V = Responds to **v**oice	Do they response to verbal stimulation?
P = Responds to **p**ain	Do they respond to pain?
U = **U**nresponsive	Do they respond at all?

Red Flag

GCS may be affected if:
- Eyes are closed due to severe swelling
- The verbal and motor responses may be absent or reduced as a result of:
  - Intubation
  - Muscle relaxants
  - Sedation or other drugs such as alcohol and recreational drugs

The AVPU can give information easily and quickly about patients' level of consciousness (see Box 34.1). Although AVPU is incorporated into the early-warning scores systems and is ideal in the initial rapid ABCDE assessment, it is not an evidence-based tool and is inadequate in assessing patients with neurological conditions and is not a replacement for the GCS.

The function of the brain, especially the cerebral hemispheres, is dependent on a continuous blood flow with unimpeded supplies of oxygen and glucose. Any process that disrupts the blood flow can cause widespread damage to the cerebral hemispheres, impairing arousal and cognition. Level of consciousness may be altered by processes that affect the arousal functions of the brain stem, the cognitive functions of the cerebral hemispheres, or both major causes are:

1. Intracranial lesions or injuries that affect the cerebral hemispheres or cause dysfunction of the RAS such as:
   - Space occupying lesions that take up space in the intracranial space such as tumour, haematomas and brain abscess
   - Cerebral oedema (brain swelling) and increased intracranial pressure (ICP)
   - Increase in cerebral spinal fluid known as hydrocephalus (dilation of the ventricular system)
   - Stroke
   - Infections – meningitis, encephalitis
   - Injury from excitatory neurotransmitters, such as glutamate
2. Extracranial causes including:
   - Blood sugar alternations hypoglycaemia or hyperglycaemia
   - Fluid and electrolyte imbalances such as hyponatraemia
   - Hypercapnia (abnormal high levels of carbon dioxide)
   - Hypotension
   - Liver dysfunction – encephalopathy
   - Drug such as opioids and benzodiazepine
   - Alcohol.

Vital signs

In the neurological patient, changes in vital signs are not consistent early warning signals. Vitals are more useful in detecting progression to late symptoms. As both respiratory and cardiac centres are located in the brain stem, compression of the brain stem due to raised intracranial pressure will cause changes in vital signs; blood pressure rises to overcome the increased ICP and reflex inhibition causes a slowing of the heart rate. This is usually a late sign and imminent death will occur if the problem is not resolved.

Temperature elevation in the neurological patient can be caused by direct damage to the hypothalamus or traction on the hypothalamus, the primary regulating centre, as a result of increased ICP, CNS infection, subarachnoid haemorrhage, etc. Cerebral tissue generates a large amount of heat due to high metabolic activity and due to the relatively high blood flow and volume, compared with other organs. Temperature is important, as a one degree increase in temperature increases the cerebral metabolic rate by 10%, which could affect neurological recovery. Pyrexia may indicate infections from surgical and or non-surgical sources.

Assessing pupillary reaction

Pupillary assessment is a vital component of neurological assessment. Changes in the size, equality and reactivity of the pupils can provide vital diagnostic information in the critically ill patient. Assessment is performed by shining a light (pen torch) from the temple into each eye in turn and observing and recording the pupillary reaction. A normal pupillary reaction to light should provide a brisk pupil constricting immediately when the light is shone into the eye in both eyes (pupils are equal and reactive to light, PEARL), this is recorded as '+', an unreactive pupils is recorded as '−'. Withdrawal of the light should produce an immediate and brisk dilatation of the pupil referred to as **direct light reflex**. A **consensual light reaction** occurs when light is shone into one pupil and causes a similar constriction to occur simultaneously in the other pupil and when the light is withdrawn from one eye, the opposite pupil should also dilate simultaneously.

The size of the pupil is recorded according to the millimetre scale (as indicated on the neurological observation chart or pen torch); average size is 2–5 mm. It is also important to note the shape of the pupil: a normal pupil should be round, abnormal pupil shapes may be described as ovoid, keyhole or irregular. It is important to record a baseline assessment of pupillary size and shape and compare subsequent assessments with the baseline; any change in reaction, shape and size of the pupil should be reported and documented immediately.

Nurses need to consider the following when performing this procedure:
- Use caution in patients who have recently had a seizures, as flashing a light in their eyes may elicit another seizure
- Certain medication may influence the size of the pupil, e.g. very small pupils (1–2 mm) may suggest the use of opiates and some eye drops, such as atropine, can dilate the pupils
- 17% of the normal population have inequality in size between the pupils, known as *anisocoria*
- Check for pre-existing irregularities in the eye, e.g. ophthalmic conditions, such as cataract, localised injury, false eye.

Red Flag

Sluggish or suddenly dilated unequal pupils are an indication the oculomotor cranial nerve is being compressed due to raised ICP or local compression, e.g. expanding aneurysm. If this is left unrelieved, the pupil will become fixed and dilated ('*blown pupil*') and the oculomotor nerve on the opposite side will also become compressed resulting in bilateral, dilated and fixed pupils.

Motor Function Assessments

Motor function assessment starts with the upper limbs and then progresses to the legs, assess each limb separately, and includes assessment of the three 'Ss':

S – **S**ymmetry observing that both sides of the body move the same

S – **S**ize of the muscle (bulk) observing for wasting atrophy and hypertrophy

S – **S**trength of the muscles (power).

In addition, the muscle tone is assessed; a soft, flabby muscle that fatigues easily is referred to as 'flaccidity', whereas an increased in tone evident by an increased resistance to passive movement is referred to as 'spasticity'. It is important to observe the patients' movements at rest (not making a purposeful movement) and during activity (making a purposeful movement) are observed for involuntary movements, e.g. tremors (rhythmic movements) and fasciculations (irregular movements).

When assessing motor function, from a neurological perspective, the assessment should focus on leg and arm movement. Assessing for symmetry is the most important consideration when identifying focal findings; comparing one side of the body to the other. Asymmetrical spontaneous movement and lateralisation (e.g. hemiparesis and hemiplegia) suggests a focal mass lesion on the side of the brain opposite the side of motor weakness.

In the unconscious patient, motor function and tone can exhibit specific abnormal motor responses and postural patterns depending upon the site of injury and motor tract interruption. These can be divided into two main patterns of posturing:

Decorticate posturing – upper arms are close to the sides; elbows, wrists and fingers are flexed; legs are extended with internal rotation; and feet are plantar flexed. Occurs with lesions of the corticospinal

Decerebrate posturing – neck is extended, jaw clenched; arms are pronated, extended and close to the sides; legs are extended straight out; and feet are plantar flexed. Decerebrate posturing occurs with lesions of the midbrain, pons or diencephalon.

The gait, posture and body positioning in the resting position and during spontaneous movement are also important considerations.

Sensory assessment

Sensory function is an important component of the neurological assessment in people with conditions or diseases affects the spinal cord or spinal nerves. Assessment involves the ability to perceive various sensations this includes:

- Touch – assessed by lightly touching both sides of various parts of the body with one or more of the following: cotton wisp, Neurotip™ (single-use neurological examination pins). Patients should be able to differentiate between soft and sharp
- Sense of position (kinesthesia) a number of tests can be performed, e.g. the assessor moves the patient's finger or big toe up or down with the patients eyes shut; the patient should be able to accurately describe the position of finger or toe when moved up or down.

Assessing the system – diagnostic tests

To enable effective neurological nursing and medical care, an accurate diagnosis is essential. Following physical and neurological examinations, a number of diagnostic tests may be ordered to investigate any abnormal findings. Commencing with the least invasive procedures and proceeding to more invasive investigations. Often the purpose of these investigations is to rule out certain diagnosis and treatment options. Diagnostic investigations may be performed in a variety of settings, such as neuro-radiology departments, day-care units, and specific procedural departments, either as an outpatient or during hospitalisation. Many neurological disorders are incurable, presenting the patients with long-term disability and thus can be anxiety provoking for both the patient and their families. Nurses need to be able to provide:

- Emotional support to patients by educating them on the procedure
- Relevant nursing care before, during and after the procedure.

Common investigations and the key nursing considerations are described in Table 34.11.

Nursing care and management of the unconscious patient

Nursing care for an unconscious person is both general and specific. For general nursing care issues, see Chapter 6. More specific nursing care considerations include the following:

Maintaining a patent airway Support of the airway and respirations is vital in the person with an altered LOC, and presents difficulties of ineffective airway clearance and risk of aspiration. A patient who is drowsy may only require an oral pharyngeal airway, such as a Guedel airway or a nasopharyngeal tube. However, more severe alterations in consciousness may require endotracheal intubation or a tracheostomy to maintain airway patency. Patients may have a depressed or absent gag and swallowing reflex due to depression of the medullary centres, this presents a high risk for aspiration, increases the risk of pneumonia. Mechanical ventilation is indicated when hypoventilation or apnoea is present. Specific nursing care includes:

- Monitoring breath sounds, rate and depth of respirations and report signs and symptoms of aspiration: crackles and wheezes, dyspnoea, tachypnoea and cyanosis
- Suctioning to clear the oropharyngeal/tracheostomy of secretion as required that might otherwise be aspirated
- Position the person to allow secretions to drain from the mouth rather than into the pharynx, e.g. lateral position
- Maintain oxygen saturation levels via prescribed oxygen therapy, monitoring oxygen levels via pulse oximetry and arterial blood gas analysis.

Maintaining hydration and nutrition The patient with reduced consciousness may not be able to maintain normal nutritional status due to reduced intake of nutrients, swallowing problems or

Table 34.11 Common investigations and the key nursing considerations.

INVESTIGATION	RATIONALE	NURSING CONSIDERATIONS
Radiological examinations		
Skull and spine X-rays: use high-energy electromagnetic radiation.	Evaluate the bones of the skull/spine to detect · Fractures · Displacement of vertebrae and tissues · Abnormal curves of the spinal	Ensure that metal hairclips and any jewellery is removed from the head and neck Reassure the patient that the procedure is painless
Computed tomography (CAT) scan: 3-dimensional (3D) pictures inside the body in grey tones correlating with tissue density, e.g. bone and blood appears white, while air appears black.	To detect: · Abnormalities and signs of diseases/conditions · Evaluate the course of some lesions postoperatively and following chemotherapy	Ensure that metal hairclips and any jewellery is removed from the head and neck Inform the patient that they will need to lie flat and still and that the procedure is painless Ensure patients' allergies are documented, in particular shellfish and iodine, inform radiology department i.v. contrast agent may be administered to provide further anatomical clarity Renal function may need to be evaluated as the contrast needs to be excreted through the kidneys Inform patient that they may experience a warm feeling when the contrast agent is injected.
Magnetic resonance imaging (MRI): uses a powerful magnetic field generated by large gradient coils that electricity passes through to create a detailed computerised image Contrast agent called 'Gadolinium' is often used to provide anatomical clarity.	To visualise the body to detect: · Abnormalities and signs of diseases/conditions	Identification of any contraindications, such as patients with medical or electronic devices (e.g. pacemakers, cochlear implants and metal pins) Ensure that jewellery, hairclips and any metal objects are removed, as they interfere with the magnetic field of the MRI scanner Inform the patient that they will need to lie flat in a large cylinder-shaped tube surrounded by the magnet, which may be claustrophobic and due to vibration of the magnet, it produces loud banging noise, which can be disturbing. Inform the patient that they will be able to talk to staff during the scan through a microphone
Cerebral blood flow tests		
Cerebral angiography: an invasive procedure carried out with or without sedation; involves the threading of a catheter via the femoral artery up into the desired vessels in the brain.	To visualise blood vessels in the brain and neck and detect an cerebrovascular abnormalities To locate surgical clips placed on blood vessels during surgery	Patients may need to be nil by mouth for a period of time before the procedure Regular neurological observations including vital signs, pre -and post-procedure Assessing the puncture site for haemorrhage and haematomas Assess the peripheral circulation via pedal pulses, and colour and warmth of extremities to detect possible embolism the femoral artery Bed-rest for a period specified according to the underlying diagnosis
CT angiography (CTA): usually involves the injection of contrast medium via a peripheral i.v. cannula and a series of images are taken of the cerebral vessels.	To investigate vascular disease or anomalies used to determine: · Vessel patency · Circulation · Provide details of vascular anomalies	As per CT scan with contrast
MR angiography (MRA): examines blood flow, involves films being taken at various time intervals. MRA can be performed with or without the injection of contrast medium.		As per MRI above

Table 34.11 (*Continued*)

INVESTIGATION	RATIONALE	NURSING CONSIDERATIONS
Neurophysiology tests		
Electromyogram (EMG): Involves inserting a very fine needle into muscles (EMG) or in the case of nerve conduction studies stimulating the nerves using small electrical pulses to record and analyse the activity of the muscle or nerve.	To test the integrity and functioning of skeletal muscles and large myelinated nerve fibres in the arms and legs Used to diagnose and evaluate neuromuscular diseases and identify nerve damage	Explain to the patient that they may experience a feeling similar to an intramuscular injection as the needle is inserted
Evoked potentials: Measure the brain's response to particular stimuli, e.g. Visual evoked responses (VEP) measure the visual pathway from the retina to the occipital cortex.	Used to diagnose and evaluate neuromuscular diseases and identify nerve damage	Encourage the patient to be still during the procedure to prevent artefacts occurring that may interfere with the recordings and interpretation of the test
Electroencephalogram (EEG): several small electrodes are applied to the scalp with skin clips and a graphic picture is obtained (similar to an ECG of the heart), over a specific period of time.	Measure the electrical activity of the brain; useful for: · In the diagnosis and management of epilepsy · Monitor brain activity in brain disease · Monitoring during brain surgery · Confirm brain death	Explain to the patient that the test is painless and the test lasts about 45–60 min Advise the patient to wash their hair prior to the procedure Certain medication may withheld prior to the test, e.g. anticonvulsants, depressants because these medication alter the EEG wave patterns Coffee, tea and other foods containing caffeine may also be withheld up to 8 hours prior to the test
Lumbar puncture (LP): involves inserting a spinal needle into the subarachnoid space of the spinal canal, usually between L3–L4 or L4–L5, once the local anaesthetic has taken effect.	To: · Measure and reduce CSF pressure · To obtain a sample of CSF for laboratory analysis · To detect blood in the CSF · Administer medication intrathecally	Normally performed while the patient is in bed with the patient lying on their left side with their knees drawn up to their chest Baseline and post-procedure observations are recorded Encouraged rest and drink plenty of fluids Assess for post-puncture headache caused by CSF leakage at the puncture site and the normal CSF mechanics is disrupted, administer analgesia as required and encourage hydration
Muscle biopsy: the procedure involves removing a small sample of muscle (e.g. top of the thigh) via a needle under local anaesthetic.	Enables the examination of muscle tissue to diagnose conditions associated with muscle weakness	Explain to the patient that during the biopsy, there is usually minimal or no discomfort; the patient may feel some pressure or 'tugging' sensations Observe and report any bleeding, swelling and haematomas and any signs of infection at the biopsy wound Assess for pain at the biopsy site; as the anaesthetic wears off administer pain relief, as required

due to cognitive inability to initiate eating. In nutritional assessments, early dietetic advice early on is crucial and enteral nutrition is important, to minimise the effect of protein catabolism and the ensuing loss of lean body mass by providing sufficient energy and protein. Patient may commence with nasogastric feeding, but longer-term enteral feeding regimes are supported with percutaneous endoscopic gastrostomy (PEG) feeding.

Maintaining mobility and skin integrity Patients who are unconscious are unable to maintain normal musculoskeletal movement and thus are at high risk for contractures related to decreased

movement and an inability to maintain skin integrity. Because the flexor and adductor muscles are stronger than the extensors and abductors, flexor and adductor contractures develop quickly without preventive measures. Passive range-of-motion motion (ROM) exercises (unless contraindicated) must be performed routinely to maintain muscle tone and function, to prevent additional disability and to help restore impaired motor function. The use of removable orthoses to hold limbs in position, for example a wrist splint or ankle foot orthosis, to prevent plantar flexion of the limbs, may be employed under the direction of the physiotherapist or occupational therapist.

Red Flag

- Do not position the unconscious person on their back: as their tongue may slide back and occlude their airway, and any vomit will not be able to drain out
- Assess the patients swallow reflex before starting any oral feeding programme

The Patient with Raised Intracranial Pressure

In the adult, the rigid, enclosed inelastic cranial cavity created by the skull is normally filled to capacity with three non-compressible interchangeable components; 85% is brain (5% extracellular fluid, 45% glial tissue and 35% neuronal tissue), 7% blood and 8% CSF account for the remaining approximate 15% of the skull contents. The pressure exerted by these three non-compressible contents of the cranium is referred to as intracranial pressure (ICP). Increased intracranial pressure (IICP) is sustained elevated pressure more than 10 mmHg or higher within the cranial cavity. Transient increases in ICP occur with normal activities, such as coughing, sneezing, straining or bending forward; these are not normally harmful. However, sustained IICP alters cerebral perfusion and oxygenation of brain cells and can result in significant tissue ischaemia and damage to delicate neural tissue. A significant number of neurological patients are at risk of developing IICP.

Pathophysiology

The *Monro–Kellie hypothesis* states that the sum of the intracranial volumes of blood, brain and CSF is constant. An increase in volume in any one of the intracranial components must be offset by a decrease in one or more of the others or be associated with a rise in ICP. The body has a limited ability to reduce the volume of these components. Early compensatory mechanism include displacement of some CSF to the spinal subarachnoid space and increased CSF absorption, venous system is also compressed, and cerebral arteries constrict to reduce blood flow. Once these compensatory mechanisms are exhausted then ICP rises, cerebral perfusion pressure (mean arterial pressure – ICP, see Box 34.2) falls, cerebral tissue becomes ischaemic, and signs and symptoms of cellular hypoxia appear.

Another important physiological mechanism is the autoregulation of cerebral blood flow (CBF). Neurones produce energy from

oxidising glucose and the brain cannot store glucose thus a constant blood supply is required to supply oxygen and glucose. Under normal conditions, the brain has the ability to auto regulate ensuring that cerebral blood flow (CBF), the amount of blood volume in the brain at any given time, remains relatively stable, despite change in blood pressure, for example if the blood pressure drops, cerebral blood vessels vasodilate, increasing CBF. CBF is affected by the following:

- Increased blood carbon dioxide levels causing vasodilation
- Decreases in arterial blood pH
- Decrease in arterial blood oxygen levels
- Changes in blood pressure; a decrease in MAP may result in a decrease CBF.

If significant ICP elevations are not aggressively treated, then severe, permanent neurological deficits or death will occur. Death occurs as a result of displaced cerebral tissue from its normal compartment through the tentorium cerebelli (double fold of dural mater), which separates the cerebrum from the cerebellum, compressing the brain stem and eventual cerebellar herniation, referred to as tentorium herniation or 'coning'. Increased ICP results from three main causes:

- A rise in cerebrospinal fluid pressure resulting in a dilatation of the ventricular system referred to as hydrocephalus ('water on the brain') due to over production, decreased absorption or obstruction of flow
- It can also be due to increased pressure within the brain matter caused by a mass (space occupying lesion, SOL), often referred to as the 'mass effect', e.g. tumour, haemorrhage, abscess
- Or swelling within the brain matter itself, due to abnormal accumulation of fluid, which subsequently impedes CBF due to the compression of the blood vessels, referred to as cerebral oedema.

Signs and symptoms

These may differ according to the speed and cause of the IICP and include:

- Headache, usually throbbing in nature and classically worse on rising in the morning due to: a rise in ICP during the night as a result of typically being flat; a rise in pCO_2 during sleep caused by respiratory depression, and a decrease in CSF absorption
- Headaches may worsen with position changes, coughing and straining
- Vomiting caused by pressure on the vomiting centre located in the fourth ventricle
- Oculomotor dysfunction – inability to move eye(s) upward; ptosis (drooping) of eyelid due to compression of the third cranial nerve (occulomotor)
- Papilloedema (swelling of the optic discs), which will eventually lead to visual abnormalities, such as decreased visual acuity, blurred vision and even blindness
- Double vision (diplopia)
- Progressive deterioration in conscious level due to displacement of the brain stem
- Late signs include: decreased level of consciousness, seizures and pupillary dysfunction – sluggish response to light progressing to fixed pupils (pupillary dysfunction is first noted on the same (ipsilateral) side)
- Other late signs include: 'Cushing response' (hypertension, widening pulse pressure, bradycardia and irregular respirations).

Box 34.2 Cerebral Perfusion Pressure

Cerebral perfusion pressure (CPP) is the pressure gradient of the mean arterial blood pressure (MAP) driving the blood into the cranial vault against the opposing pressure to keep the blood out the ICP; calculated by the following equation:

ICP – (mean arterial blood pressure) **MAP**

= **CPP** (normal CPP range 70–95 mmHg).

For example in a healthy person, ICP 10 – MAP (systolic 145 – diastolic 60 = 85) 85 = CPP of 75.

Cerebral blood flow (CBF) – normal flow is 750 mL/min, 15% of the cardiac output and fluctuates to meet the brain's constant high oxygen and metabolic demands.

Red Flag

Acutely increased intrathoracic pressure causes a significant increase in intracranial pressure and a decrease in cerebral perfusion pressure.

Increased intrathoracic pressure reduces outflow via the jugular venous system and venous return to the heart and thus cardiac output resulting in a temporary drop in blood pressure. This is followed immediately with an increase in blood pressure far beyond the original values, this increases central venous pressure which reduces venous return and increases intracranial pressure.

Increase in intrathoracic pressure can occur during the following:

- *Valsalva's* manoeuvre that accompanies straining on defecation
- Coughing (intra-abdominal pressure), sneezing, vomiting
- Bladder distention
- Extreme hip flexion.

Diagnosis and investigations

A patient presenting with signs of raised ICP requires an urgent CT scan to identify the presence of raised ICP and its underlying cause and to evaluate therapeutic options.

Nursing care and management

Primary management is directed at, if possible, removing the underlying cause of the ICP. This may involve intracranial surgical techniques to removal a mass (e.g. tumour haematoma), medical treatment of cerebral oedema associated with tumours with dexamethasome (corticosteroid) and strategies to manage hydrocephalus, such as insertion of shunts to redirect the CSF. In addition, treatment is aimed at maintaining adequate CPP, maximising venous return, reducing blood and CSF volumes.

Monitoring Multimodal monitoring to monitor changes in intracranial dynamics includes: mean arterial pressure, central venous pressure, pulse, ICP and temperature.

ICP monitoring is essential in the patients' management; facilitating early detection of increases in ICP and disease progression and monitoring of medical therapy and nursing interventions, preserving brain function and preventing secondary brain damage from raised ICP. Monitoring provides continual assessment of ICP and several monitoring devices for measuring ICP are available, including: extracranial transducers and intracranial transducers.

Treatment strategies Medications:

- Diuretics for the management of cerebral oedema, such as osmotic diuretics for example Mannitol, used to draw fluid out of the extracellular space by increasing the osmolality of the blood and loop diuretics for example frusemide
- Sedation, propofol is commonly used, when patients are receiving mechanical ventilation to control restlessness and agitation, because this can increase blood pressure, ICP, and cerebral metabolism
- Antipyretics to reduce hyperthermia, decreasing the high cerebral metabolism that contributes to ICP.

CSF drainage – a drainage catheter or shunt may be inserted into a ventricle to drain excess cerebrospinal fluid and reduce hydrocephalus known as external ventricular drain.

Hyperventilation – maintaining adequate oxygenation and control of respiratory gases preventing hypoxemia and hypercapnia, both can increase intracranial pressure.

In some circumstances, when all other measure to reduce ICP proves ineffective decompressive craniotomy is performed; this involves the removal of part of the skull to increase the intracranial volume and thus reduce ICP.

Specific nursing strategies

- Regular monitoring of conscious level and neurological status using the GCS
- Promote optimal respiratory function – regular assessment and recording of respiratory rate depth and chest symmetry, O_2 saturation and arterial blood gases, suctioning to maintain airway patency as required
- It may be necessary to mechanically ventilate to control the partial pressure of O_2 (pO_2) and CO_2 (pCO_2) to within set parameters aiming to avoid hypoxia and hypocapnia as this will increase CBF and ICP and impair CCP
- Elevation of the head of the bed to 30 degrees to promote venous return via the jugular veins
- Avoiding positions that may obstruct venous obstruction, for example tracheotomy tapes and cervical collars secured too tightly, and neck rotation and neck and head flexion
- Maintain normovolaemia through accurate fluid balance as hypovolaemia causes hypotension and a fall in CPP; avoid dextrose solutions as this increases cerebral metabolism and oedema, thus increasing ICP
- Avoid the patients being constipated by monitoring and recording bowel movement
- Monitor for signs of seizure and administer antiepileptic drugs (AEDs), seizures will result in increase in CBF which could further increase ICP
- Keep the patient comfortable and pain free to prevent rises in blood pressure and subsequent ICP
- Treat pyrexia as an increase in body temperature of 1°C increases cerebral metabolism by up to 10% and therefore an rise in ICP
- Maintain nutritional support this may require enteral feeding (N/G or PEG).

Traumatic Brain Injury (Head Injury)

Traumatic brain injury (TBI) is defined as an alteration in brain function as a result of injury from external causes. External causes include the head striking or being struck by an object, which may penetrate the brain, and the brain undergoing an acceleration/deceleration movement. Severity can range from mild concussion to coma or death. TBI is a leading cause of mortality and morbidity in young people, and is a worldwide public health problem that can cause long-term disability even in mild TBI, with impairments including physical, cognitive and psychological disabilities. It not only disrupts the patient's life but also the lives of their families/caregivers and social economic costs are high. Even though the best chance of survival is referral to a specialist neuroscience centre (NICE 2007), many TBI patients are managed in general critical care units.

Epidemiology

Epidemiological data is inconsistent and difficult to collate, partly due to the fact that the majority of TBIs are classified as mild (80%)

are not admitted to hospital and many do not seek medical assistance. However, data indicates that approximately 700 000 patients per year will attend emergency departments in the UK, with a predominance of the adolescent and young adult men and the elderly population.

The main causes of a TBI include:

- Falls, accounting for 20–30%, although severe head trauma is rare in home accidents
- Road traffic accidents, which cause the greatest severity of injury and most common cause of moderate to severe TBI in 15–25 years
- Injuries sustained at home or at work
- Other causes of TBI include sports-related trauma, for example in a contact sport, such as rugby and abuse.

Pathophysiology

Each TBI has a unique set of circumstances and consequences for the patient. Despite this, there are several ways of classifying a TBI, a common categorisation is mild, moderate and severe, which is dependent upon certain characteristics including: GCS, period of loss of consciousness and length of time (post-injury) patients remain in a post-traumatic amnesic state (PTA), which is a period of confusion and disorientation after emergence from coma (see Table 34.12).

In addition to classifying the injury according to severity, a TBI can be classified according to outcome, mechanism of injury (how it happened), the location of the injury either focal or diffuse, and whether the injury is open or closed.

Outcome Outcome can be measured by using the Glasgow Outcome Scale (GOS) (Jennet & Bond 1975) based on five categories, ranging from death to low disability; the scale predicts the long-term course of rehabilitation to return to work and everyday life.

Mechanisms of injury The mechanism of injury is often referred to as the 'primary injury' (induced by a mechanical force):

- Acceleration injury when the head is struck by a moving object, e.g. being hit a cricket ball
- Deceleration injury when the head hits a stationary object, e.g. falls

- Acceleration-deceleration injury occurs when the head hits an object and the brain 'rebounds' within the skull, e.g. road traffic accidents
- Penetrating brain injury (PBI) caused by high velocity objects, e.g. bullets, and low velocity objects, e.g. knives
- Blast-induced TBI injuries due to direct exposure to over-pressurised waves (the mechanism is not fully understood).

Location of the injury – focal or diffuse Focal:

- Scalp laceration
- Skull fractures – linear (simple) majority of skull fractures, comminuted (bone is crushed into small fragments) or depressed (inward depression of the bone)
- Contusion – a bruise on the surface of the brain occurs as a result of the patient being either struck on the head, striking his or her head against a hard surface or as a result of excessive acceleration or deceleration forces being exerted on the brain
- Intracranial haemorrhage and haematomas – extradura (in the potential space between the dural and skull), subdural (bleeding between the dural and arachnoid) or intracerebral (bleeding into the brain tissue itself).

Diffuse:

- Diffuse or global ischaemic injury involving the grey matter
- Due to hypotension, or secondary to raised ICP, resulting in reduced CBF
- Diffuse axonal injury (DAI), disruption of the axons in the white matter bundles and tracts as result of rotational forces occurring when the brain undergoes rapid acceleration and deceleration; often as result of road traffic accidents. Ranges from mild DAI, seen in concussion (mild TBI), to severe
- Brain swelling – either locally as a result of contusion or diffuse involving one or both cerebral hemispheres.

Open or closed

- Open (penetrating) injury when the outer layer of the meninges is breached (e.g. from a knife, bullet); and may result in injuries to the skull (including fractures), laceration or tears, damage to blood vessels
- Closed head injury without the integrity of the skull being compromised.

Table 34.12 Overview of classifying TBI by severity.

TBI GRADE	GCS SCORE	SYMPTOMS	MORBIDLY
Mild – often referred to as concussion	GCS 13–15	LOC <30 min PTA <1 hour Transient symptoms, e.g. dizziness, confusion, headache and vomiting	Post-concussional syndrome (PCS): · Somatic (such as headache, nausea and vomiting, dizziness, fatigue or feeling tired) · Cognitive (such as feeling like in a fog, slow reaction times, lack of concentration) · Emotional symptoms (such as lability, irritability and nervousness)
Moderate	GCS 9–13	LOC 1–24 hours PTA 30 min–24 hours Lethargic or stuporous	May have focal neurological deficits Displays a wide spectrum of physical, cognitive and behavioural impairments
Severe	GCS 3–8	LOC PTA Severe 1–7 days Very severe 1–4 weeks Extremely severe >4 weeks	Permanent neurological sequelae Functional disability

Secondary injuries Defined as the progressive events that occur after the initial (primary) injury and includes: cerebral oedema, vascular injury, seizures and infection. When the brain is injured, the response is complex and multifaceted. A neurometabolic cascade occurs, which causes neurophysiologically destruction or disruption of the neuronal network via neurone and glia death and/or damage to the axon tracts. The adult brain has a limited ability to regenerate and reorganise the CNS, referred to as *plasticity*. Although neurones cannot regenerate themselves, axonal branch growth can reactivate and functions may recover. Post-traumatic oedema is the leading prognostic factor in TBI patients, despite the current available treatment options.

Red Flag

Post-traumatic oedema is the leading prognostic factor in TBI patients and can be the result of:

- Falling from a height greater than 1 metre
- The individual lands on his or her head or feet
- Pedestrians that are hit by vehicles
- High speed injuries

(NICE 2007)

Diagnosis and investigations

Radiological examinations include; skull X-rays (to identify skull fractures and assess penetrating objects), CT scan or MRI, to detect contusions and lacerations associated with diffuse axonal injury. Other investigations include oxygen saturations and ABGs are analysed, with particular attention to oxygen and carbon dioxide levels. TBI patients are at high risk of an associated cervical spine injury and should have their neck protected; immobilised until further investigations can be carried out, e.g. cervical spine X-ray.

Signs and symptoms

Signs and symptoms are varied according to the area of the brain that has been injured. Compression of the brain tissue may result in seizure.

Red Flag

The following red flag signs and symptoms are markers of a more severe TBI:

- Loss of consciousness at any time
- GCS <15 on initial assessment
- Focal neurological deficit
- Retrograde or anterograde amnesia
- Persistent headache
- Vomiting or seizures post-injury

When the brain is injured, the response is also complex and multifaceted. The entire spectrum of TBI, from mild to severe, can change a persons' function in three major areas: physical including language, cognitive, emotional/behavioural. However, it is the unseen cognitive, behavioural and emotional sequelae that causes the most serious long-term morbidity and are most important in determining independence, social functioning and family adjustment. These difficulties can negatively impact on patients' ability to establish productive and satisfying lifestyles, and affect family members and caregivers; causing caregiver burden, distress

Table 34.13 Common physical, cognitive, emotional and behavioural problems associated with TBI.

FUNCTION	PROBLEM AND DYSFUNCTION
Physical	Somatic, such as headache, nausea and vomiting, dizziness, fatigue or feeling tired and sleep disturbances Visual changes Changes in hearing Paresis or paralysis Coordination problems Spasticity Impaired speed of movement Post-traumatic seizure disorders
Language	Verbal fluency, word finding and difficulty putting thoughts into words Concept formation Verbal comprehension Perseveration and confabulation
Cognitive	Memory, short-term, simply forgetting, can lead to repeated requests for information Poor attention and concentration Lack of insight and awareness Impaired problem-solving Poor initiation
Emotional	Depression Agitation, abusive and irritable Frustration and lack of tolerance Anxiety Anger and emotional labile (feeling up and down, emotionally) Apathy and lack of empathy
Behavioural	Confusion and disorientation Disinhibition such as swearing Impulsivity such as Restlessness Acts of aggression Excitement Change in personality (not the same person)

and a sense of loss (Braine 2011). Common physical, language and non-physical problems following TBI are summarised in Table 34.13.

Nursing care and management

The management of TBI patients is aimed at re-establishing the equilibrium of the intracranial contents and to prevent secondary injury (from ischaemia, hypoxia and cerebral compression). Neurological observations (see GCS earlier) are essential, providing a baseline for comparison for future observations and immediate evidence of any deterioration or responses to treatment strategies. Establishing the level of consciousness is an important factor in determining outcome and prognosis. The person with a TBI has or is at high risk for raised ICP (see earlier).

Early assessment and management involves:

- Assessment and stabilisation of the airway, breathing and circulation
- Assessment of neurological status
- Ascertaining the degree of the injury in order to initiate appropriate levels of care.

The **ABCDE**

A – **A**irway: intubation is required for severe TBI patients (GCS <8)

B – **B**reathing: maintain oxygenation and normocapnia

C – **C**irculation:
- Measure heart rate and blood pressure
- Treat hypotension, aiming for a target mean arterial pressure (MAP) of above 80 mmHg (NICE 2007)

D – **D**isability: assess consciousness using the GCS for baseline and to detect changes in conscious level, and assess severity of the injury

E – **E**xposure and environment: look for signs of injury, e.g. scalp wounds bleeding from ears and nose.

Surgery may include the following:

- Surgical evacuation of a clot either via burr holes made into the skull, or via a craniotomy, e.g. chronic SDH because the haematoma tends to solidify, making it difficult or impossible to remove through burr holes
- Decompressive craniectomy, the removal of part of the cranium (skull) in order to relieve pressure on the underlying brain and allowing the brain to swell upward rather than downward where it will compress the brain stem, which is critical for all of the basic vital functions, leading to brain death.

TBI provokes hypercatabolism and if left unmanaged, the ensuing malnutrition accentuates immune compromise so increasing the risk of infection. To prevent lean loss of body mass and improve outcomes (Cook *et al.* 2008), early nutritional assessment and referral to dietician for feeding regimes such as enteral feeding is critical.

As cerebral cellular respiration is entirely dependent on a constant supply of glucose, there is a risk of cell death during periods of hypoglycaemia. Thus, close monitoring of serum blood glucose is desirable during conditions of cerebral ischaemia, TBI, seizure or other severe neurological impairment, as the glucose requirements needed by the brain to heal and return to normal metabolism are thought to be enhanced (Oddo *et al.* 2008).

Red Flag

Never suction a person nasally if they have a basilar skull fracture or have CSF draining from the ears or nose, as catheters could be inadvertently advanced into the cranial cavity.

Primary care Survival with moderate and severe disability after TBI is common, even patients following mild TBI can have residual deficits for several months, and require rehabilitation and life-long care. Successful rehabilitation requires a multidisciplinary approach involving the family throughout. Adjustment following TBI is a dynamic process and changes over time. Following mild TBI, if symptoms persist beyond the typical recovery period of 3 months, the term 'post-concussion' syndrome is used. The long-term impact following moderate TBI is more variable and may result in persistent learning difficulties and the inability to develop effective social skills.

TBI affects the whole family, not just the injured person and caregiver research suggests that providing care for a family member who has suffered a TBI can be stressful, distressing, burdensome

and depressing and may exacerbate existing physiological conditions such as hypertension. Furthermore, TBI can have devastating consequences for the family as a whole, disrupting the family equilibrium of roles performed within the family unit, and families may also grieve the loss of their loved one as they knew them before the injury (Braine 2011).

Providing timely and appropriate information is an important consideration for both the patient and family and referral to other support services, such as chaplain and support organisations may be useful.

Jot This Down

Families and carers are important aspects of the rehabilitation process for a patient with a TBI. Try to identify some strategies that you might deploy to involve families and carers when providing care to patients with TBI.

Following TBI, the ability to drive again is an important indicator of recovery, and stopping a patient from driving is associated with a loss of social activities and independence. In the UK, drivers are required to inform the Driver and Vehicle Licensing Agency (DVLA) if they have any disability which is likely to last for more than 3 months and which may affect their fitness to drive. It is an offence not to inform the DVLC and the onus is on the patient to inform DVLC. Nurses should familiarise themselves with the current regulations and advice, and have a responsibility to raise awareness of the legalities of driving with a medical condition and should advise the patient to stop driving, particularly when there is concern for the safety of the patient and/or other road users.

 Link To/Go To

DVLC for leaflet D100 – What you need to know about driving licences.

http://www.dft.gov.uk/dvla/forms.aspx

Leaflet D100 is also available at the Post Office.

 Link To/Go To

Headway – The Brain Injury Association

A charity that works to improve life after brain injury, with services divided into regions throughout the UK and Channel Islands.

https://www.headway.org.uk/home.aspx

Stroke

A stroke is a preventable and treatable disease, characterised by a gradual or rapid onset of neurological deficits due to a sudden decrease in cerebral blood flow to an area of the brain. It is a major medical emergency, requiring rapid treatment in order to prevent avoidable death and long-term disability.

Epidemiology

Stroke is a major healthcare problem in the UK, and one in six people will have a stroke in their lifetime (Seshadri & Wolf 2007). Stroke remains the third-biggest killer in the UK and one of the most important causes of significant adult disability, with over 150 000 new cases of stroke per year (RCP 2012). Few stroke victims will make a full recovery; most are left with some form of disability. An estimated 20–30% of people who have had a stroke will die within 1 month. The risk of recurrent stroke is 26% within 5 years of a first stroke and 39% by 10 years (Mohen *et al.* 2011).

Pathophysiology

There are two main types of stroke: **ischaemic** and **haemorrhagic**:

- Ischaemic: up to 80–85% of all strokes caused by blockage of one of the arteries in the brain and reduced blood oxygen supply to brain cells, which can lead to irreversible brain damage and death of brain cells; known as 'infarction'
- Haemorrhagic: a bleed in the brain (burst blood vessel) known as 'cerebral haemorrhage'; (about 15–20% of all strokes).

Potential risk factors There are several risk factors for stroke and these are summarised in Box 34.3.

Transient ischaemic attack (TIA), often referred to as a 'mini-stroke', is a clinical syndrome presenting as acute loss of focal cerebral or monocular function, due to inadequate cerebral or ocular blood supply, and lasting less than 24 hours; there is rarely a loss of consciousness and a complete recovery. TIAs may be an indication that a stroke may occur.

Box 34.3 Risk Factors for Stroke

Controlling factors:

Lifestyle
- Smoking
- Being overweight
- Lack of exercise and physical inactivity
- Dietary factors, such as high saturated fats (hyperlipidaemia)
- Exceeding the recommended daily alcohol limit
- Drug abuse, e.g. cocaine can cause a rapid rise in blood pressure leading to haemorrhagic stroke.

Medical factors
- Hypertension
- Atrial fibrillation (an irregular heartbeat)
- Heart disease
- Carotid artery disease, e.g. atherosclerosis leading to stenosis (15–25% of strokes)
- High cholesterol levels
- Diabetes mellitus
- Sickle cell disease
- Oral contraceptive pill.

Uncontrolling factors:
- Age, incidences of stroke increases dramatically over the age of 55 years
- Gender, more common in men than women
- Race (higher incidences are found in South Asian, Africa and the Caribbean)
- Family history of stroke or TIA
- Fibromuscular dysplasia.

Red Flag

Ischaemic stroke and TIAs commonly are more likely to occur:

- when the blood pressure is at its lowest, i.e. waking from sleep
- when there is a sudden change in blood pressure, which may dislodge a embolism in the arterial circulation, e.g. getting out of bed.

Signs and symptoms

The constellations of signs and symptoms of the neurological deficits reflect the affected vessel along with the size and areas of the brain affected and the length of time blood flow is decreased or stopped. Signs and symptoms include:

- Loss of consciousness, nausea and vomiting
- Localised (focal) sensory and motor deficits, usually one sided
- Seizure activity
- Communication difficulties
- Visual field deficit up to 25% (Ramono 2011)
- Behavioural and emotional changes.

As the motor pathways cross at the junction of the medulla and spinal cord (decussation), loss or impairment of sensory-motor functions occurs on the side of the body opposite the side of the brain that is damaged. A stroke in the right hemisphere therefore will be manifested by deficits in the left side of the body (and vice versa). Hemiplegia that develops as a result of loss of descending motor control is may occur in two stages: initially a reduced tone with a flaccid limb (hypotonia) and if the muscle tone recovers, then this may result in a spastic (hypertonia) limb, known as spastic paralysis.

Stroke can be classified according to the vessels involved (see The Evidence Box below).

The Evidence Oxford Stroke Classification: Bamford Classification

The Bamford classification system is a relatively simple, robust, bedside method of classifying acute ischaemic strokes. It divides people with stroke into four different categories, according to the symptoms and signs with which they present:

- *Total anterior circulation (TAC)* – all of these symptoms: motor or sensory deficits, homonymous hemianopia, dysphasia and visual-spatial deficits
- *Partial anterior circulation (PAC)* – two of following: motor or sensory deficit; higher cerebral dysfunction; homonymous hemianopia
- *Posterior circulation (POC)* – any of the following: homonymous haemianopia; brain stem signs; bilateral motor/sensory deficits, cerebellar ataxia
- *Lacunar (LAC)* – pure motor and or pure sensory deficits no other impairment.

(Bamford *et al.* 1991).

Diagnosis and investigations

Early assessment and diagnosis is crucial for effective management decisions. This may begin outside the hospital when a person suddenly develops neurological symptoms, with screening using the **FAST** tool to confirm likely stroke or transient ischaemic attack (TIA) (Box 34.4). Nearly half of the stroke risk following a TIA

Box 34.4 FAST Assessment

F – Facial weakness:
  · Can the person smile?
  · Has their mouth or eye drooped?
A – Arm weakness:
  · Can the person raise both arms?
S – Speech problems:
  · Can the person speak clearly and understand what you say?
T – Time to call 999
  · If you see any single one of these signs.

(DH 2009)

Box 34.5 Post-TIA and Stroke Targeted Advice/Information

· Leading a healthy, active lifestyle aimed at preventing a reoccurrence:
  · Smoking cessation referrals/support, e.g. refer to smoking cessation groups
  · Obesity-diet advice, referrals
  · Reduced alcohol intake
  · Lack of exercise – information, referrals
  · Ethnicity – African-Caribbean/Asian – targeted information and monitoring
· Regular monitoring of blood pressure and compliance with prescribed antihypertensive therapy and salt reduction
· Raised blood cholesterol may be treated with lipid-lowering drugs, e.g. statins
· Early detection of diabetes and careful monitoring and treatment
· Carotid artery disease treatment may include:
  · Antiplatelet therapy
  · Carotid endarterectomy
· Persistent or paroxysmal atrial fibrillation – advice re anticoagulation
· Ischaemic heart disease – compliance with diet and medication.

occurs within the first 48 hours, so people who have had a TIA require urgent referral to the stroke service, so that early interventions can be implemented if necessary to reduce the risk of stroke. If confirmed, FAST-positive within 4 hours of onset of symptoms, then the patient should be transferred to a hyper-acute stroke unit (HASU), where they will undergo rapid assessment and investigations, treatment and monitoring 24 hours a day. The introduction of HASU services is to reduce death rates and long-term disability (National Stroke Strategy, DH 2007b; NICE 2008). Further assessment to determine diagnosis includes: a complete history, careful physical assessment, including a thorough neurological examination and a CT scan.

It is important to establish as much information as possible, either from the patient or the family or bystanders; this includes information on time of symptom onset, patient medication, with particular attention to identifying anticoagulant, antiplatelet and antihypertensive drugs.

Nursing care and management

Urgent assessment is particularly crucial for those who have suffered an acute ischaemic stroke and require anti-thrombolytic treatment (dissolving the thrombus), such as Alteplase, a recombinant form of human tissue plasminogen activator (rTPA), which activates intravascular fibrinolysis by converting plasminogen to plasmin, which assists in the restoration of cerebral blood supply. The window of opportunity for administration is up to 4.5 hours from onset of stroke (Lansberg *et al.* 2009). Beyond this time frame, mechanical embolectomy (debulking and aspiration of the clot) may be undertaken.

Close monitoring in the initial period following a stroke is critical. Up to 30% of all stroke patients will deteriorate within 24 hours (Adams *et al.* 2007), and monitoring for complications post-thrombolysis treatment, such as haemorrhage are also important nursing considerations. Nurses need to be able to appropriately assess the patient and recognise early signs of raised intracranial pressure (see earlier).

Red Flag

A patient receiving alteplase may develop angioedema:
· Mild, transient hemi-facial swelling starting in the tongue, usually contralateral to the ischaemic hemisphere; this may rapidly progress to cause upper airway obstruction, which may be fatal.

A central part of stroke recovery is to create a safe and therapeutic environment to ensure positive outcomes. The ultimate goal post-stroke for the patient, is to achieve as much independence as possible through learning to adapt to their disabilities. Early identification of problems and referral to relevant members of the multidisciplinary team, such as physiotherapist for exercise, posture and rehabilitation programmes; speech and language therapy for formal swallowing and speech assessments; occupational therapy for evaluation and activities to remediate performance skill deficits, body structure and function impairments, for example sitting balance/trunk control, transfers, activities of daily living.

Patients with detected or suspected visual field defects (VFD) should be referred for formal visual assessment. Patient with VFD experience difficulties with activities of living, such as eating, washing and dressing and are at increased risk of falling and bumping into objects (see Chapter 35).

Nurses can both promote and encourage participation in rehabilitation and exercise programmes to help prevent leg muscles atrophy (wasting) and restore function. At the forefront of stroke prevention is the role of nurses in initiating lifestyle changes and these are summarised in Box 34.5.

Impact on the family The impact of stroke on the family is significant, affecting their emotional well-being and physical health. It is important that healthcare professionals provide individual care and support to family members to meliorate these effects, as it is understood that the outcomes of the stroke survivor are influenced by the family functioning. After the initial shock of the typical sudden stroke event, families experience anxiety about the prognosis and uncertainty about what the future may bring. Other negative effects include high levels of strain and distress, depression, burden and a disruption in their family and social lives. These effects may change over the course of time, thus the timing of assessment to identify their needs is an important consideration.

Box 34.6 Summary of the Recommended Strategies in Supporting Families and Carers Following Stroke

- Promote active involvement in the rehabilitation process
- Identify individual family and carer's needs and reassess after the patient returns home
- Provide timely and supportive information related to:
  - stroke-related impairments, such as speech deficits
  - their role as a carer
  - how to prevent future strokes, for example lifestyle changes
  - community services and benefits and that they may be entitled to
- Provide educational training to include:
  - stroke and its consequences
  - how to provide care and support
- Help in supporting the families in asking for assistance as they may perceive this as failing as a carer
- Help the families to work with their stroke family members on pursuing their new skills to maintain as much independence as possible
- Consider appropriate referral to health and clinical psychology services.

(National Clinical Guidelines for Stroke, RCP 2012; Management of Patients with Stroke, SIGN 2010b).

Box 34.6 highlights some interventions for consideration when caring for the family members of stroke survivors.

Jot This Down
What advice and support might you offer a patient who is suffering from post-stroke depression?

Depression is a major issue post-stroke affecting approximately one-third of patients (Hackett & Anderson 2005), the highest rates reported in the first month post-stroke (Ayerbe et al. 2011). Post-stroke depression (PSD) can have a significant and negative impact on functional ability following stroke and may lead to decreased quality of care life for patient and carer (Farner et al. 2009). Early identification and treatment of PSD may enhance functional recovery. National guidelines (National Clinical Guidelines for Stroke, RCP 2012) advocate that all stroke patients are screened for mood disturbances within 6 weeks of their stroke. In the 'Jot This Down' exercise above, you may have considered the following strategies:

- Ongoing individualised contact, keeping the patient informed of the effects of stroke
- Encourage the patient to talk about their feelings
- Encourage the patient to maintain contact with family and friends and encourage the joining a support group as many people find this useful and provides an opportunity to talk to others who have experienced similar experienced
- Help identify hobbies and interest that the patient may engage in
- Encourage rest periods to maximise their periods of activity.

Neurological Oncology

Central nervous system (CNS) cancers are a group of different tumour entities with nearly 100 different types of primary tumours, with differing incidence rates, clinical behaviour and response to treatment and prognosis (Crocetti et al. 2012). Most tumours occur sporadically and are classified according to the World Health Organization's grading scheme (Louis et al. 2007). Some brain tumours can be cured by surgery, some are rapidly fatal, despite treatment and some do not require treatment (Marsh 2009).

Epidemiology

CNS tumours are rare, accounting for about 2% of all cancers of which **gliomas** are the most common; 6–8 per 100 000 per year. However, brain tumours are the fourth most common tumour, the biggest cancer killer under the age of 40 and the eighth most common under the age of 65.

The prevalence of CNS cancers is unknown, however the Vision 2012 paper (DH 2007a) suggest incidences of 15–20 per 100 000, higher than previously reported, recognising that brain tumours are grossly under-reported. This incidence is expected to rise with an ageing population and improved access to imaging and diagnosis rates.

High-grade glioma and brain metastasis occur more frequently during adulthood and especially among the elderly (Crocetti et al. 2012).

Low-grade gliomas present at a younger age than high-grade gliomas, typically between 30 and 40 years of age and commonly present with seizures. LGG are WHO Grade I–II tumours, however these tumours are not benign and the mean survival rate is approximately 10 years. Of all brain tumours, glioblastoma multiforme (GBM) (Grade IV) is the most aggressive and is characterised by rapid glial cell growth and spread throughout the CNS and is resistant to radiotherapy and chemotherapy.

Pathophysiology

Strictly speaking the term 'brain tumours' should apply only to tumours growing within and originating from the brain parenchyma, most of which are gliomas, however, it also includes tumours arising from:

- Structures adjacent to the brain, which can compress and distort it. These include tumours, such as meningiomas arising from the meninges, schwannomas from the cranial nerves and adenomas from the pituitary gland
- Metastatic tumours originate from outside the CNS; the commonest sources are carcinomas of the breast, lung and kidney and malignant melanoma.

The concept of 'benign' and 'malignant' in the brain implies simple local expansion versus brain parenchymal invasion. However, a benign tumour in areas in the brain close to vital areas may be difficult to remove completely without damage to adjacent structures. Metastatic spread of tumours from their primary site in the brain is very uncommon, but may occur via cerebrospinal fluid pathways and the spinal canal.

Glial tumours are divided and analysed in accordance with WHO classification; grading range from WHO Grade I (**pilocytic astrocytomas**) to most malignant WHO Grade IV (**glioblastoma multiforme**, GBM). Among CNS cancers, **astrocytic** tumours are the most common tumours, followed by **oligodendroglial** tumours and **ependymal** tumours.

Risk factors The cause of glioma is unknown, although previous exposure to ionising radiation is a known risk factor. Radiofrequency electromagnetic fields emitted by mobile phones have been implicated as a causative factor in gliomas in excessive users of mobile phones, however the association is unclear. Some patient groups have genetic abnormalities that give a lifelong risk of glial or other tumours (e.g. neurofibromatosis, tuberous sclerosis).

Signs and symptoms

Signs and symptoms are dependent on location rate of growth and invasiveness. The brain can be divided into 'eloquent' and 'silent' areas.

- *Eloquent* – tumour with significant neurological signs and symptoms, these include:
  - Speech areas in the temporal and frontal lobes
  - Primary motor cortex in the frontal lobe
  - Visual cortex in the occipital lobe
- *Silent* – areas where the tumour may grow to a significant size without any obvious neurological signs and symptoms; includes frontal and non-dominant temporal lobes.

Presentation may be dramatic, with seizures or focal symptoms that reflect the site of the lesion in the brain. However, tumours in *silent* may produce only subtle focal symptoms (e.g. personality change, motivational impairment). Many tumours are not suspected until a patient complains of headache, usually worse in the morning, due to raised intracranial pressure (ICP) caused by the space-occupying effect of the tumour mass and oedema, and it may be associated with vomiting. Other symptoms may include:

- Altered consciousness
- Changes in cognition, such as personality, confusion and loss of memory
- Changes in behaviour, such as increased intolerance, decreased initiation and motivation
- Epileptic seizures, very common in patients with glial tumours, reaching nearly 50% in glioblastoma patients and almost 90% in low-grade astrocytomas, due to tumour cell metabolism acting directly on neuronal network, leading to seizure susceptibility (Prakash *et al.* 2012)
- Limb weakness, hemiparesis, unsteadiness and abnormal gait
- Visual disturbances, e.g. diplopia (double vision) and loss of vision.

Diagnosis and investigations

Along with a full medical and surgical history, assessment measures appropriate to the location of the lesion and suspected type of tumour are carried out; these are summarised in Box 34.7.

Nursing care and management

Treatment options are varied and dependent on the tumour histology, grade, location and patient's functional level (assessed using the Karnofsky performance status).

Surgery

- Tumour biopsy – the removal of a sample of tissue to examine under a microscope, enabling a diagnosis to be made
- Tumour partial resection or debulking (partial removal of the tumour when it cannot be completely removed) or a total resection (complete removal of the tumour)

> **Box 34.7 Summary of the Investigations and Tests for Patients with Brain Tumours**
>
> - Karnofsky Performance Status scale (measuring the patient's functional ability and general well-being – scores range from severely impaired 10 to normal 100); may be used to determine treatment
> - MRI scan of the brain and spine, usually with intravenous injection of the contrast agent, e.g. Gadolinium
> - Whole-body CT scan for persons with metastases or PET scan (to detect primary neoplasms)
> - Chest X-ray
> - Blood tests, for example germ cell tumours (e.g. germinomas) produce chemicals (tumour markers) that can be detected in blood
> - Laboratory tests, such as haematoxylin and eosin staining (H&E stain) of tissues and cells to microscopically determine type and proliferation of tumour cells and ESR
> - Genetic screening, for example in cases of neurofibromatosis and tuberous sclerosis
> - Angiography – to visualise blood vessels near the lesion
> - Intracarotid sodium amobarbital test (WADA) pre-surgical test to determine cerebral language localisation and thus useful in deciding how much tissue can be safely removed
> - Brain stem auditory evoked responses and visually evoked responses
> - Screening for biomarker to determine distinct tumour types
>   - Loss of chromosome 1p19q in a patient with oligodendrogliomas or gliomas with oligodendroglioma component are more responsive to chemotherapy
>   - The presence of MGMT, a DNA repair protein increases the responsiveness to chemotherapy in patients with GBM.

- Methods to maximise resection of malignant gliomas include: intraoperative visualisation by means of 5-amino laevolinic acid (5-ALA), a dye that makes brain tumour cells glow red under UV light, which then helps the surgeons to check they are removing as much brain tumour as possible or intraoperative MRI)
- Insertion of biodegradable wafer, impregnated with carmustine (Gliadel°) chemotherapy drug, which slowly releases into residual tissue, placed into the resection cavity following glioma tumour removal.

Radiotherapy and chemotherapy After surgery (biopsy or resection) with external beam radiotherapy and/or chemotherapy, this is dependent on the grade and location of the tumour.

- Radiotherapy, including stereotactic radiation therapy (Gamma knife) and robotic radiation therapy (Cyberknife) often used to treat small tumours close to very important structures in the brain, and proton beam radiotherapy
- Chemotherapy, for example temozolomide, often used in conjunction with radiotherapy.

Steroids Cerebral oedema is a common feature of cerebral tumours and contributes greatly to the neurological deterioration of the patient and causes symptoms of raised intracranial pressure. Corticosteroids, such as dexamethasone, are used to treat oedema, however side-effects increase with dose and duration of treatment, thus doses are carefully considered.

Table 34.14 Treatment therapies and how these might be managed.

TREATMENT	SPECIFIC SIDE-EFFECTS	NURSING CONSIDERATIONS
Cranial radiotherapy	Worsening of presenting neurological signs and symptoms due to cerebral oedema Accumulative fatigue as the treatment progresses Hair loss (alopecia) due to the damage to the hair roots during therapy and tends to occur 2–3 weeks after treatment Hypersensitivity to taste and smell due to the stimulation of the olfactory nerve endings during treatment	Reassurance and support when the symptoms occur. Steroids may be prescribed to counter the cerebral oedema Observe for headaches and manage with analgesia, such as paracetamol Educating patients that fatigue may be long-lasting and that it is not indicative Inform the patient that they are entitled to a wig on NHS prescription Changes in taste and smell may reduce appetite, thus ensure that the patient receives adequate nutrition
Corticosteroid therapy, e.g. dexamethasone	Increased susceptibility of infections Disturbances in behaviour, e.g. irritability, insomnia, agitation Metabolic and endocrine changes, e.g. hyperglycaemia, increased appetite, Cushing's syndrome	Ensure that patient has written information regarding steroid side-effects and management of side-effects. Advise the patient that they cannot be stopped abruptly due to the suppression of the adrenal gland production of cortisol

A brain tumour diagnosis could signal the start of a long period of uncertainty and fear about the future for those involved. Additionally, patients may have neurological and cognitive, behavioural and emotional deficits, which they and their families/carers have to cope with pre- and/or post-surgery. Patients may present with disorders of consciousness (see Table 34.10). Patients may also experience side-effects from chemotherapy and following radiotherapy (these are covered in more detail in Chapter 15. More specific side-effects related to the treatment therapies and how these might be managed are described in Table 34.14.

Apart from post-surgical or radiotherapy care, the key aspects of the nursing management are the same as for the patient, with a TBI and/or raised ICP (see earlier).

Specific nursing considerations

- Observe for signs of diabetes insipidus (DI), the production of large quantity of urine with low specific gravity caused by decreased secretion of antidiuretic hormone (ADH), as a result of surgical manipulation of the pituitary gland
- Maintain an accurate fluid balance
- Assess the patient for serum electrolyte levels, urine osmolality, urine specific gravity and urine sodium level
- Observe cranial wound site for signs of infection and CSF leakage
- Assess level of pain (headache) related to stretching and cutting of the brain tissues following surgery and increase in intracranial pressure using a validated rating scale and administer analgesics as prescribed.

The diagnosis of an intracranial tumour brings anxiety and feelings of uncertainty about the future. Both the patient and family members are likely to be apprehensive and require education and emotional support. Clear, relevant and timely information is important and may include:

- An overall treatment plan, procedures and investigations along with management of deficits and/or disabilities
- Referral to a neuro-oncology specialist nurse for additional support information and guidance.

Infections of the CNS

Infections of the CNS can be categorised into three groups, depending upon the parts of the CNS tissue affected and the extent of the infection: infection of the meninges is called **meningitis**, and of brain tissue called **encephalitis**. A localised collection of pus in the brain is called a **brain abscess**. Organisms that cause these infections are varied and include viruses, bacteria, parasites and fungi.

Epidemiology

Bacterial meningitis is common worldwide, with an annual incidence rate of 5 per 100 000 and is a notifiable disease.

Brain abscesses and encephalitis is a rare condition affecting all ages and both sexes. Few epidemiological studies exist for encephalitis but studies reveal incidence rates varying between 3.5 and 7.4 per 100 000 patients per year. Despite its rarity, it is of important public healthcare importance because of its high morbidity and mortality rates; over one-third of patients may die or be left with severe disability (Granerod et al. 2010).

Pathophysiology

Meningitis infectious agents enter the CSF via fractures of the skull or breaching of the blood–brain barrier (BBB). The inflammatory response within the subarachnoid space may result in pus affecting the flow of CSF and subsequent rise in ICP. The infection may spread down the spinal cord and the sheaths of the cranial nerves.

Over 100 different infectious agents may cause encephalitis, however the aetiology of encephalitis remains unknown in most cases. The most commonly identified pathogen in the UK is herpes simplex virus (HSV or the cold sore virus). Encephalitis caused by brain cell dysfunction due to direct infective invasion and associated inflammatory changes.

Abscesses begin as a localised area of cerebritis that later evolves into a pus filled area, which then becomes encapsulated with vascularised tissue and collagen fibre; this is visible on a CT scan with contrast as a white ring.

Risk factors

Meningitis – impaired immune system caused by other diseases or patients receiving cytotoxic therapy; infection elsewhere within the body, e.g. penetrating head injury; neurosurgical procedures, e.g. lumbar punctures or epidural anaesthesia

Encephalitis – mosquito and tick-bites enhance the likelihood of encephalitis virus spread

Brain abscess – may occur singularly or in multiples and may occur following brain surgery or penetrating the head, or by haematogeneous spread of infections – the most common route of infection from nearby structures, e.g. middle ear or frontal sinuses.

Signs and symptoms

A person with meningitis may present with a variety of symptoms:

- Fever
- Restlessness, irritability and agitation
- Meningeal irritation – cervical rigidity and head retraction due to widespread muscular rigidity, photophobia
- Raised intracranial pressure
- Seizures
- Petechial rash (small spots) (in meningococcal meningitis)
- Kernig's sign and Brudzinski's signs, thought to be caused by the irritation of motor nerve roots passing through inflamed meninges, as the roots are brought under tension.
  - *Kernig's sign* with the patient supine with hips and knees in flexion, extension of the knees is attempted: the inability to extend the patient's knees beyond 135 degrees without causing pain constitutes a positive test for Kernig's sign.
  - *Brudzinski's neck sign* or Brudzinski's sign with the patient supine, flexing the patient's neck causes flexion of the patient's hips and knees.

Patient with encephalitis typically present with fever, headache and alteration of consciousness. However, the diversity of neurological symptoms can make it difficult to distinguish encephalitis from other infectious and non-infectious central nervous system conditions.

Brain abscess typically begins with fever, focal neurological signs and headaches and later raised ICP may occur due to the enlargement of the lesion and surrounding localised swelling.

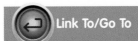

Link To/Go To

http://www.encephalitis.info/

Diagnosis and investigations

CT scan with contract may show the extent of inflammation in the brain in encephalitis and help differentiate encephalitis from other conditions, and show abscesses. Lumbar puncture, providing there are no signs of raised intracranial pressure, for identification of causative organism on CSF culture for meningitis and some cases of encephalitis. Genetic material from herpes simplex virus, varicella zoster virus (chickenpox virus) and enteroviruses can also be detected by a specific CSF test (polymerase chain reaction, PCR test).

Nursing care and management

CNS infections are associated with high morbidity and mortality early recognition and treatment is critical to preventing neurological deterioration and life-threatening complications. Patients may be extremely ill, requiring basic nursing care in addition to constant monitoring. Nursing care associated with altered LOC, IICP and seizures are also appropriate for the person with a CNS infection.

Specific nursing management

- Frequent observation of neurological function and vital signs using the GCS
- Isolation/barrier nursing considerations (if required for bacterial meningitis):
  - Seek advice from the infection control team
  - Follow local policy on isolation/barrier nursing precautions
  - Patient's emotional well-being (mental health, safety)
  - Mode of transmission of infection (air-borne, faecal/oral route)
  - Risk of spread to other service users and health workers
  - Facilities available
- Care of the intravenous site for the administration of intravenous antibiotic or anti virals
- Provision of information and prophylaxis (treatment, screening) to close family/carers, e.g. to eliminate nasopharyngeal carriage of organisms.

Epilepsy

Epilepsy is a common chronic disorder characterised by an abnormal recurrent excessive and self-terminating electrical discharge from brain neurones. This abnormal neuronal activity may involve all or part of the brain, and disturbs skeletal motor function, sensation, autonomic function of the viscera, behaviour and/or consciousness. **Epilepsy** is the name given to the diverse group of conditions all having in common the presence of at least one seizure.

Epidemiology

Epilepsy affects up to 50 million people of all ages, races, social class and ethnic backgrounds worldwide and affects 500 000 people in the UK (Joint Epilepsy Council 2011). Approximately 20% of people with learning disabilities have epilepsy (Epilepsy Society 2013). Epilepsy carries a risk to life; in the UK, approximately 1000 people every year will die due to epilepsy, with most premature deaths associated with epilepsy being related to accidents and injuries. The rate of misdiagnosis of epilepsy in adults is estimated to be 25% in adults and a significant proportion of misdiagnosis comprises 'non-epileptic seizures' (NES), which are mislabelled as epilepsy. Misdiagnosis rates of 20–31% are reported by the All-Party Parliamentary Group on Epilepsy (2007).

Pathophysiology

The full understanding of epilepsy is not known, however it is understood that it is a transient occurrence that occurs when brain neurones produce an abnormal rhythmic and repetitive hypersynchronous discharge, referred to as the 'epileptogenic focus'. This electrical discharge can be recorded with EEG scalp electrodes. Neurotransmitters play an important part of the excitation and inhibition balance in the CNS. During a seizure, metabolic needs of the brain increase dramatically, resulting in an increased demand for glucose and oxygen by as much as 60%. If cerebral blood flow cannot meet these increased needs, cellular exhaustion and cellular destruction may result. Seizures are generally self-limiting, however in some cases, generalised seizures continue for 30 minutes or more; this is termed **status epilepticus** and is a major life-threatening medical emergency, which may result in death.

Approximately 60% of epilepsies have no identifiable cause. The remaining epilepsies are caused by some form of structural or metabolic cause, for example brain damage either due to disease or injury, drug and alcohol overdose and withdrawal or genetic causes.

Diagnosis and investigations

- Clinical history from patients/eye-witnesses to the attack
- Diagnostic testing to detect any abnormal structures that may be treatable, e.g. skull X-ray, MRI or CT scan
- Electroencephalogram (EEG) to help localise the epileptogenic focus and confirm diagnosis
- Blood tests to exclude any metabolic causes, e.g. hypoglycaemia
- CSF examination for CNS infections
- Other test may be carried out to explore cardiac or psychogenic causes.

There are currently over 40 different types of epilepsies with no agreed universal classification system but three main categories can be identified: **focal or partial seizures**, **generalised** and **unclassified** seizures.

Signs and symptoms

Clinical signs of seizures depend on the brain location of the epileptogenic focus and the extent and pattern of the epileptic discharge. Typical signs include:

- Temporary changes in mental status and LOC
- Abnormal behaviour
- Sensory disturbance.

Focal or partial seizures These result from abnormal neuronal activity that is localised, causing partial or focal seizure, usually involving a restricted part of one cerebral hemisphere at the onset. Partial seizures can be further subdivided:

- Simple partial seizure, without impaired consciousness the signs and symptoms of will depend on the area of brain involved
- Complex partial seizure, usually with impaired consciousness and originating in the temporal lobe and may be preceded by an aura, such as an unusual smell, a sense of *déjà vu* or a sudden intense emotion. The person may engage in repetitive, non-purposeful activity, such as lip smacking, aimless walking or picking at clothing
- Partial seizures evolving into secondary generalised seizures. In complex partial seizures, consciousness is impaired.

Generalised seizures Generalised seizures affect both hemispheres of the brain and deep structures of the brain, e.g. hippocampus and the amygdala, and consciousness is always impaired and can be further sub-divided into six major categories:

1. Tonic-clonic seizures
2. Tonic seizures
3. Clonic seizures
4. Myoclonic seizures
5. Atonic seizures and absence seizures

Table 34.15 Different behaviours and observations during non-epileptic seizures (NESs) and epilepsy.

FEATURE	NON-EPILEPTIC SEIZURES (NES)	EPILEPSY
Response to verbal commands	Yes	No
Pupil reaction to light	Yes	No
Eyes	Shut	Closed
Attempt to open eyes when shut	Resistance	No resistance
Avoids danger	Yes	No
Synchronised movements	Yes (side-to-side head movement is common)	No

6. Tonic-clonic and absence seizures are the common forms of generalised seizure activity; they occur more frequently (especially in children) than partial seizures.

Non-epileptic seizures (NES) These are events that resemble epileptic seizures and are relatively common. There are two major types of NESs:

- *Psychogenic NES (PNES)* episodes of altered movement, sensation or experience, caused by a psychological process (NICE 2010); not caused by abnormal electrical signals in the brain or by brain damage
- *Physiological NES* caused by physiological dysfunction that may result in loss of consciousness with or without motor signs such as twitching, e.g. cardiac arrhythmias, hypotensive episodes or cerebrovascular disease.

Non-epileptic seizures can be difficult to differentiate from events due to epilepsy, and misdiagnosis leads to inappropriate treatment with antiepileptic drugs (AEDs). A correct diagnosis is important to ensure appropriate interventions and improvement in the person's quality of life. Table 34.15 illustrates the difference between non-epileptic seizures (NESs) and epilepsy.

Nursing care and management

Most people with epilepsy are treated with anti-epileptic drugs (AEDs). AEDs aim to prevent seizures from happening, without impairing cognitive function or producing undesirable side-effects, but they do not cure epilepsy. Where possible, the lowest possible dose of a single medication that will control the seizures is prescribed on an individual basis. AEDs can reduce or control most seizure activity, acting in one of two ways: by acting on the motor cortex in the brain to raise the seizure threshold or by limiting the spread of rapidly firing epileptic foci in the brain.

For some people, they may not get full control of their epilepsy, despite AEDs; alternative treatments may be offered including:

- Surgery to remove the epileptogenic focus via stereotactic radio-therapy (Gamma knife), neuro-stimulation therapy, such as deep brain stimulation or surgical resection
- Vagus nerve stimulation (VNS), designed to prevent seizures by sending regular small pulses of electrical energy to the brain via the vagus nerve.

Whether a person has established epilepsy or has been admitted having suffered their first seizure, the nurse has an important management and education role. Observing and providing a written account during an attack should include:

Before the seizure (pre-ictal)

- Was there any warning (aura)-warning that may have preceded the generalised seizure activity, e.g. sense of uneasiness or an abnormal gustatory, visual, auditory or visceral sensation; seizures often occur without auras?

During the seizure (ictal)

- Was there a loss of postural control? The patient may fall to the floor with muscle rigidity, jaw clenched
- Was there a sudden loss of consciousness?
- Was there any urinary incontinence or bowel incontinence?

Post-ictal

- Is there any confusion and/or disoriented?
- Any amnesia of the seizure and the events just prior to the seizure activity?

Seizure recognition, seizure management and awareness of the associated risks are important nursing care issues. Some considerations in the hospital setting for a patient known to have epilepsy include: call bell near to hand, bedside oxygen and suction equipment and lowering the bed to near the floor. Immediate care of a patient during a seizure includes:

- Do not restrain or put anything into the patient's mouth
- Provide a safe environment to protect the patient from unnecessary harm
- Secure airway and resuscitate administer oxygen
- Assess cardiorespiratory function
- Stay with the patient to reassure and reorientate
- Prevent the patient from injuring themselves, loosen clothing around the neck, position patients in the recovery position (after the clonic phase, suctioning if excessive salivation)
- Administer rescue AEDs, such as nasal/buccal midazolam rectal diazepam or to abort the seizure and prevent status epilepticus
- Record and report the seizure (start and stop time, activity during the seizure), on a seizure chart.

Primary care The impact may have a profound psychological, physiological and social economic consequence for the patient and their families. Hence, the National Institute for Health and Clinical Excellence (NICE 2012a) recommends all patients suspected of epilepsy should be seen by an expert in epilepsy.

Jot This Down

Julie, a 23-year-old law student with no previous medical history of note, suffers a seizure. Following tests (MRI and EEG), she is diagnosed with epilepsy. What are the long-term implications?

Helping the patient and the family adjust to a diagnosis and providing relevant information are important nursing interventions. In the 'Jot This Down' exercise above, you may have considered the following:

- General health and safety advice – safer to shower rather than bath, as this reduces the risk of drowning if you have a seizure; avoid sports activities, such as rock climbing and hand gliding.

When to call for medical assistance, i.e. when the seizure lasts for more than 5 minutes, there is slow recovery, a second seizure or difficulty breathing after the seizure and if there are signs of injury (such as bleeding from the mouth).

- Driving – the law states that you cannot drive for 1 year after a seizure (see DVLC Link To/Go To)
- Lifestyle – awareness of triggers that may precipitate a seizure, such as sleep deprivation, drinking large amounts of alcohol, general ill-health (e.g. infection), excessive stress
- Contraception – some antiepileptic medication affects oestrogen-based oral contraception; an alternative method of contraception may have to be considered
- The need to consider preconception counselling with the GP, epilepsy specialist nurse or neurologist, if pregnancy is being considered
- The importance of follow-up care, keeping medical appointments and continuing to take AEDs as prescribed, even when no seizures are experienced
- Depression is a major comorbid condition significantly affecting the patient's quality of life and recognising risk factors, such as the psychosocial effect of having or the fear of having recurrent seizures and stigma.

 Link To/Go To

The Epilepsy Society provides information about resources and support groups:
http://www.epilepsysociety.org.uk/

Headaches

Headaches are among the commonest neurological disorders and are a common occurrence. The International Headache Society (ICHS-II 2004) classifies headaches into 14 groups and lists 150 headaches, which can be broadly divided into either: **primary**, unrelated to an underlying condition and constitutes approximately 98% of all headaches or **secondary**, due to some underlying condition, for example haemorrhage, CNS tumours or infections. **Migraine** and **tension-type** headaches are the most common primary headache disorders. Many headaches are disabling, reduce the patient's quality of life and are a substantial public health problem. Tension headaches and migraine are ranked second and third globally in leading causes of years lived with a disability (Vos et al. 2012). World Health Organization (WHO 2008) weights severe migraine in the severity disability class VII (severity class I–VII).

Epidemiology

Headache affects people of all ages, races and socioeconomic status and is more common in women. Migraine is a common occurrence, affecting 1 : 7 people and most 'migraineurs' will have their first attack before they are 30 years old. Peak incidence is in the late teens and early 20s, with the vast majority of people having their first attack before the age of 35.

Tension-type headaches are common, affecting up to 80% of people from time to time and in adults, seems higher in women than men and most are episodic. Cluster headaches are rare, occurring in <1% of the UK population and men have a greater prevalence than women, with a male to female ratio of 2.5:1–3.5:1 (Fischera *et al.* 2008).

Pathophysiology

Headache is experienced when there is traction, pressure, displacement, inflammation or dilation of nociceptors in areas sensitive to pain within the cranium, including facial and scalp structures, meninges cerebral vessels.

The exact cause of tension headache is unknown but, increased muscular activity occurs around the scalp. There is no simple cause for migraine and only two migraine genes have been identified. The exact pathophysiology of cluster headache also remains unknown, however what is known is that hypothalamus dysfunction plays a significant part in its mechanism. There are a number of causes of secondary headaches:

- Vascular (subarachnoid haemorrhage, SAH), strokes
- Non-vascular
  - Tumours and other space-occupying lesions causing raised ICP
  - Benign intracranial hypertension (BIH)
  - Infections in the nasal or sinus passages and CNS infections (meningitis, encephalitis)
  - Neck and head injuries
  - Post-lumbar puncture headache
  - Substance abuse
  - Headaches related to psychiatric disorders.

Diagnosis and investigations

Studies indicate that primary headache disorders are under-diagnosed (Kernick *et al.* 2008). Diagnosis is made following a good medical history. In some cases, neuroimaging may be necessary to exclude structural causes of the headache, but for primary headache disorders (tension, migraine or cluster), this rarely reveals important intracranial pathology. A headache diary recording frequency, duration and severity of headaches may assist the doctor in the diagnosis.

Secondary headaches should be considered in those patients that present with new onset or changes in features of their usual headaches. Warning signs that require further investigations by a specialist that are suggestive of a secondary headache are highlighted in Red Flag Box below.

Red Flag

- Change in characteristics of headache, i.e. increased frequency, severity or associated symptoms
- New onset of headache in particular <10 and >50 years
- New onset of headache in patients with pre-existing cancer, HIV infection or head injury
- Progressive headache worsening over weeks or longer
- Persistent morning headache with nausea
- Headache associated with postural changes, physical exertion, coughing or Valsalva
- Thunderclap headache (intense, sudden onset).

(SIGN 2008; BASH 2010)

Signs and symptoms

Signs and symptoms of headache vary according to the cause, type and precipitating symptoms (see Table 34.16).

Nursing care and management

Chronic daily headache, consisting of chronic migraine (CM) and chronic tension-type headache (CTTH), occurs on 15 or more days per month for 3 or more months (Bigal & Lipton 2007) and is the most challenging to treat. Ultimately, the goal of treatment is to restore the patient ability to function with the minimal adverse

Table 34.16 Signs and symptoms of primary headaches (tension-type headache, migraine and cluster headache).
Adapted from NICE (2012b).

HEADACHE FEATURES	TENSION-TYPE HEADACHE	MIGRAINE (WITH OR WITHOUT AURA)	CLUSTER HEADACHE
Pain characteristics	Bilateral or generalised. Pressing and tightening like a tight band around the head	Unilateral or bilateral. Pulsing	Unilateral. Orbital and supraorbital or temporal pain. Burning stabbing like an 'ice pick'
Pain severity	Mild to moderate	Moderate to severe	Severe to very severe
Duration	30 min (continuous)	4–72 hours	15–180 min
Frequency	<15 days per month	Episodic <15 days per month	Episodic 1–8 per day with a relief period up to 1 year
		Chronic ≥15 days per month for more than 3 months	Chronic 1–8 per day with a relief period of less than 1 month in 1 year
Other symptoms	None	Unusual sensitivity to light and/or noise, nausea and vomiting. May or may not have aura. Aura symptoms may include: visual symptoms (e.g. flashing lights), sensory symptoms (e.g. numbness) and speech disturbance	Ipsilateral to the pain these include: autonomic symptoms (red watering eye, sweating over the forehead and face), nasal congestion and rhinorrhoea. Eye lid oedema, partial ptosis and constricted pupil. Restlessness

831

effects. Headache treatment is either *abortive*, aimed at managing the acute headache or *prophylactic*, aimed at reducing the frequency or severity of the attacks.

Abortive treatments include

- A triptan, e.g. sumatriptan
- Simple analgesia (aspirin, paracetamol ibuprofen)

Common prophylactic medications include:

- Anticonvulsants, e.g.
- β-blockers, calcium channel blockers
- serotonin reuptake inhibitors
- tricyclic antidepressants.

Botulinum toxin A is an effective, safe and generally well-tolerated prophylactic treatment of chronic migraine headaches, at a dose of 155 units divided among 31 injection sites and repeated as needed every 12 weeks, may improve the frequency of chronic migraine (Jackson *et al.* 2012).

Community care Encouraging the completion of headache diaries to help identify and assess triggers and how to avoid them; determine the impact of the headache and monitor the effectiveness of headache interventions may be useful for some patients, although for others this may be laborious. Providing advice and support about headache disorders, treatment options and available support groups along with reliable resources are also important to help achieve good outcomes. Refer to specialists who have the appropriate level of understanding and knowledge, for example GPSi (GP with Special interest) in headache, headache clinics and specialist neurologists.

Multiple Sclerosis

Multiple sclerosis (MS) is the most common non-traumatic disabling disease in young people in the UK. MS is incurable and unpredictable, and there is an increasing understanding that the disease is a disturbance of the immune system within the CNS. MS is both an inflammatory and a neurodegenerative disease, which is associated with brain atrophy. The needs of people with MS shift over time and they can have many disabling symptoms that result in emotional, psychological and physical burden for the patient and their families.

Epidemiology

MS affects an estimated 100 000 people in the UK and 2.5 million people globally. The worldwide prevalence of MS positively correlates with latitude (Simpson *et al.* 2011). There are wide geographical variations of MS, with the highest prevalence found in temperate zones of the world, for example Europe and North America, with a prevalence rate in the Orkney Islands of 300 per 100 000 and a low prevalence rate in Japan, and it is very rarely found in equatorial regions. Onset is usually between 20–40 years of age, with a peak age of onset at 28–31 years of age. It is more common in women than men, with a ratio of male : female 1 : 1.7.

Pathophysiology

Despite the exact cause remaining unknown, there is evidence to suggest that it involves an immune response triggered by an interaction between genetic and environmental factors (Ramagopalan *et al.* 2010). It is thought that the initial trigger involves damage to the blood–brain barrier, resulting in lymphocytes cells (T and B cells) entering the CNS and triggering an immune response in the CNS, these cells releasing substances that attack the myelin. Inflammation areas on the myelin sheath of nerves in the brain result in damage and loss of the nerve axon and the formation of localised inflammation called **plaques**, and eventual nerve death.

MS is characterised by periods of exacerbation or **relapse** (returning to old symptoms or the appearance of new ones) and periods of **remission** (recovery from relapse), during which the damaged myelin sheath undergoes remyelination. In the early stages the disease is commonly a **relapsing and remitting disease** (RR); however, over time, during the remission period, the myelin sheath is unable to repair itself completely and patients are left with residual deficits. Repeated healing and inflammation can lead to scarring (gliosis) and loss of axons, evidenced on MR scans as **black holes**. As the disease progresses, remissions become shorter and fewer, and patients' become more disabled physically and a new clinical stage called **secondary progressive MS** is initiated. There are four main types of MS:

1. Relapsing–remitting (most common type)
2. Primary progressive
3. Secondary progressive
4. Progressive-relapsing.

The Evidence

Clinically isolated syndrome (CIS) describes the first clinical episode of symptoms and signs consistent with MS; the attack lasts at least 24 hours. Up to 80% of individuals who have a first attack or CIS and who have demyelinating lesions on MRI will go on to develop MS. Clinical trials have indicated that starting disease-modifying treatment, after CIS with MRI evidence, early, delays the onset of MS.

(Comi *et al.* 2009)

Risk factors

- *Environmental risks* include:
  - Born and living in high latitude regions – reduced ultraviolet B (UVB) light radiation
  - Vitamin D deficiency
  - Infected with Epstein–Barr virus (EBV), a human herpes virus (>99.5%)
  - Smoking
- *Genetic factors* are important in causing MS, however, no specific gene has been identified, but studies consistently indicate chromosome 6 as being involved in the disease; the gene encoding 1α-hydroxylase (the enzyme that activates vitamin D) is associated with MS susceptibility
- Family history in particular maternal and 1st-degree relatives
- Female sex.

Signs and symptoms

Signs and symptoms are determined by the location and number of the demyelination plaques in the CNS and represent a balance between the inflammation, progressive neurodegeneration and the reparative processes in the brain. CIS presentations can be monofocal or multifocal and typically involve the optic nerve, brain stem/cerebellum, spinal cord or cerebral hemispheres.

Common signs of MS include:

- Visual dysfunction, such as diplopia and blurred vision due to optic neuritis (demyelination of the optic nerve)

- Brain stem symptoms including dysarthria and dysphagia
- Mobility-related symptoms
  - Spasticity is common
  - Ataxia and tremor
  - Transient muscle weakness
- Bladder, bowel and sexual dysfunction
- Fatigue, most disabling complex symptom affecting up to 74% of patients (Hadjimichael *et al.* 2008)
- Cognitive impairment is common (40–70%) especially memory, speed of information processing and mental flexibility (Chiaravalloti & DeLuca 2008)
- Psychiatric and psychological dysfunction such as depression, psychosis
- Pain, due to inflammation or neuropathic pain related to the CNS lesion or secondary to spasticity and spasms, frequently occurs (90%) (Hirsh *et al.* 2009)
- Sleep disorders.

Diagnosis and investigations

Early diagnosis, based on clinical history, examination and laboratory findings, is important in facilitating the exclusion of alternative diagnoses and early implementation of treatment. MS is diagnosed after tests to exclude alternative diagnoses have been carried out and no feature is suggestive of an alternative diagnosis, this may require repeated test before a conclusive diagnosis is given. A number of investigations that provide information to aid diagnosis include:

- MR scans may reveal plaques within the CNS
- Cerebrospinal fluid (CSF) examination via a LP to reveal the presence of oligoclonal bands (proteins called immunoglobulin suggesting inflammation of the CNS) present in over 95% of patients with MS
- Evoked response testing (visual, auditory and somatosensory), which may show delayed conduction (slowing of the nerve messages).

Nursing care and management

Management of patients with MS varies according to the acuity of exacerbations (relapses), and the presenting signs and symptoms. MS management generally is divided into treating the symptoms of the disease and those that target the disease mechanism however, both require an interdisciplinary individualistic approach.

Although there is no cure for MS disease, modifying therapies (DMT) are available, which can reduce disability and improve the quality of life of the individual. However, these therapies have only been found to be effective in preventing relapses in relapse remitting MS and for some people with secondary progressive MS. A summary of the treatment options is provided in Table 34.17.

Jot This Down

What specific aspects of medication management might need to be considered with patients receiving treatment for their MS?

In the 'Jot This Down' exercise above, you might have considered some of the following:

- Available different formulations, including injections, infusions or tablets

Table 34.17 Summary of treatment therapies for MS.

THERAPIES AND MODE OF ACTION	MEDICINES AND ADMINISTRATION ROUTES
Disease modifying therapies (DMT)	
Aimed at reducing the number of exacerbations (relapses) by reducing the production of interferon gamma thought to be involved in the formation of demyelination plaques	Beta interferon-1a (Avonex®), beta interferon-1a (Rebif®) and beta interferon-1b (Betaferon®) first-line drug of choice in relapsing–remitting MS, administered intramuscularly; common side-effects include injection site reactions, flu-like symptoms, headache and fatigue
Aimed at reducing antibody/lymphocyte activity	Glatiramer acetate (Copaxone®), administered subcutaneously; common side-effects include injection site reactions, flu-like symptoms, headache, fatigue and nasopharyngitis
Acts by preventing specific inflammatory events leading to the development of lesions in the brain	Natalizumab (Tysabri®) administered intravenously every 4 weeks at specialist centres for severe remitting–relapsing MS, recommended for those persons who are unable to tolerate or respond to another therapy
Binds to specific receptors on lymphocytes, stops cells from sensing the stimulus and prevents lymphocytes from entering the blood circulation	Fingolimod (Gilenya®) taken orally in tablet form
Disease suppressing therapies	
Given in early inflammatory phase (relapses) by suppressing the immune response	Azathioprine (Imuran®) taken orally in tablet form Methotrexate to have an effect on reducing the relapse rate, taken orally in tablet form
Corticosteroids	
Prescribed to hasten the recovery from a acute relapse	Methyl-prednisolone (synthetic steroid) administered intravenously or orally in high doses, short-term over a period of 3–5 days

- The degree of flexibility in administering the medication themselves, e.g. taking tablets or self-injections
- Understand the patient's home life; the availability and support of the family
- Ability to cope with treatment that requires administration by a healthcare professional
- Monitor the degree of compliance with medication
- Awareness of side-effects and ways to mitigate them, the importance of follow-up
- Emphasise the importance of women who are pregnant or planning to become pregnant, discussing any medications they are taking and any new medications, with their specialist.

Being diagnosed with MS may cause uncertainty about the future and worry about the possibility of becoming disabled. MS can potentially have a future impact on employment, income, relationships and activities of daily living. It is important that patients understand that early treatment can delay the development of disability but that treatment will need to be continuous and long-term. An important consideration in selecting treatment options is educating the patient and their families on their priorities and expectations, as this may impact on compliance and compromise treatment efficacy, for example invasive therapies, which may require hospitalisation. Nurses, as integral members of the multidisciplinary team, can play a major role in the education and support of the patient and their families. Nurses may be faced with adherence challenges with patients with MS and should seek strategies for optimising patient adherence; these may include:

- Patient education, including understanding of the disease, need for treatment and potential benefits of treatment
- Management of the patients' expectations
- Provide information on therapeutic options, potential side-effects and how these can be managed
- Ensure that the patient is appropriately trained, e.g. in injection technique
- The use of reminder systems, such as drug diaries, pill boxes or alarms especially for patients experiencing cognitive impairment
- Helping the patient to seek assistance from family members and/or friends
- Provide information on support networks.

It is also important that nurses remain informed about the potential risks and benefits and special considerations (e.g. long-term safety data, dosing and frequency) of all MS therapies, to ensure that patient information is accurate. Careful regular monitoring is also important, as symptoms change over the course of the disease.

Specific symptom management – spasticity (high muscle tone)
Spasticity, common in MS patients, is a motor disorder characterised by increased stretch reflexes leading to exaggerated muscle resistance (increased muscle tone) with exaggerated tendon jerks. Under normal circumstances, motor tracts have an inhibitory effect on muscle tone, however when damage occurs to the descending motor pathways from the brain to the spinal cord, muscle increases. Spasticity can range from muscle stiffness to severe painful uncontrolled muscle spasms and restricted, excessive or inappropriate movement and may be associated with pain. It can affect a single muscle or multiple muscles, for example a whole limb. Spasticity can affect an individual's ability to carry out activities of daily living and may result in complications, such as contractures as a result of prolonged spasticity and the development of pressure sores. The degree to which spasticity affects mobility is dependent upon the severity of symptoms. For example severe spasticity spasms in lower limbs results in the legs being forced into extension flexion and this poses an increased risk of falling out of chairs or bed.

Early identification and initiating referral to either hospital to community-based neurorehabilitation teams are important to prevent and manage complication of spasticity. Management requires assessment and the formulation of a management plan is dependent upon underlying pathology aimed at maximising function, relieving pain and preventing complications and injury.

Pharmacological interventions (usually in conjunction with physical interventions):

- Generalised anti-spasticity agents
  - Oral muscle relaxants (antispasmodic drugs), e.g. baclofen, dantrolene, tizanidine, diazepam (benzodiazepine)
  - Gabapentin- an anti-epileptic drugs
- Local treatments:
  - Intrathecal baclofen via a programmed pump located in the abdominal wall for lower limb spasticity
  - Injection of botulinum toxin type A (Botox or Dysport) directly into the affected muscle(s) blocking the transmission at peripheral neuromuscular junction reducing over activity
  - Intrathecal injections of phenol (carbolic acid) for large muscle groups affecting the lower limbs, e.g. femoral and sciatic nerve.

Physical interventions
- Splinting/casting regimes
- Minimising noxious stimuli that can stimulate flexor reflex afferents the may trigger spasms, for example skin irritations (tight clothing or leg bags straps, in-growing toenails), sudden movements, constipation and urinary infection and retention inappropriate moving and handling
- Passive limb exercises to prevent contractures and loss of muscle bulk
- Early involvement of the physiotherapist to assess and provide positioning and manual handling management plans
- Refer to the occupational therapist for assistive devices
- Careful positioning to maintain neural assignment to prevent primitive reflexes being triggered, which may stimulate spasms for example tonic neck reflexes when the neck or head is tilted, this may include a postural management plan
- Assessing for an treating any underlining pain
- Educating and empowering the patient to self-manage their condition. Reinforcement of safety information provided by the multidisciplinary team, e.g. physiotherapist and providing education and encouragement in self-management.

Parkinson's Disease

Parkinson's disease (PD) is a common, slow progressive neurodegenerative disorder affecting the CNS, usually affecting the older adult, which eventually leads to disability.

PD is the second most common neurodegenerative disorder after Alzheimer's disease.

Epidemiology
Approximately 1 in 500 people, approximately 127 000 people in the UK have PD (Parkinson's UK 2013). As this disease primarily affects older adults, its prevalence is expected to dramatically increase in the future. The incidence rates increase exponentially in people in their 70s and 80s. The mean age of onset is 55–60 years. PD is slightly more common in women than men, and geographically, there is an increase in the Afro-Caribbean's. Epidemiological data on PD dementia is varied, ranging from 10–80%, however it is clear that the prevalence increases with age and duration of symptoms.

Risk factors There is no cure and, in the majority of cases, the cause is not known. There is evidence that both genetics (15 genes confirmed to be linked to PD) and environmental factors play a role. Prolonged or misuse of neuroleptics (e.g. haloperidol and chlorpromazine) and anti-emetics (e.g. prochlorperazine) are also known to induce drug-induced Parkinsonism, which often resolves once the offending drug is stopped. Environmental risk factors include prolonged exposure to pesticides.

Pathophysiology

Parkinson's disease (PD) involves death of dopamine releasing neurones between the substantia nigra cells and the striatum (the connections in the basal ganglia region in the brain) and the formation **Lewy bodies** (small spherical protein deposits found in neurones). Approximately 80% of the nigra cells are lost before signs and symptoms develop. The reason for this neuronal cell loss is unknown.

Signs and symptoms

PD is a progressive development of motor and non-motor symptoms. Onset is insidious, often making it difficult for the family to notice when the signs start, and progressive. Non-motor symptoms may present well before motor symptoms occur (5–10 years), referred to as premotor phase (Hawkes *et al.* 2010), and are a key determinant in reducing functioning and quality of life (Chaudhuri *et al.* 2006). Common symptoms are summarised in Table 34.18.

Patients may experience extreme fluctuations in the severity of their symptoms, which are often difficult to predict and control, and subsequently are accompanied by a reduction in motor function. These fluctuations in symptoms are reduced psychological well-being and caregiver distress and burden. When the patient has severe worsening of parkinsonian signs and symptoms, with a very severe motor deterioration, this is considered an 'off' situation. Other common motor fluctuations are:

- Early 'wearing-off'(emergence of motor and non-motor symptoms before the next scheduled levodopa dose)

- The 'on/off' phenomenon (severe fluctuations in motor function)
- Dyskinesias.

Diagnosis and investigations

There are no specific tests that clearly differentiate Parkinson's disease from other neurologic disorders (Hickey 2009). Diagnosis is based primarily on a thorough history and physical examination, and is usually made based on the presence of two of any of the following signs and symptoms: tremor at rest, bradykinesia, rigidity, and postural instability.

Nursing care and management

Once a diagnosis of PD has been made, nursing interventions are based on a holistic assessment to include intensity, frequency and duration of symptoms and those symptoms that cause distress. This assessment will identify symptoms that need to be targeted and the necessary interventions to address those symptoms to improve disability and quality of life.

Assessing symptoms that cause distress is important, as symptom distress relates to symptoms intensity. Understanding the complete symptom experience is important so that appropriate symptoms can be targeted for interventions and help to reduce symptom distress and symptom intensity. According to Backer (2006) 'off' period, freezing gait, postural instability and sleep disturbances are some of the most distressing symptoms for the PD patient.

The aim of nursing interventions is primarily support and encouraging patients to maintain independence as far as possible. Regularly evaluating the effectiveness of these interventions on the targeted symptoms are important aspects of the nurses role in managing people with PD.

A range of medications are available to treat PD and should be prescribed on an individual basis, aiming to balance patient preference with control and management of their symptoms (NICE 2006; SIGN 2010a). PD medication, is aimed at alleviating symptoms and, if possible, slowing the progression of the disease by increasing the levels of dopamine, or mimic its effect so that they stimulate areas of the brain where dopamine works. Table 34.19 details the pharmacological management of PD.

Table 34.18 Motor and non-motor signs and symptoms in PD.

MOTOR IMPAIRMENT	NON-MOTOR SYMPTOMS
Repetitive tremor (pill rolling)	Early prodromal signs, including loss of smell (anosmia), constipation, rapid eye movement sleep disturbances
Akinesia – inability to initiate a willed movement	Sleep disturbances, up to 90% (Bonnet *et al.* 2012)
Bradykinesia – slowness of movement or difficulty in starting to move	Dysphagia
Dyskinesia – abnormal involuntary movements of the limbs, trunk or face	Excessive salivation, dribbling and drooling
Rigidity	Communication problems – voice softening, slurring and slowness of speech
Postural instability	Constipation and bladder dysfunction
Gait disturbances – shuffling and festinant gait	Apathy up to 70% (Aarsland *et al.* 2009)
Dystonia – sustained and painful muscle contractions	Cognitive impairment
	Dementia, up to 80% (Butler *et al.* 2008)
	Depression, up to 70%
	Restless leg syndrome – tingling, burning, aching or pain commonly occurring in the legs
	Pain

Link To/Go To

http://www.parkinsons.org.uk

Red Flag

Abrupt withdrawal of medications can result in:
- Sudden development of symptoms
- Increased risk of falling
- Prolonged hospital stay and may be life-threatening.

As well as ensuring that prescribed medications are administered at the prescribed time, consideration of supporting patients to self-medicate (patients control their own medication), are important aspects of nursing care, ensuring a constant therapeutic level of symptom control for PD patients.

Table 34.19 Pharmacological management of Parkinson's disease.

MEDICATIONS	POSSIBLE SIDE-EFFECTS
Levodopa therapies:	
Replace depleted dopamine Most effective drug in all stages of PD and standard initial treatment Prescribed orally in combination with dopa-decarboxylase (enzyme important in converting levodopa to dopamine), e.g. co-careldopa	Constipation, depression, postural hypotension, dyskinesia, hallucinations Impulse control disorders (ICD)
Dopamine agonists:	
Compounds that stimulate the dopamine receptors in the brain, in particular the D2/D3 receptors, e.g. Pramipexole dihydrochloride (Mirapexinde®) Continuous dopaminergic stimulation via subcutaneous injection, Apomorphine hydrochloride (APO-go®).	Nausea, postural hypotension, dyskinesia, hallucinations Impulse control disorders (ICD) Haemolytic anaemia with apomorphine
Non-ergot dopamine agonists (NEDAs):	
Stimulate the dopamine receptors in the brain in particular the D2 and D3, e.g. Ropinirole, Pramipexole and Apomorphine (cannot be given orally)	
MAO-B (Monoamine oxidase type B) inhibitors:	
Prevent the break down of dopamine in the brain by blocking the enzyme (monoamine oxidase type B) that breaks it down, e.g. Selegiline (Eldepryl®), Rasagiline (Azilect ®)	Vivid dreams and hallucinations
Catechol-O-methyl transferase (COMT) inhibitors:	
Blocks the enzyme that breaks down levodopa in the brain, prolonging its effect Used in combination with levodopa, e.g. Entacapone (Comtess®), Tolcapone (Tasmar®).	Diarrhoea, stomach cramps, and enhanced levodopa side-effects

Impulsive and compulsive behaviours, also referred to as impulse control disorders (ICD), are known side-effects of some Parkinson medications (e.g. dopamine agonists and levodopa), affecting up to 24% of PD patients (Weintraub *et al.* 2010). ICDs include pathological gambling, compulsive buying, compulsive sexual behaviour and binge eating. The impact on the patient and their families can be devastating. Nurses need to be aware of this potential side-effect of Parkinson medication and be vigilant for potential impulsive and compulsive disorders by listening to both patients and their families/carers. Any symptoms that may indicate ICD should be discussed with the PD specialist.

Other treatment options include:

- Dopaminergic stimulation therapies, such as deep brain stimulation (DBS) non-destructive surgery, which is reversible of the subthalamic nucleus (STN) or the globus pallidus interna (GPi)
- Duodenal levodopa infusions (Duodopa®), a gel pumped continuously into the small intestine, from which it is absorbed into the bloodstream, for motor fluctuations in advanced PD, with substantial improvements in quality of life (Williams *et al.* 2010)
- Restorative therapies, although still in their experimental stage, include fetal nigral transplantation and stem cell therapies.

Alzheimer's Disease and Related Disorders

Dementia is widely recognised as a major rapidly increasing epidemic and a worldwide challenge to healthcare. Dementia is a chronic progressive mental disorder and Alzheimer's disease (AD) is the most common form of pre-senile dementias and age-related cerebral disorders. Other common causes include Lewy Body dementia (accompanied by Parkinson's disease symptoms), vascular dementia and frontal lobe dementia. AD is a degenerative cerebral disease, with characteristic neuropathological and neurochemical features. Alzheimer's Disease International (ADI 2009) predicts that in 2030, there will be 66 million people worldwide with AD.

Epidemiology

Alzheimer's disease (AD) is the most common cause of dementia in the elderly. In the UK, there are approximately 496 000 people living with Alzheimer's (Alzheimer's UK 2013), and the number of cases is expected to rise with more women being susceptible to dementia than men, primarily because they live longer. A typical onset can occur from the age of 40 years and the median survival from onset has been estimated at 7 years (NICE 2011).

Risk factors Evidence from genetic linkage studies is strong enough to link defects on the amyloid precursor protein (APP) gene (β-amyloid peptide is formed from APP), and other genes of chromosomes 1, 14 and 21, in early onset familial AD (FAD) for the basis for genetic screening in suspected cases of early FAD.

Modifiable factors include:

- History of stroke, particularly in the presence of vascular risk factors (Vermeer *et al.* 2007; Brundel *et al.* 2012), although the complex interactions between cerebrovascular disease and AD is not fully understood. Disruption in cerebral blood flow following ischaemic episodes such as stroke is an important risk factor for the later development of AD
- Serious traumatic brain injury, especially repeated cerebral concussions for example, in boxers or alcoholics sometimes referred to as 'punch-drunk syndrome'.

Pathophysiology

The name 'Alzheimer's' is taken from a German psychiatrist who, in 1906, described the condition of a demented patient, in whose brain particular microscopic features called 'neurofibrillary plaques and tangles' (NTF) were discovered on autopsy. To date, a definitive diagnosis requires pathological confirmation at autopsy, with the presence of these extracellular amyloid plaques, insoluble extracellular deposits of β-amyloid peptide and intracellular neurofibrillary tangles, dense long microtubule filaments mainly composed of Tau proteins that form in the cell cytoplasm. These plaques and NTF lead to synaptic dysfunction, synapses plaques, neuronal cell death and subsequent brain atrophy (Ballard et al. 2011). Death occurs 3–15 years of onset of AD. Although the pattern of neuronal loss varies, the neuronal loss is most significant in the cerebral cortex, hippocampus amygdala and the olfactory system.

Signs and symptoms

Typically, the symptoms of AD progress from mild memory problems to severe cognitive impairment: reasoning; exercising judgement; planning and executing familiar tasks. Several behavioural symptoms are characteristics of AD, these include: apathy affecting up to 70%; agitation occurring in 60%; anxiety and depression affecting 50%. Disinhibition occurs in up to one-third of all AD patients and delusions hallucinations occur up to 25% and 10%, respectively.

The progression of AD varies but as the disease progresses, the patients exhibit a range of signs and symptoms, which are individual to the person and all do not manifest in everyone. A summary of the some common symptoms associated with each stage are summarised in Table 34.20.

Apathy is one of the first symptoms linked to alternations in frontal lobe functions distinct from depression, and correlates strongly with reduced executive functioning. Its prevalence remains high as the disease progresses.

Diagnosis and investigations

Clinical diagnosis is more difficult and as there are no specific tests for Alzheimer's, the diagnosis is based on excluding other conditions with similar signs and symptoms. This however, makes the diagnosis prone to misdiagnosis, with an estimated 10% of patients being misdiagnosed. Improving public and professional awareness and the understanding of dementia are crucial to ensure effective and timely diagnosis and care (DH 2012). As many patients present with more than one symptom, an accurate description of the

Table 34.20 Alzheimer's stages, signs, symptoms and medication. (NICE 2011)

STAGE OF DISEASE	COMMON SIGNS AND SYMPTOMS	MEDICATION TREATMENTS
Early/Initial	Mild cognitive impairment · Lapses of memory · Difficulties with planning/organising · Behavioural · Apathy – decreased interest, motivation, spontaneity, affection, enthusiasm and emotion (Levy et al. 1998). · Depression	NMDA receptor antagonist · Memantine (Ebixa)
Mid/Moderate	Cognitive · Obvious memory loss and language problems · Difficulties with simple tasks and/or instructions · Ability to perform mental challenges affected, e.g. counting backwards from 100 · Behavioural · Confusion, agitation · Aggression · Inappropriate eating and sexual behaviour · Purposeless and inappropriate activities (fidgeting, pacing, moving things around) · May have periods of irritability, paranoia, delusions and anxiety · Wandering and pacing · Sleep disturbances, e.g. insomnia	AChE inhibitors · Donepezil (Aricept®) · Galantamine · (Reminyl®) · Rivastigmine · (Exelon®) · Antipsychotic drugs (also known as neuroleptics) for agitation/ aggression · Risperidone · (Risperdal®) · Sleep may be helped by tranquillisers, e.g. Zopiclone
Late/Severe	Cognitive · Inability to manage independently · Loss of intelligible speech · Urinary and faecal incontinence · Motor problems such as inability to smile; grimaces instead · Behavioural · Psychosis, most common being delusions of thief and misidentification of a familiar person as an imposter · Wandering · Aggression · Affective disorder, e.g. anxiety and depression · Physical symptoms · Requiring support to sit up and difficulty holding head up · Neurological changes (rigidity and contractures)	NMDA receptor antagonist · Memantine (Ebixa)

patient's behaviour is crucial. The Department of Health (DH 2012) stipulates that there will be a dementia toolkit for surgeries, and a requirement of healthcare professionals to ask patients aged between 65 and 74 about their memory, as part of every standard health check. Detailed history-taking is necessary and appropriate screening, to exclude other possible causes for the patient's signs and symptoms, such as infections and side-effects of medications. Families/carers should be involved in the history-taking, as they may be extremely useful in providing information patients may have forgotten. CT scans may be useful in assessing any changes, such as atrophy, and refer to clinical psychology for more detail cognitive assessment and behavioural management strategies. In addition, genetic screening in suspected cases of early-onset FAD may be useful for some members of affected families, when there is access to appropriate genetic counselling and support.

Nursing care and management

AD is profoundly life-changing for both the individual and their family/carers. The behavioural and psychological symptoms are both challenging and a source of considerable distress, anxiety and strain for the families and carers.

Nursing care is centred on an individual approach and is summarised in Box 34.8.

Despite there being no cure for AD, if the disease is diagnosed early, medication may help to improve, slow or stabilise the symptoms and promote a better quality of life (Prince *et al.* 2011). The psychopathology of AD is thought to correlate with the low level of the acetylcholine, widely distributed throughout the CNS and PNS, which regulates behavioural and emotional responses. There-

fore, the use of acetyl cholinesterase (AChE) inhibitors, which prevent an enzyme known as 'acetylcholinesterase' from breaking down acetylcholine, resulting in a rise in acetylcholine, may result in an improvement in these symptoms (NICE 2011).

Recently, there has been increasing support for a role of diets in AD, although there is not specific diet. In Alzheimer's disease, synapses are rapidly lost, more than would normally occur, and thus there is a higher requirement to synthesise new ones; this is dependent upon a process known as 'The Kennedy Cycle', in which a number of nutrients are important. AD patients have altered dietary preferences, taste patterns and cognitive impairment, which may make it difficult to obtain a healthy diet. Thus, early nutritional screening and providing nutritional support and advice to the patient and their carer are important to prevent adverse eating behaviours that may be detrimental to the patient.

Jot This Down

During an outpatient appointment, the daughter of a 70-year-old woman with AD reports that she has difficulty in remembering things. How will you deal with this?

Peripheral Neuropathy

Peripheral neuropathy refers to a damage to the peripheral nerves, often affecting them distally. There are over 100 different conditions, each with their own specific pattern of development and prognosis.

Epidemiology

Peripheral neuropathy (PN) is common, affecting 2.4% of the population and in those 55 years and over, it affects 8% of the population (Martyn & Hughes 1997). **Charcot–Marie disease**, also known as 'hereditary motor and sensory neuropathy' is the most common inherited neuromuscular disease, affecting at least 40 per 100 000, with over 30 causative genes identified. Peripheral neuropathy occurs in 26% of patients with type 2 diabetes (Davies *et al.* 2006).

Pathophysiology

PN may be either inherited, collectively referred to as Charcot–Marie disease or acquired, with causes including:

- Chronic inflammatory demyelinating neuropathy
- Acute neuropathy, i.e. Guillain–Barré syndrome
- Physical trauma, e.g. physical damage to a nerve(s) due to accidents, falls
- Nerve entrapment; compression of the median nerve (carpel tunnel syndrome), ulnar nerve palsy or spinal nerves, as they emerge from the spinal cord, can be trapped by bony spurs or intervertebral discs and give rise to sensory and motor disturbances commonly affecting the cervical and lumbar nerves
- Disease – metabolic and endocrine, e.g. diabetes mellitus with over 60–70% of diabetic persons having some form of PND (Boulton 2005); hypothyroidism; malnutrition and vitamin deficiency, e.g. B_1 (thiamine) deficiency common among people with chronic alcoholism
- Kidney conditions, in which abnormal levels of toxins can severely damage nerve tissue
- Infectious processes, e.g. HIV, herpes simplex and syphilis
- Cancers that invade nerves

Box 34.8 Summary of the Key Points in the Nursing Management for Patients with Alzheimer's Disease

- Ensure the care plan is tailored to the individual's needs
- Regularly structured assessments, evaluation to identify, plan and meet the needs of the individual:
  - Mini mental status examination (MMSE)
  - Holistic problem-solving approach
  - Behavioural analysis using the 'ABC' (A, Antecedents, triggers and causes; B, Behaviour and C, Consequences of that behaviour) evaluation of behaviour to identify possible precipitating factors and devise effective management plans
  - Considering the possibility of maintaining a familiar environment that is stimulating and supports individual lifestyles
- Engage and work in partnership with the individual and their family/carer to:
  - Gain a comprehensive person-centred picture of the person with AD
  - Identify individual and carer's needs in a framework of respects for human rights
- Knowledge and understanding of the disease progression.
- Engage in specific training to enable:
  - Safe and effective management of problems as they occur
  - Effective management strategies to be deployed; these may include music therapy, reminiscence therapy, reality orientation, validation therapy and purposeful activity
- Multidisciplinary input and referral to relevant agencies that can offer assistance and support, e.g. Admiral Nurse Services.

- Exposure to toxins, such as heavy metals (lead, mercury), anti-cancer agents, anticonvulsants and antiviral drugs
- Medications, e.g. digoxin, phenytoin, statins.

Neuropathy can be classified according to the pattern of nerves involved and includes:

- Number of nerves involved: single (mononeuropathy), e.g. Bell's palsy; multiple (polyneuropathy), e.g. in diabetes
- Fibres affected, e.g. motor, sensory, autonomic
- Size of the fibres, i.e. large or small diameter fibres
- Proximal or distal level of involvement
- Parts of the nerves involved, e.g. soma, axons
- Pathological reaction, e.g. inflammatory, demyelinating.

Diagnosis and investigations

Diagnosis involves establishing the presence of the neurology via history (i.e. onset duration and course) and neurological examination, and tests are used to confirm the anatomical and pathological pattern of the neuropathy. The objective of the investigations is to localise the peripheral neuropathy to a part of the peripheral nervous system (PNS). Tests may include nerve conduction studies, EMG, CSF evaluation, radiological and image studies, imaging and blood tests, including fasting blood glucose, comprehensive metabolic profile and ESR thyroid stimulating hormone levels. Nerve biopsy may be considered if diagnosis remains uncertain after other tests.

Signs and symptoms

Because every peripheral nerve has a highly specialised function in a specific part of the body, the patient may present with a wide array of symptoms, depending upon the type and distribution of nerves affected. Sensory nerve damage may cause numbness, tingling, and pricking sensations (paresthesia), sensitivity to touch, or loss of position sense, inability to feel pain or changes in temperature. In the early stages of the condition, these symptoms affect the distal limbs often described as a 'glove and stocking' distribution. Others may suffer more extreme symptoms, including burning, stabbing and shooting pains. Pain is the most common presentation of PN associated with diabetes mellitus.

Motor nerve damage causes muscle wasting, paralysis or organ or gland dysfunction. Symptoms of the autonomic nerve damage are diverse, depending on the organ affected but may include; inability to sweat normally, digest food easily, maintain safe levels of blood pressure or experience normal sexual function.

Nursing care and management

Inherited PN has no specific treatment or cure. However, peripheral nerves can regenerate, thus many people have resolution of their symptoms over time but if the damage is too severe, patients may have persistent symptoms. Symptoms can often be controlled, and eliminating the causes of specific forms of neuropathy can often prevent new damage.

Peripheral neuropathy often causes neuropathic pain, due to the damage or dysfunction of the peripheral nerves and abnormal processing of stimuli, for example non-painful stimuli such as touch is painful and this is called **allodynia**. Neuropathic pain can manifest as burning, shooting, tingling, and is the most common presentation of PN associated with diabetes mellitus, and has a significant negative effect on quality of life (Davies *et al.* 2006).

Pharmacological options to treat neuropathic pain may include anticonvulsants, such as Gabapentin and antidepressants, such as amitriptyline.

The Evidence

Several screening tools are available to assist in identifying patients with pain of neuropathic origin, in particular in non-specialist settings, for example primary care. The LANSS (Leeds Assessment of Neuropathic Symptoms and Signs) Pain Scale is an internationally used tool for identifying neuropathic pain. It has also been developed into a patient self-report tool (S-LANSS). It has a maximum score of 24 and a score of 12 and above indicates neuropathic pain.

(Bennett 2001)

Primary care – supportive measure Primary prevention measures include adopting a healthy lifestyle – avoiding toxins, correcting vitamin deficiencies, limiting alcohol intake and weight reduction.

Reduced sensation in the feet may mean that friction and trauma, increasing the risk of ulceration, may go unnoticed. Advising and teaching the patient self-care skills, such as regular meticulous foot care, inspecting their feet and toes for blisters and sores that may appear on numb areas of the foot, because pressure sores or injury may go unnoticed. Advise the patient to report any changes in cuts, calluses, ulcers, etc. to their GP, practice nurse or community nurse.

Advice on suitable footwear, in particular protective footwear to protect against injury, may also be necessary, along with referral to a chiropodist or podiatrist for those patients who are at risk of trauma, for regular review. Simple physical treatments, such as the use of a bed cradle to lift the bed clothes off hyperaesthetic skin, can be beneficial, along with referral to the community physiotherapist for walking aids: sticks, frame. In the diabetic patient, the best way to prevent or delay the progression of PN is to keep blood glucose levels as close to the normal range as possible.

Conclusion

This chapter began with an overview of the organisation, structure and functions of the central and peripheral nervous system. The different cells that make up the nervous system were described along with their functions. Critical to nursing a patient with a neurological condition, is an accurate and comprehensive neurological assessment, the key principles of which have been outlined including: clinical, non-invasive and invasive assessment techniques and tools, such as the Glasgow Coma Scale. The principles of caring for a patient with raised intracranial pressure has been discussed, along with the main conditions that may present with raised intracranial pressure: traumatic brain injury, stroke, brain tumours and central nervous system infections. Common neurological conditions and disorders, such as headache, epilepsy, multiple sclerosis, Parkinson disease, dementia, and peripheral neuropathy have been outlined, along with their associated nursing care and management principles. This care is not only complex but challenging and requires the acquisition of a wide range of skills and experience. The principles of care outlines in this chapter will support a nurse in caring for a patient with any neurological condition and not just those discussed in this chapter.

Useful Links

Professional Organisations/Support Groups

Brain and Spinal Injury Charity (BASIC): http://www.basiccharity.org.uk/

Brain and Spine Foundation: http://www.brainandspine.org.uk/

Brain Tumour UK: http://www.braintumouruk.org.uk/

British Association of Neuroscience Nurses: http://www.bann.org.uk/

Multiple Sclerosis (MS) Trust: http://www.mstrust.org.uk/

The Neurological Alliance: http://www.neural.org.uk/

The World Federation of Neuroscience Nurses: http://www.wfnn.nu/

World Federation of Neurology http://www.wfnals.org/

Key Points

- The neurological system is both complex and challenging and to ensure effective and competent nursing care for neurological patients, nurses need the necessary skills and experience, especially in the utilisation of tools, such as the GCS.
- Nursing care of conditions related to the neurological system requires an understanding of the anatomy and physiology of the nervous system.
- Nursing care for this diverse, vast patient group requires a collaborative approach with other healthcare professionals, and/or their relatives/informal carers according to patients' holistic needs and goals.
- A neurological assessment is conducted to assess the function and integrity of the nervous system and should be conducted in a systematic way, with an initial assessment providing a baseline against which subsequent assessment can be compared.
- Altered level of consciousness (LOC) is a common response to intracranial disorders, and is an early manifestation of deterioration of the function of the cerebral hemispheres.
- Increased intracranial pressure is a sustained elevated pressure ($\geq 10\,mmHg$) within the cranial cavity and can result from a variety of intracranial and extracranial causes, and if untreated, can be fatal.
- Traumatic brain injury (TBI) refers to any injury of the scalp, skull or brain, and is a leading cause of death and disability worldwide. TBI affects all body systems, and may result in a constellation of deficits, including: physical, language, cognitive, behavioural and emotional.
- Central nervous system infections may be caused by a variety of organisms and the major CNS infections are meningitis, encephalitis and brain abscess.
- Intracranial tumours are named according to the tissues from which they arise and include, on or in brain tissue: the meninges, the pituitary gland, blood vessels; in addition, they are a frequent site for secondary tumours from elsewhere in the body.
- A stroke is a major healthcare problem in the UK and results from a sudden decrease in blood flow to a localised area of the brain and may be ischaemic or haemorrhagic.

- Epilepsy is a chronic disorder of abnormal, recurring, excessive and self-terminating electrical discharges from neurones – its pathophysiology is not fully understood and it is frequently misdiagnosed.
- Headaches, a common type of intracranial pain, are categorised as tension, migraine and cluster. Headaches are a sign and symptom of increased intracranial pressure.
- Multiple sclerosis (MS) is an incurable, complex, chronic demyelinating neurological disease of the CNS, commonly occurring in the young to middle-aged adults, in which inflamed areas on the myelin sheath of nerves in the brain result in damage and loss of the nerve axon and the formation of localised inflammation called 'plaques', and eventual nerve death.
- Parkinson's disease (PD) is an incurable, common, progressive neurodegenerative disorder affecting the CNS, usually affecting the older adult, which eventually leads to disability characterised by tremor, muscle rigidity and bradykinesia.
- Alzheimer's disease and related disorders is a major, rapidly increasing epidemic and a worldwide challenge to health care and, Alzheimer's disease (AD), a degenerative cerebral disease, is the most common form of pre-senile dementias and age-related cerebral disorders.
- Peripheral neuropathy refers to damage to the peripheral nerves, includes over 100 different conditions, and results in a variety of symptoms, including pain, numbness and muscle wasting.

Glossary

Acalcula: loss of the ability to write

Ageusia: loss of taste sensation

Agnosia: inability to recognise and interpret objects, people, sounds or smells; typically results from damage to the occipital or parietal lobe

Agraphia: inability to communicate ideas in written language

Akathisia: motor restlessness – inability to sit still

Anosmia: inability to smell – may be seen with lesions of the frontal lobe or early PD

Anosognosia: lack of awareness of or indifference to one's own neurological deficit

Aphasia: defective or absent language function

Ataxia: a lack of coordination and a clumsiness of movements

Aura: a symptom experienced before a migraine or seizure, e.g. flashing lights

Brudzinski's sign: flexion of the neck that causes the hip and knee to flex

Chemoreceptors: receptors that respond to changes in the chemical environment

Clonus: rhythmic contraction relaxation tremor, indicative of exaggerated stretch reflexes

Contralateral: located on the opposite side of the body (brain)

Diplopia: double vision due to lack of parallelism

Dysphonia: change in the tone of the voice seen in with paralysis of the vocal cords

Dysarthria: difficulty speaking

Dysphagia: difficulty swallowing is common with impaired blood flow to the brain

Hemiplegia: paralysis of one-half of the body, vertically

Hemiparesis: weakness on one side of the body

Hemianopia: loss of vision in one half of the visual field

Fasciculation: spontaneous firing of an axon resulting in a visible twitch of all the muscle fibres it contacts

Kernig's sign: inability to extend the knee while the hip is flexed at a 90° angle

Ipsilateral: located on the same side of the body (brain)

Ischaemia: inadequate supply of blood to an organ or part of the body as from an obstructed blood flow

Photophobia: abnormal intolerance to light, usually associated with eye pain

Prodromal: premonitory symptoms that occur hours to days before the episode

Nerve: a bundle of hundreds to thousands of axons or neurones plus connective tissue and blood vessels outside the CNS

Nociceptive: painful

Nystagmus: involuntary movement of an eye may be horizontal, vertical or rotary

Nuchal rigidity: stiff neck

Mydriasis: pupillary dilation

Myoclonus: sudden, shock-like, jerking contraction of a group of muscles

Opisthotonos: a form of extreme hyperextension of the body in which the head and heels are bent backward and the body bowed forward

Papilloedema: swelling of the nerve head in the optic discs seen in ICP

Ptosis: droopy eyelid

Syncope: sudden and temporary loss of consciousness

Tremor: involuntary, rhythmic oscillatory movements about a fixed point, due to alternating or synchronous contractions of agonist and antagonist muscles

References

Aarsland, D., Marsh, L. & Schrag, A. (2009) Neuropsychiatric symptoms in Parkinson's disease. *Movement Disorders*, 24, 2175–2186.

Adams, H.T., Brott, T.G., Furlan, A.L. *et al.* (2007) Guidelines for thrombolytic theory for acute stroke: a supplement for the guidelines for the management of patients with acute ischaemic stroke. *Circulation*, 94(5), 1167–1174.

ADI (2009) *World Alzheimer's Report*. Alzheimer Disease International. http://www.alz.co.uk/.

All-Party Parliamentary Group on Epilepsy (2007) *The Human and Economic Cost of Epilepsy in England*. All-Party Parliamentary Group on Epilepsy, London.

Ayerbe, L., Ayis, S., Rudd, A.G., Heuschmann, P.U., Wolfe, C.D. (2011) Natural history, predictors, and associations of depression 5 years after stroke: the South London Stroke Register. *Stroke*, 42(7), 1907–1911.

Alzheimer's UK (2013) *What is Alzheimer's Disease?* Fact Sheet 401, LP. http://www.alzheimers.org.uk/site/scripts/documents_info.php?documentID=100 (accessed 22 July 2013).

Backer, J.H. (2006) The symptom experience of patients with Parkinson Disease. *Journal of Neuroscience Nursing*, 38(1), 51–57.

Ballard, C., Gauthier, S. Corbett, A. Brayne, C. Aarsland, D. & Jones, E. (2011) Alzheimer's disease. *Lancet*, 377, 1019–1031.

Bamford, J., Sandercock, P., Dennis, M., Burn, J. & Warlow, C. (1991) Classification and natural history of clinically identifiable subtypes of cerebral infarction. *Lancet* 22, 337(8756), 1521–1526.

BASH (2010) *Guidelines for all Healthcare Professionals in the Diagnosis and Management of Migraine, Tension-Type Headache, Cluster Headache, Medication-Overuse Headache*, 3rd edn, 1st revision. British Association for the Study of Headache. http://www.bash.org.uk/ (accessed February 2012).

Bennett, M. (2001) The LANSS Pain Scale: The Leeds assessment of neuropathic symptoms and sign. *Pain*, 92, 147–157.

Bigal, M.E. & Lipton, R.B. (2007) The differential diagnosis of chronic daily headache: an algorithm-based approach. *Journal of Headache and Pain*, 8, 263–272.

Bonnet, A.M., Jutras, M.F., Czernecki, V., Corvol, J.C. & Vidailhet, M. (2012) Nonmotor symptoms in Parkinson's disease in 2012: relevant clinical aspects. *Parkinson's Disease*, 2012, 198316.

Boulton, A.J.M. (2005). Management of diabetic peripheral neuropathy. *Clinical Diabetes*, 23(1), 9–15.

Braine, M.E. (2011) The experience of living with a family member with challenging behaviour following acquired brain injury. *Journal of Neuroscience Nursing*, 43(3), 156–164.

Brundel, M., de Bresser, J., van Dillen, J.J., Kappelle, L.J. & Biessels, G.J. (2012) Cerebral microinfarcts: a systematic review of neuropathological studies. *Journal of Cerebral Blood Flow Metabolism*, 32, 1–12.

Butler, T.C., van den Hout, A., Mathews, F.E. *et al.* (2008) Dementia and survival in Parkinson disease: a 12-year population study. *Neurology*, 70, 1017–1022.

Chaudhuri, K.R., Healy, D.G. & Schaprio, A.H. (2006) Non-motor symptoms in Parkinson Disease: diagnosis and management. *Lancet Neurology*, 5, 235–245.

Chiaravalloti, N.D. & DeLuca, J. (2008) Cognitive impairment in multiple sclerosis. *Lancet Neurology*, 7(12), 1139–1151.

Comi, G., Martinelli, V., Rodegher, M. *et al.* (2009) Effect of glatiramer acetate on conversion to clinically definite multiple sclerosis in patients with clinically isolated syndrome (PreCISe study): a randomised, double-blind, placebo-controlled trial. *Lancet*, 374(9700), 1503–1511.

Cook, A.M., Peppard, A. & Magnuson, B. (2008) Nutritional considerations in traumatic brain injury. *Nutrition in Clinical Practice*, 23(6), 608–620.

Crocetti, E., Trama, A., Stiller, C. *et al.* (2012) RARECARE working group. Epidemiology of glial and non-glial brain tumours in Europe. *European Journal of Cancer*, 48, 1532–1542.

Davies, M., Brophy, S., Williams, R. & Taylor, A. (2006) The prevalence, severity, and impact of painful diabetic peripheral neuropathy in type 2 diabetes. *Diabetes Care*, 29(7), 1518–1522.

DH (2007a) *Cancers 2012 Vision Department of Health. Annex B Brain & Central Nervous System Cancers*. Department of Health, London.

DH (2007b) *National Stroke Strategy*. Department of Health, London. http://webarchive.nationalarchives.gov.uk/20130107105354/http://www.dh.gov.uk/prod_consum_dh/groups/dh_digitalassets/documents/digitalasset/dh_081059.pdf

DH (2009) *Stroke: Act F.A.S.T. Awareness Campaign*. Department of Health, London.

DH (2012) *Dementia Tool Kit*. Department of Health, London.

Epilepsy Society (2013) *About Epilepsy*. The Epilepsy Society, Chalfont St Peter. http://www.epilepsysociety.org.uk/AboutEpilepsy.

Farner, L., Wagle, J., Flekkoy, K. *et al.* (2009). Factor analysis of the Montgomery Aasberg depression rating scale in an elderly population. *International Journal of Geriatric Psychiatry*, 24, 1209–1216.

Fischera, M., Marziniak, M., Gralow, I. & Evers, S. (2008) The incidence and prevalence of cluster headache: a meta-analysis of population based studies. *Cephalalgia*, 28(6), 614–618.

Granerod, J., Ambrose, H.E., Davies, N.W. *et al.* (2010) Causes of encephalitis and differences in England: a multi-centred, population-based prospective study. *Lancet*, 2, 1838–1844.

Hackett, M.L. & Anderson, C.S. (2005) Predictors of depression after stroke: a systematic review of observational studies. *Stroke*, 36, 2296–2301.

Hadjimichael, O., Vollmer, T. & Oleen-Burkey, M. (2008) Fatigue characteristics in multiple sclerosis: the Northern American Committee on Multiple Sclerosis survey. *Health Quality Outcome*, 6, 100.

Hawkes, C.H., Del Tredici, K. & Braak, H. (2010) A timeline for Parkinson's disease. *Parkinsonism Related Disorders*, 16(2), 79–84.

Hickey, J.V. (2009) *The Clinical Practice of Neurological and Neurosurgical Nursing*, 6th edn. J.B. Lipponcott, Philadelphia.

Hirsh, A.T, Turner, A.P., Ehde, D.M. & Haselkorn, J.K. (2009) Prevalence and impact of pain in multiple sclerosis: physical and psychologic contributions. *Archives of Physical Medicine Rehabilitation*, 90, 646–651.

ICHS-II Headache Classification Subcommittee of the International Headache Society (2004) The International Classification of Headache Disorders, 2nd edn. *Cephalalgia*, 24(Suppl 1), 9–160.

Jackson, J.L., Kuriyama, A. & Hayashino, Y. (2012) Botulinum toxin A for prophylactic treatment of migraine and tension headaches in adults: A meta-analysis. *JAMA*, 307, 1736.

Jennett, B. & Bond, M. (1975) Assessment of outcome after severe brain damage. A practical scale. *Lancet*, 1, 480–484.

Joint Epilepsy Council of the UK and Ireland (2011) *Epilepsy Prevalence Incidence and Other Statistics*. The Joint Epilepsy Council of the UK and Ireland, Leeds. www.jointepilepsycouncil.org.uk

Kernick, D., Stapley, S. & Hamilton, W. (2008) GPs' classification of headache: is primary headache underdiagnosed? *British Journal of General Practice*, 58(547), 102–104.

Lansberg, M.G., Bluhmki, E. & Thijs, V.N. (2009) Efficacy and safety of tissue plasminogen activator 3 to 4.5 hours after acute ischemic stroke: a metaanalysis. *Stroke*, 40(7), 2438–2441.

Levy, M.L., Cummings, J.L., Fairbanks, L.A. *et al.* (1998) Apathy is not depression. *Journal of Neuropsychiatry Clinical Neuroscience*, 10(3), 314–319.

Louis, D.N., Ohgaki, H., Wiestler, O.D. *et al.* (2007) The 2007 WHO classification of tumours of the central nervous system. *Acta Neuropathologica*, 114, 97–109.

Marsh, H. (2009) Brain tumours. *Surgery*, 27(3), 135–138.

Martyn, C.N. & Hughes, R.A. (1997) Epidemiology of peripheral neuropathy. *Journal of Neurology, Neurosurgery and Psychiatry*, 62(4), 310–318.

Mohen, K.M., Wolfe, C.D.A., Rudd, A.G., Heuschmann, P.U., Kolominsky-Rabas, P.L. & Grieve, A.P. (2011) Risk and cumulative risk of stoke recurrence. *Stroke*, 42(5), 1489–1494.

Monti, M.M., Laureys, S. & Owen, A.M. (2010) The vegetative state. *British Medical Journal*, 10, 341:c3765.

NICE (2006) *Dementia: supporting people with dementia and their carers in health and social care (CG42)*. National Institute for Health and Clinical Excellence, London.

NICE (2007) *Head Injury. Triage, Assessment, Investigation and Early Management of Head Injury in Infants, Children and Adults*, 2nd edn (CG56). National Institute for Health and Clinical Excellence, London.

NICE (2008) *Diagnosis and Initial Management of Acute Stroke and Transient Ischaemic Attack (TIA) (CG68)*. National Institute for Health and Clinical Excellence, London.

NICE (2010) *TLoC*. National Institute for Health and Clinical Excellence, London.

NICE (2011) *Donepezil, galantamine, rivastigmine and memantine for the treatment of Alzheimer's disease (TA217)*. National Institute for Health and Clinical Excellence, London.

NICE (2012a) *Epilepsy (CG137)*. National Institute for Health and Clinical Excellence, London.

NICE (2012b) *Headaches. Diagnosis and Management of Headaches in Young People and Adults*. National Institute for Health and Clinical Excellence, London.

Oddo, M., Schmidt, M., Mayer, S. & Chiolereo, R. (2008) Glucose control after severe brain injury. *Current Opinion in Clinical Nutrition and Metabolic Care*, 11(2), 134–139.

Parkinson's UK (2013) What is Parkinson's. http://www.parkinsons.org.uk/about-parkinsons/what-is-parkinsons.aspx.

Prakash, O., Lukiw, W.J., Peruzzi, F., Reiss, K. & Musto, A.E. (2012) Gliomas and seizures. *Medical Hypotheses*, 79(5), 622–626.

Prince, M., Bryce, R. & Ferri C (2011) *Alzheimer's Disease International: World Alzheimer Report 2011*. Alzheimer's Disease International, London. www.alz.co.uk/worldreport2011 (accessed 22 July 2013).

Ramagopalan, S.V., Dobson, R., Meier, U.C. & Giovannoni, G. (2010) Multiple sclerosis: risk factors, prodromes, and potential causal pathways. *Lancet Neurology*, 9(7), 727–739.

Ramonon, J.G. (2011) Rehabilitation of hemianopic visual fields. *Advances in Clinical Neuroscience and Rehabilitation*, 11(1), 31–33.

RCP (2012) *National Clinical Guidelines for Stroke*, 4th edn. Royal College of Physicians, London.

Seshadri, S. & Wolf, P.A. (2007). Lifetime risk of stroke and dementia: current concepts, and estimates from the Framingham Study. *Lancet Neurology*, 6(12), 1106–1114.

SIGN (2008) *SIGN Diagnosis and Management of Headache in Adults. A National Clinical Guideline 107*. Scottish Intercollegiate Guidelines Network, Edinburgh.

SIGN (2010a) *Diagnosis and Pharmacological Management of Parkinson's Disease*. Scottish Intercollegiate Guidelines Network, Edinburgh.

SIGN (2010b) *Management of Patients with Stroke: rehabilitation, prevention and management of complications and discharge planning*. Scottish Intercollegiate Guidelines Network, Edinburgh. http://tinyurl.com/35jdq9y.

Simpson, S. Jr, Blizzard, L., Otahal, P., Van Der Mei, I. & Taylor, B. (2011) Latitude is significantly associated with the prevalence of multiple sclerosis: a meta-analysis. *Journal of Neurology, Neurosurgery and Psychiatry*, 82, 1132–1114.

Teasdale, G. & Jennett, J. (1974) Assessment of coma and impaired consciousness. *Lancet* 13, (7872), 81–84.

Vermeer, S.E., Longsteth, W.T. & Koudstall, P.J. (2007) Silent brain infarcts: a systematic review. *Lancet Neurology*, 6, 611–619.

Vos, T., Flaxman, A.D., Naghavi, M. *et al.* (2012) Years lived with disability (YLDs) for 1160 sequelae of 289 diseases and injuries 1990–2010: a systematic analysis for the Global Burden of Disease Study 2010. *Lancet*, 380, 22/29: 2163–2196.

Weintraub, D., Koester, J., Potenza, M.N. *et al.* (2010) Impulse control disorders in Parkinson Disease: A cross-sectional study of 3,090 patients. *Archives of Neurology*, 67(5), 589–595.

WHO (2008) *The Global Burden of Disease 2004 Update*. World Health Organization, Geneva.

Williams, A., Gill, S. & Varma, T. *et al.* (2010) Deep brain stimulation therapy versus best medical therapy alone for advanced Parkinson's disease (PD SURG trial): a randomised, open-label trail. *Lancet Neurology*, 9(6), 581–591.

Test Yourself

1. Which is NOT considered a major part of the brain?
   (a) Brain stem
   (b) Cerebellum
   (c) Cauda equina
   (d) Diencephalon
   (e) Cerebrum

2. This separates the two hemispheres of the cerebrum:
   (a) Flax cerebri
   (b) Falx cerebelli
   (c) Tentorium cerebelli
   (d) Tentorium cerebri
   (e) None of the above

3. This protects the brain by preventing passage of harmful substances and pathogens:
   (a) Dura mater
   (b) Arachnoid mater
   (c) Cerebrospinal fluid
   (d) Blood–brain barrier
   (e) All of the above

4. Cranial nerve II is the:
   (a) Olfactory nerve
   (b) Oculomotor nerve
   (c) Hypoglossal nerve
   (d) Optic nerve

5. Where in the brain is the speech centre for expression of speech?
   (a) Wernicke's area
   (b) Broca's area
   (c) Gustatory area nerve
   (d) Brain stem

6. What is the net-like region of white and grey matter that extends through the brain, maintaining consciousness?
   (a) Pons
   (b) Medulla oblongata
   (c) Midbrain
   (d) Reticular formation
   (e) Decussation of pyramids

7. Which structure conducts nerve impulses between gyri in different hemispheres of the cerebrum?
   (a) Association tracts
   (b) Corpus callosum
   (c) Projection tracts
   (d) Pyramids
   (e) Sulci

8. The peripheral nervous system can be divided into:
   (a) Somatic nervous system
   (b) Autonomic nervous system
   (c) Enteric nervous system
   (d) All of the above

9. Which of these contains cerebrospinal fluid?
   (a) Epidural space
   (b) Subarachnoid space
   (c) Dural space
   (d) Pia mater

10. The adult spinal cord extends from the foramen magnum to which one of the following levels?
    (a) Level of the L2 vertebra
    (b) Level of the L3 vertebra
    (c) Level of the L4 vertebra
    (d) Level of the T6 vertebra

Answers

1. c
2. a
3. d
4. d
5. b
6. d
7. b
8. d
9. b
10. a

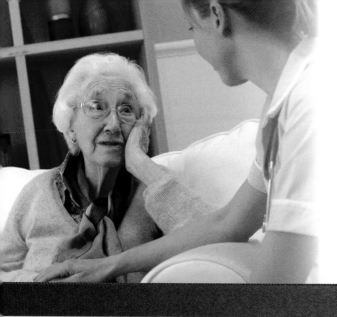

35

The Person with an Ear or Eye Disorder

Ian Peate

School of Health Studies, Gibraltar

Learning Outcomes

On completion of this chapter you will be able to:

- Discuss the anatomy and physiology of the ear and the eye
- Describe the key functions of the ears and the eyes
- Outline the various methods for undertaking an assessment of the person with an ear or eye disorder
- Discuss the skills required to undertake an effective assessment that primarily focusses on the ear or the eye
- Describe the nursing care and management of the person with an ear or eye disorder
- Discuss a range of disorders of the ear and eye

Competencies

All nurses must:

1. Possess a broad knowledge of the structure and functions of the ear and the eye
2. Provide care based on a sound evidence base
3. Undertake a comprehensive, systematic nursing assessment that considers physical, social, cultural, psychological, spiritual, genetic and environmental factors
4. Offer people care that meets their individual needs and reflects a holistic approach
5. Provide and encourage health promoting behaviour
6. Work in partnership with service users and others

 Visit the companion website at **www.wileynursingpractice.com** where you can test yourself using flashcards, multiple-choice questions and more.

Nursing Practice: Knowledge and Care, First Edition. Edited by Ian Peate, Karen Wild and Muralitharan Nair.
© 2014 John Wiley & Sons, Ltd. Published 2014 by John Wiley & Sons, Ltd. Companion website: www.wileynursingpractice.com

Introduction

Hearing and seeing are special senses: the special sense organs – the ears and the eyes – permit this to happen. These special senses are often taken for granted. The sense of smell, taste and touch are discussed in other chapters. The special sense organs respond to stimuli received using a number of pathways. These senses are key to human survival.

A disturbance in hearing, the loss of sight or a disorder of vision can impact negatively on the person's health and well-being. These two sensory organs, the ears and the eyes, are the means by which visual and auditory stimuli reach the brain. Specific structures located within the eye help the person in a number of ways, for example, from a safety perspective, and structures located in the ear assist the person with regards to the maintenance of position and equilibrium.

When malfunction of these organs occurs, this has the potential to impact on the person's ability to maintain a safe environment and can limit the person's ability to carry out the activities of living independently, temporarily or permanently. Mobility can be restricted, coupled with an impact on the person's ability to communicate, which may lead to social isolation and loneliness, safety, independence, communication and relationships with others. When the ability to receive and process information (visually and auditorily) becomes impaired, this leads to disorientation. The ability to receive and organise information orientates us to our surroundings. These two senses provide us with the ability to make known our needs and to communicate effectively with others. They provide us with the opportunity (among other things) to hear people laugh, to see the people who we love, permitting us to participate in the communication process.

When impairment or deficit occurs, the role and function of the nurse is to offer people protection, to prevent harm from occurring to them, to help them to carry out the activities of living that they are unable to carry out and above all, to help them maintain a safe environment. Following Henderson (1960), the role of the nurse when caring for people who have disorders of hearing or sight is to assist the person, sick or well, in the performance of those activities that they would ordinary perform independently.

In this chapter, the care of a number of disorders of hearing and vision will be outlined, with the person being at the centre of all that is done. An overview of the anatomy and physiology of the ears and the eyes is presented, along with the functions of these sensory organs.

The nurse will be able to offer assistance in a more competent and confident manner when they have an appreciation of the anatomy and physiology of the ears and eyes. The key aim is to provide care that is safe and effective.

Anatomy and Physiology of the Ear

Hearing is one of the major senses and, just like vision, is essential for distant warning and communication. It can be used to alert and to communicate pleasure and also fear. Hearing is a conscious appreciation of vibration perceived as sound. For this to happen, the appropriate signal must reach the higher parts of the brain. The function of the ear is to convert physical vibration into a nervous impulse. Hearing can be considered as a biological microphone. Like a microphone, the ear is stimulated by vibration: in a micro-

phone the vibration is transduced into an electrical signal; in the ear this is converted into a nervous impulse, which is then processed by the central auditory pathways of the brain. The mechanisms required to achieve this are complex.

There are two key functions associated with the ears: hearing and the maintenance of equilibrium. The anatomy and physiology of the ears, as well as both of these functions, will be discussed prior to describing a number of common ear conditions and the care required for people with ear problems.

The ears are paired organs, one on each side of the head with the sense organ itself, which technically is called the **cochlea**, buried deep within the temporal bones.

Figure 35.1 provides an illustration of the three parts of the ear:

1. **External ear**
2. **Middle ear**
3. **Inner ear.**

The External Ear

The external ear can be divided into two structures:

1. **The auricle**
2. **The external acoustic meatus**.

The auricle

Also known as the 'pinna' (Figure 35.2), the auricle is an external, lateral paired structure. Its function is to capture and transmit sound to the external auditory meatus.

The auricle has a cartilaginous framework; the lobule (lobe) is the only aspect that is not supported by cartilage. The outer curvature of the ear is known as the 'helix'. There is another curved elevation; this is parallel to the helix and is called the 'antihelix'. This divides into two aspects, the crura (singular, the crus): the infero-anterior crus and the superoposterior crus.

In the centre of the auricle is a hollow depression; this is called the 'concha' of the auricle. This continues into the skull as the external acoustic meatus. The role of the concha is to direct sound into the external acoustic meatus. Immediately anterior to the start of the external acoustic meatus there is an elevation of tissue called the 'tragus'. Opposite the tragus is the 'antitragus'.

Superficial skin innervation of the auricle comes from the greater auricular, lesser occipital and branches of the facial and vagus nerves.

The main vessels involved in the vasculature are the posterior auricular, superficial temporal and occipital arteries and veins.

The external acoustic meatus

The external acoustic meatus is a sigmoid shaped tube extending from the deep part of the concha to the tympanic membrane (Figure 35.3).

The walls are made up of cartilage from the auricle, as well as bony support coming from the temporal bone. This aspect of the external ear derives its sensory innervation from branches of the mandibular and the vagus nerves. The external acoustic meatus does not have a straight path; it travels in an S-shaped curve.

The external acoustic meatus terminates at the tympanic membrane. The tympanic membrane is a double layered structure, covered with skin on the external surface and a mucous membrane internally. At the centre of the membrane is connective tissue connected to the surrounding temporal bone by a fibrocartilaginous ring.

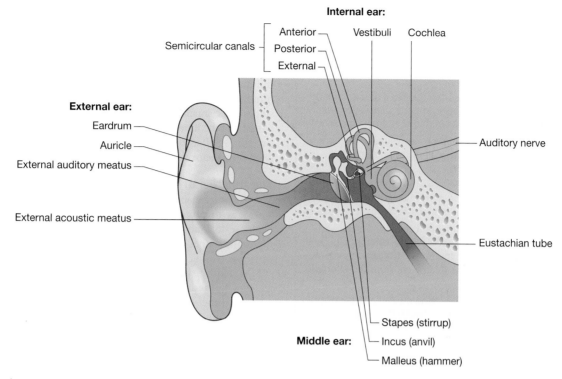

Figure 35.1 The ear.

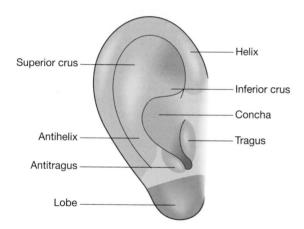

Figure 35.2 The auricle.

The tympanic membrane is translucent and, as a result of this, structures located within the middle ear can be seen. On the inner surface of the membrane, the handle of malleus attaches to the tympanic membrane at a point that is called the 'umbro of tympanic membrane'.

The handle of malleus continues superiorly and at its highest point, a small projection can be seen, called the 'lateral process of malleus'. The parts of the tympanic membrane moving away from the lateral process are called the 'anterior and posterior malleolar folds'.

The Middle Ear

The middle ear sits within the temporal bone, extending from the tympanic membrane to the lateral wall of the internal ear. The key function of the middle ear is to transmit vibrations from the tym-

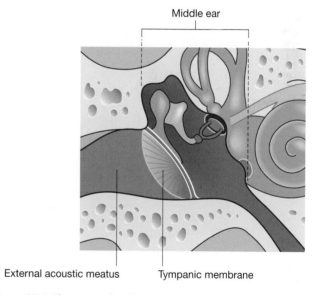

Figure 35.3 The external auditory meatus.

panic membrane (the eardrum) to the inner ear and it does this via the three bones of the ear. The middle ear can be split in two: the tympanic cavity and epitympanic membrane.

The tympanic cavity is situated medially to the tympanic membrane. It contains the majority of the bones of the middle ear. The epitympanic recess is located superiorly, close to the mastoid air cells.

The middle ear can be considered as a rectangular box, with a roof and floor, medial and lateral walls and anterior and posterior walls (Box 35.1).

847

Box 35.1 The Middle Ear and Structures

Roof	Shaped by a thin bone from the petrous aspect of the temporal bone. It separates the middle ear from the middle cranial fossa
Floor	Also known as the 'jugular wall', it is made up of a thin layer of bone that separates the middle ear from the internal jugular vein
Lateral wall	This is made up of the tympanic membrane and the lateral wall of the epitympanic recess
Medial wall	Formed by the lateral wall of the internal ear, containing a protruding bulge that is produced by the facial nerve as it passes by
Anterior wall	The anterior wall is a thin bony plate with two openings: one for the auditory tube and the other for the tensor tympani muscle. It separates the middle ear from the internal carotid artery
Posterior wall	Also called the 'mastoid wall', consisting of a bony partition between the tympanic cavity and the mastoid air cells. Superiorly, there is a hole in this partition, permitting the two areas to communicate

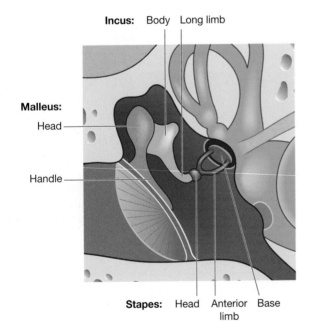

Incus: Body Long limb

Malleus:

Head

Handle

Stapes: Head Anterior Base
limb

Figure 35.4 The ossicles.

The bones of the middle ear

Also called the 'ossicles' or the 'auditory occicles', they are:

- **The malleus** (the hammer)
- **The incus** (the anvil)
- **The stapes** (the stirrup).

The bones are connected in a chain-like manner and link the tympanic membrane to the oval window of the internal ear (Figure 35.4).

The largest and most lateral of the ear bones is the malleus, attaching to the tympanic membrane via the handle of malleus. The head of the malleus lies in the epitympanic recess and here it articulates with the auditory ossicle, the incus. The incus, the next bone, consists of a body with two limbs. The body articulates with the malleus, the short limb attaches to the posterior wall of the middle ear and the long limb joins the last ossicle, the stapes. The stapes is the smallest bone in the body, joining the incus to the oval window of the inner ear. The stapes is stirrup-shaped; it has a head, two limbs and a base. The head articulates with the incus and the base joins the oval window.

The muscles of the middle ear

The tensor tympani and stapedius are two muscles that act in such a way as to protect the middle ear. These muscles contract in response to loud noise, inhibiting the vibrations of the malleus, incus and stapes and reducing the transmission of sound to the inner ear. This action is called the acoustic reflex.

The tensor tympani originates from the auditory tube and attaches to the handle of malleus; when contracting it pulls this medially. Innervation is by a branch of the mandibular nerve. The stapedius muscle attaches to the stapes and is innervated by the facial nerve.

Mastoid air cells

The mastoid air cells are located posterior to the epitympanic recess. They are a collection of air-filled spaces in the mastoid process of the temporal bone. The air cells are contained within a cavity called the 'mastoid antrum'. The mastoid antrum communicates with the middle ear via the aditus to mastoid antrum. The mastoid air cells act as a 'buffer system' of air, discharging air into the tympanic cavity when the pressure is too low.

The eustachian tube

The eustachian tube (also called the 'auditory tube') is a cartilage and bony tube connecting the middle ear to the nasopharynx. Its function is to equalise the pressure of the middle ear to that of the external auditory meatus. It extends from the anterior wall of the middle ear in an anterior, medio-inferior direction, opening onto the lateral wall of the nasopharynx.

The Inner Ear

Auditory transduction (the conversion of mechanical vibrations entering the ear canal into electrical signals) occurs in the inner ear. The inner ear is composed of several different structures (Figure 35.5).

The inner ear consists of a membranous 'labyrinth' (a complicated irregular network of passages or paths) encased in an osseous labyrinth. The system of passages makes up the two key functions of the inner ear.

- The vestibule and semicircular canals are associated with vestibular function (balance)
- The cochlea is concerned with hearing. The cochlea is a coiled tube (*cochlea* is derived from Greek, meaning 'snail').

The surface outline of the inner ear is created by a layer of dense bone that is known as the 'bony labyrinth', which refers to the network of canals. The walls of the bony labyrinth are continuous with the surrounding temporal bone. The inner aspects of the bony labyrinth closely follow the contours of the membranous labyrinth; this is a delicate, interconnected network of fluid-filled tubes in which the receptors are found.

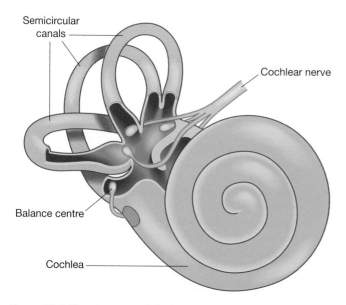

Semicircular
canals

Cochlear nerve

Balance centre

Cochlea

Figure 35.5 The structures of the inner ear.

The walls of the bony labyrinth are made up of dense bone, apart from two small areas located close to the cochlear spiral. The round window consists of a thin, membranous partition that separates the perilymph of the cochlear chambers from the air-filled middle ear. Collagen fibres connect the bony margins of the opening known as the oval window at the base of the stapes.

Perilymph, a liquid whose properties closely resemble those of cerebrospinal fluid, flows between the bony and membranous labyrinths. Another fluid, called *endolymph*, is contained in the membranous labyrinth. These fluids are in separate compartments and under normal circumstances do not mix.

The bony labyrinth can be subdivided into:

- **The vestibule**
- **Three semicircular canals**
- **The cochlea.**

The vestibule

This contains a pair of membranous sacs: the saccule (sacculus) and the utricle (utriculus). Receptors present in the vestibule provide for sensations of gravity and linear acceleration.

The semicircular canals

These enclose the slender semicircular ducts. Receptors located here are stimulated when the head moves (rotates). Together with the vestibule, this is called the vestibular complex. The fluid-filled chambers within the vestibule are usually continuous with those of the semicircular canals.

The cochlea

This structure is a bony, spiral-shaped chamber containing the cochlear duct of the membranous labyrinth. The sense of hearing is provided by receptors within the cochlear duct. Two perilymph-filled chambers can be found on either side of the duct. The cochlea is specialised for the detection of sound waves.

Blood supply to the inner ear

The internal auditory artery (a branch of the basilar artery) supplies the entire membranous labyrinth. The artery passes through the internal auditory meatus, dividing into three branches. The first is the 'vestibular artery', supplying the vestibular nerve and parts of the saccule and utricle and semicircular canals. The second branch, the 'vestibulocochlear artery', supplies the basal turn of the cochlea, the saccule, utricle and parts of the semicircular canals. The 'cochlear artery' supplies the entire cochlea via the spiral arteries.

The organ of Corti

Located in the cochlea, the organ of Corti extends from the anterior aspect of the vestibule. It is often referred to as the 'receptor organ of hearing'. Hair cells (there are approximately 16000) within the organ of Corti, sense mechanical forces. There are two kinds of hair cells – the inner and the outer hair cells. Ninety five per cent of the afferent fibres are from the inner hair cells; these are the sensory receptors that communicate with the VIIIth cranial nerve. Outer hair cells receive efferent input.

Table 35.1 provides a summary of the structures and functions of the ear.

Physiology of Hearing

The physiology of hearing is complex. It is essential to understand the anatomy and physiology of the ear prior to discussing the physiology of hearing. Hearing is the faculty of perceiving and interpretating sound.

When the molecules of a medium are compressed, resulting in a pressure disturbance, a *sound wave* is produced. The strength or loudness of sound is determined by the amplitude of the sound wave; larger amplitudes cause louder sounds. The frequency of the sound wave determines the pitch or tone; greater frequencies result in higher sounds.

Sound waves enter the external auditory canal and this then causes the tympanic membrane to vibrate at the same frequency. The ossicles (the bones in the ears) communicate the motion of the tympanic membrane to the oval window, amplifying the energy of the sound wave. As the stapes moves against the oval window, the *perilymph* (a fluid located in the vestibule) is set in motion. The increased pressure of the perilymph is transmitted to fibres of the basilar membrane and then on to the organ of Corti. The movements of the fibres of the basilar membrane cause the hair cells in the organ of Corti to be pulled up and down. This then generates action potentials that are transmitted to the VIIIth cranial nerve and then onward to the brain for interpretation (Figure 35.6) (Munir & Clarke 2013).

Equilibrium and Balance

The other function of the inner ear is to provide information concerning the position of the head; this helps to synchronise body movements with the intention of maintaining balance and equilibrium. There are two types of equilibrium:

- Static balance (influenced by alterations in the position of the head)
- Dynamic balance (influenced by head movement).

Receptors within the inner ear detect changes in the position of the head. These receptors, called 'maculae', are groups of hair cells containing protrusions that are covered with a gelatinous substance. Within this gelatinous substance are very small particles of calcium carbonate known as 'otoliths'. The function of these particles is to make the gelatin substance heavier than the endolymph that fills the membranous labyrinth.

In the membrane lining the ampulla of each semicircular canal are the 'crista' (plural cristae), the receptors responsible for dynamic

Table 35.1 A summary of the structures and the functions of the ear. (*Source:* Adapted from Munir & Clarke 2013; Jenkins & Tortora 2013; Waugh & Grant 2010)

NAME	STRUCTURE	FUNCTION
Pinna	Made up of folds of skin over cartilage	Collects sound, channelling it down the ear Helps to determine the direction of sound Protects internal aspects of the ear
Ear canal	A tube (about 2.5 cm) leading from the pinna to the tympanic membrane	Directs sound waves towards the tympanic membrane Secretes cerumen (a waxy substance) and sebum to protect and lubricate the ear
Tympanic membrane	Located between the external ear and the middle ear	Vibrates with the same frequency as the sound wave that hits it Provides air-tight protection between the external and middle ear
Ear ossicles	Three main bones in the middle ear called the malleus, the incus and stapes	Transfer the vibrations from the tympanic membrane to the middle of the ear to the oval window
Oval window	A small, thin membrane situated between the middle and inner ear	Receives the vibration from the tympanic membrane via the ossicles
Round window	Sited just below the oval window	Acts like a piston transferring the vibration from the oval window to the fluid in the inner ear
Cochlea	A long tube wound around itself and filled with liquid	The fluid in the cochlea transfers the vibrations to the hairs in the organ of Corti
Organ of Corti	Situated inside the cochlea Contains receptors and hair cells that are attached to nerves	Hairs are tuned to a certain wave frequency. When the waves pass over the hairs an electric signal is triggered
Auditory nerve	A bundle of nerve fibres	Sends the electrical signals to the brain for interpretation
Eustachian tube	A long, narrow tube that opens in the middle ear, leading to the pharynx	Equalises the pressure between the outer and inner ear

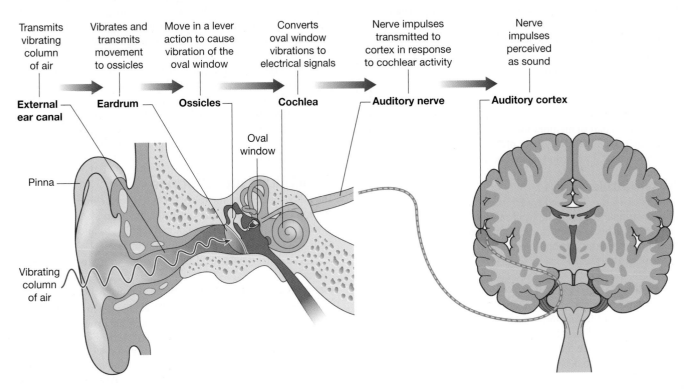

Figure 35.6 The mechanism of hearing. Source: Munir & Clarke (2013). Reproduced with permission of John Wiley & Sons Ltd.

equilibrium. The cristae are stimulated when the head is moved (up and down and side to side); head movement changes the flow of endolymph, as well as causing the movement of the thousands of hair cells in the maculae.

So far, this chapter has provided you with an overview of the anatomy and physiology of the various functions and structures of the ear, as well as a brief understanding of hearing and how equilibrium is maintained. The nurse needs to develop and hone the skills of assessment when caring for people with disorders of the ear; this takes practice and will develop over time. There are a number of ways in which the nurse can undertake a holistic assessment of the needs of people with problems associated with the ear. The use of various diagnostic tests can help the nurse gather objective data that will be essential for the planning and implementation of high quality, safe and effective care. Data collected can also help the nurse with the evaluatory stage of a systematic approach to care.

Assessing the Person with an Ear Problem

Physiological Measurement

A wide range of hearing and balance assessments may be used to determine functional ability and possible pathologies. Audiology encompasses a variety of hearing and balance assessments. Once assessment has taken place, an appropriate care pathway is selected for treatment (e.g. surgery for cochlear implant) and support, but more often for rehabilitative support strategies, for example, hearing aids, counselling and assistive listening devices to improve the ability to participate in daily activities (DH 2007).

Link To/Go To

What is physiological measurement? A guide to the tests and procedures conducted by the Physiological Measurement Diagnostic Services:

http://www.ahcs.ac.uk/wordpress/wp-content/uploads/2013/09/WhatisPhysiologicalMeasurement-dh274038.pdf (accessed May 2014)

Physiological measurement tests related to hearing are carried out in a number of care areas, generally by healthcare scientists. The nurse may be required to undertake the test or they may be involved in the delivery of some elements of the diagnostic test components (e.g. the decision to investigate, or in more complex testing or in reporting and interpreting, assisting the patient and technician). It is essential that the nurse is competent and confident if they are required to undertake these tests. Any physiological measurement that is undertaken must:

- Be patient-centred
- Make use of the benefits of new technology
- Be streamlined and efficient
- Be delivered closer to home
- Provide excellent patient information
- Be accessible from primary as well as secondary care.

Audiology services provide a number of services, which may include:

- Assessment of patient needs and selection of appropriate care pathways
- Hearing function (including pure tone audiometry) and tinnitus assessments
- Diagnostic audio-vestibular function tests (i.e. balance tests and electrophysiological tests of hearing and balance)
- Assessment for implantable devices that aid hearing and communication (e.g. cochlear implants)
- Fitting of digital hearing aids to new and existing patients
- Hearing and tinnitus patient management and follow-up
- Pure tone audiometry. This is a behavioural assessment that determines the threshold for hearing at a number of pure tone frequencies and maps them onto an audiogram in a standard manner. It requires active cooperation from the patient. Sound may be applied monaurally by means of an earphone (air conduction audiometry) or vibrations may be applied to the skull by a bone vibrator (bone-conduction audiometry).

The results of physiological tests and other diagnostic tests will support the diagnosis of a particular injury, disease process or hearing problem. The aim is to reveal information required to identify or adjust the appropriate medications or to provide hearing devices and to help monitor patient outcomes in response to treatment and care provision.

The role of the nurse when assisting people undergoing diagnostic testing, regardless of the kind of test, is to offer the person an explanation of the proposed procedure and to advise if there is any special preparation needed.

Jot This Down

Bhupi Singh is a 72-year-old gentleman who wears an analogue hearing aid. He seems rather withdrawn and less responsive than usual. How would you test if his hearing aid was working correctly?

Person-centred care

Any treatment and care must take into account people's needs and preferences. People with hearing problems should have the opportunity to make informed decisions about their care and treatment; this is in partnership with the person providing that care.

Nursing Fields Learning Disabilities

If a person with a learning disability does not have the capacity to make decisions, the nurse should follow the advice given in Chapters 5 and 10, as well as the guidance offered by the four countries' Departments of Health. Nurses must always act in the best interests of the patient.

Any information offered to people should also be accessible to those with additional needs, such as physical, sensory or learning disabilities.

Effective communication between healthcare professionals (nurses and technicians, for example) and patients is paramount. Communication should be supported by evidence-based written information that has been tailored to the individual's needs. Treatment and care and the information that people are given about it should be culturally appropriate and provision made for people who do not speak or read English.

If the person being cared for agrees, families and carers should have the opportunity to be involved in decisions about treatment and care. The nurse should also ensure that families and carers are given the information and support they need.

History-taking

History-taking may be part of an overall health assessment or it may be carried out in response to a specific complaint the person may have, for example, 'a buzzing noise in the ears'. The nurse should set out to gather as much relevant subjective data as possible that is related to the ears and hearing.

The nurse should ask when the problem started, what are features of the problem and how has it progressed; assess the severity, factors that exacerbate the condition and factors that offer relief. Ask if there are any related symptoms, noting the timing and circumstances. LeMone *et al.* (2011) suggest the following may be asked:

- Have you noted any problems hearing sounds – high-pitched or low-pitched sounds or both?
- When was it you first noticed this problem (e.g. ringing in the ears)?
- Are you exposed to extreme noise at work (e.g. working with pneumatic drills)? When at work do you need to wear protective ear equipment and if so, do you wear it?
- As the examination progresses, be aware of non-verbal responses/communication (e.g. if the person rubs at the ear or provides you with inappropriate answers) that may imply problems with ear function
- Ask the person about changes in hearing, ringing in the ears (tinnitus), pain in the ear (otalgia), drainage from the ears (otorrhoea)
- Determine if there are any vertigo or balance problems
- Does the person use a hearing aid (if so establish the type)?
- Ask about any trauma (e.g. head injury), surgery or infections of the ear and the date of the last ear examination; enquire about a history of infectious diseases, such as meningitis or mumps, as well as the use of any medications that may affect hearing (ototoxic drugs, e.g. gentamicin)
- Ascertain if there is any systemic disease, such as stroke, multiple sclerosis, cardiovascular disease, and if there is, ask about their treatment and medication
- Ear problems tend to run in families, so ask about a family history of deafness, hearing loss, ear problems or diseases that could result in such problems
- Note if the person has any allergies and if so, are these environmental or seasonal allergies or drug-related? Have they recently had an allergic response to hair dye, cosmetic products or perfumes?

Red Flag Otototoxicity

Commonly used medicines that may cause hearing loss include:
- Large doses of aspirin
- Non-steroidal anti-inflammatory drugs, such as ibuprofen and naproxen
- Certain antibiotics, especially aminoglycosides (such as gentamicin, streptomycin and neomycin). Hearing-related side-effects from these antibiotics are most common in people who have renal disease or who already have ear or hearing problems

- Loop diuretics used to treat hypertension and heart failure, such as furosemide or bumetanide
- Medicines used to treat cancer, including cyclophosphamide, cisplatin and bleomycin.

The skills required to inspect the ear are:
- Communication skills
- Inspection
- Palpation.

Inspecting the external ear

You must inspect and palpate the external structures. Observe the ears for position and symmetry. Both ears should be the same shape, and the same colour as the face. Look for obvious signs of abnormality. Consider:

- The presence of any nodules or redness
- Size and shape of the pinna
- Extra cartilage tags/pre-auricular sinuses or pits
- Signs of trauma to the pinna
- Suspicious skin lesions on the pinna, including neoplasia
- Skin conditions of the pinna and external canal
- Infection/inflammation of the external ear canal, with discharge
- Signs/scars of previous surgery.

Gently pull the helix back, determining if it is tender. Inspect and palate the mastoid area behind the auricles, noting tenderness, redness and heat.

Inspect the external ear before examination with an otoscope. Note any discharge, redness or malodour. If there is discharge, take a swab using the principles underpinned by local policy and procedure. You may need to remove any excessive wax (cerumen) prior to inspecting the ear canal and the eardrum.

Primary Care Ear Irrigation

Ear irrigation may be recommended if ear wax blockage persists, even after using eardrops. It involves using a pressurised flow of water to remove the build-up of earwax.

An electronic ear irrigator is used; the intention is to avoid damaging the ear. The irrigator has an adjustable pressure control, so that syringing can commence with the minimum pressure.

During the procedure, a controlled flow of water will be instilled into the ear canal to clean out the earwax. The water used is at body temperature.

While irrigating the ear, hold the ear at different angles to ensure the water reaches all of the ear canal.

An otoscope is used to check whether the procedure is effective.

Ear irrigation should be a painless procedure.

Red Flag

Ear irrigation is not recommended if the person:
- Has previously had problems with irrigation, such as pain in the ear or severe vertigo
- A perforated eardrum, or a perforated eardrum in the last 12 months
- A discharge of mucus from the ear

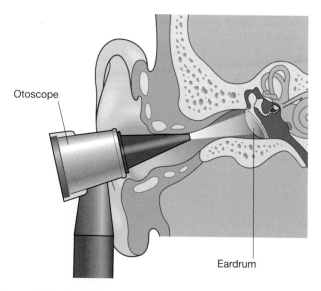

Figure 35.7 The otoscope.

- Has had a middle ear infection in the past 6 weeks
- Has a grommet
- Has had ear surgery within the last 18 months
- Has a cleft palate
- Has a foreign body in the ear
- Has otitis externa.

Inspecting the ear canal and the eardrum

To inspect the ear canal and eardrum, an otoscope with its own light source is used to perform the examination.

The otoscope (Figure 35.7) provides a good view of the tympanic membrane as it has its own magnification. Check that the batteries are fully operational in order to permit optimal light during the examination.

- The person should be asked to sit (or be supported) with the back straight and the head tilted away from the examiner
- Gently grasp the pinna, pulling posteriorly and superiorly (upwards and backwards); this helps to straighten the ear canal for inspection of the tympanic membrane.

> **Nursing Fields** Children
>
> In an infant, you should only pull the pinna posteriorly not superiorly for examination, as the shape of the ear canal is different.

- Hold the otoscope with the thumb and finger, near to the eyepiece as opposed to at the end; this helps to reduce the patient's discomfort due to hand movements, which are exaggerated in the ear
- Insert the speculum one-third of its length gently down and forward into the ear canal
- Otoscopes are designed to use a disposable speculum. Choose the correct size of speculum to achieve the best view. Note the condition of the canal skin and the presence of wax, foreign tissue, a foreign body or discharge

- The mobility of the eardrum can be evaluated using a pneumatic speculum that attaches to the otoscope. The drum should move on squeezing the balloon.

Inspecting and viewing the tympanic membrane

The otoscope should be moved in order to obtain several different views of the drum. It is not always possible to see the whole drum in one single view using an otoscope. The drum is roughly circular (about 1 cm in diameter). The tympanic membrane should be pearl grey, glistening and transparent. Observe for signs of bulging, retraction, bleeding, lesions and perforations.

Hearing acuity tests

Detailed hearing tests are usually performed in audiology clinics. People who have normal hearing should hear equally well in both ears. See Box 35.2 for an overview of three tests used to assess hearing acuity.

When the tests have been carried out, the nurse must ensure the details of the tests, the findings and any treatment are clearly documented in the person's notes. The patient should also be advised of the findings and any further treatment or tests that may be required.

Common Conditions of the Ear

Gaining an understanding of the key issues concerned with assessment of hearing can help you offer care that is safe and appropriate.

Presbyacusis

Also known as 'age-related hearing loss' or 'presbyacousia'. This condition is progressive and is usually bilateral, occurring in older people as they age. **Presbyacusis** is the most common cause of sensorineural hearing loss (see Table 35.2 for a discussion of the types of deafness). It is a multifactorial process driven by environmental factors and exacerbated by concurrent disease (Liu & Yan 2007). Presbyacusis can be used as an umbrella term that covers all causes of diminution of hearing in older people.

The condition can range from being bothersome to severely debilitating in its effects on the person. Dalton *et al.* (2003) note that when moderate to severe, it can lead to the older person becoming isolated and depressed and has the potential to significantly exacerbate age-related disability/cognitive impairment and dementia. The condition is correctable using rehabilitative measures and when treatment is successful this can improve quality of life for the older person.

When the nurse fails to communicate effectively with the deaf person, this can sometimes lead to discomfort (at best) and a break down in communication (at worst) between the patient and the nurse. Box 35.3 provides some simple steps that can be taken in order to reduce communication problems.

In the UK, it is estimated that there are more than 10 million deaf or hard of hearing people; most of these people have developed hearing loss over time. After 50 years of age, the incidence of deafness rises sharply – 55% of the over 60-year-old population have some degree of hearing impairment (Action on Hearing Loss 2011). Most people aged over 70 will have some degree of objective hearing impairment or subjective worsening compared with their youth. Gates and Mills (2005) point out that the effect of noise pollution means that hearing loss is more common in

---

Box 35.2 The Three Tests Used to Test Hearing Acuity.

A tuning fork is used to conduct these tests (Figure 35.8).

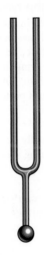

Figure 35.8 A tuning fork.

Weber's Test	Rinne's Test
This is performed in conjunction with Rinne's test. The vibrating fork is placed in the middle of the forehead and the patient is asked whether any sound is heard and, if so, whether it is equally heard in both ears or not. In a patient with normal hearing, the tone is heard centrally. If the patient has unilateral hearing loss and the sound is louder in the weaker ear, this suggests a conductive hearing loss. If the sound is louder in the better ear, it is more likely to be a sensorineural hearing loss.	Strike a tuning fork and hold it vertically with its nearest prong about 1 cm away from the patient's external auditory meatus, making sure that it is not touching any hair. Then immediately transfer it to the mastoid process and hold it firmly there (applying counter pressure to the opposite side of the head) for 2 seconds. The patient is asked to report on which of the two positions was the louder. Normally, the patient should hear the air conduction better than the bone conduction (i.e. first position better than the second). This is a positive Rinne's test. If the Rinne's test is positive and there is hearing impairment, it is a sensorineural and not a conductive problem. If there is a negative Rinne's test with hearing loss, then the problem is a conductive one.

Free Field Voice Test

Whisper from a distance of 40 cm

Table 35.2 Types of deafness. (*Source*: Adapted from Action on Hearing 2013)

CONDUCTIVE HEARING LOSS	SENSORINEURAL HEARING LOSS
Occurs when there is a problem in the transmission of sound waves from the external ear through the middle ear. The disease processes, which may be congenital or acquired, can occur at any level along this part of the ear and include conditions such as excess ear wax, trauma, otitis externa or media with effusion and otosclerosis	Refers to problems occurring in the cochlea (the most common site of disease), cochlear nerve or brain stem resulting in abnormal or absent neurosensory impulses. There are also a number of congenital and acquired conditions resulting in sensorineural hearing loss. The most common is *presbyacusis*; this may also be associated with tinnitus

---

Box 35.3 Some Simple Steps the Nurse Can Take To Enhance Communication with People Who Are Deaf

- Ask the patient how they prefer to communicate: do not assume that if the patient is wearing a hearing aid they can automatically follow what you are saying. Ask if they prefer to lip-read and have pen and paper handy
- Sit in good lighting and, if possible, away from noise and distractors
- Make sure you have the listener's attention before you start speaking
- Do not turn your face away when speaking
- Speak clearly but not too slowly or using exaggerated mannerisms
- If they do not understand what you have said, do not just repeat it but try saying it in a different way
- Do not waffle; avoid jargon and abbreviations
- Check that the person is following what you are saying
- If the patient can use British Sign Language (BSL), consider using a suitably trained interpreter or 'Sign Translate' via a computer live webcam.

---

those older people who live in urban societies, compared with rural societies.

Pathophysiology

There are many factors that contribute to hearing loss in the older person. Histological changes associated with ageing occur throughout the auditory system from the hair cells of the cochlea to the auditory cortex in the temporal lobe of the brain. The nerves or hair cells in the inner ear, where the cochlea starts to deteriorate, die off or become damaged. The loss of the hair cells makes it harder to hear. Presbyacusis can also result from changes in the middle ear as a person ages or from changes in the nerve pathways to the brain.

Risk factors There are multiple risk factors that influence the onset and severity of presbyacusis (Box 35.4).

Investigations and diagnosis

The diagnosis of presbyacusis should be suspected based upon a history of slowly progressive, symmetrical hearing loss in the older person. Screening for presbyacusis in patients aged over 60 is recommended. Ask the person 'Do you have a hearing problem?' on new-patient questionnaires or during health checks for older people. The clinically spoken voice test (whispered voice test) according to Pirozzo *et al.* (2003) is a simple and accurate test for detecting hearing impairment.

Audiometry may be used to screen patients and/or to confirm the diagnosis and to direct management. This is very effective, cost-effective and well accepted by patients and can be easily used in a community setting.

Box 35.4 Risk Factors Associated with Presbyacusis
· Noise exposure, e.g. exposure to industrial, urban, armament noise without ear protection
· Ototoxic medication, e.g. loop diuretics, non-steroidal anti-inflammatory drugs
· Family history/genetic factors
· Hypertension
· High cholesterol
· Diabetes
· Smoking
· High BMI.
(*Source:* Adapted from Gates & Mills 2005; Fransen *et al.* 2008)

A careful history of associated factors, such as family history, ototoxic medications, trauma and concurrent otological symptoms, can help explain potential aetiologies. The diagnosis of presbyacusis should be questioned if the hearing loss is asymmetric, which should lead to evaluation for other conditions such as otitis media, tumours, trauma or asymmetric noise exposure (as often occurs from firearms exposure or the long-term use of power tools on one side).

Presbyacusis develops over many years, and the rate of hearing loss progression can help to establish a diagnosis. It is often difficult for a patient or family member to give an accurate history of the onset and progression of hearing loss. However, the history of a sudden decrease in hearing (noticed over days or weeks rather than years) should raise suspicion for other aetiologies.

A physical examination would include otoscopy in addition to the whispered ear test and tuning forks for the assessment of hearing loss. The physical examination of the outer ears should be normal in presbyacusis. The otoscopic examination may be useful for assessing other potential causes of hearing loss such as cerumen impaction, infection, tympanic membrane perforation or tumours (e.g. osteoma).

Signs and symptoms
There are no definitive signs of presbyacusis. Auroscopy may reveal cerumen accumulation.

The hallmark of presbyacusis is the progressive, symmetric loss of high-frequency hearing over many years (Gates & Mills 2005). Hearing loss may also be accompanied by tinnitus, vertigo and disequilibrium, leading to falls. Presbyacusis can greatly impact on quality of life, causing low self-esteem, isolation and depression. Presbyacusis may also be associated with dementia.

Nursing care and management
Presbyacusis is not curable; however, the effects of the condition on the person's life can be alleviated. Simple recognition of the problem can be a significant positive step, as hearing loss in the older person can often be mistaken for cognitive impairment. The identification of hearing loss can be reassuring for many patients.

· *Amplification devices:* Properly fitted and working hearing aids may contribute to the rehabilitation of a patient with presbyacusis. Those with arthritis in their fingers and visual difficulties need extra help in learning to use hearing aids. Patients using hearing aids may still experience difficulties with speech discrimination in noisy situations

· *Lip reading:* Lip reading may help patients with diminished speech discrimination and may help hearing aid users who have difficulty in noisy environments
· *Assistive listening devices:* These range from a simple amplification of the telephone signal to a device on the television that sends a signal across the room to a headset worn by a patient with hearing loss. The patient can amplify the sound without disturbing other people with normal hearing who are in the same room.
· *Cochlear implants:* Some people with presbyacusis benefit from cochlear implants. Patients with cochlear changes and relatively intact spiral ganglia and central pathways appear to be most suited to this type of intervention.

The Evidence
It has been shown that proactive communication education programmes have an important role to play in the management of people with presbyacusis. This may be as an adjunct to – or even replace – more traditional interventions (such as hearing aid fitting).
(Hickson *et al.* 2007)

These measures are aimed at rehabilitating patients who already experience presbyacusis. There are efforts underway to develop therapies that treat the potential underlying causes of presbyacusis, as well as mechanisms to actually prevent the disease altogether (Darrat *et al.* 2007).

Care, Dignity and Compassion
Both speaker and listener should work at improving communication (see Box 35.3). Speakers should be face to face, reducing competing sounds where possible, and speak in a clear and unhurried manner. Listeners should repeat what was heard to allow misunderstandings to be corrected. In addition, it may help to give out written material or to give explanation to family and friends.
Patients often find it reassuring to know that they will not go completely deaf.

Health promotion
Some sensory presbyacusis is inevitable; however avoiding noise exposure and using ear protection in noisy environments will prevent some progressive damage. Gates and Mills (2005) suggest that a balanced diet, general health and fitness may reduce the cardiovascular contribution to hearing loss.

Red Flag

The nurse should remind younger people of the danger of repeated and prolonged noise exposure in clubs or at music events.

Otosclerosis
This is a disease of the bone that surrounds the inner ear. It may lead to hearing loss when abnormal bone forms around the stapes, reducing the sound that reaches the inner ear (conductive hearing loss). Otosclerosis may interfere with the inner ear nerve cells and

this can affect the production of the nerve signal (sensorineural hearing loss). It is estimated that 10% of the population will have histological evidence of otosclerosis.

Pathophysiology

Otosclerosis is a metabolic bone disease of the otic capsule, which is gradually replaced with a highly vascular type of spongy bone; this is limited to the temporal bone and the bones of the ossicles (known as an 'osseous dyscrasia'). The spongy bone interferes with the function of the stapes and immobilises it, causing disruption of the conduction of vibrations from the tympanic membrane to the cochlea.

Investigations and diagnosis

A detailed history may reveal slowly progressive, bilateral, systematic hearing loss and tinnitus. The tympanic membrane when examined (auroscopy), in the majority of people, is normal.

Audiometry is the chief investigative procedure demonstrating low tone hearing loss. Tympanometry (a test that measures stiffness of the tympanic membrane) may reveal evidence of stiffness. A CT scan may be used to determine the extent of otosclerosis.

Signs and symptoms

As there is enhanced bone conduction, this leads to the perception of the person's own speech as 'loud' and patients may have low-volume speech. Tuning fork tests (Rinne's and Weber's tests) show conductive pattern deafness in most cases.

Very rarely, otosclerosis can also cause dizziness. The person may have tinnitus.

Nursing care and management

There is no known cure for this condition. The person has a number of options available:

- Do nothing
- Be fitted with hearing aids
- Surgery.

No treatment is required if the hearing impairment is mild. Hearing aids (bilateral) may be preferred by those people who do not wish to undergo surgery or who are unfit for surgery. Hearing aids amplify sounds so that the person can hear better. The advantage is that they carry no risk to the patient. An audiologist will discuss the various types of hearing aids that are available, making recommendations based on the specific needs of the individual.

Cruse *et al.* (2010) have considered the use of sodium fluoride 20–120 mg daily as a medical therapy; the drug has an effect on bone metabolism.

Surgical intervention Effective surgical procedures are available. Stapedectomy (extraction of the footplate) or stapedotomy (a small hole is made in the stapes footplate) is carried out in order to improve the circulation of vibration of fluid within the cochlear canal. These cases are usually performed as day-cases (the procedure usually takes about an hour), utilising minimally invasive techniques that may involve the use of lasers. The majority of patients experience elimination of their conductive hearing loss; as well as improving hearing loss, there is also an increase in the quality of life (Karhuketo *et al.* 2007).

If one ear is affected, the operation may help to locate the direction of sound and enable the person to hear better when in places with noisy backgrounds. If both ears are affected, the operation is typically done on the poorer ear. The person is likely to still need a hearing aid in the opposite ear.

The procedure can be done under general or local anaesthetic. An incision is made above the ear opening or inside the ear canal. The top aspect of the stapes is removed and a small opening is then made at the base, or 'footplate', of the stapes into the inner ear. A small piece of vein may be taken from the back of the hand to use as a graft inside the ear. A plastic or metal prosthesis is then put into the ear to conduct sound from the remaining ossicles into the inner ear.

Health promotion and discharge

Prior to discharge, the person should be provided with advice that would prevent an aural infection.

Postoperatively, packing will be placed in the ear canal. In the early postoperative period, the person may experience balance disturbances and as such the nurse needs to ensure a safe environment, assisting the person as needed. They may also experience vomiting and nausea; these potential complications should be explained in the preoperative period. In order to prevent excessive air from entering the eustachian tube, the person should be advised to refrain from vigorous nose blowing, as this will increase middle ear pressure and can lead to displacement of the prosthesis (if inserted) and damage to the operative site. If the patient is sneezing, the nurse should suggest that they keep their mouth open when sneezing with the intention of relieving pressure build up in the middle ear.

Red Flag

The person should be advised not to undertake air travel until they have returned to the care setting for their follow-up appointment.

Chronic Suppurative Otitis Media

Chronic inflammation of the middle ear and the mastoid cavity is known as chronic suppurative otitis media (CSOM). While the condition primarily affects children, it can also occur in adults. CSOM is a perforated tympanic membrane with persistent drainage from the middle ear, lasting longer than 6–12 weeks (Wright & Safranek 2009).

Pathophysiology

An episode of an acute infection can cause CSOM. The pathophysiology of CSOM starts with irritation and ensuing inflammation of the mucosa of the middle ear. As a result of the inflammatory response, mucosal oedema occurs. Continuing inflammation leads to mucosal ulceration and break down of the epithelial lining. In attempting to resolve the infection or inflammation, granulation tissue forms and can develop into polyps located within the middle ear space. This cycle of inflammation, ulceration, infection and granulation tissue formation can endure, ultimately destroying the surrounding bony margins and leading to the various complications of CSOM.

Investigations and diagnosis

An audiogram will usually reveal conductive hearing loss. Mixed hearing loss may suggest more extensive disease and possible complications.

Imaging studies such as CT scanning may be useful for failed treatment and may show occult cholesteatoma, foreign body or malignancy. A fine-cut CT scan can reveal bone erosion from cholesteatoma (this is an uncommon condition where a cyst-like growth develops in the ear), ossicular erosion, involvement of petrous apex and subperiosteal abscess (areas within the middle ear).

Signs and symptoms

People with CSOM present with a draining ear of some duration and a history of recurrent acute otitis media, traumatic perforation or the placement of ventilation tubes. Usually, the person is not in pain or experiencing discomfort.

A common presenting symptom is hearing loss in the affected ear. There may be pyrexia or vertigo. A history of persistent CSOM after appropriate medical treatment may indicate the presence of a cholesteatoma.

The external auditory canal may or may not be oedematous and is usually non-tender. Discharge varies from malodorous, purulent and cheese-like to clear and serous. On examination, granulation tissue is often seen in the medial canal or middle ear space. The middle ear mucosa visualised through the perforation may be oedematous or there may be polyps; it can appear pale or erythematous.

Tuning fork examination can establish if hearing loss is present and whether it is conductive or sensorineural.

Primary Care

In the primary care setting, if there is postauricular swelling or tenderness (this may suggest mastoiditis, facial paralysis), vertigo or evidence of intracranial infection, then urgent assessment or admission by an ear, nose and throat (ENT) team is required.

Cases of CSOM should be referred for routine ENT assessment. The general practice should not initiate treatment because few non-specialists have the equipment or training to carry out aural cleaning.

The Evidence Swimming Advice

People with CSOM are often advised to avoid swimming; however, if they do swim, they should ensure they dry their ears afterwards. Evidence is limited and as a result there is no consensus among specialists. Some advise the use of ear plugs until grommets are extruded, while others do not. Similarly, there is no agreement about whether diving should or should not be permitted while grommets are *in situ*.

(Basu et al. 2007)

Nursing care and management

Conservative treatment of CSOM consists of three elements:

· An appropriate antibiotic, usually administered topically
· Regular intensive aural toilet to remove debris
· Control of granulation tissue.

Medication Aural toilet, along with the use of topical antibiotics, appears effective at resolving otorrhoea. Topical treatment is more effective at clearing aural discharge than systemic therapy (Macfadyen *et al.* 2006).

Antibiotics should have activity against Gram-negative organisms. Antibiotic failure is typically as a result of failure to penetrate the debris, rather than bacterial resistance.

Topical steroids are used to reduce granuloma formation; a combined antibiotic/steroid preparation is used.

Systemic therapy is kept for failure to respond to topical therapy. Topical therapy is continued simultaneously. This is usually done in an acute care setting with an accompanying regimen of intensive aural toilet.

Treatment should continue for 3–4 weeks after the cessation of otorrhoea.

Medicines Management

Instilling ear drops (advice for patients)
1. Wash hands
2. Gently clean the ear with a damp facecloth and then dry it
3. Warm the drops to near body temperature by holding the container in the palm of the hand for a few minutes
4. If the drops are a cloudy suspension, shake the bottle for 10 seconds
5. Check the dropper tip to ensure that it is not chipped or cracked
6. Draw the medication into the dropper or hold the dropper-top bottle with the dropper tip down
7. Tilt the affected ear up or lie on your side. Pull the ear backward and upward.

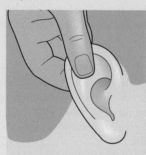

8. Place the correct number of drops in the ear. Gently press on the small skin flap over the ear to help the drops to run into the ear canal

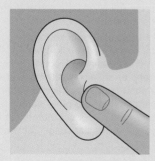

9. Keep the ear tilted up for a few minutes or insert a soft cotton plug in the ear, depending on the method recommended by your pharmacist, practice nurse or doctor
10. Replace and tighten the cap or dropper right away
11. Wash hands to remove any medication.

Red Flag

If instilling ear drops in a child younger than 3 years of age, pull the ear backward and downward to open the ear canal.

Surgery Surgical intervention and type depends on the severity of the disease process and may involve myringoplasty (repair of the eardrum perforation alone) or tympanoplasty (repair of the eardrum and surgery involving the bones of the inner ear).

If cholesteatoma is present, radical mastoidectomy, modified radical mastoidectomy or the 'combined approach tympanoplasty' (anterior tympanotomy plus extended mastoidectomy) may be used depending on the extent of cholesteatoma. The aim of surgery is to remove all disease and to give the person a dry and functioning ear.

Labyrinthitis occurs when infection has spread to the inner ear. Early surgical exploration to remove the infection reduces damage to the labyrinth. Aggressive surgical debridement of the disease (including labyrinthectomy) is undertaken to prevent possibly fatal meningitis or encephalitis.

Cochlear implants have been used in CSOM but all disease must be eradicated first. NICE (2011a) recommends:

- Unilateral implant for those who have severe or profound deafness that has not been improved by a 3-month trial of a hearing aid
- Bilateral implants for severe or profoundly deaf children who have not benefited from a 3-month trial of a hearing aid
- Bilateral implants for adults who have not benefited from a 3-month trial of a hearing aid and who have a disability such as blindness, which means they rely on hearing for spatial awareness.

Health promotion and discharge

Otitis externa has a tendency to recur. In short, the ear canal should be kept dry and the person should avoid soap, hairspray or shampoo getting in. The most important thing is to avoid scratching or poking the ear canal with fingers, towels, cotton wool buds or anything else.

What the Experts Say

I provide the following information to those people with otitis externa:

- Try not to scratch or poke the ear canal with your fingers, cotton wool buds, towels
- Do not clean your ear canal with cotton buds
- Try not to let soap or shampoo get into your ear canal. When taking a shower place a piece of cotton wool coated in soft white paraffin into your outer ear
- Do not use corners of towels or cotton buds to dry any water that does get in the ear canal. Let your ear dry naturally
- When swimming, try to keep your ears dry, wear a tightly fitting cap that covers the ears. Silicone rubber earplugs can be used, but they should only be used if they do not irritate the skin in your ear canal.

(Deeanne, Practice Nurse)

Link To/Go To

Action on Hearing Loss:

http://www.actiononhearingloss.org.uk

Action on Hearing Loss (previously known as the Royal National Institute for Deaf People) provides support for people with hearing loss and tinnitus. The website has practical advice for people who are deaf and have additional needs.

Anatomy and Physiology of the Eye

The eye is the organ that provides us with the sense of sight, letting us observe and learn more about the surrounding world, more so than we do with any of the other special senses. The eyes are used in most activities we carry out, for example reading, working, watching television, sending an e-mail or text, driving a car, etc. Sight, it could be suggested, is the sense that most people value more than the others.

The eye allows us to see and understand the shapes, colours and dimensions of objects by processing the light they reflect or emit. The eye is capable of detecting bright light or dim light.

The eye is a complex structure that has been designed to gather a substantial amount of information about the environment. Areas associated with the eye are outlined in Box 35.5.

A section of the eye is detailed in Figure 35.9.

The Protective Structures of the Eye
The orbit

The two **orbits**, sometimes called 'the sockets', which protect the eyes, are located at the front of the skull, each with a wider opening anteriorly (towards the front) narrowing to a small opening posteriorly (at the rear) where the optic nerve exits to connect through to the visual pathways and the brain (Figure 35.10). The eye is approximately 24 mm in diameter, occupying about 25% of the volume of the orbit, allowing for the extraocular muscles, blood

Box 35.5 The Eye

The protective structures of the eye

- The orbit
- The eyelids
- The eyelashes and eyebrows
- The lacrimal apparatus
- The sclera

The anterior segment of the eye

- The cornea
- The aqueous humour
- The iris
- The lens and ciliary muscle

The posterior segment of the eye

- The retina
- The vitreous humour

The visual system pathways to the brain

- The optic nerves and optic tracts
- The visual cortex

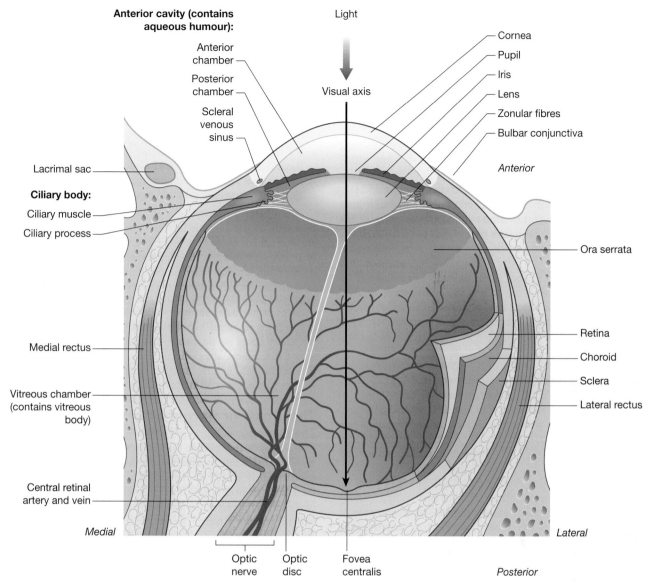

Figure 35.9 **Cross-section of the eye.**

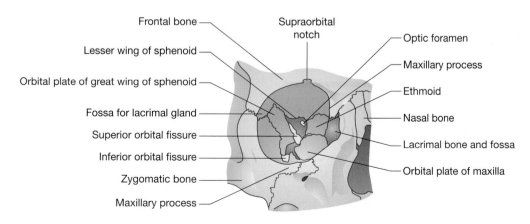

Figure 35.10 **The orbit.**

vessels, nerves, orbital fat and connective tissue that surround and support the eye. The orbit surrounds and supports most of the eye; the cornea and part of the anterior globe extend beyond the orbital rims. These structures are protected by the eyelids.

The eyelids, eyelashes and eyebrows

These structures are external to the eyeball, providing protection. Other protective structures include the conjunctiva, lacrimal apparatus and extrinsic eye muscles.

The **eyelids** (**palpebrae**) are thin, loose folds of skin covering the anterior eye, protecting the eye from foreign bodies and excessive light into the eye. They also spread tears by blinking. They contain the puncta, through which the tears flow (Figure 35.11).

The **eyebrows** provide shade and keep perspiration and other debris away from the eyes. Linstrom *et al.* (2000) have shown the eyebrows to be the most expressive part of the face.

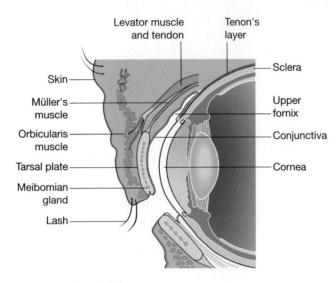

Figure 35.11 The eyelids.

Eyelashes protect the eye from foreign particles and act as sensors. They are short hairs projecting from the top and bottom borders of the eyelids. An unexpected touch to the eyelashes initiates the blinking reflex. Contact with the eyelashes can trigger an eyelid-closing reflex.

The lacrimal apparatus

The **lacrimal apparatus** (Figure 35.12) produces and drains lacrimal fluid and is composed of:

- The lacrimal gland
- The puncta
- The lacrimal sac
- The nasolacrimal duct.

The surface of the eye is continuously bathed in tears that are primarily secreted by the lacrimal gland. Conjunctival secretions are also added. These structures secrete, distribute and drain tears to cleanse and moisten the eye's surface.

Each time an individual blinks, fluid is pumped throughout the system. The tears are drained away via the nasolacrimal system. The tears have antimicrobial properties.

The sclera

The **sclera** is derived from interwoven collagen fibrils of varying widths, sitting within ground substance and maintained by fibroblasts. The sclera is made up three layers of varying thickness.

The Anterior Segment of the Eye
The cornea

The **cornea** is transparent to light; it does not contain any blood vessels. This small transparent dome at the front of the eye is approximately 11 mm in diameter and 500 μm thick in the centre, thickening to around 700 μm at the periphery. The cornea is more curved than the rest of the globe. The functions of the cornea along with the lens are to transmit and focus light into the eye. The cornea also protects the inner ocular structures.

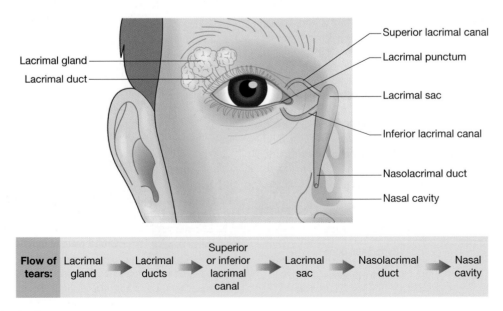

Figure 35.12 The lacrimal apparatus.

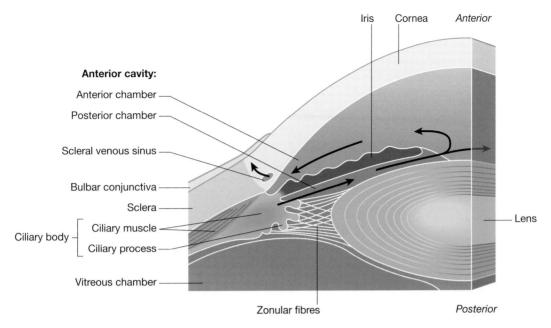

Figure 35.13 The iris and chambers of the eye.

The aqueous humour

This is a transparent fluid (the fluid that fills the anterior chamber of the eye) providing oxygen and nutrients to the lens and cornea. The area between the cornea and the front surface of the crystalline lens is called the **aqueous humour**; it continuously filters out of blood vessels in the ciliary processes of the ciliary body. The aqueous is also a part of the optical pathway of the eye.

The iris

This is the coloured aspect of the eyeball and is shaped like a flattened doughnut (Figure 35.13). It controls light levels inside the eye similar to the aperture on a camera. The round opening in the centre of the **iris** is the **pupil**. There are a number of tiny muscles embedded in the iris that dilate and constrict pupil size.

The circular sphincter muscle (innervated by the parasympathetic system) lies around the very edge of the pupil. In bright light the sphincter contracts, causing the pupil to constrict. The radial dilator muscle (innervated by the parasympathetic system) runs radially through the iris, like spokes on a wheel. This muscle dilates the eye in dim lighting. The colour, texture and patterns of each person's iris are as unique as a fingerprint.

The lens and ciliary muscle

The **lens** is posterior to the pupil and the iris, within the cavity of the eyeball. It is a transparent structure and has the ability to change its shape in order to increase or decrease the amount of refracting power applied to light coming into the eye. As we age, the lens grows. The lens provides the remaining variable focussing power and serves to further refine the focus, allowing the eye to focus on objects at different distances from the eye.

An elastic extracellular matrix known as the 'capsule' surrounds the lens. The capsule provides a smooth optical surface and is an anchor for the suspension of the lens within the eye. A meshwork of non-elastic microfibrils or 'zonules' anchors into the capsule near the equator of the lens connecting it to the ciliary muscle.

The ciliary muscle is one part of the **ciliary body**, which is divided into three parts:

- The ciliary muscle
- The ciliary processes (pars plicata)
- The pars plana.

Figure 35.14 illustrates the anatomy of the ciliary body.

The Posterior Segment of the Eye
The retina

The **retina** is a complex structure. Mostly, it is a transparent thin tissue designed to capture photons of light and initiate processing of the image by the brain. The average thickness of the retina is 250 μm and it consists of 10 layers (Figure 35.15).

There are two types of receptors in the receptor layer of the retina – 'rods and cones' (named for their shape). The outer segment of the receptor cells contains the light sensitive visual pigment molecules called opsins in stacked discs (rods) or invaginations (cones). There are approximately 5 million cones and 92 million rods in the normal adult retina. Cones provide the ability to discern colour and to see fine detail and are more concentrated in the central retina. Rods are mainly responsible for peripheral vision and vision under low light conditions and are more prevalent in the mid-peripheral and peripheral retina.

The Visual System Pathways to the Brain
The optic nerves and optic tracts

The **optic nerves** are cranial nerves and meet at the optic chiasma, anterior to the pituitary gland in the brain (Figure 35.16).

At the optic chiasma, axons from the medial half of each retina cross to the opposite side, forming pairs of axons from each eye, continuing as the left and right **optic tracts**. The crossing of the axons results in each optic tract carrying information from both eyes: the left carries visual information from the lateral half of the

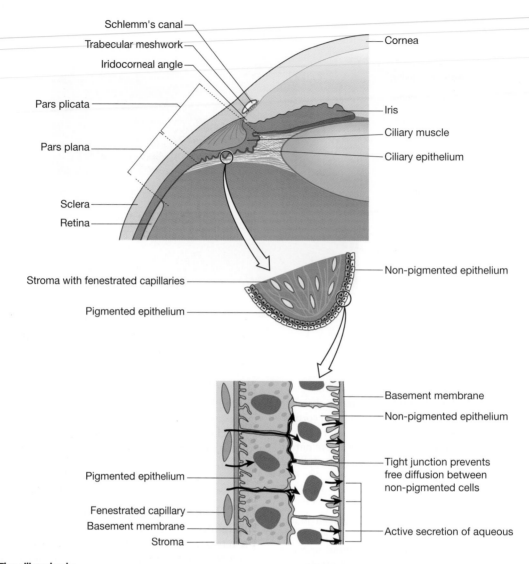

Figure 35.14 The ciliary body.

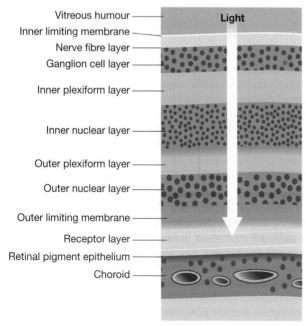

Figure 35.15 The layers of the retina.

retina of the left eye and the medial half of the retina of the right eye, whereas the right one carries visual information from the lateral half of the retina of the right eye and the medial half of the retina of the left eye (Figure 35.17).

There is an overlap of the visual fields with each eye seeing a slightly different view. As a result of this overlap, along with the crossing of the axons, information from both eyes reaches both sides of the visual cortex. The information is then fused into one image.

The visual cortex

The **visual cortex** in the occipital lobe of the brain is where the final processing of the neural signals from the retina takes place and vision occurs. The occipital lobe is in the most posterior portion of the brain (see Chapter 34). There are a total of six separate areas in the visual cortex, known as V1, V2, V3, V3a, V4 and V5.

Assessing Vision

Reaching an ophthalmic diagnosis is dependent upon a good history and detailed examination.

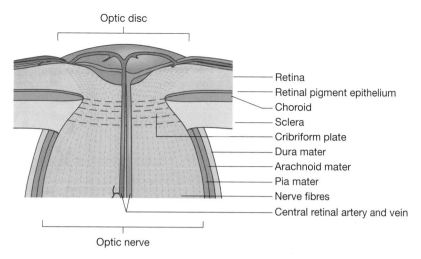

Figure 35.16 **The optic nerve.**

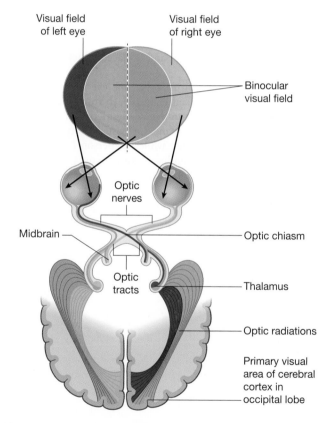

Figure 35.17 **The visual pathway.**

Red Flag

Only nurses who have demonstrated they have the competence and the confidence to take the history and undertake the examination should carry out visual activity tests.

There are a number of visual acuity tests available that measure the ability to see fine detail. Vision assessment is an organised procedure for gathering information about the health and function of the visual system. The assessments can be done in a number of venues by a number of people, for example nurses, ophthalmologists and optometrists.

General Ophthalmic History

Chapter 6 provides details concerning history-taking. With regards to a good history in the ophthalmic setting, the nurse should inspect, examine (using an ophthalmoscope) and test the eye.

Box 35.6 outlines the specific issues that need to be considered in the ophthalmic history.

Not all examinations are required for all patients. Table 35.3 provides some suggestions but examinations must be guided by the person's individual needs.

Box 35.6 Key Points and the Ophthalmic History

Think about the symptoms carefully
· Determine how long the symptoms have been present
· Are the symptoms continuous or intermittent?
· What triggered them?
· Does anything make them better or worse?
· Describe how the symptoms are changing
· Are there any related symptoms?
· Is there a previous eye or related systemic disease?
· Ascertain if there is a:
  · Past medical history (diabetes, hypertension, neurological disease, any specific eye treatment, such as laser)
  · Drug history (any drugs being taken that may cause visual disturbance, i.e. eye drops)
  · Family history (inherited visual problems, i.e. glaucoma), family history of eye symptoms, i.e. transmission of infective conjunctivitis
  · Social history (smoking, alcohol use, recreational drug use, exposure to chemicals)
· Is the person registered blind?
· Are there any adaptations in the home?
· Does the person need assistive devices, such as Braille?

(*Source*: Adapted from Gleadle 2012; James & Bron 2011)

Table 35.3 History and suggested examination in people with eye problems.

CONDITION	EXAMINATION
All patients	History and visual acuity
Red/painful eye	Lids, lacrimal system, conjunctiva, cornea, pupils, anterior chamber and intraocular pressure if possible (if not and no obvious cause, refer)
Foreign body	Lids, conjunctiva and cornea. If mechanism included high velocity, full anatomical examination of the eye is a requirement
Reduced vision	Cornea, anterior chamber and beyond, functional testing of visual field, pupils, optic nerve and macula
Double vision/orbital problems	Fundus, optic nerve function, extraocular muscle function
Headache/neurological-sounding problems in absence of red eye	Fundus, optic nerve, pupillary functions, blood pressure, full neurological examination

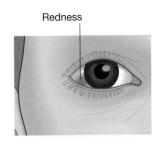
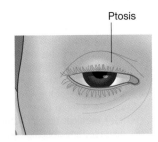

Redness   Ptosis

Pupils
- Symmetry
- Size, shape
- Reaction to light
- Reaction to accommodation
- PERRLA (pupils equal round and reacting to light and accommodation)

Figure 35.18 **Inspection of the eyes.**

Anatomical Examination

Inspect the eyes, noting any obvious abnormalities such as proptosis (an abnormal protrusion of the globe), redness, asymmetry, obvious nystagmus (involuntary, to-and-fro oscillation of the eyes) and ptosis (drooping or falling of the upper or lower eye lid). Look at the conjunctiva, the cornea, the iris, the pupils and the eyelids; note if they are symmetrical (Figure 35.18).

Note symmetry of the pupils, their size and their ability to respond normally and equally to light and accommodation. Is there ptosis? Check that the eyelids close.

Visual Acuity (Physiological Testing of the Eye)

The Snellen chart is the standard test used for testing visual acuity (Figure 35.19).

The Snellen chart contains rows of letters in varying sizes; there are standardised numbers at the end of each row. If the person is unable to read or does not read English, the E-chart (a set of random tumbling Es) can be used. The Snellen chart provides a

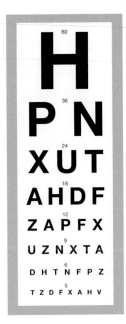

Figure 35.19 **The Snellen chart.**

standardised test of visual acuity and is placed 6 metres from the person.

The nurse asks the person to cover one eye with an opaque cover. The person is then asked to read each row of letters; they should move from the largest to the smallest letters that they can see. The same approach is used to measure visual acuity in the other eye. Visual acuity is then tested while the person has both eyes uncovered. Test the person who has glasses or contact lenses with and without the glasses or contact lenses.

Nursing Fields Children: Testing Visual Acuity

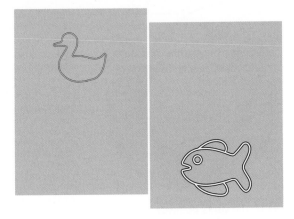

Figure 35.20 **Cardiff cards.**

- Very young children are observed to see if they can follow or pick up objects such as scattered 'hundreds and thousands' cake decorations
- A chart called the 'Cardiff card' can be used instead of the Snellen chart (Figure 35.20).
- The older child should be able to identify or match single pictures and letters on charts held in their hands with those of varying sizes presented to them at a distance.

(*Source*: Adapted from James & Bron 2011)

Other tests will include the Ishihara chart for colour vision. Visual fields are tested using a variety of methods; confrontation visual field testing is a common approach. This is a qualitative measurement but is a good starting point and can easily be carried out in a variety of settings. Usually, a hatpin with a red or white head is used to define the visual field; it is moved across the visual field to determine where it disappears.

Pupillary reactions

The pupils should be of equal size: 3–5 mm. Assess direct and consensual pupil response: ask the person to look straight ahead and shine a light obliquely into one eye at a time. Observe for constriction of the pupil in the illuminated eye. Carry out this test for both eyes. The normal direct and consensual pupillary response is constriction.

In order to test for accommodation, the nurse holds an object at a distance of about 60 cm from the person; pupils should dilate. Ask the person to follow the object as you bring it to within a few centimetres of their nose. The pupils should constrict and converge as they change focus to follow the object.

Examination with an ophthalmoscope

Examination of the internal eye, using the ophthalmoscope, should only be undertaken by a skilled practitioner. This allows visualisation of the lens, the vitreous humour and the retina. Opacity of the pupil by a cataract or a haemorrhage into the vitreous humour can be seen with an ophthalmoscope. On examination, the lens should be clear. There should be no visible haemorrhages, discharge or white patches when inspecting the retina. The optic disc should be round to oval with clear, well-defined borders. Inspecting the blood vessels of the retina can reveal glaucoma, caused by increased intraocular pressure. Hypertension can result in a narrowing of the vein. Diabetes, atherosclerosis and blood disorders can cause engorged veins to occur. The retina is usually a constant red-orange colour; it is lighter around the optic disc. The macula should be visible on the temporal aspect of the optic disc. There should be no tenderness, excessive tearing or discharge over the lacrimal glands, puncta and nasolacrimal duct.

Common Conditions of the Eye

Understanding the anatomy and physiology of the eye, along with an awareness of the various ways of assessing those with eye disorders, can assist you when you offer care to people that is person-centred.

Acute or chronic conditions can affect the eye and its protective structures. Often, eye disorders are minor and have minimal or no effect on vision, yet there are some that can cause permanent vision impairment, cause discomfort and impact negatively on a person's body image. Either temporary or permanent visual impairment can ensue after eye surgery or as a result of minor trauma.

Inflammation of the Eyelids – Blepharitis

Blepharitis is a common inflammation of the lid margins that may be acute or chronic. The true prevalence is unknown and studies trying to estimate this have been unsatisfactory (Luchs 2010).

Pathophysiology

There are several pathological causes associated with blepharitis. Direct bacterial infection can result in a response against bacterial toxins. There may be a delayed hypersensitivity reaction to bacterial antigens and an enhanced cell-mediated immunity to *Staphylococcus aureus* in those with chronic blepharitis.

There may be structural alterations and secretory dysfunction of the meibomian glands (glands located on the margin of the lid). Meibomian glands secrete meibum, the external lipid layer of the tear film responsible for decreasing tear film evaporation and preventing contamination.

Structural alteration of the glands can cause the condition 'hyperkeratinisation' that can obstruct the gland or lead to desquamation of epithelial cells into the lumen of the duct, further constricting the glands.

There may be secretory dysfunction where the composition of meibum is altered.

Investigations and diagnosis

The American Academy of Ophthalmology (AAO 2012) reports that there are no specific tests and diagnosis is made on clinical examination. Swabbing may be applicable in severe or recurrent cases and a biopsy is required where malignancy is suspected.

Signs and symptoms

The person may complain of sore eyes that are burning and gritty with crusting on waking; this is usually bilateral and chronic. The eye(s) may be red and sometimes people complain of epiphora (excess tears) or dry eye and photophobia.

Blurred vision may occur secondary to epiphora. If the person wears contact lenses, they may be unable to tolerate them. The condition can wax and wane (there may be long periods of exacerbations and remissions).

Nursing care and management

There is insufficient evidence to make definitive recommendations for the treatment of blepharitis. A cure is not possible in most cases. The American Academy of Ophthalmology (AAO 2012) suggests that the following treatments are helpful:

- Warm compresses
- Eyelid hygiene (Table 35.4)
- Antibiotics (topical and/or systemic)
- Topical anti-inflammatory agents (e.g. corticosteroids, cyclosporine)

Initially treat patients who have blepharitis with a regimen of warm compresses and eyelid hygiene, carried out twice daily during the acute phase and then daily.

A topical antibiotic such as bacitracin or erythromycin can be prescribed to be applied one or more times daily or at bedtime on the eyelids for one or more weeks for those with staphylococcal blepharitis.

For those with meibomian gland dysfunction, where chronic symptoms and signs are not adequately controlled with eyelid hygiene, oral tetracyclines can be prescribed.

A brief course of topical corticosteroids may be helpful for eyelid or ocular surface inflammation. The minimal effective dose of corticosteroid should be used and long-term corticosteroid therapy avoided.

The person should be advised to avoid contact lens wear, especially during acute inflammatory episodes. Reassurance should be given stating that the condition is seldom sight-threatening and it should not prevent all their usual activities (e.g. swimming, unless there is an acute infection). The use of make-up and eye-liner should be avoided.

Table 35.4 Lid hygiene.

ACTIVITY	TECHNIQUE	REASONING
Warm compresses	Soak a cloth or cotton wool pad with hot water – apply to each eye for 5 (ideally 10) min. Avoid excessive heat. There are commercial products available	Loosens collarettes (a narrow rim of loosened keratin) and crusting, making subsequent cleansing more comfortable. Warms the fatty content of the meibomian glands, making these easier to express during lid massage
Lid massage	Close lids and gently rotate a clean finger along lid, ending in a downward stroke (upper lid) and upward stroke (lower lid). Move along the length of each lid	Loosening meibomian gland content and expressing this through the openings that line the lid margin
Lid cleansing	Mix baby shampoo with water (a 50:50 mix and increase or decrease concentration according to effectiveness). Dip a cotton bud in the solution and run it along the margin, cleaning off debris from the lash base. Commercial lid scrubs may also be used	Aim is gentle mechanical washing, removing collarettes and debris, reducing margin inflammation

Primary Care

Early detection and appropriate treatment can reduce signs and symptoms of blepharitis and prevent permanent structural damage and possible vision loss.

Health promotion and discharge

This condition rarely fully resolves (AAO 2012). However, with careful, patient and continued adherence to lid hygiene measures (this needs to be reiterated even if the eyes are feeling comfortable), symptomatic control is good (Jackson 2008).

There are several everyday steps that the person can take to prevent blepharitis. These include:

- Keeping the hands and face clean
- Avoiding rubbing the eyes with dirty fingers or a dirty towel, for example
- Removing all eye make-up before bedtime
- Avoiding the use of eye make-up to prevent further irritation.

What the Experts Say

There is always the risk of re-infection with blepharitis and I suggest that when the patient starts to use make-up again, that they replace the products they have been using in or near the eyelids, as these may be contaminated.

(Kelly, Practice Nurse)

Box 35.7 Some of the Common Types of Conjunctivitis

Allergic
- Seasonal allergic conjunctivitis
- Vernal conjunctivitis
- Atopic conjunctivitis

Mechanical/Irritative/Toxic
- Superior limbic keratoconjunctivitis (SLK)
- Contact lens-related keratoconjunctivitis
- Floppy eyelid syndrome
- Pediculosis palpebrarum (*Pthirus pubis*)
- Medication-induced keratoconjunctivitis

Viral
- Adenoviral conjunctivitis
- Herpes simplex virus (HSV) conjunctivitis
- Varicella (herpes) zoster virus (VZV) conjunctivitis
- Molluscum contagiosum

Bacterial
- Bacterial conjunctivitis (including non-gonococcal and gonococcal)
- Chlamydial conjunctivitis

Immune-mediated
- Ocular mucous membrane pemphigoid (OMMP)
- Graft-versus-host disease (GVHD)

Neoplastic
- Sebaceous gland carcinoma.

(*Source:* Adapted from James & Bron 2011; Anderson 2007)

Conjunctivitis

Conjunctivitis and associated disorders of the conjunctiva are common causes of symptoms (James & Bron 2011). Conjunctivitis, or inflammation of the conjunctiva, is an umbrella term referring to a diverse group of diseases/disorders primarily affecting the conjunctiva. Most types of conjunctivitis are self-limited; however, some progress and can cause serious ocular and extraocular complications.

Conjunctivitis can be classified as infectious or non-infectious and as acute, chronic or recurrent. The causes of infectious conjunctivitis include viruses and bacteria. The types of non-infectious conjunctivitis are:

- Allergic
- Mechanical/irritative/toxic
- Immune-mediated
- Neoplastic.

Sometimes the causes for non-infectious conjunctivitis may overlap. Box 35.7 provides further details concerning some of the common types of conjunctivitis.

Conjunctivitis is a global condition that can affect any age group with no gender, ethnic or social preference. Generally, it is a reasonably trivial problem; however it can have a considerable impact on lost work time and, very occasionally, can result in permanent or sight-threatening sequelae (AAO 2011a).

Pathophysiology

Allergic conjunctivitis is caused by a type I immune response to an allergen. This results in the release of histamine from mast cells, as well as other mediators that immediately stimulate nociceptors, resulting in itching, increased vascular permeability, vasodilation, redness and conjunctival injection.

Infective conjunctivitis occurs as a result of reduced host defences and external contamination. Infectious pathogens invade from adjacent sites or by a blood-borne pathway, replicating within the conjunctival mucosal cells.

Investigations and diagnosis

The initial eye examination includes measurement of visual acuity, an external examination, and internal eye examination using an ophthalmoscope. The examiner should wear gloves.

The majority of cases of conjunctivitis can be diagnosed on the basis of history and clinical examination. In some cases, however, additional diagnostic tests are helpful. Cultures of the conjunctiva are indicated in all cases of suspected infectious neonatal conjunctivitis (Rapoza *et al.* 1986). Bacterial cultures may also be helpful for recurrent or severe purulent conjunctivitis if the conjunctivitis has not responded to medication.

Viral cultures are not used routinely to establish a diagnosis. Availability of these tests will vary and laboratory advice should be sought.

Suspected cases of adult and neonatal chlamydial conjunctivitis can be confirmed by laboratory testing. Immunologically-based diagnostic tests are available.

Conjunctival biopsy may be helpful in cases of conjunctivitis unresponsive to therapy. Because such eyes may hide a neoplasm, directed biopsy may be both vision-saving and lifesaving (Akpek *et al.* 1999).

Red Flag

To avoid cross-contamination in care settings, multiple-dose eyedrop containers should be discarded when inadvertent contact with the ocular surface occurs. Hand-washing procedures with antimicrobial soap and water and disinfecting ophthalmic equipment can reduce the risk of transmission of viral infection. Exposed surfaces on equipment can be decontaminated by wiping with sodium hypochlorite (a 1:10 dilution of household chlorine bleach) or other appropriate disinfectants. Local policy and procedure must be followed.

Signs and symptoms

Red eye is a key symptom that is usually generalised; frequently this is bilateral. There may be pain, irritation and discomfort. Discharge is variable in nature. Photophobia may be suggestive of corneal involvement also.

Signs of conjunctivitis can include conjunctival infection, whereby the conjunctival vessels become dilated. There may be conjunctival oedema (chemosis).

Nursing care and management

Treatment of conjunctivitis should be directed at the root cause. Indiscriminate use of topical antibiotics or corticosteroids should be avoided. Antibiotics can induce toxicity and corticosteroids can potentially prolong adenoviral infections and worsen herpes simplex virus infections. Treatment methods are described for the most common types of conjunctivitis and for those types that are particularly important to treat. Allergic and bacterial conjunctivitis are discussed here.

Mild allergic conjunctivitis can be treated with an over-the-counter antihistamine/vasoconstrictor agent or with the more topical histamine antagonists. If the condition is frequently recurrent or persistent, mast-cell stabilisers can be utilised (e.g. sodium cromoglicate, nedocromil sodium). Many new medications combine antihistamine activity with mast-cell stabilising properties and can be utilised for either acute or chronic disease. If the symptoms are not adequately controlled, a brief course (1–2 weeks) of low-potency topical corticosteroid can be added to the regimen. The lowest potency and frequency of corticosteroid administration that relieves the patient's symptoms should be used. Artificial tears can be used to promote comfort.

Mild bacterial conjunctivitis may be self-limited and resolve spontaneously without specific treatment in immune-competent adults. Use of topical antibacterial therapy is associated with earlier clinical and microbiological remission. The choice of antibiotic is usually based on empirical evidence. A 5–7-day course of a broad-spectrum topical antibiotic is usually effective; the most convenient or least expensive option can be selected, so long as care is not compromised.

Severe bacterial conjunctivitis is characterised by copious purulent discharge, pain and marked inflammation of the eye. In these cases, the choice of antibiotic is guided by the results of laboratory tests.

Saline lavage may promote comfort and more rapid resolution of inflammation in gonococcal conjunctivitis. Patients and sexual contacts should be informed about the possibility of concomitant disease and referred appropriately.

Care, Dignity and Compassion

There are a number of comfort measures that the nurse might suggest, for example reducing lighting intensity, wearing sunglasses and avoiding activities such as excessive reading while the eye is inflamed.

Topical anti-infective therapy, as eye drops or ointment, may include erythromycin, gentamicin, penicillin, bacitracin, amphotericin B or idoxuridine. If there is severe infection, these medications may be administered by subconjunctival injection or systemic intravenous infusion.

Medicines Management

Instilling of eye drops (information for patients):

1. Read the instructions carefully before using eye drops
2. Store eye drops at room temperature and away from heat, moisture and direct light (or as directed)
3. Do not use the drops if they change colour or turn cloudy
4. Do not use the drops if they have debris (bits) floating in them

(Continued)

5. Wait 10–15 minutes before using a different kind of eye drop
6. Wash hands before and after instilling eye drops
7. Gently shake the bottle
8. Do not touch the tip of the bottle to the eye
9. Tilt the head back and pull down the lower eyelid with the index finger
10. Gently squeeze the bottle to drop the correct number of drops into the eye
11. Wait 1 minute between each drop
12. Replace the cap on the bottle
13. Close the eyes. Press the index finger against the inside corner of the eye next to the nose for 1 minute
14. Gently wipe away any extra liquid with a tissue
15. Do not rub the eyes.

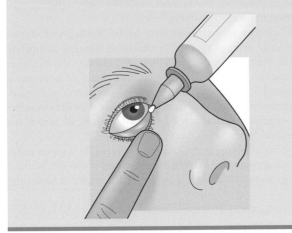

Health promotion and discharge

Individuals can protect against some chemical and toxin exposures with adequate eye protection. Those who wear contact lens can be instructed in appropriate lens care and frequent lens replacement to reduce the risk or severity. Prenatal screening and treatment of the expectant mother and prophylactic treatment of the infant at birth can prevent infectious conjunctivitis in neonates.

When conjunctivitis has been diagnosed and treatment has been initiated, the person will require follow-up care. The frequency of follow-up varies with the severity of the condition, the diversity of causes considered and the potential for ocular morbidity. Follow-up should be designed for careful monitoring of disease progression and verification that treatment choice is effective. Alteration of therapy, when needed, as well as recognition of adverse side-effects and re-evaluation of the condition and its response to treatment at regular intervals, are central to successful patient management.

Cataract Surgery

A cataract occurs when the lens of an eye becomes opaque and vision is affected. The majority of cataracts most commonly occur in the older person, developing gradually. Cataracts are usually treated as a day-case; the cloudy lens is removed and is replaced with an artificial plastic lens. However, in developing countries where treatment is not available, cataracts are a major cause of blindness.

Link To/Go To

The Royal National Institute for the Blind has produced a wealth of information concerning cataracts.

http://www.rnib.org.uk/eyehealth/eyeconditions/conditionsac/Pages/cataract.aspx

The Royal College of Ophthalmologists (RCO 2010) reported that 30% of people aged 65 years and over were found to have a visually impairing cataract in one or both eyes. Another 10% of people in this age group had previous cataract surgery in one or both eyes. The prevalence of visually impairing cataracts rose steadily with age: 16% in those aged 65–69 years; 24% in those aged 70–74 years; 42% in those aged 75–79 years; 59% in those aged 80–84 years; and 71% in people of 85 years of age or more.

Pathophysiology

Globally, cataract is the most common cause of treatable blindness. The cause of cataract is cumulative, for example ageing, smoking, ultraviolet radiation and hyperglycaemia (James & Bron 2011). Opacification of the lens of the eye occurs with cataract.

Fibres and proteins in the lens change and degenerate as the person ages. Proteins agglutinate causing clouding of the lens and reducing light transmission to the retina. As the cataract continues to develop, the whole lens may become opaque.

A cataract scatters the light as it passes through the lens, preventing a sharply-defined image from reaching the retina. As a result, the vision becomes blurred. The causes for cataract are multifactorial and include:

- Diabetes mellitus
- Sunlight (UV exposure)
- Uveitis
- Eye trauma
- Steroids
- Nutrition and socioeconomic status
- Lifestyle (smoking and alcohol)
- Dehydration/diarrhoeal crises.

Nursing Fields Children

Paediatric cataracts may be:

- Congenital: hereditary/genetic, metabolic (e.g. galactosaemia, a metabolic disorder)
- A result of *in utero* infection (e.g. rubella, cytomegalovirus, herpes simplex)
- Developmental: genetic, metabolic (e.g. galactokinase deficiency)
- Acquired: metabolic (e.g. diabetes mellitus), traumatic, post-radiotherapy
- The most common cause of congenital cataract is infection. These include rubella (this is the most common), measles, chickenpox, cytomegalovirus, herpes simplex and herpes zoster.

(RCO 2010)

The Evidence

The National Institute for Health and Clinical Excellence (NICE 2011b) has issued full guidance to the NHS in England, Wales, Scotland and Northern Ireland on implantation of accommodating intraocular lenses for cataract.

During cataract surgery, the clouded natural lens of the eye is removed and clear vision is most commonly obtained with an implanted artificial lens. The standard intraocular lens has no focussing capability, whereas an accommodating intraocular lens allows focussing on near and distant objects.

There are no major concerns about the safety of this procedure, but there are still uncertainties about how well it works. If a doctor wants to use implantable accommodating lenses for cataracts, he or she should make sure that extra steps are taken to explain the uncertainty and the likely benefits and potential risks of the procedure. This should happen before the patient agrees (or doesn't agree) to the procedure. The patient should be given written information as part of the discussion.

There should also be special arrangements for monitoring what happens after the procedure.

(NICE 2007)

Cataract management requires a multiprofessional approach that involves nurses, ophthalmologists, optometrists and technicians. Usually, only one eye at a time is operated on.

The Evidence Mono versus Bilateral Cataract

In some circumstances, bilateral simultaneous surgery is indicated, for example on anaesthetic grounds or because an infant has presented late and there may be concern for dense amblyopia developing in the second eye.

Precautions:

· The operation on each eye must be treated as a completely separate procedure
· If complications occur with the first eye, then careful consideration should be given before proceeding with surgery on the second eye
· Instructions should be given to the person on using separate drop bottles for each eye postoperatively and washing hands prior to instilling eye drops into the second eye
· Every effort should be made to reduce the possibility of infection by using instruments, fluids and intraocular lenses prepared in different batches.

(RCO 2010)

Investigation and diagnosis

Sometimes cataracts are diagnosed during a routine examination. A medical history should be obtained and the person will be asked to describe the symptoms they are experiencing.

- A visual acuity test is performed
- A slit-lamp is used to magnify and examine the eye (slit-lamp examination). This apparatus allows the practitioner to see the structures at the front of the eye under magnification. The microscope is called a slit-lamp as it uses an intense line of light, a slit, to illuminate the cornea, iris and lens as well as the space between the iris and cornea. The slit permits viewing of these structures in small sections, making it easier to detect any abnormalities. Using the slit-lamp or an ophthalmoscope provides the practitioner with the ability to examine the lens for signs of a cataract.
- Retinal examination is performed using eye drops that cause dilation of the pupils. This makes it easier to examine the retina.

Signs and symptoms

The cataract may cause painless loss of vision (a cataract does not routinely cause discomfort or pain in the eye or alter the external appearance of the eye). The person may report glare and in some instances there may be a change in refraction (this describes the bending of light rays as they pass across a particular medium).

In some people, visual acuity is reduced. There may be no symptoms with early cataracts. As the cataract develops, decrease in clarity of vision, not fully correctable with glasses, is noticed. Halos may be observed around lights. Night vision will be diminished. In some types of cataracts, diplopia may be noted in the affected eye.

Nursing care and management

Surgical removal of the cataract remains the only effective treatment available to restore or maintain vision. Non-surgical management includes counselling patients about cataract-related visual symptoms, offering reassurance concerning the cause of the visual disability and prescribing new eyeglasses where appropriate.

Chapter 14 provides detailed information concerning the role of the nurse with regards to preoperative care. The procedure can be performed on a day-case basis, using a locally injected anaesthetic or even with the use of anaesthetic eye drops.

The following should be considered prior to surgery:

- General health evaluation including blood pressure check
- Note of current medication
- Record of allergies
- Assessment of hearing and understanding of English
- Assessment of patient's ability to cooperate with the procedure and lie reasonably flat during surgery
- Identification of social problems
- Instruction on eyedrop instillation
- Clear explanation of the procedure and effect on the person
- Opportunity for person to ask questions.

It is the role of the nurse to act as the person's advocate and this may mean having to explain things concerning preoperative, perioperative and postoperative care in detail. The nurse acting on the person's behalf may need to ask the surgical team to provide the person with more details in order for informed consent to be made.

The most widely used, safest and most effective technique for cataracts is phacoemulsification (RCO 2010) (Figure 35.21).

Prior to surgery, adequate pupillary dilatation is needed (some patients can be provided with dilating drops to self-administer before they leave home).

An incision is made in the sclera approximately 3 mm in diameter. A round hole of approximately 5 mm diameter is made in the lens capsule. The hard lens nucleus is liquefied using an ultrasonic probe that is inserted through the hole and it is extracted. The soft lens fibres are aspirated. The replacement lens is placed folded into the empty capsular bag where it unfolds. No sutures are required to close the hole; the hole heals without sutures.

Complications from cataract surgery that could threaten a person's sight or require further surgery are low. The rate of

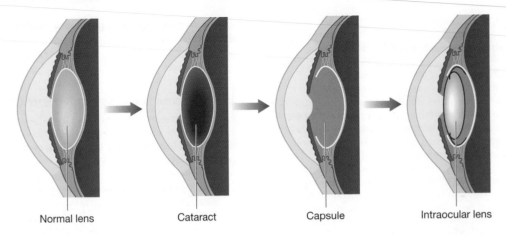

Normal lens   Cataract   Capsule   Intraocular lens

Figure 35.21 **Phacoemulsification.**

complications increases in those who have other eye diseases as well as the cataract (AAO 2011b).

Although the risk is low, surgery does involve the risk of partial to total vision loss if surgery is unsuccessful or if there are complications. Some complications can be treated and vision loss reversed; however others cannot. Complications that may occur with cataract surgery include:

- Endophthalmitis (infection in the eye)
- Swelling and fluid in the centre of the nerve layer
- Swelling of the clear covering of the eye
- Hyphaema (bleeding in the front of the eye)
- Bursting (rupture) of the capsule and loss of fluid (vitreous gel) in the eye
- Detachment of the nerve layer at the back of the eye (retinal detachment).

The following are complications that may occur some time after surgery:

- Problems with glare
- Dislocated intraocular lens
- Clouding of the portion of the lens covering (capsule) that remains after surgery
- Retinal detachment
- Glaucoma
- Astigmatism (causes blurred or distorted vision) or strabismus (squint)
- Ptosis.

Topically applied antibiotics, corticosteroids and NSAIDs may be used postoperatively but this practice varies among practitioners.

Chapter 14 discusses postoperative care in detail. When caring for a person who has undergone eye surgery, the following points should be considered:

- If possible, explain carefully to the person what the outcome of surgery was
- When approaching the person, let them know and approach from the unaffected side. This enables eye contact, enhancing communication
- Observe and assess eye dressing for bleeding or drainage, documenting your findings
- If there is an eye patch or shield in place, maintain this to help prevent unintentional injury to the operative site

- When safe to do so (i.e. physiological parameters are within normal range) elevate the head of the bed and encourage the person to lie on the unaffected side as this reduces the possibility of intraocular pressure in the affected eye. Undertake an assessment of needs, for example assess and provide analgesia as required for pain, aching
- If the person complains of sudden, sharp eye pain, this should be reported immediately as this may be an ocular emergency
- Ensure you place personal articles and the nurse call bell within easy reach
- Administer all prescribed medications
- In order to maintain normal intraocular pressures, vomiting should be prevented; offer prescribed antiemetic medication as required.

Jot This Down Assisting the Person Who Is Blind or Visually Impaired: Eating and drinking

- When serving a meal, offer to describe the location of food on the person's plate as corresponding to the numbers on a clockface. For example, tell the person that their fish is at 3 o'clock, their carrots are at 9 o'clock and their potatoes are at 6 o'clock
- This method can also be used to describe the location of other items on the table; for example, if the dinner plate is directly in front of the person, you can say that the mustard is above the plate at 1 o'clock and the person's glass is at 2 o'clock.
- Ask the person whether they would like you to refill their cup before doing so. If you refill it without telling them, it may cause a spill
- If you are filling up a person's glass or cup, do not fill it to the brim in case it spills as they lift it.

Health promotion and discharge

The person is discharged home, based on meeting certain criteria that may include:

- Vital signs are stable
- Preoperative mental state is restored
- Nausea and vomiting are controlled

- Pain is absent or minimal
- An escort is available
- Post-surgical care has been reviewed with the patient and/or escort and written postoperative instructions have been provided
- A follow-up appointment has been made.

People usually need reading glasses (for near vision) after cataract surgery but some people may choose to have different lens implants (intraocular lens) in their eyes so that one eye can be used for distance vision and the other for near vision (monovision).

The person should arrange for someone to take care of them for the first 24 hours postoperatively. Full vision may take up to 2 days to return, though sensation usually returns to the eye within a few hours. Complete healing may take several months. The nurse should ensure the person (and/or carer) understands the correct method of instilling eye drops and when they are to be administered.

The person should be advised that they can bend, carry shopping, wash their face and hair and carry on with their usual activities of living.

The person should:

- Try not to touch or rub the eye
- Keep soap and shampoo out of the eyes
- Not wear eye make-up for 1 week after surgery
- Not swim for 2 weeks after surgery
- Avoid playing sports where there is a risk of getting knocked in the eye, such as squash, for about 2 weeks
- Implement actions to avoid constipation and straining
- Wear sunglasses with side shields when outdoors.

The person will be able to read and watch television almost immediately if they have reading glasses, however vision may be blurry as the healing eye gets used to its new lens. Driving can take place when the person can read a number plate 20.5 m away. There may be a need for new glasses to be able to do this.

If the person experiences more than mild pain or loss of vision, or if the eye starts to go red, they should contact the hospital for advice. Other symptoms to report include cloudiness, drainage, floaters or flashes of light, or halos around bright objects.

Highlight the significance of attending follow-up appointments. Provide referral to the community nursing services for assistance with home care after discharge (if appropriate).

Jot This Down

Mrs Alicia Joaquin, 62, has been blind since birth. She has been admitted to your ward for surgery to her hip; understandably she is anxious. How would you help Mrs Joaquin with:

- Eating and drinking
- Mobilising
- Washing and dressing?

Conclusion

In this chapter, two of the special senses have been discussed, sight and hearing. The person who experiences problems with their sight or hearing is at risk of danger from a variety of perspectives. Hearing, for example, enables us to hear on-coming traffic or a shout that there is danger ahead; the ability to see clearly provides us with the ability to see the oncoming danger.

An overview of the anatomy and physiology of the ear and eye has been presented. The ways in which these senses function are complex and the nurse needs to have a fundamental understanding of the anatomical and physiological elements of these two organs in order to provide care that is patient-centred, safe and effective. This chapter has provided you with a brief insight concerning the care of people who may experience problems with their sight or hearing. The role of the nurse is to ensure the person, aided or independently, can maintain a safe environment.

There are several special investigations and tests related to the assessment of the person's sight and hearing. This chapter has offered an overview of some of them. It takes time to develop the knowledge, skills and attitudes that will enable you to undertake these assessments in a competent and confident manner.

A selection of common eye and ear conditions has been discussed. When a threat to a person's ability to see or hear occurs or there is potential for this to occur, the person needs the nurse to be able to offer them support and provide them with comfort. You will only be able to do this if you have developed an in-depth understanding of the person, their condition, the pathophysiology and the holistic care required.

Key Points

- The normal and altered anatomy and physiology of the ear and eye have been outlined.
- It has been noted that if the nurse is to deliver care that is patient-centred, safe and effective, there is a need to use a systematic approach.
- The nurse is required to have, or be prepared to develop, an understanding of the assessment of needs using a variety of tools, make inferences from the data collected, plan care with the person, with the person at the heart of all that is done, deliver care that is sensitive to the needs of the individual (and their family if appropriate) and undertake an evaluation of care delivered, making changes where there is a need to do so.
- There are a multitude of diagnostic tests available to help assess the function of the person's hearing and sight.
- Risk factors related to the senses of sight and hearing have been described. The nurse must have an understanding of these risk factors as preventative measures may be put in place to avoid harm or deterioration in the person's condition.
- This chapter has emphasised the need to work in partnership with the person and other healthcare professionals. At all times, the nurse should strive to practise in a holistic manner, respect the choices the individual makes, act as an advocate, support health and well-being and uphold the rights and dignity of people.

Glossary

Acute otitis media: otitis refers to an ear inflammation, media means middle. Acute otitis media is an infection of the middle ear, located behind the eardrum

Aqueous humour: the clear, watery fluid between the lens and the cornea

(Continued)

Astigmatism: a condition in which blurred vision is caused by the cornea being shaped more like a rugby ball as opposed to spherical like a basketball

Audiogram: a graph made to show hearing. An audiometer is used to obtain an audiogram

Cholesteatoma: a cyst-like structure in the middle ear (and sometimes the mastoid) filled with cheesy, skin-like material

Choroid: the layer of blood vessels between the retina and the sclera

Chronic otitis media: when infection of the middle ear persists, leading to possible ongoing damage to the middle ear and eardrum

Cochlea: the hearing part of the inner ear

Conductive hearing loss: hearing loss caused by damage to the ear's conducting system: middle and outer ear

Conjunctiva: a thin layer of tissue that lines the inside of the eyelids as well as the outer surfaces of the sclera

Conjunctivitis: inflammation of the conjunctiva (sometimes called 'pink eye').

Cornea: the clear outer layer of the eye. It covers the iris

Eustachian tube: connects the back of the nose to the middle ear and serves mainly to regulate air pressure, protect and drain the middle ear

Inner ear: receives the sound from the eardrum and ossicles in the middle ear and also houses the semicircular canals

Iris: the coloured membrane of the eye, surrounding the pupil. The iris controls the amount of light entering the pupil by expanding and contracting

Labyrinth: another term for the inner ear

Macula: the central portion of the retina; a healthy macula is critical in maintaining sharp vision

Mastoid: this is connected to and behind the middle ear, composed of many air cells

Middle ear: the space behind the eardrum, between the outer ear and inner ear and connected to the eustachian tube in front and the mastoid behind

Ophthalmologist: a doctor who specialises in the medical and surgical care of the eyes and visual system and also the prevention of eye disease and injury

Ophthalmoscope: an instrument used to examine the retina

Optic nerve: the nerve that connects the eye to the brain. It carries impulses of light from the retina to the brain, which then interprets the impulses as images

Optometrist: a doctor trained to examine, diagnose, treat and manage some diseases and disorders of the eye

Ossicles: the three smallest bones in the body, connected to each other, transmitting sound from the eardrum to the inner ear. The malleus (shaped like a hammer), incus (shaped like an anvil) and stapes (shaped like the stirrup of a riding saddle)

Otalgia: ear pain or earache

Otitis externa: means outer ear infection

Otitis media: inflammation of the middle ear

Otoscope: an instrument designed for visual examination of the eardrum and the passage of the outer ear, usually has a light and a set of lenses (also called an auriscope)

Otoscopy: otoscopy is a procedure in which the practitioner uses an otoscope to examine the ear canal and eardrum

Presbyopia: the loss of the eye's ability to change its focus to see objects that are near; it is part of the natural ageing process of the eye that affects everybody at some point in life

Pupil: the round, dark, central opening of the eye through which light enters

Refraction: the ability of the eye to bend light so that an image focusses directly on the retina

Retina: the thin layer of nerves that lines the back of the eye. The retina senses light and transmits light impulses to the optic nerve and then the brain

Sclera: the outer coat of the eyeball that forms the whites of a person's eyes

Semicircular canals: the inner ear (labyrinth); they are involved in balance

Sensorineural hearing loss: damage caused to the inner ear hearing mechanism (the cochlea), hearing nerve or hearing part of the brain

Strabismus: a condition in which the eyes are misaligned and unable to point in the same direction at the same time

Tinnitus: hearing abnormal sounds in the ear, such as ringing, buzzing, popping and snapping

Vertigo: a subjective sensation of movement of the person or the surroundings

Visual acuity: how well a person sees

Visual field: the entire range in which a person can see, including peripheral vision

Vitreous humour: the clear gel-like substance found inside the centre of the eyeball

References

AAO (2011a) *Conjunctivitis PPP*, Limited Revision, October 2011. American Academy of Ophthalmology, San Francisco.

AAO (2011b) *Cataract in the Adult Eye*. American Academy of Ophthalmology, San Francisco.

AAO (2012) *Blepharitis Summary Benchmark*. American Academy of Ophthalmology, San Francisco.

Action on Hearing (2013) *Types and Causes of Hearing Loss*. http://www.actiononhearingloss.org.uk/your-hearing/about-deafness-and-hearing-loss/types-and-cause-of-hearing-loss/conductive-and-sensorineural-hearing-loss.aspx (accessed August 2013).

Action on Hearing Loss (2011) *Fact and Figures on Hearing Loss and Tinnitus*. http://www.actiononhearingloss.org.uk/supporting-you/factsheets-and-leaflets/deaf-awareness.aspx (accessed August 2013).

Akpek, E.K., Polcharoen, W., Chan, R. & Foster, C.S. (1999) Ocular surface neoplasia masquerading as chronic blepharoconjunctivitis. *Cornea*, 18(3), 282–288.

Anderson, J.E. (2007) *Ophthalmology: a brief review*. Apollo, Texas.

Basu, S., Georgalas, C., Sen, P. & Bhattacharyya, A.K. (2007) Water precautions and ear surgery: evidence and practice in the UK. *Journal of Laryngology and Otology*, 121(1), 9–14.

Cruse, A.S., Singh, A. & Quiney, R.E. (2010) Sodium fluoride in otosclerosis treatment: review. *Journal of Laryngology and Otology*, 124(6), 583–586.

Dalton, D.S., Cruickshanks, K.J., Klein, B.E. *et al.* (2003) The impact of hearing loss on quality of life in older adults. *Gerontologist*, 43(5), 661–668.

Darrat, I., Ahmad, N., Seidman, K. & Seidman, M.D. (2007) Auditory research involving antioxidants. *Current Opinion in Otolaryngology and Head Neck Surgery*, 15(5), 358–363.

DH (2007) *What is Physiological Measurement? A Guide to the Tests and Procedures Conducted by Physiological Measurement Diagnostic Services*. Department of Health, London.

Fransen, E., Topsakai, V., Hendrisks. J.J. *et al.* (2008) Occupational noise, smoking, and a high body mass index are risk factors for age-related hearing impairment and moderate alcohol consumption is protective: a European population-based multicentre study. *Journal of the Association for Research in Otolaryngology*, 9(3), 264–276.

Gates, G.A. & Mills, J.H. (2005) Presbycusis. *Lancet*, 366(9491), 1111–1120.

Gleadle, J. (2012) *History and Clinical Examination at a Glance*, 3rd edn. Wiley, Oxford.

Henderson, V. (1960) *Basic Principles of Nursing Care*. International Council of Nursing, London.

Hickson, L., Worrall, L. & Scarinici, N. (2007) A randomized controlled trial evaluating the active communication education program for older people with hearing impairment. *Ear and Hearing*, 28(2), 212–230.

Jackson, W.B. (2008) Blepharitis: current strategies for diagnosis and management. *Canadian Journal of Ophthalmology*, 43(2), 170–179.

James, B. & Bron, A. (2011) *Ophthalmology. Lecture Notes*, 11th edn. Wiley, Oxford.

Jenkins G. & Tortora, G. (2013) *Anatomy and Physiology*, 3rd edn. Wiley, New Jersey.

Karhuketo, T.S., Lungmark, J., Vanhatalo, J., Rautiainen, M. & Sipilä, M. (2007) Stapes surgery: a 32-year follow-up. *ORL Journal for Otorhinolaryngology and its Related Specialities*, 69(5), 322–326.

LeMone, P., Burke, K. & Bauldoff, G. (2011) *Medical–Surgical Nursing. Critical Thinking in Patient Care*, 5th edn. Pearson, London.

Linstrom, C. J., Silverman, C.A. & Susman, W. M. (2000) Facial-motion analysis with a video and computer system: a preliminary report. *American Journal of Otology*, 21(1), 123–129.

Luchs, J. (2010) Azithromycin in DuraSite for the treatment of blepharitis. *Clinical Ophthalmology*, 4, 681–688.

Liu, X.Z. & Yan, X.Z. (2007) Ageing and hearing loss. *Journal of Pathology*, 211(2), 188–197.

Macfadyen, C.A., Acuin, J.M. & Gamble, C. (2006) Systemic antibiotics versus topical treatments for chronically discharging ears with underlying eardrum perforations. *Cochrane Database Systematic Review*, (1): CD005608.

Munir, N. & Clarke, R. (2013) *Ear, Nose and Throat at a Glance*. Wiley Blackwell, Oxford.

NICE (2007) *Implantation of Accommodating Intraocular Lenses During Cataract Surgery*. National Institute for Health and Clinical Excellence, London. http://www.nice.org.uk/nicemedia/live/11284/31697/31697.pdf (accessed August 2013).

NICE (2011a) *Cochlear Implants for Children and Adults with Severe to Profound Deafness*. National Institute for Health and Clinical Excellence, London. http://www.nice.org.uk/nicemedia/live/12122/42854/42854.pdf (accessed August 2013).

NICE (2011b) *Otitis Media with Effusion*. National Institute for Health and Clinical Excellence, London. http://cks.nice.org.uk/otitis-media-with-effusion#azTab (accessed August 2013).

Pirozzo, S., Papinczak, T. & Glasziou, P. (2003) Whispered voice test for screening for hearing impairment in adults and children: systematic review. *British Medical Journal*, 327(7421), 967–970.

Rapoza, P.A., Quinn, T.C., Kiessling, L.A., Green, W.R. & Taylor, H.R. (1986) Assessment of neonatal conjunctivitis with a direct immunofluorescent monoclonal antibody stain for chlamydia. *Journal of the American Medical Association*, 255(24), 3369–3373.

RCO (2010) *Cataract Surgery Guidelines*. Royal College of Ophthalmologists, London.

van der Veen EL, Schilder AG, van Heerbeek N, *et al.* (2006) Predictors of chronic suppurative otitis media in children. *Archives of Otolaryngology. Head & Neck Surgery*, 132(10), 1115–1118.

Waugh, A. & Grant, A. (2010) *Ross and Wilson Anatomy and Physiology in Health and Illness*, 11th edn. Churchill Livingstone, Edinburgh.

Wright, D. & Safranek, S. (2009) Treatment of otitis media with perforated tympanic membrane. *American Family Physician*, 79(8), 650–654.

Test Yourself

1. Another term for ear wax is:
   (a) Cholesteatoma
   (b) Cerumen
   (c) Cervix
   (d) Conjunctiva

2. The function of the eustachian tube is to:
   (a) Help with balance
   (b) Increase the pressure of the middle ear
   (c) Equalise the pressure of the middle ear
   (d) Decrease the pressure of the middle ear

3. A burst eardrum is also known as:
   (a) A perforated tympanic membrane
   (b) A perforated oval window
   (c) A perforated eustachian tube
   (d) A perforated malleolus

4. Conductive hearing loss occurs when:
   (a) There is a problem in the transmission of sound waves from the external ear, through the middle ear
   (b) There is a problem with the cranial nerve
   (c) There is a problem with the cerebellum
   (d) There is an increase in the production of cerumen

5. The key function of the middle ear is:
   (a) To transmit vibrations from the stapes to the tympanic membrane
   (b) Cushion sound
   (c) To transmit vibrations from the pinna to the inner ear
   (d) To transmit vibrations from the tympanic membrane to the inner ear

6. Cataractogenic…
   (a) Relates to or having the ability to produce a cataract
   (b) Is concerned with older people only
   (c) Is concerned with children only
   (d) Is a type of infection

7. The retina is usually:
   (a) An intermittent red-orange colour
   (b) A constant red-orange colour
   (c) A constant green-yellow colour
   (d) An intermittent green-yellow colour

8. A cataract occurs when:
   (a) There is hypertension
   (b) The person has an eye infection
   (c) The lens of an eye becomes opaque and vision is affected
   (d) The lens becomes rigid

9. A hyphema is:
   (a) A blister in the lower eye lid
   (b) Bleeding in the front of the eye
   (c) Bleeding in the back of the eye
   (d) A drooping of the upper eye lid

10. Pupillary dilatation refers to:
    (a) Contraction of the pupils
    (b) Contraction of the lens and the pupil
    (c) Widening of the pupils
    (d) Contacting and widening of the pupils

Answers

1. b
2. c
3. a
4. a
5. d
6. a
7. b
8. c
9. b
10. c

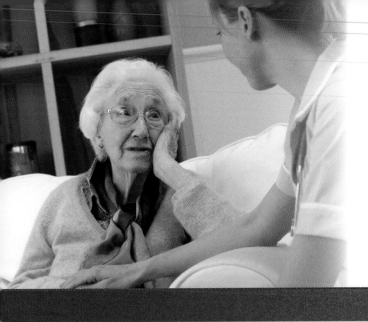

36

The Person with a Musculoskeletal Disorder

Ian Peate

School of Health Studies, Gibraltar

Learning Outcomes

On completion of this chapter you will be able to:

- Provide an overview of the musculoskeletal system
- Detail the structure of the musculoskeletal system
- Detail the function of the musculoskeletal system
- Provide an explanation for the normal and abnormal changes that can occur in the musculoskeletal system
- Describe some disorders and impairments related to the musculoskeletal system
- Use the nursing process as a framework for care provision

Competencies

All nurses must:

1. Work in partnership with patients to address their needs
2. Assess physical and psychological needs
3. Practise in a holistic manner
4. Respect individual choice
5. Support and promote the person's health and well-being
6. Offer information and advice to people relating to the musculoskeletal system

 Visit the companion website at **www.wileynursingpractice.com** where you can test yourself using flashcards, multiple-choice questions and more.

Nursing Practice: Knowledge and Care, First Edition. Edited by Ian Peate, Karen Wild and Muralitharan Nair.
© 2014 John Wiley & Sons, Ltd. Published 2014 by John Wiley & Sons, Ltd. Companion website: www.wileynursingpractice.com

Introduction

All of the bones, cartilage, muscles, joints, tendons and ligaments in the body compose what is known as the **musculoskeletal system**. The bones provide the body with a framework, giving it shape and support; they also serve as protection for internal organs, such as the lungs and liver. Muscles are fibres that help to make deliberate movement of a body part or involuntary movement within an internal organ possible. The muscles are the active part of the apparatus of locomotion. In some instances, the musculoskeletal system is seen as two body systems in one or two systems that work very closely together, with one being the muscular system and the other being the skeletal system. Without the skeleton to pull against, contracting muscle fibres could not make us sit, stand, walk or run.

Anatomy and Physiology

The Skeleton

There are 206 bones in the human adult. At birth, the number of bones is 300. The difference arises from the fact the some bones fuse over time into a single bone. The skeleton is divided into the axial skeleton and the appendicular skeleton. Bones of the axial skeleton include the skull, the ribs and sternum and the vertebral column. The appendicular skeleton is made up of all the bones of the limbs, the shoulder girdles and the pelvic girdle. The bones of the axial and appendicular skeleton can be found in Table 36.1.

Figure 36.1 shows the divisions of the skeletal system from anterior and posterior perspectives.

Bones afford a number of important functions; they provide form for the body's structure, support soft tissues, protect vital organs from injury and serve to move body parts by providing points of attachment for muscles. Bones also act as a store for minerals and serve as a site for haematopoiesis (blood cell formation). The bone also contains yellow bone marrow that stores triglycerides (fats).

Figure 36.2 provides an illustration of sections through the diaphysis of long bone.

Bone classification

Bones are classified according to shape (Figure 36.3).

Long bones These bones have a diaphysis, a medullary cavity, epiphyses, metaphyses and periosteum. The mid-portion is the 'diaphysis' and the two broad ends are called 'epiphyses'. The diaphysis is made up of compact bone, containing the marrow cavity; this is lined with endosteum (a thin layer of connective tissue). Each epiphysis is spongy bone and is covered by a thin layer of compact bone. Long bones are the bones of the toes, legs, fingers and arms (Figure 36.4).

Table 36.1 The bones that make up the adult skeletal system.

DIVISION OF THE SKELETON	STRUCTURE	NUMBER OF BONES	DIVISION OF THE SKELETON	STRUCTURE	NUMBER OF BONES
Axial skeleton	Skull		Appendicular skeleton	Pectoral (shoulder) girdles	
	Cranium	8		Clavicle	2
	Face	14		Scapula	2
	Hyoid	1		Upper limbs	
	Auditory ossicles	6		Humerus	2
	Vertebral column	26		Ulna	2
	Thorax			Radius	2
	Sternum	1		Carpals	16
	Ribs	24		Metacarpals	10
	Number of bones =	80		Phalanges	28
				Pelvic (hip) girdle	
				Hip, pelvic, or coxal bone	2
				Lower limbs	
				Femur	2
				Patella	2
				Fibula	2
				Tibia	2
				Tarsals	14
				Metatarsals	10
				Phalanges	28
				Number of bones =	126

Total bones in an adult skeleton = 206

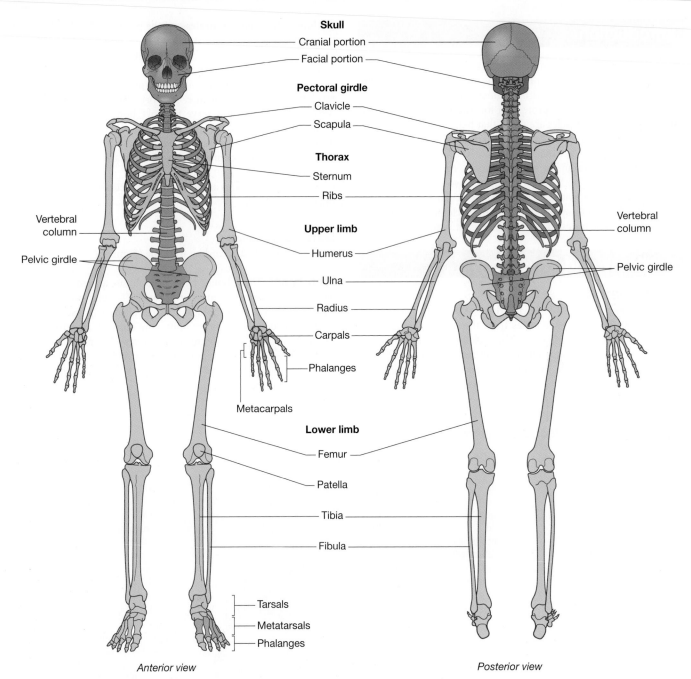

Figure 36.1 The divisions of the skeletal system.

Short bones These are also called 'cuboid'. They are spongy bone covered by compact bone. They are the bones of the wrist (carpal) and ankle (tarsal) and are about equal in length and width.

Flat bones Flat bones are usually thin and flat. Many of them are curved. They have a disc-like structure that is made up of a layer of spongy bone between two thin layers of compact bone. Flat bones are bones of the skull, the sternum and the ribs. These bones provide much protection. The cranial bones protect the brain; the sternum and the ribs offer protection to the organs located in the thorax. These bones also provide extensive surfaces for muscle attachment.

Irregular bones These are, as the name suggests, various shapes and sizes and they (like flat bones) are plates of compact bone with spongy bone between. Irregular bones include the vertebrae, the scapulae, some facial bones, the calcaneus and the bones of the pelvic girdle.

Sesamoid bone The last group, usually short or irregular bones, are imbedded in a tendon. The patella is an example, sitting within the patella or quadriceps tendon. Other sesamoid bones are the pisiform (smallest of the carpals) and the two small bones at the base of the first metatarsal. Sesamoid bones are usually present in a tendon where it passes over a joint, which serves to protect the tendon; they deal with friction, tension and physical stress.

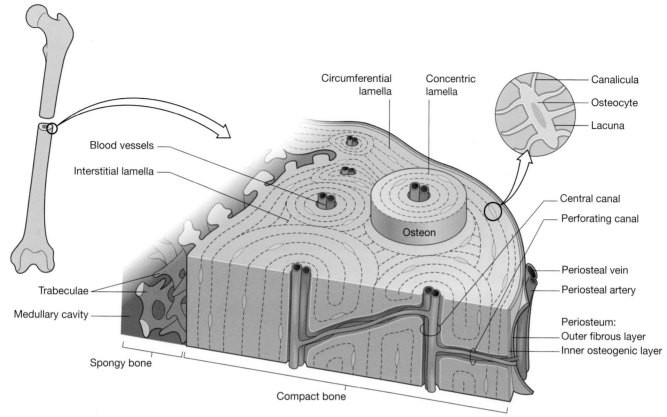

Figure 36.2 Osteons in compact bone and trabeculae in spongy bone.

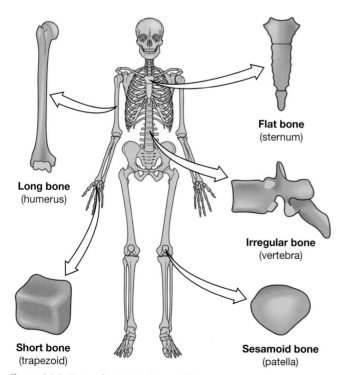

Figure 36.3 Bone shapes (not to scale).

Long bone
(humerus)

Flat bone
(sternum)

Irregular bone
(vertebra)

Short bone
(trapezoid)

Sesamoid bone
(patella)

Red Flag

Musculoskeletal disorders are the commonest cause of disability in the UK. Each year, 15% of patients on a GP's list will consult their doctor with a locomotor problem and such conditions form 20–25% of a GP's workload. About 30% of those with any physical disability and 60% of those with a severe disability have a musculoskeletal disorder as the primary cause of their problems.

(Arthritis Research UK 2011)

Bone formation is also known as ossification. Bone formation occurs during various phases of an individual's life. Tortora and Nielsen (2012) describe four principal stages in a person's life when bone formation occurs (Table 36.2).

Jot This Down

As a person ages, the action of bone breakdown and bone build-up continues. As well as breakdown and re-building, the bone also thickens and bone mass increases. Damage to joints, tissues surrounding the joints and the bones themselves can also occur as the ageing process occurs.

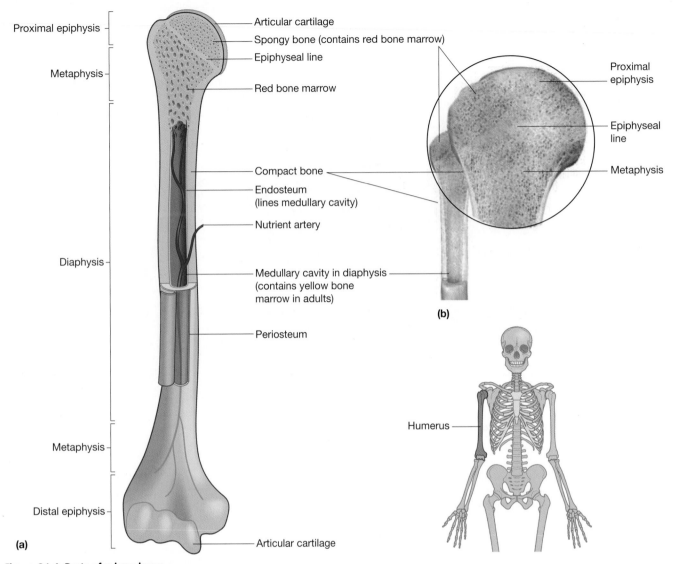

Figure 36.4 Parts of a long bone.

Table 36.2 Bone formation throughout a person's life.
(*Source*: Adapted from Tortora & Nielsen 2012)

STAGE	ACTIVITY
One	Bone is initially formed *in utero* in the fetus
Two	Bone growth during infancy, childhood and adolescence
Three	The replacement of old bone with new bone (bone remodelling) – occurring throughout an individual's life
Four	The repair of fractures that can occur throughout a person's life

Remodelling of bone

Adult bones do not normally increase in length and size; however there is continuous remodelling of bones, as well as repair of damaged bone tissue, that occurs during the person's life. Bone resorption and bone deposit occur at all periosteal and endosteal surfaces in the bone remodelling process. There are hormones and forces that cause stress on the bones and this in turn regulates this process; this includes the joint action of the osteocytes, osteoclasts and osteoblasts. Those bones that are being used are exposed to stress and when this happens they increase osteoblastic activity with the intention of increasing ossification (the development of bone). There are some bones that are inactive and these undergo increased osteoclast activity and bone resorption. Figure 36.5 shows the bone remodelling process.

Hormonal stimulus One of the stimuli for bone remodelling involves hormones. The hormonal stimulus required for bone remodelling is controlled via a negative feedback mechanism that controls calcium levels in the blood. This stimulus includes the interaction of parathyroid hormone (PTH) released from the parathyroid glands and calcitonin released from the thyroid gland. As blood levels of calcium decrease, PTH is released; the presence of PTH then stimulates osteoclast activity and bone resorption, releasing calcium from the bone matrix. The outcome is that levels of calcium in the blood increase and the impetus for PTH release

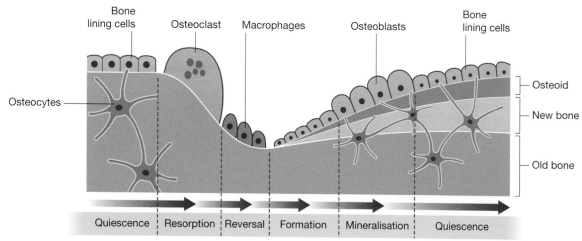

Figure 36.5 Diagrammatic representation of the bone remodelling process.

ceases. As blood calcium levels rise, the secretion of calcitonin is stimulated, inhibiting bone resorption and causing calcium salts to be deposited in the bone matrix. Calcium ions are required for the transmission of nerve impulses, the release of neurotransmitters, muscle contraction, the clotting of blood, glandular secretion and cell division. The bones therefore are needed to regulate the amount of calcium in the blood.

Mechanical stress Just as the bones require hormones to influence bone remodelling, bone remodelling also depends on, and is regulated by, the response of bones to gravitational pull, as well as to the mechanical stress resulting from the pull of muscles. The exact mechanism is not fully understood, but what is known is that those bones that undergo increased stress are heavier and larger. Bone develops and remodels itself in its attempts to resist the stresses placed on it (Wolff's law).

Joints

A joint is the point at which two or more bones come together. Joints may also be called articulations. Joints hold the bones of the skeleton together and at the same time, they permit the body to move. Joints may be classified by function:

- Synarthroses
- Amphiarthroses
- Diarthroses

    As well as by structure:

- Fibrous
- Cartilaginous
- Synovial.

Fibrous joints A fibrous (synarthrodial) joint is a joint that is held together by only a ligament. A ligament is a compact irregular tissue composed of rich collagen fibres. In this type of joint, there is no synovial cavity. These joints permit little or no movement. Examples of synarthrodial joints include where the teeth are held to their bony sockets and the radioulnar and tibiofibular joints.

Cartilaginous joints These joints are also called 'synchondroses' (the singular is synarthrosis) and 'symphyses' (the singular is sym-

physis). They are found where the connection between the articulating bones is made up of cartilage (there is no synovial cavity, e.g. the joints occurring between vertebrae in the spine). The sternocostal joints of the rib cage are also an example of a cartilaginous joint; they are composed of hyaline cartilage growths fusing together the ends of the articulating bones. These joints are immobile. In other cartilaginous joints, such as the intervertebral discs, the hyaline cartilage fuses to an intervening plate of flexible fibrocartilage. This structural feature accounts for the flexibility of the vertebral column.

The synchondroses are temporary joints. They only exist in children up until the end of puberty and at this stage the hyaline cartilage converts to bone, for example the epiphyseal plates of long bones. Symphysis joints are permanent cartilaginous joints composed of an intervening pad of fibrocartilage, for example the symphysis pubis.

Synovial joints These joints are also called diarthroses. They are the most common classification of a joint in the body. These joints are extremely flexible with a wide range of movements. They have a synovial cavity and all of them have an articular capsule encircling the whole joint, a synovial membrane (the inner layer of the capsule) that produces synovial fluid (a lubricating solution), and cartilage, known as 'hyaline cartilage', that creates a pad at the ends of the articulating bones.

The synovial fluid is a thin film that is viscous, clear or yellowish. Synovial fluid assists in preventing friction as it lubricates the joint, as well as supplying nutrients and assisting with the removal of waste products. The fluid can become gel like when the joint has become immobile for a period of time. It returns to its normal viscous consistency after the joint regains its movement.

There are a number of characteristics associated with synovial joints:

- Articular cartilage covers the articular surfaces
- The joint cavity is enclosed by a tough, fibrous, double-layered articular capsule
- Synovial fluid fills the free spaces of the joint capsule, promoting effortless movement of the articulating bones.

There are six types of synovial joints classified by the shape of the joint and the movement available (Figure 36.6).

Hinge	A convex portion of one bone fits into a concave portion of another bone. The movement reflects the hinge and bracket movement of a household hinge and bracket. Movement is limited to flexion and extension. The joint produces an open and closing motion. These joints are uniaxial.	Elbow, knee	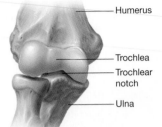	
Pivot	A rounded part of one bone fits into a groove of another bone. These joints will only permit movement of one bone around another – uniaxial movement.	Radius and ulna, the atlas and axis	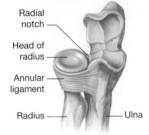	
Ball and socket	The spherical end of one bone fits into a concave socket of another bone, hence, ball and socket. Movement occurs through flexion, extension and adduction. This is a triaxial joint.	Hip, shoulder	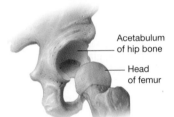	
Saddle	Similar to condyloid joints, but these joints permit greater movement. Allow flexion, extension and adduction. The joint is classed as triaxial.	The carpometacarpal joints of the thumb	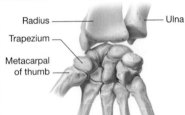	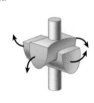
Condyloid	Where an oval surface of one bone fits into a concavity of another bone and where condyloid joints are found. Allows flexion, extension and adduction. This is a biaxial joint.	The radiocarpal and metacarpophalangeal joints of the hand	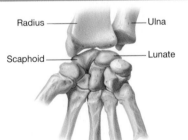	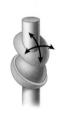
Gliding	These joints have a flat or slightly curved surface permitting gliding movements. The joints are bound by ligaments and movement in all directions is restricted. The joint moves back and forth and side to side.	Intertarsal and intercarpal joints of the hands and feet	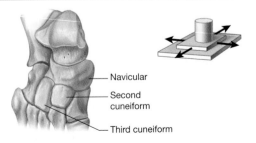	

Figure 36.6 The six types of synovial joint.

Table 36.3 Muscle types.

TYPE	DESCRIPTION	LOCATION
Skeletal	Voluntary muscle (striated). These muscles can be moved consciously	Biceps, triceps, deltoid, gluteus maximus
Smooth	Involuntary muscle (non-striated). These muscles cannot be moved consciously	Muscles in the walls of the bladder, stomach, and bronchi
Cardiac	Involuntary muscle (striated)	Only found in the heart

Muscles

The key functions of muscles are to pull bones, to contract and move the viscera and the blood vessels and to make the heart beat (cardiac muscle). Muscles turn energy into motion (locomotion) helping to propel the body. It would not be possible for us to do anything without muscles: every time we make a movement, blink, swallow, breathe, write an assignment or cry, muscle is involved. There are three types of muscle (Table 36.3).

Skeletal muscle

Skeletal muscle is the most abundant tissue in the body. This type of muscle is the type of muscle we can see, for example the biceps. Skeletal muscles are attached to and cover the bones of the skeleton. Skeletal muscles help the body to move, assist with the maintenance of posture and also produce body heat. Skeletal muscle has the ability to contract and relax and can be moved consciously. These muscles may be under voluntary control or their movement may occur as the result of reflex activity. Skeletal muscle contains approximately 80% of the body's content of water and is also a reservoir for ions such as potassium (Sambrook *et al.* 2010). Skeletal muscles make up a significant percentage of total body weight.

Skeletal muscles pull in only one direction and because of this they are paired: when bending a limb around a joint for example, one muscle moves the bone in one direction and another moves it back the other way. These muscles usually contract voluntarily (you think about contracting them and the nervous system tells them to do so). They can do a short, single contraction (twitch) or a long, sustained contraction (tetanus). Muscle cells get shorter (contract) in response to nerve impulses.

Organisation of skeletal muscle

The whole muscle (e.g. the biceps) is enclosed in a sheath of connective tissue, the 'epimysium'. This sheath folds inwards into the substance of the muscle to surround a large number of smaller bundles, the fasciculi, which are made up of even smaller bundles of elongated, cylindrical muscle cells, 'the fibres'. Each fibre is a 'syncytium' (cells that have many nuclei). The nuclei are oval in shape and located at the border of the cell, just below the thin, elastic membrane (sarcolemma). The sarcoplasm also has many alternating light and dark bands, giving the fibre a striped or striated appearance (thus the name 'striated muscle'). Each muscle fibre is made up of many smaller units, the 'myofibrils, which consist of small protein filaments, known as 'actin and myosin filaments'. The myosin filaments are slightly thicker and make up the dark band (or A-band). The actin filaments make up the light bands (I-bands) and are located on either side of the dark band. The actin filaments are attached to the Z-line. This arrangement of actin and myosin filaments is known as a 'sarcomere'. See Figure 36.7 for the gross and microanatomy of skeletal muscle and skeletal muscle fibres.

When contraction of skeletal muscle tissue occurs, the actin filaments slide inwards between the myosin filaments. Mitochondria provide the energy for this to happen. This action triggers a shortening of the sarcomeres (Z-lines come closer together), causing the whole muscle fibre to contract. This can bring about a shortening of the entire muscle, such as the biceps, depending on the number of muscles fibres stimulated. The contraction of skeletal muscle tissue is very quick and forceful.

Muscle tone

Nerve impulses from the brain cause contraction to occur that tones the muscles. The muscles are in a constant state of partial contraction; this state keeps them firm, healthy and ready for action at all times. Muscle tone is the only aspect of skeletal muscle activity that cannot be controlled voluntarily. Nerve impulses from the brain stimulate groups of muscle fibres to contract and keep muscle toned even when a muscle is relaxed. When nerve supply to a muscle is damaged or destroyed, for example as a result of trauma, the muscle fibres are no longer stimulated to contract. The result of this is that the muscle loses its tone and becomes flaccid. Ultimately, the muscle will start to atrophy (wear away).

Smooth muscle

Smooth muscle is found in the walls of hollow organs such as the intestines and stomach. These muscles work automatically (involuntary); they cannot be moved consciously. For example, the muscular walls of the intestines contract to propel food through the body. Muscles in the bladder wall contract, expelling urine from the bladder. The pupillary sphincter muscle in the eye is a smooth muscle and causes dilation of the pupil to occur. Smooth muscle functions in such a way that it changes the volume of the organ that it surrounds.

The structure of **smooth muscle** differs significantly from that of skeletal muscle. The speed of smooth muscle contraction is only a small fraction of that of skeletal muscle.

Smooth muscle tissue is made up of thin elongated muscle cells and fibres. They are pointed at their ends and each has a single, large, oval nucleus. The cells are filled with a specialised cytoplasm, the sarcoplasm, and this is surrounded by a thin cell membrane, the sarcolemma. Each cell has a number of myofibrils lying parallel to one another in the direction of the long axis of the cell. They are not arranged in a definite striped (striated) pattern, as in skeletal muscles. Smooth muscle fibres interlace to form sheets or layers of muscle tissue as opposed to bundles (Figure 36.8).

Cardiac muscle

This type of muscle is found only in the walls of the heart. The cardiac muscle shows some of the features of smooth muscle as well as some of the characteristics of skeletal muscle tissue. The fibres of cardiac muscle, like those of skeletal muscle, have cross-striations that contain a number of nuclei. Like smooth muscle tissue, this muscle tissue is also involuntary. **Cardiac muscle** differs from striated muscle: the cells are shorter, the striations are not so apparent, the sarcolemma is thinner and not as apparent, there is only one nucleus present in the centre of each cardiac fibre, and adjacent fibres branch but are linked to each other by so-called 'muscle bridges'. The spaces between different fibres are filled with

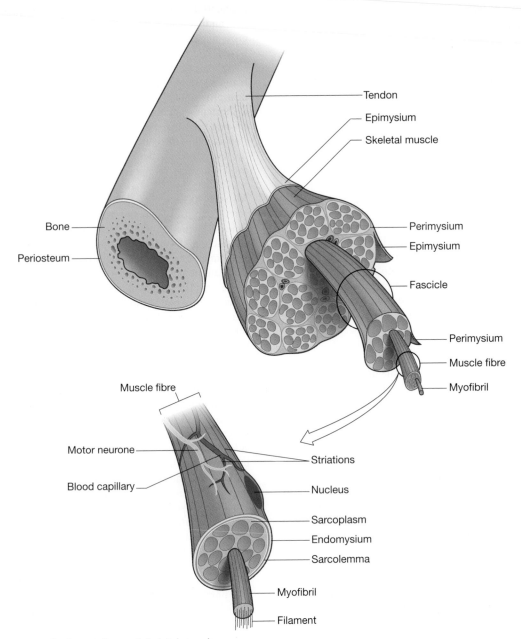

Figure 36.7 The gross and microanatomy of skeletal muscles.

areolar connective tissue; this contains blood capillaries that supply the tissues with oxygen and nutrients (Figure 36.9).

Bone Fractures

McRae and Esser (2008) define a fracture as a loss of continuity in the bone. The signs and symptoms of fracture are outlined in Box 36.1.

Types of fracture

There are several types of fracture. A fracture is often referred to as a broken bone. Fractures occur when the physical force exerted on a bone is stronger than the bone itself, and fractures are a common occurrence.

Risk of fracture is often associated with age. Children's fractures are often less complicated than those in adults. The bones of older people are more brittle and they can sustain a fracture from a fall, for example, that would not have the same affect on a younger person. As the person ages, fractures become more common (Hommel *et al.* 2012).

See Figure 36.10 for the main categories of fracture.

Bone fractures – healing

As the process of bone modelling is continuous, this ability to constantly regenerate means that bones that are fractured can fully heal. As soon as bone is broken, the inflammatory stage of healing begins and lasts for approximately 5 days.

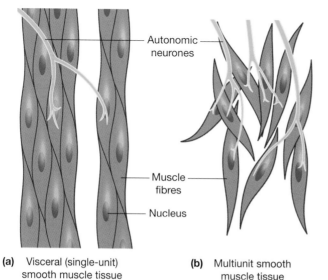

(a) Visceral (single-unit) smooth muscle tissue

(b) Multiunit smooth muscle tissue

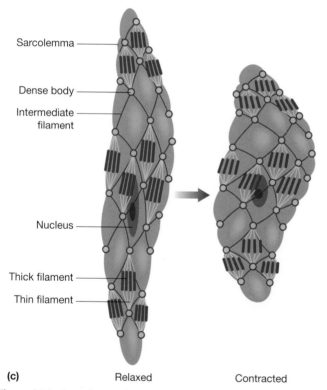

(c)   Relaxed   Contracted

Figure 36.8 Smooth muscle.

Bone has a very good blood supply (see Figure 36.11 and recall the channels within its structure), so when fracture occurs there is substantial disruption to these channels and as a result a large amount of bleeding from the fracture fragments. Because of this, immediate swelling and bruising in the area of the broken bone occurs with haematoma formation. The damaged bone tissues release cytokines which initiate the healing process. Osteoclasts remove the dead bone cells.

Within hours of the fracture, blood from the fracture fragments forms a mesh of clotted blood; this is the first link between the two fragments. The clot contains fibroblasts that begin to lay down granulation tissue between 4 and 10 days after the fracture occurs. The granulation tissue forms a 'scaffold' between the two fragments, from which the formation of a soft callus can begin.

The chemical and metabolic reactions that have produced the soft callus begin a few days after the bone is broken and the fibroblast cells present in the granulation tissue begin to form cartilage and fibrocartilage. A spongy material fills the gap between the two fracture fragments and this will remain weak to external stresses for around 6 weeks.

The soft callus provides enough stability at the fracture site for new blood vessels to begin forming and for osteoblasts at the periosteum (outer surface of bone) to begin laying down what is called 'woven bone'. This woven bone at the margins of the fracture is soft and disorganised and is the first bone contact between the two fracture fragments.

After 2–3 weeks, the soft callus is transformed completely into woven bone and the process usually continues for between 6 and 12 weeks, depending on the location and type of fracture (usually 6 weeks for the upper limb and 12 weeks for the lower limb). Hard callus formation is a complex process guided by the release of mineral compounds such as calcium and phosphate into the cartilage tissue, transforming into a bridge of hard callus over the fracture site.

When the hard callus has formed at the former fracture site, fracture union is said to have occurred and this can be seen on X-ray. Gentle weight-bearing exercise is one of the factors that encourages hard callus formation.

As normal bone healing continues, the body lays down more hard callus than is needed to unite the fracture fragments. As a result of this, the fracture site looks enlarged when viewed on X-ray. Bone remodelling may continue for several years, as a continuum of normal bone function.

As time passes, the normal shape of the bone is restored. Bone is laid down where needed by **osteoblasts** and it is removed by **osteoclasts**, depending on the stresses that are placed on the bone during everyday activities.

The loosely organised woven bone is gradually replaced by lamellar bone, which is highly organised along lines of stress and therefore as such is much stronger than woven bone. Once the fracture healing process is complete, the bone should be at least as strong as it was originally.

The Evidence Vitamin D and Calcium and Bone Health

Bentley (2013) considers vitamin D and calcium in the role of bone health. She notes that older people have less 7-dehydrocholestrol (the precursor of vitamin D) and as such, the metabolism of vitamin D and calcium becomes more complex as people age. This decline in 7-dehydrocholestrol reduces the capacity to produce vitamin D. Vitamin D deficiency adds to the demineralisation of bone and therefore osteomalacia, along with an increased risk of falls. Those adults who are over the age of 65 years and have a reduced exposure to sunlight should take vitamin D supplement (Avenell et al. 2005).

Musculoskeletal Conditions

Musculoskeletal conditions can affect muscles, joints and tendons in all parts of the body. Musculoskeletal conditions encompass over

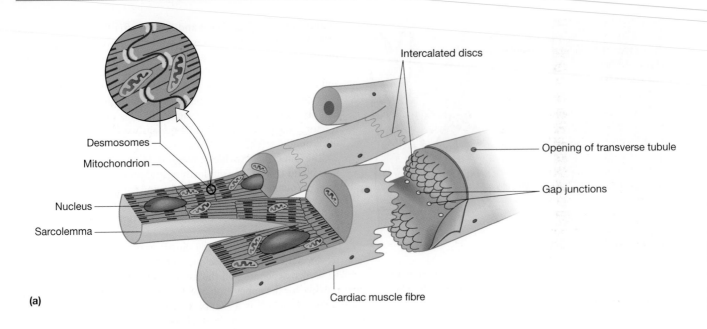

Intercalated discs

Desmosomes

Mitochondrion

Nucleus

Sarcolemma

Opening of transverse tubule

Gap junctions

Cardiac muscle fibre

(a)

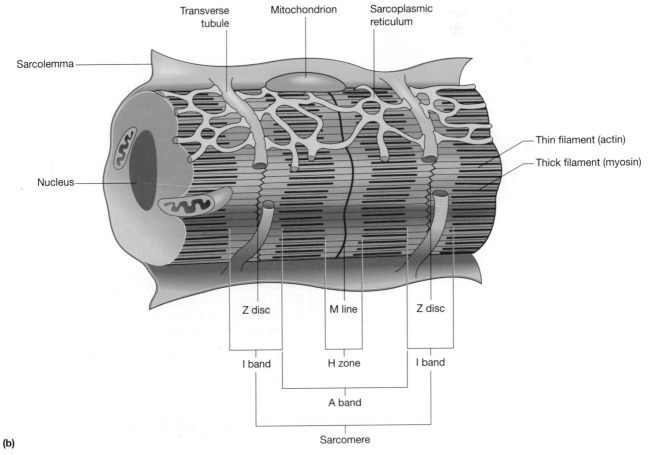

Transverse tubule

Mitochondrion

Sarcoplasmic reticulum

Sarcolemma

Nucleus

Thin filament (actin)

Thick filament (myosin)

Z disc

M line

Z disc

I band

H zone

I band

A band

Sarcomere

(b)

Figure 36.9 Cardiac muscle.

150 diseases and syndromes; these are often progressive and usually associated with pain. They can be categorised in the following ways:

- Joint diseases
- Physical disability
- Spinal disorders
- Conditions resulting from trauma.

Conditions that have the greatest impact on society include rheumatoid arthritis, osteoarthritis, osteoporosis, low back pain and limb trauma. Musculoskeletal pain is the most frequently reported complaint in health interview surveys. A number of often confusing names are given to musculoskeletal pain complaints and because of this there are several conflicting opinions and as such a lack of consensus. Musculoskeletal conditions are very common and they have important consequences for the individual and society.

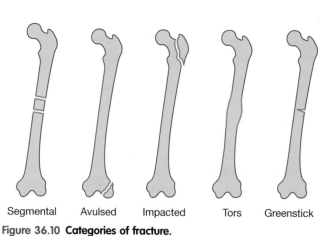

Normal Transverse Oblique Spiral Comminuted

Segmental Avulsed Impacted Tors Greenstick

Figure 36.10 Categories of fracture.

Box 36.1 Signs and Symptoms of Fracture

- Abnormal movement in a limb due to movement at the fracture site
- Crepitus or grating between the bone ends
- Deformity that can be seen or felt
- Bruising around the fracture
- Tenderness felt over the fracture site
- Pain caused by stressing the limb by bending or longitudinal compression
- Impaired or loss of function
- Swelling at the fracture site.

(*Source*: Adapted from Dandy & Edwards 2003)

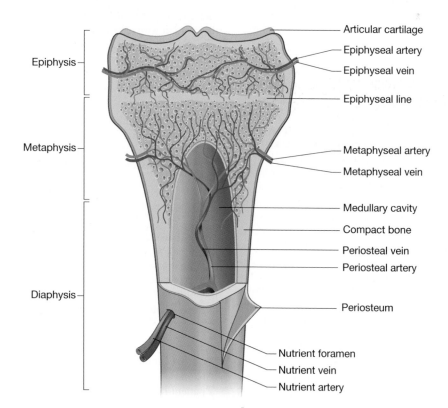

Epiphysis —
Metaphysis —
Diaphysis —

Articular cartilage
Epiphyseal artery
Epiphyseal vein
Epiphyseal line
Metaphyseal artery
Metaphyseal vein
Medullary cavity
Compact bone
Periosteal vein
Periosteal artery
Periosteum
Nutrient foramen
Nutrient vein
Nutrient artery

Figure 36.11 Blood supply of a mature long bone.

Link To/Go To

Arthritis Care exists to support people with arthritis. This is the UK's largest charity working with and for all people who have arthritis. There are a number of excellent resources available.

http://www.arthritiscare.org.uk

Nursing Fields Adult Health

Among the older population, conditions such as rheumatoid arthritis, osteoarthritis and osteoporosis often accompany a loss of independence, resulting in a need for more support in the community or admission to residential care. Total joint replacement (principally of the hip or knee) is one of the most common elective operations for older people in most European countries. There is a significant mortality associated with hip fracture.

Typically, around 50% of the population report musculoskeletal pain at one or more sites for at least 1 week in the last month. Back pain is the most common site of regional pain in younger and middle-aged adults, and knee pain in older people. The prevalence of physical disability is higher in women than men and this rises with age (Office for National Statistics, ONS 2013).

In individuals of working age, back pain and generalised widespread pain are a common cause of sick-leave and long-term work disability and, as such, have substantial economical consequences for society.

Jot This Down

How do you think the administration of medicines to control pain and inflammation can also help the person carry out their activities of living in a more effective way, promoting independence?

Musculoskeletal conditions are the most commonly reported type of work-related illness. In 2009/2010 an estimated 572 000 people in Great Britain who worked in the last year suffered from a musculoskeletal disorder caused or made worse by their current or past work. This equates to 1900 per 100 000 people (1.9%) who worked in the last 12 months in Great Britain. Of these, an estimated 248 000 suffered from a disorder mainly affecting their back, 230 000 from a disorder mainly affecting their upper limbs or neck, and 94 000 from a disorder mainly affecting their lower limbs (Health and Safety Executive, HSE 2012).

In 2009/2010, 9.2 million days were lost associated with musculoskeletal conditions: 3.6 million were related to upper limb disorders; 2.3 million to lower limb disorders and 3.3 million to disorders of the back. This amounted to, on average, 16.3 days lost per case (HSE 2012).

In the UK, hip replacements have been performed since the 1960s. Knee and ankle replacements have been performed since the 1970s. Since then, implants and techniques have developed exponentially.

In England and Wales, approximately 160 000 total hip and knee replacement procedures are carried out annually. The practice is growing rapidly. Hip and knee replacements are undertaken in around 400 hospitals; one-third of these hospitals are managed by the independent sector and the remaining two-thirds are NHS hospitals (National Joint Registry, NJR 2013).

Primary Care

Around 15–20% of consultations in the primary care setting are for musculoskeletal conditions. A large number of people with a musculoskeletal condition are referred to health professionals such as physiotherapists, occupational therapists or chiropractors; referral is also made to medical specialists such as consultant nurses, clinical nurse specialists, rheumatologists, orthopaedic surgeons or rehabilitation specialists.

Assessing the Musculoskeletal System

Assessment is the first stage of the nursing process and the nurse must be able to undertake a holistic assessment of the person's needs in a competent and confident manner. Judge (2007) notes that nursing staff need knowledge and assessment skills in order to care for patients with musculoskeletal conditions effectively and make appropriate referrals to other members of the healthcare team, as needed.

Obtaining a history from the person and undertaking an examination are central to making an accurate diagnosis and providing the person with care that is individual in meeting their needs. The nurse (with practice) will be required to inspect and palpate joints, assess a range of motion and assess muscle strength.

Arthritis Research UK (2011) suggests that there are five significant questions that need answering:

1. Does the problem arise from the joint, tendon or muscle?
2. Is the condition acute or chronic?
3. Is the condition inflammatory or non-inflammatory?
4. What is the pattern of affected areas/joints?
5. What is the impact of the condition on the patient's life?

Link To/Go To

Arthritis Research: This site helps people with arthritis to remain active. The organisation funds high quality research and provides education for healthcare professionals and information to people with arthritis and their carers.

http://www.arthritisresearchuk.org

Patient history

Chapter 6 discusses in detail patient history-taking. When taking a patient history from a person with a musculoskeletal condition, the following should also be considered:

- Patient's description of the problem
- Current health history
- Family health history
- Surgery/treatments
- Degree of impact on the ability to perform the activities of living
- Diet
- Exercise
- Weight gain/loss
- Work (occupation)
- Sporting activities
- Medications.

If the person is experiencing pain, the nurse should assess the intensity of the pain using a numerical scale (i.e. visual analogue scale). Ask about the quality of pain – is it aching, stiff, sharp or dull. Determine when the pain started (the onset, the date it started), when the pain occurs (timing). Are there any aggravating factors that are associated with the pain experience? Establish if the person has any associated symptoms. If there is joint pain, is this bilateral or unilateral? Determine if bone pain is throbbing, non-localised or aching. With complaints of muscle pain, ask the person if there is any stiffness, cramping, aching, muscle spasm or decreased flexibility.

Physical examination

When assessing gait and posture:

- Note joint and muscle symmetry
- Note extremity length and any muscle deformity
- Observe body alignment
- Is there any use of assistive devices?
- Note type of shoes being worn.

Range of movement is assessed from a passive and active perspective. A goniometer can be used to make an objective assessment of degree of movement (angles).

Joint assessment involves inspection and palpation:

Inspection:

- Size
- Contour
- Skin colour, swelling, deformities.

Palpation:

- Skin temperature
- Muscle
- Bony articulations
- Tenderness, pain, crepitations.

Muscle strength can be assessed (graded) using a six-point scale (Table 36.4).

Carrying out a competent and confident assessment of the musculoskeletal system takes much practice. The nurse should be deemed competent prior to undertaking assessment. Documentation of findings should be undertaken as soon as the assessment has been completed and should comply with local policy and procedure.

Arthritis

There are many different forms of arthritis:

- Osteoarthritis
- Rheumatoid arthritis
- Gout

Table 36.4 Grading of muscle strength. (Medical Research Council, MRC 1981)

SCORE	DESCRIPTION
0/5	Person is unable to create any visible or noticeable contraction in a specific muscle. Occurs when a muscle is paralysed, e.g. after a stroke, spinal injury. Pain can also prevent a muscle from contracting.
1/5	Occurs when muscle contraction is noted but no movement occurs. The muscle is not strong enough to lift the particular body part against gravity or move it when in a gravity-reduced position.
2/5	This muscle-strength grade is given when muscles can contract but cannot move the body part fully against gravity. When gravity is reduced or eliminated during a change in body position, the muscle is able to move the body part through its full range of motion.
3/5	This grade means that the person is able to fully contract the muscle and move the body part through its full range of motion against the force of gravity. But when resistance is applied, the muscle is unable to maintain the contraction.
4/5	Signifies that the muscle yields to maximum resistance. The muscle is able to contract and provide some resistance, but when pressure is applied to the body part, the muscle is unable to maintain the contraction.
5/5	Indicates the muscle is functioning normally and is able to maintain its position even when maximum resistance is applied.

It should not be assumed that arthritis only affects older people; arthritis can affect people of all ages.

Osteoarthritis

Osteoarthritis (OA) is associated with a clinical syndrome of joint pain that is associated with degrees of functional limitation and a reduced quality of life. OA is the most common form of arthritis and is one of the leading causes of pain and disability globally. Any of the synovial joints can develop osteoarthritis; however the most commonly affected joints are knees, hips and small hand joints (National Collaborating Centre for Chronic Conditions, NCCCC 2008).

 Link To/Go To

National Osteoporosis Society: The only UK-wide charity dedicated to improving the diagnosis, prevention and treatment of osteoporosis and fragility fractures. There are research sections on the site as well as a section for healthcare professionals.

http://www.nos.org.uk

Pathophysiology

The causes of OA are unknown – it is an idiopathic condition. The pathophysiology of OA is complex (Swift 2012a) as it involves a mixture of mechanical, cellular and biochemical processes. The interaction of these processes results in changes in the composition and mechanical properties of the articular cartilage. Cartilage is composed of water, collagen and proteoglycans (proteins).

OA is considered as a non-inflammatory disorder of the joints. Cartilage normally undergoes a remodelling process; joint movement or use stimulates this. When OA occurs, this process is changed by a combination of mechanical, cellular and biochemical processes, resulting in abnormal repair of cartilage and an increase in cartilage degradation (Hinton *et al.* 2002).

The consequences associated with deterioration and changes to the articular cartilage result in formation of new bone (osteophytes) at the surfaces of the joints (these are known as spurs). The weight-bearing joints, which include the spine, hip, knee and ankle, are the joints that are commonly affected. Other joints are affected and these are the small bone joints of the hands and the feet. During the early stages, the cartilage is frequently thicker than normal, but as the condition progresses to OA the joint surface becomes thinner and the cartilage softens; this causes disruption in the integrity of the surface and clefts begin to develop. The outcome of this is the formation of ulcers extending deep into the bones, leading to increased degenerative changes and an abnormal repair response. Repair of the cartilage does occur but the subsequent repair is substandard and as such is unable to tolerate mechanical stress. Cartilage is metabolically active and, as stress on the joints continues, the cartilage becomes hypocellular (lacking the chondrocytes to help rebuild and maintain integrity) (Figure 36.12).

The prevalence rises with age. Approximately 6% of adults aged 30 have frequent knee pain and radiographic evidence of osteoarthritis (OA). Symptomatic knee OA affects 12% of people over the age of 65 (Peach *et al.* 2005).

OA has a number of risk factors (there are only a few of these that are modifiable). Risk factors can be found in Box 36.2.

Signs and symptoms

Structural changes may occur with no associated symptoms.

Symptoms Pain is the main symptom of osteoarthritis, associated with functional impairment and disability. Usually the pain associated with osteoarthritis develops slowly. With mild to moderate osteoarthritis, the pain typically worsens with use of the joint and improves with rest.

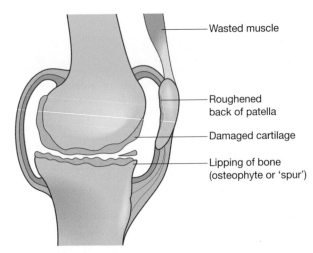

Figure 36.12 Osteoarthritis.

- Wasted muscle
- Roughened back of patella
- Damaged cartilage
- Lipping of bone (osteophyte or 'spur')

Pain in the joint is made worse by exercise and alleviated when resting. When there is advanced disease, rest and night pain may occur. If there is knee pain due to OA, this is often bilateral and is experienced in and around the knee. Hip pain due to OA is felt in the groin and anterior or lateral thigh. Hip OA pain can also be referred to the knee and, in men, to the testicle on the side that is affected.

Joint stiffness can occur in the morning or after a period of rest. There will be a reduction in function and participation in activities is restricted (NICE 2005).

Signs The person is likely to experience a reduced range of joint movement. When moving, pain in the joint or at extremes of the joint can be felt. The joints can become oedematous and there may be synovitis (the joint often feels warm and there may be an effusion and evidence of synovial thickening).

Tenderness surrounding the joint (periarticular tenderness) may be present; on palpation, there may be crepitus.

As a result of osteophyte formation, bony swelling can occur. This may be present in the fingers, occurring as swelling at the distal interphalangeal joints (called Heberden's nodes); when swelling at the proximal interphalangeal joints occurs this is known as Bouchard's nodes.

Joint instability is possible where joints can be easily displaced or dislocated leading to injury. Muscle weakness/wasting around the affected joint may be seen.

Investigations and diagnosis

There is no single test that can provide a definitive diagnosis of osteoarthritis. A medical history and physical examination will be required; diagnosis is usually based on clinical examination (NICE 2005). NICE (2005) suggests the following investigations be carried out to help make a diagnosis:

- Clinical examination
- Plain X-rays: advanced disease OA can be seen on plain X-rays. Cartilage will not show up on X-ray images; however the loss of cartilage is shown by a narrowing of the space between the bones in the joint. An X-ray can reveal bone spurs around a joint
- MRI scan can be of value to help differentiate other causes of joint pain
- Blood tests are often normal in OA. A baseline full blood count, creatinine and liver function tests should be carried out before

starting a patient on non-steroidal anti-inflammatory drugs (NSAIDs)
- Body weight and body mass index should be recorded
- Joint aspiration may be considered if the person has swollen joints. This may be done to rule out other causes, such as septic arthritis and gout.

The initial diagnostic goal is to differentiate osteoarthritis from other arthritides (other types of arthritis) such as rheumatoid arthritis. Differential diagnosis can include:

- Knee OA bursitis, referred pain from the hip or spine
- Hip OA bursitis, referred pain from the knee or spine
- OA of any joint, pseudogout, septic arthritis; viral arthritis; rheumatoid arthritis, gout, connective tissue disease.

Nursing care and management

Care provided must reflect the individual needs of the person and should be carried out after a detailed holistic health assessment has been undertaken and an individual treatment package formulated. NICE (2008) provides details about management strategies.

OA can have a significant impact on a person's ability to function, their quality of life, their ability to pursue an occupation, their mood, relationships and leisure activities. The nurse must determine how OA impacts on the individual's ability to carry out the activities of living. OA is a condition that causes pain; it is a progressive joint disorder causing stiffness, fatigue, depression and anxiety (Swift 2012b). Many people with the condition may experience difficulty with sleeping and carrying out their everyday activities, quality of life may deteriorate, the person may lose their job and they may become socially isolated.

Pharmacological interventions As pain can be responsible for the debilitating impact OA may have on a person (and their family), this should be managed using a number of techniques. Chapter 23 discusses the management of pain in detail. Pain assessment should be undertaken and the nurse should assess any self-help strategies the person is using and current drugs being used, including their doses, frequency, route of administration, timing and any possible side-effects.

Paracetamol, NSAIDs and opioids may be used (Swift 2012b) to help control the pain the person is experiencing.

Medicines Management

When taken at doses of less than 4000 mg per day, paracetamol is a relatively safe drug; however, according to Rahme et al. (2002), it may cause gastric irritation if it is taken in high doses over a long period.

The risk of adverse events related to the use of NSAIDs decreases significantly when topical gels are used as opposed to oral preparations. Topical NSAIDs according to Zhang et al. (2010) are being suggested as first-line treatment for managing osteoarthritic pain.

Opioids can be very effective in the management of pain. However, they can cause side-effects, such as nausea, vomiting, dizziness and constipation, which affect a number of people who use these drugs. A review by Turk and Cohen (2010) considered the use of extended release opioids in OA and determined that they may help to improve sleep.

Cyclooxygenase 2 (COX-2) inhibitors can be used if paracetamol and/or topical NSAIDs are not providing sufficient pain relief.

They should be co-prescribed with a proton pump inhibitor (to prevent gastric irritation). They can be prescribed in addition to paracetamol. The lowest effective dose for the shortest period of time should be prescribed. In the older person, risks and benefits should be considered: if the patient is already taking low-dose aspirin, then other analgesics should be considered prior to adding an NSAID/COX-2 inhibitor.

Exercise NICE (2008) suggests that exercise should be a core treatment for those with OA, regardless of the person's age, comorbidity, pain severity or disability. Exercise should include local muscle strengthening along with general aerobic fitness.

Maintaining fitness can help to improve endurance and suppleness, which can help to build confidence, enhance independence and improve quality of life. Pisters et al. (2010) advocate exercise, as this can help to relieve pain; fitness also has a positive influence on postoperative recovery for those people who have had joint replacements.

The nurse as a member of the multidisciplinary team working with physiotherapists can give advice about exercise. The key aim is to encourage the person to keep fit and active. Improvements in physical function and pain can lead to improvements in depression (Lim et al. 2005).

Interventions to help weight loss Turley et al. (2006) and NICE (2005, 2008) point out that obesity is a significant risk factor in OA. Weight loss advice should be offered if the person is overweight/obese. This will help to reduce the load on their joints and to improve pain. Weight reduction is one of three core interventions in NICE (2008) guidance on OA, along with information and the promotion of exercise.

Other non-pharmacological treatments Thermotherapy (locally applied heat and cold treatment) can be used as an adjunct to core treatment. The nurse must ensure that no harm from the application of heat or cold comes to the person.

Occupational therapists or disability equipment assessment centres can offer advice to people whose OA affects their activities of daily living. They may require assistive devices such as walking sticks and tap turners. A stick held in the hand of the unaffected side may reduce the load through the affected joint and help with pain relief. This can also improve function.

Jot This Down

If the occupational therapist has assessed the needs of the person and has provided assistive devices, what can you do to ensure that these are included in the person's care plan, so that they can be used appropriately?

Supports and braces can be used as an adjunct to core treatment if there is biomechanical joint pain. People with lower limb OA can be fitted for shock-absorbing shoes or insoles. Transcutaneous electrical nerve stimulation (TENS) may be used as an adjunct to core treatment for pain relief.

Surgical intervention Replacement of the hip or knee joint can be an effective management strategy. Joint surgery should be considered for those people with joint symptoms such as pain, stiffness and reduction in function if these have a negative impact on their quality of life or if they have not responded to non-surgical treatment.

Surgery can be helpful in terms of pain reduction and restoration of function, however improvement is not guaranteed. The majority of people benefit from it but around a quarter report ongoing moderate to severe pain 5–8 years after surgery, with approximately one-fifth of people saying they have not recovered sufficient function post-surgery (Jones *et al.* 2000).

Health promotion and discharge

Health promotion and prevention of OA centre on weight control, increasing physical activity and avoiding injury. It is essential to learn as much about OA as possible. The use of expert patient programmes should be considered in improving education about OA. These programmes teach people about osteoarthritis, its treatments, exercise and relaxation, patient and healthcare provider communication and ways of solving problems. People who understand more about their condition and those who participate in expert patient programmes are more likely to have positive outcomes.

What the Experts Say

Due to my age but mostly due to my arthritis, I found I was not going out much and in fact I think I was getting depressed and a little angry with the state I found myself in. I worked until the age of 55 as a physiotherapist.

My practice nurse told me about the Expert Patients Programme. This is a self-management programme for people like me who are living with a chronic condition. The aim of the programme is to support people by helping to increase confidence, improve quality of life and help manage the condition more effectively. There was a programme for people like me with arthritis.

The practice nurse said most people with a long-term condition understand the condition better than they do, as many patients become experts as they learn to cope and live with their chronic conditions. I became an expert patient and as part of a group and as an individual I can help to offer support to people with a chronic condition, and more than that, I can take the lead in managing my own condition. This has led to an improvement in my health and quality of life – I get out more, I am much happier now. Now I feel confident and in control of my life (as I was before the arthritis). I work in true partnership with the healthcare workers in managing my condition and we share responsibility for treatment. I am in a much better position now than I was before. I have my life back. I am more realistic about how my arthritis affects me and now I have hope.

(Joan, a 68-year-old woman diagnosed with arthritis 8 years ago)

Staying active and engaging in regular physical activity is a key aspect in self-care and wellness. Strengthening exercises can help to keep or increase muscle strength. Aerobic conditioning exercises improve cardiovascular fitness, help with weight control and improve overall function. Range-of-motion exercises can help reduce stiffness and maintain or increase joint movement and flexibility.

There is no specific diet that will necessarily make OA better. Eating a well-balanced diet and controlling weight can help by minimising stress on the weight-bearing joints, for example the knees and the joints of the feet.

Gout

Martinon and Glimcher (2006) suggest that gout is one of the most painful acute conditions that human beings can experience. Gout is a metabolic disease due to deposition of monosodium urate monohydrate crystals within joints causing acute inflammation and eventual tissue damage.

There are four types of gout:

- Asymptomatic
- Hyperuricaemia
- Acute gout
- Intercritical gout and chronic tophaceous gout.

The condition is classified into primary or secondary gout, depending on the cause of hyperuricaemia. Primary gout predominantly occurs in men aged 30–60 years presenting with acute attacks. Secondary gout is often due to chronic diuretic therapy. It occurs in older people, both men and women, and can be associated with osteoarthritis.

Pathophysiology

Usually, a balance exists between the production and excretion of uric acid (uric acid is the breakdown product of purine metabolism). Uric acid levels in the blood are normally maintained between 3.4 and 7.0 mg/dL in men and 2.4 and 6.0 mg/dL in women. When levels rise above 7.0 mg/dL monosodium urate crystals can form. How the crystals of monosodium urate are formed and deposited in joints is not fully understood.

The monosodium urate crystals can form in the synovial fluid or in the synovial membrane, cartilage or other joint connective tissues. It is also possible for the crystals to form in the heart and kidneys. These crystals stimulate the inflammatory system and neutrophils respond by ingesting the crystals. As a result of neutrophil activity (the release of their phagolysosomes), tissue damage can occur, continuing the inflammatory process.

Gout affects the upper and lower limbs with acute attacks. Less often it presents with painful, tophaceous deposits (with or without discharge) in Heberden's and Bouchard's nodes.

The majority of people with hyperuricaemia never develop gout, and gouty patients may not have hyperuricaemia at presentation. Patients can over-excrete uric acid, secrete normal amounts of uric acid or under-excrete. Most cases of primary gout are due to under-secretion of uric acid (Zhang *et al.* 2006). Less than 10% are as a result of over-production (Smelser 2007).

The incidence of gout is 11.9–18.0 cases per 10 000 patient-years, with a prevalence of 1.4% (years 1990–1999). In men, the prevalence increases with age and is approximately 7% over the age of 65 (Mikuls *et al.* 2005). Chen and Schumacher (2008) report that Asian populations and people of the Pacific Islands have a much higher prevalence and the disease is more severe. The male to female ratio is 9:1; the incidence increases in women after the menopause (Chen & Schumacher 2008).

Risk factors The following have been identified as risk factors by Zhang *et al.* (2006) and Mikuls *et al.* (2005):

- Male sex
- Eating meat
- Eating seafood
- Drinking alcohol
- Use of diuretics
- Obesity
- Hypertension

- Coronary heart disease
- Diabetes mellitus
- Chronic renal failure
- Chemotherapeutic drugs
- Trauma (may influence which joint is affected).

Signs and symptoms

There is synovitis (inflammation of the lining of the joints) and swelling and extreme tenderness with overlying erythema. The person may not be able to move the joint; there may be pyrexia and tachycardia.

Uncharacteristic attacks can occur with tenosynovitis (inflammation of the sheath surround the tendon), bursitis (inflammation of the synovial fluid), cellulitis (infection of the deepest layers of the skin and underlying tissue) or mild discomfort without swelling lasting a day or two.

Chronic tophaceous gout is a condition where large crystal deposits produce irregular firm nodules occurring mainly around extensor surfaces of the fingers, hands, forearms, elbows, Achilles tendons and ear. Usually, tophi are asymmetrical with a chalky appearance beneath the skin. Damage is most often found in the first metatarsophalangeal joints, mid-foot, small finger joint and wrist, with restricted movement, crepitus and deformity.

Investigations and diagnosis

A full physical examination and a patient history are required in order to ensure that an evidence-based approach to investigation is used. A clinical diagnosis can be made with reasonable accuracy for typical presentations such as inflammation of the first metatarsophalangeal joint with hyperuricaemia; however this is not definitive unless the presence of uric acid crystals can be demonstrated. Demonstration of monosodium urate (MSU) crystals in synovial fluid or tophi will confirm the diagnosis of gout.

It must be remembered that gout may present atypically. All samples of synovial fluid aspirated from joints should be analysed for the presence of MSU crystals.

The use of serum uric acid as a diagnostic test is limited, even though a raised serum uric acid level is a key risk factor for gout, as this can be normal during the acute phase of gout, while people with hyperuricaemia may never develop an attack.

Renal uric acid secretion (as detected by a 24-hour urine sample) can be helpful in diagnosis. Such patients are likely to be over-excreters of uric acid.

Radiographs may be useful in chronic gout. The first lesions usually occur in and around the first metatarsophalangeal joint. CT scanning may be helpful in less accessible areas. In early gout or during an acute attack radiography is less helpful.

Nursing care and management

The nurse's key aim (objective) in an acute attack is to relieve pain and inflammation as quickly as possible. Referral to a specialist nurse or doctor may be required.

Schlesinger and Schumacher (2002) suggest that an ice pack may help with the relief of pain and the promotion of comfort. Elevation of the limb may help to ease pain and the nurse should ensure that the limb is protected from any potential trauma.

There is a range of pharmacological therapeutic options available and these will include the administration of NSAIDs. Commencing NSAIDs within 24 hours can produce rapid relief. Consider giving the patient a stock to keep at home. Diclofenac, naproxen and indometacin are generally preferred. The dose should be tailored to meet the needs of the patient and consideration should be given to the person's age, comorbidity and interactions with other drugs. Colchicine works by reducing the number of white blood cells that travel into the inflamed areas, helping to break the cycle of inflammation (reducing swelling and pain). Colchicine is particularly appropriate when NSAIDs are poorly tolerated in patients who have heart failure and in those who are on anticoagulants (Ahern et al. 1987).

Medicines Management

Corticosteroids can be given orally, intramuscularly, intravenously or intra-articularly. They are useful where NSAIDs or colchicine are contraindicated (British Society for Rheumatology, BSR 2007). Intra-articular administration of long-acting steroids is safe and effective (Zhang et al. 2006).

Compound analgesics (a combination of two different drugs in one tablet – usually paracetamol, aspirin, codeine and dihydrochloride) may also be considered.

Colchicine and/or NSAIDs are recommended as the first-line option for acute gout (Zhang et al. 2006). Lifestyle changes should be discussed with the patient and include issues such as weight loss, exercise, diet, alcohol consumption and fluid intake.

Health promotion

The nurse should identify things that cause the person to have gout symptoms. Eliminating these triggers may reduce the chances of having gout again. Gout can be prevented from reoccurring by making changes to the diet and taking medicines if needed.

The patient should be advised to reduce the amount of foods that contain purine. Some foods are very high in purines and may increase the amount of uric acid in the blood. These include:

- Liver and kidneys
- Oily fish, such as mackerel, sardines and anchovies
- Shellfish, including mussels, crab and shrimp
- Some vegetables, such as asparagus, cauliflower, lentils, mushrooms and spinach
- Oats and oatmeal.

Eating a well-balanced diet will help to manage symptoms.

If the person drinks alcohol, they should aim to drink less and should consider cutting out beer, stout, port and fortified wines as these can have the greatest effect on causing gout symptoms. Drinking enough water every day will help to dilute blood and urine and, in so doing, lower the uric acid levels in the body. Encourage the person to drink about 2–4 L of fluid each day, with at least half being water.

As well as making changes to the diet and reducing the amount of alcohol consumed, the person may need to take medicines to prevent gout. The nurse should explain how the medications work, i.e. helping to control the levels of uric acid in the blood with the aim of preventing the person getting gout again or, if the person does get gout again, it should be for a shorter period of time and be less severe. Some medications will need to be taken daily, for example, allopurinol (or the alternative, febuxostat). These medicines prevent gout by stopping the formation of uric acid. When they are first taken, allopurinol and febuxostat may cause more symptoms of gout. NSAIDs, colchicine or steroid tablets may be prescribed along with allopurinol or febuxostat for up to 3 months.

Red Flag

In gout, the nurse must ensure the patient drinks enough fluids when taking their medicines.

Fractured Neck of Femur

The aim of fracture treatment is to achieve a solid bony union without deformity. The intention is the restoration of function so that the person can return to their previous levels of activity (McRae & Esser 2008).

It has been estimated that hip fracture in the UK (annually) costs approximately £1.4 billion. This figure can be doubled when the social care costs of hip fracture and related dependency are taken into account (British Orthopaedic Association, BOA 2010). Hip fracture is a major public health issue and is associated with an ageing population. There is an increased risk in the older population because of osteoporosis, osteomalacia and falls. There are about 70 000–75 000 hip fractures each year. Approximately10% of people with a femoral fracture will die within 1 month and about one-third within 12 months. Most of these deaths are due to related conditions and not to the fracture itself; this reflects the high prevalence of comorbidity (NICE 2011a). With an average age of over 75 years and a one in ten chance of dying within 1 month, those people with a fractured neck of femur represent some of the frailest patients the nurse may care for.

A fractured neck of femur (hip fracture) is a crack or break at the top of the femur close to the hip joint, where the leg meets the pelvis. Fractures are either intracapsular or extracapsular (Figure 36.13). Hip fractures are more common in older women and are often sustained as a result of a fall. Surgical intervention is usually needed to help mend the fracture. There are several types of operative procedures that can be used and the procedure of choice depends on where the fracture is and whether the bones have moved out of their normal position. If surgical intervention is inappropriate (e.g. if the fracture has seriously affected the person's health), further options other than surgery may be made available, for example a palliative care approach. Hughes (2012) describes how nurses can assess and manage different types of pain in older people receiving palliative care.

Jot This Down

What is the usual treatment for all types of hip fracture?

Surgical intervention is usually carried out on the day of admission or as soon as possible thereafter. Table 36.5 describes the various types of surgical procedures and Figure 36.14 shows the various devices that may be used.

The administration of analgesia is a key element in fracture care. The British Orthopaedic Association (BOA 2007) notes that good pain control, in the early stages of care, will enhance and promote comfort as well as confidence. When pain is poorly-controlled,

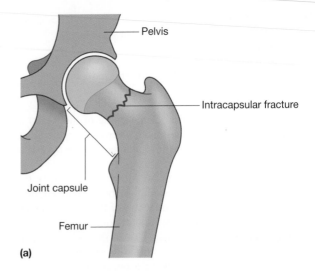

(a)

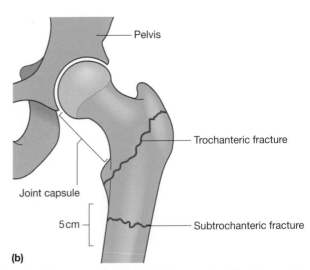

(b)

Figure 36.13 Types of fracture: (a) intracapsular; (b) extracapsular.

Walker (2013) points out that there can be a delay in mobility. Complications associated with fractures are outlined in Table 36.6.

Red Flag Acute Compartment Syndrome

This is caused by increased pressure within a closed anatomical space that compromises the circulation and function of the tissues within that space. This may result in temporary or permanent damage to muscles and nerves.

When there is increasing duration and magnitude of interstitial pressure, increasing impairment of muscle and nerve function and necrosis of soft tissues occur. Initially, venous compromise can progress to reduced capillary flow; this leads to ischaemia and can further increase the interstitial pressure, leading to a vicious cycle of increasing pressures. Arterial blood inflow is reduced when the pressure exceeds systolic blood pressure.

(Continued)

Table 36.5 Types of surgical procedure. (*Source:* Adapted from NICE 2011a)

SURGICAL TERM	DESCRIPTION	TYPE OF FRACTURE
Surgery required to replace part or all of the damaged joint		
Hemiarthroplasty	The broken part of the hip joint is replaced (half hip replacement). The femoral head at the top of the femur is removed and replaced with a metal one	The majority of displaced intracapsular fractures
Total hip replacement	Both parts of the hip joint (the femoral head at the top of the femur and the acetabulum in the pelvis) are replaced with artificial parts	Displaced intracapsular fracture. It is suitable for patients who were very fit and active before the fracture and who are well enough to have the operation
Surgery to re-position the broken bone and hold it in position as healing takes place (fixation)		
Sliding hip screw	This implant is a special screw that is mounted on a plate. It holds the broken part of the femur in place while it is healing	Most trochanteric fractures
Intramedullary nail	A device used to align and stabilise the fracture while it is healing. It is inserted into the middle of the femur for support	Subtrochanteric fractures and certain trochanteric fractures
Screws	A group of 2–4 screws used to hold the broken bone in the correct position	Undisplaced intracapsular fractures only

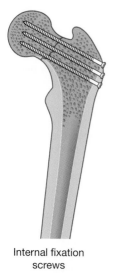

Internal fixation screws

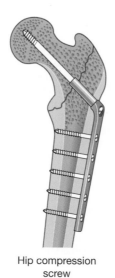

Hip compression screw

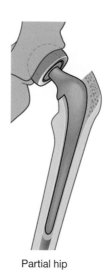

Partial hip replacement

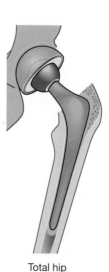

Total hip replacement

Figure 36.14 Types of fixation and implantation for hip fracture.

Table 36.6 Some complications associated with fractures. (*Source:* Adapted from Whitening 2008)

INTERMEDIATE	EARLY	LATE
Immobility	Immobility	Immobility
Damage to soft tissue	Infection	Mal-union of fracture
Nerve injury	Neurovascular complications	Delayed union of fracture
Haemorrhage	Fat and pulmonary embolism	Non-union of fracture
	Deep vein thrombosis (DVT)	Osteoarthritis
	Compartment syndrome (bleeding or swelling within an enclosed bundle of muscles)	Avascular necrosis (death of bone tissue due to a lack of blood supply)
	Pressure ulcers	
	Chest infection	

There are several causes, including:

- Fractures, especially those of the forearm and lower leg that have been internally fixed or infected
- Crush injury
- Burns
- Infection
- Prolonged limb compression, for example immobilisation in a tight plaster cast.

Presentation

Acute compartment syndromes usually present within 48 hours of injury. The nurse must be alert to the possibility of compartment syndrome, particularly in an unconscious patient following major trauma. Clinical features include:

- Increasing pain despite immobilisation of the fracture
- Sensory deficit in the distribution of nerves passing through the compartment
- Muscle tenderness and swelling
- Excessive pain on passive movement, increasing pain despite immobilisation
- Peripheral pulses may still be present.

Later features are of tissue ischaemia with pallor, pulselessness, paralysis, coolness and loss of capillary return.

Diagnosis and investigations

- Diagnosis is essentially clinical with recognition of patients at risk and recognition of early signs
- MRI scans help make the diagnosis of compartment syndrome in clinically ambiguous cases.

Management

The mainstay of treatment is prompt diagnosis and early surgery. People with a swollen limb and no clear underlying cause should be considered for urgent orthopaedic opinion.

- Urgent decompression is required to prevent severe ischaemia. Early orthopaedic referral and continuous compartment pressure monitoring are required
- All potentially constricting dressings, casts and splints must be removed. Splitting a plaster is not sufficient. The compartment pressure should be measured
- Open fasciotomy (a surgical procedure that cuts away the fascia to relieve tension or pressure) may be needed:
  ◦ The skin and deep fascia must be divided along the whole length of the compartment
  ◦ After fasciotomy, the wound should be left open. Healing may be encouraged by suturing, skin grafting or the wound left to heal by itself
- Debridement may be indicated for any muscle necrosis.

NICE (2011a) has stipulated that good postoperative care planning includes the early identification of individual goals for multidisciplinary rehabilitation to recover mobility and independence and long-term well-being. The role of multidisciplinary teams in assessing a patient and developing a care plan is vital and the provision of early multidisciplinary rehabilitation is a key standard set out by the British Orthopaedic Association (BOA 2007).

The Evidence Multidisciplinary Rehabilitation

Mobilisation strategies

- Offer a physiotherapy assessment and, unless medically or surgically contraindicated, mobilisation on the day after surgery
- Offer mobilisation at least once a day and ensure regular physiotherapy review.

Early supported discharge

- Consider early supported discharge as part of the Hip Fracture Programme, provided the multidisciplinary team remains involved and the patient:
  - Is medically stable
  - Has the mental ability to participate
  - Is able to transfer and mobilise short distances
  - Has not yet achieved their full rehabilitation potential.

Intermediate care

- Only consider intermediate care (continued rehabilitation in a community hospital or residential care unit) if all the following criteria are met:
  - Intermediate care is included in the Hip Fracture Programme
  - The Hip Fracture Programme team retains the clinical lead, including patient selection, agreement of length of stay and ongoing objectives for intermediate care
  - The Hip Fracture Programme team retains the managerial lead, ensuring that intermediate care is not resourced as a substitute for an effective acute hospital programme.

Patients admitted from care or nursing homes

- Patients admitted from care or nursing homes should not be excluded from a rehabilitation programme in the community or hospital, or as part of an early supported discharge programme.

(NICE 2011a)

Red Flag Fat Embolism

Fat embolism is a common occurrence for patients following trauma or surgery to the lower limbs. Fat from the bone marrow is able to escape into the bloodstream and form emboli (collections of fat droplets). Many patients will not even be aware that they have fat emboli as the symptoms may be minor. In a small number of people, however, these emboli block small blood vessels in the lungs, skin or brain and this triggers a cascade of events that leads to the illness known as 'fat embolism syndrome'. The most severe problem in fat embolism syndrome is acute respiratory distress syndrome – the lungs are unable to absorb oxygen properly and patients become severely hypoxic. It is this group of patients who will be admitted to the intensive care unit.

The nurse should be aware of the following.

Fat embolism syndrome is usually evident 24–72 hours after an injury and involves the lungs, the brain and the skin.

Symptoms can include:

- An altered mental state with symptoms including irritability, agitation, headache, confusion, seizures or coma
- Lung problems, including rapid breathing, dyspnoea and a low oxygen level
- A rash on the skin (petechiae) – blockages in small blood vessels lead to small pin-point haemorrhages, often in the upper torso. These haemorrhages also occur in the eye.

The nurse should report any of the symptoms immediately.

Signs and symptoms

The classic visible signs of a fractured neck of femur include shortening and external rotation of the affected leg, associated with contraction of the femoral musculature. The affected leg may be shortened, adducted and externally rotated. The person may complain of pain that may radiate to the knee, or there may be knee pain present with no pain on movement of the hip. The person may be unable to lie on the injured side. In the older person who is confused or who has other forms of cognitive impairment such as dementia there may be no history of injury. As the leg is rotated pain may be felt.

Investigations and diagnosis

X-rays, for example anteroposterior (AP) pelvic and lateral hip X-rays, are required to confirm diagnosis and type of fracture.

Magnetic resonance imaging (MRI) should be performed if a hip fracture is suspected but the AP pelvic and lateral hip X-rays are not showing a fracture. NICE (2011a) suggests that if an MRI is not available within 24 hours, or if this is contraindicated, then computed tomography (CT) should be carried out.

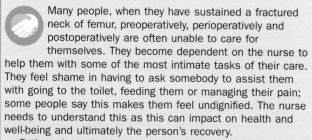

Care, Dignity and Compassion

Many people, when they have sustained a fractured neck of femur, preoperatively, perioperatively and postoperatively are often unable to care for themselves. They become dependent on the nurse to help them with some of the most intimate tasks of their care. They feel shame in having to ask somebody to assist them with going to the toilet, feeding them or managing their pain; some people say this makes them feel undignified. The nurse needs to understand this as this can impact on health and well-being and ultimately the person's recovery.

Patients have the right to be 'treated with dignity and respect in accordance with your human rights' (NHS Constitution, Department of Health 2012). Social dignity, suggests Jacobsen (2007), can be experienced through interaction and it can be lost or gained, threatened, violated or promoted. We promote dignity-of-self when we encourage self-confidence and self-respect. We convey this through interaction – the way we speak and act, letting the person know that they are of worth and that they are valued. Nurses must recognise and acknowledge the human dignity of those people we have the privilege of caring for, as well as understanding how our interactions influence their social dignity.

Throughout the person's hospital stay, the nurse should assess the person's activities of living, ensuring that needs are met and, when needed, assistance provided. Discharge planning should commence within the first 48 hours after admission (SIGN 2009).

Nursing Fields Children: Hip Fracture

In a growing child's hips and pelvis, the most common place for a fracture is the attachment point. This is the place where the muscles attach to bone. In children, the attachment point is not yet fully formed and as such it is a weak point. If a child moves the legs very suddenly and forcefully, for example during a fall or while playing sports, then the muscles that attach to the hip or pelvic bones can pull away and break the bone.

Any child can get a hip fracture, however they are rare in very young children. Hip and pelvic fractures usually happen during car or cycle accidents.

Hip fractures require surgery or a cast, sometimes both, to prevent the bones from moving and causing permanent damage. Casts alone, without surgery, are usually used only in children who are 5 years of age or younger.

Young children rarely get hip fractures as their hip bones are more flexible than the hip bones of adults and because of this they are less likely to fracture.

Preoperatively Chapter 14 discusses preoperative care. Specifically, the following based on NICE (2011a) recommendations are required prior to surgical intervention; the aim of preparing the person safely for surgery is to provide an uneventful recovery.

- Investigations include blood tests – full blood count and cross-match. Initial assessment of renal function, glucose, electrocardiograph (ECG) and chest X-ray. Depending on history and general examination, other investigations may be required
- Intravenous access and commencing intravenous infusion
- Administration of analgesia (including opiates) sufficient to allow the movements necessary for investigations and for nursing care and rehabilitation
- An early assessment is carried out of any cognitive impairment and any treatable comorbidities such as anaemia, fluid volume depletion, electrolyte imbalance, uncontrolled diabetes, uncontrolled heart failure, correctable cardiac arrhythmias or ischaemia, acute chest infection or exacerbation of chronic chest conditions.

Jot This Down

When on your next orthopaedic placement, find out what protocols exist and are being used in relation to good hip fracture care.

The nurse must ensure that the patient and the family are kept informed about what is happening during this stressful and anxiety provoking time. Nurses are ideally placed to give advice and offer information; they can offer comfort and provide explanations concerning ward routines, processes and procedures.

Nursing Fields Learning Disabilities

Good communication between healthcare professionals and patients is vital. This should be supported by evidence-based written information that has been tailored to meet the needs of the patient. Treatment and care delivery, along with the information that is given to people about it, should be culturally appropriate. This should also be accessible to those people with additional needs, for example physical, sensory or learning disabilities, and also for those who do not speak or read English.

Older people with learning disabilities may be viewed as potentially vulnerable and as such in need of safeguarding. Advocacy according to Jenkins (2012) should be part of the safeguarding process.

Surgery should be undertaken as soon as possible after the injury has occurred if the person is medically fit. Keating and Aderinto (2010) suggest that delays in surgery can cause the person distress as well as being associated with an increase in morbidity and mortality.

Postoperative care The first concern with all postoperative patients is to assess and maintain an effective airway; the use of anaesthesia has the potential to impact upon respiratory function of the older person. Chapter 14 discusses postoperative care from a general perspective. The following section of this chapter considers the specific issues associated with the care of the person who has undergone surgery related to a fractured neck of femur.

Regardless of the different types of fracture, the principles of care should remain the same (Walker 2013):

- Restore normal alignment of the bone
- Immobilise the limb so that the position is maintained until healing occurs
- Restore normal function through rehabilitation.

Postoperative care will be directed according to the type of surgery that has been performed. Depending on the nature of the facture, the nurse must act as advocate and play a key part in the multidisciplinary team approach to the care of the person with femoral fracture. O'Malley *et al.* (2011) discuss the role of the multidisciplinary team with regards to hip fracture before and after surgery.

The Evidence

The British Orthopaedic Association (BOA 2007) has produced best practice guidance for the care of people who have undergone hip fracture: *The Care of Patients with Fragility Fractures* should be considered in the light of other publications, for example the National Institute of Health and Clinical Excellence (NICE 2011a) *Hip Fracture. The Management of Hip Fracture in Adults* and The Scottish Intercollegiate Guidelines Network (SIGN 2009) *Management of Hip Fractures in Older People: A National Clinical Guideline*, as well as local policy, procedure and protocols.

Integrated care pathways (ICPs) are often used for the care of the person with a fractured neck of femur. These draw on a sound evidence base and are usually adapted to meet local needs. Tarling *et al.* (2002) suggest that the use of an ICP can enhance the overall care experience.

 Link To/Go To

The Scottish Intercollegiate Guidelines Network (SIGN) develops evidence-based clinical practice guidelines for the National Health Service (NHS) in Scotland. SIGN guidelines are derived from a systematic review of the scientific literature and are designed as a vehicle for accelerating the translation of new knowledge into action, with the aim of reducing variations in practice as well as improving patient outcomes.

http://www.sign.ac.uk

Pain relief Analgesia is an important aspect in the care and management of the person with a hip fracture. If pain is controlled in the early stages of care, this will encourage comfort and confidence; conversely, if pain is poorly controlled, then early mobilisation can be delayed and dependency can result in complications associated with prolonged bed rest.

Red Flag

 Pain is an unpleasant sensory and emotional experience associated with actual or potential skin damage or described in terms of such damage.

(International Association of the Study of Pain, IASP 2011).

The nurse must involve the wider acute pain team based in many acute care settings. It must, however, be remembered that addressing the analgesic needs of the person is the responsibility of the nurse caring for the person; the nurse must determine the presence of pain and provide analgesia (see Chapter 23).

Diagnosing pain in those people who may be cognitively impaired as a result of dementia, for example, may be difficult; therefore addressing the needs of these people requires familiarity with the person and also information from other carers (Hughes 2012).

Jot This Down

Nurses have a unique role as they can assess the pain a person is experiencing in their daily interaction with patients in a way that doctors cannot. Think about why this may be case.

In the immediate postoperative period, many people will be given opiates; these are the mainstay of treatment, given orally or intramuscularly.

Red Flag

 Intravenous opiates may be used for pain control in the older person, but they should be given only in small incremental doses due to the unpredictable response in this client group.

Regular paracetamol and other analgesia (e.g. codeine phosphate or tramadol) should be provided to all patients. The objective is to pre-empt pain control and to promote comfort when resting and during active rehabilitation. The nurse should offer analgesia in anticipation of active rehabilitation.

Wound care The most common complication of wound healing is formation of wound haematoma, with an incidence of 2–10% (BOA 2007). Some degree of bruising is to be expected for all wounds Small haematomas can be allowed to resolve spontaneously but larger collections will require surgical drainage.

Deep wound infection is defined as infection of the wound below the level of the deep fascia and invariably involves the implant (BOA 2007). Treatment usually requires surgical debridement; if an implant has been used, this may be removed. Deep wound infection that involves the implant is uncommon but devastating in its impact, with approximately half of patients dying (BOA 2007).

Superficial wound sepsis refers to infection of the wound that does not extend below the deep fascia layer. This is more common than deep sepsis and can be treated with antibiotics as well as surgical debridement if indicated. Chapter 18 discusses wound infection.

Pressure ulcer formation The nurse has the responsibility to address pressure ulcer prevention at the earliest opportunity, identifying those at risk and implementing strategies to reduce risk of pressure sore formation. The following factors contribute to pressure sore formation:

- Time spent lying on the floor at home after falling
- Delays in the accident and emergency department

- Hard surfaces on accident and emergency department trolleys
- Hard mattresses on the ward
- Poor nutrition
- Anaemia
- Delays from admission to surgery
- Prolonged surgery
- Failure to mobilise the person immediately after surgery.

Good anticipatory care has the ability to reduce the risk of pressure sore formation. Chapter 18 discusses pressure sore prevention.

Early mobilisation in the postoperative period will reduce the risk of pressure ulcer formation. A formal pressure area risk assessment is recommended for all patients, with pressure area skin inspection on admission and at least twice a day while patients are immobile. The finding of early or superficial skin damage should trigger an immediate response and the implementation of appropriate care. Risk factors such as pressure, shearing forces, friction, incontinence, pain and malnutrition should be addressed and if problems do arise, the nurse should refer the person to a tissue viability nurse.

Thromboprophylaxis The use of cyclic leg compression devices and foot pumps can help to reduce the incidence of thrombosis. Graduated stockings (compression stockings) are effective; however these are painful to put on when there is a hip fracture and also bring with them a risk of foot ulcers in those people who have fragile skin or vascular insufficiency. Chemical prophylaxis reduces the incidence of DVT and PE considerably, but this also carries the risk of introducing bleeding complications as well as increasing the rates of wound healing complications.

Link To/Go To

Venous Thromboembolism Reducing the Risk can be found at: National Institute for Health and Care Excellence (NICE 2011b)

http://guidance.nice.org.uk/CG92/NICEGuidance/doc/English

Early surgical intervention and immediate postoperative mobilisation and avoiding prolonged operations and over-transfusion will help to reduce the incidence of clinical thrombosis. The NICE guidance (2010) recommends the use of chemo- and mechanical prophylaxis. Local policy and procedure should be followed.

Jot This Down

Early mobilisation is effective in lowering the risk of clinical thrombosis. Describe the signs and symptoms of thromboembolism.

A clear, consistent protocol to prevent thromboembolism must be agreed by the nursing, surgical, medical and anaesthetic leads in the acute care setting.

Nutritional needs One of the most powerful risk factors for hip fracture is poor nutrition. Practical challenges associated with feeding pose a major threat to recovery. People with hip fracture are at risk of failing to receive the recommended daily energy, protein and other nutritional requirements. The nurse must liaise and communicate with all members of the clinical and operational services teams; nutrition is an interdisciplinary concern. The use of oral multinutrient feeds (these provide energy, protein, vitamins and minerals) can reduce the risk of death or complications (BOA 2007).

All staff caring for people who are recovering from a hip fracture should understand the importance of adequate dietary intake and ensure that specific attention is given to helping people to eat at meal times. An integral aspect of routine nursing care should include assessment of nutritional intake, using a tool such as the malnutrition universal screening tool, and where appropriate referral should be made to the dietician for specialist advice to ensure appropriate nutritional intake.

Early rehabilitation Postoperatively it is usual practice to sit the person out of bed and begin to help them stand on the day after surgery. This progress will vary significantly, depending on the individual person and the type of fracture. Those people with an extracapsular fracture tend to take longer to mobilise than those with intracapsular fractures. The care pathway can assist with early rehabilitation.

Jot This Down

Efforts to commence supervised full weight-bearing mobilisation should usually commence on the first day following surgery. Why is this important in the older person?

Weight-bearing There should be very few occasions on which weight-bearing is restricted. Most older people who sustain a hip fracture will be unable to comply with instructions on limited weight-bearing and only rarely be able to cope with the difficulties of walking 'non-weight bearing'. In practice, most people will weight-bear as pain allows and become fully weight-bearing as the fracture heals. The nurse working with the physiotherapist can help the person to weight-bear.

Hip movements Hip movements will depend on the surgical intervention. Customary practice was to restrict hip flexion after an arthroplasty in order to prevent prosthetic dislocation. This meant that the patient required a raised bed and chairs and was restricted from getting in and out of a car or bath. These measures are still used for a total hip replacement, but for a hemiarthroplasty introduced via an antero-lateral approach they should no longer be required. As surgical technique has become more refined and with a more careful repair of the hip joint capsule, the risk of dislocation is reduced, making any restrictions on hip movements unnecessary.

Discharge and community rehabilitation

Early supported discharge and community rehabilitation schemes are being implemented that will allow the more able person with a fracture to be discharged directly to their home from the orthopaedic ward. It is essential, however, that a multidisciplinary assessment of needs is undertaken with the involvement of older person consultant nurses, geriatric physicians, community nurses and community physiotherapists and occupational therapists. The multidisciplinary team will carry out a detailed assessment ensuring optimal patient selection. Such ongoing rehabilitation will allow patients to progress from using a frame to a stick, and to walking unaided if appropriate. Advice and practice about walking outside and, if appropriate, a return to driving may also be given.

Primary Care

Primary care teams are ideally placed and excel at the delivery of chronic disease management. They have much to offer concerning hip fracture, identifying the chronic underlying disease of osteoporosis. The primary care team will play an increasing role in both post-acute care and secondary prevention.

The primary care team takes over the long-term management in exactly the same way as it does for other chronic conditions, for example hypertension and heart failure. When people present with fractures, the secondary care team will manage the acute event and, if a Fracture Liaison Service is available, investigate the need for management of underlying osteoporosis. The primary care team can then undertake regular reviews to encourage adherence and persistence with therapy, referring back into secondary care if needed for advice.

(BOA 2007)

Health promotion

In early adulthood, healthy lifestyle choices can help to build a higher peak bone mass and reduce the risk of osteoporosis in later years; this may lower the risk of falls and improve overall health if adopted at any age.

The Evidence

Falls are a significant problem for older adults, and those who have sustained a fall are at risk of further falls.

This study set out to provide evidence-based guidelines of assessment and treatment to prevent falls in older people, as well as to provide researchers with tables of risk factor studies and randomised controlled trials of falls prevention.

A template for the development of practice guidelines from the Agency for Health Care Policy and Research was used. Evidence for risk factors was accepted from prospective studies with greater than 80% follow-up. Potentially modifiable risk factors were selected and a schema for evaluating the importance of each risk factor was used. Evidence for interventions was examined from randomised controlled trials and the strength of the evidence was graded. Recommendations for aspects of care where judgement was required were made by panel consensus.

The researchers developed a check list, which is provided to clinicians. They concluded that for community-dwelling older adults there is strong evidence for multifactorial specific risk assessment and targeted treatment. Balance exercises are recommended for all who have had a fall and there is evidence for a programme of home physiotherapy for females over 80 years of age, irrespective of risk factor status. For those being cared for in institutional settings, the establishment of a falls programme for safety checks, ongoing staff education and monitoring is demonstrated by research. Residents who have fallen need to be assessed for specific risk factors and clinical indicators to determine relevant management options.

(Moreland et al. 2003).

Exercise strengthens bones and improves balance. Weight-bearing exercises, for example walking, result in increased bone density. Exercise also increases overall strength, reducing the risk of falling. The nurse can suggest exercising for 30 minutes a day on most days of the week.

Drinking too much alcohol can impair balance and make the person more prone to falling. Avoiding excessive use of alcohol and not smoking preserves bone density.

The nurse can suggest an assessment of the person's home to identify any fall hazards. The following strategies may help:

- Mop up spillages straight away
- Remove clutter, trailing wires and frayed carpet
- Use non-slip mats and rugs
- Use high-wattage light bulbs in lamps and torches to help see clearly
- Organise the home so that climbing, stretching and bending are kept to a minimum and to avoid bumping into things
- Encourage the person to ask for help with things that they are unable to do safely on their own
- Avoid walking on slippery floors in socks or tights
- Do not wear loose-fitting, trailing clothes that could result in a trip
- Wear well-fitting shoes that are in good condition, supporting the ankle
- Make referral to a chiropodist about any foot problems, taking care of the feet by trimming toenails regularly
- Refer to an optician to check the eyes every other year or more often if the person has diabetes or an eye disease
- Monitor the effects of medication.

Red Flag

Be aware that the side-effects of some medicines can result in the person feeling weak and dizzy and this could increase their risk of falling.

What To Do If...

You have left Mrs Guiterrez in the bathroom as you go back to her locker to get her perfume. Upon your return you find her on the floor, conscious and in pain; you notice her left leg is externally rotated and noticeably shorter than her right leg. What do you do? How would you prevent such an incident from occurring in the future?

Caring for people with plaster casts

A cast is a rigid device applied with the intention of immobilising bones that have been injured and to encourage healing. In order to prevent the bone from moving during healing, the cast immobilises the joint above and the joint below the bone that has been fractured. A cast can also be used to apply uniform compression to soft tissue and to prevent and correct deformities. See Table 36.7 for some types of casts.

Prior to application of the cast, the fracture is first reduced manually and then the cast is applied. Casts are not used when the fracture is unstable.

Table 36.7 Some types of cast.

TYPE OF CAST	DESCRIPTION
Short arm cast	Extends from below the elbow to the palmar crease and is secured around the base of the thumb
Long arm cast	Extends from the upper level of the axillary folds to the proximal palmar creases The elbow is immobilised at a right angle
Short leg cast	Extends from below the knee to the base of the toes The foot is flexed at a right angle in a neutral position
Long leg cast	Extends from the junction of the upper and middle third of the thigh to the base of the toes The knee may be slightly flexed
Walking cast	The same as a long leg cast but reinforced for strength
Spica cast	A cast which includes the trunk of the body and one or more limbs. A hip spica includes the trunk of the body and one or both legs: one covering only one leg to the ankle or foot is a single hip spica; one covering both legs is a double hip spica. A one-and-a-half hip spica encases one leg to the ankle or foot and the other to just above the knee. The spica may extend only to the navel, allowing mobility of the spine and the possibility of walking with an aid, or may extend to the rib cage or axilla
Thumb spica	Immobilises fractures of the carpal of the navicular, thumb metacarpal and phalanges

Cast materials The cast can be made of plaster (plaster of Paris) or fibreglass and applied over a thin cushion of padding and moulded to suit the normal contour of the body. Plaster of Paris casts are made of a chalky white powder, anhydrous calcium sulphate made from gypsum. This is a cheap material that is durable. Synthetic casts can be made from fibre glass, thermoplastics or polyester–cotton weave.

Prior to any pressure being applied, the cast has to be left to dry; failure to do this can leave dents that could cause pressure ulcers. A plaster cast can take up to 48 hours to dry; a fibreglass cast, however, dries in under an hour. The type of cast applied is determined by the location of the fracture. Nursing care of the person with a cast is discussed in the 'Primary Care' box. At follow-up appointments the bone may be re-X-rayed to assess alignment and healing and perhaps the cast removed for skin assessment.

Nursing care Nursing interventions require the nurse to perform frequent neurovascular assessments. Palpate the cast for 'hot spots' that may indicate the presence of underlying infection. Report any drainage promptly.

Primary Care

- Health education for the client and family
- Do not place any objects in the cast
- If the cast is made of plaster, keep it dry
- If the cast is made of fibreglass, dry it with a blow dryer on the cool setting if it becomes wet
- Assess the injured extremity for coolness, changes in colour, increased pain, increased swelling and/or loss of sensation; report if present
- If a sling is used, it should distribute the weight of the cast evenly around the neck. Do not roll the sling as this could impair circulation to the neck
- If crutches are used, arrange for a physiotherapist to teach the correct way to walk with crutches
- Explain to the person that when the cast is removed, an oscillating cast remover is used. It has a guard on it that prevents the cast remover from penetrating past the depth of the cast; it will not cut the client. It is noisy and the person will feel vibration.

What To Do If...

A patient has had a plaster cast applied 2 hours ago. She tells you that her leg feels really hot and painful, much more painful than when the cast went on. The lady looks sweaty and says she cannot feel her toes. What do you do next?

Macpherson (2011) provides information that clarifies the legal position on driving by people who have been discharged from emergency departments or minor injury units after they have received treatment for injuries. The article discusses a literature review that had been undertaken concerning the advice given to people who have been injured and the advice they want, as well as the responsibility of nurses in providing this. The issue of driving with plaster casts is also discussed. Box 36.3 provides an overview of the guidance that can be given to drivers with injuries (including those with casts).

Conclusion

This chapter has provided you with some insight concerning musculoskeletal conditions. It has not been possible in this chapter to provide you with all of the information that you may need to care competently and confidently for people with a wide range of conditions that impact on the person's health and well-being. It has however, provided you with an overview of the anatomy and physiology of this system, along with its functions.

The nurse should aim to provide people who have musculoskeletal conditions with care that responds to their individual needs, to prevent further injury or deterioration, to reduce the risk of complications and to promote healing. The nurse working in partnership with the patient and other members of the health and social care team can minimise dependence and enhance optimal rehabilitation.

The nurse may be required to care for people with musculoskeletal conditions in a variety of settings, including primary, secondary and tertiary care, and as such, he/she will need to have some understanding of some of the common conditions that have been discussed in this chapter.

Box 36.3 Guidance for Drivers with Injuries, Including Those with Casts

Fitness to drive

- Those people who hold driving licences are accountable for their actions and the decisions they make when driving; they are also responsible for ensuring that they are fit to drive
- Drivers who are involved in accidents or stopped by the police can be asked to ascertain that they are in full control of their vehicle (this will include any form of large-wheeled land transport as well as bicycles and motor cycles)
- Those drivers who sustain an injury are not required to inform the Driver and Vehicle Licensing Agency (DVLA) unless they think that their ability to drive may be affected by their injuries for longer than 3 months
- For people who drive heavy goods or public service vehicles, the rules governing driving while injured are more stringent. These drivers must inform their employers that they have been injured or they should seek advice from the DVLA
- Drivers who have been injured should discuss their injuries with their insurance companies. There are some circumstances where insurance policies may become invalidated
- People taking medications should not drive if these medications could affect their reaction times or their ability to think clearly
- People who are deprived of sleep as a result of their injuries should not drive until they have rested
- The wearing of plaster casts and splints can reduce drivers' range of movement; this must be assessed before driving is attempted
- Drivers must assess their injuries while attempting to drive their own vehicles. Such assessments are affected by the drivers' hand dominance and by whether the vehicles have power steering and automatic or manual transmission.

(*Source*: Adapted from Macpherson 2011; Carter 2006)

Key Points

- Almost every activity we undertake will involve the musculoskeletal system. This chapter has presented an overview of the musculoskeletal system. It has detailed the structure and the functions that are associated with the system.
- Explanations have been offered concerning the normal and abnormal changes that may occur when the person has a problem related to the musculoskeletal system.
- A number of common disorders and impairments concerning the musculoskeletal system have been discussed and the nurse has been encouraged to use the nursing process as a framework for care provision in order to ensure that care delivered is safe, effective and person-centred.
- A partnership working arrangement has been advocated throughout. The nurse is encouraged to work with the multidisciplinary team to ensure that the person's care and recovery are effective.
- Partnership with the patient has also been a central thread of this chapter, working to address the person's individual needs from a physical and psychological perspective.
- The nurse must offer care that is holistic, respects individual choice and supports and promotes the person's health and well-being.

- The information the nurse provides to help to prevent illness and minimise complications associated with the musculoskeletal system must be offered in such a way that the person understands it and this will mean that various cultural nuances must be given serious consideration.

Glossary

Abduction: movement of a part away from the midline, e.g. abduction at the shoulder moves the arm away from the trunk and out to the side

Adduction: movement of a part towards the midline, e.g. adduction at the hip joint moves the leg toward the midline and adduction of both legs would press the knees together or cross the legs

Anatomical position: the reference position of the body – standing facing the observer, with the palms of the hands facing forward

Anatomical reduction: the exact adaptation of fracture fragments (hairline adjustment) in preparation for surgical fixation results in complete restoration of the normal anatomy

Ankylosis: fusion of a joint by bone or a tight fibrous union, occurring as a result of a disease

Anterior: the front aspect of the body in the anatomical position. If A is in front of B in the anatomical position, then A is said to be anterior to B

Antibiotic: any drug, such as penicillin, that can inhibit the growth of (bacteriostatic) or destroy (bactericidal) micro-organisms and is used for the prevention or treatment of infections

Antibody: a substance produced by the host's immune system, in response to the detection of an **antigen** (q.v.). The antibody is specifically elaborated to attack and destroy only the antigen which stimulated its production – antigen specific

Arthritis: an inflammatory condition of a diarthrodial (synovial) joint. It may be septic or aseptic

Articular fracture – complete: the articular surface is disrupted and completely separated from the diaphysis

Articular fracture – partial: involving only part of the articular surface; the rest of that surface remains attached to the diaphysis

Avascular necrosis: bone that has been deprived of its blood supply dies. This occurs in the femoral head and the talus more frequently than at other skeletal sites

Bactericidal: capable of killing bacteria

Callus: callus formation is the response of living bone to any irritation. Callus is a tissue complex formed at a site of bony repair

Cancellous bone: the spongy trabecular bone found mostly at the proximal and distal diaphyseal bone ends, in contrast with the dense cortical bone of the shafts. Cancellous bone has a much larger surface area per unit volume and is more readily available to the blood supply, as well as to osteoclasts for resorption

Chemotherapy: treatment of malignant lesions with drugs that impair or stop their cellular proliferation

Chondral: pertaining to cartilage. Consisting of cartilage

Chondrocytes: the active cells of all cartilage, whether articular cartilage, growth cartilage, fibrocartilage, producing the chondral matrix

Comminuted: a fracture with multiple fragments, that is more than two main fragments

Compartment syndrome: bleeding or swelling within an enclosed bundle of muscles

Complex fracture: fracture in which, after reduction, there is no contact between the main fragments

Compound fracture: a fracture in which broken bone fragments lacerate soft tissue and protrude through an open wound in the skin (also called open fracture)

Cortical bone: dense bone forming the tubular element of the shaft, or diaphysis (middle part) of a long bone

Delayed union: the failure of a fracture to consolidate within the normally expected time, which varies according to age, fracture type and location

Diaphysis: the cylindrical, or tubular part between the ends of a long bone, often referred to as the shaft

Distal: away from the centre of the body; more peripheral. For example, the hand is distal to the elbow, the phalanges are distal to the metacarpals

Dorsal: pertaining to the back or dorsum of the body in the anatomical position. An exception is the foot; the top of the foot, even though it faces forward in the anatomical position, is called the dorsum

Epiphysis: the end of a long bone that bears the articular component (the joint). The epiphysis develops embryologically from the cartilaginous element between the joint surface and the growth plate

Extension: the movement of an articulation that causes the relationship between the part above the joint and the part below the joint to straighten

Extensor: the muscles that cause extension of a part are its extensor muscles; the surface of a part where those muscles are found is sometimes called the extensor surface

Fibrocartilage: tissue consisting of elements of cartilage and of fibrous tissue

Flexion: the movement of an articulation that causes the relationship between the part above the joint and the part below the joint to become more angulated

Flexor: the muscles that cause flexion of a part are flexor muscles; the surface of a part where those muscles are found is sometimes called the flexor surface

Fracture: a loss of continuity (breakage), usually sudden, of any structure when internal stresses produced by a load exceed the limits of its strength

Haversian system: the cortical bone is composed of a system of small channels (osteons) about 0.1 mm in diameter and containing the blood vessels. These are remodelled after a disturbance of the blood supply to bone. There is a natural turnover of the Haversian system by continuous osteonal remodelling; this process is part of the dynamic and metabolic nature of bone. It is also involved in the adaptation of bone to an altered mechanical environment

Healing: restoration of original integrity. The healing process after a bone fracture lasts many years, until internal fracture remodelling subsides

Inferior: below or lesser than. In the anatomical position, if A is lower than B, A is inferior to B. The opposite is superior

Ischaemia: absence of blood flow

Lateral: toward the side. The side of the body in the anatomical position is the lateral aspect or surface. If A is nearer the side of the body than B (further from the midline), then A is lateral to B. The opposite is medial

Malunion: consolidation of a fracture in a position of deformity

Matrix: in cartilage, it is the substance between the chondrocytes, comprising a network of collagen fibres interspersed with a 'jelly' of waterlogged mucopolysaccharide macromolecules

Medial: the inner side of a part with the body in the anatomical position is the medial aspect or surface. If A is nearer the middle or centre-line than B, then A is medial to B. The opposite is lateral

Metaphysis: the segment of a long bone located between the articular end part (epiphysis) and the shaft (diaphysis). Consists predominantly of cancellous bone within a thin cortical shell

Midline: the centre-line of the body in the anatomical position

Non-union: failure of bone healing. A fracture is judged to be ununited if the signs of non-union are present when a sufficient time has elapsed since injury, during which the particular fracture would normally be expected to have healed by bony union

Opposition (anatomical): the action of opposing one part to another; if the pulp of the thumb is placed in contact with the pulp of a finger, the movement or action of the thumb is that of opposition

Osteoarthritis: a degenerative condition that affects diarthrodial (synovial) joints and is characterised by loss of articular cartilage, reactive subchondral bone sclerosis (sometimes with subchondral cysts) and the formation of peripheral bony outgrowths – osteophytes

Osteoblast: a cell that forms new bone

Osteoblastic: producing bone

Osteoclast: cell that destroys bone

Osteolytic: resorbing, destroying or removing bone

Osteomyelitis: an acute or chronic inflammatory condition affecting bone and its medullary cavity, usually the result of bacterial (occasionally viral) infection of bone

Osteon: a normal vascular structure concerned with bone remodelling, either as part of physiological bone turnover or as part of the healing process after fracture

Osteoporosis: a reduction in bone mass. It is a natural ageing process but may be pathological. It can result in pathological fracture (most fractures of the femoral neck in the older person are due to osteoporosis plus minimal trauma)

Pathological fracture: a fracture through bone that is abnormal as a result of a pathological process. Can be the result of the application of a force less than that which would be required to produce a fracture in a corresponding normal bone

Periosteum: the inelastic membrane bounding the exterior surface of a bone that plays an active part in the blood supply to cortical bone, in fracture repair and in bone remodelling. It is continuous with the perichondrium

Posterior: the back of the body in the anatomical position is the posterior surface. If A is nearer to the back of the body in the anatomical position than B, then A is posterior to B. Equivalent to dorsal, except in the foot, where the dorsum is anterior in the anatomical position

Pronation: the movement of rotating the forearm so that the palm of the hand faces backward from the anatomical position

Prophylactic: preventive

Proximal: nearer to the centre of the body in the anatomical position. The opposite of distal

Radiotherapy: treatment of pathological conditions, usually malignant, with ionising radiation

Reduction: the realignment of a displaced fracture or a dislocated joint

Remodelling (of bone): the process of transformation of external bone shape (external remodelling) or of internal bone structure (internal remodelling or remodelling of the Haversian system)

(Continued)

Resorption (of bone): the process of bone removal includes the dissolution of mineral and matrix and their uptake into the cell (phagocytosis). The cells responsible for this process are osteoclasts

Rheumatoid arthritis: a crippling, aseptic, synovial inflammatory disease, usually involving many joints (polyarthritis). Results in an intense synovitis that eventually erodes the articular cartilage and the underlying subchondral (beneath the cartilage) bone

Sagittal: bisection of the body in the sagittal plane would divide it into left and right halves, so-called because an arrow fired into the body would normally strike from the front and would pass in a sagittal direction

Simple fracture: a disruption of bone with only two main fragments

Stable fixation: a fixation which keeps the fragments of a fracture in motionless adaptation during the application of controlled physiological forces. While a mobile fracture produces pain with any attempt to move the limb, stable fixation allows early painless functional rehabilitation. Thus, stable fixation minimises irritation, which could eventually lead to fracture disease

Superior: in the anatomical position, if A is higher than, or above, B, then A is superior to B. The opposite is inferior

Supination: the movement of rotating the forearm that causes the palm of the hand to face forward, that is restoring the hand to the anatomical position

Synovial membrane: the membrane lining the interior of a synovial (diarthrodial) joint, wherever the interior surface does not bear articular cartilage

Trabecula (pl. trabeculae): a solid bony strut of cancellous bone

Transverse: across. Transverse bisection of the body in the anatomical position would divide it into upper and lower halves

Vertical: upright. Perpendicular to horizontal

References

Ahern, M.J., Reid, C. & Gordon, T.P. (1987) Does colchicine work? The results of the first controlled study in acute gout. *Australian and New Zealand Journal of Medicine*, 17(3), 301–304.

Arthritis Research UK (2011) *Clinical Assessment of the Musculoskeletal System. A Guide for Medical Students and Healthcare Professionals.* Arthritis Research UK, Chesterfield.

Avenell, A., Gillespie, W.J., Gillespie, L.D. & O'Connell, D. (2005) Vitamin D and vitamin D analogues for preventing fractures associated with involutional and post-menopausal osteoporosis. *Cochrane Database of Systematic Reviews*, (2):CD00227.

Bentley, J. (2013) Vitamin D deficiency: identifying gaps in the evidence base. *Nursing Standard*, 27(46), 35–41.

BOA (2007) *The Care of Patients with Fragility Fractures.* British Orthopaedic Association, London.

BOA (2010) *The National Hip Fracture Data Base: National Report 2010.* British Orthopaedic Association, London.

BSR (2007) *Guideline for the Management of Gout.* British Society for Rheumatology, London. http://www.rheumatology.org.uk/includes/documents/cm_docs/2009/m/management_of_gout.pdf (accessed July 2103).

Carter, T. (2006) *Fitness to Drive: A Guide for Health Professionals.* Royal Society of Medicine Press, London.

Chen, L.X. & Schumacher, H.R. (2008) Gout: an evidence-based review. *Journal of Clinical Rheumatology*, 14(5 Suppl), S55–S62.

Dandy, D.J. & Edwards, D.J. (2003) *Essential Orthopaedics and Trauma.* Churchill Livingstone, Edinburgh.

Hinton, R., Moody, R.L. & Davis, A.W. (2002) Osteoarthritis: diagnosis and therapeutic considerations. *American Family Physician*, 65(5), 841–848.

Hommel. E., Ghazi, A. & White, H. (2012) Minimal trauma fractures: lifting the specter of misconduct by identifying risk factors and planning for prevention. *Journal of the American Medical Association*, 13(2), 180–186.

HSE (2012) *Inspection Pack – Musculoskeletal Disorders 2012.* Health and Safety Executive, London. http://www.hse.gov.uk/foi/internalops/fod/inspect/msd.pdf (accessed June 2103).

Hughes, L.D. (2012) Assessment and management of pain in older patients receiving palliative care. *Nursing Older People*, 24(6), 23–29.

IASP (2011) *International Association of the Study of Pain Taxonomy.* International Association of the Study of Pain, Washington, DC. http://www.iasp-pain.org/Education/Content.aspx?ItemNumber=1698 (accessed 8 March 2014).

Jacobsen, N. (2007) Dignity and health: a review. *Social Science and Medicine*, 64(2), 292–302.

Jenkins, R. (2012) Using advocacy to safeguard older people with learning disabilities. *Nursing Older People*, 24(6), 31–36.

Jones, C.A., Voaklander, D.C., Johnson, D.W. & Suarez-Almazor, M.E. (2000) Health related quality of life outcomes after total hip and knee arthroplasties in a community based population. *Journal of Rheumatology*, 27(7), 1745–1752.

Judge, N.L. (2007) Assessing and managing patients with musculoskeletal conditions. *Nursing Standard*, 22(1), 51–57.

Keating, J. & Aderinto, J. (2010) The management of intracapsular fracture of the femoral neck. *Orthopaedic and Trauma*, 24(1), 42–52.

Lim, H.J., Moon, Y.I. & Lee, M.S. (2005) Effects of home-based daily exercise therapy on joint mobility, daily activity, pain, and depression in patients with ankylosing spondylitis. *Rheumatology International*, 25(3), 225–229.

Macpherson, J. (2011) Driving after discharge: advising injured patients. *Emergency Nurse*, 19(5), 14–18.

Martinon, F. & Glimcher, L.H. (2006) Gout: new insights into an old disease. *Journal of Clinical Investigations*, 116(8), 2073–2075.

McRae, R. & Esser, M. (2008) *Practice Fracture Treatment*, 5th edn. Churchill Livingstone, Edinburgh.

Mikuls, T.R., Farrar, J.T., Bilker, W.B. et al. (2005) Gout epidemiology: results from the UK general practice research database, 1990–1999. *Annals of the Rheumatic Diseases*, 64(2), 267–272.

Moreland, J., Richardson, J., Chan, D. et al. (2003) Evidence-based guidelines for the secondary prevention of falls in older adults. *Gerontology*, 49(2), 93–116.

MRC (1981) *Aids to the Examination of the Peripheral Nervous System*, Memorandum No. 45, Medical Research Council. HMSO, London.

NCCCC (2008) *Osteoarthritis: National Clinical Guideline for Care and Management in Adults.* National Collaborating Centre for Chronic Conditions. Royal College of Physicians, London.

NICE (2005) *Osteoarthritis: The care and management of osteoarthritis in adults.* National Institute of Health and Clinical Excellence, London.

NICE (2008) *Quick Reference Guide. Osteoarthritis: The care and management of osteoarthritis in adults.* National Institute of Health and Clinical Excellence, London. http://www.nice.org.uk/nicemedia/pdf/CG59quickrefguide.pdf (accessed June 2103).

NICE (2011a) *Hip Fracture. The Management of Hip Fracture in Adults.* National Institute for Health and Clinical Excellence, London. http://www.nice.org.uk/cg124 (accessed July 2013).

NICE (2011b) *Venous Thromboembolism Reducing the Risk.* National Institute for Health and Clinical Excellence, London. http://guidance.nice.org.uk/CG92/NICEGuidance/doc/English (accessed July 2013).

NJR (2013) *NJR Stats on Line.* National Joint Registry, Hemel Hempstead. http://www.njrcentre.org.uk/njrcentre/Healthcareproviders/Accessingthedata/StatsOnline/NJRStatsOnline/tabid/179/Default.aspx (accessed June 2103).

O'Malley, N., Blauth, M., Suhm, M. & Kates, S.L. (2011) Hip fracture management, before and beyond surgery and medication: a synthesis of the evidence. *Archives of Orthopaedic and Trauma Surgery*, 113(11), 1519–1527.

ONS (2013) *General Health*, Ch. 7. (General Lifestyle Survey Overview – a report on the 2011 General Lifestyle Survey). Office for National Statistics, London. http://www.ons.gov.uk/ons/dcp171776_302351.pdf (accessed June 2103).

Peach, C.A., Carr, A.J. & Loughlin, J. (2005) Recent advances in the genetic investigation of osteoarthritis. *Trends in Molecular Medicine*, 11(4), 186–191.

Pisters, M.F., Veenhof, C., Schellevis, F.G., De Bakker, D.H. & Dekker, J. (2010) Long-term effectiveness of exercise therapy in patients with osteoarthritis of the hip or knee: a randomized controlled trial comparing two different physical therapy interventions. *Osteoarthritis and Cartilage*, 18(8), 1019–1026.

Rahme, E., Pettitt, D., LeLorier, J., *et al.* (2002) Determinants and sequelae associated with utilization of acetaminophen versus traditional nonsteroidal anti-inflammatory drugs in an elderly population. *Arthritis and Rheumatism*, 46(11), 3046–3054.

Sambrook, P., Schrieber, L., Taylor, T. & Ellis, A. (2010) *The Musculoskeletal System*, 2nd edn. Elsevier, Edinburgh.

Schlesinger, N. & Schumacher, H.R. (2002) Update on gout. *Arthritis and Rheumatism*, 47(5), 563–565.

SIGN (2009) *Management of Hip Fractures in Older People: A National Clinical Guideline*. Scottish Intercollegiate Guidelines Network, Edinburgh.

Smelser, C. (2007) Gout. http://emedicine.medscape.com/article/389965-overview (accessed July 2013).

Swift, A. (2012a) Osteoarthritis 1: Physiology risk factors and causes of pain. *Nursing Times*, 108(7), 12–15.

Swift, A. (2012b) Osteoarthritis 2: Pain management and treatment strategies. *Nursing Times*, 108(8), 25–27.

Tarling, M., Aitken, E., Lahoti, O. *et al.* (2002) Closing the audit loop: the role of a pilot in the development of fractured neck of femur integrated care pathway. *Journal of Orthopaedic and Nursing*, 6(3), 130–134.

Tortora, G.J. & Nielsen, M.T. (2012) *Principles of Human Anatomy*, 12th edn. Wiley, New Jersey.

Turk, D.C. & Cohen, M.J. (2010) Sleep as a marker in the effective management of chronic osteoarthritis pain with opioid analgesics. *Seminars in Arthritis and Rheumatism*, 39(6), 477–490.

Turley, M., Tobias, M. & Paul, S. (2006) Non-fatal disease burden associated with excess body mass index and waist circumference in New Zealand adults. *Australian and New Zealand Journal of Public Health*, 30(3), 231–237.

Walker, J. (2013) Management of common fractures. *Nursing Standard*, 25(1), 30–36.

Whitening, N. (2008) Fractures: pathophysiology, treatment and nursing care. *Nursing Standard*, 23(2), 49–57.

Zhang, W., Doherty, M., Pascual, E., *et al.* (2006) EULAR evidence based recommendations for gout. Part I: diagnosis. Report of a task force of the Standing Committee for International Clinical Studies Including Therapeutics (ESCISIT). *Annals of Rheumatic Disease*, 65(10), 1301–1311.

Zhang, W., Nuki, G., Moskowitz, R.W. *et al.* (2010) OARSI recommendations for the management of hip and knee osteoarthritis: Part III: Changes in evidence following systematic cumulative update of research published through January 2009. *Osteoarthritis and Cartilage*, 18(4), 476–499.

Test Yourself

1. Which bone protects the brain?
   (a) The calcaneus
   (b) The calcium
   (c) The cranium
   (d) The coccyx

2. Paraesthesia refers to:
   (a) Partial consciousness
   (b) Tingling sensation 'pins and needles'
   (c) Coma
   (d) Paralysis

3. Tendons attach:
   (a) Muscles to bone
   (b) Bone to bone
   (c) The axis to the atlas
   (d) The elastic cartilage to fibrocartilage

4. Osteoblasts are responsible for:
   (a) The breakdown of bone
   (b) The formation of new bone
   (c) The destruction of tissue
   (d) The build up of tendon

5. A fat embolism…
   (a) Occurs only in obese people
   (b) Occurs after the ingestion of a fatty meal
   (c) Occurs when embolic fat macroglobules pass into the small vessels of the lung and other sites
   (d) Is harmless

6. How many thoracic vertebrae are there?
   (a) 10
   (b) 11
   (c) 12
   (d) 13

7. Arthralgia refers to:
   (a) Migraine pain
   (b) Muscle pain
   (c) Pain associated with breathing
   (d) Joint pain

8. An NSAID is:
   (a) A steroidal anti-inflammatory drug
   (b) A non-steroidal anti-inflammatory drug
   (c) A non-stiffening agent
   (d) A controlled drug

9. Falls occur more often in:
   (a) Older women
   (b) Older men
   (c) Equally in men and women
   (d) More in people with colour blindness

10. How many conditions are there that can affect synovial joints?
    (a) 50
    (b) 100
    (c) 150
    (d) 200

Answers

1. c
2. b
3. a
4. b
5. c
6. c
7. d
8. b
9. a
10. d

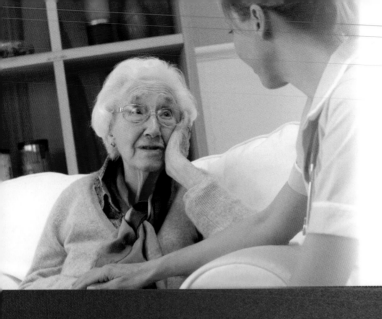

37

The Person with a Skin Disorder

Melanie Stephens

University of Salford, UK

Learning Outcomes

On completion of this chapter you will be able to:

- Review the holistic assessment of the patient with a skin disorder
- Recognise the effect of the psyche on the skin
- Explain the importance of using correct terminology in the assessment and management of skin disorders.
- Review the investigations that can be undertaken to aid diagnosis and management of skin disorders
- Recognise and review common skin conditions, their clinical management and the involvement of members of the multidisciplinary team

Competencies

All nurses must:

1. Undertake a person-centred, personalised approach to care
2. Possess a broad knowledge of the structure and functions of the human body, and other relevant knowledge from the life, behavioural and social sciences as applied to health, ill-health, disability, ageing and death
3. In partnership with the person, their carers and their families, make a holistic, person-centred and systematic assessment of physical, emotional, psychological, social, cultural and spiritual needs, including risk, and together develop a comprehensive personalised plan of nursing care
4. Evaluate the effect of interventions, taking account of people's and carers' interpretation of physical, emotional and behavioural changes
5. Make person-centred, evidence-based judgements and decisions, in partnership with others involved in the care process, to ensure high quality care
6. Promote health and well-being, self-care and independence by teaching and empowering people and carers to make choices in coping with the effects of treatment and the ongoing nature and likely consequences of a condition, including death and dying

Nursing Practice: Knowledge and Care, First Edition. Edited by Ian Peate, Karen Wild and Muralitharan Nair.
© 2014 John Wiley & Sons, Ltd. Published 2014 by John Wiley & Sons, Ltd. Companion website: www.wileynursingpractice.com

Introduction

A skin disorder can be defined as a disease affecting the skin and involves one in five babies and 54% of the population (British Association of Dermatologists, BAD 2011). Often a skin disorder has both a visible dramatic impact on the lives of the patients and their families (Changing Faces 2012). Most skin conditions are self-managed with only 24% utilising healthcare resources, such as Practice Nurse, GP, Pharmacist or Dermatologist. Often there is no cure; the condition is long term and follows periods of remission and exacerbation. Many nurses will only see patients at their worst, and therefore it is essential that those who provide care focus not only the physical aspects of care but provide psychological input too.

Anatomy and Physiology

Re-visit Chapter 18 to remind yourself of the structure and functions of the skin, hair and nails.

Jot This Down
Which groups of patients with the potential for skin disorders need extra health education on care of their nails and which members of the multidisciplinary team could provide advice and support to both the patient and each other?

Jot This Down
Take some time out and think of the different illnesses, medical problems and skin problems that could occur due to excessive production of wax, oil and sweat. What health education would you offer to the patient for each type of illness or medical problem?

Assessment

Assessment of the skin can take place using both subjective and objective data; this can take the form of a full physical assessment of a patient and an assessment interview. According to Lawton (2001), this should take into consideration four main sections: a detailed history of the patient's skin condition, a general assessment of the patient, an assessment of the patient's knowledge and a physical assessment.

Patient assessment interview

On first meeting a patient, a nurse would carry out a comprehensive, holistic health assessment, the first aspect being that of the collection of subjective data from the person with the skin disorder. There are many aspects to the collection of this data, including when did the person first notice the commencement of the skin disorder, how long has it been present, how often does it occur or recur, what are the characteristics of the skin disorder, what route the disorder has taken, is it affected by seasonal changes, the severity of the skin disorder, any precipitating or predisposing factors, for example is there a family history of the condition, what relieves the disorder if at all, pharmacological and non-pharmacological, and any related symptoms.

Jot This Down
Why would a nurse ask a patient with a skin disorder about their occupation and hobbies?

Questioning of the patient about their skin disorder would focus on skin, hair, nails and patient knowledge. Table 37.1 highlights issues a nurse would consider as part of the patient assessment interview in relation to skin, hair and nails.

It is important when carrying out the assessment that the nurse asks the patient questions in relation to their knowledge of the disorder, as this may mean that further health promotion and education is required at the end of the assessment.

The nurse would then move the focus of the interview to a full medical history, so that a holistic picture of the patient and their skin disorder can be obtained. Questions would centre on previous problems, any allergies, prior lesions or moles. Then ask questions that explore the patient's past medical and surgical history, as many skin disorders are symptoms of other disorders. Questions could focus on neurological, cardiovascular, respiratory, gastrointestinal, genitourinary, musculoskeletal, reproductive, haematological, immunological and endocrine issues. Interviewing would also focus on current and past medication and treatments and activities

Table 37.1 Questions to consider when questioning a patient about their skin disorder.

ANATOMICAL PART OF THE INTEGUMENTARY SYSTEM	QUESTIONS A NURSE WOULD CONSIDER
Skin	What recent changes in skin has occurred; have there been the development of any rashes; are they in the same place or different ones; is there any itching; is this worse at any periods during the day; have there been any changes in colour of the skin or the skin disorder; is there increased dryness or oiliness? Has the patient noticed any lesions, warts or moles; have these changed in colour or size? What might have triggered the skin disorder; has there been any changes in the use of cosmetics, soaps, skin care agents? Have they recently acquired a new pet, travelled to a different country, changed their diet or experienced recent high levels of stress?
Hair	What recent changes in hair have occurred? Is there excessive hair loss, thinning or baldness? Has the distribution of hair changed across the body? Has there been a recent change in hair products? Has the patient recently commenced a diet?
Nails	What recent changes in the nails have occurred? Is there any splitting, breakage or discolouration? Are there visible signs of infection? Have there been recent changes to the diet, dieting or exposure to chemicals?

of daily living, for example communication, work and play, sleep and how the condition affects the patient's current lifestyle.

The risk of skin cancer and malignant melanoma would also be explored, including factors such the presence and number of moles on the skin, prior exposure to radiation, X-rays, coal, tar or petroleum-based products. Record the age and gender of the patient, any previous personal or family history of skin cancer or malignant melanoma; their routine in relation to exposure to sunlight; do they have a predisposition to sunburn or an inability to tan; have they had any previous skin trauma; the presence of freckles and the colour of hair and eyes.

Examination of the skin

Examination of the skin has two components, a general assessment and a physical skin assessment, and can be part of a total assessment or a focussed assessment for those patients with a known or suspected problem, perhaps from a referral from a GP to a Dermatology Service. The place in which the examination takes place should be considered prior to the commencement of this aspect of the patient assessment. As the patient may be removing all of their clothes in front of strangers, it is necessary to ensure both that an explanation is provided to why this is necessary and that where this occurs should be an area full of bright natural light, private and warm. Consideration should be given to any religious or cultural beliefs in relation to undressing in front of others. Curtains should be closed, dignity should be maintained and, as all clothing should be removed, a gown should be worn by the patient so as not to expose unnecessarily areas of the body that do not need revealing. Depending on where the skin disorder is, the patient may be assessed standing, sitting or lying down, so equipment to accommodate all these positions is required and relayed to the patient with clear explanations and instructions. Personal protective equipment should be worn when assessing open lesions, infections, infestations or when wounds or mucous membranes are oozing discharge. Some lesions may need measuring or photographing, others visualising more accurately. Therefore, it is imperative to have torches, rulers, grids and tape measures available and consent forms for photography to hand.

General assessment A general assessment of the skin occurs when conducting a patient interview. The skin conveys a wealth of information about the patient and often reflects their health status. Often, the general appearance indicates the patient's self-caring abilities, state of mind and existence of support.

Jot This Down
What signs and symptoms from a patient's general appearance can tell us about their health status?

Physical assessment The most important aspect of a physical assessment is the opportunity to touch the patient and their skin; this should occur in a clinical area with bright natural light. This can often be embarrassing and uncomfortable on the first occasion, but the ability to touch the skin can tell the nurse a lot about the patient and their skin disorder. Vital clinical information to be gathered is the colour of the skin both in relation to race and the skin disorder; the texture and skin temperature; moisture; turgor and presence of oedema. Record other findings, such as scars, missing fingers, toes and limbs and the presence of any open wounds. As the skin tells a narrative about the patient, the nurse

Table 37.2 Questions to ask about the character, distribution and shape of lesions.

Character	Is there redness, scaling, crusting, exudate? Are there excoriations, blisters, erosions, pustules, papules? Are the lesions all the same (monomorphic), e.g. drug rash, or variable (polymorphic), e.g. chickenpox?
Shape	Are the lesions small, large, ring-shaped, linear? Does it have a border? Is it flat, fluid filled, indurated?
Distribution	Is the disorder on the hands, feet, extremities of ears and nose, in light exposed areas or mainly confined to the trunk? Is it localised or widespread? If widespread is it symmetrical and is this central or peripheral? Is the disorder linear, regional (in a groin) or following a dermatomal pattern, such as shingles?

should assess the distribution, character and shape of the lesions, the site and location (Table 37.2).

In patients with darkly pigmented skin, some disorders present differently and it is important for a nurse to be aware of these differences (Lang 2000).

Colour – lesions that appear red or brown on light skin often present as black or purple on dark skin. A good method is to assess an area of skin that is not affected by the skin disorder of the patient and compare that with the skin disorder; this will highlight any abnormalities. Mild inflammatory reactions may not be visible and the use of touch for heat to an area of skin may be the only indicator of a reaction. However, prolonged inflammation can lead to hyper- and hypopigmentation.

Pigmentation – the most obvious difference is the change in pigmentation in Asian and Afro-Caribbean patients to Caucasians. This is categorised as a normal variant, i.e. pigmentary demarcation, and midline primary conditions, i.e. vitiligo (Figure 37.1), and secondary conditions, i.e. post-inflammatory hypopigmentation and hyperpigmentation (darkening of the pigment of the skin) in atopic eczema.

Reaction patterns – darker skins show particular reaction patterns such as follicular (affecting hair follicles), papular (elevations of the skin) and annular (ring like skin conditions), and keloid scarring.

Terminology used for describing lesions

It is important for nurses to use terminology correctly when describing lesions on a body plan of care. Common terminology can include descriptions of primary lesions, those that occur at the onset of a skin disorder, and secondary lesions, those that occur over time as a consequence of the disease progressing, manipulation (scratching, rubbing, picking) and treatment. These terms can be found in Table 37.3 and Table 37.4. It is crucial that the nurse describes the lesions correctly as this may affect the general management and treatment of a patient by the nurse and other members of the multidisciplinary team. During the physical assessment, skin lesions should be palpated between the finger and thumb (unless widespread) as this helps the nurse assess if the lesion is soft, firm, hard, raised or irregular and its texture. Then the lesion should be given a colour, i.e. pink, red, purple and mauve (due to blood); brown, black and blue (due to pigment); white (due to lack of blood or pigment); or yellow and orange (due to bilirubin levels).

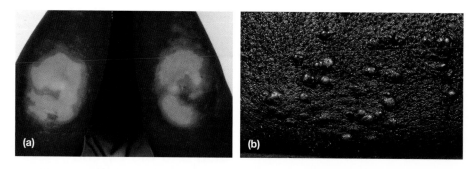

Figure 37.1 **Vitiligo.** Source: Buxton & Morris-Jones (2009). Reproduced with permission of John Wiley & Sons Ltd.

Table 37.3 **Primary lesions terminology.**

NAME	PRESENTATION	EXAMPLE
Macule	A flat circumscribed area of colour change – can be brown, red, white or tan	Vitiligo
Papule	An elevated 'spot'; palpable, firm, circumscribed, less than 5 mm in diameter	Scabies or bite from an insect
Nodule	Elevated, firm, circumscribed, palpable, larger than 5 mm in diameter	Erythema nodosum
Plaque	Elevated, flat-topped, firm, rough, superficial papule, greater than 2 cm in diameter. Papules can coalesce to form plaques	Psoriasis
Wheal	Elevated, irregular area of cutaneous oedema: red, pale pink or white	Urticaria
Vesicle	Elevated, circumscribed, superficial fluid-filled blister, less than 5 mm in diameter	Herpes simplex
Bulla	Vesicle greater than 5 mm in diameter	Bullous pemphigoid
Pustule	Elevated, superficial, similar to vesicle but filled with pus	Impetigo

Table 37.4 Secondary lesions terminology. (Adapted from Lawton 2002).

NAME	PRESENTATION	EXAMPLE
Scale	Thickened, flaky exfoliation, irregular, thick or thin, dry or oily, variable size, silver, white or tan in colour	Psoriasis
Crust	Dried serum, blood or purulent exudate; slightly elevated; size variable	Impetigo discoid
Excoriation	Loss of epidermis caused by scratching	Atopic eczema
Lichenification	Rough, thickened epidermis, accentuated skin markings due to scratching	Lichen simplex

The nurse needs to describe correctly not only the type of lesion but also its spatial relationship with other lesions on the body. Lesions can be termed as solitary (a single lesion), satellite (a single lesion in close proximity to a larger group), grouped (a cluster of lesions), generalised (total body area) and localised (a limited area of involvement that is clearly defined).

As skin disorders can be extremely distressing, the nurse needs to assess the degree of discomfort the patient may be experiencing from itching, pain and soreness from the condition. Identification and addressing of the underlying cause of the pruritus is the most important factor, with appropriate management and treatment of the condition.

Assessment of the nails, hair and mucous membranes

The nurse should complete the assessment with a review of the nails, hair and mucous membranes. This would include any blistering, scarring and erosions of the mucous membranes and colour, shape, capillary refill and pigment changes of the nails. Finally, note any hair loss, erythema and scale of the scalp.

Jot This Down

What are the most common causes of pruritus in both skin disorders and systemic diseases?

Link To/Go To

This is the link to the Quality Standards for Dermatology:

http://www.bad.org.uk/Portals/_Bad/Quality%20Standards/Dermatology%20Standards%20FINAL%20-%20July%202011.pdf

Skin and the Psyche

According to Zaidi and Lanigan (2010), emotional trauma can occur from the development of many a skin disorder. This can lead to stress, low self-esteem, social isolation, depression and even suicide. As social beings, humans need interaction with each other both verbally and physically to survive; when a factor affects this, psychological consequences can occur. Self-image and quality of life can be dramatically affected by a skin disorder as the scarring can be both physical and psychological, such as is witnessed in acne vulgaris in teenagers (Thomas 2005). However, it is also known that psychological illnesses such as depression, anxiety and stress can trigger or exacerbate a skin disorder. Due to this link between emotions and the skin, a new clinical field or subspecialty of dermatology has developed – **psychodermatology** – and within this there has been identified a four-grouping classification of disorders connecting the skin and the mind. These groupings are:

Psychophysiologic – emotional stress causing inflammatory skin reactions

Primary psychiatric – self-induced injury of the skin (iatrogenic)

Secondary psychiatric – emotional consequences such as anxiety, anger and depression developing as a result of an existing skin disease

Cutaneous sensory disorders – patients with no apparent dermatological skin or medical condition presenting with disagreeable skin sensations, such as itching, soreness and pain, and negative sensory symptoms, such as numbness and hypoaesthesia.

It is therefore imperative that the nurse assesses the patient appropriately. Does the patient have a skin disorder? Is the skin disorder having a psychological impact on the patient? Is the emotional stress suffered a constant trigger of the skin disorder itself? Is the skin disorder self-induced? Once this has been assessed, the nurse can either measure the impact the skin disorder is having on the quality of a patient's life or referrals can then be made to other members of the multidisciplinary team for psychological interventions such as relaxation, meditation, hypnosis and self-hypnosis, psychotropic medications, biofeedback and focussed psychiatric care and psychotherapy.

The effect of a skin disorder on a patient's life can be significant. A way in which nurses can assess and monitor this during a patient episode of care is through the use of quality of life tools. There are many quality of life tools for nurses to use in dermatology. Three reliable and validated tools are the Dermatology Life Quality Index, the Cardiff Tool and the SF-36, which is available for both adults and children. Using tools such as these will allow the nurse to assess the effect of the skin disorder on the patient's quality of life before, during and after treatment.

Patient-reported experience and outcome measures are also collated to allow staff to measure not only a patient's health status but also how patients feel about the care they received during their pathway of care (Department of Health, DH 2008).

Investigations

As well as collecting subjective data from the patient, the nurse may carry out further investigations in conjunction with other members of the multidisciplinary team. Investigations aid the nurse in supporting the diagnosis of a skin disease, condition or injury. This information aids management or modification of treatment used to optimise repair of the hair, nails and skin and conditions for healing. Many tests are carried out by nurses caring for patients with skin disorders. Table 37.5 highlights some of the most common tests used.

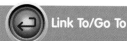

Link To/Go To

This pocket guide provides you with a simple guide to common skin conditions, their assessment, diagnosis, management and further referral:

http://www.nes.scot.nhs.uk/media/705715/dermatology _guide__amended_may_2012_.pdf

Table 37.5 Dermatological investigations.

TYPE OF TEST	REASON FOR TEST
Oxygen saturation	A test used to measure the oxygenation of a person's haemoglobin; a lack of oxygen can lead to cell death and tissue breakdown
Toe blood pressure monitoring	A test used to measure the systolic pressure of blood in the toe; aids detection of poor vascular flow
Sinogram/Fistulogram	An X-ray examination of a wound used to detect tracking, undermining and tunnelling of a wound
Urinalysis	A test used to detect and/or screen for metabolic and kidney disorders
Blood sugar	Used to determine the plasma glucose level. Mainly used as a diagnostic or screening tool for diabetes
Body mass index (BMI)	A tool to assess the weight and height of a person, which aids assessment of factors, such as nutritional status, risk of pressure ulcer development and is linked to numerous illness and child development
Blood tests	Various blood tests assess the function of the liver, kidneys and lungs and also aid screening for issues such as anaemia, infections, immune problems and platelet levels
Magnetic resonance image (MRI)	A non-invasive medical imaging technique, used to visualise the internal structures of the body
Computer tomography (CT)	A medical imaging procedure that uses computer-processed X-rays to produce tomographic images or 'slices' of specific areas of the body
Sonography	An ultrasound-based diagnostic imaging technique used for visualising subcutaneous body structures, including tendons, muscles, joints, vessels and internal organs; also used in obstetrics to visualise the unborn fetus
Phlebography	A test that provides X-ray images of the venous system when radio-opaque dye is injected into the veins of the lower limbs
Photoplethysmography	A non-invasive test used to measure blood volume changes in microvascular bed of tissues using infrared light source and transducer light probe. Often used to assess venous reflux
Duplex ultrasonography	A form of medical ultrasonography that incorporates two elements: grayscale ultrasound to visualise the structure or architecture of the body part and colour-Doppler ultrasound to visualise the flow or movement of a structure, e.g. to image blood within an artery
X-rays	A medical imaging test to detect problems such as osteomyelitis
Allergy testing	Can help confirm or rule out allergies and consequently reduce adverse reactions and limit unnecessary avoidance and medications. Tests can involve the taking of blood or skin-prick tests
Wood's lamp, immunofluorescent studies, potassium hydroxide and Tzanck test	A variety of tests used to identify infections, i.e. to look for chickenpox, fungal and bacterial infections
Cultures	A test used to identify infections from collections of tissue samples, serum, pus, exudates and drainage. In sepsis, serum will be obtained
Skin biopsy	Allows the clinician to differentiate a benign skin lesion from a cancer or to determine an infection that cannot be obtained through routine swabbing. Techniques of biopsy can be punch, incision, excision and shaving
Genetic testing	A test used to examine the structure of a person's DNA, gene products and chromosomes

Skin Infections: Viral, Bacterial and Fungal

Epidemiology

Sebum, the immune system and skin flora protect the skin from infections; however, if a breach of the skin occurs, the immune system is impaired or a potent mediator falls on to the skin, then these normal functions are weakened and the skin may be at risk of skin disorders such as viral, bacterial and fungal infections. Minor skin infestations and infections are often generally self-managed by patients; however, according to Schofield *et al.* (2011), skin conditions are major causes for consultation in primary care. Skin infections such as cellulitis affected nearly 88 000 people in 2010 (NHS 2011), all of whom required admission to hospital for intravenous antibiotics and further investigation.

Viral Skin Infections

A virus is a microorganism that is smaller than a bacterium, consisting of an RNA or DNA core, surrounded by a protein coat. It cannot grow or reproduce apart from inside a living cell. The skin lesions that occur as a consequence have attacked the keratinocyte, reproduced and caused either cell death or growth.

Common viral skin infections have recently increased and it is thought that this is due to numerous causes: antibiotics, contraceptive medication, corticosteroids and any medication that causes immunosuppression. It is the immunosuppressive properties of these medications that have affected normal body functioning and as a consequence viruses have the opportunity to multiply.

Common Viral Infections of the Skin
Warts

The human papillomavirus, of which there are over 60 types, is the cause of **warts** or **verrucae**. Often found on non-genital and genital areas of the skin and mucous membranes, warts can present as flat, tapered at both ends and round in shape, with a rough grey surface. Table 37.6 highlights the most common warts, their location and appearance.

Herpes simplex

Otherwise known as a **cold sore**, herpes simplex (HS) is a common virus that affects much of the population. An initial infection is

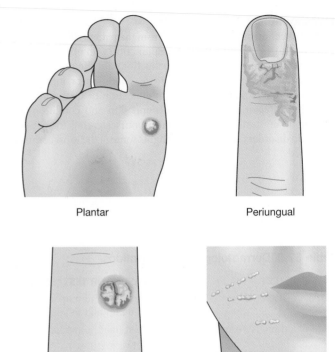

Plantar   Periungual

Common   Flat

Figure 37.2 Types of wart.

often the most severe and may be accompanied by fever and sore throat; in the under 5s HS may cause inflammation of the gums. Once a primary infection has occurred, the virus lives in the nerve ganglia and is usually reactivated by sunlight, menstruation, stress, injury or low immunity. HS is caused by two viruses:

HSV-1: most attributed to simplex lesions of the face, lips and mouth, transmitted through kissing, oral sex and physical contact

HSV-2: most commonly attributed to genital infections.

Signs and symptoms These include a tingling or burning sensation followed by reddening of the skin or membranes and formation of a painful vesicle. The vesicle advances through pustules, ulcers and crusting, and healing occurs between 10 and 14 days after the initial symptoms. If the eyes are affected, conjunctivitis can occur. Secondary infection can occur, but is mainly in patients with skin breakdown such as active eczema; in extreme cases, the ulcers can spread rapidly and affect the lungs, brain and heart (eczema herpeticum) (Lin 2011).

Nursing care For mild and uncomplicated HS, no treatment or management is necessary. An antiviral cream such as aciclovir may help ease some of the symptoms, but should be applied at the tingling stage to shorten the eruption. Patients who experience recurrent eruptions may be offered long-term antiviral therapy.

Severe infection may require hospitalisation and oral antiviral therapy. With eye infections, antiviral eye drops can be prescribed.

Health promotion Prevention is better than cure and the nurse's role is to provide education and advice in relation to the wearing

Table 37.6 Common warts (see also Figure 37.2).

TYPE OF WART	LOCATION	APPEARANCE
Verruca vulgaris (common wart)	Anywhere on the skin and mucous membranes, most common on fingers	Dome-shaped with ragged borders
Plantar warts	Pressure points on the feet	Inward growing wart due to pressure of shoes and walking; often painful
Verucca plana (flat wart)	Forehead or back of hand	Small flat lesion
Condylomata acuminate (HPV or venereal warts)	Glans of the penis, anal region, vulva and cervix	Cauliflower like, pink and purple in colour

of sunscreen, avoiding stressors that trigger the HS virus, eating a healthy diet and taking exercise – all activities that create a healthy immune system. Other advice is not to kiss or have oral sex with someone who has signs and symptoms of HS.

Herpes zoster

Most commonly known as shingles, the chickenpox (varicella zoster) virus remains dormant in the dorsal root ganglion of a nerve. Reactivation of herpes zoster triggers a reaction, a rash in the dermatome section of the skin, usually coinciding with illnesses that cause immunosuppression such as HIV or infections, malignancy such as leukaemia, lymphoma and Hodgkin's disease or during or after a course of radiotherapy or chemotherapy. Shingles can occur at any age but is most commonly seen in the over 50s and affects one in five people.

Signs and symptoms A period of hypersensitivity precedes an outbreak of shingles, with complaints of feeling under the weather, headache, fever, burning and pain; this is called **the pre-eruptive phase**. In **the eruptive phase**, blisters develop in a unilateral area, and take 3–4 weeks to clear.

Complications can occur, such as a secondary infection and post-herpetic neuralgia that can last for 3–6 months; this is named **the chronic phase**. More rare but serious complications include impairment or loss of vision if the ophthalmic division of the trigeminal nerve is affected, facial paralysis and, in the immune-compromised individual, visceral lesions and encephalitis, which potentially result in death.

Nursing care Cool tap water compresses and calamine can ease blistering and petroleum jelly aids healing. Early antiviral therapy within 72 hours of the rash developing can reduce the duration of the rash and any potential post-herpetic neuralgia. Loose fitting cotton clothing reduces the risk of irritation. Regular pain relief can be taken, such as paracetamol, paracetamol and codeine derivatives and ibuprofen. If a patient is experiencing post-herpetic neuralgia, then topical capsaicin cream and antidepressants may be prescribed. In severe cases, steroids may be prescribed. Other referrals to members of the medical team may be needed, in particular if shingles affects the eye and brain.

Health promotion Studies have shown that providing the over 60s with varicella zoster vaccine boosts immunity (Tseng *et al.* 2011) and that the vaccine prevents herpes zoster disease (Gagliardi *et al.* 2012). The person with shingles is infectious to others when the rash appears, but only if the person coming into contact has not had chickenpox. Women who are pregnant should avoid anyone with shingles until the vesicles have dried up. Patients should not share towels, play contact sports or go swimming while they have a shingles rash.

Bacterial Skin Infections

Bacterial skin infections are common infections for which patients seek advice from primary care healthcare providers. The most common are caused by Gram-positive *Staphylococcus aureus* and beta-haemolytic streptococci. Infections may be primary, caused by a single pathogen evolving from the skin, or secondary, occurring in diseased or traumatised skin. If treated quickly, the infections can be easily cleared, however severe complications such as septicaemia can occur if treatment is delayed or inadequate. Table

37.7 highlights the common different types of bacterial skin infections, the causative bacteria and their signs and symptoms. Contributing factors for the development of bacterial skin infections include no apparent cause, poor hygiene, poor nutrition, prolonged skin moisture or excessive moisture from perspiration, trauma to the skin (including trauma from shaving), systemic diseases such as diabetes mellitus and haematological malignancies and heavy fabrics on the upper legs.

Nursing care

All cases of bacterial infections need to be monitored carefully, taking vital observations, noting the spread of inflammation, and marking and measuring this clearly on a body map. In emergency situations, the ABCDE (Airway, Breathing, Circulation, Disability, Exposure) approach to patient management should be applied.

Folliculitis – No treatment is advised in mild cases, however emollients may improve the condition of the skin. Topical antibiotics may be prescribed once culture and sensitivity of the causative organism has been identified.

Furuncles and carbuncles – Warm compresses may ease the pain and draw a boil or carbuncle to a head. If they burst, cleansing with normal saline and applying of ointments and dressings may be necessary. Large boils and carbuncles may be lanced by a trained nurse who has extended their skill in this area. Antibiotics are often not necessary unless the inflammation extends around the boil or carbuncle, or lymphadenopathy, fever or multiple boils are present. A urinalysis for glucose levels should be performed in cases of patients who return with frequent boils.

Cellulitis – Mild or moderate cellulitis is treated with antibiotics for 7 days. More serious cases may need hospitalisation. Orbital cellulitis is a medical emergency that can lead to loss of sight and cerebral complications.

Erysipelas – This is a medical emergency and the patient would receive antibiotics for the first 7 days; often patients are hospitalised.

Health promotion

Any health education should be related to contributing factors of the bacterial infection. Advice should be given on personal hygiene, nutritional intake, weight management and choice of clothing a patient might wear.

Link To/Go To

Scarlet fever is a bacterial skin infection common in children. This link provides information on the condition:

http://www.nhs.uk/conditions/Scarlet-fever/Pages/Introduction.aspx

Fungal Skin Infections

Dermatophytoses, candidiasis and mycoses are all fungi that cause superficial skin infections in humans. Many people have a fungal infection without even knowing it and it is often only when they access healthcare resources that the infection is identified and treated (Nazarko 2011). Common fungal infections are caused by two main groups of fungi: **dermatophytoses** (tinea or ringworm)

Table 37.7 Common types of bacterial skin infections.

BACTERIAL INFECTION OF THE SKIN	COMMONEST CAUSATIVE BACTERIA	SIGNS, SYMPTOMS AND COMPLICATIONS	SITE
Folliculitis – bacterial infection of the hair follicle	*Staphylococcus aureus* and *Pseudomonas aeruginosa*	Inflammation, pustules and lesions seen at the hair follicle. Discomfort ranging from slight burning to intense itching. Complication of abscess formation	Scalp, face of bearded men (sycosis-barbae), eye (stye) and extremities on the legs of women who shave
Furuncles (boils) inflammation of the hair follicle	*Staphylococcus aureus*	Deep, firm, red, painful nodule 1–5 cm in diameter. After few days the nodule changes to large painful cystic nodule draining infected, purulent pus	Any part of the body that has hair, particularly neck, face, flexures and buttocks
Carbuncles – group of infected hair follicles	*Staphylococcus aureus*	Firm mass located in the subcutaneous tissue and lower dermis. Mass becomes painful and swollen and has multiple openings to the skin surface. Patient may experience chills, fever and malaise	Neck, back and lateral thighs
Cellulitis – localised infection of the dermis and subcutaneous tissue	*Streptococcus pyogenes*	Red, swollen and painful area. Vesicles may form over the cellulitic area, accompanied by chills, fever, malaise, headache and swollen lymph glands	Anywhere on the body. Common areas lower legs in adults and eye and peri-anal area in children
Erysipelas – infection of the skin	*Streptococcus pyogenes*	Chills, fever and malaise (4–20 hours) precede a skin lesion appearing. Lesion(s) appear as firm red spots enlarging to form a circumscribed, bright red, raised, hot lesion. Petechiae, necrosis and blistering can occur if not treated early	Face, ears and lower legs

and **candidiasis** (yeasts). Patients most at risk of developing a fungal infection are those who take antibiotics, either orally or intravenously, as antibiotics not only treat the invading infection but kill the bacteria and disturb the normal flora on the body. Increased risk exists with those patients who already have an underlying medical condition, such as diabetes mellitus, leukaemia or HIV, and the elderly. Fungi love a moist environment so areas of the skin where moisture is prevalent and high, such as between the toes and under folds of skin, are at risk. Patients who have poor nutritional status, are obese, take oral contraception, are pregnant, iron-deficient or immune-suppressed are equally at risk.

Candidiasis

Candida albicans is the yeast-like infection generally found on mucous membranes, the skin, vagina and gastrointestinal tract. *Candida* intertrigo (sweat rash) occurs due to perspiration being trapped in skin folds or tight clothes and the skin not being able to allow the sweat to evaporate.

Signs and symptoms

The first sign of *Candida albicans* is a pustule that extends under the stratum corneum. The pustule habitually burns, causes itching, and has a red and swollen base. As the infection develops, a white curd-like substance appears. This is the shedding of the surface cells and accumulation of inflammatory cells, such as white blood cells. Satellite lesions can be seen outside of the boundaries of the original site.

Candida intertrigo, however, occurs in folds of skin under the breasts, in the groin or in the apron (overhang of skin from the abdomen).

Dermatophytoses (Tinea and Ringworm)

Fungal infections that are superficial in nature are often known as **dermatophytoses** and can be identified by the body part that they are invading (Table 37.8). The organism can come from direct contact from an animal, another person or an inanimate object. However, contact can occur from the sharing of towels, pillowcases and combs. As does candidiasis, dermatophytoses like most environments.

Nursing care

Local fungal infections are treated with topical antibiotics either as a cream, powder or solution. The length of time the antibiotic should be used for depends on the type of infection the patient has; this can vary from 1 to 4 weeks and can continue for an extra week once the infection has cleared. If the infected area is very sore, red

Table 37.8 Signs and symptoms of dermatophytoses.

NAME OF DERMATOPHYTOSES	AREA AFFECTED	SIGNS AND SYMPTOMS
Tinea pedis (athlete's foot; Figure 37.3)	Sole of foot, space between the toes and toe nails	Lesions that can appear as scaliness to fissures with drainage, accompanied by pruritus and foul smelling odour. Occurs more frequently in summer due to feet perspiring
Tinea capitis (infection of the scalp)	Scalp	Grey, round, bald spots with erythema and crusting. Temporary hair loss. More common in children than adults
Tinea corporis (infection of the body)	Anywhere on the body	Large circular patches with raised red borders; can include vesicles, papules or pustules. Very itchy
Tinea versicolor (infection of the upper chest, back and arms)	Upper chest, back and arms	Yellow, pink or brown lesions that are like sheets of scaling skin. The patches of skin contain no pigment and do not tan in sunlight
Tinea cruris (infection of the groin, thigh and buttocks)	Groin, thigh and buttocks (jock itch)	Signs and symptoms as tinea pedis. Occurs in the physically active, obese and who wear tight clothing

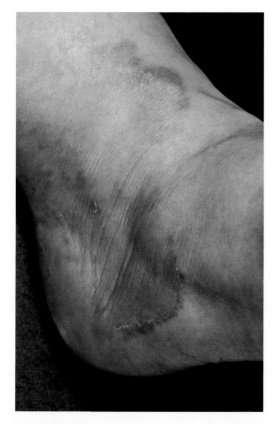

Figure 37.3 Tinea pedis. *Source*: Buxton & Morris-Jones (2009). Reproduced with permission of John Wiley & Sons Ltd.

and painful, topical steroids can be used in conjunction with the antibiotic treatment, treating and soothing the skin.

Health promotion

As fungal infections are often embarrassing and uncomfortable, it is important to promote preventative methods such as weight loss, attention to personal hygiene, such as washing and drying folds and creases well, and the wearing of clothes made of natural fibres such as cotton and linen as this enables perspiration and evaporation, keeping the skin dry and cool.

Infestations

Skin irritations and disorders can often be a result of infestations. They can affect anyone, regardless of social class or standing, but are often associated with crowded or unsanitary conditions. The most common types of infestations seen in the UK are lice, scabies, fleas and bedbugs.

Lice

An infestation of lice is known as **pediculosis**. Lice are parasites that live on humans or animals and feed off their blood. There are three types of lice infestation, named according to the part of the body affected; *pediculosis corporis* (body lice), *pediculosis pubis* (pubic lice) and *pediculosis capitis* (head lice). A typical louse is 2–4 mm in length and oval in shape. It possesses a stylet that enables it to pierce the skin to be able to feed on the host; an anticoagulant is contained within the louse's saliva to prevent clotting. While living on the host, the female louse lays eggs on the shaft of hair. These eggs are pearl-grey or brown in colour. Once hatched, the louse quickly reaches the reproductive stage of adulthood, lays eggs and then dies. The normal lifecycle of a louse is 30–50 days. The spread of lice requires hair to hair contact. Signs and symptoms include:

Head lice – an itchy scalp; on closer observation the scalp may contain sores and the eggs and the louse may be seen, especially behind the ears and on the nape of the neck

Body lice – itching, scratch marks, eczema, discoloured skin and urticaria

Pubic lice – itchy, small red spots in the pubic area and the hair matts.

Secondary infections can occur in all cases.

Scabies

The scabies mite, *Sarcoptes scabiei*, burrows into the skin to lay eggs each day for a month; 3–5 days later, the eggs hatch, travel to the surface of the skin and then burrow back down for food and security. Back in the safety of the skin, the mites lay larvae and the cycle repeats itself. Scabies tend to leave lesions 2 mm in length that are small and reddish brown in colour and often found in webspaces of the fingers, the wrists and elbow, the axillae, the nipple, the penis, belt line and gluteal crease. Common signs and symptoms include pruritus that is exacerbated at night and urticaria (an allergic response to the scabies droppings). Immunocompromised elderly patients are at risk of developing Norwegian scabies where thousand of mites are present in the body. If this is diagnosed, the Health Protection Agency is to be notified. The spread of scabies requires skin-to-skin contact.

 Link To/Go To

This link is to the advice from the Health Protection Agency regarding the management of scabies infection in the community, in particular an outbreak of Norwegian scabies:

http://www.hpa.org.uk/webc/HPAwebFile/
HPAweb_C/1194947308867

Fleas

There are many different types of flea (*Siphonaptera*), however those that most commonly affect humans are *Ctenocephalides* (cat and dog flea) and *Pulex irritans* (human flea). A flea, like lice, feeds on the blood of humans by piercing the skin and sucking on the blood. The female lays eggs on bedding, soft furnishing or carpets. After 2 weeks, the eggs hatch into larvae that feed on organic matter around them. They then pupate into a cocoon and then the flea hatches. The flea has the ability to leap some distance to source its host. The lifecycle of a flea is 3–4 weeks. Signs and symptoms include a clustering of irritating, inflamed papules, which if consistently scratched can become infected. On assessment of the skin, especially the skin folds of the waist and flexures (knees and elbows), a darkened red spot with a surrounding reddened area is seen.

Bed Bugs

Cimicidae, otherwise known as the bed bug family, spend most of their life in dark places near hosts, for example the settee, chair or bed. They do this so that at night they are then near to feed on the host, either animal or human. Bed bugs are 6–9.5 mm in size. Their bodies are flattened, oval in shape and rust coloured and they possess small wings. Once mature, a female bed bug will lay 2–3 eggs per night, The eggs take 10–20 days to hatch and this cycle is then replicated. To mature, a bed bug has to pass through five moults, which occur commonly after a feed. The bite of a bed bug leaves a firm white swelling. Signs that bed bugs are present are small spots of blood on the sheets in the morning and an almond-like smell in the room if there is a large infestation.

Nursing care

The nursing care of infestations is as follows:

Head lice – Wet combing can be done every 4 days for 4 weeks, with each wet comb taking 30 minutes per occasion, although this is not considered reliable as a standalone treatment. Parasiticidal preparations may be applied to the hair, following manufacturer's guidance and repeated after 7 days. Dimethicone, a silicone oil, can be rubbed into the hair or scalp and left for 8 hours. It coats, suffocates and kills the lice, but has no effect on the nits, so treatment has to be repeated after 7 days, when they have hatched (Burgess *et al.* 2005).

Body lice – Washing clothes and bedding in a hot wash and tumble drying kills body lice and their eggs. Close family members and partners need treating with a parasiticidal preparation, which is repeated after 7 days. Oral antihistamines should be prescribed to help reduce itching and damage to the skin.

Pubic lice – The affected area, once diagnosed with pubic lice, should be shaved or groomed with a fine comb. A pediculicide is used following manufacturer's instructions and repeated 7 days later.

Scabies – How scabies is managed depends on whether it is a single case or outbreak. Usual treatment is to apply to the whole body, paying particular attention to areas to which the scabies tend to migrate but avoiding the eyes, either a 5% permethrin cream or a lotion containing 0.5% malathion, which kills the scabies. The preparation is left on the skin as per manufacturer's instructions and then showered off. Treatment is repeated 7 days later to kill any eggs that survived and hatched into mites. Clothes, bedding and towels are washed in a hot wash and tumble-dried. Antihistamines may be prescribed to reduce the itching and damage to the skin.

Fleas – Antiseptic soaps and creams are used to prevent a secondary infection. Calamine lotion or 1% hydrocortisone may be used to ease the itching. Other treatments are aimed at killing the fleas, so spraying an insecticide (following manufacturer's guidance) and then vacuuming the carpets, beds, chairs, settee and soft furnishings and throwing away the Hoover bag when finished. This is to kill the eggs and pupae. Animals may need to be treated and veterinary advice should be sought.

Bed bugs – Advice from the pest control unit can help decide which company to use to treat the house. Cleanliness is paramount, so laundering of all bed linen, meticulous cleaning of cupboards, drawers and bed frames with hot water and vacuuming of carpets and soft furnishings is advised.

Health promotion

Household cleanliness is a key factor in the prevention of many infestations; however some infestations occur from touching or sitting close to another person who owns pets. Advice should be provided to patients and their significant others about personal hygiene, household maintenance and care of animals.

Acne

One of the most common skin disorders in the UK, acne can cause significant psychological distress. However it is both treatable and preventable if managed early. A skin condition most commonly found on the face, back and chest, acne is the partial or total obstruction of pilosebaceous ducts from hypercornification of cells (atypical accumulation of keratinocytes) lining the ducts (Figure 37.4). Acne can be both non-inflammatory and inflammatory. Non-inflammatory acne is thought to arise from the movement of melanin into the duct from adjacent epidermal cells, leading to the development of lesions called **comedones**, which can be open, such as blackheads, or closed, such as pimples and whiteheads. Inflammatory acne on the other hand consists of lesions called comedones, erythematous pustules and cysts. These are thought to develop from the obstructed ducts being colonised by bacteria, in particular *Propionibacterium* which produces substances along with the fatty acid constituents of sebum that irritate the skin. Cytokines (inflammatory mediators) are released which attracts white cells, such as polymorphs and lymphocytes, to the area and pus formation occurs as a consequence. Rupture of the comedones can occur. There are many forms of acne: the most common are

Atopic dermatitis (eczema)

- Erythema, wet 'weeping' areas, dry scaly, thickened skin
- Intensely itchy
- Risk of secondary bacterial (staphylococcal) and viral (herpes zoster) infection
- Often linked with other atopic problems, e.g. asthma and hay fever
- Some cases linked with food and environmental allergens
- Breast-feeding may reduce risk of eczema
- Treat with moisturizing creams to prevent skin drying
- Cream (water based) to wet areas
- Ointment (oil based) to dry areas
- Wet wraps to prevent drying and reduce scratching
- Topical steroids to persistent inflamed areas
- Topical (tacrolimus) and oral (ciclosporin) immunomodulators if severe
- Family support and follow-up important for chronic condition

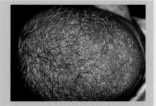

Seborrhoeic dermatitis

- Dry, scaly and erythematous
- Cradle cap in infancy
- Affects face, neck, axillae and nappy area
- May look like psoriasis

Contact dermatitis

- Erythema and weeping
- Itching
- Caused by irritants such as saliva, detergents and synthetic shoes
- Looks like atopic dermatitis

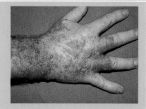

Psoriasis

- Erythematous plaques
- Silver/white scales
- Extensor surfaces
  —scalp, knees, elbows
- Guttate psoriasis—linked to streptococcal tonsillitis (antibiotic may improve skin)
- Pitting of nail bed
- Guttate psoriasis—multiple tiny psoriatic plaques over large area of body
- Treat with topical vitamin D analogues (calcipotriol), coal tar

Henoch–Schönlein purpura

- Vasculitic illness of uncertain aetiology, often follows viral illness
- Purpuric rash to buttocks and legs
- +/– Arthritis
- +/– Abdominal pain with gastrointestinal vasculitis, risk of intussusception
- +/– Nephritis (haematuria, proteinuria, hypertension) rarely renal failure
- Some evidence steroid helpful if abdominal pain severe

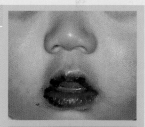

Acne*

- Very common at puberty
- Linked to androgen hormones
- Pustular erythema to face, scalp and trunk
- Treat with antibiotic erythromycin or tetracyclines (over age 12)
- Hormonal treatment with antiandrogen sometimes used
- Isotretinoin for severe cases under dermatology

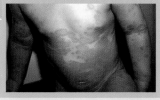

Kawasaki disease*

- Acute inflammatory systemic disorder
- Many features of infectious illness
- Fever > 5 days
- Macular erythematous rash
- Peeling skin typically at fingers and toes
- Lymphadenopathy
- Mucosal changes (cracked lips, strawberry tongue)
- Conjunctivitis
- Risk of coronary artery aneurysms
- Treat with immunoglobulin and aspirin

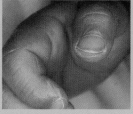

Urticaria

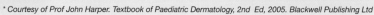

Courtesy of Prof John Harper. Textbook of Paediatric Dermatology, 2nd Ed, 2005. Blackwell Publishing Ltd

Figure 37.4 Acne.

Table 37.9 Common signs and symptoms of acne.

TYPE OF ACNE	SIGNS AND SYMPTOMS
Acne vulgaris	Common in teenagers and young to middle-aged adults Cause unknown but possible androgenic influence on sebaceous glands Can be: · Mild – a few scattered comedones and occasional papules · Moderate – presence of comedones, macules, papules and pustules · Severe – comedones, papules and pustules, painful nodules and cysts that scar and cause pigment changes
Acne conglobata	Occurs in middle years Cause unknown Serious skin lesions occur, with discharge ranging from serous to purulent. Has a foul odour

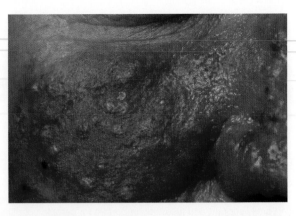

Figure 37.5 Rosacea. Source: Buxton & Morris-Jones (2009). Reproduced with permission of John Wiley & Sons Ltd.

acne vulgaris and *acne conglobata*. Table 37.9 highlights the common forms and signs and symptoms.

Nursing care

Nursing care requires a full assessment of the severity of the acne. Many dermatology specialists use the Leeds Acne Scale (Cunliffe 1994), medical photography and a quality of life indicator. General principles of care include washing twice daily with a mild cleanser or antiseptic wash. Spots should not be picked or scratched. If the pustules are tense, the traffic light guide should be used: red pustules means stop; yellow means get ready and squeeze gently; green means go to the doctor. Oral antibiotics may be ineffective if patients do not follow and take the full course. Early topical treatment can prevent scarring. Advise the patient to avoid irritant oils and non-comedogenic cosmetics and that all acne treatments are slow to respond and improvements may not be seen until 2–3 months later.

Referrals to other members of the multidisciplinary team may be advisable for further support – counselling and therapies, both skin and psychological.

Health promotion

Health promotion that would coincide with the general management advice above would be to consider a healthy nutritious diet, take exercise and avoid triggers such as stress. There is an increasing link between aggravation of acne and a diet with a high glycaemic load and dairy products (Smith *et al.* 2007).

Rosacea

Rosacea is a persistent reddening or flushing of the skin, accompanied by visible superficial facial capillaries (telangiectasia) (Figure 37.5). It is often mistaken as a side-effect of the excess consumption of alcohol. It is an under reported skin disorder, mainly affecting middle-aged and older adults. It is a chronic skin condition that affects women more than men, usually aged between 36 and 50 years, and more often than not with fair skin. Its cause is unknown but suggestions include damage to dermal connective tissue caused by the sun, which may result in damage to the endothelium of

blood vessels or abnormal vascular reactivity, and an association with those who suffer with migraine (Berth-Jones 2010). Rosacea has many subtypes and the characteristics. Symptoms and areas affected are as follows:

Erythematotelangiectatic – Signs of redness and visible superficial blood vessels, stinging and soreness around the central zone of the face.

Papulopustular – Signs of redness, flushing, papules, pustules and transient oedema. The face stings, has a burning sensation and is sore and sensitive to facial products and topical creams. This can appear on the face, chest, ears and scalp (bald men).

Phymatous – The patient has a visibly distorted shaped nose, redness and pustules on the face. The symptoms are the same as erythematotelangiectatic, however only the nose is affected.

Ocular – Only the eye is affected and this is often sore, red and can have conjunctivitis and blepharitis. The patient complains of a gritty feeling in the eyes, with blurred vision. Often, eye problems can occur before a flare-up of the skin.

Nursing care

Like all dermatological conditions that affect the face, rosacea can be very distressing and have a dramatic affect on a patient's mental well-being. With a full assessment and the completion of a dermatology quality of life index, care should then focus around factors that trigger and exacerbate the skin disorder. This can include keeping the face cool, avoiding overheating from warm rooms, baths and showers and protection of the face all year with a good sun block no less than factor 30. The nurse should also discuss the limiting of alcohol and spicy food. Skincare would focus around gentle washing with emollient face washes, avoiding soap products and the application of light non-greasy moisturisers in between treatments. Any oil-based products, both skin care and cosmetic, should be avoided. Treatment usually takes 3 months before any visible changes are noted, but is effective in the long term; topical treatments such as metronidazole and azelaic acid are prescribed and used as per dermatologist guidance. Oral antibiotics may also be prescribed.

Referrals may be made to other members of the multidisciplinary team, in particular cosmetic camouflage, dermatologists who offer laser therapy, plastic surgery for severe rhinophyma, and ophthalmology if keratitis (eye pain, sensitivity to light and blurred vision) is suspected.

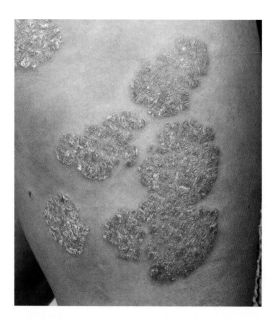

Figure 37.6 Psoriasis. Source: Buxton & Morris-Jones (2009). Reproduced with permission of John Wiley & Sons Ltd.

Health promotion

Health promotion focusses around general skin care and guidance for patients with rosacea. However the nurse must explore the side-effects of the topical agents, treatments and options to ensure informed consent. Changing Faces is a charity that can offer support to patients and their families affected by rosacea.

Psoriasis

Affecting 2–3% of the population, psoriasis is a common non-infectious, inflammatory skin disorder, that, according to Ryan (2008), offers the patient and nurse many challenges due to its unpredictable periods of exacerbation and remission.

The phase of epidermal cell proliferation is hastened in psoriasis, reducing from 28 days to only four. This acceleration does not allow the cell to mature; the nucleus remains and keratinisation does not occur. A build up of keratin transpires and the classic scales seen in a patient with psoriasis result (Figure 37.6). As the epidermis becomes thickened, blood flow to the subcutaneous layer increases and gives the psoriasis the reddened appearance that accompanies the scaly plaque. The cause of psoriasis is unknown; however, causative factors can include genetic predisposition and environmental triggers such as trauma, infection, stress, smoking, hormones, medication and sunlight. The psychological impact of psoriasis cannot be understated: not only are the plaques and scales visible to others, but when they fall off on bedding, clothes and furniture they are a constant reminder of the chronic condition. Psoriasis can occur anywhere on the body, either as a single lesion or multiple – the areas most commonly affected are elbows, knees and scalp. The nail and gluteal cleft can also be affected. The different presentations of psoriasis are outlined in Table 37.10.

Nursing care

The treatment of psoriasis is generally classified according to the severity of the skin disorder: topical for mild to moderate disease,

Table 37.10 Different presentations of psoriasis.

PRESENTATION OF PSORIASIS	SITE OF PRESENTATION	CLINICAL APPEARANCE
Plaque psoriasis	Elbows, knees and scalp	Red well-defined plaques with silver scales
Guttate psoriasis	Upper trunk and extremities, usually preceded by a throat infection	Small erythematous plaques in the shape of a raindrop
Scalp psoriasis	Scalp	Dry scaly skin to thick plaques
Flexural psoriasis	Axillae, submammary area and groin	Well-demarcated smooth plaques
Erythroderma	Entire skin	Reddening all over the body. A medical emergency as the patient will feel generally unwell
Localised pustular psoriasis	Palms and soles	Inflamed skin with yellow pustules that dry to form brown patches
Generalised pustular psoriasis	Entire skin	Inflamed skin with clusters of pustules that join together. A medical emergency. The patient may appear toxic with severe pain. Often precipitated by a course of high dose steroids (topical or systemic)

phototherapy for moderate to severe disease and systemic for severe disease. However, often patients receive a combination of treatments.

Topical treatments include the use of emollients, vitamin D analogues, tar, dithranol and topical steroids. Patients often find topical treatments messy and offensive smelling. A good nurse will discuss and support the patient undergoing this level of treatment.

When there is poor response to topical treatments, phototherapy and photochemotherapy are advised. Phototherapy entails irradiation with UVB, whereas photochemotherapy necessitates the use of a photoactive drug (psoralen) in combination with UVA irradiation (Van Onselen 2001). During this treatment, patients will attend hospital 2–3 times per week for 6 weeks. During this type of therapy, a nurse must document the patient's lifetime of exposures, as there is a risk of cutaneous malignancy with this treatment.

Patients who require systemic treatment include those who, for example, have had repeated hospital admissions, pustular psoriasis and extensive disease.

Health promotion

Health promotion centres on reducing trigger factors for the exacerbation of psoriasis and encouraging the patient to apply the topical therapies and attend for phototherapy. Keeping the skin soft and moist can offer comfort as well as avoiding itching and the use of irritating cosmetics and soaps.

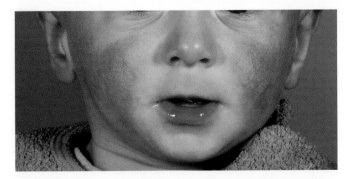

Figure 37.7 **Eczema.** Source: Buxton & Morris-Jones (2009). Reproduced with permission of John Wiley & Sons Ltd.

Eczema

Eczema (Figure 37.7) is reported to affect one in nine of the population. It is often described as an itchy, inflammatory skin disorder and it can have unfavourable affects on the sufferer and their significant others. There are many different types of eczema, each caused by different factors. **Atopic eczema** (AE) has no known cause, however scientists believe that there are genetic links; the patient has a predisposition to develop an allergic response to various substances (DermNet NZ 2011). Many patients with atopic eczema have asthma and/or hay fever: 15–20% of children and 2–10% of adults are affected. Flare-ups can often be triggered by allergies, the seasons, infection and even teething in small children (BAD 2009). Other types of eczema include irritant eczema, allergic contact eczema, food allergy, xerosis (dry skin), lichen simplex from repeated scratching, gravitational eczema, discoid eczema and seborrhoeic eczema.

Age causes the signs and symptoms of atopic eczema to differ: early in the acute phase of eczema the rash can be inflamed, weeping and blistering, in the sub-acute phase dry, scaly and burning, and in the chronic phase the skin becomes dry, thickened, fissured and excoriated. Atopic eczema can start as early as 4 months of age and can commence as a dry scaly rash on the face that may well be on the rest of the body. BAD (2009) have developed guidance on diagnosing AE and suggest that the patient can present with three of the following in conjunction with a dry, itchy rash:

- Previous history of rashes to the back of the knees and elbows
- Family history or medical history of asthma and or hay fever
- Tendency to dry skin
- Onset under 2 years of age.

Nursing care

A full history is required when assessing a patient with eczema. This will help identify the type of eczema, the triggers and causative factors in order to focus treatment and management. The nurse should also be aware of the possibility of complications resulting from a secondary infection from bacteria, a virus or fungi, as this can often become a medical emergency. Once the type and cause has been ascertained, then the treatment will focus on removing the trigger factors, keeping nails short and avoiding scratching.

The most important aspect of management is regular use of emollients to moisturise the skin. This can be supplemented with topical steroids to reduce inflammation, antibiotics to treat infection and antihistamines to reduce pruritus. More serious cases may need referral for immunomodulatory treatments, phototherapy and immunosuppressive drugs. Patients may need other therapies in relation to body image and psychological issues.

Health promotion

Health promotion focusses around removing the causative factors, moisturising of the skin, a well-balanced diet and self-help and support.

What the Experts Say

Having eczema on her hands really affected my 9-year-old daughter's life. Previously she was a really happy child, apparently always putting her hand up at school and joining in activities. One day, I was rung by the school who were asking what had happened to my daughter. They had noticed a dramatic change in her behaviour, she was now quiet, did not get involved in activities and was always tucking her hands in her jumper or cardigan; they asked if anything was going on at home and wanted me to come in to speak with them about her. We agreed on a group meeting and she just blurted it out; she was ashamed of her hands and wished they would heal up. I could not believe that I had missed something so simple.

(Scarlett Taylor, mother of Matilda who is 9)

Jot This Down

What advice can you give to patients with a skin disorder in relation to nutrition? Which nutrients are essential to optimise the skin's condition and why?

Skin Tumours

Often, some lesions found on the skin are malignant in aetiology; this is frequently due to long-term exposure to the environment and sun. The three main types of malignant lesions are **actinic keratosis, non-melanoma skin cancer** and **melanoma**.

Actinic Keratosis

Premalignant epidermal lesions that occur due to long-term exposure to the sun are known as actinic keratosis. The lesions are small, shiny but scaly, erythematous rough macules found on the face, upper trunk, forearms and dorsa of the hands in patches. They are considered as premalignant lesions and signs that suggest transformation include enlargement or ulceration.

Non-melanoma Skin Cancer

Basal cell and squamous cell cancer are malignant tumours of the skin. They are mainly found in adults over the age of 30, in men more than women, and in those with fair hair and blue eyes. Rates of new cases are rising rapidly and it is suggested that almost 100 000 new cases of these types of skin cancers occur each year (Cancer Research UK 2013). Other risk factors include red hair, freckles, green eyes, family history of skin cancer, unprotected or repeated exposure to the sun, radiation treatment, occupational exposure (coal, tar, pitch, asphalt), sunburns as a child and lowered immunity due to medication.

Basal cell cancer

Basal cell cancer is the most common form of skin cancer, and most likely to recur, but it is the least aggressive; 75 out of every 100 cases of skin cancer are basal cell in origin (Cancer Research UK 2013). Basal cells are found in the basal layer of the epidermis and the cancer that originates from them is thought to develop from the cells having an impaired ability to mature into keratinocytes. This causes a solid neoplasm to grow, destroying around it skin, nerves, blood vessels, lymphatic tissue, cartilage and bone. Although this type of cancer rarely metastasises it can destroy body parts such as the nose or eyelid. There are different types of basal cell cancer: nodular, superficial, pigmented, morpheaform and keratotic.

Nodular cancers are the most common and initially look like a smooth pimple that is itchy. This papule progressively grows, doubling its size every 6–12 months. The epidermis thins but remains intact as the cancer grows, often with the skin having a pearly white appearance that is shiny with visible telangiectasia. As the cancer grows, ulceration may occur either in the centre or at the periphery. This may bleed when knocked; it has well-defined borders.

Superficial cancers appear as flat erythematous papules or plaques. These too can ulcerate and can appear covered with crusts or erosions. They are often found on the trunk and extremities.

Pigmented basal cell cancer occurs on the face, neck and head and concentrates the melanin pigment from the skin into the centre of the lesion, thus the appearance of this form of skin cancer is dark brown, blue or black with a shiny well-defined border.

Morpheaform basal cell cancer is very rare; it resembles a flesh-coloured scar along a tissue plane and is usually found on the head and neck.

Keratotic basal cell cancer is a square-like lesion located on the groove at the front of and behind the ear.

Squamous cell cancers

Squamous cell carcinoma develops from proliferating keratinising cells of the squamous epithelium. It permeates the epidermis, over-runs the dermis and grows into irregular-shaped lesions. Pre-existing skin disorders such as scars and actinic keratosis can develop into squamous cell carcinoma. Metastases are common via the lymphatic system and the development of secondaries is dependent on the size and site of the initial tumour.

Skin that is exposed to sunlight and weather such as on the legs, arms and face is most commonly where squamous cell cancers occur. This malignant cancer of the squamous epithelium (either skin or mucous membranes) is more aggressive than its basal cell counterpart and has the potential to metastasise. It can also occur on skin that has been burned or had periods of chronic inflammation. The cancer initially starts as a small red nodule, which may or may not have crusts on it; as the cancer develops it can bleed and become painful and indurated.

Malignant Melanoma

Melanocytes, cells that produce the pigment melanin in the basal layer of the skin, are where melanomas occur – a third of them originating in pre-existing moles. The characteristics of a melanoma are a slow developing, symmetrical, flat lesion, more than 6 mm in diameter. Initially, they are classified as malignant melanoma *in situ*. These are considered benign but have the potential to infiltrate the dermis and metastasise by spreading through the blood and lymph network. The melanoma's characteristics change to a raised nodular appearance with satellite lesions around the margins.

Table 37.11 Types and clinical presentations of malignant melanomas.

TYPE OF MELANOMA	CLINICAL PRESENTATION
Superficial spreading melanoma	2 cm in diameter, flat, scaly and crusty lesions, found on the trunk and back of men and legs of women. Begins as mixture of tan, brown and black in colour in the radial phase and to red, white and blue in the vertical phase
Nodular melanoma	Raised, dome-shaped, blue, black or red nodules found on the head, neck and trunk. Looks like a blood blister, which can ulcerate and bleed. Only has a vertical growth phase, which makes this an aggressive form of melanoma, and metastasises usually before diagnosis
Acral lentiginous melanoma	Usually commences as a flat tan, brown or black coloured lesion to an elevated nodule approximately 3 cm in diameter. Found on the soles of the feet, palms of the hands, mucous membranes and nail beds. Affects men and women equally, usually in their 50s and 60s.

People with fair skin are 10 times more at risk of melanoma than those with dark skins and those who have had prolonged exposure to the sun. Strangely, those who are middle-class and predominantly work indoors are more at risk than others, usually because of the number of occasions they have suffered repeated sunburn with blistering, sunburn as a child and holidays in countries with powerful sun exposure. Nevertheless, melanomas can occur in those patients who do not over expose themselves to the sun, or in skin covered by clothes and lesions already present on the body. Other risk factors include people with lots of freckles and precursor moles, regular use of sunbeds, family history, previous history of skin cancer, lowered immunity, being a woman over 50, higher body mass index in men and working with chemicals.

Melanomas account for 10% of all skin cancers and 79% of skin cancer deaths (Cancer Research UK 2013). Several factors determine the prognosis for patients with a melanoma; these include tumour thickness, presence of ulceration, site, age, gender and metastasis.

Malignant melanomas are classified using Clark's 5 levels of staging, from level 1, where the melanoma grows parallel to the skin surface, to grade 5, where there is invasion of the epidermis, dermis and subcutaneous tissue increasing the risk of metastasis (vertical growth phase). Table 37.11 highlights the types of melanoma and their clinical presentations.

Nursing care

Treatment for skin cancers depends on whether the skin cancer is diagnosed at an early, medium or advanced stage (Cancer Research UK 2013). All patients undergo a thorough medical examination and assessment and are then offered treatment options as follows:

Early stage (Clark's level 1) – wide local excision of the lesion under local or general anaesthetic, depending on how large the lesion is, with or without sentinel lymph node biopsy where a small amount of dye is or radioactive substance is injected into where the cancer was removed. The dye drains away into the lymph glands and the surgeon can see when the dye reaches the lymph glands or measure the radioactivity of the glands with a scanner. These nodes that are visible or measurable are called sentinel nodes and are excised and sent for testing to see if they contain melanoma cells. If the results are positive other lymph nodes are removed at a later date.

Medium stage (Clark's levels 2 and 3) – same surgery as level 1 (wide local excision and sentinel node biopsy with potential lymph node removal), with adjuvant treatment such as chemotherapy, radiotherapy and biological therapy (the use of interferon only in rare instances because of the side-effects).

Advanced stage (Clark's levels 4 and 5) – the treatment and management of these stages of cancer will depend on the spread of metastasis, symptoms currently experienced by the patient and prior treatments. Surgery and adjuvant therapies may be offered, however palliation may be the only plan with symptom control. Other members of the multidisciplinary team would be involved including the Specialist Nurses (Skin cancer, Macmillan, District), GP and oncologist. Plans for end of life care may need to put in place with support for the family and significant others.

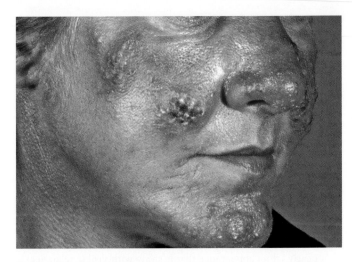

Figure 37.8 Haemangiomas and naevi. Source: Buxton & Morris-Jones (2009). Reproduced with permission of John Wiley & Sons Ltd.

Link To/Go To

The British Association of Dermatologists has produced guidance on the management of basal cell and malignant melanomas:

http://www.bad.org.uk/site/622/default.aspx

Health promotion

Health promotion in the care of patients with skin cancer will focus around attending for follow-up, checking the skin on a regular basis for other moles, lesions, growths and swellings and checking lymph nodes. A nurse would also discuss the importance of care of the skin in the sun, eating a well-balanced diet, taking exercise, returning to work or social activities, giving up any habits that impact on the patient's health and well-being and offering support and referral to others for emotional well-being. For advanced stages of melanoma, health promotion will focus around quality of life and symptom management issues.

Vascular Disorders (Including Naevi)

Benign vascular skin disorders are much more common than malignant ones, so it is imperative that a nurse is able to recognise and differentiate between the various types of lesions in order to offer support and guidance to patients. Many require identification and the reassurance that no clinical treatment is required.

Angiomas

Angiomas, otherwise known as 'haemangiomas' (abnormal proliferation of capillaries), and naevi (moles), flat or raised macules and papules with well-rounded and defined borders, commonly appear on child and adult skin (see Figure 37.8) in various forms:

Venous lakes, found on the back of the hands, ears and lips of older adults, present as small, flat, blue blood vessels.

Spider angiomas (small red papules with radiating lines) occur on the face, neck and upper chest. They are superficial dilated arteries and are usually associated with puberty, pregnant women, those take the contraceptive pill and patients with hepatic disease.

Telangiectases appear like broken veins on the nose and cheeks. They are commonly found in older adults and are the result of photoaged skin.

Cherry angiomas occur at any age and appear as small, red to purple, rounded papules. They are most common in the over 40s and increase in number the older a person gets.

Naevus flammeus (port-wine stain) is a vascular lesion that develops congenitally. The light red to dark purple lesion appears on the face or upper body as macular patches, is often present at birth and grows proportionately with the child.

Mongolian blue spot is a variant of a blue naevus and resembles a large bruise over the lumbo-sacral area of babies, especially from Asian and Afro-Caribbean families. Most fade by injury but they can be mistaken for accidental injuries.

Blue naevus begins from melanocytes in the basal layer of the epidermis. It appears as a smooth, round, raised, blue, black lesion in late childhood on the hands, face or feet and is only 1 cm in diameter. These remain for the life of the patient.

Spitz naevus is a fast growing lesion that appears on the face of children or pregnant women. The lesion is single, red or orange in colour and, because of its rapid growth, is almost always excised.

Becker's naevus affects the skin of men in puberty on the chest and shoulders. It is visible as a faint pigment with hypertrichosis (abnormal amount of hair growth) and often occurs after being burnt by the sun.

Strawberry naevus is a raised haemangioma that grows rapidly in the first year of life. There are two types: *capillary*, superficial, which fades and disappears by the age of 5–7 years; and *cavernous*, which can impair organ functions such as the eye, nose, mouth and genitals, and can often itch or bleed.

Nursing care

Nursing care is often just supporting and educating patients to understand that many of the lesions are benign and do not require any treatment. If the lesions are unsightly, causing emotional and psychological distress and affecting the patient's quality of life, then referral to a dermatologist, cosmetic camouflage team or psychologist may be of benefit. Occasionally some benign vascular lesions do require further management and this can be surgical excision, cryosurgery, laser therapy, cold point cautery and shave biopsy.

Health promotion

The main focus of health promotion for the nurse for patients with vascular lesion is to offer advice on skin protection in the sun and support from other services in relation to cosmesis and body image.

Disorders of the Hair and Nails

Nails

When assessing a patient in clinical practice it is considered good practice to always take note of their nails, as an underlying condition or problem may be highlighted. Common conditions that affect the nail bed are listed in Table 37.12 and shown in Figure 37.9.

Table 37.12 Common conditions and the effect on the nail bed.

CONDITION	EFFECT ON NAIL BED
Anxiety, depression or compulsive disorders	Nail biting, paronychia, periungual warts
Median nail dystrophy usually caused by an underlying psychological condition	Longitudinal depression along the nail bed with an enlarged lunula
Psoriasis	Pitting of the nail plate, onycholysis (separation of the free edge of the nail plate which whitens) and dystrophy (thickened, opaque and discoloured nail)
Alopecia areata, eczema, Reiter's syndrome and pemphigus	Pitting of the nail plate
Eczema, lichen planus, periungual warts, fungal infections of the nail, iron deficiency anaemia, thyrotoxicosis and sarcoidosis	Onycholysis
Psoriasis acrodermatitis continua of Hallopeau	Dystrophy
Eczema	Nail shedding
Trauma, rheumatoid arthritis and bacterial endocarditis	Splinter haemorrhages
Systemic lupus, erythematosus, dermatomyositis, sarcoidosis and HIV	Periungual erythema
Terry's half and half-nail (proximal part whitens)	Renal failure, liver cirrhosis, congestive cardiac failure, type 2 diabetes

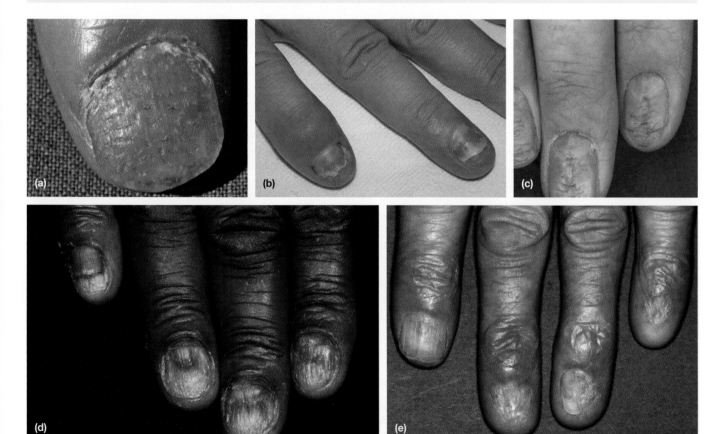

Figure 37.9 Nail disorders: (a) pitting of nail, (b) nail psoriasis, (c) nail eczema, (d) lichen planus and (e) dystrophy due to lupus. Source: Buxton & Morris-Jones (2009). Reproduced with permission of John Wiley & Sons Ltd.

Hair

During a normal lifecycle, hair is constantly falling out and new hairs growing. However, when changes to the hair occur, the consequences can make the patient both embarrassed and upset and having the potential of significant psychological problems, as the potential to have healthy hair has been dramatically affected. There are many hair problems that can occur, from disproportionate oiliness to a dry flaky scalp. Some are due to infections, others allergic responses, but all have some level of inflammation; hair loss can occur as a consequence. Table 37.13 highlights common diseases and disorders of the scalp.

Nursing care

Nursing care of hair and nails will always concentrate around treating and managing the causative factor. This may require the taking of nail clippings for further investigation, treatments varying from topical applications, phototherapy and systemic treatments, referral to other members of the multidisciplinary team for advice and psychological support for the patient and, in some instances, the obtaining of wigs and hairpieces. General care of hair and nails in most skin disorders is to ensure that hair is kept clean and styles are altered accordingly, and nails are kept short.

Health promotion

The nurse would focus on promoting the eating of a well-balanced diet, avoiding trigger factors and ensuring that the patient concords with treatment options.

Connective Tissue Disorders

Connective tissue disorders comprise a wide range of autoimmune diseases and are often associated with specific autoantibodies

Table 37.13 Common disorders of the scalp.

NAME OF HAIR DISORDER/DISEASE	SIGNS AND SYMPTOMS
Seborrhoea – excessive production of sebum	Excessive oiliness of hair and scalp
Seborrhoeic dermatitis – dermatitis of the scalp	Seen as cradle cap in babies. Flaking of whitish to brown scales from the scalp, greasy crusts on the scalp that turn yellow brown when they fall off, inflamed boggy patches under the crusts, extension of inflammation to ears, eyebrows, eyelids, cheeks and nostrils, and pruritus
Tinea capitis – a fungal infection of the scalp (see Figure 37.10)	Non-inflammatory – where hairs are made to appear grey because of the dusting of fungi, the scalp has reddish patches and scaling, hairs break just above the follicle. Inflammatory – hair follicles are inflamed with moist patches and broken hairs; discharge and pus may be visible, itching is intense Black dot – black dots of infected hairs are seen in the scalp, these are broken hairs just above the follicle; accompanied by inflammation
Bacterial and viral infections of the scalp	Bacterial infections – abscesses can occur, the scalp is inflamed and painful; folliculitis can be present Viral infections – can be caused by herpes simplex or zoster and inflamed oozing lesions can appear
Head lice	Red swollen patches in areas. Louse may be visible as may brown or silvery white nits attached to the hair shaft, particularly around the nape of the neck and ears
Psoriasis	Red, scaly, silvery white lesions and plaques to the scalp
Lichen planus – inflammatory disorder of the mucous membranes and skin	Violet papules, 2–10 mm in size, that are intensely itchy, thicken over time and become dark red and form hypertrophic lichen planus
Lupus erythematosus – autoimmune condition of the skin and organs	Patchy skin inflammation, scaling of the skin, plugging of the follicles and telangiectasia
Alopecia areata – an autoimmune disorder of the scalp	Small localised patches of hair loss to scalp and beard to complete hair loss, including eyebrows
Androgenic alopecia – male and female pattern hair loss	Begins with thinning of the hair with a receding hairline at the frontotemporal area
Trauma traction alopecia – alopecia developing at the site of a hairstyle that constantly pulls on the hair	Bald areas between plaits and ponytails
Trichotillomania – self-inflicted hair loss	Patches of hair loss which are geometrical, small or single patches without scarring. Usually psychological cause to the hair pulling
Telogen effluvium – hair loss following childbirth, chemotherapy or drugs	Can vary from thinning to complete hair loss of all body hair
Acne	The scalp may be affected by acne that is: Mild – a few scattered comedones and occasional papules Moderate – presence of comedones, macules, papules and pustules Severe – comedones, papules and pustules, painful nodules and cysts that scar and cause pigment changes
Allergic or irritant dermatitis of the scalp	Itchy inflammation of the scalp caused by a reaction to an external agent

(blood proteins) that aid their diagnosis. They occur when the body's own immune system mistakenly attacks the body tissues, causing an inflammatory reaction. Connective tissue is found in all body organs and its role is to support the organs, as it is made from elastin and collagen. If attacked by the immune system, the tissue becomes inflamed and can consequently result in cell death.

The most common connective tissue disorder that affects the skin is discoid lupus erythematosus (DLE).

Discoid lupus erythematosus (Figure 37.11) is considered a chronic long-term condition and affects 12–48 people per 100 000. It is most common in women aged between 20 and 40 years of age and is thought to be triggered by underlying genetic factors, smoking, exposure to UV light and certain drugs such as non-steroidals. Of patients with DLE, 5% may develop SLE.

At the outset, the patient presents with symptomless erythematous plaques or papules that can spread and merge, to sun-exposed areas of the skin. The lesions then become thickened and scaly, often with hypopigmentation, follicular plugging and hyperpigmentation of the lesion's edges; the lesions can then become itchy and painful. Once the lesions resolve, they leave scars.

Nursing care

Care of the patient with DLE concentrates on controlling the rash and preventing spread and recurrence by reducing exposure to the triggering factors. Topical steroids are prescribed, usually beginning with quite potent levels and reducing these on a sliding scale over weeks of treatment to moderate and then mild steroids. Antimalarial drugs such as hydroxychloroquine (200 mg daily) should also be offered as first-line treatment, increasing to twice daily when tolerated, reminding the patient that any visible change will not be noticed for 4–6 weeks. It is important for the nurse and patient to look out for potential side-effects of the medication such as retinal toxicity and visual disturbances and inform the doctor of these immediately.

Red Flag

The use of topical steroids should be confined to the affected areas of skin and under the instructions of a doctor or nurse specialist as they can have serious side-effects if used long term or incorrectly. The amount applied to the skin should be according to the finger tip unit rule, using the patient's finger tip size as the rule, not your own, if you are applying the topical steroids for them.

Affected Body Area	Quantity of Cream/Ointment
Both sides of one hand	1 finger tip unit
One foot	2 finger tip units
One arm	3 finger tip units
One leg	6 finger tip units
Chest and abdomen	7 finger tip units
Back and buttocks	7 finger tip units

Health promotion

Health promotion is aimed at reducing the trigger factors, such as smoking cessation, avoiding exposure to UV rays by wearing protective clothing, using factor 30 sunscreen and avoiding going outdoors when it is sunny between 11 a.m. and 3 p.m. As with most dermatological conditions, consider referral to other members of the multidisciplinary team such as psychologists and the cosmetic camouflage team.

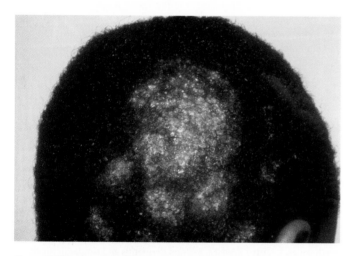

Figure 37.10 Tinea capitis. Source: Buxton & Morris-Jones (2009). Reproduced with permission of John Wiley & Sons Ltd.

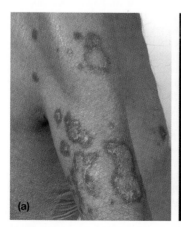
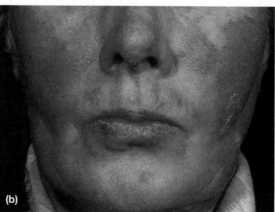

(a) (b)

Figure 37.11 Lupus erythematosus. Source: Buxton & Morris-Jones (2009). Reproduced with permission of John Wiley & Sons Ltd.

Conclusion

Dermatology conditions are a major part of the primary care workload, and the incidence of skin conditions is rising. Skin conditions affect all age groups and although problems such as eczema and acne can be considered minor in biomedical terms they actually present the patient with considerable psychological challenges (Rumsey *et al.* 2002). The role of the nurse in caring for patients with skin disorders involves the use of the nursing process, in particular a thorough assessment, planning and implementation of smart realistic and patient-centred care and regular evaluation.

Key Points

- This chapter has provided the reader with an overview of the structures of the skin, hair and nails.
- An understanding of the processes involved in the way wounds heal has been offered.
- The nurse is required to undertake a holistic assessment of the patient with a skin disorder in order to provide care that is safe and effective, as well as meeting the individual needs of the person and recognising the effect of the psyche on the skin.
- An emphasis has been made with regard to the importance of using correct terminology in the assessment and management of skin disorders.
- There are a number of investigations that can be undertaken to aid diagnosis and management of skin disorders and the nurse should assist the person pre, peri and post investigation, explaining the rationale for the investigations and the care required after the investigation has been completed.
- This chapter has provided a review of common skin conditions, the care required, clinical management and the involvement of members of the multidisciplinary team.
- High quality care requires the nurse to promote health and well-being, self-care and independence, by teaching and empowering people and carers to make choices in coping with the effects of treatment.

Glossary

Acral: acral distribution of a dermatosis means it affects distal portions of limbs (hand, foot) and head (ears, nose)
Annular: annular distribution refers to lesions grouped in a circle
Atrophy: atrophy occurs when some component of the skin has shrunk
Crusting: crust occurs when plasma exudes through an eroded epidermis and dries on the skin surface. It is rough on the surface and is yellow or brown in colour. Bloody crust appears red, purple or black
Dermatologist: the medical specialist in diseases of skin, hair and nails
Distribution: the distribution of a dermatosis refers to how the skin lesions are scattered or spread out
Flexural distribution: flexural distribution of a dermatosis involves the flexures, i.e. the body folds
Follicular: follicular distribution of a dermatosis refers to individual lesions arising from hair follicles, e.g. acne

Hyperpigmentation: darkening of the pigment of the skin
Hypopigmentation: lightening of the pigment of the skin
Induration: induration is skin that feels hard and thickened
Lesion: a lesion is any single area of altered skin. It may be solitary or multiple
Macule: a macule is a small area of colour change, often defined as less than 1.5 cm diameter. The surface is **smooth**
Nodule: a nodule is an enlargement of a papule in three dimensions (height, width, length). It is a solid lesion more than 1 cm in diameter
Papule: papules are small palpable lesions. The usual definition is that they are less than 1 cm diameter. They are raised above the skin surface, and may be **solitary** or **multiple**
Plaque: a plaque is a palpable flat lesion usually greater than 1 cm diameter
Polymorphic: a polymorphic eruption means the lesions may have varied shapes
Pustule: a pustule is a collection of pus. It is filled with neutrophils, and may be white, or yellow. Not all pustules are infected
Scaling: scaling or hyperkeratosis is an increase in the dead cells on the surface of the skin (stratum corneum)
Telangiectasia: telangiectasia is the name given to prominent cutaneous blood vessels. They are red or purple in colour
Vesicle: vesicles are small fluid-filled blisters less than 1 cm in diameter. They may be single or multiple. The fluid may be clear or blood-stained

References

BAD (2009) *Guidelines for the Management of Atopic Eczema.* British Association of Dermatologists, London. http://www.pcds.org.uk/images/stories/pcdsbad-eczema.pdf

BAD (2011) *Quality Standards for Dermatology.* British Association of Dermatologists, London. http://www.bad.org.uk/shared/get-file.ashx?itemtype=document&id=795

Berth-Jones, J. (2010) Rosacea, perioral dermatitis and similar dermatoses. In: T. Burns, S. Breathnach, N. Cox & C. Griffiths (eds) *Rook's Textbook of Dermatology,* 8th edn., pp. 1–6. Wiley-Blackwell, Oxford.

Burgess, I.F., Brown, C.M. & Lee, P.N. (2005) Treatment of head louse infestation with 4% dimethicone lotion: Randomised controlled equivalence trial. *British Medical Journal* 330(7505), 1423.

Cancer Research UK (2013) *Skin Cancer Diagnosis and Treatment Statistics.* http://www.cancerresearchuk.org/cancer-info/cancerstats/types/skin/treatment/

Changing Faces (2012) *Look at Me: integrated care for people with skin conditions.* Preliminary Report. https://www.changingfaces.org.uk/downloads/Look%20at%20Me%20preliminary%20report%202012%20final.pdf

Cunliffe, W. (1994) *New Approaches to Acne Treatment.* Martin Dunitz, London.

DermNet NZ (2011) *The Causes of Atopic Dermatitis (Eczema).* http://www.dermnetnz.org/dermatitis/atopic-causes.html (accessed 25 August 2013).

DH (2008). *Guidance on the Routine Collection of Patient Reported Outcome Measures (PROMs).* For the NHS in England 2009/10. Department of Health, London.

Gagliardi, A.M., Gomes Silva, B.N., Torloni, M.R. & Soares, B.G. (2012) Vaccines for preventing herpes zoster in older adults. *Cochrane Database Systematic Reviews,* (10):CD008858.

Lang, P.G. (2000) Dermatoses in African-Americans. *Dermatology Nursing*, 12(2), 87–98.

Lawton, S. (2001) Assessing the patient with a skin condition. *Journal of Tissue Viability*, 11(3), 113–115.

Lawton, S. (2002) *Assessing the Patient with a Skin Condition*. World Wide Wounds. http://www.worldwidewounds.com/2002/may/Lawton/Skin-Assessment-Dermatology-Patient.html (accessed 21 August 2013).

Lin, C. (2011) *Eczema herpeticum*. DermNet NZ. http://www.dermnetnz.org/viral/eczema-herpeticum.html (22/08/13)

Nazarko, L. (2011) Fungal skin infections and HCAs: identify, treat and act. *British Journal of Healthcare Assistants*, 4(11), 551–553.

NHS (2011) *Hospital Episode Statistics. Primary diagnosis: summary*. NHS Information Centre, NHS Statistics, London.

Rumsey, N., Clarke, A., & Musa, M. (2002) Altered body image: the psychosocial needs of patients. *British Journal of Community Nursing*, 7(11), 563–566.

Ryan, S. (2008) Psoriasis: characteristics, psychosocial effects and treatment options. *British Journal of Nursing*, 17(5), 284–290.

Schofield, J.K., Fleming, D., Grindlay, D. & Williams, H. (2011) Skin conditions are the commonest new reason people present to general practitioners in England and Wales. *British Journal of Dermatology*, 165(5), 1044–1050.

Smith, R.N., Mann, N.J., Braue, A., Mäkeläinen, H., & Varigos, G.A. (2007) A low-glycemic-load diet improves symptoms in acne vulgaris patients. *American Journal of Clinical Nutrition*, 86(1), 107–115.

Thomas, D.R. (2005) Psychosocial effects of acne. *Journal of Cutaneous Medicine and Surgery*, 8(Suppl 4), 3–5.

Tseng, H.F., Smith, N., Harpaz, R., Bialek, S.R., Sy, L.S., & Jacobsen, S.J. (2011) Herpes zoster vaccine in older adults and the risk of subsequent herpes zoster. *Journal of the American Medical Association*, 305(2), 160–166.

Van Onselen, J. (2001) Psoriasis. In: E. Hughes & J. Van Onselen (eds) *Dermatology Nursing: A Practical Guide*. Churchill Livingstone, Edinburgh.

Zaidi, Z. & Lanigan, S.W. (2010) *Dermatology in Clinical Practice*. Springer-Verlag, London.

Test Yourself

1. What percentage of the population is affected by a skin disorder?
   (a) 10%
   (b) 50%
   (c) 80%
   (d) 54%

2. What components are necessary in the assessment of a patient as according to Lawton?
   (a) A general assessment of the patient, an assessment of the patient's knowledge and a physical assessment
   (b) A general assessment of the patient, an assessment of the patient's emotional state and a physical state
   (c) A general assessment of the patient, an assessment of the skin and assessment of the emotional state
   (d) A general skin assessment, an assessment of the patient's knowledge and a physical assessment

3. What information should be collated about the lesions when assessing the patient's skin?
   (a) The lesions' shape, colour, site and texture
   (b) The lesions' distribution, pigmentation, site and location
   (c) The lesions' colour, texture, site and personal opinion of the patient
   (d) The distribution, character and shape of lesions, the site and location

4. What is hypopigmentation?
   (a) Darkening of the pigment of the skin
   (b) Lightening of the pigment of the skin
   (c) Linear pigmented marks of the skin
   (d) Stretch marks

5. What is a bulla?
   (a) A flat circumscribed area of colour change that can be brown, red, white or tan
   (b) An elevated, circumscribed, superficial fluid-filled blister less than 5 mm in diameter
   (c) A vesicle greater than 5 mm in diameter
   (d) A vesicle greater than 10 mm in radius

6. What is a crust defined as?
   (a) Thickened, flaky exfoliation, irregular, thick or thin, dry or oily, variable size, silver, white or tan in colour
   (b) Dried serum, blood or purulent exudate; slightly elevated; size variable
   (c) Loss of epidermis caused by scratching
   (d) Rough, thickened epidermis, accentuated skin markings due to scratching

7. What bacteria cause folliculitis?
   (a) *Pseudomonas* and *Streptococcus*
   (b) *Pseudomonas* and coliforms
   (c) *Staphylococcus* and *Streptococcus*
   (d) *Staphylococcus aureus* and *Pseudomonas aeruginosa*

8. How long does the lifecycle of a louse last?
   (a) 30–50 days
   (b) 35–50 days
   (c) 20–40 days
   (d) 30–40 days

9. What other two conditions do sufferers of atopic asthma commonly have?
   (a) Asthma and psoriasis
   (b) Asthma and dermatitis
   (c) Asthma and hayfever
   (d) Hayfever and psoriasis

10. What staging system is used to grade the severity of skin cancer?
   (a) John's
   (b) Wood's
   (c) Clark's
   (d) Smith's

Answers

1. d
2. a
3. d
4. b
5. c
6. b
7. d
8. a
9. c
10. c

Appendix A Reference Values in Venous Serum (Adults)

Analysis	Reference range	
	SI units	Non-SI units
Albumin	36–47 g/L	3.6–4.7 g/100 mL
Alkaline phosphatase	40–125 U/L	–
Amylase	<100 U/L	–
Bilirubin (total)	2–17 μmol/L	0.12–1.0 mg/100 mL
Calcium	2.12–2.62 mmol/L	4.24–5.24 mEq/L or 8.50–10.50 mg/100 mL
Chloride	95–107 mmol/L	95–107 mEq/L
Cholesterol (total)	<5.5 mmol/L	–
HDL-cholesterol		
Male	0.5–1.6 mmol/L	19–62 mg/100 mL
Female	0.6–1.9 mmol/L	23–74 mg/100 mL
Copper	13–24 μmol/L	83–153 μg/100 mL
Creatine kinase (total)		
Male	30–200 mmol/L	–
Female	30–150 mmol/L	–
Creatinine	55–120 μmol/L	0.62–1.36 mg/100 mL
Ferritin		
Male	17–300 μg/L	17–300 ng/mL
Female	14–150 μg/L	14–150 ng/mL
Glucose (fasting)	3.6–5.8 mmol/L	65–104 mg/100 mL
Glycated haemoglobin (HbA$_1$)	5.0–6.5%	–
Immunoglobulin A	0.5–4.0 g/L	50–400 mg/100 mL
Immunoglobulin G	5.0–13.0 g/L	500–1300 mg/100 mL
Immunoglobulin M		
Male	0.3–2.2 g/L	30–220 mg/100 mL
Female	0.4–2.5 g/L	40–250 mg/100 mL
Iron		
Male	14–32 μmol/L	78–178 μg/100 mL
Female	10–28 μmol/L	56–156 μg/100 mL
Magnesium	0.75–1.0 mmol/L	1.5–2.0 mEq/L or 1.82–2.43 mg/100 mL
Osmolality	280–290 mmol/kg	280–290 mosm/L

Nursing Practice: Knowledge and Care, First Edition. Edited by Ian Peate, Karen Wild and Muralitharan Nair.
© 2014 John Wiley & Sons, Ltd. Published 2014 by John Wiley & Sons, Ltd. Companion website: www.wileynursingpractice.com

Analysis	Reference range	
	SI units	Non-SI units
Phosphate (fasting)	0.8–1.4 mmol/L	2.48–4.34 mg/100 mL
Potassium (plasma)	3.3–4.7 mmol/L	3.3–4.7 mEq/L
Potassium (serum)	3.6–5.1 mmol/L	3.6–5.1 mEq/L
Protein (total)	60–80 g/L	6–8 g/100 mL
Sodium	132–144 mmol/L	132–144 mEq/L
Total CO_2	24–30 mmol/L	24–30 mEq/L
Transferrin	2.0–4.0 g/L	0.2–0.4 g/100 mL
Triglycerides (fasting)	0.6–1.7 mmol/L	53–150 mg/100 mL
Urate		
Male	0.12–0.42 mmol/L	2.0–7.0 mg/100 mL
Female	0.12–0.36 mmol/L	2.0–6.0 mg/100 mL
Urea	2.5–6.6 mmol/L	15–40 mg/100 mL
Zinc	11–22 μmol/L	72–144 μg/100 mL
Haematological values		
Bleeding time (Ivy)	Less than 8 minutes	–
Body fluid (total)	50% (obese) to 70% (lean) of body weight	–
Intracellular	30–40% of body weight	–
Extracellular	20–30% of body weight	–
Blood volume		
Male	75 ± 10 mL/kg	–
Female	70 ± 10 mL/kg	–
Coagulation screen		
Prothrombin time	8.0–10.5 seconds	–
Activated partial thromboplastin time	26–37 seconds	–
Erythrocyte sedimentation rate[a]		
Adult male	0–10 mm/h	–
Adult female	3–15 mm/h	–
Fibrinogen	1.5–4.0 g/L	0.15–0.4 g/100 mL
Folate		
Serum	1.5–20.6 μg/L	1.5–20.6 ng/mL
Red cell	95–570 μg/L	95–570 ng/mL
Haemoglobin		
Male	130–180 g/L	13–18 g/100 mL
Female	115–165 g/L	11.5–16.5 g/100 mL
Leucocytes (adults)	$4.0–11.0 \times 10^9$/L	$4.0–11.0 \times 10^3$/mm³
Differential white cell count		
Neutrophil granulocytes	$2.0–7.5 \times 10^9$/L	$2.0–7.5 \times 10^3$/mm³
Lymphocytes	$1.5–4.0 \times 10^9$/L	$1.5–4.0 \times 10^3$/mm³
Monocytes	$0.2–0.8 \times 10^9$/L	$0.2–0.8 \times 10^3$/mm³
Eosinophil granulocytes	$0.04–0.4 \times 10^9$/L	$0.04–0.4 \times 10^3$/mm³
Basophil granulocytes	$0.01–0.1 \times 10^9$/L	$0.01–0.1 \times 10^3$/mm³
Packed cell volume (PCV) or haematocrit		
Male	0.40–0.54	–
Female	0.37–0.47	–
Platelets	$150–350 \times 10^9$/L	$150–350 \times 10^3$/mm³

(Continued)

Analysis	Reference range	
	SI units	Non-SI units
Red cell count		
Male	$4.5–6.5 \times 10^{12}$/L	$4.5–6.5 \times 10^{6}$/mm^3
Female	$3.8–5.8 \times 10^{12}$/L	$3.8–5.8 \times 10^{6}$/mm^3
Red cell lifespan (mean)	120 days	–
Red cell lifespan $T_{\frac{1}{2}}(^{52}Cr)$	25–35 days	–
Reticulocytes (adults)	$25–85 \times 10^{9}$/L	$25–85 \times 10^{3}$/mm^3
Vitamin B$_{12}$	130–770 pg/mL	–

[a]Higher values in older patients are not necessarily abnormal.

Appendix B List of Units

cm	centimetre
mm	millimetre
L	litre
mL	millilitre
kg	kilogram
g	gram
mg	milligram
μg	microgram
ng	nanogram
pg	picogram
mol	mole
mmol	millimole
μmol	micromole
mEq	milliequivalent
mosm	milliosmole
mmHg	millimetres of mercury
kcal	kilocalorie

Nursing Practice: Knowledge and Care, First Edition. Edited by Ian Peate, Karen Wild and Muralitharan Nair.
© 2014 John Wiley & Sons, Ltd. Published 2014 by John Wiley & Sons, Ltd. Companion website: www.wileynursingpractice.com

Index

Nursing Practice: Knowledge and Care, First Edition. Edited by Ian Peate, Karen Wild and Muralitharan Nair.
© 2014 John Wiley & Sons, Ltd. Published 2014 by John Wiley & Sons, Ltd. Companion website: www.wileynursingpractice.com